Masseter	Occipitalis
Sternomastoid	Splenius capitis
Trapezius	Levator scapuli
Spine of scapula	Acromion (process)
Infraspinatus	Deltoid
Triceps long head	Teres minor
Triceps lateral head	Teres major
Triceps medial head	Latissimus dorsi
Brachioradialis	External oblique of abdomen
Extensor carpi radialis longus	Olecranon (process)
Extensor digitimini	Anconeus
Extensor pollicis brevis	Subcutaneous border of ulna
Gluteus medius	Extensor carpi ulnaris
Gluteus maximus	Extensor carpi radialis brevis
Position of greater trochanter	Extensor digitorum
Semitendinosus	Abductor pollicis longus
Iliotibial tract	Extensor pollicis longus
Biceps femoris (short head)	1st Dorsal interosseous
Plantaris	Extensor retinaculum
Gracilis	Adductor magnus
	Biceps femoris (long head)
Tibialis posterior	Semimembranosus
Calcaneal tendon (Achilles)	Popliteal surface of femur
Flexor digitorum longus	Sartorius
Medial malleolus	Gastrocnemius lateral head
	Gastrocnemius medial head
	Soleus
	Peroneus longus
	Peroneus brevis
	Calcaneal tendon (Achilles)
	Lateral malleolus

Major Muscles of the Body—Posterior View

Brief Contents

PART 1 FOUNDATIONS FOR MASSAGE THERAPY PROFESSIONALS 1

Chapter 1 Massage Therapy Profession 2
Chapter 2 History of Massage as a Vocation 25
Chapter 3 Professional and Personal Development 45
Chapter 4 Physical Skills, Fitness, Self-Care for the Massage Therapist 73
Chapter 5 Ethics and the Therapeutic Relationship 91

PART 2 FOUNDATIONS OF PLANNING AND GIVING MASSAGE SESSIONS 119

Chapter 6 Effects of Massage and Research Literacy 120
Chapter 7 Clinical Applications of Massage 151
Chapter 8 Endangerment Sites, Contraindications, Cautions 166
Chapter 9 Medical Terminology, Goal-Oriented Planning, Documentation 188
Chapter 10 Hygiene, Equipment, Environment 226
Chapter 11 Body Mechanics, Table Skills, General Guidelines 245

PART 3 TAPPAN'S GUIDE TO HEALING MASSAGE 267

Chapter 12 Swedish Massage Techniques 268
Chapter 13 Joint Movements 290
Chapter 14 Full-Body Swedish Massage 310
Chapter 15 Regional Massage Applications—Upper Body 339
Chapter 16 Regional Massage Applications—Lower Body 376
Chapter 17 Hydrotherapy and Temperature Therapies 400

PART 4 TAPPAN'S GUIDE TO SPECIAL APPLICATIONS 419

Chapter 18 Special Populations and Adaptations 420
Chapter 19 Spa Treatments 465
Chapter 20 Seated Massage 496

PART 5 TAPPAN'S GUIDE TO CONTEMPORARY MASSAGE AND BODYWORK 511

Chapter 21 Myofascial Massage 512
Chapter 22 Trigger Point Therapy 526
Chapter 23 Lymphatic Facilitation 539
Chapter 24 Reflexology 558
Chapter 25 Asian and Energy-Based Bodywork 576

PART 6 FOUNDATIONS OF CAREER AND PRACTICE DEVELOPMENT 631

Chapter 26 Career Plans and Employment 632
Chapter 27 Private Practice and Finances 647
Chapter 28 Business Ethics 667

APPENDICES

Appendix A Organizations and Publications A-1
Appendix B Code of Ethics and Standards of Practice for Massage Therapists A-3
Appendix C Goal-Oriented Planning A-8
Appendix D Performance Evaluation Forms A-10
Appendix E References and Additional Resources A-54

Interactive Glossary G-1
Index I-1

Tappan's
Handbook *of* Massage Therapy

Blending Art with Science

Sixth Edition

Patricia J. Benjamin
PhD, LMT

PEARSON

Boston   Columbus   Indianapolis   New York   San Francisco   Hoboken
Amsterdam   Cape Town   Dubai   London   Madrid   Milan   Munich   Paris   Montreal   Toronto
Delhi   Mexico City   São Paulo   Sydney   Hong Kong   Seoul   Singapore   Taipei Tokyo

Publisher: Julie Levin Alexander
Publisher's Assistant: Sarah Henrich
Executive Editor: John Goucher
Program Manager: Nicole Ragonese
Editorial Assistant: Amanda Losonsky
Development Editor: Lynda Hatch
Director of Marketing: David Gesell
Marketing Manager: Brittany Hammond
Marketing Specialist: Michael Sirinides
Project Management Lead: Cynthia Zonneveld
Project Manager: Patricia Gutierrez
Operations Specialist: MaryAnn Gloriande

Art Director: Maria GuglielmoWalsh
Text & Cover Designer: Studio Montage
Cover Art: Mark Segal Photography
Media Director: Amy Peltier
Lead Media Project Manager: Lorena Cerisano
Full-Service Project Management: Patty Donovan, Laserwords, Inc.
Composition: Laserwords, Inc.
Printer/Binder: Courier/Kendallville
Cover Printer: Courier/Kendallville
Text Font: 10/12 Times LT Pro Roman

Credits and acknowledgments for content borrowed from other sources and reproduced, with permission, in this textbook appear on appropriate page within text and below.

Chapter opener icons: Camellias/Fotolia; Rosinka79/Fotolia; Naluwan/Fotolia. *Critical Thinking icon:* Giuseppe Porzani/Fotolia. *Case Studies icon:* Somchaij/Fotolia. *Practical Applications icon:* Saiva_l/Fotolia. *Practical Sequence icon:* Aleksander1/Fotolia. *Reality Check photos:* Pearson Education, Inc.

Library of Congress Control Number: 2015934397

10 9 8 7 6 5 4 3 2 1

ISBN-13: 978-0-13-408269-1
ISBN-10: 0-13-408269-9

Welcome!

Welcome to *Tappan's Handbook of Massage Therapy,* Sixth Edition, the book that "started it all" when it was first published in 1980 and became the first major textbook to present a broad collection of massage therapy techniques. With her landmark publication, Frances Tappan began a tradition of excellence that has spanned decades and touched thousands of therapists and clients alike. Tappan's Handbook is a learning tool for a new generation, but it results from years of experience, wisdom, and research on the part of the author and countless therapists who have molded this book with their suggestions, feedback, and original writings. Truly this represents the culmination of great ideas from the world's massage community. In crafting this text, we aimed to reflect the needs of students and educators alike. Here are our basic premises.

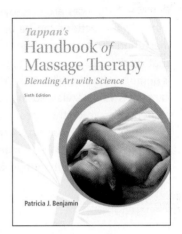

- **Students are visual and kinesthetic learners.**   We have designed this book with a wealth of beautiful anatomical illustrations and clear, step-by-step sequences that zero in on techniques. Our goal is to provide an engaging visual link between the book and hands-on practice.

- **Video is a dynamic way of demonstrating techniques.**   We produced a complete video library in connection with this book. The videos will bring the study of the techniques and professional aspects of massage into three dimensions.

- **Instructors can shine when provided with world-class resources.**   We have invested in a full battery of instructional support materials to facilitate dynamic presentations, well-organized lectures, and successful testing experiences.

- **Online learning is a viable option.**   With this book and the component resource materials, we have built a program that can support online instruction. This book is available as an e-text, and all support materials are available for instructor download via the web.

This is a comprehensive text for entry-level massage therapy programs. It covers the wide variety of competencies and prepares you for employment in a range of settings when you graduate. The book's title conveys that successful massage therapists excel at blending the art and science of the profession. Massage therapists must be knowledgeable about the human body in health and disease, skillful in interpersonal relationships, ethical in their behavior, and shrewd in building their careers. This is in addition to mastering theory, physical skills, and finally putting it all together in applications that accomplish client goals. Our text reflects the highest curricular standards, the expectations of employers, and the demands of a growing profession. It provides the foundations, guidance, and the know-how that you will need in order to master the essential task of *blending art with science* and becoming an outstanding massage therapist.

Tappan's Handbook of Massage Therapy takes a holistic approach by addressing many different learning styles to maximize your potential. You will use your mind, hands, and heart in acquiring the fundamental skills needed to start your new career. Professional knowledge and skills cannot be downloaded like a computer software program. It will take effort to transform yourself from the inside out. This book is your guide for that transformation.

Now please turn the page to get a glimpse of what makes this book an ideal guide to the fundamentals, techniques, and profession of massage therapy.

A "NEXT-GENERATION" LEARNING TOOL

Tappan's Handbook of Massage Therapy prepares therapists for careers in today's world. This edition features several important elements that will foster a successful, engaging, and interactive teaching and learning experience. Here are some exciting features:

Practice Sequences with Corresponding Videos

Practice Sequences are step-by-step suggested applications. These sections can be used as starting points for mastering the techniques and coming up with routines that work best for each student. Each *Practice Sequence* is demonstrated in full, vibrant detail on video. The video segments can be viewed in class or at home. So that students can track their progress, Appendix D provides *Performance Evaluation Forms* for every *Practice Sequence*. Videos and Performance Evaluation Forms can be found at www.myhealthprofessionslab.com

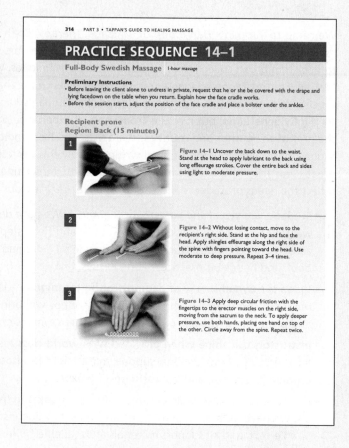

PRACTICE SEQUENCE 14–1

Full-Body Swedish Massage 1-hour massage

Preliminary Instructions
• Before leaving the client alone to undress in private, request that he or she be covered with the drape and lying facedown on the table when you return. Explain how the face cradle works.
• Before the session starts, adjust the position of the face cradle and place a bolster under the ankles.

Recipient prone
Region: Back (15 minutes)

1 Figure 14–1 Uncover the back down to the waist. Stand at the head to apply lubricant to the back using long effleurage strokes. Cover the entire back and sides using light to moderate pressure.

2 Figure 14–2 Without losing contact, move to the recipient's right side. Stand at the hip and face the head. Apply shingles effleurage along the right side of the spine with fingers pointing toward the head. Use moderate to deep pressure. Repeat 3–4 times.

3 Figure 14–3 Apply deep circular friction with the fingertips to the erector muscles on the right side, moving from the sacrum to the neck. To apply deeper pressure, use both hands, placing one hand on top of the other. Circle away from the spine. Repeat twice.

A LOGICAL FORMAT FROM START...

Each chapter begins with a consistent set of features that help readers set their goals.

- **Chapter Outline** provides an organized overview of the material to be covered.
- **Learning Outcomes** points readers toward intended goals.
- **Key Terms** identifies essential words and concepts.

...TO FINISH

Each chapter concludes with a built-in study guide that helps prepare students to succeed in their training and beyond.

Chapter Highlights summarizes each chapter's information in a user-friendly, bulleted outline.

Exam Review presents several different tools to help readers confirm their mastery of the content. Features include:

- **Key Terms** – a matching exercise for studying and applying essential vocabulary
- **Memory Workout** – a fill-in-the-blank review of main concepts
- **Test Prep** – a multiple-choice mock exam
- **Video Challenge** – a quiz based on selected segments of the videos.
- **Comprehension Exercises** – a series of short-answer questions that key in on important ideas.
- **For Greater Understanding** – suggested field-based activities that employ various learning styles to help readers apply chapter concepts

A WEALTH OF LEARNING TOOLS ON EVERY PAGE

Photoreal Illustrations

Over 880 full-color illustrations provide first-class reinforcement for visual learners. The photoreal style is clear, focused, and detailed, without background distractions.

FIGURE 11–28 Draping for massage of arm. A. Hold arm to side and tuck drape at ribs. B. Lift arm across chest and tuck sheet underneath the shoulder. C. Place the arm on table ready for massage.

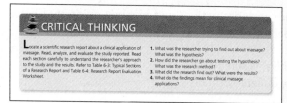

Case for Study

Real-world, critical-thinking scenarios that challenge readers to analyze a situation and solve the problem.

Practical Application

Activities that involve observation, role play, creativity, and planning.

Critical Thinking

Situations that students can analyze and evaluate on a deeper level, by contemplating thoughtful questions, asking intelligent questions, broadening their knowledge base, and making informed decisions.

Reality Check

A report-from-the-real-world feature, in which a new massage therapist asks for advice from a more experienced colleague who provides an insightful view into the profession by responding to questions, feelings, and doubts often left unmentioned.

ORGANIZED FOR STUDENT SUCCESS

Tappan's Handbook of Massage Therapy is divided into six parts covering the essential competencies.

PART 1: FOUNDATIONS FOR MASSAGE THERAPY PROFESSIONALS

An overview of the massage therapy profession and its history, important elements of personal and professional development, and ethical considerations. It addresses foundation knowledge apart from hands-on skills.

> *Chapter 2: History of Massage as a Vocation* looks at who went into the occupation, how they were trained, what types of skills and knowledge they had, their work conditions, and their status in society. It describes differences in various times and locations, how situations changed over the years, and what factors influenced the work of massage practitioners, while providing a better understanding of today's massage therapy profession.

PART 2: FOUNDATIONS OF PLANNING AND GIVING MASSAGE

Background specific to planning effective and safe massage therapy sessions and coverage of the physical setup for massage. It takes the view that no matter where massage therapists work, they owe it to clients to provide a safe environment and to tailor sessions to meet client expectations and goals.

PART 3: TAPPAN'S GUIDE TO HEALING MASSAGE

An introduction to basic Swedish massage and joint movement techniques, regional applications, and hydrotherapy and temperature therapies. It presents essential hands-on skills and applications.

> *Chapter 14: Full-Body Swedish Massage* explains how individual techniques are organized logically into massage routines that address the entire body. It presents a suggested full-body Practice Sequence that can be used to demonstrate basic principles, or as a starting point for learning full-body massage.

PART 4: TAPPAN'S GUIDE TO SPECIAL APPLICATIONS

Provides approaches for enhancement of basic Swedish massage and adaptations to address needs of special populations, an overview of spa treatments, and planning and giving seated massage.

> *Chapter 19 Spa Treatments* presents common spa applications. Detailed instructions are provided for applying herbal wraps, skin treatments, temperature therapy, and massage sessions common in spa settings.

PART 5: TAPPAN'S GUIDE TO CONTEMPORARY MASSAGE AND BODYWORK

Introduces myofascial massage, trigger point therapy, lymphatic facilitation, reflexology, and popular forms of energy-based bodywork from Asia.

PART 6: FOUNDATIONS OF CAREER AND PRACTICE DEVELOPMENT

This section describes what it takes to get started in a successful massage therapy career—from envisioning a future practice to making that dream come true. It covers career planning, finding employment, developing a private practice, and the ethics of the business side of massage.

A COMPLETE VIDEO LIBRARY IN YOUR HANDS

The massage videos provide a dynamic learning tool. They can be viewed at home as a study tool and review of chapter material; in class to illustrate concepts and spark discussion; or prior to practicing hands-on skills in technique classes.

Videos may be accessed at www.myhealthprofessionslab.com

- Healing Massage: Wellness and Workplaces
- History of Massage
- Professionalism
- Emotional Intelligence
- Social and Communication Skills
- Holistic Self-Care Plan
- Foundation of Ethics
- Therapeutic Relationship
- Goal-Oriented Planning
- Documentation
- Hygienic Hand Washing
- Body Mechanics
- Positioning and Draping
- Overview of Swedish Massage Techniques
- Effleurage
- Petrissage
- Friction
- Tapotement
- Touch without Movement
- Joint Movements

- Full-body Massage: Back
- Full-body Massage: Lower Limbs and Buttocks
- Full-body Massage: Turning Over and Lower Limbs
- Full-body Massage: Arms, Shoulders, and Chest
- Full-body Massage: Abdomen
- Full-body Massage: Face and Head
- Head and Face Massage
- Massage of Neck Region
- Upper Back and Shoulder Massage
- Low Back Massage
- Massage for Upper Extremities
- Chest and Abdominal Massage
- Hip and Buttocks Massage
- Thigh and Lower Leg Massage
- Foot Massage
- Hot Application on Upper Back
- Cold Application for Knee
- Ice Massage for Elbow

- Postevent Sports Massage
- Pregnancy Massage
- Infant Massage
- Massage for the Elderly
- Gentle Hand and Arm Massage
- Seated Massage
- Myofascial Massage
- Trigger Point Therapy
- Lymphatic Facilitation for the Head and Neck
- Lymphatic Facilitation for the Lower Extremity
- Reflexology
- AMI for the Back
- AMI for Anterior Arm
- AMI for Neck–Head–Face
- Qi Gong for Self Care
- General Session of Polarity Therapy
- Career Plans and Employment
- Private Practice and Finances
- Business Ethics

MyHealthProfessionsLab™

The ultimate personalized learning tool is available at **MyHealthProfessionsLab.com**. This online course correlates with the textbook and is available for purchase separately or for a discount when packaged with the book. MyHealthProfessionsLab is an immersive study experience that reinforces concepts learned within the text through, quizzes, videos, and other self-study challenges. The system allows learners to track their own progress through the course and use a personalized study plan to achieve success.

MyHealthProfessionsLab saves instructors time by providing quality feedback, ongoing individualized assessments for students, and instructor resources all in one place. It offers instructors the flexibility to make technology an integral part of their course, or a supplementary resource for students.

Visit **MyHealthProfessionsLab.com** to log in to the course or purchase access. Instructors seeking more information about discount bundle options or for a demonstration, please contact your Pearson sales representative.

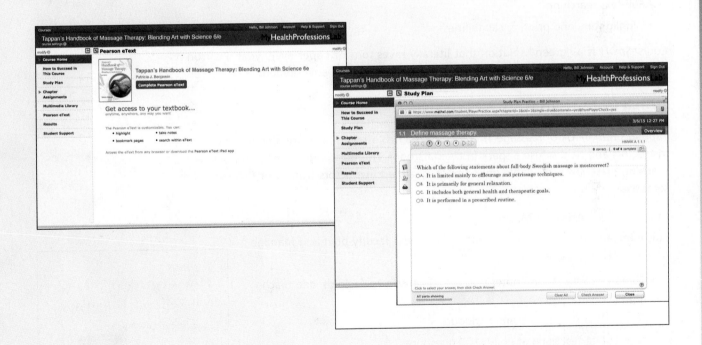

COMPREHENSIVE INSTRUCTIONAL PACKAGE

Perhaps the most gratifying part of an educator's work is the "aha" learning moment when the light bulb goes off and a student truly understands a concept—when a connection is made. Along these lines, Pearson is pleased to help instructors foster more of these educational connections by providing a complete battery of resources to support teaching and learning. Qualified adopters are eligible to receive a wealth of materials designed to help instructors prepare, present, and assess. For more information, please contact your Pearson sales representative or visit **www.pearsonhighered.com/educator**.

ONLINE RESOURCES AT YOUR FINGERTIPS

No massage therapy textbook has as extensive a selection of web-based resources as *Tappan's Handbook of Massage Therapy*.

Instructor Resource Center

All instructional ancillary resources are available online for instant download by educators at **www.pearsonhighered.com**. Here instructors will find an instructor's manual, PowerPoint lecture slides, an electronic test bank, and an image library.

CourseSmart e-text

We realize that massage therapy students are conscious about avoiding placing undue strain on their bodies. We also know that students are often on tight budgets. Introducing CourseSmart, a value-priced e-text option that relieves the stress of carrying an extra book. Students can download this textbook for a reduced price at **www.coursesmart.com** and they can begin taking advantage of these benefits:

- Instant access
- Full-text searching
- Highlighting and printing capabilities

CourseSmart is a "green" solution that literally saves tons of paper every year. Pearson is proud of this initiative as a measure of our commitment to the environment.

TOOLS TO HELP INSTRUCTORS SHINE

Tappan's Handbook of Massage Therapy offers a rich array of ancillary materials to benefit instructors and help infuse a spark in the classroom. The full complement of supplemental teaching materials is available online to all qualified instructors from your Pearson representative.

Instructor's Resource Manual

This manual contains a wealth of material to help faculty plan and manage their courses. It includes:

- Comprehensive lecture notes that contain abstracts, factoids, and teaching strategies.
- A wealth of worksheets and handouts.
- A complete test bank of nearly 600 questions.

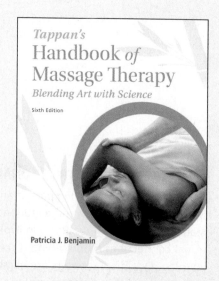

Test Bank

A complete test bank of nearly 600 questions that allows instructors to generate customized exams and quizzes.

PowerPoints

A comprehensive, turn-key lecture package in PowerPoint format containing discussion points, with embedded color images.

Image Library

Every photograph and illustration contained in the textbook.

A WORD ABOUT BOARD CERTIFICATION

Through our Vue division, Pearson is pleased to provide a variety of massage therapy certification and licensing exams. While this book is not directly correlated to these exams, it can serve as a useful study reference. Visit **http://www.vue.com/fsmtb/** or **http://www.vue.com/ncbtmb/** for information.

To help prepare you for any of these important certification exams, you may wish to purchase our bestselling test prep book, *SUCCESS! in Massage Therapy* by Jane Garofano. The book is organized based on the national exam format and contains review content and a variety of mock exams. Order online or at your local bookstore (ISBN: 0135072220)

Acknowledgments

How can one even begin to acknowledge all those who have contributed to *Tappan's Handbook of Massage Therapy: Blending Art with Science*? Producing a comprehensive textbook like this involves many people both known and unknown to the primary author. Everyone who touched this project in any way has my gratitude for their efforts. A few who stand out will be acknowledged here.

First is Frances M. Tappan (1917–1999), who many years ago invited me to join her on the adventure of writing massage therapy textbooks. She provided the spark that started me on the journey that has led to this point.

Thanks to all those who contributed to *Pearson's Massage Therapy*, *Tappan's Handbook of Healing Massage Techniques*, and *Professional Foundations for Massage Therapists*. These three textbooks laid the groundwork for *Tappan's Handbook of Massage Therapy*.

Various people have lent their expertise and knowledge and provided a depth of understanding and accuracy that would otherwise be missing from this text. They include Beverly Shoenberger, Polarity Therapy; Will Parks, Acupressure Massage Integration; Xie Ling Welch, Qi Gong; Christopher Alvarado, Myofascial Massage; Dale Perry, Lymphatic Facilitation; Paula Stone, Reflexology; and Ann L. Mihina and Sandra K. Anderson, Spa Applications.

Massage therapists who appear in the video massage segments include Christopher Alvarado, Bobbe Bermann, Danielle Bianchi, Annette Chamness, Larry Clemmons, Maria D. Cooper, Wayne Hussey, Connie Love, John Magruder, Will Parks, Dale Perry, Xie Ling Welch, and Patricia Vater, who coordinated the demonstrations. Other massage therapists appearing in the videos include Joli Behr-Cook, Jennifer van Dam, Caleb Edmond, Julie Favaro, and Jeff Mann. Appearing in recently updated illustrations are Maria D. Cooper, Andrea Black, and Nathan Bell.

Reviewers who made thoughtful criticisms and suggestions on draft pages have added greatly to the quality and relevance of the book. This includes official reviewers as well as colleagues who offered their opinions on different aspects of this text. It is a better book because of your comments.

Thanks to the production staff at Pearson—especially John Goucher, Executive Editor, Health Professions, and to Development Editor, Lynda Hatch, who has kept me more or less on schedule and who improved the text in so many ways.

Last, but not least, I want to acknowledge the support and encouragement of family and friends. Special appreciation is reserved for Martha Fourt who stepped up whenever I needed a model, photographer, editor, gofer, or any other task—usually on short notice.

Thanks to all.

Patricia J. Benjamin

About the Author

Patricia J. Benjamin, PhD, LMT, is a massage therapist, educator, author, and appreciative massage and bodywork client. She has a deep respect for massage therapy as an art, science, and wellness practice. She has studied its traditions and watches for trends in the massage therapy profession today.

Building on her earlier background in sports and fitness, Dr. Benjamin graduated from the Chicago School of Massage Therapy in the mid-1980s. She was drawn to massage as an active, hands-on therapy whose foundations dovetail with her former career in health, physical education, and recreation. After having a full-time massage therapy practice, she gravitated back to education, first as an association education director, and then as a teacher and massage school administrator. Over the years, she has served on various committees involved in the development of ethical standards and national certification for massage therapists, and the accreditation of massage programs.

Dr. Benjamin has taught at the high school and college levels and enjoys developing curriculum materials for the career-oriented courses offered in vocational programs. She holds master's and advanced study degrees in education with a specialty in curriculum development from Northern Illinois University. A doctorate in recreation and leisure studies from Purdue University has deepened her appreciation of the many facets of wellness and grounded her in a variety of research methods.

Frances Tappan approached Pat Benjamin to join her as coauthor of *Healing Massage Techniques* for its 3rd edition (1998). After Dr. Tappan's passing in 1999, Dr. Benjamin continued to update and improve *Tappan's Handbook of Healing Massage Techniques* (2010), which remains a standard in the field. Dr. Benjamin authored *Professional Foundations for Massage Therapists* (2009) to address related professional competencies and combined that information with basic massage skills and applications in *Pearson's Massage Therapy: Blending Art with Science* (2011). This latest edition of *Tappan's Handbook* combines all three of its predecessors for the most comprehensive and up-to-date presentation of the theory and practice of massage therapy available today. *Tappan's Handbook of Massage Therapy: Blending Art and Science*, sixth edition, remains true to Frances Tappan's vision of healing massage as holistic manual therapy that contributes to the well-being of humanity in so many ways.

In her leisure time, Dr. Benjamin enjoys reading historical fiction and nonfiction, gardening, tai chi and qi gong, and table tennis. Her outdoor pursuits include hiking, canoeing, and birding. She currently resides in Chicago, Illinois.

Our Development Team

The fresh and unique vision, format, and content contained within the pages of *Tappan's Handbook of Massage Therapy: Blending Art with Science* comes as a result of an incredible collaboration of expert educators from all around. This book represents the collective insights, experience, and thousands of hours of work performed by members of this development team. Their influence will continue to have an impact for decades to come. Let us introduce the members of our team.

CONTRIBUTORS

Text

Ann L. Mihina—Spa Applications,
    Tucson, AZ
Sandra K. Anderson—Spa Applications,
    Tucson, AZ
    Chapter 19, Spa Treatments, is adapted from their
        book, *Natural Spa and Hydrotherapy* (2009).
Christopher Alvarado—Myofascial Massage
    Licensed Massage Therapist
    Evanston, Illinois
Will Parks—Acupressure Massage Integration
    Connecticut Center for Massage Therapy
    Newington, Connecticut
Dale Perry—Lymphatic Facilitation
    Center for Natural Wellness School of Massage
        Therapy
    Albany, New York
Beverly Shoenberger—Polarity Therapy
    Psychotherapist and Physical Therapist
    Malibu, California
Paula Stone—Reflexology
    The Stone Institute
    St. Charles, Missouri
    Chapter 24, Reflexology, is adapted from her book,
        Therapeutic Reflexology (2011).

Video

Christopher Alvarado
Joli Behr-Cook
Dr. S. C. Benanti
Bobbe Berman
Danielle Bianchi
Annette Chamness
Larry Clemmons
Maria D. Cooper
Cheryl Coutts
Christopher Coutts
Jennifer van Dam
Selene DelValle
Caleb Edmond
Julie Favaro
Wayne Hussey
Theresa Cecylija Leszczynski
Connie Love
John Magruder
Jeff Mann
Abby Nickerson
Will Parks
Dale Perry
Patricia Vater
Xie Ling Welch

REVIEWERS

William G. Connell, MA, LMT
John A. Logan College
Carterville, IL

Jodi Gootkin, PT, MEd
Edison State College
Fort Myers, FL

Carol Gott, BS, CMT
Ivy Tech Community College
Evansville, IL

Karen Hobson, MS, LMT
Miller Motte College
Greenville, NC

Dr. Steven Koehler, ND, LMBT
Lenoir Community College
Kinston, NC

Walter Lopez, LMT
Milan Institute
Las Vegas, NV

Sheri Manthei, NBCMTB, LMT, MS-IDT, BBA, AAS MSG, AAS
Baker College
Allen Park, MI

Vajra Matusow, MA, CMT, CHT
Diamond Light School of Massage and Healing Arts
San Anselmo, CA

David Merlino, LMT, NCETM
Milan Institute
Sparks, NV

Marek Sawicki, BA, CAyur, LMBT, eRYT 500
AB Tech Community College
Weaverville, NC

Kathleen Wellman, CPA, LMT
Moraine Valley Community College
New Lenox, IL

A Commitment to Accuracy

As a student embarking in health care you probably already know how critically important it is to be precise in your work. Clients and coworkers will be counting on you to avoid errors on a daily basis. Likewise, we owe it to you—the reader—to ensure accuracy in this book. We have gone to great lengths to verify that the information provided in *Tappan's Handbook of Massage Therapy: Blending Art with Science* is complete and correct.

To this end, here are the steps we have taken:

1. *Editorial Review*   No fewer than 12 content experts have read each chapter for accuracy. In addition, some members of our developmental team were specifically assigned to focus on the precision of each illustration that appears in the book.

2. *Accurate Ancillaries*   The teaching and learning ancillaries are often as important to instruction as the textbook itself. Therefore, we took steps to ensure accuracy and consistency of these components by reviewing every ancillary component. The author and editorial team studied every PowerPoint slide and online course frame to ensure the context was correct and relevant to each lesson.

Although our intent and actions have been directed at creating an error-free text, we have established a process for correcting any mistakes that may have slipped past our editors. Pearson takes this issue seriously and therefore welcomes any and all feedback that you can provide along the lines of helping us enhance the accuracy of this text. If you identify any errors that need to be corrected in a subsequent printing, please send them to:

Pearson Health Editorial
Massage Therapy Corrections
221 River Street
Hoboken, NJ 07030

Thank you for helping Pearson reach its goal of providing the most accurate textbooks available.

Massage Practice Sequences

Find the Practice Sequences in the text and on video at MyHealthProfessionsLab.com.

PRACTICE SEQUENCE 10-1
Hygienic Hand Washing

PRACTICE SEQUENCE 14-1
Full-Body Swedish Massage

PRACTICE SEQUENCE 15-1
Head and Face Massage

PRACTICE SEQUENCE 15-2
Massage of the Neck Region

PRACTICE SEQUENCE 15-3
Upper Back and Shoulder Massage

PRACTICE SEQUENCE 15-4
Low Back Massage

PRACTICE SEQUENCE 15-5
Massage of the Upper Extremities

PRACTICE SEQUENCE 15-6
Chest and Abdominal Massage

PRACTICE SEQUENCE 16-1
Hip and Buttocks Massage

PRACTICE SEQUENCE 16-2
Thigh and Lower Leg Massage

PRACTICE SEQUENCE 16-3
Foot Massage

PRACTICE SEQUENCE 17-1
Hot Application on Upper Back

PRACTICE SEQUENCE 17-2
Cold Application for Knee

PRACTICE SEQUENCE 17-3
Ice Massage for Elbow

PRACTICE SEQUENCE 18-1
Postevent Sports Massage for Run/Walk Event

PRACTICE SEQUENCE 18-2
Pregnancy Massage in Side-Lying Position

PRACTICE SEQUENCE 18-3
Infant Massage

PRACTICE SEQUENCE 18-4
Massage for the Elderly in a Semireclining Position

PRACTICE SEQUENCE 18-5
Gentle Hand and Arm Massage

PRACTICE SEQUENCE 20-1
Seated Massage

PRACTICE SEQUENCE 21-1
Myofascial Massage of the Back

PRACTICE SEQUENCE 22-1
Trigger Point Therapy for Tension Headaches

PRACTICE SEQUENCE 23-1
Lymphatic Facilitation for the Head and Neck

PRACTICE SEQUENCE 23-2
Lymphatic Facilitation for the Lower Extremity

PRACTICE SEQUENCE 24-1
General Reflexology Session

PRACTICE SEQUENCE 25-1
AMI for the Back

PRACTICE SEQUENCE 25-2
AMI for the Anterior Arm

PRACTICE SEQUENCE 25-3
AMI for the Neck-Head-Face

PRACTICE SEQUENCE 25-4
General Session of Polarity Therapy

Contents

Welcome!   iii
Acknowledgments   xii
About the Author   xiii
Our Development Team   xiv
A Commitment to Accuracy   xvi
Massage Practice Sequences   xvii
Fast Track to Success   xxvi

PART 1   FOUNDATIONS FOR MASSAGE THERAPY PROFESSIONALS   1

Chapter 1   Massage Therapy Profession   2

Learning Outcomes   2
Key Terms   2
The Journey   3
Massage Defined   3
Wellness Profession   3
Trends   4
Typical Work Settings   6
   Personal Care   6
   Sports, Fitness, and Recreation   6
   Health Care   7
   Private Practice   8
Becoming a Massage Therapy Professional   8
Body of Knowledge and Skills   10
Education   10
   Continuing Education   11
Credentials   12
   School Diploma   12
   Board Certification   12
   Specialty Certification   12
   Occupational Licensing   13
Organizations   14
   Professional Associations   14
   Member Services Organizations   15
   Specialty Associations   16
Scholarship and Publications   16
Research   17
Ethical Standards   17
Recognition by the Public and Health
  Professionals   17
   Recognition from Other Professionals   18
Chapter Highlights   19
Exam Review   21

Chapter 2   History of Massage as a Vocation   25

Learning Outcomes   25
Key Terms   25
History of a Vocation   26
Personal Grooming and Rejuvenation   26
   Public Baths   27
   Salons and Spas   28
Sports and Fitness   29
   Rubbers and Athletic Masseurs   29
   Fitness/Health Service Operators and Expert
      Masseuses   30
Health Care   31
   Western Medicine   32
Natural Healing and Drugless Doctors   36
   Massage in the Natural Healing Tradition   36
Massage Therapy Revived in the United States   37
Massage Therapists and Bodyworkers   38
   Unified Profession   40
Chapter Highlights   41
Exam Review   42

Chapter 3   Professional and Personal Development   45

Learning Outcomes   45
Key Terms   45
Professionalism in Massage Therapy   46
   Service   46
   Work Ethic   46
Professional Image   46
   Dress   47
   Grooming   48
   Posture   48
   Image Detractors   48
Professional Boundaries   48
Ethics for the Massage Student   49
Intellectual Skills   50
   Higher-Level Thinking   51
   Concentration   52
Intuition   53
Emotional Intelligence   53
   Self-Awareness   54
   Managing Emotions   54

Motivating Yourself 55
Recognizing Emotions in Others 55
Handling Relationships 55
Social Skills 55
Courtesy and Good Manners 56
First Impressions 56
Greeting a First-Time Client 56
Introductions 57
Conflict Resolution 57
Communication Skills 59
Verbal Skills 59
Body Language 60
Listening 62
Presentations 63
Written Communication 64
Chapter Highlights 67
Exam Review 69

Chapter 4   **Physical Skills, Fitness, Self-Care for the Massage Therapist** 73

Learning Outcomes 73
Key Terms 73
The Physical Side of Massage 74
Body Awareness 74
Skilled Touch 75
Contact 75
Qualities of Touch 76
Communication 76
Palpation 76
Physical Fitness 76
Cardiovascular Fitness 76
Muscular Strength and Endurance 77
Flexibility 77
Body Composition 80
Self-Care Practices 80
Body–Mind Practices 80
Stress-Control Strategies 82
Time Management 82
Nutrition 84
Holistic Self-Care Plan 86
Chapter Highlights 87
Exam Review 88

Chapter 5   **Ethics and the Therapeutic Relationship** 91

Learning Outcomes 91
Key Terms 91
Overview 92
Nature of Ethics 92
Values, Rights, and Duties 92
Values 92
Rights 93
Duties 93
Vulnerability to Unethical Behavior 94
Ethical Codes and Standards 94

Ethics and Law 95
Ethical Decision Making 96
Ethical Questions and Dilemmas 96
The Ethical Decision-Making Model 96
Development of Ethical Judgment 98
The Therapeutic Relationship 99
Transference and Countertransference 100
Defense Mechanisms 100
Roles and Boundaries 101
Dual Relationships 102
Evaluating Dual Relationships 102
Sexual Relationships 103
Sexual Misconduct 104
Informed Voluntary Consent 105
Sexual Misconduct by a Client 106
Intervention Model 106
Relationships in School 107
Scope of Practice 108
Staying in Bounds 109
Education and Home Care 110
Confidentiality 111
Chapter Highlights 112
Exam Review 114

PART 2   **FOUNDATIONS OF PLANNING AND GIVING MASSAGE SESSIONS** 119

Chapter 6   **Effects of Massage and Research Literacy** 120

Learning Outcomes 120
Key Terms 120
Effects of Massage Overview 121
Massage Techniques and Effects 121
Time, Dose, and Effects 121
Holistic View of Effects 121
Knowledge of Effects 124
Research 124
Research Literacy 125
Scientific Method 125
Levels of Evidence 125
Locating Research Studies 127
Reading Research Reports 127
A Closer Look at the Effects of Massage 129
Physiological Effects—Tissue level 129
Tissue Repair 129
Connective Tissue 130
Physiological Effects—Organ System Level 131
Integumentary System 131
Skeletal System 132
Muscular System 132
Nervous and Endocrine Systems 135
Cardiovascular System 136
Lymphatic System and Immunity 138
Respiratory System 139

Digestive System 139
Urinary System 139
Reproductive System 140
Physiological Effects—Organism Level 140
Growth and Development 140
Pain Reduction 140
Stress Reduction 141
Psychological Effects 141
Mental Clarity 142
Reduced Anxiety and Depression 142
Character Armor and Emotional Release 142
Feelings of General Well-Being 143
Limbic System 143
Mechanisms of Massage 144
Mechanical Effects 144
Physiological Effects 144
Reflex Effects 144
Body–Mind Effects 144
Energetic Effects 145
Benefits of Wellness Massage 145
Chapter Highlights 145
Exam Review 147

Chapter 7   Clinical Applications of Massage 151
Learning Outcomes 151
Key Terms 151
Clinical Massage Therapy 152
Evidence-Based Practice 152
Client-Centered Massage 153
Therapeutic Outcomes 153
Musculoskeletal Applications 154
Fibromyalgia Syndrome 154
Cardiovascular and Lymphatic Applications 156
Edema and Lymphedema 156
Immune Function 156
Respiratory Applications 156
Back Massage for Hospitalized Patients 157
Massage for Cancer Patients 157
Pediatric Applications 158
Preterm Infants 158
Additional Pediatric Applications 159
Psychological Clinical Applications 160
Therapeutic Touch 160
Complement to Chiropractic Care 161
Case Reports 161
Chapter Highlights 162
Exam Review 163

Chapter 8   Endangerment Sites, Contraindications, Cautions 166
Learning Outcomes 166
Key Terms 166
Do No Harm 167
Endangerment Sites 167
Head and Face 167
Anterior Neck 167

Vertebral Column 167
Thoracic Cage 169
Shoulder and Axilla 169
Elbow and Wrist 169
Torso 169
Inguinal Area 171
Popliteal Area 171
Major Veins in Extremities 171
General Principles for Safety Around Endangerment Sites 173
Contraindications 173
Principles for Contraindications and Cautions 173
Medications 178
Person-Centered Massage 182
Resources for Reliable Information 183
Chapter Highlights 184
Exam Review 185

Chapter 9   Medical Terminology, Goal-Oriented Planning, Documentation 188
Learning Outcomes 188
Key Terms 188
Medical Terminology 189
Prefixes 189
Word Roots/Combining Forms 191
Suffixes 191
Singular and Plural Endings 191
Abbreviations and Symbols 195
The Importance of Planning 197
Goal-Oriented Planning 197
Steps in Goal-Oriented Planning 198
Long-Term Planning 199
Individual Session Planning 200
Treatment Planning 201
Collecting Subjective Information 202
Health/Medical History 202
Intake Interview 203
Collecting Objective Information 205
General Observations 205
Palpation 205
Range of Motion Evaluation 206
Posture Analysis 208
Biomechanical Analysis 210
Gait Analysis 211
Orthopedic Tests 211
Importance of Documentation 212
Soap Note Overview 212
SOAP Note Format 213
SOAP Note Content 213
Writing Soap Notes 214
Guidelines for Writing SOAP Notes 214
Simplified Documentation 216
Designing a System of Documentation 217
Legal and Ethical Issues 219
Chapter Highlights 221
Exam Review 222

Chapter 10 Hygiene, Equipment, Environment 226

Learning Outcomes 226
Key Terms 226
Introduction 227
Personal Hygiene and Hand Washing 227
    Personal Hygiene 227
    Hand Washing 227
Massage Equipment 230
    Massage Tables 230
    Massage Chairs 231
    Equipment Setup and Care 233
    Alternatives to Tables and Chairs 233
Supplies for Massage 233
    Bolsters and Pillows 233
    Sheets, Blankets, and Towels 235
Topical Substances 236
    Uses of Different Topical Substances 236
    Sanitation and Topical Substances 237
Physical Environment for Massage 237
    Room Setup 237
    Floors, Walls, and Windows 237
    Lighting and Color 238
    Temperature, Humidity, and Fresh Air 238
    Music and Sound 238
    Safety 238
    Maintenance Schedule 239
Infection Control 239
    Universal Precautions 239
    MRSA 240
Chapter Highlights 240
Exam Review 242

Chapter 11 Body Mechanics, Table Skills, General Guidelines 245

Learning Outcomes 245
Key Terms 245
Principles of Hand and Body Mechanics 246
Preventing Injury and Overuse 246
    Hand and Wrist Care 246
Hand Mechanics for Different Techniques 247
Body Mechanics for Table Massage 248
Body Mechanics for Seated/Chair Massage 251
Table Skills 253
    Assistance Getting Onto and Off of the Table 253
    Assistance Turning Over 254
Positioning 254
    Supine 254
    Prone 254
    Face Cradle Adjustment 254
    Side-Lying and Semireclining 255
    Seated 256
Draping 256
General Guidelines for Massage 258
    Length of Sessions 258
    Amount of Lubricant 260

    Sequence of Techniques and Routines 261
    Specificity and Direction 261
    Pressure, Rhythm, and Pacing 261
Chapter Highlights 263
Exam Review 264

PART 3 TAPPAN'S GUIDE TO HEALING MASSAGE 267

Chapter 12 Swedish Massage Techniques 268

Learning Outcomes 268
Key Terms 268
Swedish Massage Overview 269
Swedish Massage Techniques 269
Effleurage 270
    Variations of Effleurage 270
Petrissage 274
    Variations of Petrissage 274
Friction 277
    Variations of Friction 277
    Friction Used in Rehabilitation 279
Tapotement 279
    Variations of Tapotement 280
Vibration 282
    Variations of Vibration 282
Touch Without Movement 283
    Passive Touch 283
    Direct Pressure 284
Chapter Highlights 285
Exam Review 286

Chapter 13 Joint Movements 290

Learning Outcomes 290
Key Terms 290
Overview of Joint Movement 291
    Categories of Movements 291
    Joint Movement Techniques 291
Methods of Stretching 292
Safety 292
    Cautions and Contraindications 294
General Guidelines for Joint Movement Techniques 295
Regional Applications of Joint Movements 295
    Neck 295
    Shoulder Girdle 297
    Elbow 298
    Wrist 299
    Hand 299
    Chest 300
    Hip 301
    Knee 303
    Ankle 303
    Foot 304
Chapter Highlights 306
Exam Review 307

Chapter 14 Full-Body Swedish Massage 310

Learning Outcomes 310
Key Terms 310
Overview 311
Guidelines for Full-Body Swedish Massage 311
  Draping 312
  Sequence of Body Regions 312
  Order of Techniques 312
  Continuity and Flow 312
  Rhythm, Pacing, Specificity, Pressure 313
Full-Body Swedish Massage Practice Sequence 313
Chapter Highlights 336
Exam Review 336

**Chapter 15 Regional Massage Applications—
                Upper Body** 339

Learning Outcomes 339
Key Terms 339
Regional Massage 340
  Interconnections and Meaning 340
  Regional Practice Sequences 340
Head and Face 340
  Anatomy of the Head and Face 341
  Applications of Massage for the Head and Face 341
Neck 347
  Anatomy of the Neck 347
  Applications of Massage for the Neck 348
Back 353
  Anatomy of the Back 353
  Applications of Massage for the Back 354
Upper Extremities 359
  Anatomy of the Upper Extremities 359
  Applications of Massage for the Upper Extremities 361
Chest and Abdomen 367
  Anatomy of the Chest and Abdomen 367
  *Applications of Massage for the Chest and
    Abdomen* 367
Chapter Highlights 372
Exam Review 373

**Chapter 16 Regional Massage Applications—
                Lower Body** 376

Learning Outcomes 376
Key Terms 376
Regional Massage of the Lower Body 377
Hips and Buttocks 377
  Anatomy of the Hips and Buttocks 377
  *Applications of Massage for the Hips and
    Buttocks* 378
Lower Extremities 383
  Anatomy of the Lower Extremities 383
  *Applications of Massage for the Lower
    Extremities* 386
Chapter Highlights 397
Exam Review 397

**Chapter 17 Hydrotherapy and Temperature
                Therapies** 400

Learning Outcomes 400
Key Terms 400
Introduction 401
History of Hydrotherapy 401
  The Water Cure 401
  Hydrotherapy versus Hydropathy 401
Healing Properties of Water 402
Hydrotherapy Facilities 403
Hot Applications 405
  Hot Packs and Massage 405
Cold Applications 409
  Cold Packs and Massage 410
  Ice Massage 412
Chapter Highlights 414
Exam Review 415

**PART 4   TAPPAN'S GUIDE TO SPECIAL
            APPLICATIONS** 419

**Chapter 18 Special Populations and
                Adaptations** 420

Learning Outcomes 420
Key Terms 420
Introduction 421
Athletes 421
  Techniques and Knowledge 421
  Recovery 422
  Remedial Massage and Rehabilitation 422
  Maintenance 422
  Events 422
Pregnant Women 429
  Contraindications 429
  Pregnancy Massage Application 430
  Labor, Delivery, and Recovery 435
  Women with Infants and Toddlers 436
Infants 436
  Infant Massage Application 436
The Elderly 441
  Physiological Age 442
  Positioning Options for the Elderly 442
  Guidelines for Massage of Older Adults 443
  Cautions and Adaptations 444
  Massage in Semireclining Position 444
The Terminally Ill 451
  Adaptations for the Terminally Ill 452
  Self-Care 456
Impairments and Disabilities 456
  Visual Impairment 456
  Hearing Impairment 457
  Speech Impairment 457
  Size Issues—Large and Small 457
  Mobility Challenges 458

Amputees and Prostheses   459
Internal and External Medical Devices   460
   Pacemakers and Defibrillators   460
   Colostomy Bag   460
Rewards and Challenges   461
Chapter Highlights   461
Exam Review   462

Chapter 19   Spa Treatments   465

Learning Outcomes   465
Key Terms   465
Overview   466
Equipment and Supplies   466
   Equipment   466
   Supplies   466
   Sanitation   467
Helping Clients Choose Spa Treatments   467
   Practitioner's Role   467
   Health and Medical Considerations   468
   Other Considerations   468
Exfoliation   469
   Methods of Exfoliation   469
   Manual Exfoliation   469
   Preparing for a Scrub Treatment   472
   Performing a Scrub Treatment   473
   Chemical Exfoliation   474
Body Wraps   475
   Muds and Clays   475
   Peat   476
   Moor Mud   476
   Seaweed and Sea Mud   477
   Preparing for a Body Wrap Treatment   477
   Performing a Body Wrap Treatment   478
   Herbal Wraps   481
Aromatherapy   481
   Essential Oils   482
   How Essential Oils Work   482
   Classification by Notes   484
   Ten Foundational Essential Oils   484
   *Using Essential Oils in a Spa or Massage Therapy
      Practice*   487
Stone Massage   488
   Preparing for Stone Massage   488
   Performing Hot Stone Massage   489
   When to Use Cold Stones   490
Chapter Highlights   491
Exam Review   492

Chapter 20   Seated Massage   496

Learning Outcomes   496
Key Terms   496
Seated Massage Overview   497
History of Seated Massage   497
Benefits of Seated Massage   497
   Public Places and Events   497

   In the Workplace   498
   Popularity of Seated Massage   498
Body and Hand Mechanics   498
Screening for Seated Massage   498
Positioning for Seated Massage   499
Seated Massage Sessions   500
Preparing for Different Venues   505
Chapter Highlights   506
Exam Review   507

**PART 5   TAPPAN'S GUIDE TO
           CONTEMPORARY MASSAGE
           AND BODYWORK**   511

Chapter 21   Myofascial Massage   512

Learning Outcomes   512
Key Terms   512
Myofascial Massage Overview   513
History of Myofascial Massage   513
Fascia and Fascial Anatomy   513
   Depths of Fascia   513
   Fascial Structures   514
Guidelines for Myofascial Applications   515
   Contraindications   515
Basic Myofascial Techniques   516
   Skin Lifting Techniques   516
   Fascial Stretching Techniques   516
   Fascial Mobilizations   517
Myofascial Massage Techniques on the Back   518
Chapter Highlights   522
Exam Review   523

Chapter 22   Trigger Point Therapy   526

Learning Outcomes   526
Key Terms   526
Trigger Point Therapy Overview   527
History of Trigger Point Therapy   527
Trigger Points   527
   Origin of TrPs   528
Referral Patterns   528
Locating Trigger Points   529
   Palpation of TrPs   530
Deactivation Techniques   530
   Direct Pressure Techniques   530
Trigger Point Therapy for Tension
   Headaches   532
Chapter Highlights   535
Exam Review   536

Chapter 23   Lymphatic Facilitation   539

Learning Outcomes   539
Key Terms   539

Overview of Lymphatic Facilitation 540
History of Lymphatic Massage 540
*Lymphatic Facilitation Compared to Manual
    Lymphatic Drainage* 540
The Lymphatic System 540
Homeostasis 540
Lymph 541
Interstitial Matrix 542
Lymphatic System Vessels 542
Initial/Terminal (I/T) Lymph Vessels 542
Collector Vessels 543
Transport Vessels 543
Cisterna Chyli 543
Terminus 543
Lymph Nodes 544
General Drainage Patterns 544
Indications and Contraindications 544
Contraindications 544
Lymphatic Facilitation Attributes and Strokes 545
L Stroke and Long Stroke 546
Lymphatic Facilitation Applications 547
Integration of Lymphatic Facilitation into a Massage
    Session 553
Chapter Highlights 554
Exam Review 555

Chapter 24 Reflexology 558
Learning Outcomes 558
Key Terms 558
Overview 559
History of Reflexology 559
Ancient Roots 559
Reflexology in Europe 559
Reflexology in America 561
Modern Professional Reflexology 561
Zone Therapy and Guidelines 561
Theories about Reflexology 562
Reflexology Research and Application 563
Sensation During and after Reflexology 563
*Possible Reasons for Tenderness
    and Pain* 563
After the Reflexology Session 564
Positioning the Receiver 564
Body Mechanics 564
Reflexology Techniques 564
Walk and Roll 565
Hook-and-Backup 565
Press-and-Flex 565
Direct Pressure and Friction 565
Dorsal Fulling 566
Joint Movements 566
Adjuncts to Reflexology 566
Reflexology Session 567
Chapter Highlights 572
Exam Review 573

Chapter 25 Asian and Energy-Based Bodywork 576
Learning Outcomes 576
Key Terms 576
Energy-Based Bodywork 577
Eastern Bodywork Forms 577
Traditional Chinese Medicine Overview 577
Yin and Yang 577
Qi 578
The Five Elements 578
Energy Channels 580
Acupoints 580
*Assessment and Treatment in Traditional Chinese
    Medicine* 583
Acupressure Massage Integration 584
Basic AMI Approach 585
Principles for Applying Pressure to Acupoints 585
*AMI Practice Sequences for the Back, Arm,
    and Neck–Head–Face* 585
Qi Gong 607
Qi Gong Forms 607
Ayurveda 607
Ayurvedic Health Practices 608
*The Physical Body—Koshas, Doshas, and
    Chakras* 609
Marma Points 611
Ayurvedic Massage 611
Varieties of Ayurvedic Massage 612
Massage Oils 613
Massage Applications 613
Hatha Yoga 614
Thai Massage 614
Polarity Therapy 615
Polarity Therapy Theory 615
Principles of Polarity Therapy 618
Basic Polarity Movements 619
Notes on the Practice Sequence 625
Some Final Thoughts on Polarity Therapy 625
Chapter Highlights 626
Exam Review 628

**PART 6   FOUNDATIONS OF CAREER
AND PRACTICE
DEVELOPMENT** 631

Chapter 26 Career Plans and Employment 632
Learning Outcomes 632
Key Terms 632
Follow Your Dream 633
Vision 633
Part-Time or Full-Time Work 633
Employment or Private Practice 633
Mission Statement 636
Income Goal 636

Identity   637
  Business Name and Logo   637
  Credentials   637
  Résumé   638
  Business Cards and Stationery   639
  Brochures and Websites   640
Getting Employment   640
  Successful Job Interviews   641
Chapter Highlights   643
Exam Review   644

Chapter 27 Private Practice and Finances   647

Learning Outcomes   647
Key Terms   647
Private Practice   648
Business Plan Overview   648
Description of the Business   648
  Legal Structure   648
  Location   648
Marketing   649
  Market Research   650
  Building a Client Base   650
  Advertising and Promotions   650
Management   651
  Licenses and Insurance   652
  Contracts   652
  Practice Policies   653
  Massage Practice Office Space   654
  Appointments   654
  Client Records   655
Finances   655
  Startup Costs   656
  First-Year Budget   656
  Income Taxes   657
  Bookkeeping   660
  Banking   660
Health Insurance Billing and Reimbursement   661
  Standardized Forms and Billing Codes   662
Chapter Highlights   663
Exam Review   664

Chapter 28 Business Ethics   667

Learning Outcomes   667
Key Terms   667
Business Ethics   668
Local and State Regulations   668
Advertising   669
  Professional Image   669
  Guarantees and Endorsements   670
  Prices and Bait Advertising   671
Claims for Massage Therapy   671
Copyrights, Trademarks, and Patents   672
Fees and Pricing   673
Tips and Gifts   673
Selling Products   674
Referrals   675
Client Base   675
Defamation   676
Safety and Welfare of Clients   677
Reporting Unethical Behavior   677
Beyond Graduation—An Invitation   678
Chapter Highlights   678
Exam Review   679

APPENDICES

A   Organizations and Publications   A-1

B   Code of Ethics and Standards of Practice for Massage
    Therapists   A-3

C   Goal-Oriented Planning   A-8

D   Performance Evaluation Forms   A-10

E   References and Additional Resources   A-54

Interactive Glossary   G-1
Index   I-1

Fast Track to Success

Before you begin, we encourage you to read this brief section to help you get off to a great start in your studies and test-taking.

STUDY TIPS

Knowing your own learning style is a key to success in school. Are you primarily a visual, auditory, or kinesthetic learner? Do you learn best alone or in a study group? Do you study better in the morning or at night? Do you have a learning disability, and if so, have you gotten help to learn compensation techniques? Develop a learning strategy that works best for you, and take responsibility for using it in school and beyond.

Big Picture versus Details

Research indicates that learners fall into two camps: "right-brained" learners who process information by focusing on the big picture and relationships between ideas, and "left-brained" learners who process information in a sequential step-by-step fashion focusing on details. Each style of learning has strengths and drawbacks. For example, right-brain learners can miss important details, whereas left-brain learners may get so bogged down in details that they miss the big picture. Be aware of your natural style, but incorporate methods that help you get both the big picture as well as the details.

Better Study Habits

Here are some simple things you can do to improve your study habits:

- Understand the learning outcomes for a class, and keep your attention on material that helps you achieve them. Be selective and focused.

- Read assigned material before a lecture so that you are not hearing about the subject for the first time in class. The lecture will sink in more deeply if you are already somewhat familiar with terminology and concepts presented. You will be less likely to get lost in class.

- Underline, highlight, and write in the margins of reading material to identify important terms and concepts. Be selective in finding the most important ideas. Mark passages directly related to topics from classes. Don't highlight too much.

- Pick out key terms, and write out their definitions. Identify related concepts and subtopics.

- Become familiar with the features in your textbooks. The table of contents, figures, tables, appendix, glossary, and index provide valuable information and help you find what you are looking for more quickly.

- Within 24 hours after a class, review and rewrite your class notes. Write summaries of major topics in your own words, noting where ideas covered in class are found in your textbooks.

- If you learn best by hearing (auditory learner), ask permission to tape lectures so that you are not distracted from what the teacher is saying by taking notes. Replay the tapes after class, and then make notes of the most important ideas.

- If you learn best by doing (kinesthetic learner), write out concepts and definitions, draw pictures and diagrams, and outline chapters in your textbooks. Do things like handle bones of the skeleton when learning anatomy, palpate muscles as you memorize their locations and attachments, and combine doing massage techniques with memorizing their effects.

- In study groups, explain basic concepts to each other, ask each other questions, and discuss important topics. Listen to what others have to say, and also practice saying your ideas out loud to others. This helps you clarify your thoughts.

- Use study guides and supplemental materials that come with your textbooks.

Take Time

Set aside enough time to read, discuss, think about, and test yourself on material you are learning. The more you review the material and interact with it in different ways, the better your grasp of it will be. A general rule is to study 3 hours for every hour you are in class. Finally, tell the instructor or a counselor if you are getting lost or behind in class. Be open to suggestions and to trying new learning methods.

Remember the old adage "You can lead a horse to water, but you can't force him to drink." The school and teachers are responsible for setting up a good learning environment, but you must do your part for learning to take place.

TAKING TESTS

Written examinations are a fact of life in school and in attaining certification and licensing. Some people find exams a positive experience. They enjoy testing their knowledge and approach them like game shows on TV. Others find exams anxiety provoking and decidedly unpleasant. Following some simple guidelines can maximize the chances that your test results will truly reflect what you have learned.

Get Focused

First, arrive early and get organized and settled into your seat. Get out your pencil and other items you will need for the test. Put your other things away and out of sight so that you have a clear space to work and think. Do whatever works for you to calm down, focus, and concentrate, for example, quiet sitting or deep breathing.

If you get distracted easily, find a quiet place in the room away from doors and windows. Sit in the front row near a wall if possible. Ask the monitor if you can wear earplugs to muffle distracting sounds.

Understand the Test

Read and understand the test directions before you start. Ask the monitor for an explanation of directions you do not understand. Quickly look over the entire test to see how long it is and what types of questions are on it, so that you can plan your time.

Read each question carefully before answering. Reading too quickly can cause you to miss important words. Be sure you fully understand what the question is asking.

Don't panic if you have a momentary lapse of memory. If you draw a blank on a question, skip over it, and go back to it later. Don't be disturbed if others finish before you do. Focus on what you are doing, and take the time allowed to finish. If you have extra time, check over your answers to catch careless mistakes, or reread and improve essay answers.

Answer Questions Thoughtfully

ESSAY QUESTIONS   First, determine what level of knowledge the question requires. Action words like *list*, *define*, *compare*, *analyze*, and *explain* tell you how to approach your answer. Outline your answer on a scratch sheet to organize your thoughts and identify important points.

Do not write everything you remember about the topic. Be sure that your answer addresses the specific question asked. Be concise and direct in your answer. Don't ramble. Write legibly and in complete sentences. Use good grammar and correct spelling. Come back to your answer later if you have time to recheck for accuracy, completeness, clarity, and to correct grammatical and spelling errors.

If you run out of time, quickly outline an answer. Providing some information is better than leaving the question blank.

OBJECTIVE TEST QUESTIONS   The most common objective test questions are multiple choice, true/false, and matching. Answer the questions in order, marking the ones you are not sure of in the margin. Do not spend too much time on any one question. Give it your best guess and move on. You can go back to it later if you have time.

Watch out for negative wording such as *not* or *least*, "double negatives," and qualifying words like *always*, *seldom*, *never*, *most*, *best*, and *largest*. Read each question thoroughly for full understanding of what it says.

Multiple-choice questions are designed so that only one choice is correct. A good strategy is to find the correct answer by the process of elimination of the incorrect ones. Grammatical inconsistencies may tip you off to the right answer or to a wrong one. Read the question and your choice together to make sure it makes grammatical sense.

True/false questions need to be read very carefully. One incorrect detail makes the whole statement false. If a sentence has two parts (a compound sentence), both parts need to be true for the whole question to be true.

For matching questions, use one column as your reference. For each item in that column, go through all items in the second column until you find a match. Match all the ones you are sure of first, and then go back to match the others with your best guess.

Do not change your answers without good reason. First "guesses" tend to be better than "second guessing." If you are not guessing, but have a good reason to change your mind, go ahead and change an answer.

YOUR RESOURCE FOR LEARNING

Tappan's Handbook of Massage Therapy: Blending Art with Science is intended to be your resource for learning. Every feature is designed to lead you to success in laying the foundations for your career in massage therapy. By keeping your career goals in sight, you can find motivation to do what it takes to get the most out of your time in school.

Getty Images/Bruce Ayres

Chapter 1

Massage Therapy Profession

Chapter 2

History of Massage
as a Vocation

Chapter 3

Professional and Personal
Development

Chapter 4

Physical Skills, Fitness, Self-
Care for the Massage
Therapist

Chapter 5

Ethics and the Therapeutic
Relationship

PART

1

Foundations for Massage Therapy Professionals

Pearson Education, Inc.

CHAPTER

1 Massage Therapy Profession

CHAPTER OUTLINE

Learning Outcomes

Key Terms

The Journey

Massage Defined

Wellness Profession

Trends

Typical Work Settings

Becoming a Massage Therapy
   Professional

Body of Knowledge and Skills

Education

Credentials

Organizations

Scholarship and Publications

Research

Ethical Standards

Recognition by the Public and
   Health Professionals

Chapter Highlights

Exam Review

LEARNING OUTCOMES

After studying this chapter, you will have information to:

1. Define massage therapy.
2. Explain the scope of massage therapy using the Wellness Massage Pyramid.
3. Identify trends related to massage therapy.
4. Summarize the variety of career opportunities for massage therapists.
5. Describe the unique knowledge base of massage therapy.
6. Discuss education standards for massage therapists.
7. Describe the types of credentials available to massage therapists.
8. Distinguish among various kinds of professional organizations.
9. Identify major sources of information about massage therapy.
10. Describe the state of massage therapy research.

KEY TERMS

Accreditation

Board certification

Complementary and
   alternative medicine
   (CAM)

Continuing education (CE)

Credentials

Ethical standards

Health care settings

Home visit practice

Integrative medicine center

Massage

Massage therapy

Occupational licensing

Personal care settings

Private practice settings

Professional associations

Sports, fitness, and
   recreation settings

Wellness Massage Pyramid
   (WMP)

Wellness profession

THE JOURNEY

Welcome! You have begun the journey to becoming a successful massage therapist. The next several months will be a period of transformation as you learn to be a competent and caring professional. Your education will be a holistic experience as you physically master massage techniques, mentally absorb the science and theory of massage therapy, and practice the social skills needed for good relationships with clients. You will exercise your memory, develop reasoning skills, and internalize the principles of ethical behavior. You will learn about employment opportunities and how to start and maintain your own massage therapy practice.

The first step on this journey is to survey the landscape of massage therapy, that is, to get the big picture of the career that you have chosen. That means understanding what massage therapy is, its broad scope as a wellness profession, trends related to its use, and where massage therapists work. The next step is to get an overview of the massage therapy profession, such as education, certification, licensing, research, and the organizations and publications available to massage therapists.

MASSAGE DEFINED

Massage is the intentional and systematic manipulation of the soft tissues of the body to enhance health and healing. Massage is performed with or without lubricating substances such as oil and lotion. Joint movements and stretching are commonly performed as part of massage. Adjunct modalities within the scope of massage include the use of hot and cold packs and hydrotherapy in the form of the whirlpool bath, sauna, and steam room.

Simple hand tools are sometimes used to apply pressure during massage, as are machines that mimic massage techniques. However, massage is primarily manual therapy; that is, it is performed by hand. It is the person-to-person touch essential to massage that gives it a unique healing potential.

The most common system of massage in North America is traditional European massage, often called *Swedish massage*. Swedish massage is based on an understanding of anatomy, physiology, pathology, and other biosciences. The seven technique categories of Swedish massage consist of the following:

- Effleurage
- Petrissage
- Tapotement
- Friction
- Vibration
- Touch without movement
- Joint movements

Swedish massage techniques are applied to improve overall functioning of the body systems, to enhance healing, and for relaxation of body and mind.

In addition to Swedish massage, massage therapy today encompasses a variety of specialized techniques and alternative approaches. Specialized systems of soft tissue manipulation include manual techniques that affect specific body systems, for example, myofascial massage, trigger point therapy, and lymphatic facilitation. Other types of manual therapy, like reflexology and polarity therapy, have gone outside Western science and encompass alternative theories of health and healing.

Traditions of manual therapy are found all over the globe. Major traditions include folk and native practices from different areas of the world, the more developed systems of European massage, Ayurvedic massage from India, and Asian bodywork therapies based in Chinese medicine. Some eclectic approaches combine theory and techniques from several systems.

Massage therapy is a general term used to describe all the different systems of soft tissue manipulation. *Bodywork* is a term coined in the late twentieth century to encompass a wide variety of manual therapies including massage, movement integration, structural integration, and energy balancing. The terms *massage* and *bodywork* are often used together to describe the occupational field of massage therapy, as in *therapeutic massage and bodywork*.

WELLNESS PROFESSION

Massage therapists apply massage and related modalities to help clients on their quest for high-level wellness. This includes massage therapy for stress reduction, for treatment and recovery from illness and injuries, as a simple healthy pleasure, and for many other purposes. The broad scope of the field is evident in the **Wellness Massage Pyramid (WMP)** in Figure 1–1 ■.

The WMP illustrates the major goals of massage therapy and its many applications. The goal at the top is high-level wellness, a condition of optimal physical, emotional, intellectual, spiritual, social, and vocational well-being. The concept of wellness is holistic at its core, encompassing the whole person.

The three levels at the base of the pyramid address *deficiency* needs related to illness and injury. These include applications of massage therapy for treatment of, recovery from, and prevention of illness and injury. Satisfying those needs brings one to the *neutral zone*, which is the old definition of health as the absence of disease.

Next in the WMP are the *growth* levels. These include massage therapy applications for health maintenance, personal growth, and enjoyment of life to its fullest—all aiming toward a state of high-level wellness. The upper part of the pyramid contains massage therapy for purposes such as optimal body system functioning, developing greater awareness

FIGURE 1–1
Wellness Massage Pyramid.

of the inner self, feeling integrated in body and mind, and enjoying the healthy pleasure of caring touch.

Massage therapy is included in the broad category of **complementary and alternative medicine (CAM)**. CAM therapies are healing systems or modalities generally outside mainstream allopathic medicine, for example, herbal remedies, acupuncture, naturopathic medicine, biofeedback, and music therapy. The White House Commission on CAM Policy (2002)[1] cited therapeutic massage, bodywork, and somatic movement therapies as a major CAM domain. Massage therapy as a CAM domain generally refers to applications of massage at the base of the WMP.

In its fullest sense, massage therapy is best thought of as a **wellness profession** because the work of massage therapists spans the entire wellness massage paradigm. Because of its broad scope, there are a wide variety of career opportunities for massage therapy practitioners. These include developing general practices, or more narrow specializations such as personal care, sports and fitness, or health care.

Some massage therapists focus on a particular client group, such as the elderly, children, athletes, people with a certain disease or disability, or other special population. Over time, massage and bodywork practitioners learn new skills, deepen their knowledge, take advanced training, and change work settings. Because it is a wellness profession, a career in massage therapy opens many opportunities for satisfying individual interests, talents, and strengths.

TRENDS

Consumer surveys reveal trends in the popularity of massage and the reasons people seek it out. Recent studies indicate an increased use of massage overall. A 2012 survey showed that a high percentage of consumers (68%) received their massage in spas and independent massage therapy offices. Other places mentioned were hair salons, hotels, and medical practices. The majority of massage recipients were women (60%) according to survey results.[2]

CRITICAL THINKING

Think about your current state of well-being. Note where improvements can be made, and formulate some wellness goals for yourself. Now determine how massage might fit into a plan to meet those goals.

1. Consider the broad scope of wellness, including physical, emotional, intellectual, spiritual, social, and vocational well-being.

2. Use the Wellness Massage Pyramid to identify areas of personal deficiency (e.g., illness or injury) and areas for personal growth.

3. Explain how massage might fit into a plan to help you meet your personal wellness goals.

4. Compare the benefits you might expect from massage to others in the class. Notice how each person's needs and desires are unique.

FIGURE 1–2

Ten most common CAM therapies used by adults.

Source: Data from *CDC National Health Statistics Report #12 Complementary and Alternative Therapy Use Among Adults and Children: United States, 2007.* Published December 2008.

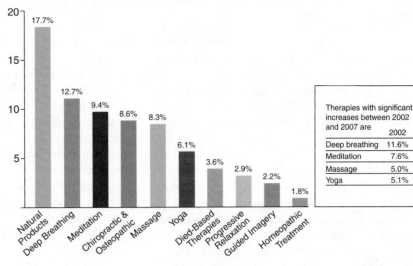

10 Most Common CAM Therapies Among Adults - 2007

Therapies with significant increases between 2002 and 2007 are		
	2002	2007
Deep breathing	11.6%	12.7%
Meditation	7.6%	9.4%
Massage	5.0%	8.3%
Yoga	5.1%	6.1%

A different study conducted in 2014 noted that 77% of the people surveyed who got a massage in the past 12 months said that their primary reason for receiving massage was either medical (54%) or stress related (23%). Medical reasons cited for receiving massage included soreness, stiffness or spasms, injury recovery, migraines, prevention, and general well-being. Of those surveyed, 91% viewed massage as beneficial to overall health and wellness and 92% believed it effective for reducing pain. A majority of consumers surveyed (74%) agreed that massage therapy should be considered a form of health care.[3]

The popularity of massage has grown at the same time that consumers are using more complementary and alternative therapies. These trends are undoubtedly related. The annual National Health Interview Survey in 2007 found that "38.1 million adults made an estimated 354.2 million visits to practitioners of CAM," and that "about three-quarters of both visits to CAM practitioners and total out-of-pocket costs spent on CAM practitioners were associated with manipulative and body-based therapies" including massage.[4] A similar survey a few years earlier found that women were more likely to use CAM than men, that CAM use increased with age and education level, and that those who had been hospitalized in the past year were more likely to turn to CAM.[5]

CAM therapies are also being used more often in hospital settings. A 2010 survey sponsored by the American Hospital Association found that 42% of responding hospitals offered one or more CAM therapies, up from 37% in 2007. According to the survey, patient demand was the main reason hospitals provided CAM (85%), followed by clinical effectiveness (70%). Massage therapy ranked fifth among the top 10 most common CAM therapies among adults. Massage therapy was one of the top two services provided in both outpatient and inpatient settings.[6] See Figures 1–2 ■ and 1–3 ■.

These surveys indicate a trend of increased utilization of massage therapy in the future in a variety of settings. The growth in availability of massage in spas for relaxation

and rejuvenation, and in medical settings as a CAM therapy, are particularly significant. It is not surprising, then, that according to the U.S. Department of Labor, employment for massage therapists is expected to increase 20% from 2010 to 2020, faster than the average for all occupations.[7]

FIGURE 1–3 Top six hospital outpatient and inpatient CAM therapies.

Source: Data from *Complementary and Alternative Medicine Survey of Hospitals 2010: Summary of Results,* by Samueli Institute and Health Forum: An American Hospital Association Company.

TYPICAL WORK SETTINGS

Massage therapists work in a variety of settings, reflecting the broad range of the benefits of massage. Four categories of typical work settings include personal care; sports, fitness, and recreation; health care; and private practice. Table 1–1 ■ lists examples of places where massage therapists typically work. Part 6 of this text, *Foundations of Career and Practice Development*, explores the options for a massage practice in more detail.

Personal Care

Personal care settings focus on personal grooming, relaxation, and rejuvenation. They include beauty salons and barbershops and day, destination, and specialty spas. In these settings, massage is just one of several services offered. Chapter 19, *Spa Treatments*, describes several of the services a massage therapist working in a spa might perform after receiving additional training, such as aromatherapy, body wraps, exfoliations, and hot stone massage.

Beauty salons and barbershops offer cosmetic services related to hair, nails, and skin care. These establishments are found in storefronts, shopping malls, department stores, hotels, and other commercial spaces. Cosmetologists, beauticians, barbers, and estheticians are licensed professionals providing services in these businesses. Massage may be part of their services as allowed within their scope of practice; for example, cosmetologists are usually permitted by law to perform facials and pedicures that include massage. In this setting, massage therapists usually offer full body massage for relaxation.

Spas are establishments that focus on improving overall well-being by offering a variety of personal care services. Their aim is to help patrons renew mind, body and spirit.

Seven major kinds of spas include club spa, cruise ship spa, cruise ship spa, day spa, destination spa, medical spa, mineral spring spa, and resort/hotel spa. The intent of the spa experience is expressed in the 4Rs—relax, reflect, revitalize, and rejoice.[8]

Day spas offer many of the same services as beauty salons and barbershops, plus special services such as herbal wraps, various kinds of hydrotherapy (e.g., whirlpool, sauna, steam room), mud baths, mineral baths, exercise facilities, and therapeutic massage and bodywork. See Figure 1–4 ■. Patrons come for one or more services, staying a short time or the entire day. Massage therapists are sometimes trained to perform services in addition to massage, for example, herbal wraps.

Destination spas are places with overnight accommodations, which immerse guests in a healthy environment. Services include fitness activities, nutritious meals, lifestyle education, and the day spa services listed earlier, including massage.

Other types of spas are distinguished either by focus or location. For example, club spas are fitness facilities that also offer spa services. Medical spas integrate spa services with conventional and complementary therapies for healing mind and body. Cruise ship spas are located aboard cruise ships, and mineral spring spas at mineral and hot springs. Resort and hotel spas cater to business and vacation travelers staying at their establishments. The range of services offered in different spas varies, but their common purpose is renewal and rejuvenation through personal care. Massage is an integral part of the modern spa scene.

Sports, Fitness, and Recreation

Sports, fitness, and recreation settings are facilities whose main purpose is to provide opportunities for physical exercise and sports, but that also provide support services such as

TABLE 1–1	Typical Work Settings for Massage Therapists		
Personal Care	**Sports, Fitness, and Recreation**	**Health Care**	**Private Practice— Self-Employment**
• Beauty salon or barbershop	• Nonprofit community center	• Conventional health care center	• Massage therapy office or clinic
• Spa	• Commercial health club	*Medical office or clinic*	• Storefront business
Club spa	• Specialty exercise studio	*Hospice service*	• Home-based practice
Cruise ship spa	• Sports club or team	*Hospital*	• Home visit practice
Day spa		*Skilled nursing or extended care facility*	• On-site chair massage
Destination spa		*Outpatient rehabilitation centers*	
Medical spa		• Integrative medical center	
Mineral spring spa		*Integrative medical clinic*	
Resort/hotel spa		*Sports medicine clinic*	
		Medical spa	
		Wellness center	
		• Alternative health care center	
		Chiropractic office	
		Naturopathic clinic	
		Chinese medicine clinic	

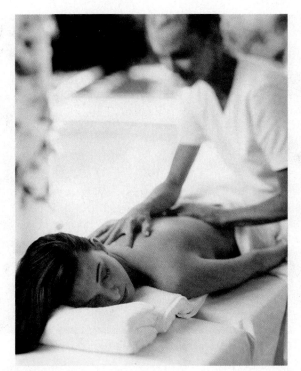

FIGURE 1–4 Personal care setting.

Source: Getty Images/Bruce Ayres.

massage. These include nonprofit community centers such as the YMCA, commercial health clubs, and specialty exercise studios such as yoga centers. Some massage therapists work with professional or amateur sports teams at their own training facilities and on the road. See Figure 1–5 ■.

Massage is offered in these settings as an adjunct to fitness and sports programs. Massage therapists interact with other health professionals working in these facilities, including coaches, personal trainers, exercise physiologists, and athletic trainers. The focus of massage here is to help clients achieve their fitness goals, improve athletic performance, and enhance healing from minor injuries.

Health Care

Health care settings are places where patients are treated for illnesses and injuries. They include conventional Western medical facilities such as doctors' offices and clinics, hospitals, hospice facilities, skilled nursing and extended care facilities, and rehabilitation centers. Integrative medical settings offer both conventional and complementary and alternative healing methods as options, based on the greatest potential benefit for the patient. Health care settings also include alternative medicine venues such as chiropractic clinics, naturopathic offices, and Chinese medicine and acupuncture clinics.

In conventional medical settings, massage therapists work in conjunction with doctors, nurses, physical therapists, and other health care professionals within the tradition of Western medicine. Hospital-based massage is a specialty in which massage is integrated into the regular hospital framework, such as in the pediatric ward, cancer unit, or cardiac care (Figure 1–6 ■). Conventional health care centers may take an integrative approach by having alternative healing practitioners, including massage therapists, available to patients. An **integrative medicine center** goes one step further by offering a team approach among a variety of Western medical health care providers, traditional and indigenous healers, and CAM practitioners in a collaborative effort. Massage therapists in these environments are an integral part of a health care team.

Integrative medical settings take different forms. In sports medicine centers, massage therapists team up with physical therapists and athletic trainers for rehabilitation of athletic injuries and improvement of sports performance. In medical spas, conventional and complementary therapies are available in a spa environment. Wellness centers connected to hospitals offer fitness activities, rehabilitation programs, massage therapy, and classroom instruction in preventing disease and developing a healthy lifestyle.

Chiropractors hire massage therapists to work with their patients in conjunction with regular chiropractic treatment.

FIGURE 1–5

Sports, fitness, and recreation setting.

Source: Pearson Education, Inc.

FIGURE 1–6 Health care setting.

Source: Pearson Education, Inc.

FIGURE 1–7 Private practice setting.

Source: Pearson Education, Inc.

Massage may be given before or after a chiropractic adjustment or at a different time as part of an overall treatment plan. Chiropractors also lease space to massage therapists to whom they refer patients for ongoing massage for prevention of problems and general well-being.

Naturopathic physicians sometimes refer patients for massage as part of a treatment strategy. They also hire massage therapists to work in their clinics, or they may lease space to massage therapists so that they are on-site at the naturopathic office.

Chinese medicine clinics often employ practitioners skilled in massage and Asian bodywork therapies. Asian bodywork systems that complement traditional healing practices such as acupuncture and herbs include tuina, amma, shiatsu, acupressure, and Jin Shin Do®.

Private Practice

Private practice settings are the most varied. Massage therapists in private practice are self-employed and develop their businesses to suit their own interests and talents and to respond to current consumer demands.

The most common private practice setting is the one-room massage office, or massage clinic with two or more rooms, in an office building. A storefront massage business might be on a commercial street, in a shopping mall, or at an airport. A dedicated massage room can be set aside in a residence for a home-based practice where not prohibited by zoning laws (Figure 1–7 ▪). Clients come to the massage therapist's space for appointments in these settings.

An alternative is for the massage therapist to travel to the client's home, sometimes called a **home visit practice**. There the massage therapist creates a setting for massage in an appropriate space provided by the client. The home visit practice is convenient for busy working clients and the homebound elderly and disabled.

With the invention of the special massage chair, settings for massage have expanded to the workplace and various public places. Seated massage settings have been created in such places as parks, inside grocery or department stores, and at trade shows and conferences. The traveling or *on-site massage practice* can be set up temporarily in a small space using portable equipment suitable for the situation.

Many massage therapists develop eclectic practices, for example, combining an office practice with making home visits or part-time employment at a spa or chiropractic office. Specialized or advanced training may be required to work in certain settings; however, the examples described here demonstrate the broad and diverse range of career opportunities for massage therapists in today's world.

BECOMING A MASSAGE THERAPY PROFESSIONAL

Massage therapists contribute to the overall health and well-being of their clients and their communities. As the benefits of massage therapy become better appreciated and the demand for massage therapy grows, there are corresponding expectations that massage therapists become increasingly professional. That means being better educated, having valid credentials, adhering to a code of ethics, and generally being held to a higher standard. Massage therapy is considered an emerging profession in that some of the hallmarks of a mature profession are still in development.

The benchmarks of mature professions include having a unique body of knowledge and skills and intensive entry-level education. It also includes continuing education throughout a career and having valid credentials. The theoretical and scientific information underlying a profession

PRACTICAL APPLICATION

Prepare an informal survey of the availability of massage in your community and the varieties of career opportunities for massage therapists there.

1. Make a list of the places in your community where massage is available.
2. Look at the types of settings, for example, personal care, sports and fitness, health care, and private practice.
3. Indicate the name and address of the business, and what type of massage they offer. Note the environment, for

example, if massage is one of many services offered like at a spa, or is unique like chair massage at a health food store, or a separate massage office.

4. Divide the list according to how close the places are to where you live. Are they within a half-mile, one mile, more than one mile?
5. Comment on the accessibility of massage in your community and the potential for career opportunities for massage therapists there.

develops through scholarship and research, as well as experience, and is published in professional journals. Professionals form associations that support their members, set standards, represent the profession to the public, and promote professional interests overall.

Ethical codes and standards of practice describe expectations of excellence and good conduct. They are the foundations of self-determination and self-regulation for a profession. The overall focus of all professions is commitment to service and the good of humanity. This latter commitment sets professions apart from other businesses and occupations. The public trust afforded to professionals is based on an expectation of honesty, integrity, and selfless service.

All the benchmarks mentioned here set the stage for acceptance by other professionals and recognition by the general public. The professionalizing of massage therapy has occurred at a steady pace since the 1980s. Box 1–1 ■ summarizes the foundational characteristics of a profession.

Because organizations have such a significant role in professions, it is important to know the major organizations in the profession you have chosen. They are typically known by their acronyms or initials, and the "alphabet soup" of organizations can be confusing. Use Table 1–2 ■ as a reference for the organizations mentioned in this chapter. Some of the important aspects of professionalism in massage therapy today are explored in the following paragraphs.

CASE FOR STUDY

Sarah and Finding the Right Massage

Sarah has read a lot about the benefits of receiving massage and has decided to try it for herself. She sees massage advertised in different places in her community and wonders where the best place to go for massage would be for her. Sarah has been feeling stressed out lately and somewhat sore from her new fitness program. She has a few health problems like mild asthma and allergies. She has a busy schedule and values convenience highly, but also wants a high-quality massage experience.

Question:

How should Sarah go about finding the right place to receive massage for herself?

Things to consider:

- What might Sarah's initial goals be for her massage session?
- What might her priorities be in terms of location and setting?
- What types of settings might she explore for a massage that meets her current needs?

Where might Sarah go for massage in your community?

Using the information from the preceding Practical Application exercise in this chapter, determine the two best places for Sarah to go for massage in your community. (Assume she lives near you.)

_____

_____

_____

| BOX 1–1 | Characteristics of a Profession |

- Specialized knowledge and skills
- Intensive entry-level education
- Accreditation of schools and programs
- Continuing education
- Valid credentials
  - Board certification
  - Specialty certification
  - Occupational licensing
- Professional associations
- Ethical codes and standards of practice
- Acceptance among other professionals
- Recognition by the general public
- Commitment to public service and the good of humanity

with one-on-one interaction with clients and patients. The communication skills involved in health history taking and documentation are also required in other professions.

Massage skills are part of the scope of other professionals (e.g., estheticians, physical therapists, athletic trainers). However, soft tissue manipulation is only a small part of other professions, whereas it is the defining modality for massage therapists. Massage therapists apply massage through the entire range of wellness applications as depicted in the Wellness Massage Pyramid (WMP)—from treatment, recovery, and prevention of illness and injury to health maintenance, personal growth, and enjoyment of life.

This unique body of knowledge is found in the increasing number of books and journals written specifically for massage therapists. It is also reflected in massage therapy program curriculum standards, core competencies, job analyses, and licensing examinations for massage therapists.

BODY OF KNOWLEDGE AND SKILLS

The body of knowledge and skills that defines the massage therapy profession is unique in many respects, while sharing some things with other professions. The uniqueness of massage therapy lies in the primacy of touch and soft tissue manipulation in its skill base and the broad range of applications throughout the entire Wellness Massage Pyramid. The knowledge base for massage therapy, although occasionally borrowing from other professions, is uniquely focused on the use of soft tissue manipulation to improve the well-being of recipients. The profession is rooted in the tradition of natural healing and maintains a holistic and wellness perspective.

Examples of shared knowledge are the sciences of anatomy, physiology, and pathology that are basic to all health professions. Concepts such as the therapeutic relationship and related ethical principles are common to professions

EDUCATION

Entry-level education lays the foundation of knowledge and skills needed to perform massage therapy competently. The curriculum typically includes basic massage and bodywork techniques; sciences of anatomy, physiology, kinesiology, and pathology; assessment skills; client communication skills; hygiene and safety; professional standards, ethics, and law; and business practices. Basic massage techniques and their applications are learned in hands-on classes (Figure 1–8 ■).

The Commission on Massage Therapy Accreditation (COMTA) has identified core competencies for massage therapists. Competencies define education in terms of what a practitioner can actually do, rather than just having completed a number of hours in certain subjects.

TABLE 1–2	Guide to Major Massage Therapy Organizations in the United States*	
Acronym	Name	Type
ABMP	Associated Bodywork & Massage Professionals	Member Organization (Student membership available)
AMTA	American Massage Therapy Association	Professional Association (Student membership available)
AOBTA	American Organization for Bodywork Therapies of Asia	Specialty Association (Student membership available)
COMTA	Commission on Massage Therapy Accreditation (USDE recognized)	School Accreditation
FSMTB	Federation of State Massage Therapy Boards	Licensing Boards, Licensing Exam
MTF	Massage Therapy Foundation	Research, Education, Outreach
NCBTMB	National Certification Board for Therapeutic Massage and Bodywork	Board Certification

*Many other massage therapy organizations have been founded to serve the profession, and many others are located in countries outside the United States. This is a sample of the largest and most influential organizations in the United States.

FIGURE 1–8
Hands-on class in a massage therapy program.

Source: Pearson Education, Inc.

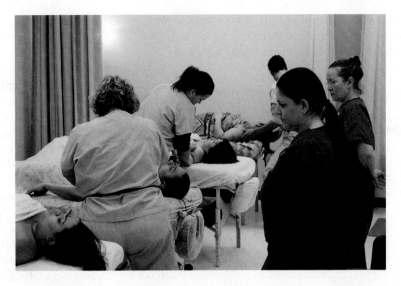

COMTA competencies for entry-level massage therapy programs include the following:

- Plan and organize an effective massage and bodywork session
- Perform massage therapy for therapeutic benefit
- Develop and implement a self-care strategy
- Develop ethical relationships with clients
- Develop a strategy for a successful practice
- Identify strategies for professional development

A more extensive list of standards can be found on the COMTA website (see Appendix E, *References and Additional Resources*).

Most massage therapy programs are offered in private vocational schools and community colleges, and award a diploma or certificate, associate degree, or, in a few cases, an academic bachelor's degree. The length of entry-level programs in the United States generally varies from 500–1,000 clock hours. COMTA requires 600 clock hours of classroom instruction.

Massage programs in the United States are required to be approved by the state government agency that oversees vocational, academic, or other school programs. This ensures minimal standards of operation. In other countries, a provincial or national education agency typically approves school programs. For example, in Canada, education is a responsibility of the individual provinces.

Massage schools, and massage programs within larger institutions such as community colleges, may seek additional recognition through **accreditation**. Accreditation is awarded by a nongovernmental organization whose mission is to uphold high educational standards. Accreditation organizations develop evaluation criteria and conduct peer evaluations to confirm that their standards are met. For example, the Integrative Massage and Somatic Therapies Accreditation Council (IMSTAC), a division of ABMP, is a body that sets standards for massage programs.

The U.S. Department of Education (USDE) publishes a list of nationally recognized nonprofit accrediting commissions determined by their criteria to be reliable. Some USDE-recognized authorities that accredit massage programs include the Accrediting Bureau of Health Education Schools (ABHES), Accrediting Commission for Career Schools and Colleges of Technology (ACCSCT), and the National Accrediting Commission of Cosmetology Arts and Sciences (NACCAS). The Commission on Massage Therapy Accreditation (COMTA) is the only accrediting agency focused exclusively on massage therapy programs and recognized by the USDE. A complete list of USDE recognized accrediting agencies can be found on the USDE website (see Appendix E).

Massage schools and programs may also join member organizations that provide forums for discussion of education-related issues, publications, liability insurance, and other resources. ABMP and AMTA both provide assistance to schools affiliated with them. The Alliance for Massage Therapy Education (AFMTE) is an independent nonprofit organization dedicated to improving the quality of massage therapy education. Membership in these organizations does not mean that a school or program is accredited by them.

Continuing Education

Continuing education (CE) is education beyond entry-level training. Continuing education keeps massage therapy professionals up-to-date and offers the opportunity to gain a higher level of knowledge and skills. A certain number of hours of continuing education are generally required for occupational license and certification renewals and by some membership organizations.

Continuing education is provided by massage schools, individual teachers, and professional associations. CE providers may be required to be approved for license or certification renewal. The National Certification Board for Therapeutic Massage and Bodywork has a list of their Approved CE Providers and the criteria for approval on their website (see Appendix E). If your state or local government licenses massage therapists, check with them for their approved providers of continuing education.

CREDENTIALS

Credentials testify to the accomplishments of the person holding them. They are a method for the general public, other professionals, and employers to evaluate a person's background in a given field. Credentials are awarded by a school, organization, or government agency to a person meeting their criteria for the credential. Using the language of credentials properly is important as massage therapists take their place in the larger world of health professionals. Presenting credentials honestly is a basic ethical principle. Four types of credentials available to massage therapists are a school diploma or certificate, board certification, specialty certification, and occupational licensing.

School Diploma

A school diploma or certificate is a statement that a person has graduated or successfully completed a course of study. It is the piece of paper hung on the wall to show the public the education a massage therapist has had. It designates the school name, location, course of study, number of hours completed, and date of graduation and is signed by school officials (Figure 1–9 ■). A *transcript* is a more detailed record of a student's performance while in school, including specific subjects studied, grades, and attendance, in addition to the information on the diploma. An original transcript carrying the school seal is usually required for official purposes such as obtaining a license to practice.

Board Certification

Board certification is a term usually reserved for a credential given by a nongovernmental nonprofit organization that attests to a person's competency and experience in a given profession. It involves qualifying by virtue of education and/or experience and passing a written examination and/or performance evaluation based on an objective analysis of job requirements. Those certified agree to abide by a specific code of ethics. Board certification is renewed periodically, which usually requires a certain amount of continuing education. It is sometimes referred to as *national certification*. Do not confuse *voluntary board certification* with a governmentally issued license to practice, which is called *certification* in some jurisdictions.

How does one know if a board certification credential is based on accepted standards and will be respected by other professionals? The National Commission for Certifying Agencies (NCCA) accredits certifying programs that comply with their standards. Many certification programs in the health professions seek NCCA recognition. A list of NCCA-accredited programs can be found on their website (see Appendix E). Two NCCA-accredited programs apply to massage and bodywork practitioners.

The National Certification Board for Therapeutic Massage and Bodywork (NCBTMB) is an organization that offers recognized credentials for massage therapists. It currently offers the title *Board Certified in Therapeutic Massage and Bodywork (BCTMB)*. Eligibility criteria and content outlines for their exams can be found on their website (see Appendix E).

The National Certification Commission for Acupuncture and Oriental Medicine (NCCAOM) offers a credential called *Diplomate in Asian Bodywork Therapy (Dipl. A.B.T.–NCCOAM)*. Information about this certification and others in oriental medicine, acupuncture, and Chinese herbology can be found on their website (see Appendix E).

Specialty Certification

To be certified in a specific massage and bodywork system (e.g., polarity therapy, reflexology, or shiatsu) involves some combination of education, skill development, internship, written and performance tests, ethical code, continuing education, and/or periodic renewal. Specialty certifications can be as rigorous as a 1,000 clock-hour program

Plainville School of Massage

Let it be known that

Mary Ann Smith

Has graduated with distinction from the
Professional Massage Therapy Program with 650 hours of instruction
and is thereby awarded this diploma.

On this 23rd day of August 2015

Plainville School of Massage
Plainville, Wisconsin

Leanne Binette
Director of Education

FIGURE 1–9
A diploma or certificate is proof of education completed.

with internship and written and performance exams, or as minimal as a weekend workshop. Therefore, determining what a specialty certification really means requires some information about who is offering it and what is involved in getting it.

Because massage therapy is an emerging profession and retains some entrepreneurial aspects, the terms *certification* and *certified* are sometimes used with ambiguity. For example, a course of study is sometimes called a *certification program* when it would be more correctly referred to as a *certificate program* for which a *certificate of completion* is given. In established professions, the term *certification* is more commonly reserved for credentials with more extensive education, examinations, continuing education, and renewal.

Some massage and bodywork systems are protected by trademark, and the name is registered with the U.S. Patent and Trademark Office. These systems use the registered trademark symbol®. Practitioners may not use a trademarked name to describe their work unless certified by their organization and properly authorized to do so. Examples are Jin Shin Do®, Rolfing®, and Bonnie Prudden Myotherapy® (see Appendix E).

Occupational Licensing

When deemed in the public interest, governments may choose to regulate a profession. A growing number of governments are licensing massage therapists. The main purposes of **occupational licensing** are consumer protection and the assurance of a minimal level of competence of practitioners. However, in the case of massage, an underlying motivation may also be to weed out practitioners using massage as a cover for prostitution.

In the United States, occupational licensing is done at the state level. In some unlicensed states, jurisdictions like big cities or counties may choose to license massage therapists. In Canada, occupational licenses are administered at the provincial level, and in some other countries at the federal or national level of government.

Occupational licensing is permission granted to qualified practitioners to accept compensation for massage in a specific governmental jurisdiction. Licenses are awarded by the government agency that regulates professions in the jurisdiction. It is required to practice, unlike the board or specialty certifications described earlier, which are voluntary. Table 1–3 ■ compares and contrasts diplomas, board certification, occupational licensing, specialty certification, and accreditation.

The details vary, but massage licenses typically require being a certain age (usually 18 years of age or older), having a minimum level of general education (usually a high school diploma), completing massage therapy education of a defined length (usually from 500–1,000 clock hours), passing a designated written and/or practical test, having no criminal record, abiding by a code of conduct, and paying fees. People practicing without a license are subject to fines, and, in some cases, criminal prosecution.

A few states have created their own licensing exams. Most states, however, accept a standardized exam developed to test minimum competency. The most widely used exam for massage therapists is the Massage & Bodywork Licensing Examination (MBLEx) developed by the Federation of State Massage Therapy Boards.

Occupational licensing may be called certification or registration in some jurisdictions. Variations of licensing include a form of government regulation called *registration*, in which only those meeting certain requirements can call themselves massage therapists, but other practitioners are not prohibited from working.

TABLE 1–3	Guide to Credentials in Massage Therapy				
Type of Credential	Voluntary/Required	Given To	Given By	Purpose
Accreditation	Voluntary	School	Nongovernment Accreditation Commission	Testify that school meets commission standards
Certificate	Voluntary	Individuals	Schools/Instructors	Proof of education completed
Continuing Education Approval	Required	Schools/Instructors	Credentialing Body	Approval of education programs for credential renewal
Diploma	Voluntary	Individuals	Schools/Instructors	Proof of education completed
Board Certification	Voluntary	Individuals	Nongovernment Certification Board	Attest to competency in the profession
Occupational License*	Required	Individuals	Government	Permission to practice in jurisdiction
Specialty Certification	Voluntary	Individuals	Nongovernment Organization/Instructor	Attest to competency in specialization

*Exact terminology for occupational licensing may vary in a specific jurisdiction, and certain states have adopted variations of regulation of the massage therapy profession. Check with your instructor about the situation in your location.

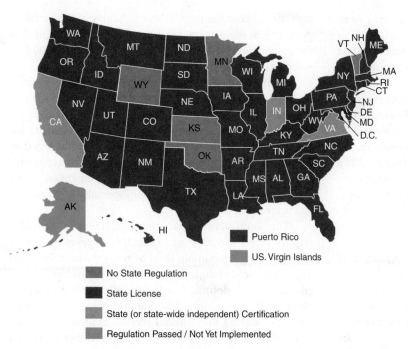

FIGURE 1–10 States that require licensing or certification.

Source: Graphic provided by Associated Bodywork & Massage Professionals.

■ Puerto Rico

■ US. Virgin Islands

■ No State Regulation

■ State License

■ State (or state-wide independent) Certification

■ Regulation Passed / Not Yet Implemented

In the United States today, 44 states plus the District of Columbia regulate massage therapists, and licensing bills are pending in several other states. Figure 1–10 ■ shows the states that require licensing or certification. The most current information on licensing can be found at professional organizations' websites, such as the sites sponsored by the AMTA and ABMP.

The Federation of State Massage Therapy Boards (FSMTB) was established in 2005 to facilitate communication among boards that regulate massage therapy in the United States. FSMTB concerns include standardizing license requirements and promoting portability of massage licenses from state to state.

A different type of license called an *establishment license* might also be required for a massage practice at a specific location. This is a business license to operate a commercial space where customers come for massage. Also for public protection, establishment licenses typically require revealing the business ownership, maintaining a certain level of hygiene and safety, posting services and prices, and that all practitioners in the establishment have the required occupational licenses.

ORGANIZATIONS

Massage and bodywork practitioners have formed several organizations to address their needs and promote the profession. They can be categorized as general membership organizations and specialty organizations. General membership organizations welcome practitioners of different forms of massage and bodywork and can be further categorized into professional associations and member services organizations. Specialty associations are composed of practitioners of a particular style of bodywork such as polarity therapists,

or those who work in a particular setting like the nurse massage therapists.

Professional Associations

Professional associations are nonprofit organizations run by elected leadership, whose mission is to promote their profession, to represent their members and the profession in the larger world, and to offer services to members. They set standards for the profession by developing codes of ethics and standards of practice. They typically have an IRS designation as 501(c)(6) corporations, that is, a nonprofit professional association.

The mission of the association, its goals and plans, position statements, and services are determined by an elected board and implemented by volunteers and staff. Involvement in the work of committees, special projects, and activities of the association help develop the present and future leadership of the profession. All the money generated by the association is reinvested in its mission.

Association services typically include providing information via official publications and websites, offering professional liability insurance and group insurance plans, hosting referral services, and selling products related to the profession. Associations raise public awareness of the profession and conduct consumer and other surveys to collect information about the field. At annual conventions, members get together for board and committee meetings, education sessions, exhibits of the latest equipment and supplies, and networking with other members (Figure 1–11 ■).

Governments consult with professional associations as representatives of the profession in developing legislation such as licensing and establishment laws. They also turn to associations when seeking participants in studies and policy development. For example, professional associations participated in preparing the 2002 report of the White House

FIGURE 1–11
Professional association conventions provide opportunities for networking with other massage therapists.

Source: Pearson Education, Inc.

Commission on Complementary and Alternative Medicine Policy (see Appendix E).

Organizations also look to professional associations for participation in multidisciplinary projects. An example of this is the participation of massage organizations in the Integrated Healthcare Policy Consortium (IHPC) of the Collaboration for Healthcare Renewal Foundation (see Appendix E).

Some professional associations have local chapters to address the needs of members in a particular state or other local jurisdiction. Chapters provide opportunities for leadership development and networking closer to home. They are important in the United States where regulation of massage therapy occurs at the state and local levels.

The American Massage Therapy Association (AMTA), founded in 1943, is the oldest and largest professional association for massage and bodywork therapists in the United States. Its mission is "to develop and advance the art, science and practice of massage therapy in a caring, professional and ethical manner in order to promote the health and welfare of humanity." Its core purpose is "to promote, advance and provide innovative thinking in the field of massage therapy while facilitating, supporting and serving AMTA members." It currently has over 56,000 members in 27 countries and chapters in all 50 states.

Member Services Organizations

Member services organizations are general membership organizations whose major mission is to provide benefits such as professional liability insurance, group health insurance, and publications. They also provide information of interest to their members in newsletters and on websites. These organizations may also act to protect the interests of members, for example, related to licensing and legislation. They differ from professional associations in that they may be for-profit businesses, and if so, the owner sets policy and determines the direction of the organization. They typically do not hold conventions nor have elected leadership.

The Associated Bodywork and Massage Professionals (ABMP), founded in 1987, is the largest member services organization for massage and bodywork practitioners in the United States, with over 80,000 members. Its stated goal is "to provide massage, bodywork, skin care and somatic therapies practitioners with professional services, information, and public and regulatory advocacy. ABMP is devoted to promoting ethical practices, protecting the rights of practitioners, and educating the public regarding the benefits of massage and bodywork."

 PRACTICAL APPLICATION

Explore student membership in a major professional organization. Use the organization's website and promotional materials for information.

1. Write a brief description listing the specific benefits offered with student membership.

2. Discuss with a classmate or study partner the potential value to you of joining a professional organization while still a student.
3. Answer the question: How might student membership in a major professional organization give me a head start in my career?

Specialty Associations

Massage therapy, like many other professions, can be divided into subgroups of practitioners with special knowledge and skills. They may focus on a particular form of massage and bodywork, a specific population of clients, or in a particular setting. Specialty groups often form their own associations to address their unique needs and interests. They offer members many of the same benefits as general membership organizations. The following are examples of different types of specialty associations for massage and bodywork practitioners.

The American Organization of Bodywork Therapies of Asia (AOBTA) is a professional association founded in 1989. It represents over 1,100 practitioners of different forms of bodywork based in traditional Chinese medicine as developed in China, Japan, Korea, and other Asian countries. The AOBTA provides members with educational and networking opportunities and promotes their professional development and success.[9]

The American Polarity Therapy Association (APTA) was founded in 1984 as an educational and charitable nonprofit organization. Its members include practitioners, teachers, and students of Polarity Therapy as developed by Randolph Stone. It promotes practitioner standards, approves education programs, sponsors education events, and publishes a newsletter and other materials.

The Rolf Institute® of Structural Integration was established in 1971 as an educational and scientific nonprofit organization. Its purpose is to promote a form of myofascial bodywork called Rolfing®, provide quality training programs in Rolfing®, certify Rolfing® practitioners, provide continuing education, and promote research and public awareness of the value of Rolfing®.

The International Association of Infant Massage (IAIM®) was formed in 1980 and incorporated in 1986. The organization promotes infant massage as a vehicle for nurturing touch and communication. It offers training to parents, caregivers, and health professionals, and also supports research on the importance of touch to the proper development of children. The organization trains and certifies *Certified Infant Massage Instructors (CIMI®)* who in turn teach parents and caregivers to massage their babies.

Most of the organizations described here were founded in the late twentieth century, when the field of massage and bodywork experienced a period of growth and expansion. Many other specialty organizations have been formed since that time. Their websites (see Appendix E) contain descriptions of their missions, membership, and programs.

SCHOLARSHIP AND PUBLICATIONS

Scholarship in therapeutic massage and bodywork has been increasing in volume and quality over the past 25 years. Vehicles for this information have evolved from a few self-published manuals in the 1970s to a variety of

REALITY CHECK

MANUELA: Remembering all of the massage organizations and credentials seems impossible. I'm not even sure why it's important. I just want to get a job doing massage after graduation.

ROB: There's a difference between seeing massage therapy as a job and thinking about it as a career. A career in massage therapy opens the door to a future doing meaningful work and options for any number of jobs or a private practice. The organizations and credentials related to massage therapy may seem confusing at first, but over time you'll become familiar with them. You'll read about them in publications for massage therapists, and you may want to join an organization as a student member. And building a résumé includes decisions about what organizations to join and what credentials you need for your dream job. Knowing all that's available to you as a massage therapist will help you make better choices.

well-documented and illustrated texts published by major publishing houses today.

The depth of scientific knowledge in anatomy, physiology, kinesiology, and pathology required by today's practitioners has spawned a number of books written specifically for massage and bodywork practitioners. Authors with extensive academic backgrounds in human sciences, who are also massage therapists, have provided a depth of knowledge absent in the past. The same can be said for the areas of pharmacology, psychology, and professional ethics.

As the profession of massage therapy matures, and experienced practitioners become teachers and authors, the understanding of massage therapy theory and principles deepens. In addition, massage therapists who have come from more established professions have enriched massage therapy scholarship. Nurses, physical therapists, physical and health educators, athletic trainers, psychologists, pharmacologists, and other professionals who have come into the field have helped transform massage theory and practice in a number of areas.

For example, information from other professions related to things such as the therapeutic relationship, assessment skills, effects of medications, documentation, and ethics have been integrated into the massage therapy knowledge base. The result is a more developed body of knowledge for massage therapists.

A variety of publications disseminate information about massage and bodywork to practitioners and the general public. The *Massage Therapy Journal* is the official publication of the AMTA, and ABMP publishes *Massage & Bodywork*. Although intended for a general audience, *Massage* magazine also provides information about the massage and bodywork profession. *Massage Today* is a monthly publication in newspaper format that contains news about the field, as well as informative articles on a variety of related subjects.

Peer-reviewed publications that report research related to massage therapy are *The Journal of Bodywork and Movement Therapies* and the free online journal *International Journal of Therapeutic Massage & Bodywork* (IJTMB) sponsored by the Massage Therapy Foundation. Peer review is a more rigorous process than editorial review used by most trade magazines. Peer reviewed means that a panel of massage therapists with expertise in the subject of an article evaluates the article for accuracy, reviews any research for validity, and approves the article for publication.

RESEARCH

A research base for massage therapy is developing gradually. Scientific studies about massage therapy are now conducted primarily within more established health professions and in connection with universities and hospitals. Although the emphasis of past research has been on clinical applications of massage, current research has expanded to include studies on the physiological effects of massage and benefits for special populations. Basic research on fascial tissue has revealed some of its amazing properties not previously known.

Two obstacles to the growth of massage therapy research are lack of an academic infrastructure to support it and inadequate funding. Private vocational schools and community colleges, where most massage therapy education takes place, do not ordinarily have the resources to conduct research. Neither do they have faculty with advanced training in experimental design and statistics to conduct the studies. The limited number of peer-reviewed research journals specifically for massage therapy means that reports of massage research are scattered among journals from other health professions.

There are, however, some developments to advance research in the profession. The Touch Research Institute (TRI) at the University of Miami School of Medicine was founded by Tiffany Field, MD, in 1992. It was the first center in the world devoted to the study of the use of touch and massage in the treatment of various ailments. Its website (see Appendix E) has information about many studies sponsored by TRI.

The Massage Therapy Foundation (MTF) was founded in 1992 to promote massage therapy research, education, and outreach. It funds experimental studies and encourages the writing of case reports related to massage therapy. The MTF published the *Massage Therapy Research Agenda* in 2002 that identified goals for the future. The first was to build an infrastructure to support massage research and increase research literacy among massage therapists. The

agenda also called for more funding for studies about the safety and efficacy of massage, physiological and other mechanisms of massage, massage in a wellness paradigm, and the massage therapy profession. MTF holds conferences that bring together researchers from all over the world to network and present the latest studies about massage and bodywork. It also maintains a free, online, peer-reviewed journal called the *International Journal of Therapeutic Massage and Bodywork: Research, Education, and Practice.*

Research about the effectiveness of massage is becoming more important as it is integrated into mainstream health care. It provides the "evidence" in evidence-based approaches to treatment, confirms what massage therapists know from experience, and reveals important information that advances the field.

ETHICAL STANDARDS

Knowledge of ethics and ethical behavior are essential competencies for massage therapists. There is a growing body of literature about ethical behavior in the profession.

Ethical standards in massage therapy are reflected in the codes of ethics and standards of practice of professional organizations. Licensing laws also require adherence to ethical codes and standards and often mandate continuing education in professional ethics as a condition of license renewal. Professional organizations and licensing boards also have disciplinary procedures for censoring those practitioners not in compliance with their ethical standards. Further discussion of professional ethics can be found in Chapter 5, *Ethics and the Therapeutic Relationship*, and Chapter 28, *Business Ethics*.

RECOGNITION BY THE PUBLIC AND HEALTH PROFESSIONALS

Evidence of public acceptance of massage therapy is found in the many positive articles appearing in newsstand magazines and health and fitness publications. Massage therapy is also a popular service at spas and health clubs.

Consumer surveys confirm the growing acceptance of massage therapy by the general public. According to a recent consumer survey, only 29% of respondents viewed massage therapy as only a form of pampering, while 74% agreed that it is a form of health care. The majority of massage recipients were women, and spas now appear to be the most popular place to get a massage. The public seeks massage for stress relief, pain management, injury rehabilitation, headache relief, and overall health and wellness.[10] Two stereotypes that have negatively affected the level of public acceptance of massage therapy in the past are diminishing. These are the association of massage with prostitution and with quackery and pseudoscience. As massage therapists achieve greater degrees of professionalism, these stereotypes will continue to decrease in the future.

Recognition from Other Professionals

There is ample evidence of the recognition of the massage therapy profession by the government and by other professionals. For example, manual therapies, including massage, were included in a report on alternative medicine to the National Institutes of Health (NIH) in 1992. The White House Commission on Complementary and Alternative Medicine Policy (WHCCAMP) cited therapeutic massage, body work, and somatic movement therapies as a major CAM domain in its Final Report (2002).

More doctors and health care providers are recommending massage therapy to their patients than in the past. In a 2014 consumer survey, 59% of respondents reported that their physicians recommended they get a massage, and 14% were referred to a massage therapist by their doctor.[11]

Representatives of the massage therapy profession have been asked to participate in a variety of professional activities. For example, a massage therapist has been appointed to the CPT® Committee of the American Medical Association. CPT®, or Current Procedural Code, lists the numerical codes for official reporting of medical services and procedures to insurance companies. Massage therapy is also represented on the Academic Consortium for Complementary and Alternative Health Care (ACCAHC).

The formal activities cited earlier, along with countless referrals and inclusion in integrative health care settings, attests to the growing acceptance of massage therapy and massage therapists as professionals.

CRITICAL THINKING

Think about the effect that negative stereotypes have had on the acceptance of the massage therapy profession by the general public and by other health professionals.

1. Identify those stereotypes.

2. Write a brief explanation of why you think the stereotypes developed and why they still exist.

3. What factors related to massage therapy as an emerging profession are likely to lessen negative stereotypes about massage?

CASE FOR STUDY

Huang and Explaining Massage Therapy as a Profession

Huang enrolled in a massage therapy program after high school to learn a marketable skill so he could eventually have his own business. He liked to work with his hands and was interested in health and fitness. He had received massage while recovering from a sports injury and thought he would like to be a massage therapist. He saw many career opportunities for his future in massage therapy. Huang's old high school friends could not understand the attraction of massage therapy as a career, nor did they think one had to go to school to learn something that seemed so simple.

Question:

What can Huang tell his friends to explain the profession of massage therapy to them and its growing importance as a health practice?

Things to consider:

- What can he say about the growing acceptance of massage by the general public and other health professionals?
- How can he explain the extent of his education and the skills he is learning?
- What other occupations or professions might he compare to being a massage therapist?
- What can he point out about the credentials he is working toward obtaining?
- How might he describe professional associations he may join or has joined?
- What publications can he show them to illustrate what massage therapy is all about?
- How would mentioning massage therapy research help explain the profession and its place in health and healing?

What three things could Huang focus on to best explain the massage therapy profession to his friends?

1. _____

2. _____

3. _____

CHAPTER HIGHLIGHTS

- The journey to becoming a successful massage therapist is a holistic experience requiring development of physical, mental, and social skills.
  - The first step on the journey is to survey the landscape to get the big picture of massage therapy as a career choice.

- Massage is the intentional and systematic manipulation of the soft tissues of the body to enhance health and healing.
  - Massage and bodywork is a term often used to describe the occupational field of massage therapy.

- Massage is performed with or without oil and may include joint movements and stretches, as well as hydrotherapy.

- Massage is primarily a manual therapy, and the person-to-person touch essential to massage gives it a unique healing potential.

- The Wellness Massage Pyramid (WMP) illustrates the broad scope of massage therapy. In this schematic, the goal for the client is achieving high-level wellness.
  - The three base levels of the pyramid include deficiency needs related to treatment, recovery from, and prevention of illness and injury. Satisfying these needs gets one to the neutral zone.
  - Above the base levels are growth levels related to health maintenance, personal growth, and enjoyment of life.

- As wellness professionals, massage therapists work within the entire wellness massage paradigm, although individuals may focus on a specific level of the WMP or with a certain client population.

- Recent surveys reveal a trend in increasing popularity of massage at spas and as a CAM therapy.
  - In hospital settings, massage is used for stress reduction in patients and staff, for pregnant women, and for pain management.

- Typical work settings for massage therapists include
  - Personal care (e.g., beauty salons and spas)
  - Sports, fitness, and recreation (e.g., health clubs, exercise centers, sports teams)
  - Health care (e.g., conventional Western medical centers, integrative health care centers, chiropractic offices, naturopathic centers, and Chinese medicine clinics)
  - Private practice (e.g., commercial office or storefront, home visit practice, and on-site business)

- Massage therapists often develop eclectic practices working in a variety of settings.

- Massage therapy, a modern profession with a tradition as old as time, has evolved into a wellness profession, with corresponding expectations that massage therapists be increasingly professional.

- Massage therapy is an emerging profession that has achieved some of the benchmarks of a mature profession.

- The body of knowledge and skills that defines the massage therapy profession is unique in many respects, while sharing some things with other professions.
  - The uniqueness of massage therapy lies in the primacy of touch and soft tissue manipulation in its skill base and the broad range of applications throughout the entire Wellness Massage Pyramid.
  - The profession is rooted in the tradition of natural healing and maintains a holistic and wellness perspective.

- Curriculum standards for entry-level education in massage therapy range from 500–1,000 clock hours of instruction and include the knowledge and skills required for competency in the field.

- Accreditation is a voluntary, nongovernmental process for massage schools and programs that ensures compliance with established standards.
  - The U.S. Department of Education recognizes agencies that accredit massage programs and meet their standards.

- Continuing education beyond initial training is often required for renewal of certifications, licenses, and by some general membership organizations.

- Four types of credentials available to massage therapists include a school diploma or certificate, board certification, specialty certification, and occupational licensing.
  - A diploma or certificate is evidence of having completed a particular course of study.
  - Board certification is a nongovernmental voluntary credential that shows competency and experience in the field.
  - Specialty certification attests to education and competency in a specific form of massage and bodywork.
  - An occupational license is a permission to practice in a certain jurisdiction, and massage therapy is regulated in 44 states plus Washington, DC, in the United States and some provinces in Canada.

- Massage therapists have founded a number of professional organizations that include general membership organizations (i.e., professional associations and membership services organizations) and specialty associations.
- Scholarship in therapeutic massage and bodywork has been growing in volume and quality over the past 25 years.
  - An increasing number of textbooks and journals have been published specifically for massage therapists.
  - Professionals from other fields, who are also massage therapists, have enriched the scholarship in the field.

- The Massage Therapy Foundation, established in 1992, has developed a research agenda, funds scientific research, and publishes a free electronic peer-reviewed research journal that can be found on its website.
- Ethical standards for the profession are embodied in codes of ethics and standards of practice developed by professional associations.
- Many accomplishments in the massage therapy profession in recent years have led to greater acceptance by the general public and recognition by other health professionals.

EXAM REVIEW

Key Terms

Match the following key terms to their descriptions. For additional study, look up the key terms in the Interactive Glossary and note other terms that compare or contrast with them.

_____ 1. Accreditation
_____ 2. Board certification
_____ 3. Complementary and alternative medicine (CAM)
_____ 4. Continuing education (CE)
_____ 5. Credentials
_____ 6. Ethical standards
_____ 7. Health care settings
_____ 8. Home visit practice
_____ 9. Integrative medicine center
_____ 10. Massage
_____ 11. Massage therapy
_____ 12. Occupational licensing
_____ 13. Personal care settings
_____ 14. Private practice settings
_____ 15. Profession associations
_____ 16. Sports, fitness, and recreation settings
_____ 17. Wellness Massage Pyramid (WMP)
_____ 18. Wellness profession

a. Awarded by a school, organization, or government agency to a person meeting their criteria
b. Offers a team approach to healing, including a variety of conventional health care providers, traditional healers, and CAM practitioners in a collaborative effort
c. Awarded to a school or program by a nongovernmental organization whose mission is to uphold high educational standards
d. General term used to describe the many systems of soft tissue manipulation
e. Provides consumer protection and the assurance of a minimal level of competence of practitioners
f. Education beyond entry-level training
g. Healing systems or modalities generally outside mainstream allopathic medicine
h. Can be a one- or two-room office space, a storefront in a mall or airport, or a dedicated room in a residence
i. The massage therapist travels to the client's home to perform massage therapy
j. Focus on personal grooming, relaxation, and rejuvenation and include beauty salons, barbershops, and spas
k. Illustrates the major goals of massage therapy and its many applications
l. Reflected in the codes of ethics and standards of practice of professional organizations
m. Nonprofit organizations run by elected leadership, whose mission is to promote their profession, to represent their members and the profession in the larger world, and to offer services to members
n. Facilities whose main purpose is to provide opportunities for physical exercise and sports, but that also provide support services such as massage
o. Term that reflects the broad scope of the massage therapy profession
p. Credential given by a nongovernmental nonprofit organization that attests to a person's competency and experience in a given profession
q. Intentional and systematic manipulation of the soft tissues of the body to enhance health and healing
r. Places where patients are treated for illnesses and injuries

Memory Workout

To test your memory of the main concepts in this chapter, complete the following sentences by circling the most correct answer from the two choices provided.

1. Massage is the (intuitive and orderly) (intentional and systematic) manipulation of the soft tissues of the body.
2. Massage is primarily a (manual) (digital) therapy, meaning it is performed by hand.
3. There are (seven) (nine) technique categories of Western massage.
4. The occupational field of massage therapy is often called (professional) (therapeutic) massage and bodywork.
5. Because the work of massage therapists spans the entire Wellness Massage Pyramid, massage therapy is best thought of as a (wellness) (medical) profession.
6. Spas with overnight accommodations, which immerse guests in a healthy environment, are referred to as (day) (destination) spas.
7. The focus of massage therapy in (sports) (personal care) settings is to help clients achieve their fitness goals, improve sports performance, and enhance healing from minor injuries.
8. In (conventional) (integrative) health care settings, both allopathic and CAM therapies are available.
9. Massage therapists in private practice are (self-employed) (employees).
10. The term *profession* is used to describe an occupation with a higher level of (ethical standards) (potential income).
11. A specific number of hours of (continuing) (entry-level) education is often required for renewal of occupational licenses, certifications, and membership in some professional organizations.
12. A diploma or certificate is a statement of (registration) (completion) of a course of study.
13. The main purpose of occupational licensing is (massage therapist) (consumer) protection.
14. (Alternative) (Specialty) associations are formed by practitioners who focus on a particular form of massage and bodywork.
15. Two stereotypes that have negatively affected massage therapists in the past and that are (increasing) (diminishing) today are the association of massage with quackery and prostitution.
16. Ethical standards in massage therapy are reflected in the (standards of practice) (membership requirements) developed by professional associations.

Test Prep

The following multiple-choice questions will help to prepare you for future school and professional exams.

1. Which of the following is not within the scope of massage therapy as practiced in the United States?
   a. Soft tissue manipulation
   b. Joint movements
   c. Spinal adjustments
   d. Use of hot packs

2. Which of the following would appear nearest the top of the Wellness Massage Pyramid?
   a. Prevention of illness
   b. Enjoyment of life
   c. Recovery from illness
   d. Neutral zone

3. Herbal remedies, acupuncture, music therapy, and massage therapy are considered:
   a. Allopathic medicine
   b. Mainstream medicine
   c. Conventional medicine
   d. Complementary and alternative medicine

4. "Enhancing overall well-being through a variety of professional services that encourage renewal of mind, body and spirit" is the main focus of which type of setting?
   a. Health club
   b. Naturopathic physician office
   c. Spa
   d. Private practice

5. Health care settings that use a collaborative approach to healing by including a variety of Western medical health care providers, traditional and indigenous healers, and/or CAM practitioners, are referred to as:
   a. Integrative
   b. Comprehensive
   c. Conventional
   d. Alternative

6. Facilities connected to hospitals that offer fitness activities, rehabilitation programs, massage therapy, and classroom instruction in developing a healthy life-style are called:
   a. Sports medicine centers
   b. Medical spas
   c. Wellness centers
   d. Chiropractic offices

7. A massage practice in which seated massage is given on special massage chairs at the workplace or at events such as health fairs is called:
   a. Home visit practice
   b. On-site practice
   c. Sports massage practice
   d. Integrative practice

8. Combining a massage office with some home visits and part-time employment at a spa or chiropractic office is called:
   a. Environmental practice
   b. Ecological practice
   c. Eclectic practice
   d. Eccentric practice

9. A specific position of employment is called a:
   a. Career
   b. Profession
   c. Job
   d. Calling

10. Which of the following statements about massage therapy today is *not* true?
    a. It is rooted in the tradition of natural healing.
    b. It is narrowly focused on medical applications.
    c. It maintains a wellness perspective.
    d. It is holistic at its core.

11. Recognition given to a school by a nongovernmental organization for upholding high educational standards is called:
    a. Accreditation
    b. Certification
    c. Licensing
    d. Approval

12. A detailed record of a student's performance while in school is called a:
    a. Diploma
    b. Certificate
    c. Resume
    d. Transcript

13. A credential given by a nongovernmental nonprofit organization that attests to a person's competency and experience in a given profession is called:
    a. Specialty certification
    b. Board certification
    c. Accreditation
    d. Licensing

14. In the United States, what level of government typically regulates professions such as massage therapy by issuing occupational licenses?
    a. Town
    b. County
    c. State
    d. Federal

15. Nonprofit organizations run by elected leadership, whose mission is to promote their profession, to represent their members and the profession in the larger world, and to offer services to members are called:
    a. Professional associations
    b. Member services organizations
    c. Specialty associations
    d. Certification boards

16. The growing acceptance of massage therapy by the general public is confirmed in:
    a. Hospital surveys
    b. Licensing laws
    c. Consumer surveys
    d. Government reports

Video Challenge

Watch this video, which can be found at MyHealthProfessionsLab.com, Chapter 1, and then answer the following questions.

Healing Massage: Wellness and Workplaces

1. Give examples from the video of massage therapists working at different levels of the Wellness Massage Pyramid.

2. Can you see yourself working in any of the settings shown in the video? Which settings appeal to you the most, and why?
3. What credentials are available to massage therapists as shown in the video?

Comprehension Exercises

The following short-answer questions test your knowledge and understanding of chapter topics and provide practice in written communication skills. Explain in two to four complete sentences.

1. Define massage therapy. What are its essential characteristics? What is its intent?
2. Describe the variety of settings in which massage therapists work today. Discuss which settings are best suited for your interests and talents as you currently see them.

3. Who licenses massage therapists, and why? What are the benefits of occupational licensing for massage therapists? What are the penalties for practicing without a license?

For Greater Understanding

The following exercises are designed to take you from the realm of theory into the real world. They will help give you a deeper understanding of the subjects covered in this chapter. Action words are underlined to emphasize the variety of activities presented to address different learning styles and to encourage deeper thinking.

1. Interview a successful massage therapist, and describe his or her practice in terms of the types of clients served and the setting in which the therapist works. Write a report, and present it to a study partner or to a class.
2. Find the most recent massage therapy industry information reported by a professional organization.

Analyze the data to see what it says about the massage therapy profession and the acceptance of massage therapy by the general public and other health professionals. The information is based on what factual sources? Discuss the implications of the findings with the class.

3. Attend a state, regional, or national convention sponsored by a professional association for massage therapists. Take advantage of all the opportunities offered at the event, including education, networking, massage equipment and supplies vendors, and organizational meetings. Report to the class about your experience.

MyHealthProfessionsLab™

MyHealthProfessionsLab.com is a premium online homework management system that includes a host of features to help you study. Registered users will find:

- Powerful tools that track and analyze your results—allowing you to create a personalized learning experience
- Videos, flashcards and other learning tools to help enrich your progress
- Streaming lesson presentations and self-paced learning modules
- A space where you and your instructors can view and manage your assignments

History of Massage as a Vocation

From Massage and Training by Andrews, 1910.

CHAPTER OUTLINE

Learning Outcomes

Key Terms

History of a Vocation

Personal Grooming and Rejuvenation

Sports and Fitness

Health Care

Natural Healing and Drugless Doctors

Massage Therapy Revived in the United States

Massage Therapists and Bodyworkers

Chapter Highlights

Exam Review

LEARNING OUTCOMES

After studying this chapter, you will have information to:

1. Trace the history of massage related to personal care services.

2. Describe the use of massage for athletes from ancient times to the present.

3. Explain how massage has been used over the centuries in Western medicine.

4. Identify aspects of today's massage therapy that can be traced to the natural healing philosophy.

5. Name important figures in the history of massage and describe their contributions.

6. Discuss factors leading to the revival of massage as a popular health practice in the 1970s.

7. Describe important developments in the massage profession in recent decades.

KEY TERMS

Aleiptes

Ammashi

Bath attendant

Health service operator

Massage operator

Masseurs/masseuses

Medical gymnast

Rubbers

Sobardoras

Trained masseuses

HISTORY OF A VOCATION

The term *vocation* means the work a person has chosen to do for his or her livelihood, especially one for which the individual has talent or is drawn to. It comes from the Latin *vocare,* to call, and refers to the concept of having "a calling" to a particular type of work. Over the centuries, many have been called or have chosen to be massage practitioners.

Like other vocations, massage therapy has its own history. Massage practitioners of the past include servants and slaves, tribal and village healers, rubbers and masseurs, doctors and nurses, medical gymnasts, natural healers, Swedish masseuses, and 1970s bodyworkers. Today's massage therapists are the latest in the line of countless massage practitioners that have gone before. Each generation received knowledge and skills from its predecessors and shaped the future for those who followed.

The history of massage as a vocation looks at several different aspects of the work, for example, who went into the occupation, how they were trained, what types of skills and knowledge they had, their work conditions, and their status in society. This history describes differences in various times and locations, how situations changed over the years, and what factors influenced the work of massage practitioners. It offers a better understanding of today's environment and the outlook for massage therapists in the future.

There are four major threads to the history of massage as a vocation:

- Personal grooming and rejuvenation
- Sports and fitness
- Health care
- Natural healing

They roughly parallel today's work settings. Each thread has its own story and cast of characters that woven together create the tapestry of massage therapy as a vocation over time.

The following sections take a closer look at each thread individually and trace important developments through time to the present day. The major events in each section are highlighted in accompanying tables. Note that each strand ends with the massage therapist. All four threads came together in the late twentieth century in the United States and each contributed to the formation of the massage therapy profession today.

PERSONAL GROOMING AND REJUVENATION

Massage has been part of personal care from time immemorial. As people groomed themselves by bathing, cleaning and cutting their hair, and trimming their nails, the pleasurable and rejuvenating effects of rubbing their skin were obvious. People in dry climates learned to rub vegetable and mineral oil on their skin to keep it moistened and healthy.

This practice would have been natural for mothers caring for infants and children, those caring for the frail and elderly, and people grooming themselves and family members.

In ancient civilizations, it was often slaves or domestic servants who provided personal care services, including massage, in the private sphere or home. These servants had low social status, were uneducated, and learned their skills from family members or others performing massage.

In ancient Greece, friction and rubbing with oil was a daily practice. The ancient historian Plutarch reported that Alexander the Great (356–323 BCE) traveled with a personal attendant who rubbed him and prepared his bath. Other nobles of that time also "used fragrant ointment when they went to their inunction [application of skin moisturizer] and bath, and they carried about with them rubbers (triptai), and chamberlains."[1]

In ancient India, royalty and nonroyalty alike enjoyed a similar practice. The Greek geographer Strabo (63 BCE–24 CE) described how Indian royalty rubbed their skin with staves or flat sticks, "and they polished their bodies smooth by ebony staves." He also mentions that the king received foreign ambassadors while being rubbed, and "there are four rubbers standing by."

In the 1800s, the British used the English word *shampooing* to describe massage practices seen in India, China, and the Middle East. The word is thought by some to come from the Sanskrit word transliterated as *tshampua,* meaning body manipulation. Shampooing was a full-body experience that often involved a hot, soapy bath, followed by a form of bodywork involving percussion and friction massage, joint cracking, and applying scented oils or perfume. It was said to give "ineffable happiness and energy" and that "the Indian ladies seldom pass a day without being thus shampooed by their slaves."[2]

In China in the 1800s, barbers set up shop in markets and parks offering grooming services and a type of bodywork (Figure 2–1 ■). Patrons sat on stools while the barbers cut hair, shaved or trimmed beards, cut nails, cleaned ears, or gave a percussive type of massage. As itinerant tradesmen, these Chinese barbers also were part street performers who played "a thousand tricks to please and amuse their customers, to whom and the surrounding audience they tell their gossiping stories."[3]

The blind masseurs or **ammashi** of Japan have their own unique story. In the 1800s, the government of Japan decreed that the occupation of ammashi (amma = traditional Japanese massage; shi = practitioner) be reserved for blind persons as a welfare measure. As a result, government programs for training ammashi were created, and blind amma practitioners were licensed and enjoyed public respect. See Figure 2–2 ■. These blind ammashi walked the streets announcing their presence: "Formerly they used to blow a small flute as they went about, and people used to call them in as they heard the sounds."[4] It is said that at the outbreak of World War II in the 1940s, 90% of the ammashi in Japan were blind. After the war, blind ammashi were found mainly in rural districts.

FIGURE 2–1 Chinese barber performing a form of percussion on a seated patron in China in the 1790s.

Source: Picturesque Representations of the Dress and Manners of the Chinese by Thomas M'Lean, 1814.

Public Baths

Public bathhouses are community centers for personal hygiene, grooming services, pleasure and rejuvenation, and social interaction. They are found all over the world. In the past, they were sometimes operated by the government, as in ancient Rome, but most were commercial bathhouses. Today, massage continues to be an integral part of the public bath tradition in its latest form, day and destination spas.

Ancient Greece and Rome, ancient China and Japan, Medieval Europe, and the Middle East all had public baths. In times and places where individual homes did not have indoor plumbing, public baths provided bathing and grooming facilities and services, as well as community gathering places.

The Roman bath is the prototype public bath in Western civilization. These bathhouses provided by the state were built all over the Roman Empire, which extended from Asia Minor in the East to the British Isles in the west (27 BCE–476 CE). In addition to exercise courts, warm rooms (tepidarium), steam rooms (caldarium), and a cold pool (frigidarium), there were spaces for manual therapy. The providers of the manipulations would have been slaves or servants to individuals, or possibly slaves or employees of the state that operated the bath. See Figure 2–3 ■.

After the fall of the Roman Empire, public baths remained popular in Medieval Europe until the sixteenth century, when the spread of communicable diseases and promiscuous behavior made common bathing undesirable.

The Turkish bath, also called a *hammam,* based on the Roman prototype, became popular in the Middle East and reached Europe in the 1800s. After bathing, and perhaps a haircut and a shave, patrons received a vigorous type of manipulation from a practitioner called a *telltack.* It involved gripping and pressing the muscles, stretching, and cracking the joints.[5] The telltack would have learned his trade by informal apprenticeship and was unlikely to have had anything other than a practical knowledge of human anatomy learned on the job. The Turkish bath was popular in the cities of Europe and North America through the first half of the twentieth century and is still found in the Middle East.

The Chinese bathhouse tradition appears very similar in nature to those found elsewhere. An example can be seen in a Chinese film called *Shower* in English. The film is set in a late twentieth-century Chinese bathhouse that is slated to be torn down to make way for modern buildings. Local men come to the bathhouse to take hot baths and showers, sleep on cots, listen to music, get their hair and nails trimmed, gossip, play board games, hold cricket fights, and drink tea—the Chinese version of the Turkish bath. The bathhouse owner serves as bath attendant and manual therapy practitioner. A brief scene shows a patron lying on a bench and the bathhouse owner applying percussion techniques such as slapping and cupping with open hands. A little later he resets a patron's shoulder that had gone out of joint.[6]

FIGURE 2–2 Blind Japanese masseur or ammashi, c.1880.

Source: The Art of Massage by Kellogg, 1895.

FIGURE 2–3 A Roman bath.

Source: Haven/Getty Images.

The occupational designation of **bath attendant** stems from ancient traditions of servants or attendants giving rub-downs or rubbing in scented oils after a bath. In the nineteenth century, attendants were assistants to doctors of hydropathy, and some worked in public baths and spas giving treatments such as cold mitt rubs. The low-skilled friction and rubbing applied by bath attendants hardly equated with the more highly skilled massage that evolved later for health and heal-ing. Nevertheless, bath attendants were misleadingly equated with massage therapists in government occupational codes until the 1980s. Bath attendants at a late nineteenth-century European spa are shown in Figure 2–4 ∎.

Salons and Spas

In the early 1900s, women went to salons or parlors for per-sonal care services. *Beauty culture* was the term used for the art and science of grooming women's hair and nails, applying makeup or cosmetics, and other beauty treatments to enhance appearance. Massage for rejuvenation, reduc-ing, and bust development were part of beauty culture in the early twentieth century.

In large urban areas in the United States, upscale salons such as Elizabeth Arden and Helena Rubenstein enjoyed downtown locations, whereas smaller beauty salons (also known as beauty parlors and beauty shops) dotted local neighborhoods. Specialists in hair, skin, and nail groom-ing learned their trade in vocational schools and became licensed as beauticians or cosmetologists in most states. In their scope of practice, massage was largely limited to the head, neck, and shoulders; hands and arms up to the elbow; and feet and lower leg up to the knee.[7] These were superfi-cial massage applications done during personal grooming at the salon. The first U.S. licenses for barbers and beauticians appeared around 1900.

Full-body massage remained part of the beauty culture scene and was offered in salons for relaxation and rejuve-nation. The general Swedish massage, an amalgamation of Pehr Henrik Ling's medical gymnastics (or Swedish move-ment cure) and Johann Mezger's massage, became the sig-nature massage of salons. By the 1930–1940s, colleges of Swedish massage were training **masseurs** (men) and **mas-seuses** (women) to work in a variety of places, including personal care settings. See Figure 2–5 ∎.

Graduate masseuse or graduate masseur was the title for a practitioner trained in a school, as opposed to someone who learned massage by apprenticeship or on the job, and served as a kind of credential. Careers as graduate masseuses were extolled in college catalogs. Massage students had courses in anatomy and physiology, dietetics, hydrotherapy, light therapy, electrotherapy, and massage.[8]

Swedish masseuses were also trained in *reducing massage,* a form of massage erroneously thought to help women slim down. Swedish masseuses at reducing salons offered reducing massage, as well as nutritional advice, exercise, and steam room and steam cabinets. Many mas-seuses also taught exercise classes. Breast massage was advertised as developing "firmness and plumpness of the bust."[9]

FIGURE 2–4 Bath attendants, c.1890.

Source: The Natural Method of Healing, Vol. 2, Bilz Sanatorium in Germany, 1898.

FIGURE 2–5 Swedish masseuse, c. 1935.

Source: The College of Swedish Massage Catalogue, Chicago, 1939.

PRACTICAL APPLICATION

Find some historical objects or pictures that you could use for decoration or conversation pieces in your future office. Old massage machines, oil and liniment bottles, books, drawings, and photos can spark the interest of people who see them. Having one or more historical objects around can also offer you a special depth of connection to your chosen field.

Several well-respected massage programs in the 1930s–1940s were correspondence courses. The knowledge base was learned through the mail, followed by a week of more intensive training at the school to learn the physical skills. This arrangement, called distance learning today, was ideal for people who did not live in big cities where schools were readily available. Most people still lived in small towns prior to World War II, and transportation was difficult. These correspondence courses gave people who did not live in big cities the opportunity to receive massage training.

Massage technician or **massage operator** was considered a good career option in the 1930s–1940s for those wanting to develop a private practice—much like today. Graduate masseurs and masseuses formed professional associations, such as the American Association of Masseurs and Masseuses established in 1943, and worked to upgrade standards for education and ethical behavior.

Over sixty years later, day spas and full service salons continue to offer personal grooming services, and some modern establishments are incorporating hydrotherapy facilities such as those found in European spas. Swedish massage and other forms of massage therapy continue to be provided in these settings by graduate, and in most states, licensed massage therapists. See Box 2–1 ■ for a personal grooming and rejuvenation timeline.

SPORTS AND FITNESS

From ancient Greek times, massage has been associated with sports and fitness. The Greek gymnasia were places where freeborn citizens went to train their bodies and minds. Athletes were rubbed with oil by practitioners called **aleiptes,** "whose business it was to anoint the wrestlers before and after they exercised, and took care to keep them sound and in good complexion."[10] The last part of the gymnasium exercises was called *apotherapeia,* or a routine for recovery. Its purpose was ridding the body of waste products and preventing fatigue. It consisted of bathing, friction, and inunction or applying oil.[11]

Paidotribes in ancient Greece were like the trainers in Western sports many centuries later. They were often former athletes and served in many capacities, including coach, nutritionist, masseur, physiotherapist, and hygienist. Although the paidotribes were self-taught or trained by apprenticeship, they would have been exposed to theories about diet, exercise, muscle physiology, and therapies of Greek medicine.[12]

Rubbers and Athletic Masseurs

When amateur sports regained popularity in the eighteenth to nineteenth centuries, the rubdown after a bath was a mainstay of the care of athletes. It consisted of rubbing and friction of the limbs. It was performed by the trainers themselves, but also by specialists called **rubbers.** Rubbers were unschooled massage practitioners who might have been athletes themselves and had a knack for rubbing. They learned their skills on the job or from other rubbers. When describing the treatment for sore shins, trainer and early Olympic track coach Michael Murphy noted, "If the runner has the services of a trainer and rubber he will be properly cared for."[13]

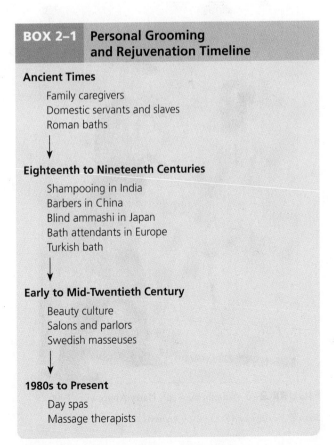

BOX 2–1	Personal Grooming and Rejuvenation Timeline

Ancient Times

  Family caregivers
  Domestic servants and slaves
  Roman baths

Eighteenth to Nineteenth Centuries

  Shampooing in India
  Barbers in China
  Blind ammashi in Japan
  Bath attendants in Europe
  Turkish bath

Early to Mid-Twentieth Century

  Beauty culture
  Salons and parlors
  Swedish masseuses

1980s to Present

  Day spas
  Massage therapists

As in the Greek gymnasium, athletic facilities such as the YMCA and sports centers also had pools, showers, and steam rooms. The bath attendant was a familiar figure there who might also be skilled in a rubdown-style massage. In 1902, a trainer named Pollard commented that "in all cases vigorous rubbing should follow the use of water; a bath attendant who knows something about massage is invaluable, for how to rub down a man or a horse is an art."[14]

Early twentieth-century trainers were multitalented and helped athletes with sports skills, conditioning, motivation, and injury rehabilitation. Many had been athletes themselves and were drawn to training, or had "good hands" and became masseurs. In professional sports such as boxing and club sports like track and field, athletic masseurs were either self-taught or apprenticed. Their knowledge of anatomy consisted of what they learned around the gym. A trainer–masseur from the early 1900s named Harry Andrews is shown in Figure 2–6 ■.

The specialty of massage for athletes became more sophisticated in the mid-twentieth century. Although many trainers had learned through experience on the athletic field, others were starting to be trained in colleges and universities. The term *athletic masseur* was used to indicate a higher level of training and knowledge than that of the rubbers of the past.

In the 1930s–1940s, some athletic masseurs were graduates of colleges of Swedish massage. Working with athletes and professional sports teams was one of the career paths for graduate masseurs. Others were trained in physical education programs in colleges and universities, where they learned basic sciences, musculoskeletal anatomy, kinesiology, sports injuries, and other sport sciences—as well as massage applications for athletes.

This affiliation with physical education departments in colleges eventually led to a separate profession for athletic trainers. The National Athletic Training Association (NATA) was formed in 1950. Athletic trainers soon dropped massage as used in training athletes in the past and patterned their new profession on physical therapy, focusing almost exclusively on injuries.

For about 20 years, the old skills of the athletic masseurs were not available to college and professional athletes in the United States except where the old-school rubbers and athletic masseurs continued their work. This was not the case in many European countries, where the tradition of athletic massage remained strong.

Then in the 1970s in the United States, within the emerging profession of massage therapy, the tradition now called *sports massage* was revived. Athletes who had been turned on to massage as a training aid because of the success of European athletes sought specialists in this old art. The knowledge and skills of massage for athletes had fallen out of the realm of the modern professions of coach and athletic trainer, and so it made sense that massage specialists with an affinity for athletics would respond to the call.

Trained massage therapists, like the graduate masseurs and masseuses before them, already had knowledge of muscular anatomy and physiology and highly developed hands-on skills. Work with athletes, or sports massage, continues to be a specialty for massage therapists.

Fitness/Health Service Operators and Expert Masseuses

In the first half of the twentieth century, masseurs and masseuses worked in athletic clubs, private gymnasia, and YMCAs providing massage for health and fitness buffs. As early as 1915, a rubdown by a bath attendant was an established part of the routine at the YMCA. R. Tait McKenzie described a workout at the Y as a mixture of Swedish and German gymnastics and games, "ending with a bath and a rub down."[15]

Commercial health clubs for office workers and businessmen were popping up in cities across America. A December 1917 advertisement for Postl health club in Chicago featured a photo of 14 trainers and masseurs who have "adequate experience and know the laws of health through long service with us." See Figure 2–7 ■. They promised to give "physical and mental health, strength, and vigor," and "steal your weak stomach and tired nerves, sending you away vibrating with glowing health and ambition."

An ad for Burke's Gymnasium from 1932 boasted "the finest and most completely equipped health institution in

FIGURE 2–6 Athletic masseur, Harry Andrews c. 1900.

Source: Massage and Training by Andrews, 1910.

FIGURE 2–7
Masseurs and trainers from the Postl Heath Club in Chicago.

Source: A "Physical Training for the Tired Business Man," ad in *Chicago Tribune Pictorial Weekly,* December 9, 1917.

San Francisco." There were graded classes for ladies and their children, handball and tennis courts, and acrobatics for girls. The ladies' Turkish bath, with its cabinet baths, blanket sweats, hot room, and steam room, offered a course of baths and reducing treatments. It was under the management of "expert masseuses."

By 1943, 274 YMCAs in the United States were operating health service departments that offered massage. The scope and methods of these YMCA massage operators was described by Frierwood in 1953: "The technician uses massage, baths (shower, steam, electricity cabinet), ultraviolet irradiation (artificial and natural sunlight), infrared (heat), instruction in relaxation and in some cases directed exercises. The adult members secure a relief from tensions, gain a sense of well-being, give attention to personal fitness and develop habits designed to build and maintain optimum health and physical efficiency throughout the lifespan."[16]

The **health service operator** was trained in the familiar cluster of natural health and healing methods sometimes called physical therapeutics or physiotherapy. These were massage, hydrotherapy, electrotherapy, light, relaxation techniques, and exercise. The goals, however, were not medical, but were focused on health, fitness, and general well-being.

Health service operators and masseurs were trained in YMCA colleges in physical education departments, as well as in colleges of Swedish massage. The Dayton YMCA in Ohio established a School of Health Service and Massage in 1937. A professional association called the Health Service Operators Society was established in 1942 "to combat the abuses of commercial bathhouses and the unethical conduct of 'cure-all' agents in the health field."[17] The association was active through the 1950s.

Health clubs today have adopted the YMCA format of exercise, hydrotherapy (steam room, sauna, whirlpool), and massage. It is the same format as the ancient Greek gymnasium. See Box 2–2 ■ for a sports and fitness timeline.

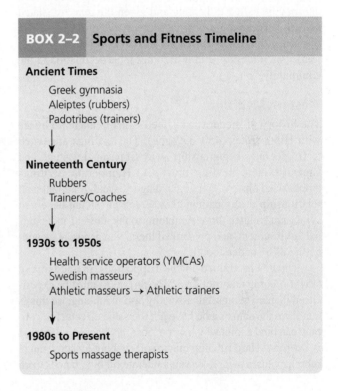

BOX 2–2 Sports and Fitness Timeline

Ancient Times
Greek gymnasia
Aleiptes (rubbers)
Padotribes (trainers)
↓

Nineteenth Century
Rubbers
Trainers/Coaches
↓

1930s to 1950s
Health service operators (YMCAs)
Swedish masseurs
Athletic masseurs → Athletic trainers
↓

1980s to Present
Sports massage therapists

HEALTH CARE

In its broadest sense, health care encompasses all the arts and sciences of healing. Rubbing, friction, and pressing of the soft tissues have been a mainstay of health care across time and place. In native cultures, massage was performed in the treatment of a variety of ailments by shamans and traditional healers, as well as by family members. It was often the domain of women.

Captain James Cook, on an expedition to Tahiti in the 1770s, gives a firsthand account of how the mother and sisters of a native named Tu used massage to treat "rheumatick pain" in his hip and leg. Cook relates, "I was desired to lay down in the midst of them, then as many as could get around me began to squeeze me with both hands from head to foot, but more especially the parts where the pain was, till they made my bones crack and a perfect Mummy of my flesh. . . . I found immediate relief from the operation. They gave me another rubbing down before I went to bed."[18] These women were not "professionals" in the sense of having an occupation, but performed massage as part of everyday family care skills.

On the other hand, traditional Hispanic healers called **sobardoras** are trained by apprenticeship to use massage in treating ailments of those in the community who call on their services. They also use ritual, herbal remedies and bone-setting manipulation techniques in their work. Sobardoras are part of the healing tradition of *curanderas,* who combine folk traditions from Spain and Mexico. It is believed that curanderas inherit their power to heal, although an individual may be called to healing and given the *don,* translated as "gift." These traditional healers are like professionals in the sense that they feel called to the work, go through a long apprenticeship, and it becomes their occupation in the community.[19]

Western Medicine

The history of modern medicine begins in ancient Greece with Hippocrates (450–377 BCE). The writings attributed to Hippocrates began a shift away from magic, ritual, and superstition in healing practices. Hippocratic writings emphasized observation, logic, diagnosis and treatment, and relationship to the patient. The Greek physician observed symptoms, related those symptoms to the internal and external environment, and prescribed therapy in accordance with nature as he understood it.

Physicians trained in the Hippocratic methods were taught rubbing and frictions: "The physician must be experienced in many things, but assuredly also in rubbing; for things that have the same name have not the same effects. For rubbing can bind a joint which is too loose, and loosen a joint that is too rigid. Hard rubbing binds; soft rubbing loosens; much rubbing causes parts to waste; moderate rubbing makes them

grow" (Hippocrates, "Peri Arthron" quoted in Graham).[20] The implication is that practitioners must be skilled in different rubbing techniques to elicit different effects.

Those in ancient Greece who specialized in rubbing were called *triptai.* Massage and bodywork was called the *anatriptic art.* Anatriptic meant to "rub up" or toward the body's center, presumably when rubbing the arms and legs.

Ancient physicians began to identify the most effective soft tissue technique applications for various conditions. For example, Hippocrates advised "to rub the shoulder gently and smoothly" after resetting a dislocated shoulder. Celsus (25 BCE–50 CE), a Roman physician, said to stroke "the chest with a gentle hand" for a cough, and use "soft and long continued rubbing of the affected part" for a spasm. Galen (130–230 CE) advised physicians to warm the body with moderate rubbing with a linen cloth before applying oil and compressing tissues, and that "one should first rub quietly, and afterwards gradually increasing it, push the strength of the friction so far as evidently to compress the flesh but not to bruise it."[21] Obviously, skilled massage applications took more knowledge and skill than mere rubbing.

The more recent tradition called medical rubbing began to emerge in eighteenth-century Europe. Douglas Graham's *A Treatise on Massage* (1902) devoted two chapters to the history of massage and names several physicians who used soft tissue manipulation in medical treatments during this and earlier periods. One of these was Dr. J. B. Zabludowski of Berlin, Germany, shown in Figure 2–8 ■ performing massage of the ankle, c.1910.

Much earlier, in 1780, a well-known French professor of clinical medicine named Simon Andre Tissot wrote about massage and exercise called *gymnastique medicinale et chirurgicalein.* An English physician named William Balfour published a book on the subject in 1819. Other English physicians of the time, such as the surgeon Mr. Grosvenor of Oxford, developed medical rubbing systems. In 1859, Mr. Beveridge of Edinburgh published a pamphlet called, "The cure of disease by manipulation, commonly called medical rubbing."

FIGURE 2–8

Dr. J. B. Zabludowski of Berlin, Germany, performs massage of the ankle, c. 1910.

Source: Zabludowski's Technik der Massage by Eiger, 1911.

But medical rubbing did not catch on at the time in mainstream English medicine, "and from that time to this [1866] rubbing has been left almost wholly in the hands of unprofessional persons . . . some of whom used simple rubbing . . . while others employed various kinds of liniments and ointments."[22] By the end of the nineteenth century, the practice of medical rubbing would evolve into a budding profession for trained masseurs and masseuses.

TRAINED MASSEUSES

About a century ago, the word *massage* replaced *medical rubbing* to describe the treatment of illness and injury with soft tissue manipulation. The French had developed soft tissue manipulation skills they called *massage,* and the term was later popularized by Johann Mezger, a physician from Amsterdam. The word *massage* stuck as the generic term for soft tissue manipulation and is used to this day. The terms *massotherapy* and *manual therapeutics,* once used to describe skilled massage, are not used anymore.

Johann Mezger (1838–1909) developed a system of soft tissue manipulation that is the basis for today's traditional Western massage. Using French terminology, Mezger called the work massage, and its practitioners, masseurs and masseuses. He categorized massage techniques as effleurage, petrissage, friction, and tapotement; vibration was added later. The place where massage was given was called a parlor or salon. Mezger's massage became popular throughout Europe and North America.

Although a number of physicians championed massage as a treatment modality, most assigned the actual massage work to assistants. Some training schools for nurses gave general instruction in massage. Graham thought that *manipulators,* or massage practitioners, should have "a natural tact, talent, and liking for massage, with soft elastic, and strong hands and physical endurance sufficient to use them, together with abundance of time, patience, and skill acquired by long and intelligent experience."[23]

That there were many untrained massage practitioners is mentioned in textbooks from the early 1900s. Graham lamented that "it is not to be wondered at that many a shrewd, superannuated auntie, and others who are out of a job, having learned the meaning of the word massage, immediately have it printed on their card and continue their 'rubbin,' just as they have always done."[24]

On the other hand, **trained masseuses** took courses of study in private schools and hospital programs. *A Manual for Students of Massage,* written by Mary Anna Ellison (1909), outlines a typical turn-of-the-century massage curriculum. After an overview of anatomy, topics include massage techniques, how to give a general massage, vibration treatment, Schott treatment for heart disease, treatment for locomotor ataxia, Weir-Mitchell treatment for neurasthenia, and the Swedish system of medical gymnastics, which was considered a specialty.

Trained masseuses were valued by the doctors who employed them. Weir Mitchell, who developed the famous Rest Cure, which included general massage, found many benefits from the manipulations themselves. He also valued observations about his patients by "practiced manipulators." He found that "their daily familiarity with every detail of the color and firmness of the tissues is often of great use to me."[25] The level of professionalism expected of trained masseuses is evidenced by the "hints to masseuses" given by Ellison. She admonishes students to cease treatment "if you have real cause for believing that it or your personality is in any way prejudicial," and to concentrate their attention on the patient "having her mind full of healthfulness and hope regarding . . . her work."[26] A list of *don'ts* include "don't discuss the doctor's methods with the patient, and don't mention the names of other patients in conversation."[27] Other hints are listed in Figure 2–9 ■ and offer good advice 100 years later, particularly Ellison's comment: "One thing I am assured of—that is, the absolute necessity for a masseuse . . . to keep her mind in as well-balanced condition as possible, and during her treatment to concentrate her attention (as fully as circumstances permit) on the patient and her needs, not necessarily speaking much, but having her mind full of healthfulness and hope as regards the ultimate issue of her work. She follows up *mentally,* as it were, the results she is trying to achieve *manually.*"[28] The Society of Trained Masseuses was formed in England in 1894 to raise professional standards for massage specialists working in the medical field.

As mainstream health care developed in the United States through the twentieth century, massage became a minor modality within the scope of other professions such as nursing and physical therapy. The occupation of masseuse and masseur never rose to the level of a separate profession within institutionalized medicine. Massage specialists were relegated to natural healing settings and deemed "alternative." That is why although massage therapy has a long tradition as a healing agent, massage is considered an alternative therapy in today's health care system.

MEDICAL GYMNASTS

A separate but related tradition of manual therapy was known variously as medical gymnastics, mechanotherapy, and physical therapeutics. This was the curing of diseases through movement, that is, active and passive exercises. Although the Swede, Pehr Henrik Ling (1776–1839) is perhaps the most famous individual who developed a system of medical gymnastics, others preceded him. In the sixteenth century, Mercurialis wrote *De Arte Gymnastica* or the science of bodily exercise, including movements for the cure of diseases. An English physician, Thomas Fuller, published *Medicina Gymnastica* in 1704, and a French physician, Clement Tissot, wrote *Gymnastique Medicinale* in 1781.

Ling's system was comprehensive and included educational gymnastics for building strong healthy bodies, military gymnastics for hand-to-hand and small weapons combat, and medical gymnastics for treating diseases. Ling

Hints for Masseuses, c. 1909

- ೦೩ Don't take a case without medical permission, at least, if not supervision. Fatal results have sometimes followed massage of unsuitable cases.
- ೦೩ Don't discuss the doctor's methods with the patient, and don't mention the names of other patients in conversation.
- ೦೩ Don't talk scandal to your patients, and, on the other hand, avoid shop talk.
- ೦೩ Don't speak as if you were the one competent masseuse to be had.
- ೦೩ Don't undertake more cases than you have energy and vitality for, or both you and the patients will suffer.
- ೦೩ Don't accept any stimulants at a patient's house.
- ೦೩ Don't abuse any confidence reposed in you, or publish abroad private matters that come to your knowledge.
- ೦೩ Don't continue your attendance a day longer than is necessary, or if you see that massage is not providing beneficial results.
- ೦೩ Don't forget that you have come on business, and don't give the impression that massage is an act of condescension on your part.
- ೦೩ Don't neglect to study your patient's individuality, and if you can in any way rest her mind as well as her body, do so.
- ೦೩ Don't give the servants more trouble than you can help, whilst maintaining your position with dignity.
- ೦೩ Don't allow a patient to experience the discomfort of feeling your breath.
- ೦೩ Don't wear rings or bracelets.
- ೦೩ Don't sweep the patient's skin with your sleeve or any part of your dress.

FIGURE 2–9

Hints for Masseuses.

Source: A Manual for Students of Massage 3e by Mary Ellison, Bailliere Tindall.

based his exercises on knowledge of anatomy and physiology as he understood them and so is credited with putting the practice on a rational or scientific basis. Physical educators, physical therapists, and massage therapists all consider Ling a "father" of their profession.

The Swedish system of medical gymnastics was considered an alternative therapy. Whereas allopathic medicine relied on drugs and surgery as its major modalities, Ling's system was an alternative for treating a variety of chronic diseases from asthma to spinal curvature to headaches. In its heyday, before strict medical licensing, movement cure practitioners were considered primary health care providers and accepted patients for diagnosis and treatment.[29] Many were also physicians, but there were many lay practitioners too.

One of Ling's greatest contributions was the development of **medical gymnast** as an occupation. Whereas others wrote books and taught individual students, Ling founded a school that gained international fame and trained thousands of practitioners from all over the world in his system. His school, the Royal Gymnastic Central Institute, was established in 1813 in Stockholm. It was open to men and women, and the curriculum included anatomy, physiology, pathology, hygiene, diagnosis, principles of the movement treatment, and the use of exercises for general and local development.[30]

CRITICAL THINKING

Analyze the "Hints to Masseuses" made in 1909 by Mary Anna Ellison listed in Figure 2–9.

1. What do the hints reveal about masseuses of one hundred years ago?

2. Which ones are still applicable today?

3. What do they tell you about the historical development of ethics for massage therapists?

Graduates of Ling's program, and spin-off programs in the United States and Europe, found employment as physical education teachers in the schools (educational gymnastics) and as medical gymnasts at Swedish movement cure institutions. In places such as the Swedish Cure Institute in New York, founded by Dr. George Taylor, medical gymnasts led patients through active movements and applied passive movements or soft tissue manipulations. Medical gymnasts assisting a patient through a movement prescription are shown in Figure 2–10 ■.

By the late nineteenth century, medical gymnasts adopted Mezger's system of massage as a complement to Ling's system. Eventually, Ling's and Mezger's systems of manual therapy were so identified together that they became known in the United States as Swedish massage.

Many colleges that adopted the Swedish system for physical education classes also began training physical educators in the tradition of Ling. The location of these training programs within colleges influenced the direction of the development of the athletic training and physical therapy professions.

Physical therapy began to form as a separate profession around World War I when practitioners, called *reconstruction aides,* were trained to help rehabilitate wounded soldiers. Many reconstruction aides were trained in departments of physical education in colleges, where they learned to apply corrective exercise and massage. In fact, up to World War II, a prerequisite for many physical therapy (also called physiotherapy) programs was a degree in physical education. A photograph of a corner of the general massage department of an army hospital in the 1920s shows soldiers receiving massage in chairs as well as on tables (Figure 2–11 ■).

Physical therapists formed their first professional association in 1921, the American Women's Physical Therapeutic Association. The name was changed in the 1940s to the American Physical Therapy Association. Occupational licensing for physical therapists in the 1940s–1950s anchored the profession to mainstream medicine. Today, physical therapists have their own associations and training programs at the bachelor's and master's degree levels.

The distinction between massage therapists working in medical settings and physical therapy professionals was not crystal clear in the 1940s–1950s. Many physical therapists had been initially trained in colleges of Swedish massage where Ling's work was also taught. In fact, the American Association of Masseurs and Masseuses (AAMM), founded in 1943, changed its name to the American Massage & Therapy Association in 1958 to reflect that some of its members identified themselves as massage practitioners and some as physical therapists.

By the 1960s, those who wanted to work in medical settings were grandfathered into physical therapy licenses. The professions of physical therapy and massage therapy were now going their separate ways. As the distinction between the professions became clearer, the "&" was dropped from the AM&TA, and it became the American Massage Therapy Association (AMTA) in 1983. See Box 2–3 ■ for a health care timeline.

FIGURE 2–10 Medical gymnasts assist patient in performing movements, 1909.

Source: Handbook of Medical and Orthopedic Gymnastics by Wide, 1909.

FIGURE 2–11 A corner of the general massage section of an army hospital.

Source: A Practice of Physiotherapy by Sampson, 1926.

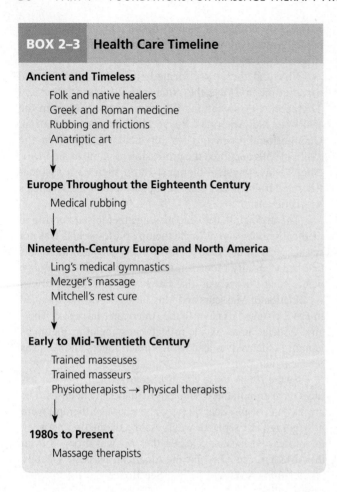

BOX 2–3	Health Care Timeline

Ancient and Timeless

Folk and native healers
Greek and Roman medicine
Rubbing and frictions
Anatriptic art

↓

Europe Throughout the Eighteenth Century

Medical rubbing

↓

Nineteenth-Century Europe and North America

Ling's medical gymnastics
Mezger's massage
Mitchell's rest cure

↓

Early to Mid-Twentieth Century

Trained masseuses
Trained masseurs
Physiotherapists → Physical therapists

↓

1980s to Present

Massage therapists

Naturopaths, drugless healers who utilized a number of different natural methods, had begun to organize their profession in 1902 with the founding of the Naturopathic Society of America. It was reorganized as the American Naturopathic Association (ANA) in 1919. *The Naturopath,* a magazine focused on the "interests of all schools of drugless healing," and "the Art of Natural Living," also "devotes itself especially to the defense of the individual drugless practitioner persecuted by the Medical and Osteopathic Trust" (advertisement 1925). Today, the profession of naturopathic physician is licensed in 17 of the 50 states in the United States.[32]

Massage in the Natural Healing Tradition

Massage and the Swedish movements were important natural healing methods. Dr. P. Puderbach, director of the Brooklyn School for Massage and Physiotherapy and author of *The Massage Operator,* wrote that massage "has taken its rank as the equal of other sanative [healing] methods, and thus we see in the Massage that is applied correctly by experienced hands, a powerful means for the rejuvenation of mankind, the beautification of the human body, the alleviation of innumerable weaknesses, and the cure of many diseases that have been the curse of humanity."[33]

Dr. Puderbach's school trained massage specialists to work in natural healing environments. Figure 2–12 ■ shows an operator massaging the shoulders and using a heat lamp or radiant rays. These lamps were used to relax muscles and

NATURAL HEALING AND DRUGLESS DOCTORS

The natural healing movement began in the late 1800s. Natural healing practitioners rejected the allopathic methods of drugs and surgery and instead used natural remedies to treat ailments. They were known as the *drugless doctors.* They relied on medicinal herbs, mineral waters, hydrotherapy, colonic irrigation, therapeutic massage and movement, hypnosis, meditation, and electrotherapy. They promoted healthy practices such as rest, exercise, good nutrition, deep breathing of fresh air, sunbathing, singing, and laughter. Many were vegetarians. They recognized that true health is a matter of body, mind, and spirit.

Fundamental to the natural healing philosophy is a belief in the innate healing power of nature, or "the inherent restorative power for health that resides in every organism."[31] The job of the natural healing practitioner is to facilitate that natural process and avoid "heroic" or intrusive methods. Preventing illness and promoting healthful natural living were also essential to this philosophy. The natural healing movement was a precursor to today's wellness movement and gave birth to the profession of naturopathic physician.

FIGURE 2–12 Masseuse performs massage of the shoulder under heat lamp, c. 1925.

Source: The Massage Operator by Puderbach, 1925.

increase local circulation, "producing the most favorable conditions for effective massage."[34]

Several well-known natural healing centers appeared at the turn of the century in the form of country resorts. Benedict Lust (1872–1945), a German immigrant, was considered a "father" of naturopathy. Lust operated two such places called *Yungborn* in Butler, New Jersey, and Tangerine, Florida. Yungborn in New Jersey, established in 1896, was billed as the "original nature cure resort and recreation home," and "the parent institution of naturopathy in America." An advertisement for Yungborn lists massage, Swedish movements, and mechanotherapy as some of many treatments available at the nature resort.

Perhaps the most famous natural healing center was the Battle Creek Sanitarium in Michigan run by J. Harvey Kellogg (1852–1943). Kellogg, who is widely known for Kellogg cereals, had a great interest in health and nutrition and was especially interested in massage. He wrote a classic on the subject titled *The Art of Massage: Its Physiological Effects and Therapeutic Applications* (1895). The manual was intended for medical and nursing students, but also became a standard text for masseurs and masseuses. Kellogg employed 10 to 20 masseurs and masseuses at the "San" at any one time.

Kellogg numbered the descriptions of different massage techniques and applications so that physicians could prescribe the exact methods they wanted the massage practitioner to perform on an individual patient. But the experienced masseur and masseuse were also expected to modify the application for each case and not follow the written prescription "slavishly."

Kellogg makes reference to the work of Ling in the preface to *The Art of Massage* (1895). He states that "it is rare that the most perfect results can be obtained without supplementing the treatment by massage with a judiciously conducted course of gymnastics." He suggests that a translation of Ling's work on medical gymnastics "ought to be in the hands of every masseur."[35] So just as medical gymnasts at that time were adopting massage to complement their work, masseurs and masseuses were adopting the Swedish movements as a natural complement to massage.

A popular version of natural healing was promoted by Bernarr Macfadden (1868–1955), which he called *physical culture.* Macfadden opened physical culture resorts and a Physical Culture Training School in Chicago that graduated "doctors" of hydropathy, kinesitherapy, and physcultopathy. Physcultopathists were essentially medical gymnasts trained in Macfadden's school. This is an early example of an entrepreneurial enterprise in massage therapy.[36]

Today's massage therapy profession is a direct outgrowth of this natural healing tradition. This is evident in the affinity of massage therapists for natural healing methods, in the adoption of the wellness model to define our scope, and in our identity as a complementary and alternative medicine (CAM) therapy. Issues related to differences in philosophy and the mistrust of mainstream medicine, as well as the push for freedom of choice in medical treatment, stem from this heritage.

The first convention of the American Association of Masseurs and Masseuses in 1946 included a lecture on zone therapy (i.e., reflexology) by Eunice Ingham, a lecture on massage and multitherapy by John Granger, an equipment demonstration by a representative of the Therm-Aire Corporation, and a talk on "cradepathy." Their first president, Clark Cottrell, said about this event, "I am sure we are on the right track to the natural methods of healing."[37]

It is important to understand this connection to the natural healing tradition as the profession of massage therapy interfaces with mainstream medicine in the twenty-first century. This history is especially important to remember as massage therapists work to maintain their integrity while they find their place in integrative medical settings. The fundamental identity of massage therapy as a natural healing agent is a primary strength it brings to integrative health care today. See Box 2–4 ■ for a natural healing timeline.

MASSAGE THERAPY REVIVED IN THE UNITED STATES

The 1950s were a dark time for the massage profession in the United States. Physical therapists and athletic trainers were developing their own professions and were being educated in colleges and universities. Most of the old colleges of Swedish massage were closing. Mainstream America considered natural healing the province of "health nuts" or akin to quackery, and massage was being used blatantly as a cover for prostitution. "Massage parlor" had become permanently associated with houses of ill repute.

During this time, massage was kept alive by natural healers working out of their homes, in private practice, and

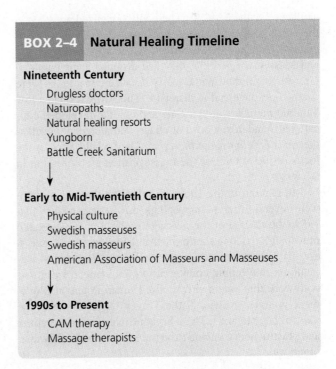

BOX 2–4   Natural Healing Timeline

Nineteenth Century

Drugless doctors
Naturopaths
Natural healing resorts
Yungborn
Battle Creek Sanitarium

↓

Early to Mid-Twentieth Century

Physical culture
Swedish masseuses
Swedish masseurs
American Association of Masseurs and Masseuses

↓

1990s to Present

CAM therapy
Massage therapists

REALITY CHECK

SHANNON: A newspaper article I read a few days ago featured a local spa and called the massage therapist working there a "masseuse." I know the writer had good intentions because he talked about the benefits of massage, but calling her a masseuse sounded like she worked in a red light district. Don't people know the difference?

BARBARA: Masseuse is just an old term used decades ago to describe women who did Swedish massage. Some people haven't caught up with changing times and still call massage therapists "masseuses." And they confuse "masseuse" with "masseur," which is even worse. "Masseur" is the correct term for a male. A good approach might be to contact this writer and politely educate him about how using the term "masseuse" affects massage therapists negatively by its current association with prostitution, and that the correct term today is "massage therapist" for both men and women. We can be proud of our heritage as masseurs and masseuses, but still ask others to use the more correct name today.

at places like the YMCAs. Their only organized presence in the 1950s was in the American Massage & Therapy Association, formerly the American Association of Masseurs and Masseuses. In 1958, they had dropped "masseurs and masseuses" in their name partly because those terms were deemed obsolete and in disrepute. The AM&TA had a few hundred members at that time and quietly developed educational standards, a code of ethics, and a credential called the *registered massage therapist*. They would later be the locus of the revival of the massage therapy profession in the 1980s.

Beginning in the 1960s and through the 1970s, there were several different happenings in American society that led to the revival of the massage profession. Two related movements based in California that reintroduced massage as a valuable health practice were the Human Potential Movement and the hippie counterculture movement. Forms of bodywork that emerged from the Human Potential Movement included Rolfing®, the Trager® approach, and the Feldenkrais Method®. These became trademarked therapies, and practitioners continue to be trained and certified by their organizations.

A simplified form of massage was developed at the Esalen Institute in Big Sur, California. Called Esalen massage, it incorporated simple Western massage techniques and emphasized sensual aspects using scented oils, candle lighting, incense, and new age music. Draping of the body was optional. Its purpose was to help the giver and receiver alike get in touch with their senses. At first, Esalen massage was adopted as a tool for personal growth and learned in meditation and self-improvement centers. It was associated with the hippie counterculture.

Some hippies who learned Esalen massage recognized its potential for health and healing and aspired to do the work for their livelihood. Some of those joined the natural healers in the AM&TA, giving the organization and the profession an influx of people and new energy. Mistrust of "establishment" health care, openness to non-Western health and healing practices, ambivalence toward regulation, and awareness of the psychological and spiritual aspects of massage are some of the values that they reinforced in the field.

Other factors that contributed to a revival of massage therapy in the 1970s were an interest in Eastern philosophies and health practices, particularly from India, China, and Japan. Yogis founded ashrams in the United States that promoted ancient Indian health practices such as meditation, deep breathing, vegetarianism, and massage. Trade with China was reopened in the 1970s, leading to an exchange of information about medical practices such as acupuncture and *tuina*. Shiatsu and amma practitioners from Japan came to the United States and trained people in their arts.

A new fitness craze called *aerobics* also emerged in the 1970s. Ordinary people began taking aerobic exercise classes and participated in jogging and in local fun runs and marathons. The success of European athletes who received massage revived an interest in sports massage in the United States. The wellness movement gained ground in the field of health and physical education and introduced the concept of high-level wellness. The movement urged people to take responsibility for their own well-being and emphasized a holistic approach to health for body, mind, and spirit.

All these factors led to consumer demand for massage therapy and to the establishment of vocational schools to train massage practitioners. New schools of massage based on the holistic and wellness perspectives appeared in the early 1980s. The ranks of massage therapists and bodyworkers swelled, as did membership in professional organizations. See Box 2–5 ■ for a modern massage therapy timeline.

MASSAGE THERAPISTS AND BODYWORKERS

In the 1970s, massage therapy was largely unregulated, entrepreneurial, and alternative. Only a few states regulated massage in the 1970s, notably Arkansas, Hawaii, Nebraska, New York, Ohio, Oregon, Rhode Island, Washington, Florida, and North Dakota.

Modern Massage Therapy Timeline

1950s

> Dark ages for massage

1970s

> Human potential movement
> Hippie counterculture
> Esalen massage
> Asian health practices
> Fitness and aerobic exercise
> Wellness movement
> Bodywork specialties

1980s to 1990s

> Massage and bodywork
> Increased consumer use of massage
> Increased number of massage schools
> Increased professionalism

1990 to Present

> Massage therapists
> Licensed massage therapists

Regardless of what the practitioners were called, more and more consumers were looking for massage and bodywork services. And the benefits of massage touted by practitioners and their organizations were beginning to be accepted by the general public. Graduates of massage programs in the 1980s opened private practices that attracted a diverse population of clients (Figure 2–13 ■). The momentum for massage that began in the 1970s carried over into the 1980s and beyond to the present time.

Some indication of the growth of the profession can be seen in the steady increase in the number of members in professional organizations. In 1960, AMTA had 359 members; 1,051 members in 1970; 1,405 in 1980; and 3,183 in 1985.[38] AMTA had grown to over 56,000 members by 2012. ABMP, founded in 1986, has over 80,000 members today.

Professional challenges during the 20-year period 1980–2000 ranged from winning the respect of the general public to gaining acceptance as health professionals by the health care community to establishing educational and competency standards. Appropriate dress, draping standards, and the ethics of the therapeutic relationship were hashed out in professional publications and meetings.

Many of the benchmarks of a profession listed in Box 1–1, have been achieved in the last few decades. The early 1990s were particularly busy with the first National Certification Examination for Therapeutic Massage and

Many who became massage therapists at that time were looking for a second career, an alternative to corporate life, and/or a more holistic approach to health care. Many were escaping what they considered soulless overregulated professions and were drawn to the independent, nonstandardized field of massage and bodywork.

The term *massage* was still tainted, and so the term *massage therapy* was adopted to distinguish legitimate massage from massage as a cover for prostitution. It was also accepted as the designation for the field as a whole, including traditional Swedish massage and other forms of manual therapy. Some practitioners who had been trained in distinct forms of manipulation (e.g., Rolfing® and Polarity Therapy), and who did not wish to be associated with massage, coined the term *bodywork* to describe the larger occupational field.

Unlike physical therapists and athletic trainers, practitioners of the manipulative arts are not in agreement on one name for the profession. This ambivalence is seen in the various names of organizations such as the American Massage Therapy Association (AMTA), the Associated Bodywork & Massage Professionals (ABMP), and the National Certification Board for Therapeutic Massage and Bodywork (NCBTMB). Most, however, use various combinations of *massage* and/or *bodywork* with or without references to therapy. *Somatic therapy* (i.e., body therapy) and *touch therapy* are less used terms for the field as a whole.

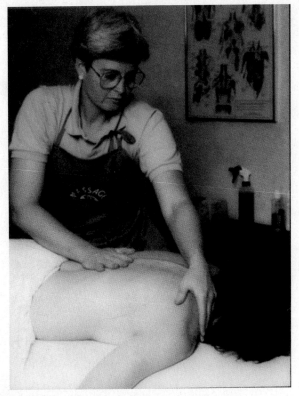

FIGURE 2–13 Massage therapist, c. 1985.

Source: Pearson Education, Inc.

Bodywork, the incorporation of the Massage Therapy Foundation, the founding of the Touch Research Institute at the University of Miami, and the establishment of the Office of Alternative Medicine at the U.S. National Institutes of Health. The Commission on Massage Therapy Accreditation (COMTA) received U.S. Department of Education recognition in 2002. The number of states licensing or certifying massage therapists has grown from about six in 1985 to 44 plus the District of Columbia in 2014 with licensing laws working their way through the legislative process in several states today.

Unified Profession

The trend in the early twenty-first century is toward a more unified profession of massage therapy. Although there are notable exceptions, most massage and bodywork practitioners find common ground in entry-level educational standards, licensing requirements, and board certification. They are comfortable with diversity, and just as medical gymnasts of the nineteenth century embraced the new massage treatment, massage therapists today incorporate different techniques of soft tissue manipulation in their work.

Many of the image problems of the past have been resolved with the creation of recognized credentials identifying legitimate massage practitioners and the adoption of codes of ethics. Some states, such as Illinois, prohibit the use of the word *massage* by anyone except licensed massage therapists.

The profession is becoming more standardized as more massage therapists enter the field through educational programs that meet accreditation and licensing requirements instead of through trademarked systems. Many techniques and approaches that were originally trademarked in the 1970s–1980s have been absorbed into massage therapy in generic form. For example, myofascial massage, trigger point therapy, and various styles of shiatsu were originally introduced in trademarked systems, but are now integrated into many basic massage therapy programs.

There has been some discussion of splitting the field into levels or tiers, thereby distinguishing between so-called relaxation massage and medical massage. The intent of this proposal is to resolve issues related to minimum education standards. Perhaps this is a reflection of the historical tension between medical and natural healing models and the use of massage for personal care. A better option might be to hold fast to the wellness model and embrace the whole scope of the field as outlined in the Wellness Massage Pyramid. Educational standards could be resolved by adopting entry-level standards for everyone, with additional knowledge and skills needed for those working in specialty areas or specific settings. This is an issue to resolve in the years to come.

 # CASE FOR STUDY

Alex and Researching Historical Background for a Legislative Issue

Alex, a massage therapist, is on the law and legislation committee of a professional organization that is preparing comments on a change in the definitions and scope of practice sections of the massage therapy licensing law. His task is to provide historical background on the issues involved.

Question:

Where would Alex look for relevant historical information that would provide a broader understanding of the issues his committee is investigating?

Things to consider:

- History of the passage of the licensing law and amendments made over the years.
- Definitions and scope of practice statements in current and old versions of the licensing law in question, as well as similar laws in other states.

- Identification of issues that have arisen over the years related to definition and scope of practice; note individuals and organizations involved.
- Definitions and scope of practice statements in current and old versions of licensing laws for cosmetologists, estheticians, physical therapists, and other relevant occupations.
- Historical relationships among professionals who use massage within their scope, for example, cosmetologists, physical therapists, and athletic trainers; focus on similarities and differences; local issues; and organizations and people involved.
- Advances in the massage therapy profession throughout recent history, including advances in education and research.

Important historical information you have learned about massage laws in your geographic area:

_____

_____

_____

CHAPTER HIGHLIGHTS

- Over the centuries, many have been called or have chosen to be massage practitioners; their stories form the history of massage as a vocation.
- The four major branches of this history are (1) massage for personal grooming and rejuvenation, (2) sports and fitness, (3) health care, and (4) natural healing.
- In ancient civilizations, domestic servants and slaves performed many personal care services, including helping with bathing, rubdowns, and applying scented oils.
- In China in the 1800s, street barbers performed a type of seated massage, and in Japan at the same time, blind masseurs called ammashi traveled the streets blowing a flute to attract customers.
- Forms of manipulation have been available in public bathhouses all over the world. The occupational designation of bath attendant stems from this ancient tradition.
- In the early 1900s, massage was part of personal care services called beauty culture.
  - A limited use of superficial massage continues in the scope of practice of barbers and cosmetologists, who began to be licensed around 1900.
  - Full-body massage for rejuvenation and reducing, and breast massage were performed by Swedish masseuses in the 1920s–1940s in beauty culture settings.
  - Practitioners trained in schools were called graduate masseuses and masseurs.
- Massage for athletes has a long tradition.
  - Massage with oil by aleiptes and paidotribes was part of the routine at the ancient Greek gymnasium.
  - Bath attendants and rubbers provided massage to amateur athletes in the eighteenth to nineteenth centuries in Europe and North America.
  - In the twentieth century, athletic masseurs were trained in schools.
  - By 1950, athletic trainers had developed their own profession specializing in sports injuries, and athletic massage in America largely died out.
  - Sports massage was revived in the United States in the 1970s within the growing profession of massage therapy.
- In the early twentieth century, masseurs and masseuses provided massage in health clubs in American cities.
  - Health service operators and masseurs offered massage and related services in YMCAs.
  - The Health Service Operators Society was established in 1942.
- Massage has been used for healing from time immemorial by families and tribal and community healers.
  - At the beginning of Western medicine, massage was used by Greek and Roman physicians.

- Some European physicians of the eighteenth to nineteenth centuries utilized soft tissue manipulation in medical treatment.
- American physicians of the early twentieth century prescribed Mezger's massage to be performed on patients by assistants.
- The occupation of trained masseuse was formed as a greater level of skill and professionalism was required to work with patients.
- Practitioners of Ling's system of medical gymnastics applied active and passive movements to treat various chronic diseases.
  - Ling founded a school in Stockholm, Sweden, in 1813 to train educational and medical gymnasts.
  - Medical gymnasts, also known as movement cure practitioners, were alternative medical providers in the late nineteenth century. They eventually adopted Mezger's massage into their work, which then became known in America as Swedish massage.
- By the 1950s, a separate profession of physical therapy was formed for physiotherapists working in mainstream medical settings.
  - The American Women's Physical Therapeutic Association was founded in 1921.
- Massage was an important part of natural healing systems of the late nineteenth and early twentieth centuries.
  - Naturopaths began to organize their profession of drugless healers in 1902 with the founding of the Naturopathic Society of America.
  - Massage operators were trained in schools to work in natural healing resorts.
  - In 1895, Kellogg wrote *The Art of Massage,* which became a classic massage textbook.
  - A popular version of natural healing called physical culture, with practitioners called physcultopathists, was promoted by Bernarr Macfadden.
- Swedish massage practitioners working within a natural healing framework founded the American Association of Masseurs and Masseuses in 1943, changed to the American Massage & Therapy Association in 1958, and known as the American Massage Therapy Association today.
- Today's massage therapists are part of the natural healing tradition as evidenced in their attraction to natural healing methods, adoption of the wellness model, identity as a CAM profession, wariness of mainstream medicine, and champions of choice in medical treatment.

- An understanding of the tradition of massage within natural healing is important to massage therapists as they find their places today in integrative medical settings.

- The use of massage in the United States declined in the 1950s.

- Massage was revived in the 1970s due to a variety of factors including the human potential movement, counter culture movement, interest in Asian health practices, fitness craze, and wellness movement.

- An increased number of people seeking massage therapy, and the founding of new massage training schools, helped increase the number of massage practitioners in the 1980s.
  - The 1980s–1990s were a period of growth and the professionalizing of massage therapy.

- In the early twenty-first century, massage therapy has become a more unified profession comfortable with diversity in approaches and moving toward generally recognized standards.

EXAM REVIEW

Key Terms

Match the following key terms to their descriptions. For additional study, look up the key terms in the Interactive Glossary and note other terms that compare or contrast with them.

_____ 1. Aleiptes
_____ 2. Ammashi
_____ 3. Bath attendant
_____ 4. Health service operator
_____ 5. Massage operator
_____ 6. Masseurs/masseuses
_____ 7. Medical gymnast
_____ 8. Rubbers
_____ 9. Sobardoras
_____ 10. Trained masseuses

a. Specialists who rubbed and frictioned athletes in the early twentieth century

b. Terms for male and female massage therapists in the mid-twentieth century

c. Traditional Hispanic healers trained to use massage for treating ailments of those in their communities

d. Those who rubbed athletes with oil in ancient Greek gymnasia

e. Women massage therapists who studied in private schools and hospital programs in the early part of the twentieth century

f. Blind masseurs of Japan

g. Term for massage therapist in the natural healing tradition in the 1920s

h. Occupation stemming from the ancient traditions of servants or attendants giving a rubdown, or rubbing in scented oils, after a bath.

i. Worked in YMCAs in the early twentieth century offering physical therapeutics or physiotherapy and focused on health, fitness, and general well-being

j. Practitioners trained in the system of bodywork developed by Pehr Henrik Ling of Sweden in the nineteenth century.

Memory Workout

To test your memory of the main concepts in this chapter, complete the following sentences by circling the most correct answer from the two choices provided.

1. The four major branches of the history of massage as a vocation roughly parallel today's (approaches to bodywork) (work settings).
2. A British delegation to China in the 1790s described street (barbers) (performers), who offered grooming services, including a form of seated bodywork.
3. (Deaf) (Blind) masseurs of Japan walked the streets announcing their presence by playing a small flute.
4. The occupational designation of (masseur) (bath attendant) stems from ancient traditions of servants or other assistants giving a rubdown, or rubbing scented oils into the skin after a bath.
5. As early as 1915, (a rubdown) (medical rubbing) by a bath attendant was an established part of the routine at the YMCA.
6. Traditional Hispanic healers called (sobardoras) (ammashi), specialize in massage to treat a variety of ailments.
7. In the eighteenth century, the general name for soft tissue manipulation as used in medical settings was (medical rubbing) (drugless healing).
8. The Society of Trained Masseuses was formed in (United States) (England) in (1894) (1943) to raise professional standards for massage specialists working in the medical field.
9. In the 1950s, massage was being used as a cover for prostitution in the United States, and the term massage (parlor) (establishment) had become permanently associated with houses of ill repute.
10. In the 1970s, a movement in the field of health and physical education encouraged people to take responsibility for their own well-being and emphasized a holistic approach to health. This was known as the (human potential) (wellness) movement.

Test Prep

The following multiple-choice questions will help to prepare you for future school and professional exams.

1. In ancient civilizations, who typically provided personal care services like grooming and bathing in the home?
   a. Well-paid employees
   b. A class of priests and priestesses
   c. Slaves and domestic servants
   d. Older family members

2. The name used by the British to describe a practice from India that involved a hot soapy bath, followed by a form of bodywork involving percussion and friction massage, joint cracking, and applying scented oils or perfume is:
   a. Anatriptic art
   b. Shampooing
   c. Padshah's bath
   d. Ammashi

3. The prototype public bath in Western civilization and forerunner of today's day spa is the:
   a. Greek gymnasium
   b. Roman bath
   c. Mineral bath
   d. Beauty salon

4. Women massage practitioners working in beauty and reducing salons in the early 1900s were typically called:
   a. Manipulators
   b. Health service operators
   c. Swedish masseurs
   d. Swedish masseuses

5. In the 1940s, massage practitioners who worked with athletes and who were well trained in the massage field were typically called:
   a. Athletic masseurs
   b. Paidotribes
   c. Rubbers
   d. Bath attendants

6. In the United States in the late 1800s, Ling's medical gymnastics used to treat chronic diseases was known as:
   a. Physical culture
   b. Mechno-manipulation
   c. Swedish massage
   d. Swedish movement cure

7. The doctor from Amsterdam who developed a system of soft tissue manipulation in the mid-1800s that is the basis for today's European-style massage is:
   a. Pehr H. Ling
   b. Johann Mezger
   c. J. Harvey Kellogg
   d. Douglas Graham

8. In the United States in the 1970s, a simplified form of massage was developed in California that incorporated simple Western massage techniques and emphasized sensual aspects using scented oils, candle lighting, incense, and "new age" music. It was called:
   a. Swedish massage
   b. Esalen massage
   c. Shampooing
   d. Anatriptic art

Video Challenge

Watch this video, which can be found at MyHealthProfessionsLab.com, Chapter 2, and then answer the following questions.

History of Massage

1. Identify the various settings in which massage practitioners of the past worked, giving examples from the video.
2. Describe the dress of massage practitioners of the past as shown in the video. Explain how their dress, even though outdated today, shows a sense of professionalism.
3. Look closely at the photos of massage shown in the video. Do you notice anything that would probably be done differently today, for example, draping or techniques? Is there anything that would be done exactly the same today?

Comprehension Exercises

The following short answer questions test your knowledge and understanding of chapter topics and provide practice in written communication skills. Explain in two to four complete sentences.

1. Name the four branches of the history of massage as a vocation. Give examples of settings today that correspond to these historical branches.
2. Briefly trace the history of sports massage, and identify the names used over the centuries for massage practitioners specializing in working with athletes.
3. What do the terms *massage parlor* and *masseuse* mean in the context of the history of massage?

For Greater Understanding

The following exercises are designed to take you from the realm of theory into the real world. They will help give you a deeper understanding of the subjects covered in this chapter. Action words are underlined to emphasize the variety of activities presented to address different learning styles and to encourage deeper thinking.

1. Imagine that you are walking around a village in ancient China, and describe the different forms of massage and bodywork that you might see there. Repeat for the cities and towns of ancient Rome, Medieval Europe, 1880 Europe, and then 1920, 1950, and 1990 United States. Note that at any one time and place, massage and bodywork can be found in a number of settings and performed by practitioners with different backgrounds.
2. Visit a day or destination spa, and note the services on the menu. Receive a massage or other spa services if possible. Compare and contrast your experience to bath houses and natural healing resorts of the past. Report your findings to the class.
3. Locate a historical facility in your community where massage has been available for a long time or was offered in the past (e.g., old YMCA, Turkish bath, athletic club, beauty salon, resort, mineral spring spa). Look for an ad for the facility from the past, especially one that mentions massage. Share your discovery with the class. (Variation: Report on a place you visited on vacation that had historical connections to massage.)

MyHealthProfessionsLab™

MyHealthProfessionsLab.com is a premium online homework management system that includes a host of features to help you study. Registered users will find:

- Powerful tools that track and analyze your results—allowing you to create a personalized learning experience
- Videos, flashcards and other learning tools to help enrich your progress
- Streaming lesson presentations and self-paced learning modules
- A space where you and your instructors can view and manage your assignments

Professional and Personal Development

CHAPTER OUTLINE

Learning Outcomes

Key Terms

Professionalism in Massage Therapy

Professional Image

Professional Boundaries

Ethics for the Massage Student

Intellectual Skills

Intuition

Emotional Intelligence

Social Skills

Communication Skills

Chapter Highlights

Exam Review

Pearson Education, Inc.

LEARNING OUTCOMES

After studying this chapter, you will have information to:

1. Describe the importance of personal growth for professional development.
2. Understand *service* as an important value for massage therapists.
3. Develop a strong work ethic.
4. Look and behave professionally.
5. Develop intellectual skills and concentration.
6. Develop greater emotional intelligence.
7. Use basic courtesy and good manners.
8. Communicate well and be a good listener.
9. Resolve conflicts peacefully and positively.
10. Present yourself to the public with confidence.

KEY TERMS

Body language

Compassion

Concentration

Conflict resolution

Critical thinking

Emotional intelligence

Ethics

Intellectual skills

Intuition

Listening

Problem solving

Professional boundaries

Professional image

Service

Social skills

Work ethic

PROFESSIONALISM IN MASSAGE THERAPY

Becoming a successful massage therapist is a journey of transformation. Part of that journey is learning to be a professional. What is professionalism? It is more than knowing the Latin names of muscles and bones and performing massage techniques skillfully.

> Professionalism is a state of mind, a way of "being," "knowing," and "doing" that sets you apart from others. It gives you direction to how you look, behave, think, and act. It brings together who you are as a person, what you value, how you treat other people, what you contribute in the workplace, and how seriously you take your job. . . . To *be* a professional, you must *feel like* a professional.[1]

Feeling like a professional comes from the inside, but it manifests in the image you present by your appearance and behavior. Likewise, by presenting a professional image, you cultivate feeling like a professional. When you finally become a professional, the inside and outside are totally in sync, and your professional presence is genuine.

Attitude is the sum of how a person presents him- or herself to the world—a way of acting, thinking, and feeling. To have a professional attitude is to embody all that it means to be a professional.

Becoming a professional massage therapist inevitably involves change and personal growth. Some of the key growth areas are dedication to service, developing a strong work ethic, establishing a professional image, cultivating intellectual skills, improving concentration, developing intuition, and nurturing emotional intelligence. Social and communications skills are essential to a massage therapist.

Service

The essence of the massage therapy profession is serving others. Dedication to **service** means that we hold clients' well-being above our own desire for money, power, and worldly recognition. It means that the primary motivation for being a massage therapist is to help people achieve their personal wellness goals.

Dedication to service helps keep priorities in order. It focuses attention on the well-being of our clients rather than on us. It guides our way and offers a higher and more satisfying motivation than merely making money. It spurs us to being the best that we can be. It provides a moral compass for ethical decision making.

There are much easier, more prestigious, and more lucrative ways to make a living than being a massage therapist. But using massage therapy to help others live healthier, happier, and more stress-free lives provides great satisfaction to those who choose this work.

Many start on the road to becoming a massage therapist for other reasons. But those who stay and find satisfaction in their work realize that the ultimate motivation is to be of service to those who come to us for massage therapy.

Work Ethic

A strong work ethic provides a firm foundation for all other aspects of professionalism. **Work ethic** is described as "positioning your job as a high priority in your life and making sound decisions about how you approach your work."[2] It means taking your work seriously, staying focused, and applying yourself to doing a good job.

A strong work ethic is reflected in good attendance and punctuality, reliability and accountability, positive attitude and enthusiasm, and taking responsibility for doing the highest quality work of which you are capable. It starts when you are a student and carries on into your professional life. It is a trait that employers value highly and an essential characteristic for success in private practice.

Good attendance means showing up when expected or when scheduled, and punctuality means showing up on time. Punctuality also entails getting to school or work early enough that you are settled in and ready to go when the class starts or when the client arrives. Running in late or at the last minute prevents you from preparing, centering, and focusing yourself. It shows disrespect for your classmates, teachers, and clients.

Reliability is a related trait that means people can depend on you to do what you say you are going to do, when you are supposed to do it. If you are reliable, people will have trust and confidence in you. Accountability means that you accept responsibility for your actions, and do not make excuses for repeated mistakes. You apologize sincerely for and correct mistakes that you have made.

A positive attitude and enthusiasm shows in how you speak about your work and the energy you put into it. The word *enthusiasm* comes from the Greek language and means possessed or inspired by the gods. If you have enthusiasm, you exhibit keen interest and eagerness for your work. You value it and look forward to studying, practicing, and learning more about it.

With a strong work ethic, you take responsibility for doing your highest quality work every time. Regardless of whatever else is going on in your life, you strive for quality in your work. You exhibit competence in applying the knowledge and skills of your profession for the good of your clients.

PROFESSIONAL IMAGE

Your appearance reflects your inner state of professionalism. A **professional image** makes a favorable impression on your clients, and identifies you as someone they can have confidence in and trust. Your appearance should be clean, neat, modest, and appropriate for the setting in which you work. Establishing a professional presence involves attention to dress, grooming, posture, and language.

PRACTICAL APPLICATION

Analyze your own work ethic as reflected in your behavior so far in massage school and your attitude toward class work and homework. Concentrate on attendance, punctuality, behavior in class, and getting assignments in on time, as well as good attitude and enthusiasm.

1. Do you see areas for improvement?
2. Can you pick out three things you can start doing today that show a commitment to your massage training and enthusiasm for massage therapy?
3. How will that help you in your career as a massage therapist?

Dress

The way you dress sets the tone of your relationship with clients—respectful, nonsexual, and trusting. It also helps set boundaries by saying to the client that this is a professional relationship. Remember that as a professional massage therapist you are not dressing to impress your friends or attract a romantic date (Figure 3–1 ■).

Many massage therapists adopt a uniform look such as loose pants and polo shirt, hospital scrubs, sports clothes, or a martial arts outfit. A spa might have a required uniform such as a smock with the company logo. With a little thought and creativity, you can find work clothes that are attractive, practical, and express who you are as a professional.

Some guidelines for professional dress are

- Have work clothes that are separate from your everyday clothes.
- Choose clothes that are conservative and modest.

- Choose clothes that can be cleaned easily.
- Wear clothes that allow the freedom of movement you need for your work.
- Wear clothes appropriate for your work setting and in compliance with your employer's dress code.
- Wear closed-toed shoes, or other coverings that enclose the feet (e.g., socks with sandals).
- Keep clothes clean, neat, and odor-free.

Some generally accepted *don'ts* for professional dress are

- Don't wear tops that show cleavage or breast tissue (e.g., low-cut tops or sleeveless shirts with large armholes).
- Don't wear tops with large or long sleeves that may touch the client.
- Don't wear pants that are tight or provocative (e.g., show the navel).
- Don't wear short shorts or short skirts.
- Don't wear denim jeans, either long or short.
- Don't wear sandals without socks or go barefoot.
- Don't wear T-shirts with advertising or sayings that may be offensive.
- Don't wear jewelry that is likely to touch the client (e.g., dangling necklaces and rings). Rings can also be unsanitary if dirt and skin cells collect around and underneath them.
- Don't wear clothing that suggests a social setting rather than a professional setting.

An employer may have a mandatory dress code. Ask about it in your job interview so you are clear about what is expected. Most dress codes identify acceptable and unacceptable attire and indicate whether a uniform is required. They specify rules about jewelry and body decoration such as tattoos and body piercings.

FIGURE 3–1 Your appearance reflects your professionalism.

Source: Pearson Education, Inc.

Grooming

Grooming is an important part of appearance that includes nails, hair, and skin. Your hands, the instruments of massage, should receive special attention. Keep fingernails clean and short, that is, below the line of the fingertips. If you hold up the palm of your hand and look at the fingers, the fingernails should not be visible. Keep cuticles neat and trimmed.

Rough spots on the hands can be softened and cracks prevented with the application of healing lotions and creams. Because you will be washing your hands frequently, it is important to use soap with lotion added and to dry your hands thoroughly to prevent chapping. Chapped hands with cracked skin provide an entry point for germs and can feel rough on the client's body.

Use face makeup conservatively. Applying makeup to enhance appearance in a professional setting is appropriate. Being "made-up" to make a trendy statement or as you might for a date or social event is not appropriate.

Body piercing and tattoos may be all right if within the norms acceptable to your employer and clients. Cover any tattoo that you think might be offensive to clients. Consider removing potentially offensive tattoos that you might have had done before your professional life as a massage therapist.

Wash your hair regularly using unscented or lightly scented products. Adopt a hairstyle that prevents the hair from falling forward when bent over or from touching the client in any way. Men with facial hair should keep it clean and trimmed.

Body odor can be a problem in a profession such as massage that involves physical activity and close contact with clients. Always use an underarm deodorant. Those who do not shave under the arms should be aware that hair retains sweat, and that unpleasant odor develops faster there than on shaved areas. If necessary, wash under the arms during the day, and change your shirt after a few massage sessions.

Breath odor is another potential trouble spot. If you like to eat spicy foods or smoke, adopt strategies to eliminate the resulting odor. Breath mints can be effective for normal instances of "stale breath." Smokers must also consider the smell of smoke on their hands, clothes, and hair. Nonsmokers are more sensitive to cigarette and cigar smoke, so they can often smell odors that smokers cannot. Remember that when working around your client's head and face, he or she will be very aware of the smell of your hands. Here is a summary of guidelines for good grooming:

- Keep nails trimmed and manicured below the tips of the fingers; avoid nail polish.
- Keep hair clean and in a style that prevents it from touching the client.
- Keep skin on hands healthy and soft.
- Take precautions to prevent offensive body odor.
- Take precautions to prevent offensive breath odor.
- Keep areas around body piercing jewelry clean.

Posture

Good posture is not only healthy, but it also enhances your professional presence. Keep your back and neck in good alignment, head up, and muscles relaxed. Good posture should feel balanced and uplifting. Avoid slouching, leaning, tilting, and other poor postural habits. By correcting poor postural habits, you set a good example for clients. Chapter 11, *Body Mechanics, Table Skills, General Guidelines* outlines the elements of good sitting and standing posture in greater detail.

Image Detractors

Needless to say, annoying habits detract from a professional image. Nervous habits such as finger tapping, nail biting, knuckle cracking, leg bouncing, and hair twirling are best left to private moments. Other detractors include noisy jewelry, chewing gum, smoking, and eating or drinking in a client's presence.

PROFESSIONAL BOUNDARIES

Boundaries communicate limits or borders that define personal and professional space. They are the fences we place around ourselves to preserve our integrity as individuals. Good boundaries allow two individuals to meet with integrity and without violation of the other's space, but close enough to make connection.

CRITICAL THINKING

Visit three different places where massage therapists work, and evaluate the level of professionalism you see there.

1. Report your findings to the class or study group, noting specific details of dress, grooming, posture, speech, and image detractors on which you base your evaluation.

2. Compare what you see in different settings, and notice whether there is more than one way to look and be professional.

3. Determine which elements you find essential to presenting a professional image and those that are a matter of choice.

Professional boundaries clarify the nature of the therapeutic relationship and help us to differentiate the roles of massage therapist and client. Such boundaries communicate to the client that the relationship is professional, not personal, and define ethical behavior for both parties. It is the responsibility of massage therapists to establish and maintain professional boundaries in their practices through their communications with clients.

Boundaries are the heart of how we protect ourselves and our clients. A boundary is like a protective circle drawn around ourselves and our clients; it defines what goes on within that circle and the ways practitioners will and will not treat each other.[3]

There are five types of boundaries according to Benjamin and Sohnen-Moe[4]:

1. Physical

2. Emotional

3. Intellectual

4. Sexual

5. Energetic

Setting appropriate professional boundaries in these five areas is a matter of ethics as well as social propriety.

How far we sit or stand from each other sets physical boundaries for personal space. Invading people's space by getting too close to them can make them nervous and uncomfortable. Clothes also serve as physical boundaries, as does draping during a massage session. Physical boundaries limit where and when it is appropriate to touch a client and vice versa. Leaving the room when clients are dressing and undressing gives them personal space and preserves their boundaries.

The physical space for massage, that is, office and massage room, should be free of personal property such as family photos or collections of objects. If practicing in a home, segregate the reception area, bathroom, and massage room from personal and family space as much as possible, especially from bedrooms.

Emotional boundaries limit disclosure about feelings. Because massage therapists are not professionals in psychology, too much emotional disclosure on the client's part may cross the line of a massage therapist's scope of practice. Emotional disclosure by the massage therapist may turn the tables in the therapeutic relationship by seeming to call for help from the client.

Intellectual boundaries demand respect for other people's beliefs and restrict forcing our beliefs and opinions on others. For example, some massage therapists who are health conscious may try to indoctrinate their clients regarding their eating habits, such as their belief in vegetarianism. This is not only an intellectual boundary violation, but also a scope-of-practice problem.

Sexual boundaries in a professional relationship are absolute. They protect both massage therapists and clients. Sexual boundary violations by massage therapists are unethical and illegal.

Energetic boundaries are less obvious; for example, not letting a client's bad mood or "negative energy" affect your state of being. Clients who seek massage are frequently stressed and carry a lot of nervous energy. Helping clients disperse this energy without permeating the massage therapist's boundaries is an important self-care consideration.

Professional boundaries are also defined by routine office procedures and policies. These include policies for clients arriving late for sessions, not showing up for appointments, standards of hygiene, and payment due dates. Communicating policies clearly reduces misunderstanding and increases satisfaction when expectations are met.

Keeping good professional boundaries is a key factor in maintaining ethical massage therapy practices. Common boundary violations are discussed further in Chapter 5, *Ethics and the Therapeutic Relationship*.

ETHICS FOR THE MASSAGE STUDENT

Ethics is the study of the nature of moral behavior, of right and wrong. It examines choices for behavior and uses critical thinking and problem solving skills to determine the degree of morality of certain actions.

Ethics have a positive aspect related to *what to do,* and a negative aspect related to *what not to do.* Common values on which ethical choices are made include honesty, integrity, compassion, quality care, respect for persons, privacy and confidentiality, abiding by the law, keeping professional ethical standards, and doing no harm.

Professional ethics looks at common ethical situations that arise within a specific occupation such as massage therapy. Codes of ethical behavior and standards of practice are developed by professional associations as the collective standard for the profession. Chapter 5, *Ethics and the Therapeutic Relationship*, is devoted to ethics for massage therapists and presents guidelines for ethical behavior within the profession. In addition, Chapter 28, Business Ethics, discusses ethical behavior in the operation of a massage therapy practice.

Massage therapy students have their own unique circumstances that require ethical consideration. Some are the same for all students, but others are unique to massage therapy students. The following standards for massage students are a good a start to learning professional ethics for massage therapists.

Standards for massage students include

Professionalism

1. Dress professionally for school.

2. Practice good hygiene.

CRITICAL THINKING

We have many professional relationships in our lives, for example, doctors, dentists, lawyers, teachers, school administrators, and more. We also have relationships with service providers such as hairstylists, personal trainers, and car mechanics.

Choose one such person in your life and analyze your relationship with him or her. Write a short essay answering the following questions:

1. What is your role and the other person's role in the relationship?
2. What boundaries can you identify in the relationship?
3. How were those boundaries established? Are they implicit or explicit?
4. How do the established boundaries enhance the relationship? Do you think there are adequate boundaries, or would you feel more comfortable if the boundaries were clearer?

Now, consider your relationship with practice clients. Write out a plan for establishing professional boundaries with them. Include physical, emotional, intellectual, sexual, and energetic boundaries. Continue your essay by answering the following questions:

1. What professional boundaries will you establish as a student of massage with your practice clients?
2. What are some polite but clear methods you can employ to communicate those boundaries effectively?
3. Explain why such boundaries are important to practice now while you are still in training to be a massage therapist.

3. Bring equipment and supplies needed for class.

4. Avoid offensive language and behavior with classmates.

5. Come to class on time and sober.

Class Work

6. Meet or exceed attendance requirements.

7. Put your best efforts into class, homework, and tests.

8. Devote adequate time to study and practice.

9. Present your own work in class, homework, and on tests (do not plagiarize or cheat).

Relationship with Classmates

10. Respect all classmates regardless of gender, ethnic background, religious tradition, sexual orientation, disability, or other distinguishing characteristic.

11. Respect the powerful effects of a relationship based on touch.

12. Refrain from a sexual relationship with a current classmate.

13. Take precautions to prevent the spread of disease in school.

14. Keep personal information about classmates confidential.

15. Practice informed consent with classmates.

Professional Boundaries

16. Change clothes modestly during hands-on classes.

17. Practice proper draping in class.

18. Keep good professional boundaries when practicing on family and friends.

19. Never engage in sexual behavior in the context of practicing massage therapy.

Relationship with the School

20. Treat your teachers and school administrators with respect.

21. Abide by school policies.

22. Represent your school professionally at public events.

23. Take good care of school equipment and use it safely.

The topic of relationships at school is discussed further in Chapter 5, *Ethics and the Therapeutic Relationship*. That discussion expands on the introduction presented in this chapter and includes a detailed list of ethical principles regarding relationships with classmates that promote trust, respect, and harmony.

INTELLECTUAL SKILLS

Massage therapy is performed with the head, heart, and hands. **Intellectual skills**, or thinking skills, play an important part in being a professional massage therapist. From learning about the human body to planning massage sessions to making ethical decisions, the ability to use your head is essential.

Intellectual or cognitive skills can be thought of as having six levels.[5]

Level 1: *Knowledge* of terms, concepts, principles, facts, and methods. At this level the massage therapist can recall or remember things such as the names of bones or different massage techniques.

Level 2: *Comprehension*, in which the massage therapist can reorganize, paraphrase, or explain the material beyond mere recall. For example, the therapist can describe in his or her own words how a synovial joint works, or why a specific massage technique has a certain effect.

Level 3: *Application*, in which knowledge is used in real-life situations. For example, when giving a massage for stress reduction, the massage therapist applies principles learned previously, such as using long flowing strokes and avoiding stimulating techniques such as tapotement.

Level 4: *Analysis*, or breaking down a communication or situation into its parts and identifying specific elements, relationships among parts, patterns, and overall organization. Analysis is an important skill in assessing a problem a client is having or in considering an ethical question.

Level 5: *Synthesis*, or putting the pieces together to create a whole, or arrive at a solution. For example, after an analysis of a problem presented by a client, a massage therapist takes all that he or she knows about massage therapy and creates a session plan to achieve certain goals.

Level 6: *Evaluation*, such as judging to what extent a certain massage application was successful in achieving session goals.

These last three levels (analysis, synthesis, and evaluation) are the foundations of goal-oriented session planning explained in Chapter 9, *Medical Terminology, Goal-Oriented Planning, Documentation*. The six levels of intellectual skills are summarized in Table 3–1 ■.

Higher-Level Thinking

There will be many situations in your career that call for higher-level thinking. Two types of higher-level thinking useful to massage therapists are critical thinking and problem solving, as well as related applications such as planning sessions for clients and making ethical choices. Higher-level thinking involves all six levels of intellectual skills described earlier.

CRITICAL THINKING

Critical thinking helps you get at the truth and avoid being deceived. A childhood learning specialist noted that "Noncritical thinkers accept far too much at face value. They may be more concrete and have trouble looking beneath the surface, analyzing and evaluating that which is more than meets the eye."[6] Noncritical thinkers tend to be naïve and gullible. Be careful though not to go too far and risk becoming cynical, doubting everything and trusting nothing. Asking pertinent questions to discover the truth is a sign of healthy skepticism.

Critical thinking weighs reasons to believe against reasons to doubt. It looks for objective evidence, confirmation of claims, errors, distortions, false information, and exaggerations. It looks beneath the surface for authenticity and honesty. It takes into consideration the thinker's own prejudices and beliefs, which is an exercise in self-reflection.

Critical thinking is bolstered by communicating the thought process to another person. In explaining their thinking, people clarify their ideas and test their logic and conclusions. Listening to others can add information and opinions and provide valuable insights from another perspective.

An example of critical thinking about a product being sold involves a series of questions:

- What are the claims about this product?

- Is there any objective evidence for the claims?

- How good is that evidence?

- Who is presenting the claims, and do they have a personal stake (e.g., monetary interest) in the situation?

- What do others say about this product?

- What is the basis for their thinking?

- Have I used the product, and do the claims ring true, given my experience?

TABLE 3–1	**Six Levels of Intellectual Skills**	
Level	Intellectual Skill	Description
1	Knowledge	Recall or remember terms, concepts, principles, facts, and methods.
2	Comprehension	Reorganize, paraphrase, or explain the material beyond mere recall.
3	Application	Use information in real-life situations.
4	Analysis	Break down a communication or situation into its parts, and identify specific elements, relationships among parts, patterns, and overall organization.
5	Synthesis	Put together the pieces to create a whole, or a solution.
6	Evaluation	Form a judgment; determine the worth, value, or quality.

- Is there anything that might influence my perception of the product, for example, knowledge of similar products or attractive packaging?

- Do I have likes or dislikes, prejudices or beliefs that might influence my evaluation?

- What is the level of risk involved in believing or not believing the claims?

- If I buy the product, how will I benefit from it, and do I really need it?

Critical thinking is important to massage therapists in situations such as spending money on equipment and supplies and deciding whether to believe a claim made for massage or other healing practice. It is useful in choosing continuing education in a particular form of massage therapy and for evaluating a contract for a business partnership. Important issues in the profession call for critical thinking, such as whether to support a certain provision in a licensing law or a position taken by a professional association. Critical thinking is a good habit for a mature professional.

PROBLEM SOLVING

Problem solving in its various forms is a systematic approach to finding a solution to a problem using critical thinking skills. The starting point for problem solving is some issue, question, or dilemma for which there are response options. Time and effort are taken to gather the information needed to make an informed choice or formulate a solution. Gathering information involves listing the facts, soliciting opinions, understanding the history of the situation, and recalling similar situations. Decisions made in similar circumstances, and their results, are important to note. Information gathered is then analyzed and evaluated, and finally a choice or decision is made.

A significant aspect of problem solving is self-reflection as found in critical thinking. Things that may color your thinking, such as fears, prejudices, habits, past experiences, and feelings, are taken into consideration in a conscious way. This is not to negate them, but to put them into the equation with other information. Self-reflection promotes greater objectivity.

Evaluation involves weighing the pros and cons of choices for action, or clarifying the priority of values involved. The conclusion or final choice of action is based on some criteria such as highest values (ethical decisions), legal considerations, good business principles, or meeting client goals (goal-oriented session planning).

Systematic problem solving leads to better decisions because the process helps avoid common pitfalls like jumping to conclusions, narrow thinking, and lack of clarity about reasons for choices. It allows thoughtful consideration of complex situations. Critical thinking and problem-solving skills are summarized in Table 3–2 ■.

The basic elements of problem solving are found in its specific applications. For example, goal-oriented session planning described in Chapter 9, *Medical Terminology, Goal-Oriented Planning, Documentation*, and ethical decision making described in Chapter 5, *Ethics and the Therapeutic Relationship*, are variations on the basic process of problem solving.

Concentration

Concentration is the ability to sustain attention on something for a period of time. *Attention span* is the length of time a person can concentrate before becoming distracted. Concentration is a mental skill that can be developed with practice.

The ability to concentrate is important to massage therapists for several reasons. For students, it makes learning easier and attending classes more productive. You can hear what the teacher is saying in class, pay attention to details, and make connections between facts and concepts. You can attain a greater depth of understanding.

TABLE 3–2	Higher-Level Thinking Skills Used in Massage Therapy
Critical Thinking	<ul><li>Process for discovering the truth and avoiding deception.</li><li>Weigh reasons to believe against reasons to doubt.</li><li>Look for objective evidence, confirmation of claims, errors, distortions, false information, and exaggerations.</li><li>Look beneath the surface for authenticity and honesty.</li><li>Take into consideration the thinker's own prejudices and beliefs, which is an exercise in self-reflection.</li></ul>
Problem Solving	<ul><li>Systematic approach to finding a solution to a problem using critical thinking skills.</li><li>Starting point is an issue, question, or dilemma for which there are choices for responding.</li><li>Information needed to make an informed choice or formulate a solution is gathered.</li><li>List the facts, solicit opinions, understand the history of the situation, and recall similar situations.</li><li>Information gathered is analyzed and evaluated, and finally a choice or decision is made.</li><li>Solution based on some criteria such as highest values (ethical decisions), legal considerations, good business principles, or meeting client goals (goal-oriented session planning).</li></ul>

Massage therapists are more present while talking to clients and during massage sessions if they focus their attention. An aware client can feel when the massage therapist's mind is wandering, much the same way you can tell if someone in front of you is not listening to what you are saying. A wandering mind interferes with the essential connection or presence with a client.

Details also tend to get lost if the mind is jumping from one thing to another. For example, it takes time to absorb sensations from your hands and interpret them as you perform massage techniques. If your mind is not present, even if your hands are working, a lot of information will be lost.

Letting the mind wander in activities such as daydreaming, ruminating about the past, worrying, or looking forward to a future event are barriers to good concentration. Being easily distracted by sights and sounds in the environment shortens the attention span. The mind goes off somewhere and is not paying attention to the task at hand.

IMPROVING CONCENTRATION

Concentration can be improved through minimizing attention disruptors, single-tasking, creating a more distraction-free environment, and practicing focusing the mind through meditation techniques.

Stressful situations, lack of sleep, illness, and overuse of stimulants such as caffeine can temporarily disrupt the ability to concentrate. Conversely, relaxation techniques, getting enough sleep, taking care of health problems, and proper nutrition improve the ability to concentrate. Recreation activities and light entertainment can offer a break from work, helping to calm and focus the mind. As mentioned previously, massage itself is known to improve mental alertness and focused attention.

Single-tasking, or doing one thing at a time, is a prerequisite for concentration. Its antithesis, *multitasking,* or doing more than one thing at a time, is a modern stress producer. Watching television while trying to study, reading email while on the phone, and planning a grocery list in your mind while doing massage, are examples of multitasking. The quality of one or both activities suffers as a result of split attention. Single-tasking is a practice in concentration.

Simple uncluttered space minimizes visual distracters. Silence, "white noise," or quiet background music also help concentration. Students can cut down distracters by sitting in the front of the classroom and eliminating behavior such as eating and drinking, doodling, and talking during class time. Electronic devices are perhaps the biggest distracters of modern times. During periods of concentration, turn off all electronic appliances such as cell phones, pagers, and personal digital assistants. Being constantly interrupted breaks concentration.

Massage therapists create distraction-free environments for themselves and their clients. Dim lights, soft music, and minimal talking allow concentration on the massage itself. Using meditation to increase your powers of concentration is discussed in Chapter 4, *Physical Skills, Fitness, Self-Care for the Massage Therapist.*

INTUITION

Intuition is defined as "a direct perception of the truth, independent of any rational process . . . [it] lets us see and respond to our environment without calling rational problem-solving into play. There is an organic knowing at work." Intuition is related to *instinct,* which has been called "the hardware of intuition."[7] Our instincts help guide us through complex situations without having to stop and think everything through.

Instincts come in handy when we are faced with unfamiliar situations, don't have all the facts, or have to act quickly. "Trust your instincts" is good advice when safety is involved. The terms *common sense* and *horse sense* have this same connotation (i.e., knowing through an inner voice). Intuition is like a sixth sense. People with developed intuition can sense things, or have hunches about things they cannot fully explain.

Intuition has its place in the practice of massage therapy. Massage therapists who work intuitively are not thinking through every move they make. Their hands "know" where to go and what to do. These are called *intelligent hands,* as if the hands themselves were doing the work disconnected from the brain.

Of course, just because the brain is not consciously thinking doesn't mean it is not involved. All the stored knowledge and experience are available in the brain and working on an unconscious level as skills are performed. If something doesn't seem right according to intuition, the thinking brain becomes engaged to do rational problem solving as the situation requires.

A case can be made for the value of adding intuition to the massage therapist's tool chest of knowledge and skills. Intuition is developed by quieting the mind and letting go of conscious thinking. When a student is first learning massage techniques, he or she thinks about every move, but after a while and with practice, the mind can loosen its grip and intuition be given more rein. Such a massage is felt by the receiver as smooth and effortless.

EMOTIONAL INTELLIGENCE

Emotional intelligence is the "heart" in the familiar triumvirate—head, heart, and hands. Emotional skills work hand in hand with intellectual and physical skills for full maturity as a massage therapy professional.

Neuroscientists are exploring the complex connections between the limbic structures of the brain, which are the seat of emotions, and the neocortex, or thinking brain. It turns out that rather than being totally independent, these two "minds" interact continuously. The head and heart work together for best results:

In a sense we have two brains, two minds—and two different kinds of intelligence: rational and emotional. How we do in life is determined by both. . . . Indeed, intellect cannot work its best without emotional intelligence. . . . The new paradigm urges us to harmonize head and heart.[8]

Emotional intelligence is defined in Goleman[9] by a set of skills related to five domains:

1. Knowing one's emotions

2. Managing emotions

3. Motivating oneself

4. Recognizing emotions in others

5. Handling relationships

Emotional skills are important in laying the foundation for success, for example, maintaining a positive outlook, building healthy relationships with clients, dealing with conflict, and making good decisions. They are essential for success in school and building thriving practices afterward.

Like mental IQ, everyone is born with brain circuitry that provides a starting point for emotional intelligence. And like thinking skills, emotional skills are first learned in childhood and developed throughout a lifetime.

Self-Awareness

The keystone of emotional intelligence is self-awareness, that is, recognizing a feeling as it happens and its accompanying emotion or impulse to act. Understanding the difference between a feeling and an emotion is a good starting point for self-awareness.

Although these are often equated, there is a subtle difference between *feelings* and *emotions*. The verb *feel* comes from an old English word related to sensation and perception, whereas *emotion* comes from an old French word related to movement and behavior. "Emotions are the outward expressions we use to either display or disguise an underlying feeling, matching or masking our inner state."[10] People described as *emotional* freely display their feelings outwardly.

There is no agreement about which emotions are primary. However, some common emotions and their variations can be identified: enjoyment (happiness, joy, amusement, sensual pleasure, satisfaction); love (friendliness, kindness, devotion, adoration, infatuation, selfless love or *agape*); surprise (shock, astonishment, amazement, wonder); anger (outrage, resentment, annoyance, irritability, hatred, violence); sadness (grief, sorrow, loneliness, self-pity, depression); fear (anxiety, nervousness, dread, fright, phobia, panic); disgust (contempt, disdain, scorn, aversion, revulsion); shame (guilt, embarrassment, remorse, humiliation, regret, contrition). Figure 3–2 ■ depicts the broad range of emotions of which humans are capable.

Temperament is a term for a person's basic disposition, or tendency toward certain moods or emotions. Extremes of temperament can be a negative factor in being a massage therapist. For example, being excessively shy or sad can interfere with developing a practice. Being excessively bold can result in poor judgment about behavior toward clients. Recognizing our basic temperament and learning to improve aspects that interfere with our life and work is part of developing emotional intelligence. An added incentive to become more self-aware is that the more we understand ourselves, the more we'll understand and have empathy for clients.

Naming our moods and emotions is an empowering step. Naming requires the ability to pause and look at emotion from the thinking brain. Humans have a unique capability of self-reflection that allows us to look at ourselves with some outside perspective. This provides the separation necessary to recognize the difference between emotions and our reactions to them. Naming emotions lays the foundation for identifying their causes and learning to manage them.

Managing Emotions

Once there is self-awareness, managing emotions becomes possible. Managing emotions involves learning to handle emotions so they are healthy expressions of our feelings and appropriate for the setting. This means recognizing them and responding in ways that benefit self and others. A balance must be struck between suppressing emotions and letting them get out of control.

Two examples of managing emotions related to being a massage therapist are dealing with annoyance with a client and continuing to work while feeling sad about a recent loss. In the first instance, being direct with the client about the cause of annoyance (e.g., habitual lateness) is appropriate, whereas allowing feelings of anger to fester is not. In the second instance, something simple like having fresh flowers

Enjoyment	Love	Compassion	Surprise	Sadness	Fear	Disgust	Shame	Anger
Happiness	Friendliness	Empathy	Shock	Grief	Anxiety	Contempt	Guilt	Outrage
Joy	Kindness	Sympathy	Astonishment	Sorrow	Nervousness	Disdain	Embarrassment	Resentment
Amusement	Devotion	Pity	Amazement	Loneliness	Dread	Scorn	Remorse	Annoyance
Sensual Pleasure	Adoration		Wonder	Self-Pity	Fright	Aversion	Humiliation	Irritability
	Infatuation				Phobia	Revulsion	Regret	Hatred
Satisfaction	Selfless Love				Panic		Contrition	

FIGURE 3–2 The broad range of human emotions.

in the room may cheer you up, whereas ruminating about your situation would not help.

A basic aspect of managing emotions is controlling impulses. Emotion is by definition an impulse to action. Being overcome with emotion can short-circuit the rational brain, leading to actions regretted later. Anger management is an example of learning impulse control. Strategies include walking away, counting to 10 before reacting, and taking a cooling-off period. Chronic anxiety may be managed by learning relaxation and mind-calming techniques.

Delayed gratification is also possible when a person has impulse control. That means resisting an impulse today for a greater reward at a later date. The ability to delay gratification is a sign of maturity and makes many things possible, such as staying with an exercise routine, studying for classes, saving money for a new massage table, or responding ethically to a client.

Motivating Yourself

Two useful skills for self-motivation are nurturing an optimistic outlook and learning to get into the flow of peak performance. Taking responsibility for cultivating these abilities is part of emotional intelligence.

Optimism is a known contributor to success in school, sports, and even healing. Being optimistic means expecting that things will turn out all right in the end, despite setbacks and difficulties. An optimistic attitude helps a person persevere when the going gets rough. Being pessimistic, or expecting failure, leads to giving up when there are bumps in the road.

Optimism may be part of inborn temperament; however, a positive outlook can be nurtured. It is related to what psychologists call *self-efficacy,* the belief that you have the skills to meet the challenges you will face. A sense of self-efficacy can be nurtured by challenging yourself within your current abilities and building on those abilities by making the challenges progressively more advanced. Once a person knows this principle, he or she can work on developing a sense of self-efficacy and, therefore, a sense of optimism.

Flow, or being in the *zone,* refers to a state of complete harmony during peak performance. There is a fluidity, sense of ease, and mastery that makes the performance a joyful experience. Performers get lost in the action as they become totally absorbed in what they are doing. Flow is a state that can be accessed. It involves quieting and focusing the mind on the task at hand and experiencing the sheer joy of the activity. It occurs most easily when the activity is challenging, but not too hard. Flow can be experienced in learning something new, practicing a skill, or during a challenge such as a test. Flow is thwarted by worry, boredom, or too much thinking.

Recognizing Emotions in Others

Empathy, or recognizing emotions in others, is an important social skill for massage therapists. It is essential for good communications with clients and developing effective therapeutic relationships. It is the basis for creating rapport and is the root of caring.

The ability to read someone else's emotions is based primarily on nonverbal cues. It means noticing things such as tone of voice, facial expression, and gestures and then matching emotions accurately to what is observed. Reading emotions can be very subtle, that is, interpreting *how* things are said, not just the words that are said. For example, a person with empathy can detect underlying sadness, anger, or anxiety in a client's words or actions. Empathy is emotional attunement with clients.

Empathy does not mean taking on someone else's pain as your own. It differs from *sympathy,* which is defined as a relationship in which whatever affects one person correspondingly affects the other, and *pity,* which is feeling sorrow for someone else's misfortune. Sympathy and pity result from a lack of emotional boundaries with others and can lead to burnout for practitioners in the caring professions.

Compassion takes empathy one step further. **Compassion** is the "deep awareness of the suffering of another coupled with the wish to relieve it."[11] Compassion combines empathy with a dedication to service to others. Compassion within the context of the massage therapy profession means the wish to relieve the suffering of others with the work of our hands.

Handling Relationships

The fifth domain of emotional intelligence is handling interpersonal relationships. The fundamental relationship between a massage therapist and client is called the *therapeutic relationship.* Elements of a healthy therapeutic relationship include clarity about the nature of the relationship, understanding of individual roles within the relationship, and establishing clear boundaries related to roles.

For the massage therapist, it means taking responsibility for the relationship and being honest, trustworthy, and ethical. For the client, it involves confidence in the therapist's abilities, trust and respect for the therapist, and satisfaction with the service provided. The massage therapist takes the lead in resolving conflict, responding to a client's anxiety or anger, and keeping good professional boundaries.

Examples of situations calling for skill in interpersonal relationships include resolving a misunderstanding about a cancellation policy, counseling a client with a body odor problem, or showing concern for a grieving client. Massage therapists might also have to respond to clients who use offensive language, come for massage under the influence of alcohol, or make romantic or sexual advances. The therapeutic relationship is discussed further in Chapter 5, *Ethics and the Therapeutic Relationship.*

SOCIAL SKILLS

Massage therapy practices are built and maintained on a foundation of good social skills, resulting in successful relationships. These include relationships with clients, other health professionals, and people encountered in a place of employment or while managing a private practice. Massage therapy is a person-to-person profession, and even the most skillful massage techniques cannot make up for poor people skills. Social skills are essential abilities for massage therapists.

Social skills encompass behaviors between people that promote harmony, understanding, and connection, while peacefully solving problems like disagreements, misunderstandings, and reconciliation after harm has been done. The primary goal of social skills is building good relationships. The social skills described in this chapter are specific to massage therapists and the situations they encounter daily.

Courtesy and Good Manners

Courtesy and good manners are behaviors that are expected in social situations, such as saying "please" and "thank you," listening when someone is speaking to you, and introducing newcomers to a group. Courteous behavior shows respect for others and exhibits thoughtfulness about their feelings, comfort, and safety. It is essential for client satisfaction and good customer service.

The unwritten rules of good manners vary in different societies and in specific situations, and they change over time. Today, good manners include turning off audible signals on cell phones and other electronic devices in places where silence is appreciated, such as theaters, classrooms, and massage rooms. Good manners also include not having personal conversations on the phone, checking email, or "texting" when clients are present.

Good manners in school show respect for teachers, classmates, and yourself. Disturbing class by talking when the teacher is talking, eating during class, letting a cell phone ring, fidgeting, and leaving a mess where you were working are examples of bad manners in school.

Courteous, respectful language goes along with good manners. Use of offensive slang, crude sayings, and angry or demeaning words are especially out of place in school and professional settings.

Whereas good manners open the door to good professional relationships, bad manners can slam the door shut. People have certain expectations about how they will be treated, and showing disrespect can evoke feelings of anger, disappointment, or annoyance. Having good manners is a sign of emotional intelligence and thoughtfulness.

Because what is considered good manners varies by culture and changes over time, professionals working in diverse environments become very aware of their behavior toward others. Business is particularly sensitive to this as it expands into a global marketplace. Professionals remain aware and flexible, adapting to times and circumstances to support building good relationships.

Courtesy and good manners can become second nature, but awareness and practice are prerequisites. Many of the social and professional skills described in this chapter are considered good manners and are expected of trained professionals.

First Impressions

It is a truism that you only get one chance to make a first impression. When you greet clients, potential employers, and others for the first time, they get an immediate impression of your professionalism.

Whenever we walk into a room, our clothing, manners, and mannerisms are on display. Others assess our self-confidence and our ability to present ourselves based on 60 seconds of information. Each of us has our own signature of professional presence—an indelible statement that we make the instant we show up.[12]

Because massage therapy is based on touch and close contact, it is especially important to establish good rapport right away, as well as confidence, trust, and a certain comfort level. In addition to projecting a professional image as described earlier in this chapter, the manner of greeting is also part of a first impression.

Greeting a First-Time Client

The elements of greeting a client are to make eye contact, say the person's name, introduce yourself, shake hands, and give further directions. In the therapeutic relationship, the massage therapist is in charge, so it is her or his responsibility to take the initiative in greeting and helping the client feel comfortable.

Ten minutes before a client is expected, check your dress and grooming. Clean and organize your office space to make sure it projects a professional image. Review the available client information. If possible, greet the client in a reception area.

When the client arrives, stand up, make friendly eye contact, and smile. Really look at the person to gauge his or her state of being and comfort level. Does the individual seem happy or sad, in pain, nervous, shy, or tired? Your assessment of the client for planning the massage session starts now. Then say the client's name to continue to make a connection and introduce yourself. Say, for example, "Hello Dennis, my name is Debra and I will be your massage therapist today." You would have learned the client's name from checking the appointment book. Now shake hands, and invite the client to sit down (Figure 3–3 ■). All this takes place in a matter of seconds.

The handshake is the first time you touch your client, so it is especially important in establishing good rapport. Try not to reach over a barrier, like a desk or counter, when you shake hands. Extend your hand to the client first. Meet the client's grip palm to palm with good-quality contact as you would during the massage. Squeeze firmly, but not too hard, for about 3 seconds and then release the hand. A general rule is to meet the other person's force, and squeeze more gently if the person is weak or injured.

Avoid the "bone crusher," "limp noodle," and "two-finger wiggle" handshake styles. Variations of the handshake include the "handshake sandwich" with your two

FIGURE 3–3 Greet a first-time client with a firm handshake.

Source: Pearson Education, Inc.

hands around the client's one hand, which may be perceived as overpowering or patronizing; and the handshake with the left hand on the other person's forearm or shoulder, which is more intimate. Do not use these variations, or perhaps use them only later in the relationship as a comforting gesture in special circumstances. If a person is missing the right hand, or has a prosthetic arm, extend your left hand instead. The handshake should not feel rushed, but also should not linger too long, suggesting familiarity.

Hugs are a gesture used frequently in American society and may be appropriate in certain situations. However, when establishing professional boundaries, the handshake is a clearer statement of the business nature of the relationship and is safer for first-time clients. Use your judgment about hugs before or after subsequent appointments. Do not feel that you must hug a client to appear friendly or caring. Hug only if you have clear professional boundaries with a particular client, if you want to express particular affection for some specific reason, if it is acceptable to the client, and if it fits your personality. Remember that hugs may seem invasive to certain clients.

There are cultural differences in what is considered acceptable for greetings. For example, in some Asian and Middle Eastern countries, direct eye contact shows disrespect. Or touching at any time outside the massage may seem too intimate. These are judgment calls that will become easier with more awareness and experience.

After the handshake, a client needs direction about what to do next. It could be, "Please sit down while we go over your goals for the session," or "Let's take a moment to go over your health history," or whatever you would like the client to do next. Be clear in your direction when pointing to a chair, or leading the client to the massage room. Clients receiving massage for the first time will need more guidance and assurance.

Introductions

Making introductions is a basic social skill used during the regular business day and at meetings or conferences. Introductions help people feel comfortable and welcome, as well as transmit useful social information. They are an essential networking tool.

The golden rule of introductions is to mention the name of the most honored person first. Other considerations are rank, gender, and age. If people are of equal rank, the woman's name is mentioned first. In a professional practice, the client is always the most honored person, but in other situations, determining the most honored is a judgment call.

The first person's name is followed by a phrase like, "I'd like you to meet [second person's name]," or simply, "This is [second person's name]." If possible, follow up the second person's name with a comment containing information about one or the other person. Ideally the comment would be something to further identify a person, or acknowledge his or her relationship to the situation. Say, for example, "John is a massage therapist at the Marian Hospital Integrative Health Care Center," or "Deidre works with me at the Rejuvenation Spa in Centerville," or "Kristin is going to the workshop on sports massage next month." This opens the door to further conversation and a sense of connection.

Here are some examples of brief introductions:

"Mary, I'd like you to meet Bill. Bill has a massage therapy practice in Milwaukee specializing in orthopedic massage. Mary is in from Minneapolis."

"Dr. Hernandez, this is Jerry Black, a massage therapist. Jerry has a question about a possible contraindication for one of his clients. Would you mind talking to him about it?"

"Dylan Smith, I'd like you to meet Reuben Jones. You two have something in common as fellow reflexologists."

Name tags that are worn prominently and can be read clearly are valuable social devices. Wear yours so that others can readily identify you, call you by name, and introduce you to other people more easily. If you work in a clinic or spa with other employees, a name tag identifies you to clients. Name tags worn at conferences facilitate networking.

There are times when introductions are not necessary. For example, if other massage therapists or clients are in the reception area, you would not ordinarily be expected to introduce everyone to everyone else as you would in a social situation. Your business is with your client, and no other introductions are expected.

Conflict Resolution

Conflicts can arise in any relationship. Conflicts occur when personalities or styles clash, or when people trying to work together have different goals or expectations. Differences of perception, belief, opinion, values, or understanding of facts can cause strife and disharmony. Conflicts often manifest as arguments, disappointment, anger, annoyance, or frustration. They involve two or more people at odds with one another.

Conflict resolution means resolving conflicts amicably and begins with a conscious desire to do so. It involves setting aside competitiveness and the need to win, and focusing on goals rather than obstacles. Five basic approaches to dealing with conflict are the following:[13]

1. *Collaboration*—Taking the time to find a solution together is the way to go when building a long-term relationship, when goals are too important for compromise, or when you need to work together for the greater good.

2. *Force*—Demanding that your way be followed is only acceptable in an emergency, when the stakes are high and the relationship nonessential, or when a higher principle is at stake and you have the power to enforce your will.

3. *Avoidance*—Not acknowledging a conflict is risky because unresolved conflicts seem to grow worse rather than go away. Avoidance may be all right if it is a temporary situation, and the issue is minor.

4. *Accommodation*—Letting the other person have his or her way is best when keeping harmony in the relationship is most important, when the issue is more important to the other person than to you, when you cannot win, or when you realize that you are wrong.

5. *Compromise*—Both people adjusting their original positions works best when a quick resolution is the goal, when the problem is temporary, or when a complete solution is impossible after much negotiation.

The approach that is most appropriate for a given situation depends on the importance of two factors: (1) Concern for others versus concern for your own needs and desires, and (2) importance of the relationship. Box 3–1 ■ explains when each approach is most appropriate.

BOX 3–1	Choosing the Best Conflict Resolution Approach	

Method of Conflict Resolution	Relationship Importance	Need or Desire to Win
Collaborate	Very High	Equal
Accommodate	Very High	Low
Compromise	High	Moderate
Avoid	Low	Low
Force	Low	High

Special Situation	Method
When building long-term relationships:	Collaborate
When you need their support to reach goals:	Collaborate
When harmony is more important than the issue:	Accommodate
When you realize you are wrong:	Accommodate
When you cannot win:	Accommodate
When time is short:	Compromise
When an issue has low importance:	Compromise
When the conflict is a one-time thing:	Avoid
When the conflict is trivial:	Avoid
When you need to act fast in an emergency:	Force
When the issue is ethical or legal:	Force

Minor conflicts occur all the time in therapeutic relationships with clients. Because the relationship is of such high importance, accommodation and collaboration are the usual modes of resolution, followed in order by compromise, avoidance, and force. Force would rarely be used and only in cases of emergency.

An example of a midlevel conflict is a client who misses an appointment once and does not want to pay the cancellation fee. If keeping the client is important, then accommodation may be the answer; that is, waiving the fee for this time. Avoidance, or not bringing the issue up, is a bad idea because it does not call attention to the policy, and the client may think that it is unimportant. If the client misses again, then the stakes are higher, and you might want to insist on charging the cancellation fee.

Another example is a conflict with a fellow massage therapist who shares a massage room with you at a clinic. She always leaves the massage room messy, and you have to come along afterward and clean up before your client arrives. Given that the relationship and your needs are both important, as well as the principle of the situation, your best choice is an attempt at collaboration. That would involve confronting the other person with the facts as you see them and asking her to be more conscientious about cleaning up. You may be surprised to find out that she thought other workers at the spa or clinic were supposed to clean up, or maybe she has to rush out to another job and forgets about cleaning up. Collaboration involves listening and coming to agreement on a solution.

Major conflicts are uncommon but do happen occasionally. There may also be ethical situations such as a client who wants to date you, or expects treatment outside your scope of practice, or asks for sexual favors. For this type of conflict, insistence on ethical behavior is the only way to go.

Tips for successful conflict resolution include the following:

• Being respectful in language and demeanor

• Keeping a positive attitude

• Looking for the win–win situation

• Finding a way for everyone to save face

• Staying open to options

• Being a good listener

• Finding common goals

Resolution barriers are the following:

• Needing to win

• Taking things personally

• Letting hostility fester

• Giving orders

Phrases such as "you must," "you should," and "you have to" are sure to rankle the other person. Remember that conflicts

CASE FOR STUDY

Elise and a Conflict in Appointment Times

Elise has a steady client who recently changed jobs and is now on a different schedule. The times he prefers for massage appointments are now outside Elise's regular hours. She sees clients from 10:00AM–4:00PM on Tuesday–Saturday. Elise would like to keep the client, but needs to resolve this conflict in their schedules.

Question:
Can Elise find a satisfactory appointment time for this steady client?

Things to consider:
- How important is it for Elise to continue with this client?
- How much outside her regular hours would the new appointment time have to be?
- Does he have time for appointments outside his "preferred" times?

- How flexible is he willing to be?
- How firm do her work hours need to be?
- Does she have family or other obligations that limit her availability?
- How willing is each person to compromise? Accommodate the other? Collaborate to find a solution?
- Is there a point at which dissolving the relationship is the only option?

Write examples of different scenarios for resolving this conflict.

1. **Accommodation:** _____
   _____

2. **Compromise:** _____
   _____

3. **Collaboration:** _____
   _____

---

are inevitable among people working together. Approach conflict resolution as an opportunity to practice your social skills rather than as a chore to be avoided.

COMMUNICATION SKILLS

Communication skills facilitate information exchange between people, and include verbal (i.e., speech and writing) and nonverbal (i.e., body language and facial expression) methods. Good communication avoids misunderstanding, confusion, and lack of clarity that can produce social friction. Social and communication skills are polished through awareness, learning, experience, and practice.

Verbal Skills

Speech or verbal communication is the primary medium of delivery during telephone calls and for important tasks such as greeting and interviewing clients, explaining policies and procedures, networking with other health professionals, and giving presentations. The delivery of the spoken word in verbal communication can sometimes be more important than the content. It is estimated that in a spoken message, body language accounts for 55% of the communication, voice for 38%, and the words for 7%.[14]

A good general rule is to speak with moderate speed in a calm, steady, strong voice. Vary the energy, rhythm, and inflection to make the delivery more interesting. Articulate clearly and avoid mumbling. Try to modulate accents unfamiliar to listeners.

Talk more slowly to people who have a different native language than the one you are speaking. Learn a few key words in the language of your regular clients; for example, words for *hello, pressure, pain, turn over,* and *good-bye.* If speaking a language that is not your own, be more conscious of using your voice quality, hand gestures, and body language to clarify your meaning.

When speaking to persons with hearing challenges, face them directly so they can read your lips. Speak slowly with good articulation, but do not exaggerate your words. Turn up the volume on your speech a little, but do not shout, especially to a person wearing a hearing aid. Learn some sign language if you work in a situation where you have regular clients who are hearing impaired.

Voice quality is also important. Lower-pitched voices sound more confident and competent. Avoid seeming harsh or being overly loud or soft. Be aware that your tone of voice can type you; for example, a whining, nasal voice sounds like a complainer; a high-pitched, quavering voice sounds nervous; a breathy, slow voice sounds seductive. To add volume and richness to your voice, breathe deeply and relax your neck muscles and vocal cords. Your voice should come from the diaphragm rather than the throat.[15]

Poor speech habits include using sounds like "uh" as space fillers, constantly clearing the throat, pausing too long between words, and speaking too fast. Ending sentences with a high inflection, as in asking a question, sounds uncertain and unconfident.

Avoid street slang and use good grammar. Call adult females "women" and adult males "men." Do not use terms of familiarity such as "sweetie," "dear," "doll," or "dude" when talking to clients. Also avoid overly formal language and use of technical terms that clients might not understand. It is not appropriate to "show off" by using anatomical terms unfamiliar to the general public. For example, the term *thigh* will do just as well as *femur* in most cases. Using anatomical terms when educating the client about what you are doing is acceptable if done in moderation and the client is able to understand what you are saying.

Speech is a product of experience and habit and can be improved with practice. Become aware of your speech and develop speaking habits that enhance your verbal communications with clients and other social contacts.

TELEPHONE USE

Telephones and answering machines are essential communication tools for massage therapy practices. Clients usually call via telephone for their first appointments, so it is important to have good phone skills. Use the good speech habits as described earlier in this chapter.

REALITY CHECK

MARIA

DAVID: I'm really shy around strangers and don't have a lot of confidence in my social skills. I never seem to know what to say. I'd rather just do the massage and not have to talk to anyone. How can I learn to relate professionally to clients when I don't know where to start?

MARIA: What you say and how you treat clients sets the stage for the massage experience itself. It won't matter how good your massage skills are if you don't have good people skills. Acknowledging your current limitations is a good first step. That's self-awareness. Now try observing people you think have the confidence and social skills you want to develop. What is it exactly that gives them that image? Notice their body language and the actual words that they use. Develop a professional persona in your mind's eye—the person you want to be. Try using that persona when you're in the role of massage therapist—like playing a part in a drama. Ask a friend to role-play meeting new clients with you to practice being your professional self. Remember that you are not being someone different from who you are. You are just being yourself in your new professional role.

Chances are that in private practice, a prospective client's first encounter with you will be via an answering machine. Script your answering machine message to be clear and concise. For example: "Hello. You have reached Green Fields Massage Therapy. I am unable to take your call at this time. Please leave a short message including your name and telephone number, and I will return your call as soon as possible. Please wait for the beep to record your message." Rerecord your message until you are satisfied that it sounds open, inviting, and professional.

When answering your telephone, visualize a prospective client at the other end. In other words, be friendly and relaxed (Figure 3–4 ■). If you feel hurried or stressed, pause and take a deep breath to calm yourself down before you answer. Identify yourself right away. For example: "Hello. This is Thomas Alter of Green Fields Massage Therapy. How may I help you?"

Here are some other tips for telephone use:

- Have a phone line dedicated to your practice.

- Do not make client calls on a cell phone while driving or in public places.

- Do not accept other incoming calls (e.g., call waiting) when on the phone for business.

- Turn off ringers and cell phones when in a massage session.

- Do not interrupt a massage session to answer a phone call.

- Avoid distractions or multitasking while on the phone.

- Smile while on the phone. It can project a friendly impression.

Return calls promptly within 24 hours, if possible. If you will be unavailable to return calls for more than a day, change your message to alert callers when you will return their calls. This shows that you are reachable and reliable.

Body Language

Body language speaks volumes. Your posture, how close you stand to others, hand gestures, eye contact, and facial expression communicate your mood, interest, and even respect for a person you are talking to. As a massage therapist, knowing some of the common meanings of body language can help you project the meaning that you want and also understand others better.

Good upright, aligned posture commands respect and confidence. On the other hand, slouching, tilting, looking around, and a drooping head can communicate disinterest, evasion, or boredom.

The comfortable distance between people who are talking varies somewhat with culture. Be aware of your own comfort level and how it might differ from a client's preferred distance. Moving closer can indicate an interest in

FIGURE 3–4
Be friendly and relaxed when talking on the phone to clients.

Source: Pearson Education, Inc.

the subject, friendliness, or just difficulty hearing. Moving uncomfortably close is a type of physical boundary violation.

Arms crossed in front convey a sense of protection or distancing, whereas arms uncrossed and relaxed convey openness. Legs crossed can project the same sense as crossed arms. Hands on the hips signal impatience or anger. Fidgeting or habits such as tapping a pencil or doodling project boredom, nervousness, or distraction.

Hand gestures are particularly communicative. In some cultures people seem to "talk with their hands" as they accentuate the meaning of their words with gestures. Putting a hand over the heart area or placing a hand lightly on another person's arm expresses sympathy and is a way of "reaching out" or making a connection. On the other hand, putting a hand out in front with palm facing the other person implies "stop" or "wait a minute." A common gesture to avoid is finger pointing, which seems accusatory and scolding.

Eye contact is extremely important. Looking at someone when you are speaking or being spoken to makes an essential connection. Knowing when to break eye contact is also important. Staring, looking too intently or too long, can be uncomfortable to a recipient. Break eye contact every so often and then come back. Looking away or around the room when someone is speaking to you is taken as a sign of disrespect or dismissal.

The eyes can also communicate such things as friendliness, concern, annoyance, anger, pleasure, confusion, questioning, flirting, and seduction. Eyes communicate best along with other aspects of facial expression. The massage therapist in Figure 3–5 ■ displays openness to the client through body language and a friendly smile. Having an expression that is hard to decipher, the so-called poker face, might be useful in some circumstances, but tends to make people distrustful and uncomfortable.

The smile is perhaps the most universally recognizable sign of friendliness. A warm smile when greeting someone is welcoming. But beware—a genuine smile is hard to fake.

Remember that body language is only one piece of the communication puzzle. It is part of the whole communication package, along with facial expression, voice quality, words,

FIGURE 3–5
Relaxed posture and a friendly smile communicate an open and welcoming attitude toward clients.

Source: Pearson Education, Inc.

PRACTICAL APPLICATION

Situations in which the words, voice quality, and body language are not in sync can lead to miscommunication. When this happens, one or both parties may feel uncomfortable, misunderstand what is being communicated, or even look for a way to end the conversation. This awkward, out-of-sync interaction is the kind of communication you want to avoid having with your massage clients.

With a study partner, role-play situations in which what is intended to be communicated does not match the voice quality, inflection, or body language used. For example, try greeting a client with arms folded and frowning. Next, try playing a client who claims to feel fine and have no pain, while the body language clearly portrays discomfort, pain, or unease. Then correct the out-of-sync elements to communicate your message clearly. Switch roles with your partner a few times and be creative.

For a variation, try role-playing using different types of eye contact. Include not looking at the other person, staring too long without a break, or looking around the room. Switch roles.

1. What can you learn about a client from voice quality and body language? Can you learn even more than his or her words alone convey?
2. What messages might you inadvertently communicate to a client through your body language? How might you ensure that your communication is clear?
3. What degree of eye contact is the most comfortable? What does your study partner communicate by having little or no eye contact with you when you are conversing?

and the general situation. People's personal habits (e.g., they might always fold their arms) must also be taken into consideration. The better you know someone, the easier it is to "read" him or her. Piece all the parts together to understand the full meaning being projected by a person's body language.

Listening

Listening involves taking in and trying to understand what someone else is communicating to you. "I hear you" is a familiar expression that means "I understand (or empathize with) what you just said."

Listening is an essential communication skill for building relationships, discussing important issues, planning massage sessions, solving problems, resolving conflicts, and negotiating contracts. It also plays a big part in learning and critical thinking. Listening allows you to gather information, understand others better, and take in new ideas. Being a good listener begins with the intention to hear what others are really saying and overcoming poor listening habits.

Poor listening habits include letting the mind wander and formulating replies while others are speaking. Other bad habits are interrupting speakers, tuning out different points of view, jumping to conclusions, finishing people's sentences for them, and talking while others are speaking. People also tend to hear what they want to hear and tune out what they don't want to deal with. Do not try to talk over environmental noise such as street sounds or music playing in the background. Background noise interferes with hearing someone else's words.

Really listening involves focusing on what a speaker is saying (the words), feeling, and meaning. Know that people sometimes have trouble expressing in words what they mean. The Chinese character for *listen* consists of four characters: the heart, the mind, the ears, and the eyes.[16]

When "listening" for feelings, pay attention to how the words are said, that is, inflection and voice quality. Watch body language and facial expressions as well. Listening for feelings is important for developing *empathy,* or recognizing emotions in others, as discussed earlier in this chapter in the section on emotional intelligence.

Listening for the context is also important for understanding what someone is really trying to say. Getting the full picture helps you respond appropriately. Listen for what is not being said, and ask questions to "fill in the blanks." Summarize what you think you heard, and check out your accuracy. This is an important interviewing skill, as discussed later in this chapter.

AFFIRMATIVE LISTENING

This type of listening involves letting the speaker know that you are paying attention. This is accomplished by occasional verbal cues and body language. These affirming cues by the listener include nodding, saying "uh-huh" or "I see" or "yes," and repeating a word or key phrase or idea. Body language such as leaning slightly forward toward the speaker and orienting your body to face the speaker also indicates attention. Eye contact, too, is important.[17]

Affirmative listening allows someone to say all that they have to say without interruption. However, active listening is better for promoting true understanding of someone's ideas and feelings and is an important communication skill for massage therapists.

ACTIVE LISTENING

Active listeners become more engaged in the communication process by reflecting back to the speaker what they think was said. This is not done by parroting the words exactly, but by paraphrasing or restating the words to clarify their meaning. Reflective listening is useful because "by paraphrasing their views, you give talkers a chance to reflect on what they just said, to make sure that's what they mean, maybe even to change what they think or feel after hearing it again."[18]

These lead-in phrases are useful for active listening:

"You seem to be saying . . ."

"If I understand you correctly, you're saying . . ."

"Let me see if I get where you're coming from. You think that . . ."

"Am I hearing this right? You think . . ."

"Help me sort this out. You feel that . . ."

Notice that some lead-ins refer to the factual meaning of what was said, and some are geared toward the feelings behind the words. They are statements, not questions. By paraphrasing, you are neither agreeing nor disagreeing with what was said. You are just checking out the meaning.

Five guidelines for reflective (active) listening are[19]

1. When several points are made, summarize the one that you want to focus on. This will help you keep the conversation pointed in the direction you want to take.

2. When several emotions are expressed, reflect the final one, as this is usually the most accurate.

3. Keep your reflective listening restatement short to keep the focus on the speaker.

4. Only reflect what's there—don't start guessing.

5. Wait out thoughtful silences.

Active listening is useful for drawing out information, understanding new ideas, being clear about statements, and clarifying your understanding. It can also be used in conflict situations to defuse emotion (yours or the speaker's), allow the speaker to express the emotions underlying his or her words, and show empathy. Some have suggested not using reflective listening if you don't like or respect the speaker. This avoids the possibility of unintentionally displaying your negative feelings. Also, do not use reflective listening as a substitute for stating your own thoughts and feelings on a subject.

Presentations

Massage therapists make presentations in a variety of informal and formal ways. One-to-one, informal presentations include explaining policies and procedures to new clients and showing clients self-massage techniques to use at home. More formal presentations may include talking to local community groups about the benefits of massage, or to a governing body in favor of or opposing legislation that affects massage therapists. Explaining, demonstrating, and persuading are useful communication skills in these situations.

Because presentations are essentially teaching opportunities, the audience receiving the presentation can be thought of as a group of learners. Include as many facets of learning as you can, for example, auditory, visual, and kinesthetic elements.

The first rule in making presentations is to know your goals. Why are you making the presentation? What do you expect to gain from it? Second is to know the audience and their expectations. Knowing the audience includes understanding their level of knowledge and experience with what you are presenting. Knowing their expectations helps you plan your presentation to meet their goals as well as yours. Then organize and plan what you want to say.

Explanations are verbal descriptions telling the what, how, and/or why of something. For routine tasks such as explaining policies and procedures to new clients, develop a loose script with an opening statement, points to emphasize, and an ending such as "Do you have any questions?" Use props such as a copy of the policies that you can read together. Give yourself a time limit, and stick to it.

It might be useful to explain to clients why you are using particular techniques to address their goals for a massage session. For example, you might explain that "Given that our goal today is to reduce your postexercise soreness, I'll be doing a lot more stroking, kneading, and stretching to improve circulation and elongate those tight muscles. I'll be paying more attention to your legs because that's where you're feeling the soreness most." Do not explain more than the client needs to know, and gear the explanation to his or her current knowledge of the human body and experience with massage. Anatomy charts and models are handy props for reinforcing verbal explanations of what is happening in the body during massage.

Demonstrations involve showing an audience how something is done or how something works by actually performing the action while giving a verbal description or explanation. Demonstrations enhance learning by giving the audience the opportunity to watch actions that would take many words to describe. A demonstration is worth ten thousand words. For example, demonstrating self-massage or stretching techniques to clients is more effective than verbal explanations alone. Performing massage techniques while explaining the effects of massage adds a valuable component when making a presentation to a community group or other health professionals.

When doing a demonstration, keep things simple. Avoid the urge to expound on everything you know about a topic or things that you find interesting. Tell your audience what you will show and why it is important to them, followed by a step-by-step explanation as you perform the actual demonstration. Allow for questions from the audience either during or after the demonstration.

The room setup is particularly important for demonstrations because the audience needs to see what you are doing. Be aware of how far away they are from you and their angle of viewing. For larger groups, having a video camera that can project the demonstration onto a screen is useful.

The art of persuasion comes into play when you are trying to convince an audience to behave a certain way, take a specific course of action, agree on a particular solution to a problem, or accept a certain fact or belief. For example, you might persuade a client to allow you to massage a tight area even though it will be uncomfortable at first, or persuade legislators to vote for a massage licensing bill, or convince an audience that getting massage regularly is a good idea.

The first concern in persuasion is establishing credibility, trust, and confidence in you, the persuader. Informing the audience of your training and experience is useful, as is presenting a confident and professional appearance.

An organized presentation of ideas is next. The four steps in a persuasive presentation are[20]

1. Get the audience's attention.

2. Present the conclusion, action, or decision that you are looking for and its key benefits.

3. Build your case in detail.

4. Call for a specific action or decision.

To build your case, establish a need or goal, and then show how your plan can meet it. Anticipate objections, and answer them in your presentation. Clear thinking is persuasive in itself. Avoid being too pushy or demanding. Invite others to your way of thinking.

A word of caution is in order here. Persuading clients to accept a certain approach to their therapeutic goals or to allow you to perform specific techniques when they would really rather not, is more coercion than persuasion and is considered unethical. In Chapter 5, *Ethics and the Therapeutic Relationship*, the idea of *informed consent* is explained as a way of giving clients choice while presenting your case.

All presentations should end with an opportunity for the audience to ask questions for clarification. For a client, you might say "Was that clear?" "Do you have any questions?" For a formal presentation, you might invite questions during the talk, or leave time for a short question-and-answer period at the end.

Written Communication

Written communication is a statement of who you are and a reflection of your level of professionalism. There is a greater likelihood that you will be listened to and understood, and your goals achieved, if your written correspondence is well formatted, grammatically correct, neat, and clearly stated.

Memos, emails, and business letters are the most common types of written correspondence for massage therapists and demand basic writing skills such as correct spelling, punctuation, and grammar. Simple sentence construction, clear organization of thought, and brevity are hallmarks of good business correspondence.

MEMOS

Memos are informal notes used to communicate information in short form to clients, coworkers, and colleagues. They dispense with some of the formalities of the business letter, but can retain a professional look by being printed on business stationary. All the elements of a memo are important, especially the date, which is often overlooked. The block format makes skimming the memo content easier for the recipient.

Memos are appropriate for short notes, unofficial business, and other informal correspondence. Note that memos are still business correspondence and should project a professional image using professional language. The memo format and an example are found in Figure 3–6 ■.

EMAIL

Email is essentially an electronic memo. The email format varies with the computer program used, but usually contains all the elements of a standard memo. Email is becoming the preferred method of correspondence in both personal and professional settings. Delivery is fast and inexpensive, and email is easy to respond to. However, there are some pitfalls to watch out for when using email for business purposes.

First is your email address. Have separate personal and professional email addresses if possible. Use a professional-sounding address, such as your own formal name or the name of your practice (e.g., jonesmassagetherapy@email.com). Avoid abbreviations and trendy email jargon. Leave out "emoticons" for more professional correspondence, for example, smiley face :) sad face :(or perplexed :/. Remember that using all capital letters is like SHOUTING at the recipient—never do it.

State your message concisely and clearly. People are being overwhelmed by the volume of emails they receive, and the messages you send are more likely to be read if they are short. Always put an informative title in the subject line. Use a phone call, paper memo, or letter if the message is lengthy. Memos and letters can be faxed or sent electronically if speed of delivery is desirable.

BUSINESS LETTER

Formal business letters are used for official correspondence with government agencies, insurance companies, vendors, employers, and clients. When corresponding for the first time with other health professionals, use the business letter format. They are also preferred for legal matters. The formal business letter format, and the use of official stationary, lends a more serious tone to a document.

Business letters have more identification and introductory information than memos and usually longer paragraphs. There are several different acceptable formats, and it is advisable to choose one to use for your practice and stick to it.[21] The basic business letter format in Figure 3–7 ■ uses a modified block style, that is, aligned with the left-hand margin.

FIGURE 3–6
Memo format and example.

MEMO

Date

To
From
Subject

Main message (1–3 sentences)
Closing (1–2 sentences)

Signature/Initials

Example

MEMO

October 22, 2015

To: Jose Rodriquez
From: Timothy Kim, Massage Therapist
Re: Presentation at Rotary Club Meeting

Hello Jose—This is a note to confirm that I will give a 30-minute presentation on the benefits of massage at the Rotary Club luncheon on November 15, 2015, at 12:00 noon at the Bebop Café in Brenton. I understand that you will have a microphone and overhead projector available for my use.
Thank you again for the invitation to speak to the club.

Jim

WRITTEN CORRESPONDENCE GUIDELINES

Remember that business correspondence has a different function than social correspondence and is more formal. Some general guidelines for written correspondence related to a massage therapy practice are

- Choose the appropriate format for the correspondence (memo, email, or letter).

- Use official printed stationary for memos and letters.

- Type business correspondence; memos may be written or printed legibly.

- Use correct grammar, punctuation, and spelling.

- Keep sentences simple and organization logical.

- Use a more formal tone, and avoid slang and jargon.

- Do not put anything in writing that you would not like to see in a court of law.

- Keep a file of all of your written correspondence in chronological order.

Business/Practice Name
Address/P. O. Box
City, State, Zip Code
Phone/E-Mail

Date: Month-Day-Year

Recipient Name
Address/ P. O. Box
City, State, Zip Code

Dear [Title] First name, middle initial, last name:

Introductory paragraph

Middle paragraph

Closing paragraph

Sincerely,
Signature

Printed name, title

FIGURE 3–7
Business letter format and example.

Example

Anita Davis, Licensed Massage Therapist
1234 Box Street
Everytown, CA. 44444
(123) 456-7890 / adavis@email.com

June 14, 2015

Mineral Water Spa
567 South Street
Watertown, CA. 44445

Dear Ms. Edie Giacomo:

Thank you for the opportunity of interviewing for the position of full-time massage therapist at the Mineral Water Spa last Wednesday. I enjoyed seeing your facility and meeting other spa staff members. I was impressed by the level of professionalism and care for guests that I saw there.

I have enclosed the additional information you requested. This includes a copy of my license to practice massage therapy, my massage school transcript, and a list of my continuing education for the past five years.

Please let me know if you need anything else for your review of my credentials. I would welcome the opportunity to be a massage therapist at the Mineral Water Spa.

Sincerely,
Anita Davis

Anita Davis, Licensed Massage Therapist

CHAPTER HIGHLIGHTS

- The journey to becoming a professional massage therapist involves personal growth and change.
- To have a professional attitude is to embody a professional way of acting, thinking, and feeling.
- Dedication to service means that the client's well-being is held above the massage therapist's own desire for money, power, and worldly recognition. This provides a moral compass for ethical decision making and the motivation to be the best that you can be.
- Having a good work ethic means giving work a high priority in your life and is reflected in good attendance, punctuality, reliability, accountability, positive attitude, and enthusiasm.
- Projecting a professional image means dress that is modest, is clean, and allows freedom of movement and good personal grooming, posture, and speech.
- Professional boundaries clarify the nature of the therapeutic relationship and the roles of both massage therapist and client.
  - Five types of professional boundaries are (1) physical, (2) emotional, (3) intellectual, (4) sexual, and (5) energetic.
- Keeping good professional boundaries is a key factor in maintaining ethical massage therapy practices.
- Ethical standards for massage students lay the foundation for ethical practice after graduation and include the areas of professionalism, class work, relationship with classmates, professional boundaries, and relationship with the school.
- Intellectual skills needed by massage therapists span the range from knowledge to comprehension, application, analysis, synthesis, and evaluation. Higher-level thinking skills include critical thinking and systematic problem solving.
- The ability to concentrate makes studying more productive and performing massage better focused.
  - Concentration is improved through minimizing attention disruptors, single-tasking, creating a more distraction-free environment, and learning to focus the mind.
- Intuition is direct perception of the truth without using rational problem solving and is useful for performing smooth, effortless massage.
- Emotional intelligence is defined by self-awareness, managing emotions, self-motivation, recognizing emotions in others, and handling relationships. It is essential for developing healthy and ethical therapeutic relationships with clients.
- Good social and communication skills are essential for success as a massage therapist.

- Social skills promote harmony and connection between people, and resolve disagreements and misunderstandings.
- Verbal and nonverbal communication skills facilitate the exchange of information and are polished through awareness, learning, experience, and practice.
- Courtesy and good manners are the foundation of customer service.
  - What is considered good manners varies by culture and can change over time.
- First impressions are important to establish rapport with new clients.
- Greeting clients involves making eye contact, saying the person's name, introducing yourself, shaking hands, and giving further directions.
  - The handshake is the first time you touch your client, so it is important to have good, firm contact.
  - Use good judgment in hugging clients to maintain professional boundaries and avoid violating the client's comfort level.
- Introductions help people feel comfortable and welcome, as well as transmit useful social information.
  - In introducing two people, say the most honored person's name first.
- Five basic approaches to conflict resolution are (1) collaboration, (2) accommodation, (3) compromise, (4) avoidance, and (5) force.
  - Choose the best approach to any specific conflict, taking into consideration the priority of your own needs versus the other person's needs and the importance of the relationship. Try for a win–win resolution.
- Verbal communication is improved through practice.
  - Speak in a calm, steady, strong voice; vary energy, rhythm, and inflection to make delivery interesting; articulate clearly and avoid mumbling.
- Telephones and answering machines are essential communication tools.
  - Use a clear and concise answering machine message, and return calls within 24 hours.
  - Turn off ringers and cell phones when in a massage session.
  - Avoid distractions and multitasking while on the phone.

- Body language speaks volumes.
  - Use good upright, aligned posture, and avoid slouching, tilting, and a drooping head.
  - Use welcoming and friendly posture and gestures; communicate with your eyes and smile.

- Being a good listener begins with the intention to hear what others are really saying and to overcome poor listening habits.
  - Focus on what the speaker is saying (words), feeling, and meaning. Avoid letting the mind wander and formulating replies while others are speaking.
  - Affirmative listening lets the speaker know that you are paying attention through verbal cues and body language.
  - In active listening, you reflect back to the speaker in your own words what you think he or she said.

- Massage therapists make presentations in a variety of informal and formal ways to both individuals and groups.
  - Know your goals and your audience, and then organize and plan what you want to say.
  - Explanations are verbal descriptions telling the what, how, and/or why of something.
  - Use loose scripts and props for routine explanations to clients.

- Demonstrations involve showing an audience how something is done or how something works by performing the action while giving a verbal description.
  - Keep descriptions clear and simple, and be sure the audience can see the demonstration well.

- In making persuasive presentations, first establish your credibility, then get the audience's attention, present your point and build your case for it, and call for action.
  - Always provide an opportunity for listeners to ask questions.

- Written correspondence reflects your level of professionalism.
  - Use correct spelling, punctuation, and grammar, as well as simple sentence construction and brevity.
  - Memos and business letters are written in a more formal tone on printed stationary using the correct format.
  - Email is an electronic memo and follows rules of any other business correspondence.
  - Keep a file of all written correspondence in chronological order.

EXAM REVIEW

Key Terms

Match the following key terms to their descriptions. For additional study, look up the key terms in the Interactive Glossary, and note other terms that compare or contrast with them.

_____ **1.** Body language
_____ **2.** Compassion
_____ **3.** Concentration
_____ **4.** Conflict resolution
_____ **5.** Critical thinking
_____ **6.** Emotional intelligence
_____ **7.** Ethics
_____ **8.** Intellectual skills
_____ **9.** Intuition
_____ **10.** Listening
_____ **11.** Problem solving
_____ **12.** Professional boundaries
_____ **13.** Professional image
_____ **14.** Service
_____ **15.** Social skills
_____ **16.** Work ethic

a. Primary motivation is to help others
b. Taking your work seriously, staying focused, and applying yourself to doing a good job
c. Attention to dress, grooming, posture, and language
d. Sets limits or borders that define personal and professional space
e. The study of moral behavior, of right and wrong
f. Thinking or cognitive skills
g. Type of higher-level thinking that helps you get at the truth and avoid being deceived
h. The ability to sustain attention on something for a period of time
i. Set of skills important for self-awareness, self-motivation, and building healthy relationships with clients
j. Deep awareness of the suffering of another coupled with the wish to relieve it
k. A direct perception of the truth, independent of any rational process
l. Behaviors that promote harmony, understanding, and connection, while peacefully solving problems such as disagreements, misunderstandings, and reconciliation after harm done
m. Posture, hand gestures, eye contact, facial expression
n. Trying to understand what someone else is communicating to you.
o. Resolving differences amicably
p. Systematic approach to finding a solution to a problem using critical thinking skills

Memory Workout

To test your memory of the main concepts in this chapter, complete the following sentences by circling the most correct answer from the two choices provided.

1. Dedication to (service) (self-development) offers a higher and more satisfying motivation than merely making money and provides a moral compass for ethical decision making.
2. (Accountability) (Reliability) means that people can count on you to do what you say you are going to do, when you say you will do it.
3. Have work clothes that are (separate from) (similar to) your everyday clothes.
4. (A work ethic) (Boundaries) communicate(s) limits that define personal and professional space.
5. Intuition is a direct perception of the truth, independent of any (thought) (meditation) process.
6. Recognizing a feeling in oneself and its accompanying impulse to act as it happens is called (self-awareness) (self-motivation).
7. Good (intellectual) (social skills) promote harmony, understanding, and connection between people.
8. A general rule when shaking hands is to (match) (exceed) the other person's force

9. Wearing name tags at professional conferences facilitates (networking) (listening).
10. The delivery of the spoken word is usually more important than (content) (voice quality).
11. (Lower-) (Higher-) pitched voices sound more confident and competent.
12. Good upright, aligned posture commands respect and projects (compassion) (confidence).

13. Poor listening habits include letting the mind wander and formulating (replies) (interruptions) while others are speaking.
14. Presentations are essentially (teaching) (motivational) opportunities.
15. Business correspondence has a different function than personal correspondence and is more (legal) (formal).

Test Prep

The following multiple-choice questions will help to prepare you for future school and professional exams.

1. Taking your work seriously, staying focused, and applying yourself to getting the job done right is known as having a good:
   a. Service orientation
   b. Punctuality
   c. Work ethic
   d. Sense of ethics

2. Which of the following is considered professional dress?
   a. Short shorts
   b. Denim jeans
   c. Closed-toe shoes
   d. Dangling jewelry

3. Nervous habits such as finger tapping, nail biting, knuckle cracking, leg bouncing, and hair twirling can be:
   a. Stress reducers
   b. Image detractors
   c. Image enhancers
   d. Grooming problems

4. Using knowledge in real-life situations is an example of intellectual skill at the following level:
   a. Comprehension
   b. Application
   c. Analysis
   d. Synthesis

5. What type of higher-level thinking weighs reasons to believe something against reasons to doubt it?
   a. Logical thinking
   b. Problem solving
   c. Clinical reasoning
   d. Critical thinking

6. Which of the following does *not* improve the ability to concentrate?
   a. Single-tasking
   b. Multitasking
   c. Meditation
   d. Distraction-free environment

7. A deep awareness of the suffering of others coupled with a desire to relieve it is called:
   a. Empathy
   b. Sympathy
   c. Compassion
   d. Appreciation

8. Which of the following directions for greeting a first-time client is *not* correct?
   a. Make eye contact.
   b. Offer your hand to shake.
   c. Wait for the client to speak before introducing yourself.
   d. Smile.

9. When introducing two people, whose name is said first?
   a. The oldest
   b. The youngest
   c. The most honored
   d. The woman's

10. In terms of body language, arms crossed in front of the body can convey a sense of:
    a. Protection and distancing
    b. Welcome and openness
    c. Confidence and trust
    d. Friendliness and invitation

11. The type of listening that lets a speaker know that you are paying attention is:
    a. Attentive listening
    b. Distracted listening
    c. Active listening
    d. Affirmative listening

12. What type of conflict resolution is most appropriate when building long-term relationships, or when you need to work together with someone for the greater good?
    a. Force
    b. Collaboration
    c. Accommodation
    d. Compromise

13. Which of the following statements about phone use in your private practice is *not* good advice?
    a. Try to return phone calls within 24 hours.
    b. Keep phone ringers on low volume during massage sessions.
    c. Do not interrupt a massage session to answer the phone.
    d. Do not interrupt a phone call with a client to answer another call, for example, with call waiting.

14. The first rule in making presentations is to know:
    a. How much time you have
    b. Your goals
    c. Your audience
    d. The room setup

15. The most appropriate form of written correspondence for official business is:
    a. A memo
    b. An email
    c. A brief note
    d. A business letter

Video Challenge

Watch these videos, which can be found at MyHealthProfessionsLab.com, Chapter 3, and then answer the following questions.

Professionalism

1. What do the massage therapists interviewed in the video say about clothes and projecting a professional image?
2. What advice do the massage therapists give about greeting clients?
3. Which of the image detractors discussed in the video do you recognize in yourself?

Emotional Intelligence

4. Identify ways that the massage therapists interviewed in the video show a high level of emotional intelligence. How is that important to a successful massage therapy practice?
5. What do the facial expressions of massage therapists in the video convey to their clients? What similarities do you see in the massage therapists' expressions? Do you see any differences?

6. What do the massage therapists in the video say about establishing good relationships with their clients?

Social and Communication Skills

7. Review the scenes in the video in which massage therapists are greeting clients. Identify ways that professionalism, competence, and confidence are communicated.
8. In what ways do the massage therapists in the video create professional boundaries with their clients? Comment on the different kinds of boundaries established.
9. What principles of good communication do you see in video scenes showing client interviews? How do the massage therapists create a sense of openness to encourage client response?

Comprehension Exercises

The following short-answer questions test your knowledge and understanding of chapter topics and provide practice in written communication skills. Explain in two to four complete sentences.

1. What are some important elements of a good work ethic? Why is this important for success in school and as a future massage therapist?

2. What are professional boundaries? Give some examples of physical, emotional, and intellectual boundaries with clients.
3. In addition to words, what are you listening for when talking to clients? What is the difference between affirmative and active listening?

For Greater Understanding

The following exercises are designed to take you from the realm of theory into the real world. They will help give you a deeper understanding of the subjects covered in this chapter. Action words are underlined to emphasize the variety of activities presented to address different learning styles and to encourage deeper thinking.

1. Choose a dilemma related to massage therapy for an exercise in critical thinking; for example, whether you should buy a certain a product (e.g., type of oil, table, or massage tool); or take a certain elective class; or spend time and money on a particular certification program; or support a proposed licensing provision (e.g., hours of continuing education for license renewal). Analyze the situation listing pertinent questions, evaluate the situation, and decide on a course of action. What influenced your final decision?

2. Create and practice a routine for greeting regular clients to make them feel welcome, comfortable, and confident in you. Take into consideration your body language, voice quality, and words. Have a study partner help you develop this professional "persona." (Variation: Videotape your greeting and analyze it with classmates. Modify it as needed to project what you want.)

3. Practice affirmative and active listening with a partner. Listen to how his or her day went yesterday, and at first simply nod and give affirmative signals that you are listening. Then practice active listening by reflecting back what you thought the person said for clarification.

MyHealthProfessionsLab™

MyHealthProfessionsLab.com is a premium online homework management system that includes a host of features to help you study. Registered users will find:

- Powerful tools that track and analyze your results—allowing you to create a personalized learning experience
- Videos, flashcards and other learning tools to help enrich your progress
- Streaming lesson presentations and self-paced learning modules
- A space where you and your instructors can view and manage your assignments

Physical Skills, Fitness, Self-Care for the Massage Therapist

CHAPTER OUTLINE

Learning Outcomes

Key Terms

The Physical Side of Massage

Body Awareness

Skilled Touch

Physical Fitness

Self-Care Practices

Holistic Self-Care Plan

Chapter Highlights

Exam Review

LEARNING OUTCOMES

After studying this chapter, you will have information to:

1. Develop good body awareness.
2. Describe the elements of skilled touch needed by massage therapists.
3. Summarize the basic elements of physical fitness.
4. Evaluate your overall level of physical fitness.
5. Explain how body–mind practices develop coordination.

6. Improve concentration through meditation.
7. Plan a personal stress-management strategy.
8. Create a time-management plan.
9. Describe the basics of good nutrition.
10. Develop a holistic self-care program.

KEY TERMS

Body awareness

Body–mind practices

Centered

Communication through touch

Contact

Grounded

Holistic self-care plan

Nutrition

Palpation

Qualities of touch

Self-care

Skilled touch

Stress-control strategy

Time management

THE PHYSICAL SIDE OF MASSAGE

Massage therapists bring their whole selves to their work—body, mind, emotions, and spirit. They need the intellectual, emotional, social, and communication skills described in Chapter 3, *Professional and Personal Development*. But perhaps most fundamental are the physical abilities and fitness that allows them to apply massage skillfully and continue to perform massage day after day. Developing physical skills and fitness is an important part of being a massage student, and implementing a self-care plan lays the foundation for years of success in the profession.

Massage is performed with the whole body, not just the hands and arms. Being a massage therapist requires a certain level of body awareness, touch skills, and physical fitness. Self-care practices related to the physical body not only develop the physical conditioning necessary to perform massage, but also help prevent repetitive strain injuries that can cut short a massage therapy career.

BODY AWARENESS

Learning physical skills begins with body awareness. **Body awareness** is the ability to sense where your body is in space while at rest and in motion and to coordinate movement with mind. It entails an integration of body and mind so that a person exists as a unified organism.

People who lack body awareness have difficulty following instructions for good body mechanics and for performing techniques because they are not "in their bodies." There is a disconnect between body and mind, as expressed in this James Joyce quote from *Dubliners*: "Mr. Duffy lived a short distance from his body."

Body awareness is one of the beneficial effects of receiving massage and bodywork, and it is a wellness goal for clients. Body awareness is also essential for learning massage techniques and skillful implementation of massage sessions. Athletes and dancers, artists and craftsmen, musicians, and others who use their bodies in their work and leisure pursuits develop good body awareness over time. It is an awareness that can be developed through movement exercises. It can only be learned by actually performing movements and paying attention to how they feel.

Being centered and grounded are two basic concepts related to body awareness. *Center* has a physical and psychological dimension and refers to a focal point or point of organization from which being and movement occur. Its opposite is being scattered, off balance, and moving from the periphery. Being **centered** refers to finding your center and staying there while you move about.

Center of gravity is a biomechanical concept indicating the point at which body weight is equally balanced in all directions. Think of the point at which your body is balanced from top to bottom, front to back, and left to right. Your exact center of gravity depends on your body shape and how tall you are. The center of gravity for most women is in the hip region and higher toward the chest for most men.

Asian health practices also talk about the center as an important concept. In Chinese, the center is called the *dan tian* (pronounced *dan tyen*) located about 1.5 inches below the navel and one third of the way from front to back. In Japanese, it is called *hara*. The hara is not only a place of physical centering, but also a point of organization on many levels. This center is "a state of unity in which effective action, emotional balance, mental alertness, and spiritual vision are in a harmonious balance. When we are centered our actions are coherent with what we care about."[1] You can begin to find this centered state by learning to move from the physical center.

The tai chi stance and walk are simple exercises that give you a sense of moving from the center. They can also be the foundation of learning good body mechanics for applying massage therapy. Figures 4–1 ■ and 4–2 ■ describe these useful exercises for developing good body awareness.

Ground refers to the firmness of the earth. Being **grounded** refers to establishing a connection and being rooted to the earth through the legs and feet. The meaning can be extended to having a stable base and connection to a foundation whether standing or sitting. This idea becomes important as you learn to move from and use the power of your legs in performing massage. The energy of the movement comes up from the ground through the legs, into the center, and then into the upper body. This concept will be explored further in Chapter 11, *Body Mechanics, Table Skills, General Guidelines*.

FIGURE 4–1 Tai chi stance with front foot pointing straight ahead and back foot at 45° angle, heels in line, and feet shoulder width apart. Shift weight back and forth feeling the movement from the hara or center.

FIGURE 4–2 Tai chi walk along straight line. From tai chi stance, shift weight to the back leg and turn the front foot 45° degrees outward. Then shift weight to front leg while bringing the back leg to the front along the straight line; the new front leg receives the weight. Shift weight back and repeat the walk. Keeping hands near the hara helps you feel the movement from the center.

SKILLED TOUCH

Touch is the basis of massage, therefore **skilled touch** is essential for success as a massage therapist. Skilled touch has four dimensions important to massage therapists:

1. Contact

2. Qualities of touch

3. Communication

4. Palpation

Contact

Contact refers to the sense presence of the massage therapist's hands on the client's body. When contact is good, the client feels a full, confident, deliberate, and warm connection with the massage therapist (Figure 4–3 ■). Poor contact feels tentative, hesitant, unsure, fearful, or distracted.

Good contact is achieved by purposeful touch applied with precision and sensitivity. The massage therapist meets the client's tissues with awareness and performs manual techniques skillfully and with intention. The hand softens to conform to the contour of the client's body rather

FIGURE 4–3
Good contact feels full, confident, and deliberate and establishes a warm connection between massage therapist and client.

Source: Pearson Education, Inc.

than moving on top of the structures and tissues. Slower movement of the hands during massage enhances the sense of contact.

Being fully present mentally and physically heightens the sense of presence with the client. Thinking about something else or daydreaming while giving massage diminishes the feeling of connection. On the other hand, too much thinking about what you are doing can cause tension in your hands and detract from the feeling of good contact. Confident touch comes with experience and loosening up and letting the technique flow.

Qualities of Touch

Qualities of touch are related to contact and vary from soft and gentle to firm and forceful. Qualities might also be described as delicate, firm, deep, energetic, forceful, brisk, or robust. The ability to vary the quality of touch is important for the skilled massage therapist. You may have a personal manner in everyday life related to softness or toughness, but as a massage therapist your quality of touch should always be respectful of the client and appropriate for the situation. The quality of touch in massage should never be weak, shaky, limp, halfhearted, or hard and rough.

Human beings are capable of many nuances in quality of touch, and massage therapists become more conscious of how they are touching their clients and what is called for in a given situation. For example, athletes often prefer a firmer, deeper, and more vigorous massage, whereas a person who is ill requires a gentler touch. As you practice your hands-on skills, try varying your quality of touch when applying certain techniques. Get feedback from your practice partner and adjust as needed to improve your contact and quality of touch.

Communication

Communication through touch is achieved by the contact and different qualities of touch applied during massage, or before or after the session when greeting or saying good-bye to a client. Be conscious of what you might be communicating when you touch your clients. Caring and openness are examples of what can be communicated through touch. Touch during massage should be caring, but never personal, sexual, or aggressive.

Respect for your clients' boundaries is a significant aspect of skilled touch. Know what is off limits for everyone (e.g., touching genitals), and for each individual client (e.g., ticklish feet or an old injury site). Obtaining informed consent for permission to touch is an important communication skill discussed in Chapter 5, *Ethics and the Therapeutic Relationship*.

Palpation

Palpation involves sensing information about the client through touch and by the feel of tissues and movement at joints. Palpatory literacy includes the ability to locate specific anatomical structures and distinguish normal and abnormal conditions in tissues. It is essential for detection of

changes in the client during massage. Palpatory sensitivity is developed through hands-on experience and is sharpened by verbal descriptions of what you feel during hands-on applications. The nature and importance of palpation skills is discussed in more detail in Chapter 9, *Medial Terminology, Goal-Oriented Planning, Documentation*.

PHYSICAL FITNESS

In addition to being good role models for their clients, having a good level of physical fitness allows massage therapists to work without harmful stress and strain. Learning the fundamentals of fitness is also good for better understanding the health of clients. Basic fitness includes cardiovascular function, strength, flexibility, and body composition.

Testing by a fitness professional using the latest methods will give the most accurate results. However, the simple tests described in the following sections offer a general fitness profile and demonstrate the concepts involved. Elements of a physical fitness profile are shown in Figure 4–4 ■.

Cardiovascular Fitness

A basic cardiovascular (CV) fitness profile includes resting heart rate, blood pressure, and cardiovascular endurance. Measurements of these three aspects of CV fitness give an indication of how efficient and strong the heart is and the level of stress on the blood vessels and the system as a whole.

Take your resting heart rate (RHR) either at the wrist below the base of the thumb or on the anterior neck (carotid artery). The best time to measure your RHR is in the morning just after waking up and before any activity. As an alternative, sit still for 10 minutes and then find your pulse with your index and middle fingers, not the thumb. Count the number of beats for 1 minute (or number of beats per 15 seconds × 4). Normal resting heart rate is 60–80 beats per minute.

Blood pressure (BP) is measured with a device called a sphygmomanometer or blood pressure machine. Blood pressure readings have two numbers (e.g., 120/80). The first or top number is the *diastolic pressure*, that is, the pressure of the blood on the vessels when the heart contracts. The second number is the *systolic pressure*, that is, the pressure on the blood vessels between beats. Anyone with BP over 140/90 is considered hypertensive and should see a doctor about it. High blood pressure puts stress on blood vessels and can lead to stroke and other serious health problems.

Cardiovascular endurance refers to the heart's capacity to keep up with a certain workload and its ability to recover afterward. A simple test to demonstrate this concept is the 3-minute step test. This test is performed by stepping on and off a 12-inch-high bench for 3 minutes and then immediately checking your heart rate (HR) (see Figure 4–5 ■). Check the HR again at 1-minute intervals to see when it starts to drop

FIGURE 4–4
Physical fitness profile form.

Name _____ Date _____

♥ **Cardiovascular Fitness**

Resting Heart Rate (RHR)	_____			
Blood Pressure (BP)	_____ / _____			
Cardiovascular Endurance	poor	fair	good	excellent

🏋 **Muscular Strength/Endurance**

Abdominal/Sit-Ups	poor	fair	good	excellent
Upper Body/Push-Ups	poor	fair	good	excellent

( ) **Flexibility**

Sit and Reach	poor	fair	good	excellent

△ **Body Composition**

Body Mass Index (BMI)	underweight (less than 19)	healthy (19-24.5)	overweight (25-29.9)	obese (30+)

Waist Measurement (inches)* _____

Note: Fitness test results tables can be found in books like *Fitness for Dummies* by S. Schlosberg and L. Neporent (Wiley Publishing).

*Waist measurement as an indication of healthy body composition is discussed in *You on a diet: The owner's manual for waist management* by M. F. Riozen and M.C. Oz (Free Press). Recommended is 32.5 inches or less for a woman and 35 inches or less for a man.

back to the RHR. The lower the HR after the exercise, and the faster the recovery, the better the CV endurance is.

Good CV endurance increases the capacity to work longer without fatigue and offers protection against heart disease. Cardiovascular endurance is improved by participating in exercises like walking, running, or cycling for at least 30 minutes 5 days per week. The activity should be vigorous enough to get the heart rate elevated and the body sweating, but not so high that you cannot carry on a conversation. As your CV endurance improves, it will take more effort to feel like you're working hard.

Muscular Strength and Endurance

Overall muscular strength and endurance is developed naturally as the time spent performing massage gradually increases. However, by increasing muscular fitness beyond what is needed to perform massage, less of the muscles' total capacity is used up when working, so there is less stress and fatigue at the end of the day.

Muscular strength refers to a muscle's ability to move a maximum amount of resistance once, whereas *muscular endurance* indicates the capacity to move against resistance for a number of repetitions over time. Strength and

endurance are related because the stronger a muscle is the less effort it has to exert to complete a task. Simple tests for muscular endurance include the number of push-ups or squats you can do, or the number of sit-ups in one minute (Figure 4–6 ■). These tests taken together evaluate the major muscle groups of the body.

In addition to strength in large muscle groups, massage therapists benefit from having exceptional strength in the shoulders, arms, wrists, and hands. Resistance exercises for the upper body can help build strength in those important areas. Use of resistance bands offers a convenient way to increase strength in muscles used most in massage.

Flexibility

Flexibility is the ability to flex or the possible range of movement at joints. Range of motion at each joint can be assessed by performing simple stretches or measured precisely using an instrument called a goniometer, which works like a protractor used in geometry to measure angles. For example, normal range of motion for the wrist joint is determined by assessing how much movement can be achieved starting from the neutral position and then taking the wrist into flexion, extension, and radial and ulnar deviation. See Figure 4–7 ■.

FIGURE 4–5 Step test for cardiovascular endurance.

Source: Pearson Education, Inc./Segal Photography.

A simple test for overall body flexibility is the sit-and-reach test, which is really a test of lower back, hamstring, and shoulder flexibility. Sit with the bottoms of your feet flat against a stair or low box. With no warm-up tries, reach forward as far as you can toward your toes and hold the position (Figure 4–8 ■). Note how far you reach, that is, how far short of your toes or past your toes your fingers extend. For good flexibility, you should be able to reach past your toes.

FIGURE 4–6 One minute sit-up test for abdominal muscle strength and endurance.

Source: Pearson Education, Inc./Segal Photography.

Neutral position

Extension   Flexion

Radial deviation   Ulnar deviation

FIGURE 4–7 Range of motion at the wrist.

Flexibility is maintained by regular stretching. Getting into the habit of stretching every day and between client appointments can protect you from tight, shortened muscles. A regular stretching routine should include stretches for the legs and hips, arms and shoulders, and wrists and hands. Figure 4–9 ■ shows a variety of stretching techniques for massage therapists to address the shoulders, arms, and hands.

FIGURE 4–8 Sit-and-reach test for overall flexibility.

Source: Pearson Education, Inc./Segal Photography.

A

D

B

E

C

F

FIGURE 4–9

A. Palm stretch by hyperextending the fingers.
B. Forearm and palm stretch by hyperextending the wrist.
C. Shoulder stretch by horizontal flexion of arm.
D. Shoulder and pectoral muscles stretch by reaching behind.
E. Triceps and side stretch with arm overhead.
F. Shoulder and torso stretch by twisting and looking behind.

Source: Pearson Education, Inc./Segal Photography.

Body Composition

Body composition refers to your body-fat percentage; that is, how much of your body is composed of fat tissue in comparison to other tissues (muscle, bones, organs, etc.). It is a general indication of health and a signal for health risk factors. Tests like skin-fold calipers, underwater weighing, bioelectrical impedance analysis (BIA), and other methods have been developed to measure body composition with varying levels of accuracy.

The BMI (body mass index) is a method that compares your height and weight to come up with an index number to determine your weight status. Some BMI calculations also factor in chest and waist measurements. BMI is not as accurate a measurement as the more technical methods mentioned earlier, but offers a general indication of healthy body composition and is used here for demonstration purposes. Knowing your BMI can help you make informed decisions about your diet and exercise habits.

A simple BMI calculation is: weight ÷ (height in inches × height in inches) × 705. BMI categories are underweight (less than 18.5), healthy (18.5–24.9), overweight (25–29.9), and obese (30 or greater).[2] Visit the National Institutes of Health website (www.nhlbi.nih.gov/guidelines/obesity/BMI/bmicalc.htmsupport.com/bmi/bmicalc.htm) for a quick calculation of your BMI and to see BMI tables for adult men and women.

Body type and shape are determined by heredity and affect body composition. But genetic predisposition can be managed with a program of good nutrition and exercise. It is important to maintain a BMI that allows for the level of endurance necessary for activity as a massage therapist.

SELF-CARE PRACTICES

It can be a challenge to balance family and friends plus work and school while training to become a massage therapist. It takes a comprehensive, realistic plan. **Self-care** is a term used by massage therapists to describe how they take care of their own well-being while they fulfill their career goals and are of service to clients.

Body–Mind Practices

Some physical exercises do not fit neatly into the strength, flexibility, and cardio fitness categories described earlier. Yet they are useful for improving various aspects of physical fitness with the added benefit of developing coordination, body awareness, and concentration. And they are performed in a way that promotes relaxation. These can be thought of as **body–mind practices** or "any type of exercise that requires a conscious effort to link how (what) you are feeling to what your body is doing."[3]

Body–mind practices popular today include yoga, tai chi, qi gong, and Pilates. Although the first three practices stem from larger systems of philosophy and health practices in India and China, they can be found today adapted and simplified for Westerners. It is not necessary to know or accept the entire philosophical context to benefit from the exercises themselves.

Yoga is an ancient practice from India that concentrates on holding various postures thought to balance energy as understood in Ayurveda, and which improve bodily strength, flexibility, and body awareness. Yoga also includes meditation and breathing exercises.

 ## CASE FOR STUDY

Robin and Getting into Shape for Massage

Robin started massage school about 2 months ago and is now noticing that she has difficulty getting through technique classes without feeling extremely tired and sore. She always thought of herself as being in good shape, but now realizes that doing physical work such as massage might require a higher fitness level. She knows that to be successful in school and in a massage practice afterward, she must get into better physical condition.

Question:

What can Robin do to get into better physical condition for doing massage?

Things to consider:

- Current physical fitness profile
- Areas (e.g., muscles, joints) that feel stressed after practicing massage

- Current types and level of exercise (e.g., CV, strength, flexibility)
- Quality of body mechanics while practicing massage techniques
- Related health practices:
  ○ Amount of sleep each night
  ○ Eating habits
  ○ 3Rs (rest, relaxation, recreation)
- Areas for improvement
- Possibilities for fitness activities

Now put yourself in Robin's place. What three things can you do to improve your physical fitness for performing massage?

1. _____

2. _____

3. _____

The Chinese developed exercises to stimulate the flow of life energy or Qi (also *chi*). *Qi gong* (chi-*gong*) literally means *energy exercises* and focuses on the mind, posture, breathing, and movement. Qi gong is a very useful supplement to Asian bodywork therapy because it has the same goal, which is to improve the flow of Qi in the body's energy channels.[4] Chapter 25, *Asian and Energy-Based Bodywork*, contains examples of yoga and qi gong exercises.

Tai chi (ti-*chee*), another ancient practice from China, was originally based on martial arts. Tai chi involves movements that promote balance, coordination, control, and strength. The movements are performed alone or in movement routines called forms. The quality of movement in the popular Yang style is slow and flowing. Tai chi stances and locomotion, weight transfer, and quality of movement are ideal for learning good body mechanics for performing massage.

Pilates (pih-*lah*-teez) is a modern system of exercise developed by Joseph Pilates, who created the movements to treat injured dancers. Pilates emphasizes the body's core; that is, the abdominal muscles, upper and lower back, and hips and thighs. The exercises focus on using good alignment and strengthening muscles used for good posture (Figure 4–10 ■). Pilates is eclectic, borrowing from yoga, ballet, and standard strengthening exercises. Its uniqueness and benefit lies in its concentration on core muscles, good posture, and correct form. It increases body awareness and control as it promotes good body mechanics.

There are many styles or spin-offs of these systems of exercise. Doing a little homework and critical thinking about them will help you choose one or a combination of practices appropriate for your wellness goals.

MEDITATION

Meditation techniques are designed to quiet the mind and enhance the ability to pay focused attention. The essence of modern meditation techniques is choosing something like a word or object to place attention on, and when the mind wanders as it invariably does, bringing it back to the object of attention. It is that simple—and that difficult—because the mind likes to wander.

Learning focused attention is like trying to teach a puppy to sit and stay. You place the puppy into a sitting position and tell him to stay. He stays for a few seconds, then sees something interesting and wanders off. You gently bring him back to the same spot, sit him down, and tell him to stay. This routine is repeated again and again, and gradually his ability to stay improves. Similarly, a person's concentration ability improves with meditation practice.

A good posture for practicing meditation is seated in a comfortable chair or cross-legged on a cushion. Keep the back upright and in alignment, and let the hands rest on the thighs. If in a chair, feet are flat on the floor. Meditation can be practiced with the eyes closed or open slightly (soft eyes) looking 6–10 feet ahead. Good meditation posture is demonstrated in Figure 4–11 ■.

The surroundings should be quiet and free of distractions. Although meditation can be practiced at any time, many find the early morning or late evening more conducive for calming the mind. Set aside 10–30 minutes daily

FIGURE 4–10 Pilates exercises strengthen the body's core muscles.

Source: Pearson Education, Inc./Segal Photography.

FIGURE 4–11 A good posture for practicing meditation is seated in a chair with the back upright and in alignment, the hands resting on the knees, feet flat on the floor, with soft eyes looking 6–10 feet ahead.

Source: Pearson Education, Inc./Segal Photography.

for best results. Consistency is important for developing concentration ability over time.

A simple form of meditation is called *peaceful abiding*. The object of attention in peaceful abiding is the breath. "In peaceful abiding, we ground our mind in the present moment. We place our mind on the breath and keep it there."[5] By having a focal or reference point like the breath, we can better detect when concentration is broken and bring it back as we practice focused attention. The end result is a clear, focused, uncluttered mind.

Another form of meditation is called *quiet sitting*. This is the practice of taking time to calm your mind, collect your thoughts, and center yourself. It is taking a break from the distractions of life and sitting quietly for a moment. The idea is to find a comfortable place to sit, close your eyes, and calm your breathing and your thoughts. Keep your thoughts centered on this quiet moment, and let go of unnecessary thinking. After a few moments, resume activity keeping the calmness you have created.[6]

In *active meditation*, an activity like walking, knitting, or even doing the dishes can be used as a practice for focusing the mind. The point here is to focus on thoughts relevant to what you are doing, and let go of unrelated thoughts. If your mind drifts into other thoughts, gently bring it back to the task at hand. By raising awareness of when the mind is wandering and learning to bring it back to the object of attention, you are increasing your ability to concentrate.

Athletes try to improve their powers of concentration for better sports performance. Zen practices like kyudo (archery), flower arranging, and tea ceremony are ancient forms of active meditation. Eventually, massage itself becomes an active meditation in the sense that you are concentrating on what you are doing without distraction.

Many massage therapists do a variation on quiet sitting before going into a massage session. They take a few moments to stand outside the door to the massage room and collect and focus their thoughts. This prepares them to be present and to give the massage session focused attention.

Stress-Control Strategies

Massage therapists appreciate the major role that stress can play in undermining health and fitness. Students are under special circumstances that increase the stress in their lives and therefore need **stress-control strategies** to help maintain

good health. Good stress-control habits developed while in school can continue throughout your life.

Consequences of stress overload for students include problems like inability to pay attention in class (distraction), poor attendance and lateness, test anxiety, and chronic emotional upset. Stress-control plans include strategies like good time management, adequate rest and relaxation, and anxiety-reduction techniques, including massage.

Poor time management is perhaps the biggest stress producer for students. Developing a good time management plan as described later in this chapter is the cornerstone of a stress-control strategy.

Adequate rest, relaxation, and recreation are essential stress-control strategies. Getting 7–9 hours of sleep per night and having at least 30 minutes of "downtime" or quiet time per day are good goals. Recreation (think of *re-creation*) activities offer a break from work and revive the spirit. The three Rs should be scheduled into your time management plan.

Massage therapists, who are looked to as experts in stress reduction, accumulate a number of different methods to promote relaxation. These include relaxation music, physical practices like yoga and tai chi, meditation and quiet sitting, and massage itself. The more students practice relaxation techniques, the better able and more credible they will be when helping clients who come to them to reduce the stress in their lives.

Time Management

Time management involves planning a workable schedule. It is a matter of priorities, which means making time for what matters most and letting go of the rest. A common mistake of students is to try to fit school into an already crowded schedule. Being rushed or late, eating on the run, cramming for classes and exams, and suffering from sleep deprivation are symptoms of poor time management. You have to *make* time for what you value most.

So the first step in time management is to identify goals and priorities for the time under consideration. That could be for a week, a month, a year. It might be defined by your life at the moment, such as the time you are in school or for the semester. If priorities are not clear, it is difficult to make good choices about the use of time. Students who start with school as a top priority are more likely to produce a time management plan that leads to success.

PRACTICAL APPLICATION

Practice some form of sitting meditation for 10–15 minutes every day for 2 weeks. Evaluate how regular meditation affects you and your experience with learning massage.

1. What method of meditation most appeals to you?
2. Can you find a regular time and place for meditation?

3. Does it become easier with practice to minimize distracting thoughts?
4. Can you focus better in class and with practice clients at home?

REALITY CHECK

LUTHER

CHERISE: I know cardiovascular fitness is important, but I'm not the marathon runner type. And I don't have the time or money to join a gym. Isn't there something simple I can do to get more fit?

LUTHER: Running really isn't necessary. Walking at least 30 minutes 5 days a week will get you on the road to cardiovascular fitness. That doesn't mean a stroll, but a moderate to fast-paced walk. Your breathing will be a little faster, and you may sweat a little if you are moving at a good pace. You can combine your walks with your stress-management strategy. Either walk by yourself for some alone time, or walk with a friend for some relaxing social time. You also can include the time spent walking to and from the bus or train in your total for the day, or you might try taking a walk at lunchtime. Fifteen minutes twice a day would also count. After a few weeks of walking, you'll see a boost in your fitness level.

Plotting out a weekly schedule is the next step toward getting your use of time under control. The time management chart in Figure 4–12 ■ is an example of planning adequate time for regular activities.

A time management plan for students includes the following: work, school (classes and homework/practice), commuting, regular appointments and meetings, family time, sleeping, eating, rest/relaxation, and recreation. A good rule of thumb is to plan 60% to 75% of your time and leave 25% to 40% for unplanned or spontaneous activities. Working while attending school tends to decrease "spontaneous" time, but may be manageable for a short period.

A good time management tip is to identify *time wasters* and eliminate them from your life. A time waster would be something that does not contribute to your high-priority goals. Delayed gratification and learning to say "no" to yourself, with sights on a higher goal, are important signs of emotional maturity.

Reserve your prime time for high-priority tasks. For example, plan to study when you are most awake and full of energy. Also figure in adequate travel time between scheduled events. For example, list 7:30AM—leave for school, as well as 8:30AM—anatomy class begins.

Plan enough time for homework and practicing massage skills. For each hour of lecture class allot 2–3 hours of study time. Practice massage as required in your program for at least 4–6 hours per week outside class time. Practice is not only for doing your homework and honing your massage skills, but also for building the strength and stamina to make a living as a massage therapist after graduation.

Time Period September – December (Fall Semester)			**Class Time:** 24 hrs			**Study/Practice Time:** 20 hrs	
Time	**Monday**	**Tuesday**	**Wednesday**	**Thursday**	**Friday**	**Saturday**	**Sunday**
5:00 am	sleep	sleep	sleep	sleep	sleep	sleep	sleep
6:00	sleep	sleep	sleep	sleep	sleep	sleep	sleep
7:00	up & eat	up & eat	up & eat	up & eat	up & eat	up & eat	sleep
8:00	travel	travel	travel	travel	travel	travel	up & eat
9:00	class	class	class	class	work	work	recreation
10:00	class	class	class	class	work	work	recreation
11:00	class	class	class	class	work	work	recreation
12 noon	lunch	lunch	lunch	lunch	work	work	lunch
1:00 pm	class	class	class	clinic	lunch	lunch	study/practice
2:00	class	class	class	clinic	work	study/practice	study/practice
3:00	class	class	class	clinic	work	study/practice	study/practice
4:00	travel	travel	travel	travel	work	study/practice	study/practice
5:00	dinner	dinner	dinner	dinner	work	study/practice	dinner
6:00	work	study/practice	work	read/study	dinner	dinner	read/study
7:00	work	study/practice	work	read/study	recreation	recreation	read/study
8:00	work	study/practice	work	read/study	recreation	recreation	recreation
9:00	read/study	study/practice	read/study	read/study	recreation	recreation	recreation
10:00	relax/meditation	relax/meditation	relax/meditation	relax/meditation	recreation	recreation	relax/meditation
11:00	sleep	sleep	sleep	sleep	sleep	sleep	sleep

FIGURE 4–12 Sample time management planning chart for a massage student.

CRITICAL THINKING

Analyze the level of stress in your life. Develop a strategy for minimizing harmful stressors and for including more stress-reducing activities.

1. What are the biggest stress-producing aspects of your life right now?

2. Which stressors are under your control, and which are outside your control?

3. Do you have adequate time for rest, relaxation, and recreation?

4. Can better time management help manage your stress level?

By graduation, you should be comfortably performing the number of hours of massage (class plus practice time) that you are aiming for in your practice start-up.

Get in the habit of using a daily or weekly planner to keep track of regular and special appointments, events, and deadlines. Check your schedule at the beginning of each month, week, and day for an overview of the time period. Refer to your planner when making appointments so that you don't double schedule a time period.

Good time management while at school will naturally spill over into postgraduate employment and private practices. Build good habits in school that will serve you well afterwards.

Nutrition

Nutrition refers to the intake of food and drink to nourish the body and mind. Eating healthy food in appropriate amounts lays the foundation for all-around well-being. Nutrition and physical activity go hand in hand in maintaining a healthy lifestyle. The U.S. Department of Agriculture (USDA) maintains the Food and Nutrition Information Center (FNIC) that publishes dietary guidelines for healthy eating based on the latest research. They created the MyPlate program in 2011 (replacing MyPyramid) "to help consumers adopt healthy eating habits by encouraging them to build a healthy plate" consistent with current dietary guidelines. MyPlate is now the government's primary food guidance symbol. See Figure 4–13 ■. The latest USDA Dietary Guidelines can be found at www.dietaryguidelines.gov.

Giving nutritional advice to others is not within the scope of massage therapy, but healthy eating is an important aspect of self-care for everyone. A basic knowledge of nutrition provides a starting place for learning more about choosing the right foods and developing good eating habits.

Nutrients are substances in food used by the body to generate energy and to promote normal growth, maintenance, and repair. Six major categories of nutrients are carbohydrates, lipids, proteins, vitamins, minerals, and water. Broadly speaking, carbohydrates are composed of sugars and starches, lipids are fats, and proteins are amino acids found in fish, meat, seeds, nuts and legumes. Vitamins are organic nutrients and minerals are inorganic substances that the body needs in small amounts. Water is especially

important because about 50%–60% of a healthy adult's body weight is water, and fluid balance is essential for many physiological processes.[7]

Food is the familiar form of plant and animal products that we eat to obtain nutrients. When planning meals, it is easier to think in terms of food groups to include in different amounts. There are six major food groups: grains, vegetables, fruits, oils, milk, and meat and beans. Different foods contain a variety of nutrients in combination. For example, vegetables contain carbohydrates, water, vitamins, and minerals. Fish and legumes typically contain protein, lipids, vitamins, and minerals. Table 4–1 ■ identifies some of the major nutrients found in different foods.

Calories measure the energy value of food. The number of calories in a particular food is a measurement of how much energy that food can produce when used in the body. For example, 2 tablespoons of almond butter contains about 190 calories, whereas 8 fluid ounces of orange juice provides about 110 calories. Some foods are "empty calories," that is, they add to the total calories consumed per day, but have little or no nutritional value.

FIGURE 4–13 MyPlate encourages healthy eating by recommending that people fill half their plates with fruits and vegetables.

Source: U.S. Department of Agriculture and U.S. Department of Health and Human Services.

TABLE 4–1	Basic Food Groups and Their Major Nutrients

Source: Shutterstock/Jovan Nikolic.

Group	Examples	Nutrients *Supplied by all in food group*	Nutrients *Supplied by some in food group*
Fruits	Apples, bananas, grapes, oranges, pears, kiwi, pomegranate, mango, tomatoes	Carbohydrate Water	Vitamins: A, C, folic acid Minerals: Iron, potassium Fiber
Vegetables	Broccoli, leafy greens, eggplant, green beans, peas, lettuce, potatoes, sweet potatoes, squash	Carbohydrate Water	Vitamins: A, C, E, K, B vitamins except B_{12} Minerals: Calcium, magnesium, iodine, manganese, phosphorus Fiber
Grain products	Breads, cereals, pasta, crackers, tortillas, cookies *Sources*: wheat, oats, rice, quinoa, spelt, amaranth (whole grains are best)	Carbohydrate Protein Vitamins: Thiamin (B_1), niacin	Water Fiber Minerals: Iron, magnesium, selenium
Dairy products	Milk, cheese, yogurt, kefir, ice cream *Sources*: cow, goat, or sheep's milk	Protein Fat Vitamins: Riboflavin, B_{12} Minerals: Calcium, phosphorus Water	Carbohydrate Vitamins: A, D
Meat and vegetarian protein sources	Beef, poultry, fish, eggs, seeds, nuts, soybeans, tofu, legumes (beans)	Protein Vitamins: Niacin, B_6 Minerals: Iron, zinc	Carbohydrate Fat Vitamins: B_{12} thiamin (B_1) Water Fiber

The number of calories needed per day varies for different people depending on their gender, age, height, activity level, and other health factors. For example, if you are 30 years old, female, 5'6" tall, and engage in 30 to 60 minutes of physical activity per day, your energy needs are about 2200 calories per day. If you are a 25-year-old male, 5'11" tall, and engage in moderate exercise, your energy needs are about 2800 calories per day. A calculator for determining the number of daily calories needed by individuals based on relevant factors can be found at the FNIC website (www .fnic.nal.usda.gov/fnic/interactiveDRI/).

If you consume more calories than you use each day, you gain weight. If you consume fewer calories than you need each day, you lose weight. To maintain your ideal weight, the number of calories you consume each day should match the number you use for energy. Charts have been developed that show ideal weight for people of different ages. Body mass index (BMI), as described earlier in this chapter, is also a method of determining if you are underweight, normal, overweight, or obese.

The U.S. government has developed a program to help people reach and maintain their ideal weight, while eating a nutritionally balanced diet. It is based on U.S. Dietary Guidelines and can be found online at www.ChooseMyPlate.gov. The program helps you to determine your ideal weight and to plan healthy meals. Worksheets include suggestions for amounts of food to eat from different food groups (grains, vegetables, fruits, milk, meat and beans) and space for tracking what you actually eat each day. Tracking your daily progress can be done online at www.supertracker.usda.gov/default.aspx.

Practicing good nutrition and maintaining a healthy weight are important for massage therapists. Performing massage and keeping a full schedule of appointments are easier if you are in optimal physical condition. In addition, being a good role model for clients is an important aspect of being in a health profession.

HOLISTIC SELF-CARE PLAN

A **holistic self-care plan** includes those activities that support your development as a massage therapist and that minimize factors that lead to illness and injury. It means having a plan for physical, mental, and emotional health and fitness and avoiding undue stress and burnout. Even though self-care plans are as unique as the individuals involved, they have some common elements.

Self-care plans include healthy nutrition, physical fitness, rejuvenation, and stress control. Good body mechanics while performing massage is essential to prevent injury and increase longevity as a massage therapist. Quiet sitting or some other form of meditation helps maintain mental alertness and emotional calm. Taking time for recovery, rest, and relaxation prevents burnout. Good time management is the foundation of putting it all together and making it happen.

Keeping a journal or logbook, especially while putting a self-care plan into place, can help track progress and identify aspects that need to be strengthened. Figure 4–14 ■ is an example of a page from a journal for tracking a holistic self-care plan.

FIGURE 4–14
Sample daily log for holistic self-care plan.

CHAPTER HIGHLIGHTS

- Being a massage therapist requires having good body awareness.
  - Body awareness is the ability to sense where your body is in space while at rest and in motion and to coordinate movement with mind.
  - Being centered and grounded are two important aspects of body awareness.

- Skilled touch has four dimensions important to massage therapists: contact, qualities of touch, communication, and palpation.
  - *Contact* refers to the sense presence of the massage therapist's hands on the client's body.
  - *Qualities of touch* are related to contact and vary from soft and gentle to firm and forceful.
  - Caring and openness are examples of what can be *communicated* through touch.
  - *Palpation* is sensing information about the client through touch and by the feel of tissues and movement at joints.

- Physical fitness includes cardiovascular health, muscular strength and endurance, flexibility, and body composition.
  - A basic cardiovascular (CV) fitness profile includes resting heart rate, blood pressure, and cardiovascular endurance.
  - *Muscular strength* refers to a muscle's ability to move a maximum amount of resistance once, whereas *muscular endurance* indicates the capacity to move against resistance for a number of repetitions over time.
  - Flexibility is the "ability to flex" or the possible range of movement at joints.
  - Body composition can be measured using the body mass index (BMI) to determine if you are underweight, normal, overweight, or obese.

- Self-care is taking care of your own well-being while fulfilling family, work, and school responsibilities.
- Body–mind practices such as yoga, tai chi, qi gong, and Pilates develop coordination, body awareness, and concentration.
- Meditation techniques are designed to quiet the mind and enhance the ability to pay focused attention; methods include peaceful abiding and quiet sitting.
- Stress-control strategies include the 3 Rs: adequate rest, relaxation, and recreation; help prevent overload and burnout.
- Time management involves planning a workable schedule; includes setting priorities and eliminating time wasters.
  - Plotting out a weekly schedule, and using a daily or weekly planner to keep track of regular and special appointments, events, and deadlines helps get your use of time under control.

- Nutrition refers to the intake of food and drink to nourish the body and mind; includes concepts of nutrients, food groups, and calories.
  - Good nutrition and healthy weight result from balanced eating habits and adequate physical activity.
  - The U.S. government publishes dietary guidelines and sponsors a healthy eating program at www.ChooseMyPlate.gov.

- A holistic self-care plan encompasses the many aspects of well-being, including the physical, mental, emotional, and social.
  - Keeping a self-care log or journal tracks progress and is motivating.

EXAM REVIEW

Key Terms

Match the following key terms to their descriptions. For additional study, look up the key terms in the Interactive Glossary, and note other terms that compare or contrast with them.

_____ 1. Body awareness
_____ 2. Body–mind practices
_____ 3. Center
_____ 4. Communication
_____ 5. Contact
_____ 6. Ground
_____ 7. Holistic self-care plan
_____ 8. Nutrition
_____ 9. Palpation
_____ 10. Qualities of touch
_____ 11. Self-care
_____ 12. Skilled touch
_____ 13. Stress-control strategy
_____ 14. Time management

a. The firmness of the earth; having a stable base and connection to a foundation whether standing or sitting
b. The basis of massage; skill in physical contact with clients
c. Related to contact and varies from soft and gentle to firm and forceful
d. Taking care of your own well-being
e. Planning a workable schedule
f. The ability to sense where your body is in space while at rest and in motion and to coordinate movement with mind
g. Exercises that require a conscious effort to link what you are feeling to what your body is doing
h. Includes good time management, adequate rest and relaxation, and anxiety-reduction techniques
i. Achieved by the contact and different qualities of touch applied during massage
j. Includes all activities that support your development as a massage therapist and minimize factors that lead to illness and injury
k. A focal point or point of organization from which being and movement occur
l. The intake of food and drink to nourish the body and mind
m. Sensing information about the client through touch and by the feel of tissues and movement at joints
n. The sense presence of the massage therapist's hands on the client's body

Memory Workout

To test your memory of the main concepts in this chapter, complete the following sentences by circling the most correct answer from the two choices provided.

1. Knowing where your body is in (space) (time) while it is at rest or in motion is called body awareness.
2. Establishing a connection to the earth through the legs and feet is called being (centered) (grounded).
3. A basic cardiovascular fitness profile includes (regular) (resting) heart rate (RHR).
4. Flexibility is maintained by regular (walking) (stretching).
5. Sensing information about the client through touch and by the feel of tissues and movement at joints is referred to as (intuition) (palpation).
6. (Body–mind) (Cardiovascular) practices such as yoga and tai chi help improve coordination, body-awareness, and concentration.
7. A good meditation posture is sitting in a chair with your back upright and hands resting on the (thighs) (knees).
8. The three Rs of (stress-control) (time management) strategy are rest, relaxation, and recreation.
9. Carbohydrates are composed of sugars and (starches) (fats).
10. In developing a time management schedule, a good rule of thumb is to leave (25–40) (5–20) percent of your time for unplanned or spontaneous activities.

Test Prep

The following multiple-choice questions will help to prepare you for future school and professional exams.

1. The point of organization in your body from which being and movement occur is referred to as your:
   a. Body awareness
   b. Physical fitness
   c. Ground
   d. Center

2. The sense of presence of the massage therapist's hands on the client's body during massage should feel:
   a. Deliberate and nervous
   b. Confident and warm
   c. Hesitant and fearful
   d. Full and unsure

3. The capacity to move against resistance for a number of repetitions over time is called:
   a. Cardiovascular endurance
   b. Muscular strength
   c. Muscular endurance
   d. Grounding

4. Palpatory literacy involves the ability to:
   a. Locate specific anatomical structures
   b. Detect normal tissue conditions
   c. Feel abnormal tissue conditions
   d. All of the above

5. The essence of modern meditation techniques is choosing something like a word or object to place attention on, and when the mind wanders, to:
   a. Bring it back to the object of attention
   b. Let it wander
   c. See where it takes you
   d. Change the object of attention

6. Grains, vegetables, fruits, oils, milk, and meat and beans are the basic:
   a. Nutrient categories
   b. Empty calorie sources
   c. Food groups
   d. Amino acids

7. Organic nutrients that the body needs in small amounts are called:
   a. Carbohydrates
   b. Vitamins
   c. Minerals
   d. Sodium

8. Body–mind exercises require a conscious effort to link what your body is doing to:
   a. Verbal instructions
   b. Written instructions
   c. Role models
   d. What you are feeling inside

9. A self-care plan that includes goals for physical, mental, and emotional well-being is called:
   a. Fitness
   b. Focused
   c. Nutritional
   d. Holistic

10. Planning a workable schedule for good time management is a matter of:
    a. Setting priorities
    b. Instant gratification
    c. Finding time wasters
    d. Luck

Video Challenge

Watch this video, which can be found at MyHealthProfessionsLab.com, Chapter 4, and then answer the following questions.

Holistic Self-Care Plan

1. What methods of developing physical fitness are shown in the video? How do they compare with your physical fitness activities?

2. Identify the different methods of stress control and relaxation shown in the video. How do they compare with your stress-control strategy?

3. What aspects of time management are mentioned in the video? How can you improve time management in your life?

Comprehension Exercises

The following short-answer questions test your knowledge and understanding of chapter topics and provide practice in written communication skills. Explain in two to four complete sentences.

1. Define being *centered* and being *grounded*. Why are these concepts important for massage therapists?

2. Describe the basic components of physical fitness. Give an example of how each component can be evaluated.

3. Explain what the body mass index (BMI) measures. What is your BMI score, and what does it mean?

For Greater Understanding

The following exercises are designed to take you from the realm of theory into the real world. They will help give you a deeper understanding of the subjects covered in this chapter. Action words are underlined to emphasize the variety of activities presented to address different learning styles and to encourage deeper thinking.

1. Evaluate your level of physical fitness, and fill out the Physical Fitness Profile Form in Figure 4–4. Identify your areas of strength and weakness, and set some physical fitness goals.

2. Fill out a time management chart for the rest of this semester or the next. Use the chart in Figure 4–12 as an example. Discuss your plan with a study group or classmate, and evaluate it according to the priorities you set for yourself. Note how well it supports your success in the massage school program.

3. For at least 2 weeks, keep a daily log of your self-care activities. Use the form in Figure 4–14. Use your increased awareness of holistic self-care to build good habits for a healthier life.

MyHealthProfessionsLab™

MyHealthProfessionsLab.com is a premium online homework management system that includes a host of features to help you study. Registered users will find:

- Powerful tools that track and analyze your results—allowing you to create a personalized learning experience
- Videos, flashcards and other learning tools to help enrich your progress
- Streaming lesson presentations and self-paced learning modules
- A space where you and your instructors can view and manage your assignments

Ethics and the Therapeutic Relationship

5

CHAPTER OUTLINE

Learning Outcomes
Key Terms
Overview
Nature of Ethics
Values, Rights, and Duties
Vulnerability to Unethical Behavior
Ethical Codes and Standards
Ethics and Law
Ethical Decision Making
Development of Ethical Judgment

The Therapeutic Relationship
Roles and Boundaries
Dual Relationships
Sexual Relationships
Sexual Misconduct
Relationships in School
Scope of Practice
Confidentiality
Chapter Highlights
Exam Review

LEARNING OUTCOMES

After studying this chapter, you will have information to:

1. Explain values, rights, and duties as the basis of ethics.
2. Describe ethical standards for massage therapists.
3. Understand the consequences of unethical behavior.
4. Use a decision-making model to address ethical questions.
5. Establish appropriate roles in the therapeutic relationship.
6. Avoid all levels of sexual misconduct.
7. Obtain informed voluntary consent when appropriate.
8. Stop inappropriate client behavior using the intervention model.
9. Stay within the scope of practice of massage therapy.
10. Keep client information confidential.

KEY TERMS

Boundary crossing
Codes of ethics
Confidentiality
Defense mechanisms
Dual relationship
Duties
Ethical decision-making model

Ethical dilemmas
Ethical judgment
Ethical questions
Ethics
Informed voluntary consent
Intervention model

Personal boundary
Personal temptations
Power differential
Professional ethics
Rights
Scope of practice
Sexual misconduct

Standards of practice
Therapeutic relationship
Transference
Values

OVERVIEW

The concept of ethics was introduced in Chapter 2, *Professional and Personal Development*, along with ethical standards for the massage student. Although some of the principles presented there apply to all students (for example, those related to classwork), others are unique to learning to be massage therapists. Acting ethically with classmates provides the practice and reflection necessary to internalize ethical principles in the process of becoming a professional. It lays the foundation for being ethical massage therapists after graduation. Professional boundaries in particular are such an important aspect of good ethical behavior that the idea was worth exploring earlier in the context of personal integrity and coming back to again in this chapter, in which professional ethics are explored in more detail.

Being a responsible massage therapist goes beyond having good hands-on skills. Employers and clients expect their massage therapists to behave with honesty and integrity and to uphold the ethical standards of their profession. Clients especially want the people who touch them to be trustworthy and to act in their clients' best interests. But knowing the right thing to do in different situations can be challenging, especially in professional relationships based on touch. The roles and responsibilities are very different from more familiar relationships with family and friends and in other types of work.

The study of ethics, specifically ethics for massage therapists, complements the physical, intellectual, and social skills needed by well-rounded professionals. Understanding the nature of ethics sets the stage for examining ethical standards for massage therapists.

NATURE OF ETHICS

Ethics is the study of moral behavior; that is, determining the *right* thing to do in a specific situation. Ethical behavior conforms to certain values such as honesty and fairness, upholds human rights such as privacy and safety, and reflects the duties inherent in being in a position of power. Ethical codes and standards translate moral values into guidelines for decisions made every day.

Laws are sometimes enacted by governments to enforce ethical behavior. These laws are passed for the protection of the public. However, many behaviors considered unethical are perfectly legal. For example, gossiping about a client may not land you in jail, but it is considered unethical.

Professional ethics is the study of moral behavior relative to a specific occupation such as massage therapist. Because massage therapy falls into the categories of service, helping, and therapeutic professions, standards of behavior are high. Although the first rule is "to do no harm," professional standards also take into consideration what is best therapeutically for the client.

Such standards specify those behaviors which have proven counter-therapeutic and are therefore considered unacceptable by the professional community. In other words, sets of ethical guidelines *encourage* behavior that is most effective therapeutically and *discourage* behavior that is ineffective or therapeutically harmful.[1]

Professional organizations develop codes of ethics and standards of practice to clarify the values of the group and serve as references for ethical decision making. These documents contain the collective wisdom of the profession regarding ethical behavior among its members. "Establishing an ethical code is an exercise in self-reflection and clarification of values for those who write, review, and approve such documents."[2] See Appendix B for the *National Certification Board for Therapeutic Massage and Bodywork (NCBTMB) Code of Ethics and Standards of Practice*.

Business ethics concern the commercial aspects of being a massage therapist and the treatment of clients as customers. Business ethics encompass the areas of advertising, payment policies and procedures, keeping proper licenses, and other business-related matters. It can be thought of as that part of professional ethics that has to do with having a private practice. Chapter 28, *Business Ethics*, specifically focuses on ethical issues concerning the commercial side of massage therapy.

VALUES, RIGHTS, AND DUTIES

Ethical principles are founded on the values, rights, and duties deemed important in society. Professionals apply these factors in determining acceptable conduct in the practice of their work.

Values

Values are principles, traits, or qualities considered worthwhile or desirable. Ethical codes and standards are developed to protect the values that give meaning and direction to the profession. For example, the standard that massage therapists represent their qualifications truthfully stems from the value of *honesty*.

Values that have come to the forefront in the massage and bodywork profession include *compassion*, or the wish to relieve suffering, and *selfless service*, or giving clients' well-being top priority. For example, "refuse any gifts or benefits intended to influence a referral, decision, or treatment that are purely for personal gain and not for the good of the client."[3]

Honesty is speaking the truth and avoiding deception, whereas *integrity* is living up to our values consistently. Being *trustworthy* includes being reliable, honest, and principled.

Equality, fairness, and *nondiscrimination* entail treating others with equal respect and not playing favorites.

Unconditional regard for others calls for being nonjudgmental and giving our best efforts to everyone, regardless of who they are. An item in the *NCBTMB Code of Ethics* (2008) directs massage therapists "to respect the inherent worth of all persons."

For every positive value, there is an opposite or negative, which is often the thing that catches our attention. People have inner voices or consciences that tell them that something is wrong. For example, you might have an uncomfortable feeling when talking about one of your clients to a friend. Knowing about the principle of *confidentiality* helps you sort out which actions are ethical and which are not.

A better sense of important values can be cultivated by study and discussion. Some values, like honesty, are widely recognized and deeply ingrained. But how these values are applied in a specific profession may not be so obvious at first, like applying the concept of honesty to making health claims for the benefits of massage therapy.

Values provide a moral compass to point the way when we are lost or confused. Having an awareness of the values held by the profession is a prerequisite for making ethical decisions as massage therapists.

Rights

Rights also come into play when discussing ethical behavior. **Rights** are claims to certain treatment or protection from certain treatment. Rights are expected to be honored by others and enforced by standards or laws if necessary. For example, clients have a right to privacy, which is the basis for draping practices and confidentiality policies. They also have a right to freedom from personal violations such as sexual misconduct. Client rights that play an important part in ethical standards for massage therapists are the rights to privacy, self-determination, and safety (Figure 5–1 ■).

The client's *right to privacy* is the root of several ethical standards. Draping procedures and the custom of leaving the room when clients are undressing preserve their privacy. Prohibitions against revealing information about clients to others, or *confidentiality*, also protects their privacy. Confidentiality rights related to medical records are protected by law through the Health Information Portability and Accountability Act (HIPAA). HIPAA is discussed in greater detail later in the chapter.

The client's *right to self-determination*, also called *autonomy*, asserts that clients should have the opportunity to make informed choices about what happens to them. Self-determination is protected by standards about massage therapists obtaining informed voluntary consent from clients to perform certain massage techniques or to work in certain body areas. Another is "the client's right to refuse, modify, or terminate treatment regardless of prior consent given."[4]

The client's *right to safety* is the basis of hygiene standards and regulations. Clients have a right to expect cleanliness and a germ-free environment in a massage

FIGURE 5–1 Clients have certain rights like the rights to privacy, self-determination, and safety.

Source: Pearson Education, Inc./Segal Photography.

room, as well as that tables and other equipment be in good repair. Also related is the standard that massage therapists "provide only those services which they are qualified to perform."[5]

In recent years, the consumer rights movement has led to a crackdown on deceptive business practices and the enactment of a number of consumer protection laws. How these relate to massage therapists is discussed in Chapter 28, *Business Ethics*.

Massage therapists have rights, too; for example, the right to fair compensation for their work and the right to a safe environment. They have the right to create and enforce policies for their practices. The *NCBTMB Code of Ethics* recognizes the right "to refuse to treat any person or part of the body for just and reasonable cause."

Duties

Duties or *responsibilities* are obligations to act in a particular way. Duties arise out of being in a certain position in relationship to others or as the result of some action. Massage therapists have duties related to their clients, colleagues, coworkers, employers, and others. Duties reflect moral bonds that are generally recognized in a society and deeply felt as obligations or things that we "ought to" do by individuals. They are intricately related to the values and rights discussed earlier.

A basic duty of massage therapists is to maintain professional boundaries that clarify and preserve the roles inherent in the therapeutic relationship. It is the massage therapist's responsibility to establish good boundaries regardless of what the client wants. This potential dilemma is discussed later in the chapter.

Duties can arise out of the rights of others; that is, if individuals have a right to something, and a massage therapist is in a position to influence what happens to them, then that massage therapist has a duty to protect those rights.

TABLE 5-1	The Basis of Ethical Principles for Massage Therapists	
Values	**Rights**	**Duties**
Compassion	**Client**	Beneficence
Equality	Personal respect	Avoid harm
Fairness	Privacy	Professional boundaries
Honesty	Self-determination	
Integrity	Safety	Gratitude
Nondiscrimination	Fair treatment	Veracity
Selfless service	Honest advertising	Reparation
Unconditional regard for others	Best effort of massage therapist	Fidelity
		Trustworthy
	Massage Therapist	
	Fair compensation	
	Respect	
	Safe environment	
	Practice policies	

For example, given that clients have a right to a safe environment when receiving massage, massage therapists have a duty to keep their spaces clean and remove potential safety hazards.

Duties related to being a health professional include *nonmaleficence* (refraining from harming anyone), *beneficence* (doing good for those in our care), *fidelity* (keeping promises—explicit or implicit), and *veracity* (telling the truth). Causing harm or wrong to someone else calls for *reparations*, whereas *gratitude* is due when someone is good to us.[6]

Just as with values and rights, there is no finite list of duties for massage therapists. However, the concept of duties is useful when discussing ethical behavior for two reasons. First, duties have the weight of moral obligations. Second, when values, rights, and duties are in conflict, creating an ethical dilemma, critical thinking about such a situation calls for consideration of all sides of the issue, including the duties involved. Table 5-1 ■ lists many of the foundation values, rights, and duties on which ethical principles are based.

VULNERABILITY TO UNETHICAL BEHAVIOR

Almost everyone considers him- or herself a moral, ethical person. However, if people are honest with themselves, everyone can think of instances when they didn't live up to ethical standards, or, in retrospect, would have acted differently (i.e., more ethically) in a given situation. Admitting our human vulnerability and making a conscious commitment to be ethical massage therapists is the first step on the path to building ethical practices.

The next step is to learn about ethical standards in the profession and take them seriously. Ignorance of ethical standards leaves one vulnerable to unethical behavior. Codes of ethics and standards of practice are documents that open the door to discussion of ethical issues in the profession. They should be familiar to all massage and bodywork practitioners. Codes of ethics and standards of practice are discussed further in the next section.

A key principle for behaving ethically is to hold your client's well-being above your own personal gain. This principle is sometimes expressed as "selfless service." This does not mean that you work for free because you have a right to make a living as a massage therapist. It means that when making decisions that might affect your clients' well-being, you do nothing that has the potential to cause them harm, even if for you it means a loss of money, power, or other desirable gain. For example, you do not expose your clients to illness by dragging yourself to work when you are contagious with the flu.

For personal ethical development, it is important to know your weaknesses as well as your strengths. Issues related to money, power, and sex are the usual culprits in unethical decisions. But less obvious roots of unethical behavior might be found in a need to feel loved and accepted, a need to be right, a lack of assertiveness, or even sloppy bookkeeping. Unexamined personal issues may also trip you up in the therapeutic relationship, for example, transference and countertransference, in which negative or positive feelings toward someone in a person's past are brought into the therapeutic relationship by either the client or therapist. Transference and countertransference are discussed in greater detail later in this chapter.

Self-care in all facets of life lessens vulnerability to unethical behavior. Wellness in the physical, mental, emotional, social, spiritual, and financial realms is a foundation for clear, ethical thinking. Even good time management plays a role because caregiver burnout can lead to poor judgment when making decisions.

Lack of skill in ethical decision making also leaves one vulnerable. Knowing standards and possessing the ability to apply them in specific situations are very different. It is also harder to think clearly when in the midst of difficult or emotional circumstances. Practicing the steps in ethical decision making in simpler situations is good preparation for the more difficult and complex issues that come up. The process of ethical decision making is explained in more detail in a later section.

ETHICAL CODES AND STANDARDS

Most major professional organizations for massage therapists have published codes of ethics, and some have developed standards of practice. **Codes of ethics** are usually stated in broad terms as general principles that reflect commonly held values. **Standards of practice** are longer, more detailed documents that go into specifics in interpreting ethical principles. These documents can be found on organization websites.

Ethical codes and standards are the products of the collective thinking of a group of professionals. They take into consideration the traditional values and recognized clients' rights related to the profession. These ethics documents are updated from time to time to reflect current issues and new awareness. As ethical understanding evolves, so do the documents that codify the latest thinking on the subject.

Professional organizations organize and display their codes of ethics differently. Some go into more detail than others in a combined codes/standards document. However, the values and clients' rights contained in the codes are very similar. The summary of ethical principles for massage therapists found in Box 5–1 ∎ is based on the major common themes from current massage therapy organization codes of ethics.

The summary of ethical principles is a good overview for discussing ethics for entry-level massage therapists. Some items present general principles that can be expanded (e.g., "Give your best effort to each client"), and others describe specific behavior (e.g., "Refrain from alcohol and recreational drugs when performing massage") to give more pointed direction. This list can be used along with other codes and standards in ethical decision making.

ETHICS AND LAW

Ethics and law are related but are not the same. Both ethics and law are based on values, rights, and duties recognized by a community, but they are enacted and enforced in different ways by different entities.

Professional ethics are the province of associations, which adopt codes of behavior related to the practice of the profession. These are enforced within the group, usually by disciplinary action against members who violate the accepted code of behavior. Disciplinary actions for ethical code violations generally range from letters of reprimand, to probation, to suspension of membership for a period of time, to cancellation of membership in the organization. The decision usually follows a hearing in which the accused is given the opportunity to defend him- or herself. This enforcement of values within the group is referred to as *self-regulation* within a profession.

Laws, on the other hand, are passed by governmental bodies at the local, state, and federal levels to protect the public from harm or to ensure fair practices. Laws are usually only passed when there is a compelling public reason. Violations of law are determined by a judge or by trial and are punishable by fines, community service, or time in jail.

Some of the ethical principles recognized by professional associations have been given the force of law. An example is the federal HIPAA privacy law that ensures confidentiality of medical records. This law lifts the ethical principle of confidentiality to a legal status and specifies what that means under federal law.

BOX 5–1   Summary of Ethical Principles for Massage Therapists

Massage Therapist

1. Give your best effort to each client.
2. Hold your clients' well-being above your own personal gain.
3. Present a professional image.
4. Present your credentials honestly.
5. Perform only those services for which you are trained and qualified.
6. Stay within your legal scope of practice.
7. Refrain from alcohol and recreational drugs when performing massage.
8. Keep licenses to practice massage therapy current.
9. Stay up-to-date in your field through continued education.

Therapeutic Relationship

10. Set clear professional boundaries with clients.
11. Treat all clients equally with courtesy and respect.
12. Honor your clients' physical, intellectual, and emotional boundaries.
13. Practice good draping skills for client privacy and comfort.
14. Get clients' informed voluntary consent for all massage therapy performed and for touching sensitive body areas.
15. Do not perform massage when it is contraindicated for a client.
16. Acknowledge your limitations, and refer clients to other health care professionals as appropriate.
17. Keep your professional and social lives separate.
18. Do not engage in sexual activities with clients or sexualize a massage session in any way.
19. Keep your clients' information confidential.

Business Practices

20. Do not make claims for massage therapy that are not true or that you cannot reasonably defend.
21. Do not sell or recommend health products or services outside your area of expertise.
22. Develop written policies about time and money, and make sure clients understand them.
23. Keep the massage room, equipment, and yourself sanitary.
24. Do not solicit tips directly.
25. Keep accurate client and financial records.
26. Abide by all local and state laws related to your practice.

Note: Based on the codes of ethics of major massage therapy organizations (American Massage Therapy Association—AMTA; American Organization for Bodywork Therapies of Asia—AOBTA; Associated Bodywork and Massage Professionals—ABMP, National Certification Board for Therapeutic Massage & Bodywork—NCBTMB).

In addition, laws licensing massage therapists usually have sections dealing with ethical issues. For example, the Illinois Massage Licensing Act, Section 45, Grounds for Discipline, prohibits "advertising in a false, deceptive, or misleading manner," and "making any misrepresentation for the purpose of obtaining a license." If convicted of an offense, a massage therapist licensed in Illinois can be assessed a fine, be put on probation, or have his or her license suspended or revoked. Disciplinary actions are matters of public record. Currently 44 states plus Washington, DC, in the United States have similar provisions for regulating massage therapists. Whereas violations of an association's code of ethics can result in censure by the organization, violations of the law can lead to losing a license, paying fines, and/or spending time in jail.

Another connection between professional ethics and law is found in legal cases where the standard of behavior is based on the accepted practices in the profession. An example would be a massage therapist who is being sued for injury to a client during a massage session. If by professional standards the massage therapist should have known about a contraindication for the massage technique used, or if it was outside the therapist's scope of practice, then the judgment may be in favor of the person making the complaint. In other words, the judge may use a recognized professional standard to decide a case when no specific law pertains to the situation.

ETHICAL DECISION MAKING

Massage therapists make ethical decisions every day. Most are small, uncomplicated issues such as keeping client records secure, staying within the scope of practice, and giving their best effort to each client. Other situations can be complex and pose a dilemma about the best way to act. The ethical decision-making model explained next provides a step-by-step method of sorting out the answers to ethical questions and dilemmas.

Ethical Questions and Dilemmas

Ethical issues are most often framed like questions; for example, "Is it ethical to . . . .? **Ethical questions** are frequently followed by qualifiers; for example, "Is it ethical to (do something), if (this is the situation)? Many ethical questions can be answered by reviewing a code of ethics or standard of practice to find the profession's view of the subject. However, as in all complex human interactions, the variables of the situation can influence a decision and make it a judgment call.

It is important to distinguish between ethical questions and legal questions. As mentioned before, something

may be quite legal, but unethical by professional standards. However, if something is illegal, it is automatically unethical because an all-encompassing ethical principle is to abide by all local, state, and federal laws related to the practice of massage.

Ethical dilemmas occur "when two or more principles are in conflict, and regardless of your choice, something of value is compromised."[7] Put another way, no matter what you do, some harm will result or some good not happen. The solution to an ethical dilemma is in selecting the lesser harm or greater good.

Ethical dilemmas are in a different league than **personal temptations** to act unethically. For example, it may be a personal temptation to mix your social and professional lives, and that may be a personal dilemma ("What am I going to do?"), but it is not an ethical dilemma ("What is the most ethical action to take?"). Those are two different questions.

Temptations often involve time and/or money. Working when sick, skimping on hygiene, not completing session notes, constantly arriving late for appointments, and keeping a client who should be referred to another health professional are all personal temptations. These should take a backseat to doing what is best for the client.

The Ethical Decision-Making Model

The **ethical decision-making model** is a step-by-step process of thinking through an ethical question or ethical dilemma. It involves critical thinking because you are analyzing the situation and taking into consideration your own motivations and biases. Both external standards, like codes of ethics and laws, and internal standards, like your own sense of right and wrong, play a part. It is essentially a problem-solving process for an ethical situation.

A 10-step ethical decision-making model is summarized in Box 5–2 ■. Although the model is listed in steps, implying a linear sequential process, it is best thought of as a logical process that proceeds in an orderly manner. Information may be gathered, and steps revisited, at any time. For Step 9, selecting the course of action, it is useful to review the information gathered in Steps 1 through 8 to have a full picture of the situation.

The first step in ethical decision making is to define the ethical question or ethical dilemma. Remember that some choices are not ethical questions if no moral principle is involved. It might simply be a business decision or choice

CRITICAL THINKING

Examine a code of ethics or standards of practice document for massage and bodywork therapists. Analyze the underlying values, rights, and duties for each item.

1. Do some values, rights, or duties appear more than others?

2. Are there any relationships among these values, rights, and duties?

3. What does your analysis say about the ethical principles most important to massage therapists?

between two plans of action. Frame the situation by filling in the blanks: "Is it ethical to . . . (do something), if . . . (this is the situation)?" or "Is it more ethical to . . . (do something), or to . . . (do something else)?"

BOX 5–2   Ethical Decision-Making Model

Step 1   Define the ethical question or ethical dilemma.
"Is it ethical to . . . (do something), if . . . (if this is the situation)?"
"Is it more ethical to . . . (do something), or to . . . (do something else)?"

Step 2   Determine if this is also a legal issue.
Consumer protection laws
Privacy laws (e.g., HIPAA)
Licensing laws
Other laws (e.g., zoning)

Step 3   Identify values, rights, and professional standards that apply.
What values or rights are involved?
Is this situation mentioned in a code of ethics or standard of practice?
Does an employer policy apply to the situation?

Step 4   List the people who might be affected by the outcome of the decision.

Step 5   List alternative courses of action.

Step 6   Identify the most important values, rights, standards, and other considerations.
Is there an overriding principle that applies (e.g., do no harm, selfless service, abide by laws)?

Step 7   Identify your own motivations or interest in the outcome, and any personal temptations.

Step 8   Consider advice from others.
Consult colleagues or former teachers or an association
Consult coworkers or work supervisors
Consult a professional supervisor

Step 9   Select the course of action that maintains the highest values, or that results in the greatest good with the least harm. Do the right thing.

Step 10   Evaluate the consequences of your decision, and learn from your experience.

Next, determine if this is also a legal issue. Some situations are covered by consumer protection, privacy, licensing, zoning, or other laws. The overriding principle of abiding by local, state, and federal law may apply.

Identify the values, rights, and professional standards relevant to the situation. For example, is it a matter of honesty, integrity, beneficence, fairness, or privacy? Look through the professional codes of ethics and standards of practice for massage therapists to see if the ethical question is covered. If the situation is not specifically mentioned, is there a relevant principle, value, or right that can be applied in this case?

List the people who might be affected by the decision. They might include yourself, the client, the client's family or friends, your family and friends, coworkers, employers, or landlords. Remember that actions can have ripple effects.

List alternative courses of action. Include all possibilities even if you reject them later; they may suggest new approaches you had not thought of at first. Consider creative solutions to the problem that preserve important values or rights.

Identify the most important values, rights, standards, and other considerations. This is especially important in ethical dilemmas where competing values or rights are at stake. An overriding principle, such as "do no harm" or "abide by the law," may apply.

Before you choose an action, identify your own motivations or interest in the outcome. Look at your personal temptations related to time, money, power, or social advantage. Remember the overriding principle to "hold the client's well-being above your own personal gain."

Consult with others to get a more objective view of the situation, generate more options for actions, and check your own biases and temptations. Sometimes just talking it through with someone else can help you see things more clearly. People familiar with professional ethics and who have experience in the field are especially good to consult. They may have dealt with similar problems in the past and can help you sort out alternatives.

In the end, you have to decide what to do. Base your choice on the action you think will maintain the highest values, or that will result in the greatest good with the least harm. Then do the right thing. Knowing what to do and actually doing it are two different things. Get emotional support if you need it.

PRACTICAL APPLICATION

An important way to learn ethical behavior and how to navigate ethical issues is by observing others who model ethical conduct. Interview a practicing massage therapist about his or her most memorable ethical issue or dilemma. Not only listen to the massage therapist's narrative, but also observe the body language while this person describes the ethical decision and its consequences.

Questions to consider:

1. What was the ethical question?
2. What were the most important factors in the situation?
3. What were the consequences of the therapist's actions?
4. Do you think this massage therapist handled the issue appropriately and made the best ethical decision? Why?

CASE FOR STUDY

Twila and the Flu

Twila works as a part-time massage therapist at a day spa. She woke up on Tuesday feeling weak and sick to her stomach. She was running a mild fever. Several people in her family had the flu over the past week, and she thought she might be coming down with it, too. Twila is a responsible person and did not want to miss the four massage appointments scheduled for the day. She also did not want to lose the income if she stayed home from work.

Question:

Is it ethical for Twila to take some over-the-counter medicine to reduce her symptoms and help her get through her massage appointments?

Things to consider:

- Is this situation covered in a code of ethics or standard of practice for massage therapists?
- What is Twila's responsibility to her clients in terms of their health and safety?
- Who might be affected by Twila's decision?
- What are the "worst-case" and "best-case" scenarios?
- What are her alternative courses of action?
- What would her supervisor advise her to do?
- What are the most important considerations in this situation?
- What decision would result in the greatest good with the least harm?

Your Reasoning and Conclusions:

_____

_____

_____

_____

Finally, learn from the outcome. The end result will help you judge whether your decision was the best. Analyze the consequences of your decision. Did it uphold the values or rights as you thought it would? Was there something you didn't take into consideration that you should have? Were there any surprises? Would you do it differently next time?

Learn from your successes and your mistakes. You will get better at making ethical decisions with experience. Examples of ethical decision making related to the therapeutic relationship are discussed later in the chapter.

DEVELOPMENT OF ETHICAL JUDGMENT

The development of **ethical judgment**, that is, consistency in making good ethical decisions, is a lifelong process. Just being aware that decisions might have ethical consequences is important. Ethical behavior is strengthened by continued learning, including learning from successes and mistakes. Ethical judgment improves with critical thinking and evaluating results. See Figure 5–2 ■.

Codes of ethics can be framed and hung in offices to show a commitment to ethics in a practice. Keeping a code of ethics and standards of practice for massage therapists on file for reference makes it easier to consult when an issue arises.

Some licensing laws and certification programs require continuing education in ethics for renewal. Classes in ethics are offered through massage schools and by professional associations. Classes in ethics for health professionals and business ethics classes offer a wider perspective on the subject.

Networking with other massage therapists in professional associations increases awareness of ethical issues that come up in practices and consequences of certain actions. Reading professional journals helps massage therapists keep up-to-date on the latest thinking about ethical issues. Reports on individual cases dealing with ethics can be instructive.

Clinical supervision involves consultation about different issues that come up in the therapeutic relationship. It is

FIGURE 5–2 Good ethical judgment comes from both learning and experience.

Source: Pearson Education, Inc./Segal Photography.

done in a formal setting with a specially trained supervisor. Clinical supervision is an idea borrowed from mental health professionals that is catching on in the massage and body-work community. Supervision sessions are an opportunity for massage therapists to process what is happening in their practices and their experiences with clients.

Group supervision of practitioners in similar circumstances can be especially useful. "In a group setting clinical supervision undertakes four functions: (1) addressing the relationship issues that arise between clients and practitioners; (2) functioning as a support group for the participants; (3) serving as a forum for didactic instruction on important psychological concepts (such as projection, transference, countertransference); and (4) training the participants in supervisory skills so that they feel confident continuing this helpful type of coaching by themselves at a later date without a supervisor."[8]

Good ethical judgment comes with learning and experience. Mistakes will most likely happen along the way. There might be errors in judgment or lapses of moral behavior. The important thing is to make a commitment to ethical behavior as a massage therapist, learn from successes and failures, and reenergize your ethical sense from time to time throughout your career.

THE THERAPEUTIC RELATIONSHIP

The **therapeutic relationship** begins when a client seeks greater well-being through massage from a particular massage therapist, and the massage therapist agrees to provide that service. It is a special relationship based on specific roles and responsibilities.

In nonmedical settings such as spas and health clubs, the relationship is *therapeutic* in a more general sense in that the goals are the improved health and well-being of the client. In clinical settings, the therapeutic relationship may be part of the treatment itself and a key to the healing process. "The most healing aspect of a series or course of massage therapy sessions, especially in the longer term, can be the relationship between client and therapist. The massage therapist can facilitate this through building a trusting relationship by being non-judgmental, reliable, and supportive."[9]

Therapeutic relationships are very different from social relationships (e.g., between friends) and have a deeper dimension than simple business transactions. The therapeutic relationship in massage therapy is more intimate and personal than relationships in most commercial settings because clients are seeking help for their personal well-being from a service based on touch.

The intimacy in massage therapy is *physical* because it involves caring touch; *emotional*, as feelings of support and closeness develop; and *verbal* because there is disclosure of personal information. However, the appropriate intimacy in the therapeutic relationship is one-way.

Practitioners physically touch their clients, allow them to disclose thoughts and feelings, and offer both verbal

and physical support. The therapeutic relationship's function is not for the clients to do the same for the practitioner.[10]

There is also an inherent **power differential** between massage therapists and their clients in therapeutic relationships. That is, massage therapists have more power in the relationships by virtue of their training and experience, and by their being in a position of authority (Figure 5–3 ■). It is similar to other familiar relationships such as teacher–student, boss–employee, and nurse–patient. "Even if the massage therapist does not want or seek out power, clients still ascribe power to the therapist because power *is an intrinsic element in the therapist–client relationship*."[11]

Our clients come to us in pain or in need of help. Just by showing up at our offices, they make themselves vulnerable. They are hurting, and we are the authority. Even though they may not be conscious of it, we can become a doctor/parent figure in their eyes. Our responsibility is to meet that vulnerability with respect and kindness.[12]

The massage therapist, therefore, has a fiduciary responsibility in the therapeutic relationship. *Fiduciary* is a legal term used to describe a relationship in which person A has placed a special trust in person B, who is then obligated to watch out for person A's best interests. In other words, the client puts a special trust in the massage therapist, who is then obligated to look out for the client's best interests.

There are both explicit and implicit agreements in the therapeutic relationship. Explicit agreements are spoken or written and include things such as pricing information, payment policies, cancellation policies, and the type of massage and bodywork provided. Implicit agreements are those commonly understood for this type of relationship, which may be unspoken and unwritten. These include being on

FIGURE 5–3 There is an inherent power differential between massage therapists and their clients.

Source: Pearson Education, Inc.

time, doing no harm, acting in the best interest of the client, keeping client information confidential, providing a safe environment, and staying within the scope of practice.

When a client comes for massage, there is an implicit understanding that the massage therapist is upholding the standards of the profession. These standards are found in codes of ethics and standards of practice documents that outline what is expected of competent and ethical massage therapists.

As in any relationship, human interactions in the therapeutic relationship can be influenced by psychological factors. Massage therapists can learn to recognize those factors at work in their relationships with clients. In addition to improving the quality of their therapeutic relationships, awareness of the potential influence of psychological factors can help massage therapists make better ethical choices. Two factors with great potential to influence therapeutic relationships are transference and countertransference.

Transference and Countertransference

Transference occurs when a client transfers negative or positive feelings toward someone from his or her past into the therapeutic relationship. The feelings transferred would typically be about an authority figure such as a parent, teacher, or other person important to the client when he or she was growing up. Transference has been called "a kind of spell generated by one's own psyche," with the result that the client "cannot see the therapist and/or the therapy as they actually are."[13]

A client who is experiencing *positive transference* projects good feelings toward the massage therapist. Positive transference can contribute to the therapeutic relationship by opening the door to acceptance, cooperation, and trust.

However, positive transference can also blind the client. For example, the client might place the massage therapist on a pedestal, thinking the therapist to be more knowledgeable than he or she actually is, or try too hard to please the therapist, or be overly submissive. A client in positive transference might give inappropriate gifts, or want to step over the line into a social or romantic relationship. The danger in positive transference is the temptation for massage therapists to relax professional boundaries, or to lose sight of who they (the massage therapists) really are.

Negative transference, or the projection of negative or bad feelings into the therapeutic relationship, can cause more obvious problems. A client thinking that the massage therapist doesn't like her, feeling like she just can't please the massage therapist, trying to argue with the massage therapist, or thinking that the massage therapist doesn't know what he or she is doing, all work against the massage therapy itself. If it is a case of transference, these negative thoughts and feelings have nothing to do with the reality of the situation with the massage therapist, but have been transferred from another relationship in the past.

Because massage therapists are not trained as psychotherapists, cases of positive and negative transference may be hard for them to identify. Suspect transference if you are uncomfortable with a client's behavior, and you can say to yourself, "Her reaction doesn't make sense," or "This is not about me," or "This is not about this therapeutic relationship." When going through an ethical decision-making process as described earlier in the chapter, take the possibility of transference into consideration.

The best strategy when faced with a client's transference is to maintain your objectivity through critical thinking and getting someone else's viewpoint. Do not try to analyze your client's behavior, which is outside your scope of practice. Keep good professional boundaries.

Countertransference occurs when massage therapists transfer positive or negative feelings toward others from their pasts into the therapeutic relationship. In this case, the massage therapists do not see the clients or the therapeutic situations as they really are; their judgment is clouded. Trying too hard to please clients, relaxing professional boundaries against better judgment, and feeling more knowledgeable or powerful than they really are exemplify countertransference by massage therapists.

Being confident in your role as a massage therapist, and in your own thoughts and feelings, helps minimize the effects of countertransference. Because it is an unconscious response, however, countertransference is difficult to detect in ourselves. Personal awareness, peer advice, and professional supervision can help sort out issues of transference and countertransference.

Defense Mechanisms

Defense mechanisms are behaviors or thoughts that help us cope with unwanted feelings such as fear, anxiety, guilt, and anger. Both massage therapists and clients bring their defense mechanisms into the therapeutic relationship. These defenses can be amplified when receiving bodywork. Common defense mechanisms are projection, denial, repression, displacement, and resistance. Although there are subtle differences in these mechanisms, their common purpose is to protect the psyche from unwanted feelings.

Projection occurs when someone imputes to someone else a behavior that they themselves are doing or a feeling that they are having. For example, a massage therapist who is attracted to a client might suppress that feeling within him- or herself and instead perceive the client as seductive. Or a client may think of a massage therapist as a "know-it-all" instead of acknowledging his or her own feelings of superiority.

Denial is blocking out the existence of an unwanted feeling or refusing to recognize the reality of a situation. For example, a massage therapist may not recognize that a valued client is taking advantage of him or her by frequently canceling at the last minute. Fear of losing the client may create a situation of denial. Or because of fear, a client may be unwilling to admit to him- or herself the pain he or she is feeling and therefore not give useful feedback about pressure during a massage session.

Repression involves burying unwanted feelings, for example, by erasing them from conscious memory or not allowing them to be felt. Repressed feelings can cause anxiety and depression unless and until they surface and are resolved. Either the massage therapist or client may have repressed feelings from past events or trauma.

Displacement is reacting to a feeling generated by a person or situation by acting out toward someone else or in different situation. For example, bringing anger from something that happened at home or in your private life into the workplace is displacement. You're angry with your best friend, and you take it out on a coworker—that is displacement.

Resistance occurs when a client refuses to cooperate or fails to participate in plans for his or her well-being. Resistance is usually unconscious and can take many forms, such as being unable to relax during a massage, missing appointments, or forgetting suggestions for self-massage at home. Resistance would be something that comes up with regular clients, or those coming for a series of massage sessions as treatment for a condition.

The resistance might have nothing to do with the massage therapist, but could be due to some other factor, such as failure to commit to the therapeutic process. It is not massage therapists' place to judge their clients' behavior, but just noticing resistance and bringing up observations with clients can be enough to bring it to a conscious level for resolution.

Defense mechanisms can cause problems in therapeutic relationships because they tend to deflect attention from the reality of a situation. The key is not to eliminate them (a near impossible task because they are habitual behaviors), but to recognize them when they surface and minimize their negative impact. Seeing through defense mechanisms can help massage therapists build healthier therapeutic relationships and avoid unethical behavior.

ROLES AND BOUNDARIES

Both massage therapists and clients have specific roles to play in the therapeutic relationship. The massage therapists' general role is to apply their training and experience within their scope and standards of practice to help clients meet their health goals. The clients' general role is to provide relevant information, participate cooperatively in massage therapy sessions, abide by policies and procedures, and pay the fees.

Professional boundaries maintain these roles within therapeutic relationships. As explained in detail in Chapter 3, *Professional and Personal Development*, these include physical, emotional, intellectual, sexual, and energetic limits on what will and will not happen between the massage therapist and client. It is the massage therapist's responsibility to create the framework that defines these boundaries, for example, with policies, rules, procedures, and the whole massage environment into which clients walk.

Practical aspects of maintaining professional boundaries are discussed further in sections on dual relationships, sexual misconduct, and scope of practice found later in this chapter.

In addition to professional boundaries, massage therapists and clients have personal boundaries that must be respected. A **personal boundary** is a limit established by a person to maintain his or her own integrity, comfort, or well-being. For example, a client may ask a massage therapist not to touch his feet or not to use oil with a fragrance. Or a massage therapist may prefer handshakes to hugs or refuse to use petroleum-based oil. These are legitimate personal boundaries.

The *NCBTMB Code of Ethics* (see Appendix B) directs massage therapists to "respect the client's boundaries with regard to privacy, disclosure, exposure, emotional expression, beliefs, and the client's reasonable expectations of professional behavior. Practitioners will respect the client's autonomy." That includes the client's right to set personal boundaries.

"Stepping over the line," or boundary crossings and violations, can be ethical matters if they harm the therapeutic relationship or the individuals involved. A **boundary crossing** has been defined as "a transgression that may or may not be experienced as harmful," whereas a *boundary violation* "is a harmful transgression of a boundary."[14] So whether a boundary transgression is a crossing or a violation is a matter of degree and a matter of consequences. If a boundary crossing is not experienced as harmful, then it does not rise to the level of a violation, although it can be problematic. Boundary crossings can be annoying, intrusive, hurtful, or just uncomfortable. For example, a client answering a cell phone during a massage session might be annoying. A massage therapist may ask a client a question that seems intrusive or too personal. Or a client may be uncomfortable with a massage therapist massaging her neck but says nothing about it. These are examples of boundary crossings but probably not violations.

Violations leave one with a sense of being *violated*, a much stronger feeling than just feeling annoyed or uncomfortable. Integrity is compromised in some way, and the agreement within the therapeutic relationship is broken. Examples of boundary violations include a client who learns that the massage therapist talked to someone else about his or her medical condition without permission; a massage therapist whose client calls him or her at home to ask for a date; or a massage therapist touching a part of the body he or she was asked not to touch or for which there is an implicit agreement to avoid, such as a woman's breasts.

All professional and personal boundary violations are unethical because some harm has been done. Even unintentional harm is still harm and may have adverse consequences. At minimum, there will be negative consequences to the therapeutic relationship, and there may also be personal, professional, employment, or legal repercussions.

The majority of client complaints about massage therapists typically fall into two general categories of boundary violations: (1) blurring professional and social roles, and (2) going beyond their expertise and training.[15]

DUAL RELATIONSHIPS

A **dual relationship** means that in addition to the therapeutic relationship, there are other social or professional connections between a client and a massage therapist. This applies to clients who are also family members, friends, coworkers, neighbors, fellow organization members, service providers such as accountants and plumbers, or any other additional relationship.

In some cases a dual relationship can enhance a therapeutic relationship. This works if the two people involved are emotionally mature and able to keep their roles in different situations separate. For example, the familiarity between friends can give the massage therapist greater insight into what the client–friend is experiencing. However, a friend who becomes a client would have to agree to the role of a client during massage sessions and be comfortable with the appropriate professional boundaries set for that time. The same would apply to the massage therapist, who would have to set aside his or her own needs and wants and keep to a professional role during the massage time.

In reality, most dual relationships have problematic dimensions. Issues are magnified if the power differential between the client and massage therapist varies in different situations. For example, in a client–neighbor dual relationship, the massage therapist holds a power role during massage sessions, but is an equal outside the sessions. Or in a client–family member situation, family dynamics may come into play and affect the therapeutic relationship.

Financial or economic arrangements outside the massage therapy relationship have their own potential problems. Two common scenarios involve bartering and employment. Bartering for services, such as accounting or website design, can be a mutually beneficial arrangement as long as both parties feel that they are getting a fair deal and follow through on their agreement. The exchange might be hour for hour, or session for session, regardless of time involved. Or for an accountant, it might be six massage sessions for doing the massage therapist's taxes for the year. A verbal contract for bartering needs to be crystal clear to avoid someone feeling taken advantage of. Exchanging invoices for services can reduce the potential for misunderstandings.

Being a massage therapist to a boss or an employee also calls for very clear boundaries because the power differential changes with the different roles. In the boss–client scenario, the boss is in a position of authority in the workplace, whereas during massage therapy, the practitioner is in charge. As long as both people can accept their roles in the different situations, the arrangement can work. However, it can become awkward if something happens that crosses boundaries, such as your boss asking you for information about your coworker while he or she is getting a massage.

Perhaps the most difficult lines to draw are those about socializing with clients. Degrees of socializing range from a cup of tea before a massage session, to meeting for coffee outside the massage setting, to belonging to the same club or organization, to attending events together. Ethical issues that might come up during socializing are failing to protect other clients' confidentiality and offering too much self-disclosure about the massage therapist's personal life.

As mentioned previously, when people known in social settings become clients, strong professional boundaries can minimize problems. However, when a current client initiates a social invitation, a massage therapist must take into consideration the possibility of transference and consequences for the therapeutic relationship. The risk may outweigh any benefits, and romantic or sexual socializing would be unethical, as is explained in more detail later in this chapter. A massage therapist whose personal social circle is heavily populated by clients is taking advantage of his or her practice for the wrong reasons. It is obvious that the variety of dual relationships is endless, and each one needs to be thought through carefully.

Evaluating Dual Relationships

For a massage therapist, deciding whether to enter into a dual relationship with a client, or to continue one already established, requires evaluating the potential benefits and risks. As the person in authority in the therapeutic relationship, it is the massage therapist's responsibility to make decisions in the best interest of the client. It is unethical to enter into or continue a dual relationship if there is high potential of harm to either party or if the therapeutic relationship will be compromised.

One factor for consideration is the nature of the relationships involved. Are there conflicting power differentials? Do they involve money, friendship, love? Are they of short or long duration? Another factor is the maturity of the people involved. Are they good at keeping boundaries and cooperative in respecting limits? Do both parties understand the complexities involved? Experience says that both people involved must agree to the arrangement, understand the potential pitfalls, and be willing to end the dual relationship if necessary.

Motivations for entering into the dual relationship need to be scrutinized. Does one party benefit at the possible expense of the other? Is there a possibility of transference or countertransference clouding the reality of the situation? Professional standards can help in certain situations, for example, the special case of sexual relationships, which is discussed in the next section.

The potential effects of the dual relationship on the therapeutic relationship are important to consider. Can both parties maintain their respective roles as massage therapist and client in relation to massage sessions?

"Worst-case" and "best-case" exercises are useful for making decisions about dual relationships. For example, a best-case scenario for a dual relationship in which the massage therapist hires a mechanic/client to repair his or her car is that the car gets fixed satisfactorily, and the therapeutic relationship continues unaffected. A worst-case scenario might be that the mechanic damages the engine and refuses to make fair compensation. Negative feelings from that scenario are likely to affect the therapeutic relationship and possibly damage it permanently. The question to ask is this: Is hiring the client worth the risk, or can someone else do the job just as well without the complicating factor?

A good question for a massage therapist to ask him- or herself is, "If this dual relationship does not work out . . . am I willing to lose this person as a client? Or, am I willing to lose this person as a beautician (or accountant, friend, etc.)? Am I willing to jeopardize my other job (or membership in an organization, etc.)?" It is important not to underestimate the possible consequences of the dual relationship, but to enter into such relationships with thoughtfulness and clear vision. This is another case where discussing the situation with someone familiar with the complexities of dual relationships would be useful, for example, with a colleague, supervisor, or other professional.

SEXUAL RELATIONSHIPS

There are two general scenarios for professional relationships involving sexual partners. One is when a current client wants to become romantically or sexually involved with the massage therapist (and vice versa), and the other is when a current spouse or romantic friend becomes a client. These are two very different situations with different ethical considerations.

First of all, it should be noted that sexual activity with a client is strictly prohibited by professional standards and by massage therapist licensing laws. The *NCBTMB Code of Ethics* states that massage and bodywork practitioners should "refrain, under all circumstances, from initiating or engaging in any sexual conduct, sexual activities, or sexualizing behavior involving a client, even if the client attempts to sexualize the relationship."

REALITY CHECK

DENISE

YOLANDA: I find it hard to stick to boundaries in my relationships with clients. I'm just an outgoing person who wants to be friends with people. A client asked me out for coffee the other day because we're both interested in environmental issues. If I didn't already have other plans, I might have gone. How do you handle this kind of situation?

DENISE: I really try to keep my professional and personal lives separate. I've learned from experience that socializing with clients isn't best for my practice or my social life either. When clients walk in the door, I focus on meeting their needs and goals within massage therapy. It's true that sometimes you pass up the opportunity to know some really interesting people better, but keeping good boundaries helps me stay clear about what I am doing here as a massage therapist. And I've found plenty of other friends outside of my professional life. Think of a polite way to refuse this kind of invitation like "Thank you for asking, but this isn't a good time."

CASE FOR STUDY

Rebecca and the Movie Invitation

Rebecca graduated from massage school and got a job at a local health club working part-time. She likes to exercise and stay fit, so the setting was perfect for her. Dan comes to the health club to work out several times a week and gets a massage regularly. He enjoys Rebecca's massage, so lately he has been going to her exclusively. They are both single and like each other. Dan asked her to go with him to a movie they both wanted to see.

Question:

Is it ethical for Rebecca to go with Dan to the movie?

Things to consider:

- Does the health club have a policy about staff dating members?
- Is this situation covered in a code of ethics or standards of practice for massage therapists?

- Who might be affected by this decision?
- What are the "worst-case" and "best-case" scenarios?
- What are alternative courses of action?
- What are the most important considerations in this situation?
- What might Rebecca's motivation be for accepting the invitation? Declining it?
- What would a former teacher advise Rebecca to do?
- What decision would maintain the highest standards?

Your Reasoning and Conclusions:

_____

_____

_____

_____

That means no dating or even socializing with clients who have romantic intentions. The power differential in the therapeutic relationship and the possibility of transference or other psychological factors having an influence make it unethical to enter into such a relationship. It can be dangerous emotionally for one or both parties and distorts the therapeutic relationship.

The *NCBTMB Standards of Practice*, however, offers a solution for special cases that would minimize the dangers involved (see Appendix B). It states that the massage practitioner should "refrain from participating in a sexual relationship or sexual conduct with a client, whether consensual or otherwise, from the beginning of the client/therapist relationship and for a minimum of six months after the termination of the client–therapist relationship." It also makes allowances for preexisting relationships. The general ethical principle is to end the therapeutic relationship and wait for a period of time before beginning the romantic/sexual relationship. Waiting clearly separates the roles in time and provides perspective on the situation.

Developing a romantic relationship with someone special, who just happens to be a former client, can be perfectly ethical. However, dating a current client or regularly dating former clients is clearly considered unethical by professional standards.

If someone who is *already* a spouse, significant other, boyfriend or girlfriend, or a romantic or sexual partner later becomes a client, clear boundaries are a must. In addition to power issues coming into the therapeutic relationship, there is the potential for the association of massage therapy with sexual activity. During time set aside for massage therapy, there is no place whatsoever for sexual activity.

Engaging in sexual behavior during a time set aside for massage therapy, and especially on a massage table or in a space set aside for massage practice, is confusing on many levels even if the person is a spouse. Why? For the massage therapist, his or her professional role strictly prohibits sexual activity with a client, and so the situation is a blurring of roles. For the client–spouse, the association is made between massage therapy and sex, so he or she may feel uneasy, often unconsciously, about what his or her partner–therapist is doing with other clients. A clear separation of massage therapy and sexual activity in time and space is the only workable approach.

SEXUAL MISCONDUCT

Sexual misconduct involves any sexualizing of the relationship between a massage therapist and a current client. Sexual misconduct can occur before, after, or during a massage session and can be perpetrated by the massage therapist or by the client.

Forms of sexual misconduct range from those involving speech and body language to inappropriate touch to sexual contact to sexual assault. Box 5–3 ■ lists categories and examples of sexual misconduct encountered in massage practices.

BOX 5–3   **Forms of Sexual Misconduct**

Categories of sexual misconduct that grow progressively more serious:

- No touch involved: suggestive speech and body language
- Inappropriate touch involved
- Direct sexual contact
- Sexual assault

Examples of sexual misconduct of clients and massage therapists that grow progressively more serious:

Client

Flirting
Use of slang or crude words referring to the genitalia
Jokes with sexual content or innuendo
Talk about personal sexual experiences or problems
Seductive speech
Exposes his or her genitalia; woman exposes her breasts
Asks for sexual favors
⇓

Touches the massage therapist on thigh or buttocks seductively
Stimulates him- or herself sexually during massage
⇓

Assaults the massage therapist sexually; rape

Massage Therapist

Flirting
Use of slang or crude words referring to the genitalia
Jokes with sexual content or innuendo
Talk about personal sexual experiences or problems
Seductive speech
Exposes client through improper draping
Watches client dress or undress
Sexual fantasies about a client
⇓

Touches sensitive areas (e.g., upper thigh) without informed consent
Positions or braces the client using face or front of pelvis
Uses chest, head, face, lips, hair, pelvis, or breasts to massage a client

Outside of massage session

Dating or romantic socializing with a client
Sexual activity outside of massage setting

During massage session

Touches client's genitals or nipples
Fails to intervene when client sexually stimulates him- or herself
Stimulates him- or herself sexually during massage
Sexually stimulates client during massage
⇓

Assaults the client sexually; rape

The degree of severity of sexual misconduct ranges from relatively minor to very severe. How serious the offense is depends on the intentions of the initiator, the experience of the victim, whether physical contact is involved, and the resulting physical or psychological harm.

The most common forms of sexual misconduct involve flirting, suggestive comments about a person's body or appearance, and off-color jokes or innuendo. Discussion of the sexual performance, preferences, or problems of either party sexualizes the situation. Seductive behavior is an open invitation to misconduct.

Sexual misconduct by a massage therapist also includes exposing clients' genitals or women's breasts. Good draping technique can prevent accidental exposure. Watching a client undress or dress, except in cases of advanced age or disability when assistance is needed, is also inappropriate. Respecting a client's privacy is essential.

Because of the physical contact involved, misconduct related to touch is especially harmful. Inappropriate touch by a massage therapist is a serious violation of the therapeutic relationship. Guidelines for appropriate touch include the following:

- Use only hands, forearms, elbows, or feet to massage a client.

- Never use the chest, head, face, lips, hair, pelvis, or breasts to massage a client.

- Use only knees, shoulders, lateral hip, and lower leg for bracing or stabilizing.

- Never use the face or front of the pelvis for bracing or stabilizing.

- Never massage in the nipple or genital areas.

- Never touch any part of your body to the client's genital area.

- Get informed consent to massage high on the thigh, around breast tissue, the buttocks, anywhere near the genitals, and on the abdomen.[16]

Informed Voluntary Consent

Informed voluntary consent is a process used by massage therapists to get the client's permission to touch areas that may have sexual associations (e.g., high on the thigh, buttocks, abdomen), or areas out of the scope of general care (e.g., ear canal, nasal passages, mouth, anal canal, and breast tissue). For some areas, the *NCBTMB Standards of Practice* further require *written* consent and that the treatment be part of a plan of care (Standard VI: Prevention of Sexual Misconduct).

The words used to describe this process tell the story of its key elements. It is *informed* in that the client receives information about the proposed action and the reasons for it. It is *voluntary* in that the client freely agrees to the proposal. Finally, there is *consent* or permission by the client who exercises his or her right to self-determination.

The process of informed voluntary consent has five parts. First, the massage therapist informs the client about the nature and duration of the proposed action, that is, the body part to be touched, the technique to be used, or other relevant factors. Second, the massage therapist gives reasons for the proposed action. Third, the massage therapist describes what the client should expect. Fourth, the massage therapist gives the client the option to say no, either before beginning or at any time during the application. Fifth, the massage therapist explicitly asks permission to touch the area. This process is summarized in Box 5–4 ■.

For areas that are generally within the scope of a regular massage, but that may have sexual associations, verbal consent is usually adequate. Informed voluntary consent in these cases may be simple. For example, to an athlete complaining of tight thigh muscles, you might say, "I'd like to work the tendons to the muscles in your thighs closer to their points of insertion. That's a little higher than you're used to me working. But it should help those muscles loosen up better. I'll adjust the drape to make sure you're covered. The inner thigh can be sensitive so it may feel a little strange to you. If it gets uncomfortable at any time, just let me know. Is that all right with you? Shall I go ahead and start?" If the client says yes, remain aware of nonverbal communication such as facial expression and muscle tightening that may signal discomfort. That could also signal "no" or "I changed my mind."

BOX 5–4   Informed Voluntary Consent

Obtain permission to touch areas with sexual association (e.g., buttocks, inner thigh) and areas outside the norm for massage (e.g., nasal passages, mouth). Touching the genitals is never allowed even with consent.

Step 1   Inform the client about the nature and duration of the proposed action; for example, the body part to be massaged, the massage techniques to be used, the amount of time involved.

Step 2   Explain the reasons for the proposed action; for example, the goals and therapeutic benefits expected.

Step 3   Describe what the client should expect to feel.

Step 4   Invite the client to agree to the goals and methods for the proposed action; the client has complete freedom to accept or reject the proposed action, or any part of it, before the massage is applied or anytime during the application.

Step 5   Ask permission to touch the area, and to begin the massage application; client signs written consent if applicable.*

*Written consent is advised for all massage treatments involving nasal passages, mouth, ear canal, anal canal, and women's breasts.

For body areas out of the general scope of massage, the ethical requirements are stricter. Special training is necessary to enter body orifices like the nose, mouth, and anus, and to massage the breasts. In addition, written consent must be obtained. Massage techniques for these areas are not usually taught in entry-level programs in the United States or may be advanced treatments taught in longer, medically oriented programs. Working in these areas may also be outside a massage therapist's legal scope of practice under his or her license.

The *NCBTMB Standards of Practice* require that massage treatments in these sensitive areas be performed within a *plan of care*. That means that there should be a medical reason for the special massage techniques, and the massage is part of an overall treatment plan. This also implies that other medical professionals may be aware of the massage treatment. The standards stop short of requiring a prescription from a doctor. However, such a prescription would validate the therapeutic necessity of the procedure and provide justification if needed. There are legal as well as ethical issues to consider.

Sexual Misconduct by a Client

Although the vast majority of clients respect the professional nature of massage therapy, massage therapists should be prepared to handle sexual misconduct by a client. This is a matter of safety as well as ethics for the massage therapist.

The importance of establishing a professional setting and boundaries cannot be emphasized enough. If the massage therapist is fuzzy about his or her boundaries, the client will also be unclear about where to draw the line on behaviors like flirting, jokes, and more overt sexual behavior.

Depending on where you work (e.g., spa, health club, clinic, office at home), and the amount of confusion in your city, town, or local area about the difference between legitimate massage and sexual massage, you may want to be more explicit about your standing. For example, when making appointments, you may want to state up front, "You understand that this is therapeutic and not sexual massage." Or you may wish to highlight a similar statement in the policy document that clients sign at their first appointment.

Client misconduct on any of the levels shown in Box 5–3 should be addressed with directness and assertiveness. A client intent on sexualizing the massage will often begin testing the waters with minor misconduct such as flirting and then escalate the sexual behavior over time. Stopping the misconduct early will clearly draw the boundary of acceptable behavior.

Minor misconduct can be addressed by clarifying boundaries. For example, "Seth, this is a professional setting. Please don't tell a joke like that again." Or "Barbara, I appreciate the invitation, but I am declining because socializing like that with clients can lead to problems in our relationship here." Or "Ricardo, you understand that as your massage therapist, I cannot go on a date with you. It is against our professional standards." If the client is mature and respects your professionalism, then that should be enough.

Clients looking for sexual gratification might come right out and ask for it. They might use euphemisms such as "Do you give a *full* massage?" (with a vocal emphasis on *full*). Or "Do you give the 'happy ending'?" If that comes up before the massage, an assertive statement about your professional standards will usually send the client looking somewhere else. If it happens during the session, use the intervention model explained in the next section.

A client, either male or female, may become sexually aroused during a massage session with no prior intention of that happening. This might occur either in a cross-gender or same-gender session. Although there is no exact formula for dealing with the situation, there are some guidelines to consider.

One possibility is that a technique that the massage therapist is performing, the body area he or she is massaging, or a combination of the two is causing an arousal response. If this is the case, changing the technique, tempo, or area being massaged can interrupt the process and the arousal may subside. Whether to talk to the client about the incident is a judgment call. It may be an opportunity to explain that sexual arousal can be a short-lived physiological response, and it need not be interpreted as deliberate or improper. However, it should be avoided if possible, interrupted if it occurs, and never acted on during massage therapy.

If a man has a partial or full erection during a massage session, it may or may not be necessary to intervene. If he shows no signs of embarrassment or sexual intent, it may be an innocent physiological response as described previously, and no formal intervention is necessary at that time. If he acts uncomfortable or embarrassed, even though he has not behaved inappropriately in any way, it is best to talk to him about it and assure him that you understand the physiological response involved. However, if he has made suggestive comments or other sexual overtures, touches himself, or asks you to touch him inappropriately, then you are ethically obligated to intervene and stop the session.

More extreme forms of sexual misconduct may also be illegal. Cases of assault, battery, gross indecency, and threatening behavior by clients should be reported to the local police. Massage therapists who have been victims of illegal client misconduct have been known to take their clients to court. This helps protect massage therapists and others in the community from becoming future victims of the perpetrator.

Intervention Model

The **intervention model** is a useful tool to address misconduct or suspected misconduct by clients. A seven-step approach is presented in Box 5–5 ■. For minor misconduct, an abbreviated version of the model may be all that is necessary. For more severe misconduct, all seven steps are recommended.

First, stop the massage session or interrupt the behavior, using assertive verbal and body language. Assertive behavior signals that you are competent and in charge. If misconduct occurs during a massage session, remove your hands from the client's body, and step away from the table. You want

BOX 5–5 **Intervention Model—Response to Client Misconduct**

Step 1   Stop the session using assertive behavior.
Step 2   Describe the behavior you are concerned about.
Step 3   Ask the client to clarify the behavior.
Step 4   Restate your intent and professional boundaries.
Step 5   Evaluate the client's response.
Step 6   Continue or discontinue the session as appropriate.
Step 7   Document the situation and discuss it with a trusted colleague.*

*Assault, battery, gross indecency, and threatening behavior should also be reported to the local police.

the client's full attention. Address the client calmly but firmly by name, and make a statement about why you are intervening. For example, say something like, "Peter, we need to talk about what just happened." Or "Vanessa, I'd like to talk about what you just said."

Next, describe the behavior you are concerned about. Be as specific as possible. For example: "That was the second time your hand brushed my leg. It seems to be intentional." Or "You keep removing the drape and exposing yourself." Or "You continue talking about your sexual relationship with your husband."

Ask the client to clarify his or her behavior, if appropriate. For example: "Are you trying to sexualize this massage?" Or "Are you looking for professional help with your sexual problems with your spouse?"

Restating your intent and professional boundaries may be all that is needed to get things back on track. For example, you can state, "This is a nonsexual massage, and you must stay draped at all times." Or "Sexual problems are outside the scope of massage therapy, and I am not a psychotherapist. Please keep the conversation related to massage." Or "Touching me that way is not all right with me. Please stop."

Then evaluate the client's response. If you believe that the client will keep the reinforced boundaries, and you are comfortable and feel safe, you may continue the massage. If the

client repeats the misconduct, or despite what he or she says, you still feel uncomfortable or unsafe, you should terminate the session. Trust your intuition. This is a judgment call. You have a right to a professional, safe, and comfortable environment.

If you are in a public facility such as a spa or clinic, you are less vulnerable to misconduct. If you have a private practice in an office or in your home, or are at a client's home or in a hotel, you are more vulnerable. Have an emergency plan in place including contacts, phone numbers, and an escape route. If you fear for your safety, leave the office or house, and go somewhere people can help you.

Finally, document your experience either in the client's file or in a separate incident report file. Remember that clients have a right to see their personal files, and anything written in them should be descriptive (not interpretive) and professional. Other massage therapists who are scheduled with the client will appreciate knowing about what happened.

In terms of self-care, massage therapists who have experienced an incident of sexual misconduct by a client, especially one involving the intervention model, should talk about it with a trusted friend, colleague, or supervisor. Talking helps a person analyze and process the situation, which may have been upsetting. Getting it out in the open also helps to objectify the incident and use it as a learning experience.

RELATIONSHIPS IN SCHOOL

Massage therapy students have the potential for dual relationships with classmates, teachers and administrators, practice clients, and clients in student clinics and at outreach sites. Each of these situations deserves some careful thought. Although some of these ideas were introduced in Chapter 3, *Professional and Personal Development*, they are discussed more fully here.

Classmates often get to know one another well during the course of a massage program. Relationships among classmates have some similarities to relationships with clients. Although these are not therapeutic relationships by a strict definition, they are special relationships based on giving

 PRACTICAL APPLICATION

The following client situations involve setting professional boundaries. With a friend or study partner, practice what you would say in these situations to maintain professional boundaries. Responding to a client who:

● Invites you out for social time
● You want to hire to do your taxes
● Is habitually late
● Talks throughout the whole massage session
● Asks about another client's health
● Tells off-color or ethnic jokes or uses profanity

1. How did you feel during each role-playing exercise?
2. Was your verbal and nonverbal communication about your professional boundaries clear?
3. How could you modify what you said to make it clearer?
4. What are some other boundary-setting situations in which it would be useful to rehearse your response?

and receiving massage and involve knowledge of personal information about the people in class. Classmates become somewhat vulnerable to one another, and a level of trust is established. Friendships also develop among classmates, and these are dual relationships with their own dimensions. Being a student of massage therapy is very different from other vocational and academic programs because of the intimate contact inherent in the learning situation.

There are implicit agreements among classmates involving confidentiality, trust, and respect just like in the therapeutic relationship. Box 5–6 ■ lists some of the important ethical aspects of relationships among classmates. It is a matter of integrity that ethical principles related to the therapeutic relationship carry over into massage school classmate relationships.

As in any school setting, friendships and socializing between students and teachers or school staff is a double-edged sword. Learning may be enhanced through informal interactions; on the other hand, the inherent power differential can cause problems similar to problems in dual relationships between clients and massage therapists. In this case, students are in a position of lesser power. It is the teacher's or staff member's responsibility to maintain appropriate

---

BOX 5–6 Ethical Principles Regarding Relationships with Classmates

To promote trust, respect, and harmony, and to avoid unethical behavior, classmates agree to

1. Treat all classmates with equal respect, and avoid cliques and exclusive social groups during class time.
2. Keep personal information, including medical information, about classmates confidential, and refrain from gossiping about classmates with other classmates and with family and friends.
3. Respect classmates' privacy and modesty in hands-on technique classes while dressing and undressing and by using proper draping.
4. Practice massage therapy techniques with care and attention to classmates' well-being, and respond promptly to their feedback about pressure, pain, and other concerns.
5. Observe precautions and contraindications with classmates regardless of a technique assignment, and consult with the teacher for necessary modifications to practice with a specific classmate.
6. Use informed voluntary consent as with any client.
7. Seriously consider the possible impact of transference and other psychological factors in relationships with classmates, and refrain from a sexual relationship with a classmate until after graduation.
8. Report to school personnel about personally experienced or suspected cases of unethical behavior, especially inappropriate touching, intentional nudity, and other sexual misconduct of classmates during class time and practice sessions outside class.
9. Do not ask or expect a classmate to lie, cheat, or cover up unethical behavior for you or another classmate.

---

social boundaries with students. Students can also recognize and avoid problems by limiting such socializing to official school events and group activities.

Another dual relationship situation occurs when students become massage therapy clients of teachers. These relationships can be problematic, especially for the teacher–massage therapist, who may have conflicting roles in the two settings. The positive and negative aspects of such a relationship need to be weighed before entering into it.

It is helpful to remember that after graduation, the relationships between graduates and teachers and school staff are more equal. Waiting to develop other relationships with teachers and school staff is much safer after graduation. It is wise to know and obey school policies about dual relationships between teachers and students.

A third type of dual relationship encountered by students is with family and friends who agree to be practice clients. Thinking of these people as special kinds of clients, rather than as "practice dummies" or "guinea pigs," will help students understand how they should be treated. Practice clients should receive all the respect and care due to paying clients in the future. Practice time offers the opportunity to learn how to maintain professional boundaries and to internalize professional standards. Your practice clients will appreciate and respect the level of professionalism that you show during practice sessions.

Finally, providing massage therapy to the general public at outreach sites and in student clinics is usually a student's first encounter with "real" clients. Even though students may not be paid for these services because the experience is part of their education, these are real clients in every sense of the term, and all professional standards apply.

SCOPE OF PRACTICE

Massage therapists are required by their ethical standards and by law to stay within their scope of practice. **Scope of practice** means the range of methods and techniques used in a profession or by a professional, which may also include their intention in performing them (e.g., relaxation or treatment of a medical condition). Scope of practice is defined by professional organizations and licensing laws, often in their official definitions of massage therapy.

The scope of practice for massage therapists generally includes various soft tissue manipulation techniques, joint movements, and hydrotherapy. Different systems or modalities fall under the general scope of massage therapy, for example, trigger point therapy, polarity therapy, and lymphatic massage. A more broadly defined scope of practice might also include massage with mechanical and electronic devices, energy-based bodywork, relaxation techniques, and physical exercises.

The scope of massage therapy as taught in the United States today does not include "chiropractic adjustments" of the spine and other joints. It also does not cover psychotherapy, nutrition, and methods designated exclusively for other professions by law (e.g., skin care by estheticians). Scope of practice can change over time; for example, colon therapy (colonics) was once within the scope of Swedish massage, but is now a separate profession.

A massage therapist's personal scope of practice is limited ethically by the extent of his or her training, that is, massage therapists "will provide only those services which they are qualified to perform."[17] For example, it would be unethical to accept clients for physical rehabilitation if a massage therapist's training was primarily relaxation oriented.

Scope of practice in any particular state, province, or country is defined by licensing or other laws. Massage therapists are prohibited from diagnosing medical conditions. For example, according to the Illinois licensing law, the purpose of massage is "to enhance the general health and well-being of the mind and body of the recipient" and "does not include the diagnosis of a specific pathology."[18] Even if massage therapists are well trained in a certain method, it might be outside their legal scope of practice under their particular licensing law.

In its grounds for discipline, the Illinois Massage Licensing Act includes "practicing or offering to practice beyond the scope permitted by law or accepting and performing professional responsibilities which the licensee knows or has reason to know that he or she is not competent to perform" (Section 45). Massage therapists could face probation or lose their massage licenses if it is determined that they are practicing beyond their scope.

It is noteworthy that massage is within the legal scope of practice of several other licensed professions. Nurses, physical therapists, and athletic trainers typically use a limited amount of massage as part of the scope of their work. Cosmetologists and barbers are allowed to use massage during facials, manicures, and pedicures. However, the title *massage therapist* is usually restricted to those with professional training and credentials in massage therapy.

Some massage therapists are trained and licensed in more than one profession, for example, nurse–massage therapists. Other common professional combinations are massage therapist and chiropractor, athletic trainer, physical therapist, physical therapy assistant, psychotherapist, colon therapist, esthetician, or cosmetologist. Individuals with more than one license need to keep good boundaries about which "hat" they are wearing (i.e., which role they are playing) in a specific setting or with a specific client. When working under a license, a professional must keep within that particular license's legal scope of practice.

Staying in Bounds

To stay within their scope of practice, massage therapists need to understand two things. First, the legal scope for massage therapy in the specific jurisdiction, and second, the personal scope dictated by their training and experience. Keep a copy of the licensing law under which you practice handy for reference. Read the definition of massage therapy or scope of practice section carefully to understand what is allowed and not allowed under the law in your area.

Do not give advice to clients in areas outside that scope, and refer clients to the appropriate professionals when their goals or conditions are outside your scope. Three areas that massage therapists need to be especially clear about are their limits related to treating clients with musculoskeletal injuries and other pathologies, giving nutritional advice, and psychotherapy.

When clients come for massage with physical complaints such as pain or limited movement, it is the massage therapist's responsibility to determine if massage is indicated or contraindicated. Remember that the first principle is to "do no harm." Always ask clients if they have seen medical providers for diagnoses of their complaints. A medical diagnosis can tell you whether massage might do some good, or whether it should be avoided.

For undiagnosed musculoskeletal injuries accompanied by severe pain, deformity, or acute inflammation (redness, swelling, pain), it is best to refer clients to their health care providers or to an emergency room for evaluation. Symptoms for other pathologies that might be detected by massage therapists include skin diseases such as cancerous moles, tumors, and misaligned vertebrae or ribs.

Do not verbally speculate about what you think is going on, especially using medical terms. Although it is acceptable to observe things like swelling, redness, limited movement, or a client's level of pain, it is inadvisable to use diagnostic terms like *second-degree sprain*, *plantar fasciitis*, or *cancer*. Putting a label on a set of symptoms is considered diagnosis, and medical diagnosis is not within the scope of practice of massage therapists.

When clients' needs are within the scope of massage therapy, but not within your personal scope, refer clients to another massage therapist who does have the appropriate training and experience. Remember that you can widen your personal scope by getting advanced training and certifications.

Giving nutritional advice, including suggestions about food supplements such as vitamins is outside the scope of massage therapy. It may be tempting to share with clients your personal beliefs and practices in the area of nutrition. But remember that to clients, you are a person of authority, and they may take what you say as expert advice. Do not say things like "You should try this . . ." or, "Take two of these each day, and your joints will feel better."

You could use a qualifier like, "You might want to ask your doctor about . . . ," or "You might want to read the research about . . . ," or "Other clients have reported good results with . . . ," to point them in a direction that you think might be helpful. You can also share information such as an article or pamphlet, but avoid seeming like you are telling a client to do something specific outside your area of expertise.

Massage therapists sometimes increase their incomes by selling food supplements or other products. It is unethical to pressure massage clients to buy anything you are selling, especially if it has the appearance of a prescription.

Mental and emotional wellness is another area in which scope of practice is important to define. When does listening to clients' emotional problems, which may also relate to their physical stresses and illnesses, step over the line of scope of practice? Or as Deane Juhan puts it in the Foreword to *Beyond Technique: The Hidden Dimensions of Bodywork*, what is the difference between "practicing professional psychology and the responsible handling of a range of psychological issues that are likely to emerge in the course of any bodywork practice?"[19]

The massage therapist's role is to provide massage, which is fundamentally a hands-on therapy. As clients relax during massage and let down their defenses, buried emotions may surface. In the course of a massage session, massage therapists may provide emotional support, listen to a client's concerns, or just be there when a client becomes emotional during a session.

The proper approach is to be supportive while not becoming too involved or trying to help the client resolve his or her feelings by talking. When discussing the client's emotional or mental issues becomes the focus of massage sessions, or the client looks to the massage therapist to resolve psychological issues, the scope of practice has been exceeded. Boundaries must be drawn "between intelligent, compassionate support on the part of the bodyworker and the recognition of the need for further discussion, clarification, and possible referral to various other forms of therapy."[20]

Similar to not diagnosing physical pathologies, massage therapists should not diagnose psychological pathologies such as posttraumatic stress disorder, depression, bipolar disorder, disassociation, and psychotic episodes. These are specific medical diagnoses. Massage therapists can, however, recognize symptoms and refer clients to mental health professionals when appropriate.

Some forms of bodywork (e.g., Hakomi and Rosen Method) are specifically designed to help clients resolve psychological issues. These certified practitioners are highly trained in their approaches, and mental and emotional problems are within their scope of practice. If you are interested in expanding your scope and practicing psychologically focused bodywork, it will be necessary to get additional education beyond your initial massage training program.

Education and Home Care

It is outside the scope of practice of massage therapists to give prescriptions, sometimes abbreviated *Rx*. *Prescription* is a medical concept that implies a command on the part of the person making the prescription. Rx implies "do this" or "take this medication" and is sometimes called an "order." Prescriptions are written instructions that patients take to the pharmacy or to another health care professional. Doctors typically prescribe medications and sometimes physical therapy or even massage therapy. Prescriptions are given by doctors for medical conditions and may be paid for by insurance companies.

Massage therapists, on the other hand, provide information and education. They make suggestions to clients about home care for conditions within their scope of practice. For example, a massage therapist might show a client a self-massage technique for recovery after running, or a stretch to help relax and elongate a certain muscle group. Therapists may suggest an ointment for stiff joints or taking advantage of the whirlpool at the health club. Massage therapists do

CASE FOR STUDY

Samantha and the Nutritional Supplements

Samantha is a massage therapist who works in a spa and has built a regular clientele among the spa customers. She has a side business selling nutritional supplements, some of which are advertised as aids to losing weight. Sara, one of Samantha's regulars, is overweight and has expressed an interest in finding a good weight-loss plan.

Question:

Is it ethical for Samantha to mention the nutritional supplements and offer to sell them to Sara?

Things to consider:

- Does selling nutritional supplements fall under Samantha's scope of practice as a massage therapist?
- Are there different roles for Samantha as massage therapist and Samantha as sales representative for the supplements?

- How does the power differential in the therapeutic relationship impact this situation?
- Does the spa have a policy about staff selling their own products?
- Is this situation covered in a code of ethics or standards of practice for massage therapists?
- Is there potential for causing harm? For doing good?
- What are alternative courses of action?
- What are the most important considerations in this situation?
- What might Samantha's motivation be for selling the product to Sara?
- What would a former teacher advise Samantha to do?
- What decision would maintain the highest standards?

Your Reasoning and Conclusions:

_____

_____

_____

_____

not give prescriptions for topical applications or anything taken internally.

This careful use of words is very important for clarity about scope of practice. Massage therapists do not prescribe, but do offer information, education, and suggestions for home care.

CONFIDENTIALITY

Confidentiality is an implicit agreement between massage therapist and client; that is, there is an unspoken understanding and trust that the massage therapist will not reveal personal or medical information about the client to others without the client's permission. This principle is based on the client's right to privacy.

Confidential information includes what is written on health history forms, what is discussed in massage sessions, and observations about the physical, mental, and emotional health of the client. Even mentioning to someone else that a certain person is a client can be considered a breach of confidentiality. It is unethical to use people's names in advertising without their permission, especially celebrities or people prominent in the community. Gossiping about a client's personal life is a serious breach of trust.

The *NCBTMB Code of Ethics* states that practitioners must "safeguard the confidentiality of all client information, unless disclosure is required by law, court order, or is absolutely necessary for the protection of the public." Licensed massage therapists in some states may have a legal responsibility to report the abuse of minors and the aged. Exceptions to the ethical duty related to confidentiality include knowledge of abuse of a child or a dependent elder, or if clients reveal information indicating that they pose serious threats to themselves or others. This is an ethical dilemma that requires reasoned evaluation and good ethical judgment to resolve. Reviewing the situation with a trusted colleague may also be helpful.

Confidentiality of health records in this age of electronic information has important legal implications. In 1996, the U.S. Congress passed the Health Insurance Portability and Accountability Act (HIPAA) to protect the privacy of medical records. HIPAA rules apply to "covered entities" including health care providers who electronically transmit claims, benefit eligibility inquiries, referral authorization requests, and other information transfers. If your practice or a company you work for are covered entities, you are legally, and therefore ethically, bound to comply with all regulations that apply. HIPAA is administered by the U.S. Department of Health & Human Services (DHHS), and enforcement and complaints are handled by the DHHS Office of Civil Rights (OCR). Information about HIPAA can be found on the HHS website (www.hhs.gov/ocr/hipaa).

Client records in massage therapy offices may or may not fall under HIPAA. More clinically or medically oriented practices, and those that keep records electronically and that take insurance payments, are more likely to be subject to HIPAA requirements. In any case, HIPAA offers practical guidelines for ensuring client confidentiality, and massage therapists are encouraged to follow their general guidelines, even if not required to do so by law. HIPAA rules and methods of keeping client records secure are discussed in more detail in Chapter 27, *Private Practice and Finances*.

CASE FOR STUDY

Jason and His Former Teammates

Jason has accepted some of his former teammates from high school as massage clients. They have kept in touch over the years and get together periodically to watch basketball games. One of these clients, Bill, is a very sociable person. During every appointment, Bill wants to talk to Jason about what's going on with the others. Bill knows some of them come for massage and that Jason has probably seen them more recently than he has.

Question:

Is it ethical for Jason to discuss his other clients with Bill?

Things to consider:

- Is this situation covered in a code of ethics or standards of practice for massage therapists?
- What is Jason's responsibility to his other clients in regard to confidentiality?

- What aspects of this dual relationship are problematic?
- Who might be affected by Jason talking to Bill about other clients during massage sessions?
- What if he just listened to what Bill had to say?
- What are the "worst-case" and "best-case" scenarios?
- What are alternative courses of action?
- What are the most important considerations in this situation?
- What might Jason's motivation be for talking about their mutual friends to Bill?
- What would a former teacher advise Jason to do?
- What decision would maintain the highest standards?

Your Reasoning and Conclusions:

_____

_____

_____

_____

PRACTICAL APPLICATION

It is the responsibility of massage therapists to protect their clients' rights to confidentiality, privacy, and safety. The following three activities explore ways that you might protect clients' rights in your practice.

1. Analyze samples of privacy statements that are used in massage therapy businesses. What purpose do they serve? Is there a place for the client's signature in each one? Identify key elements, and locate provisions related to confidentiality and legal requirements such as HIPAA. Develop a written privacy statement for your future practice.
2. Research the legal responsibility of licensed massage therapists in your state to report suspected cases of child, spousal, or elder abuse. Discuss your ethical responsibility in these cases. Identify the agencies to which these reports would be made. How does the principle of confidentiality relate to these situations?
3. Research how and to whom to report a massage therapist whom you suspect is doing something unethical. When is it appropriate to make such accusations? What steps do you take to ensure that you approach the situation ethically and protect yourself legally? After you've developed your answers in writing, discuss them with a group of classmates or a study partner.

CHAPTER HIGHLIGHTS

- Ethics is the study of moral behavior; that is, determining the "right" thing to do in a specific situation.
  - Professional ethics is the study of moral behavior relative to a specific occupation such as massage therapist.
  - Business ethics concern the commercial aspects of a massage practice.
- Values, rights, and duties provide the foundation for ethical principles.
  - Values are principles, traits, or qualities considered worthwhile that serve as a moral compass.
  - Rights are claims to certain treatment or protection from certain treatment.
  - Duties are obligations to act in a particular way.
- Building ethical practices starts with acknowledging human vulnerability to unethical behavior. This vulnerability can be minimized by making a commitment to ethical practices and learning about ethical standards in the profession.
- A key ethical principle is selfless service or holding your client's well-being above your own personal gain.
- Two overriding ethical principles are *do no harm* and *obey the law*.
- Professional organizations develop codes of ethics and standards of practice that are updated periodically to reflect current thinking in the field related to ethics.
  - Ethical standards are enforced within organizations through disciplinary action against members who violate the standards.
- Some ethical principles are given the force of local, state, or federal law.
  - Violators of laws can be fined, lose their licenses, or end up in jail.
- Ethical questions can be framed in this way: "Is it ethical to . . . (do something), if . . . (this is the situation)?"
- An ethical dilemma occurs when two values or rights conflict.
  - Personal temptations to act unethically should not be confused with true ethical questions or dilemmas.
- The ethical decision-making model is a step-by-step process of thinking through an ethical question or dilemma. It involves critical thinking, making ethical choices, and analyzing the consequences of the final decision.
- Development of ethical judgment is facilitated through having professional standards ready for reference, continuing education classes, professional networking, and clinical supervision.
- The therapeutic relationship between a massage therapist and client is based on specific roles and responsibilities.
  - There is an inherent power differential between massage therapists and their clients, with the massage therapist in the position of authority and trust.
  - Massage therapists have a fiduciary responsibility to act in the client's best interests.

- The therapeutic relationship involves both explicit and implicit agreements, and the massage therapist is expected to uphold the standards of the profession.
- Psychological factors can influence the therapeutic relationship.
  - Transference and countertransference.
  - Defense mechanisms such as projection, denial, repression, displacement, and resistance.
  - Being aware of these psychological factors and their impact helps build healthier therapeutic relationships and avoid unethical behavior.
- It is the massage therapist's responsibility to ensure that professional and personal boundaries are respected.
  - Boundary crossings may be annoying or uncomfortable.
  - Boundary violations are crossings that cause harm.
- Dual relationships between massage therapists and clients should be avoided or entered into only after evaluating the potential benefits and risks. They can work only if both parties are emotionally mature and able to maintain appropriate roles in the therapeutic relationship.
- When an already established sexual partner becomes a client, it is important to enforce professional boundaries during massage sessions.
- Sexualizing the relationship with a current client is highly unethical. Professional standards require ending the therapeutic relationship and waiting for a period of time before beginning a sexual relationship with a former client.
- Sexual misconduct ranges in severity from relatively minor to severe and includes flirting, suggestive comments, jokes, discussing sex, seductive behavior, inappropriate touching, and sexual contact.
- Use the intervention model to deal with suspected sexual misconduct by a client.
  - The intervention model includes interrupting the behavior, describing it, asking for clarification, restating your nonsexual intent, evaluating the client's response, and deciding whether to continue the session or to end it.

- Afterward, the massage therapist documents the incident in writing, and for self-care, discusses it with a friend or colleague.
  - Illegal misconduct by clients should be reported to the local police.
- Informed voluntary consent is used to get a client's permission to touch him or her in certain areas.
  - Five parts of informed voluntary consent are informing, explaining, describing, agreeing, and consenting.
- Relationships in school include those with classmates, teachers and administrators, practice clients, and student clinic clients. Ethical principles related to the therapeutic relationship may carry over into these relationships as well.
- The scope of practice of massage therapists is defined by professional organizations and by law.
  - Massage therapists' personal scope of practice is limited by their training and experience.
  - Massage therapists should know their legal scope of practice and stay within that scope.
  - Three areas to be especially clear about are limits on treating clients with illness and injuries, giving nutritional advice, and psychotherapy.
  - Massage therapists do not give prescriptions (Rx) to clients, but do provide information, education, and suggestions for home care.
- Massage therapists are bound to keep client information confidential. Confidentiality is expected unless disclosure is required by law or necessary to protect the public.
  - HIPAA was enacted in 1996 to protect the privacy of medical records, and some massage therapy practices may be required to abide by HIPAA regulations.

EXAM REVIEW

Key Terms

Match the following key terms to their descriptions. For additional study, look up the key terms in the Interactive Glossary, and note other terms that compare or contrast with them.

_____ **1.** Boundary crossing
_____ **2.** Codes of ethics
_____ **3.** Confidentiality
_____ **4.** Defense mechanisms
_____ **5.** Dual relationship
_____ **6.** Duties
_____ **7.** Ethical decision-making model
_____ **8.** Ethical dilemmas
_____ **9.** Ethical judgment
_____ **10.** Ethical questions
_____ **11.** Ethics
_____ **12.** Informed voluntary consent
_____ **13.** Intervention model
_____ **14.** Personal boundary
_____ **15.** Personal temptations
_____ **16.** Power differential
_____ **17.** Professional ethics
_____ **18.** Rights
_____ **19.** Scope of practice
_____ **20.** Sexual misconduct
_____ **21.** Standards of practice
_____ **22.** Therapeutic relationship
_____ **23.** Transference
_____ **24.** Values

a. The study of moral behavior; determining the *right* thing to do in a specific situation

b. Principles, traits, or qualities considered worthwhile or desirable

c. Claims to certain treatment or protection from certain treatment enforced by standards or laws

d. The study of moral behavior relative to a specific occupation

e. Way of framing an ethical situation

f. List of general principles that reflect commonly held values in a profession

g. Urge to act in a way that is unethical for your own personal gain

h. Defined by specific roles assumed by the massage therapist and the client

i. Obligations to act in a particular way

j. Documents that go into detail in interpreting ethical principles

k. Differences of perceived power within a professional relationship

l. Occurs when a client injects negative or positive feelings toward someone from his or her past into the therapeutic relationship

m. When two or more principles are in conflict, and regardless of your choice, something of value is compromised

n. Step-by-step process of thinking through an ethical question or ethical dilemma

o. Behaviors or thoughts that help us cope with unwanted feelings like fear, anxiety, guilt, and anger

p. Stepping over personal or professional limits within the therapeutic relationship

q. Other connections between a client and a massage therapist in addition to the therapeutic relationship

r. Consistency in making good ethical decisions

s. A process used to get the client's permission to touch areas that may have sexual associations, or areas out of the scope of general care

t. A limit established by a person to maintain his or her own integrity, comfort, or well-being

u. Tool to address misconduct or suspected misconduct by clients

v. Implicit agreement that the massage therapist will not reveal personal or medical information about the client to others without the client's permission.

w. Range of methods and techniques used by a professional; may be legally defined

x. Sexualizing of the relationship between a massage therapist and a current client

Memory Workout

To test your memory of the main concepts in this chapter, complete the following sentences by circling the most correct answer from the two choices provided.

1. Ethics is the study of (moral) (social) behavior.
2. Speaking the truth and avoiding deception is called (honesty) (integrity).
3. The principle of *confidentiality* stems from a client's right to (fairness) (privacy).
4. That clients get to make informed choices about what happens to them is based on their right to (safety) (self-determination).
5. Issues related to money, sex, and (respect) (power) are the usual culprits in unethical decisions.
6. The ethical decision-making model is an (intuitive) (orderly) process of thinking through an ethical question or dilemma.
7. Before making a final ethical decision, examine your own (motivation) (logic) or interest in the outcome.
8. Ethical (supervision) (judgment) refers to developing consistency in making good ethical decisions.
9. Consulting with others about an ethical issue offers a more (knowledgeable) (objective) view of the situation.
10. Clinical supervision is done in a(n) (informal) (formal) setting with a specially trained supervisor.
11. The therapeutic relationship is a special relationship based on specific (roles and responsibilities) (rules and regulations).
12. Failure or refusal of a client to cooperate in the therapeutic process is called (denial) (resistance).
13. A limit established to maintain a person's own integrity, comfort, or well-being is called a (professional) (personal) boundary.
14. Bartering for services can be (mutually) (morally) beneficial if both parties feel that they are getting a fair deal.
15. Sexual activity with a client is strictly (prohibited) (discouraged) by professional standards.
16. When massaging areas outside the general scope of massage (e.g., inside the mouth), a plan of care and (verbal) (written) consent is required.
17. After an intervention with a client related to sexual misconduct, (document the incident in writing) (report incident to licensing board).
18. Time with (paying) (practice) clients offers students the opportunity to learn early about how to maintain good professional boundaries.
19. To stay within their scope of practice, massage therapists need to understand the (legal) (professional) scope in their governmental jurisdiction.
20. When discussing a client's emotional issues becomes the focus of sessions, the massage therapist's scope of practice has been (exceeded) (achieved).
21. Client information may be ethically disclosed if required by law, or is absolutely necessary for public (safety) (information).
22. According to HIPAA rules, medical records must be kept confidential, and only those who (want) (need) to see them should have access.

Test Prep

The following multiple-choice questions will help to prepare you for future school and professional exams.

1. Values are:
   a. Principles, traits, or qualities considered worthwhile
   b. Claims to certain treatment or to protection from certain treatment
   c. Obligations to act in a certain way
   d. Moral bonds with society

2. Integrity means:
   a. Telling the truth
   b. Keeping your promises
   c. Living up to your values consistently
   d. Learning from your mistakes

3. Unconditional regard for others calls for giving our best efforts to everyone and being:
   a. Honest
   b. Critical
   c. Judgmental
   d. Nonjudgmental

4. In contrast to a code of ethics, standards of practice are:
   a. Shorter
   b. More general
   c. More detailed
   d. Stated in broad terms

5. How do professional organizations typically enforce ethical standards?
   a. Criminal prosecution
   b. Disciplinary action such as probation or revoking membership
   c. Jail time
   d. Filing lawsuits

6. An ethical dilemma occurs when:
   a. Values, rights, or ethical principles are in conflict
   b. An overriding ethical principle is violated
   c. There is personal temptation to act unethically
   d. An ethical question is unclear

7. Which of the following is the *least* important consideration in making an ethical decision?
   a. Determining what will maintain the highest values
   b. Judging what will result in the greatest good overall
   c. Judging what will result in the least harm overall
   d. Determining what will produce the best monetary outcome for myself

8. Which of the following is an important reason to discuss an ethical situation with a colleague?
   a. To get a more objective view of the situation
   b. To generate more options for action
   c. To check my own biases and temptations
   d. All of the above

9. Which of the following statements about the power differential in the therapeutic relationship is correct?
   a. The power in the therapeutic relationship is equal between adults.
   b. Clients have greater power in the therapeutic relationship because they are paying for the massage.
   c. Massage therapists have greater power by virtue of their perceived authority.
   d. Power is not an important factor in the therapeutic relationship.

10. Behaviors or thoughts that help us cope with unwanted feelings such as fear, guilt, and anger are called:
    a. Offense mechanisms
    b. Defense mechanisms
    c. Boundary crossings
    d. Self-disclosure

11. When a massage therapist transfers positive or negative feelings about someone in his or her past into the therapeutic relationship, it is called:
    a. Countertransference
    b. Repression
    c. Projection
    d. Denial

12. A boundary transgression experienced as harmful is called a:
    a. Boundary collapse
    b. Boundary violation
    c. Boundary crossing
    d. Faulty boundary

13. Which of the following factors is *least* important in determining the potential success of a dual relationship with a client?
    a. The emotional maturity of each person
    b. The ability of each person to maintain their proper role in the therapeutic relationship
    c. The power differential within the relationship outside the therapeutic relationship
    d. How often you socialize outside the therapeutic relationship

14. Before massaging an area that may cause the client embarrassment or discomfort, the following procedure should always be followed:
    a. Informed voluntary consent
    b. Intervention
    c. Informed intervention
    d. Written consent

15. What is the most ethical response for a massage therapy student to give to a student clinic client who asks him/her out for a dinner date?
    a. "Call me later this week when I am not working in the student clinic."
    b. "Yes, but don't let anyone here know about it."
    c. "Yes, but only as friends."
    d. "No thank you. I prefer to keep my social and professional lives separate."

16. Which of the following is an example of a massage therapist who has clearly exceeded his or her scope of practice?
    a. One who refers a client to another health professional for a condition beyond her training
    b. One who gives advice about taking certain vitamins to improve a client's health
    c. One who listens to a client's concern about her situation at work
    d. One who instructs a client on how to give herself self-massage for home care between appointments

Video Challenge

Watch these videos, which can be found at MyHealthProfessionsLab.com, Chapter 5, and then answer the following questions.

Foundation of Ethics

1. What everyday ethical situations are mentioned in this video segment?
2. How did the massage therapist in the video handle the situation of a client who asked her out on a date?
3. What ethical decision-making steps are presented in the video?

Therapeutic Relationship

4. Locate the situation involving informed voluntary consent depicted in the video. Identify the essential aspects of informed voluntary consent that are illustrated.
5. What steps in the intervention model are outlined in the video? Give examples of sexual misconduct by clients that may call for using the intervention model.

Comprehension Exercises

The following short-answer questions test your knowledge and understanding of chapter topics and provide practice in written communication skills. Explain in two to four complete sentences.

1. Contrast codes of ethics and the law. What are they based on? Who develops them? How are they enforced?

2. Explain how a therapeutic relationship is different from a social relationship. Include the concept of *power differential* in your explanation.

3. Explain the process of *informed voluntary consent*. When is it used?

For Greater Understanding

The following exercises are designed to take you from the realm of theory into the real world. They will help give you a deeper understanding of the subjects covered in this chapter. Action words are underlined to emphasize the variety of activities presented to address different learning styles and to encourage deeper thinking.

1. Locate an article about ethics in a professional journal for massage therapists. What ethical question or ethical dilemma is addressed? What values, rights, or duties are involved? What factors were considered in decision making? What did you learn from the situation presented?

2. Examine the massage licensing law in your state or a neighboring state for the section on ethics and discipline. What is the defined scope of practice for massage therapists? What ethical principles are reinforced in the law? What are the consequences for violations of the law?

3. Discuss in small groups or with a study partner, any boundary issues that you are having with practice clients. Define the problem, and discuss how you are currently handling the issue, and how you might approach it better in the future.

MyHealthProfessionsLab™

MyHealthProfessionsLab.com is a premium online homework management system that includes a host of features to help you study. Registered users will find:

- Powerful tools that track and analyze your results—allowing you to create a personalized learning experience
- Videos, flashcards and other learning tools to help enrich your progress
- Streaming lesson presentations and self-paced learning modules
- A space where you and your instructors can view and manage your assignments

arson Education, Inc.

PART

2

Foundations of Planning and Giving Massage Sessions

Chapter 6
Effects of Massage and Research Literacy

Chapter 7
Clinical Applications of Massage

Chapter 8
Endangerment Sites, Contraindications, Cautions

Chapter 9
Medical Terminology, Goal-Oriented Planning, Documentation

Chapter 10
Hygiene, Equipment, Environment

Chapter 11
Body Mechanics, Table Skills, General Guidelines

Pearson Education, Inc.

6 Effects of Massage and Research Literacy

CHAPTER OUTLINE

Learning Outcomes

Key Terms

Effects of Massage Overview

Knowledge of Effects

Research Literacy

Physiological Effects—Tissue Level

Physiological Effects—Organ System Level

Physiological Effects—Organism Level

Psychological Effects

Mechanisms of Massage

Benefits of Wellness Massage

Chapter Highlights

Exam Review

LEARNING OUTCOMES

After studying this chapter, you will have information to:

1. Discuss the effects of massage and its benefits for well-being.

2. Describe the holistic nature of clients' responses to massage.

3. Identify sources of knowledge about the effects of massage.

4. Locate and analyze experimental research about the effects of massage.

5. Explain the effects of massage at the tissue level.

6. Explain the effects of massage at the organ system level.

7. Explain the effects of massage at the whole organism level.

8. Describe the psychological effects of massage.

9. Discuss various mechanisms for the effects of massage.

10. Describe how different massage techniques are applied for different effects.

KEY TERMS

Body–mind effects

Conventional wisdom

Effects of massage

Empirical knowledge

Energetic effects

Long-term effects

Mechanical effects

Multiple-dose effects

Physiological effects

Randomized control trial (RCT)

Reflex effects

Research literacy

Scientific method

Short-term effects

Single-dose effects

Systematic review

EFFECTS OF MASSAGE OVERVIEW

The client's response to different massage techniques and applications is at the heart of massage therapy. This is true whether a massage therapist is giving a set routine for relaxation or designing a massage session to achieve a client's personal health goals. Every time you touch and move a client's physical body, changes occur in that person's whole being. Your effectiveness as a massage therapist is increased when you understand the potential responses to massage.

The term **effects of massage** refers to the physiological and psychological changes that typically take place in response to soft tissue manipulation and movement. For instance, increased local circulation, relaxation, and pain reduction are common reactions to massage. The generally accepted effects of massage at the tissue, organ system, and organism levels are summarized in Table 6–1 ■.

These changes can be beneficial or detrimental depending on the circumstances. They are benefits if they have a positive impact and lead to healing or to a higher state of wellness. Illustrations of positive outcomes of massage include stress reduction, improved health of tissues, and increased feelings of well-being.

The term *indication* is used in the context of medical treatment, if the effects of massage contribute to healing, alleviate symptoms, or increase the patient's comfort. For example, massage is generally *indicated* for relieving tension headaches or as an adjunct to cancer treatment. These medical applications of massage are discussed in more detail in Chapter 7, *Clinical Applications of Massage*.

The term *contraindication* is used if the effects of massage would be harmful to the recipient. For example, increased blood and lymph circulation are effects of massage that are beneficial most of the time. However, for someone with congestive heart failure or an acute infection, increased fluid circulation might make matters worse. Massage would be *contraindicated* in those cases and should not be given. Contraindications for massage are covered in Chapter 8, *Endangerment Sites, Contraindications, Cautions*.

The overall effects of massage for an individual client or patient are complex and depend on a number of factors. Among these are the manual techniques applied, their immediate and accumulative effects, and how often sessions are received.

Massage Techniques and Effects

Different types of massage techniques produce different effects, and how they are applied influences the eventual outcomes. For example, percussion or tapotement techniques have a stimulating effect if received for a short period of time or a sedating effect if received for a long time. Effleurage applied slowly, rhythmically, and with moderate pressure usually has a relaxing effect, but applied briskly can feel invigorating.

Articles and reports about the effects of massage sometimes speak of massage in general as if all applications were the same. To really understand the effects, especially when reading research, it is important to know which techniques or approaches the author is talking about. Only then are conclusions about the application and its effects useful on a practical level.

Practitioners who know how to combine massage techniques to obtain specific effects will be more successful in achieving session and treatment goals. They will be able to plan effective sessions and avoid harming their clients. As the effects of massage are laid out in this chapter, the techniques that produce them will be discussed as well. More information about Swedish massage techniques and how to apply them for specific effects is also found in Part 3, *Tappan's Guide to Healing Massage*.

Time, Dose, and Effects

It is useful to distinguish between the short- and long-term effects of massage. **Short-term effects** are changes that occur during a massage session. They may last for the time of the session and for a brief period afterward, perhaps a few hours or a day. Examples of potential short-term effects are decreased heart rate, muscle relaxation, and a more positive mood.

Long-term effects are changes that start during a massage session and last for a longer period of time, such as a few days or weeks. Long-term can also refer to more enduring changes that occur from massage received regularly over a period of time. For example, regular relaxation massage can lead to a decrease in a person's general state of stress and anxiety in the long term.

The dosage, or how often and how many massage sessions are received, can also influence their effects. **Single-dose effects** refer to those changes that happen from one application of massage. **Multiple-dose effects** happen over time from repeated massage applications.

Combining the concepts of time, dose, and effects makes matters more interesting and reveals the complexity of massage in practice. For example, a single dose of massage can have a long-term effect such as relief from a tension headache. In contrast, it usually takes multiple doses of massage, each with a shorter-term effect for rehabilitation of an injury such as a muscle strain.

How long the effects of massage last can be affected by what happens to the recipient after the massage session. For example, the relaxation benefits of a massage might wear off sooner if a person returns to a stressful environment. Or the benefits might be prolonged if he or she takes time to relax further by having a restful walk or soaking in a warm bath. Time and dose illustrate the complexity of discussing the effects of massage.

Holistic View of Effects

Later in the chapter, the effects of massage on specific tissues and organ systems are examined. This is appropriate as a starting point for understanding the human biological response to touch and movement. However, certain effects are best explained by viewing human beings as whole

TABLE 6–1	Summary of the Effects of Massage*
Body Level	**Effects of Massage**
Tissue Level	
	Enhance tissue repair and scar formation.
	Improve connective tissue health.
	Improve pliability of fascia.
	Release adhesions and separate tissues.
Organ System Level	
Integumentary System	Stimulate sensory receptors in skin.
	Increase superficial circulation.
	Remove dead skin.
	Add moisture with oil or lotion.
	Increase sebaceous gland secretions.
	Facilitate healthy scar formation.
Skeletal System	Promote smooth joint function.
	Promote optimal joint flexibility and range of motion.
	Promote proper skeletal alignment.
Muscular System	"Milk" metabolic wastes into venous and lymph flow.
	Elicit specific muscle relaxation.
	Promote general muscle relaxation.
	Enhance connective tissue health and pliability related to muscles and joints.
	Relieve myofascial trigger points.
	Release myofascial adhesions.
Nervous System	Stimulate parasympathetic nervous system (relaxation response).
	Reduce pain (e.g., neural-gating mechanism).
	Sharpen body awareness.
Endocrine System	Reduce stress and anxiety:
	• Increase dopamine level.
	• Lower cortisol level.
	• Lower norepinephrine/epinephrine level.
	Elevate mood:
	• Increase serotonin level.
Cardiovascular System	Increase general and local circulation.
	Enhance venous return.
	Reduce blood pressure and heart rate.
	Increase red blood cells in circulation.
Lymphatic System and Immunity	Increase lymph fluid movement.
	Improve immune function.
	• Reduce cortisol level.
Respiratory System	Encourage diaphragmatic breathing.
	Relax muscles of respiration.
	Promote good structural alignment and rib cage expansion.
Digestive System	Improve digestion.
	Facilitate bowel movement.
Urinary System	Enhance circulation to kidneys.
	Increase urinary production and bladder tension.
Reproductive System	Improve reproductive function with relaxation.
	Promote general breast health.

Body Level	Effects of Massage
Organism Level	
Growth and Development	Promote growth and development in infants.
Pain Reduction	Relieve muscle pain from tension and poor circulation.
	Deactivate myofascial trigger points.
	Activate neural-gating mechanism.
	Increase endorphins and enkephalins.
	Increase serotonin.
Stress Reduction	Trigger relaxation response:
	• Increase dopamine and serotonin levels.
Psychological Level	
	Increase mental clarity.
	Reduce anxiety.
	Facilitate emotional release.
	Promote feelings of general well-being.

*These effects do not occur during every massage session. The massage techniques used and the qualities of movement (e.g., rhythm, pacing, pressure, direction, duration) help determine which effects are likely to occur. The physical, mental, and emotional conditions of recipients and their openness to massage might also have impact on which effects occur.

organisms. These might be changes that involve more than one body system or that influence the mind and emotions. This holistic view recognizes that we live as whole persons, and that a change in one aspect of our being can affect all other aspects in complex ways. Therefore, small changes induced by massage locally can produce an overall effect that is greater than the sum of its parts. This holistic phenomenon deserves a closer look.

The body and mind are indivisible and function as a single unit. Their connection begins in the embryonic stages of life when the basic components of the major organ systems appear. In the third week after fertilization occurs, the human embryo is comprised of three layers of cells; the outer layer, called the *ectoderm*, eventually develops into the skin, brain, and nervous system. Therefore, the physical structures that make sensation possible (skin and nerves) come from the same cellular material as the brain, which is the center for coordination and integration of the whole organism. These structures stay functionally interconnected for the life of the person. It has been observed that "depending on how you look at it, the skin is the outer surface of the brain, or the brain is the deepest layer of the skin."[1]

This connection between the skin and nervous system has profound implications when studying the effects of massage. When massage therapists touch the outermost surface of the physical body, they simultaneously touch the innermost parts of their clients' whole being. Research on touch has borne out this connection. For example, a well-documented effect of massage is that it reduces anxiety, which is a mental state. Massage has also been used successfully to help premature infants gain weight and generally thrive. Many more organism-level and body–mind effects are described throughout this chapter.

Massage is sometimes referred to as a *body-centered therapy*. That is, it produces its effects primarily through touch and movement of the client's body. In the broad scope of bodywork, this includes the energetic as well as the physical body. This is in contrast to mind-centered therapies, such as psychotherapy, that primarily involve talking, or music therapy, which relies on listening.

This is not to say that verbal communication between the massage therapist and client is unimportant. On the contrary, listening and talking are necessary for things such as establishing rapport, giving directions, asking for feedback,

PRACTICAL APPLICATION

"Learning by doing" is particularly useful in a vocational program. In the case of massage, "learning by receiving" can be equally valuable. Receive two professional massages within a period of 2 weeks to see what beneficial effects it has on you.

1. What effects did you notice on your organ systems?
2. Did you experience any psychological effects?
3. Did the type of massage you received or the setting have particular effects?

and getting informed consent. However, the primary therapeutic benefits of massage come from hands-on applications of touch and movement. In fact, some of the most important communication during massage happens through skillful and caring touch.

An observer can see the massage therapist performing techniques such as kneading, sliding, and vibrating to the client's body. However, the recipient experiences changes that are unseen and involve his or her whole being. For example, calming the nervous system, relaxing muscles, and pleasurable touch are felt on many levels unknown to others outside the recipient. These are largely unobservable effects.

Massage therapists encounter the unity just described in many ways. For example, a practitioner may be focused on some physical aspect such as relaxing tense muscles, but the recipient might talk about something emotional such as painful memories of the accident that caused the trauma. Or a massage therapist may witness the physical effects of stress on a client in the form of tension headaches. A holistic view recognizes that even though massage is body centered in application, its effects are felt by the recipient on many different levels as a whole person.

KNOWLEDGE OF EFFECTS

Two basic questions stand out in relation to the effects of massage: *What happens? Why does it happen?* Or to expand a little: *How does a person receiving massage (or a certain technique or application) respond physically, mentally, and holistically? What is the mechanism that creates that response?* Those key questions have typically been answered in the past either by tradition, experience, and/or rational thinking. More recently, systematic observations in the form of research are making greater inroads into understanding the various effects of massage.

Traditions are beliefs and practices passed from one generation to another. Traditions had more credence in the past when massage practitioners learned by apprenticeship, and old authorities were rarely questioned. Traditions can be problematic, though, because they may be based in outdated knowledge and practices. As scientific knowledge advances and new information about the body and how it functions arises, theories and practices need to be updated.

Experience offers more solid footing for discussing effects. Massage therapists can see responses in their clients with their own eyes and feel changes with their own hands. These observations are the basis of **empirical knowledge**. This type of observation-based knowledge is practical and priceless for developing skill in massaging clients. Much of what is currently accepted about the effects of massage comes from the empirical knowledge accumulated by countless massage practitioners in the past. Experience alone, however, can be incomplete and influenced by personal biases and limitations.

A different kind of knowledge is required when the discussion enters the realm of explanation for the effects observed. Usually the theories about what is happening are framed in terms of anatomy, physiology, pathology, or psychology. Sometimes conjectures involve references to energy. Reasoning proceeds from science or a particular philosophy to logical interpretations of the chain of events leading to the outcome being explained. These rational explanations are as good as the information on which they are based and the logic employed. Taken together, the accumulated experiential knowledge of massage practitioners and rational explanations for outcomes observed make up much of the **conventional wisdom** related to the effects of massage. Conventional wisdom consists of generally accepted beliefs regardless of their basis.

Conventional wisdom needs to be updated periodically when new information becomes available. For example, it was conventional wisdom not too long ago that massage was absolutely contraindicated for people with cancer. That principle was based on a misunderstanding of both cancer and the effect massage might have on it spreading to other parts of the body. The buildup of experience with cancer patients and recent research studies showed this to be a false belief, and now massage is viewed as a valuable complementary therapy for patients receiving cancer treatment.[2]

Research

Research is the systematic examination of a phenomenon based on careful observations using measurements. It is empirical in the sense that it is knowledge gained through the physical senses. However, it differs from the hands-on experience acquired through years of practice in that it offers a more methodical, objective, and focused study of a particular subject or question.

Basic research is the in-depth study of a phenomenon without a specific practical application in mind. For example, recent basic research has looked at the surprising properties of fascial tissue, information that will undoubtedly be valuable for manual therapists in the future. More sophisticated scientific instruments have allowed scientists to study the human organism in ways not possible before.

Over a century ago, research methods began to be used to study manual therapy. This early research was conducted to determine the effects of massage techniques on biological processes such as blood and lymph circulation and recovery after muscle exertion. These studies were trying to verify explanations for the success of massage applications popular at the time. Experiments involving dissection were done on animals to measure the effects of selected massage techniques directly. Advocates of massage were eager to explain claims made for the manual treatment of various pathologies (i.e., why they worked) and to prove that massage had a scientific basis.[3]

Doctors who advocated for massage in the late nineteenth century assumed that it was effective from their own clinical observations. Books and journals of the time contained many stories or anecdotes about how patients were healed using massage. When the stories were detailed and included measurements, they became the precursors to case studies as we know them today. Some doctors, especially those connected to universities in Europe, began to apply the scientific method to cases and compare the results from different patients. They occasionally compared massage to conventional treatments of the time like immobilization of injuries or use of electrical stimulation. The amount and quality of research conducted about massage therapy has varied over the past century, with periods of plenty alternating with periods of scarcity. The upsurge in the number of massage research studies since the 1990s has increased the need for research literacy among today's massage therapists who want to stay up-to-date and advance their knowledge and skills.

RESEARCH LITERACY

Massage therapists today should be fluent in the language of research, at least at a practical level. Some of the fundamental concepts are presented in this chapter, and a research terminology list can be found in Table 6–2 ■. **Research literacy** includes understanding the scientific method, appreciating the strength of different types of studies, locating and evaluating studies on a specific topic, and gleaning practical information from research reports.

Scientific Method

The **scientific method** was initially developed to test whether certain medical treatments were truly effective. The famous American businessman, politician, and scientist Benjamin Franklin is credited with vastly improving the scientific method in the late eighteenth century. When Franklin was investigating a dubious treatment called "mesmerism," he introduced the ideas of using a control group and blinded (i.e., blindfolded) subjects. The tools for statistical analysis of results were refined in the early twentieth century, which was a leap forward for testing cause-and-effect relationships. The scientific method has proved so useful that it has been adopted in a number of professions, including health-related disciplines such as massage therapy.

The scientific method goes beyond merely observing clinical results; it involves comparing patients who receive a specific treatment to those who do not, or to those who get a different treatment altogether. This type of experimental research began being applied to massage in the late nineteenth century, but was dropped for many decades until interest in complementary and alternative medicine (CAM) therapies was revived in the 1990s. Since then an increasing number of experimental studies have looked at the effectiveness of massage as a health and healing measure.

The scientific method is a systematic procedure for collecting and analyzing information relevant to answering a research question. It is based on measured observations

of what actually happens in a well-defined situation and involves a large number of subjects. The results of a well-done study are more applicable to the general population than anecdotal reports of something that occurred in an individual case.

Experimental studies start with a research question that defines the topic of the study broadly; for example, "Is massage an effective treatment for tension headaches?" The *hypothesis* reframes the question for the study as a theory about what will happen in a specific situation. Hypotheses make a statement about the relationship between two or more variables. For example, a hypothesis might be that a certain massage application will reduce the frequency and severity of chronic tension headaches. The variables here are the massage application (variable #1), frequency of headaches (variable #2), and severity of headaches (variable #3).

Measurement of relevant variables before and after a particular massage application is an essential part of the research design. Measurements offer an objective and verifiable way to describe changes that might be attributed to massage. In the earlier example, measuring the frequency of tension headaches provides a quantitative assessment of improvement after massage. The severity of headaches is a more subjective variable, but it can be assessed using a qualitative measure, for example, on a scale of 1 (mild) to 10 (most severe). Comparing pre- and posttreatment measurements provides evidence that real change took place due to the massage application.

Pilot studies are preliminary studies made with a small number of subjects to test the usefulness of measurements or some other aspect of research design. Pilot studies are sometimes conducted to assess the desirability of investing in a larger, more costly study, such as one on massage and tension headaches.[4]

The best evidence for cause and effect requires what is called a **randomized control trial (RCT)**. These experiments randomly divide subjects of the study into an experimental group and a control group. The experimental group receives the massage application being studied. The control group usually gets nothing at all or an alternative or *sham* treatment. The research design tries to control for variables that might affect the outcomes, for example, consistency in the treatment given. Subjects are *blinded*, that is, neither group knows if they are getting the treatment being studied or the sham treatment. The pre- and posttreatment measurements are then compared within each group and then between the groups. Statistical analysis subsequently determines if differences in the outcomes of the two groups could have happened by chance, or if the treatment really did have the effect hypothesized. Basic experimental research design elements are illustrated in Figure 6–1 ■.

Levels of Evidence

The strength of evidence for cause and effect, or whether a certain massage application actually played a part in the

TABLE 6–2	Research Terminology
Term	**Definition**
Anecdote	General descriptive story about the treatment of a condition and the outcomes for one patient.
Blinded	Single—subjects do not know who is getting the treatment being studied.
	Double—neither subjects nor people giving the treatment know which group is getting the treatment being studied.
Case report	Detailed observation and analysis of the treatment of a condition and the outcomes for one patient.
Case series	Multiple case reports about a specific treatment for a particular condition.
Control group	Subjects who do not receive the treatment being studied, or who receive a placebo, or a different treatment than the experimental group.
Empirical	Based on observation and/or measurement.
Experimental group	Subjects who receive the treatment being studied.
External validity	Degree to which the results of a study can be generalized to the larger population.
Hypothesis	Statement about the relationship between one or more variables.
Internal validity	Degree to which the study design and execution is capable of determining cause and effect.
Intervention	Application given to subjects in a study; same as treatment.
Pilot study	Preliminary study to test a research design.
Posttest	Measurement of relevant variables *after* the application of the treatment.
Pretest	Measurement of relevant variables *before* the application of the treatment.
Qualitative	Measurement of variables using word-based assessments.
Quantitative	Measurement of variables using numerical data.
Random assignment	Subjects are assigned to control groups by chance.
Randomized control trial (RCT)	Study that uses experimental and control groups to examine possible cause and effect relationships among variables.
Research question	The topic of a study stated as a broad question.
Results	Analysis of changes measured in pre- and posttests.
Scientific method	A systematic procedure for collecting and analyzing information relevant to answering a research question.
Statistical	Use of numerical computations to analyze the relationship among variables.
Subjects	People participating in a research study.
Systematic review	Analysis of a number of experimental research studies to determine the strength of evidence for use of a particular treatment for a certain condition.
Treatment	Application given to subjects in a study; same as intervention.

changes observed, varies with different types of studies. Studies also differ as to whether the results can be reasonably applied to the population at large or only to a special group. The major types of studies, in order of their rigor as evidence for cause and effect (from low to high), are the following:

- Case studies
- Case series
- Experimental study with no control group
- Randomized control trial
- Systematic review

Case studies are measured observations of the results of massage therapy given to improve the health of a single client. This is valuable information as far as it goes, but does not tell us if the results would be the same in others. A *case series* or number of similar cases would provide stronger evidence for cause and effect. However, they lack a control group and the consistency of a well-planned experimental study. Case studies and case series are sometimes precursors to experimental studies and might show that a certain treatment has promise. Case studies will be discussed further in Chapter 7, *Clinical Applications of Massage*.

Basic Research Design Elements

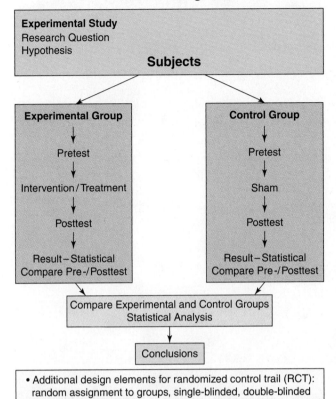

FIGURE 6–1 Elements of experimental design.

An *experimental study* with no control group has a number of subjects getting exactly the same treatment and statistical analysis of pre- and posttest results. These studies can establish that a significant change in certain variables did occur during the study. However, with no control group, they do not verify that the change occurred from the application and not from some other common factor.

The *randomized control trial (RCT)* described earlier and illustrated in Figure 6-1 is considered the "gold standard" for research study design. It is basically an experimental study that includes a control group.

A **systematic review**, or meta-analysis, of a number of well-designed research studies on the same topic provides an even more credible basis for evidence of a treatment's effectiveness. Systematic reviews are used in health care to make evidence-based decisions about treatment.

Locating Research Studies

Locating research studies about massage has become easier in recent years. Research reports are listed in a number of online databases, as well as in professional publications. *Peer-reviewed journals* are credible sources of information about research studies. Peer-reviewed journals only publish research that meets certain standards and that has been evaluated by experts in the field. This is in contrast to reports on websites or in trade journals by those with monetary interests

in the outcomes of the studies and to anecdotal stories about massage often found in popular magazines.

The Massage Therapy Foundation (MTF) funds research studies, promotes research literacy among massage therapists, and disseminates information about current studies related to massage and bodywork. MTF also publishes a peer-reviewed, open access, quarterly online journal called the *International Journal of Therapeutic Massage & Bodywork: Research, Education, & Practice* (see Appendix E, *References and Additional Resources*).

Research studies about massage can be found on *PubMed*, a website of the National Institutes of Health that has citations for biomedical literature from a variety of sources. PubMed often provides abstracts or summaries of research reports and sometimes access to entire reports. (www.ncbi.nlm.nih.gov/pubmed).

Systematic reviews of studies about the effects of massage for specific pathologies can be found on The Cochrane Collaboration website (see Appendix E). The Cochrane Database of Systematic Reviews contains reports that include a summary of research on some topic, for example, massage for promoting mental and physical health in infants under age 6 months. The reports also present the conclusions of a committee of experts about how strong the evidence is for the effectiveness of massage in those cases based on the available research. Other topics on the Cochrane website include massage for people with HIV/AIDS, for promoting growth and development of preterm and/or low-birth-weight infants, for mechanical neck disorders, for people with dementia, and for low back pain. Systematic reviews are necessarily limited to topics for which a significant amount of research exists. These reviews of research are used in health care as support for evidence-based practice.

Another source for locating research studies is the Touch Research Institute (TRI) at the University of Miami School of Medicine (see Appendix E). Their website contains information about studies they have sponsored, including topics such as massage, weight gain in preterm infants, enhanced attentiveness, alleviation of depression, pain reduction, stress reduction, and improved immune function.

National and international conferences on massage research are held periodically. Some are focused specifically on massage therapy, such as those sponsored by the Massage Therapy Foundation. Studies on massage and bodywork are also presented at conferences on alternative and integrative medicine research. These meetings provide opportunities for researchers to network and to report on the latest studies related to the effects and applications of massage therapy.

Reading Research Reports

Reading and evaluating research reports requires an understanding of their basic elements. Typical research reports include six sections: abstract, introduction, methods, results, discussion, and references. Research reports lay out the reasons for the study, describe the methods used, discuss the results, and identify references used. Abstracts summarize the main elements

TABLE 6–3	Sections of a Research Report
Section	**Contents**
Abstract	Quick overview of background, methods, results, and conclusion. Keywords (for database searching).
Introduction	Overview of the study topic. Relevant literature review. Reasons massage could be beneficial. Rationale for treatment procedure and measurement of variables.
Methods	Description of study subjects. Description of massage application used, measurements, and other factors, such as session frequency and timing. Statement of hypothesis. Description of the research design.
Results	Case study: narrative summary of treatment and outcomes. Clinical trial: summary of outcome measurements. Organized display of results/findings.
Discussion	Connects results back to Introduction. Speculates on why the massage application worked or did not work as hypothesized. Comments on implications for practice. Provides ideas for future studies.
References	Main sources of ideas and facts mentioned in the report. Citations of past research about the research topic. Establishes confidence in approach to the study.

of the study and are useful for identifying studies you would like to know more about. Full reports give much more detailed information. Descriptions of methods, measurements, and results are especially interesting to practitioners. Table 6–3 ■ summarizes the typical sections of a research report.

It is important to remember that research studies can have flaws that make their conclusions less valid. *External validity* is "the capacity of the findings to be generalized to a larger group than the one that participated in the study." *Internal validity* involves elements within the study design or execution that make the findings more or less credible.[5] Careful reading of research reports allows you to evaluate them and their usefulness for real-life therapeutic situations. Table 6–4 ■ provides an example of a research report evaluation worksheet.

TABLE 6–4	Research Report Evaluation Worksheet	
Steps		**Your Analysis**
1. State the general research question.		
2. Describe the research design and methods.		
• Hypothesis		
• Subjects demographics		
• Intervention/Treatment		
• Control: sham, different treatment		
• Variables observed		
• General procedure: pre- and posttest, number of treatments, spacing of treatments, etc.		
3. Describe the measurement tools used for specific variables.		
4. Summarize the results (statistics).		
5. Summarize the study conclusions.		
6. Note strengths and weaknesses of the study.		
7. Explain how well the study did or did not answer the research question.		
8. Give suggestions for future research designs for this topic.		
9. Discuss implications of this study for your practice.		

It has been argued that the nature of massage as a holistic therapy makes it unsuited for scientific inquiry. For example, some practitioners dismiss the fixed protocols used in many studies that don't take into account individual differences in clients. Others believe that there are many immeasurable factors that cannot be accounted for, or that it is difficult to translate research findings into practical information. Those are valid criticisms that researchers in other complementary and alternative therapies share, and innovative research designs have been proposed to address these issues in the future. Nevertheless, reading research reports about massage can broaden your knowledge and stimulate critical thinking about the work you are engaged in.

A CLOSER LOOK AT THE EFFECTS OF MASSAGE

Now that you understand a little better how knowledge about massage is generated, it is time to return to the discussion of the effects of massage. The following sections take a closer look at the physiological effects of massage at the tissue, organ system, and organism levels, and in the psychological domain. The discussion in each section outlines the conventional wisdom concerning the responses of the body–mind to touch and movement. Relevant research studies are described as examples of how the scientific method has advanced knowledge in the areas examined. Keep in mind that new

REALITY CHECK

KELLY

ALLISON: I don't plan on going into clinical massage therapy so research seems irrelevant to me. Did you ever read a research report once you graduated from school? Have you ever found it useful?

KELLY: When I graduated from school there wasn't much massage research to read. Now I find that some of the research being conducted is quite relevant to my practice and pretty interesting too. For instance, articles written in mainstream magazines about massage as a stress reducer and for relief from low back pain and tension headaches often cite recent research on the subject. Research on infant massage is often reported, too. Some of my clients have read about these benefits and come looking for that from me. I read the reports to see what massage application was used, what the study measured, and the results. Sometimes I pick up practical tips that I use in my massage sessions.

studies are continually being published and often bring fresh insights regarding the effects of massage. Students are encouraged to delve deeper into topics they are curious about and check out the latest research in areas of interest.

You will notice that even though the effects are divided into different areas for purposes of study, the recipient experiences the massage as a whole integrated person. Effects are often related, and some might trigger other effects in a sort of chain reaction. The complexities will stand out as you examine the effects of massage more closely.

PHYSIOLOGICAL EFFECTS—TISSUE LEVEL

Massage improves the overall health of cells and tissues of the body, primarily by increasing blood and lymph circulation. The "milking" action of petrissage techniques and the sliding movements of effleurage are very effective in moving body fluids to facilitate natural processes. Increased fluid circulation improves delivery of oxygen and nutrients to tissue cells and helps in removal of metabolic wastes and by-products of the inflammatory process.[6] Two topics of special interest to massage therapists are tissue repair and the nature of connective tissue.

Tissue Repair

Healing from soft tissue injuries such as burns, bruises, sprains, and wounds involves three physiological phases. The tissue repair process consists of *inflammation* to stabilize the injured area, *regeneration* to restore the tissue structure, and *remodeling* for healthy scar formation. Massage can play an important role in the tissue repair process. See Figure 6–2 ■ for a schematic rendering of the tissue repair process.

The initial reaction to injury, called inflammation, is designed to stabilize the situation and prepare damaged tissues for repair. Inflammation results in increased blood flow to the area causing redness, warmth, swelling, pain, and decreased function. The lymphatic system plays an important role in the resolution of inflammation by removing fluid that creates swelling and inspecting that fluid for harmful microorganisms. The length of the inflammatory phase varies depending on the severity of the initial trauma and the strength of the individual's immune system.

Massage is contraindicated in the immediate location of an injury during the inflammatory phase, especially in the presence of infection. If there is no infection associated with an injury, lymphatic massage techniques may be used in some cases to reduce swelling in an area. Once the signs of inflammation subside, standard massage techniques can be applied safely around the injury site.

In the regeneration phase, the tissue structure is rebuilt and restored. New tissue replaces damaged tissue of the same type. This involves removing damaged cells, excess fluids, and other by-products of inflammation, as well as delivering the building blocks for new tissue formation. By improving general and local circulation, massage

FIGURE 6–2 Three phases of the tissue/wound repair process.

can facilitate this regeneration process. Gentle, passive stretching techniques around the wound area can also contribute to general tissue health. The amount of pressure used at this phase of healing is limited to what the tissues can withstand without further damage. Aggressive techniques should be avoided.

Massage can also play a role in the remodeling phase of tissue repair by encouraging healthy scar formation. Deep transverse friction is used in rehabilitation to help form strong mobile scar tissue. Deep friction helps break inter-fiber adhesions by mechanically broadening the tissues. This in turn helps produce more parallel fiber arrangement and fewer transverse connections in the tissue that may inhibit movement. Subcutaneous scar tissue may be loosened by careful and persistent friction.[7] Other goals for the remodeling phase of tissue repair are reduction in swelling, pain and itching, and maintenance of mobility around joints in the area. Swedish and lymphatic massage, fascial release techniques, and passive stretching support healing in this phase of repair. Clinical experience suggests that once a scar is mature, massage may reduce the sensation of tightness and improve the softness and color of the scar.[8]

A less understood role for massage in tissue repair is related to its promotion of stress reduction. A study reported in *Lancet*, a British medical journal, showed that wounds healed more slowly in people suffering from chronic stress. Researchers found that the stressed group had lower levels of interleukin-1 beta, an immune system substance known to play a role in wound repair.[9] To the extent that massage reduces stress, it may help wounds heal faster.

Connective Tissue

Connective tissue is the most pervasive tissue in the body. It fills internal spaces, provides structural support, and is a vehicle for fluid transportation and energy storage.

Classifications of connective tissue include fluid (e.g., blood and lymph); supporting (e.g., cartilage and bone); dense (e.g., tendons, ligaments, dermis), loose (e.g., fascia), and adipose tissue (i.e., fat). Figure 6–3 ■ shows common types and locations of connective tissue of interest to massage therapists. Some general connective tissue considerations and the nature of fascia are discussed briefly in the following section.

TENDONS, LIGAMENTS, FASCIA

The connective tissue in tendons, ligaments, and fascia has a property called *thixotropy*, which means that it becomes more fluid and pliable when it is mobile and firmer when it is immobile. Pressing, friction, stretching, and other movements of massage raise the temperature and the energy level of the tissue slightly and create a "greater degree of sol (fluidity) in organic systems that are already there but are behaving sluggishly."[10]

In addition to promoting healthy function, massage helps to prevent some connective tissue abnormalities and dysfunction. For example, massage techniques such as kneading and deep friction have been found to help prevent the formation of abnormal collagenous connective tissue called *fibrosis*.[11]

Fascia is a type of connective tissue that surrounds all muscles, bones, and organs and helps to give them shape. Fascia literally holds the body together and can be thought of as continuous sheets of supportive tissue, which envelop the entire body and its parts. A theory of physical structure used by some bodyworkers views connective tissue, not bones, as the main support of the body and thus the foundation of good posture. Recent studies have revealed that fascial tissue has the ability to contract, much like smooth muscle, and is therefore more dynamic in posture and movement than previously thought.[12]

FIGURE 6–3
Types and locations of
connective tissue.

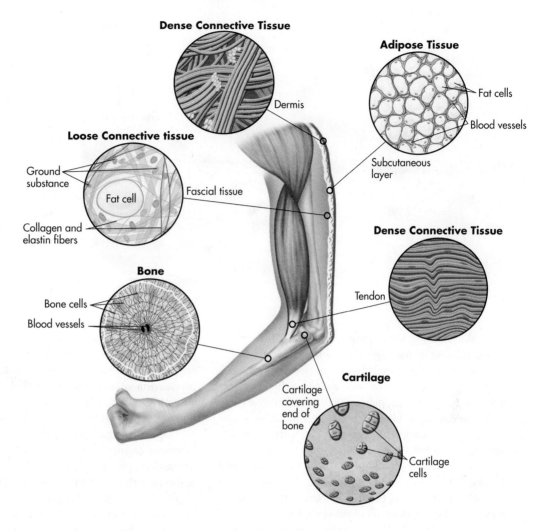

In healthy bodies, fascial tissues are pliable and move freely. With chronic stress, chronic immobility, trauma, or disease, connective tissue may become thickened and rigid or may stick to other tissues, forming adhesions. Adhesions result in restricted movement and impair the ability of the affected tissues to conduct exchanges of nutrients and cellular wastes. Massage can improve tissue function by helping to restore tissue pliability and eradicate adhesions.

Certain massage techniques remove adhesions formed when fascial tissues stick to each other or to other tissues. The simple mechanical action of some massage techniques separates tissues, for example, lifting, broadening, and applying a shearing force across the parallel organization of fibers. Kneading, skin rolling, deep transverse friction, broadening techniques, and myofascial techniques are examples of effective methods for separating and "unsticking" adhering tissues.

Chapter 21, *Myofascial Massage*, provides more detailed information about myofascial techniques applied to improve the condition of fascial tissues. The discussion of increased joint mobility and flexibility in the *Muscular System* section of this chapter has further information on connective tissue and massage.

PHYSIOLOGICAL EFFECTS— ORGAN SYSTEM LEVEL

Massage has specific effects on the different organ systems of the body. In addition to keeping the organ tissues healthy and enhancing healing, massage can also improve the function of the system as a whole. And because organ systems interact in myriad ways, the effects of massage on any one system impacts others as well. Overlapping function is especially obvious in certain system pairings, such as muscular–skeletal, circulatory–lymphatic, nervous–endocrine, and respiratory–circulatory–muscular.

Integumentary System

The integumentary system includes the skin and its accessory structures such as hair, nails, and sebaceous and sweat glands. The skin has three layers: the epidermis or outermost layer, dermis, and subcutaneous fascia. Sensory receptors in the skin detect touch, tickle, pain, traction, heat, cold, and pressure and relay that information to the nervous system. See Figure 6–4 ■.

Touch   Tickle   Pain   Traction   Heat   Cold   Pressure

FIGURE 6–4
Common touch sensations.

The skin is the primary point of contact between the giver and receiver of massage. One of the major effects of pressure to the skin is stimulation of the sensory receptors found there. This stimulation may have beneficial effects such as general relaxation, pain reduction, and body awareness. By increasing a client's body awareness, massage enhances a person's sense of integrity and wholeness, which is important for good mental and emotional health.

For the exocrine glands in the skin (sebaceous and sweat glands) to work properly, skin pores must be free from blockage. Pores may become blocked with substances such as dirt, makeup, dried oils, and sweat, or the accumulation of dead skin cells. Bathing with soap and water and hydrotherapy—such as whirlpool, steam room, and sauna—help open pores. Exfoliating, or removing dead skin cells by scraping or friction (e.g., with a loofa, brush, or coarse towel) is an old health and beauty practice. Read more about exfoliation in Chapter 19, *Spa Treatments*.

The friction of massage also increases superficial circulation and raises the temperature of skin. This promotes perspiration and increases sebaceous oil secretions. Oil and lotion applied to the skin during massage add moisture needed to prevent further drying or cracking. This is especially beneficial in dry climates, on aging skin, and with certain dry skin conditions.

Massage can facilitate the formation of healthy scar tissue on the skin surface following lacerations, surgery incisions, or burns. Applying cross-fiber and with-fiber friction techniques to scars during the remodeling phase helps form strong mobile scars, remove adhesions to underlying tissues, and reduce scar thickness. Skin lifting and rolling techniques stretch underlying fascia and remove superficial adhesions.

Skeletal System

The skeletal system includes the bones of the skeleton, associated cartilage, ligaments, and other stabilizing connective tissue structures. In addition to general tissue health promoted by good circulation, massage and related joint movements help maintain good joint function and range of motion. Movement of the joints stimulates production of synovial fluid that keeps joints moving smoothly. The major bones and joints of the skeletal system are shown on the back inside cover of this textbook.

Optimal range of motion is achieved when the bones are in proper alignment and the tissues surrounding the joints are healthy, pliable, and relaxed. Joint flexibility (i.e., flexability) is enhanced with massage and stretching movements (Figure 6–5 ■). Flexibility is discussed in greater depth in the *Muscular System* section of this chapter.

Proper body alignment is necessary for optimal functioning of the skeletal system. Maintaining good posture is a function of the combined muscular, skeletal, and nervous systems and is discussed in more detail in the section that follows.

Muscular System

The muscular system includes skeletal muscles, associated connective tissue (i.e., fascia and tendons), and motor and sensory neurons related to movement. Proprioceptors, important sensory neurons that monitor the movement and position of the body in space, are located in the skeletal muscles and related connective tissue. Major muscles of the body are illustrated on the inside front cover of this textbook.

The importance of muscular system health for overall well-being cannot be overestimated. It is through the musculature and the movement it produces that so many other health benefits derive, for example, good circulation, body heat, metabolism, kinesthetic awareness, and even emotional balance. Adequate exercise has been named in numerous research studies as one of the most powerful prevention measures for a number of chronic diseases that plague sedentary humans.

Problems in the musculature can cause severe pain and reduce quality of life. It is not surprising that massage

Ball and Socket Joint

FIGURE 6–5 Passive stretching enhances joint function.

therapy is valued so highly for its role in maintaining good health and function of the muscular system.

CELLULAR LEVEL ACTIVITY

Muscles maintain normal cellular level activity and balance through movement. Muscle contraction puts mechanical pressure on the veins and lymphatic vessels, thereby pushing fluids along and carrying away metabolic by-products. As the muscles relax, fresh blood flows into them, bringing nutrients to the area. This balancing action is disturbed through underactivity or overactivity.

Underactivity disturbs balance because the muscle contractions that provide the "milking" effect are less than needed for good fluid circulation. Waste products then accumulate in the muscle tissue, and the arrival of nutrients is slowed. When illness or injury results in muscular inactivity, massage techniques such as petrissage mimic the action of muscle contraction, thereby improving fluid circulation.

Overactivity (e.g., from strenuous exercise or work) also disturbs balance at the cellular level. Insufficient time between contractions decreases the inflow of nutritive products and oxygen to muscle tissues. In addition, metabolic waste products are formed faster than they can be eliminated. Muscle tension increases, and muscles shorten due to reduced cellular nutrition. Muscle tension worsens the situation by further limiting fluid circulation.

Massage given immediately after strenuous physical activity relieves muscle stiffness and soreness. Several research studies have concluded that massage also lessens the discomfort felt the day after such activity, known as *delayed-onset muscle soreness (DOMS)*.[13, 14] A combination of effleurage (i.e., sliding) and petrissage (i.e., kneading or compression) flushes metabolic wastes, brings oxygen and nutrients to the area, and enhances tissue repair. These are important benefits of postevent, interevent, and recovery sports massage. For more information, see the discussion on increased blood circulation in the *Cardiovascular System* section of this chapter.

MUSCLE RELAXATION

Massage is often used to relax hypertonic or tense muscles. There are several ways that muscle relaxation may be achieved. Reduction of general muscle tension may result from stimulation of the parasympathetic nervous system via relaxation massage (Figure 6–6 ■). There may also be a conscious letting-go of muscle tension by the higher brain centers as the recipient assumes a passive state during a massage session.

General muscle relaxation may also be traced to increased sensory stimulation that accompanies the application of massage techniques. Yates reasons that massage causes a massive increase in the sensory input to the spinal cord, which results in readjustments in reflex pathways, which leads to spontaneous normalization of imbalances of tonic activity between individual muscles and muscle groups. Residual muscle tension left over from past activity

FIGURE 6–6 Massage reduces muscle tension and promotes relaxation.

or emotional stress is released as the system balances itself.[15] Thus, muscular relaxation results from the general application of a variety of basic massage techniques such as effleurage, petrissage, friction, tapotement, and vibration.

Manual techniques may be applied to relax specific muscles. For example, in a technique called *muscle approximation* the combined action of the muscular and nervous systems is utilized to reduce muscle tone. In this technique, the practitioner slowly and forcibly draws the attachments of the muscle closer together. This decreases stretch of the muscle spindles, which are composed of nerve filaments coiled around specialized muscle fibers (Figure 6–7 ■). Muscle spindles cause contraction when muscles are suddenly elongated (i.e., stretch reflex). Approximation causes slack in the muscle and is held until the muscle spindles stop firing and the muscle fibers relax. Approximation is useful for treating muscle spasms.

Another muscle relaxation method called the *origin and insertion technique* is useful when direct work on the muscle belly is too painful. In the origin and insertion technique, cross-fiber and with-fiber friction is performed on the attachments of the targeted muscle in small segments until the muscle fibers relax. Eventually, overall muscle tone is reduced. This works by stimulating sensory receptors called Golgi tendon organs, located in tendons near muscle attachments (Figure 6–8 ■). When Golgi tendon organs fire, they inhibit contraction of the associated muscle. Several other manual techniques for promoting muscle relaxation are discussed throughout the text because muscular relaxation is one of the more common goals of massage. The major muscles of the muscular system are shown on the front inside cover of this textbook.

INCREASED JOINT MOBILITY AND FLEXIBILITY

Flexibility refers to the degree of range of motion in a joint. It is a function of the combined muscular and skeletal systems with some nervous system involvement. Hypertonic muscles, scarring in muscle and connective tissues, myofascial adhesions, trigger points, and general connective tissue thickening and rigidity may all restrict movement at joints. Massage and passive joint movements can be used effectively to help maintain joint mobility and normal range of motion by addressing any abnormal conditions found in the soft tissues surrounding the joint.

In a study conducted by sport physical therapists and a massage therapist, massage was found to significantly increase range of motion in the hamstrings. The massage techniques used in the study were light and deep effleurage, stretching effleurage, petrissage (kneading), and friction (deep circular and deep transverse). Increased flexibility lasted for at least 7 days after the massage.[16] Additional information on improving flexibility through joint movements may be found in Chapter 13, *Joint Movements*.

FIGURE 6–7
Muscles spindles.

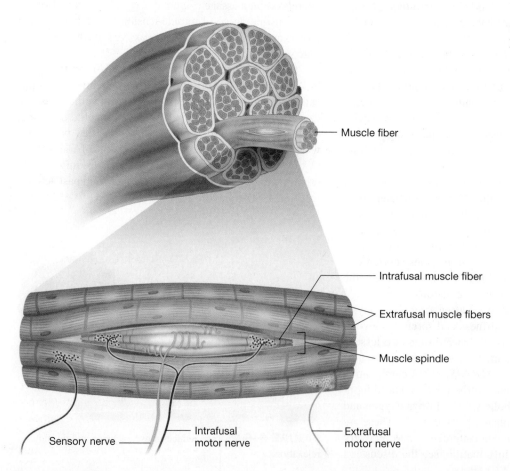

Muscle fiber

Intrafusal muscle fiber

Extrafusal muscle fibers

Muscle spindle

Sensory nerve — Intrafusal motor nerve — Extrafusal motor nerve

FIGURE 6–8
Golgi tendon organs.

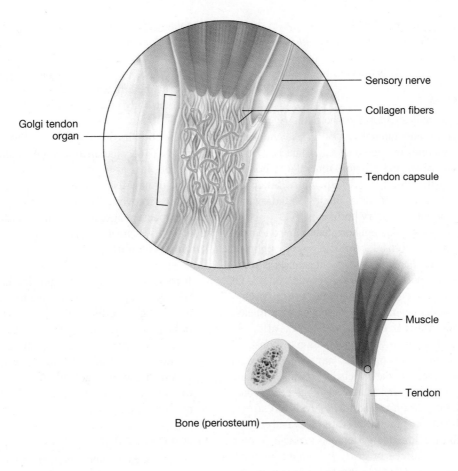

Sensory nerve

Collagen fibers

Golgi tendon organ

Tendon capsule

Muscle

Tendon

Bone (periosteum)

POSTURE

Proper body alignment or good posture is the combined function of the muscular, skeletal, and nervous systems. Poor posture usually results from a combination of factors such as ergonomically inadequate workstations or tools, injuries, and unhealthy postural habits such as slouching. Misalignment of the physical structure leads to imbalances between muscle groups, hypertonic and shortened muscles, fascial adhesions, trigger points, and other problem conditions. Or vice versa: muscle imbalances or pathologies may result in poor posture.

Some forms of massage and bodywork specifically focus on helping clients improve their body alignment. After analyzing the client's posture and identifying the probable cause of misalignment, massage and related joint movements are applied with the goal of proper alignment. This might involve strategies such as relaxing and elongating muscles with massage, lengthening muscle groups with stretching, or removing fascial adhesions with myofascial techniques. Posture analysis is described in detail in Chapter 9, *Medical Terminology, Goal-Oriented Planning, Documentation.*

Nervous and Endocrine Systems

The nervous and endocrine systems work together to coordinate organ system functions and respond to environmental stimuli. The nervous system controls relatively swift responses such as those related to movement, whereas the endocrine system regulates slower responses such as metabolic rate.

NERVOUS SYSTEM

Nervous system anatomy consists of the central nervous system (i.e., brain and spinal cord) and peripheral nervous system (i.e., sensory receptors and motor neurons). The division of the nervous system that regulates the activity of smooth muscle, cardiac muscle, and glands is called the *autonomic nervous system*, which plays an important role in relaxation massage.

Some of the effects of massage related to the nervous system have already been discussed. For example, stimulation of sensory receptors in the skin enhances body awareness and plays an important role in muscle relaxation and pain reduction. The effects of massage on growth and development in infants are directly related to stimulation of the nervous system via the skin and through body movement.[17, 18]

Some massage and movement techniques use the nervous system to stimulate the desired results. For example, some assisted stretching techniques deliberately activate proprioceptors in muscles to effect relaxation and elongation.

One of the most important effects of massage is its ability to elicit the relaxation response. This combined autonomic nervous system and endocrine system response is discussed in more detail in the *Physiological Effects—Organism Level* section of this chapter because it involves many organ systems, as well as mental and emotional states.

ENDOCRINE SYSTEM

The endocrine system is composed of the pituitary, thyroid, parathyroid, thymus, and adrenal glands. These endocrine glands secrete hormones that regulate important body processes such as cell growth and division, general metabolism, water loss, blood calcium levels, and immunity. Some tissues in the kidneys, heart, pancreas, and testes and ovaries also produce important regulatory hormones.

Noteworthy endocrine system hormones related to massage include dopamine, cortisol, serotonin, norepinephrine, and epinephrine. The secretion of these hormones is regulated in conjunction with the central nervous system. Of particular interest for massage is the effect of the parasympathetic nervous system in increasing or reducing the release of these hormones. Massage can be understood as affecting the levels of these hormones via the relaxation response.

Levels of these five hormones have been used in research studies to measure the effects of massage on stress and anxiety levels. For example, massage has been linked to elevated levels of dopamine and lower levels of cortisol, which provides evidence of reduced stress. Elevated cortisol levels also inhibit the immune system, so massage is seen to reduce the negative effects of stress on immune function. Massage has also been linked to increased serotonin levels, which reduces pain and elevates mood. In addition, massage helps decrease levels of norepinephrine and epinephrine, as a result of turning off the fight-or-flight response.[19, 20]

A recent exploratory study posed the question: Does a single session of Swedish massage have a positive effect on immune function? The hypothesis was that Swedish massage would increase hormones that enhance immune function and reduce hormones that inhibit it. The control group received a sham treatment of light touch. Measurements of hormone levels were taken prior to administration of treatment and afterwards at spaced intervals of time. The results for the group that received Swedish massage showed changes in hormone levels consistent with improved immune function, as well as an increase in the number of circulating lymphocytes. The conclusion was that Swedish massage did have measurable biologic effects, which may have implications for managing inflammatory and autoimmune conditions. Because of the promising results, a larger replication study was called for.[21]

Cardiovascular System

Cardiovascular (CV) system anatomy includes the heart, blood vessels (i.e., arteries, veins, and capillaries), and blood, which is considered a fluid connective tissue. It is essentially a fluid transportation system for nutrients, waste products, dissolved gases, hormones, and cells and molecules for body defense. The CV system teams up with the lymphatic system for important functions related to fighting infection and disease.

The cardiovascular and lymphatic systems are transport systems that rely specifically on the movement of fluids to carry out their functions. Good fluid circulation in these important body systems is a key to health at the cellular level.

The benefits of enhanced circulation include improved nutrient delivery and increased metabolic waste removal via the blood. It is also important for tissue repair, as building blocks for new tissues are brought to an area and damaged cells are removed. When pathogens enter the body, fluids deliver macrophages to attack the invaders and help prevent disease. The team action of these two body systems has been succinctly described by Yates:

> Increases in blood and lymph circulation are the most widely recognized and frequently described of the physiological effects of massage therapy. Changes in blood and lymph circulation are appropriately discussed together because they have effects in common on the clearance of metabolic wastes, and the byproducts of tissue damage and inflammation, the absorption of excess of inflammatory exudate, and on the delivery of oxygen and nutrients to tissue cells.[22]

BLOOD CIRCULATION

Massage increases blood circulation particularly in the area receiving the massage (Figure 6–9 ■). Even light pressure was shown to have an effect.[23] The benefits of increased circulation include improved nutrient delivery and increased metabolic waste removal.

Superficial friction, effleurage, and petrissage in particular produce hyperemia or increased local circulation in the skin and underlying connective tissue. As a result the skin appears red and feels warm. One study that examined this effect asked the research question: *Does massage increase peripheral blood flow?* Skin temperature was taken as a sign of peripheral blood flow and was measured using dynamic infrared thermography. Measurements were taken before and after massage of the neck and shoulders. The study found an increase in surface temperature in the area treated and in adjacent nonmassaged areas. Skin temperature stayed above baseline for more than 60 minutes. The study concluded that massage did measurably increase peripheral blood flow.[24] One theory for explaining this effect is that a release of the chemical *histamine* triggers dilation of capillaries in the area.

Recent research using Doppler ultrasound technology has challenged the common belief that massage also increases blood flow in the larger vessels. Studies failed to detect an increase in arterial blood flow in the limbs after massage, although one did confirm increased blood flow in the skin.[25, 26] The researchers reasoned that blood might be diverted away from the muscles and to the skin with massage. Although these findings do not diminish the known

FIGURE 6–9
Massage increases blood
circulation.

general effects of massage, they do call for a rethinking of what is happening in terms of blood circulation. For example, massage is still known to have benefits for recovery after exercise, although circulation may play a different role than previously thought.

The relaxation response of the parasympathetic nervous system is known to promote circulation to the internal organs and away from the larger muscle groups. Relaxation massage therefore might be said to improve general circulation for better overall health. There will be further discussion of the relaxation response in relation to the nervous system.

VENOUS RETURN

The mechanical action of deep effleurage enhances venous flow in the limbs. This technique physically pushes blood through venous circulation.

The structure of veins dictates the direction of the application of deep stroking on the limbs. A dictum in classic Swedish massage states that deep stroking should always be "toward the heart," or moving distal (away from) to proximal (near the center).

Veins are low-pressure tubes. Movement of blood through them is aided by muscle contraction and by valves that prevent pooling due to the effects of gravity. Deep effleurage in the direction of the natural movement of blood enhances the flow. Conventional wisdom holds that applying deep massage in the opposite direction puts pressure on the valves and could possibly damage them.

Damage to valves results in a condition known as varicose veins (see Figure 8–23). In varicose veins we find static, pooled blood. The constant pressure of pooled blood weakens the vein walls even further, causing a vicious cycle of pooling and weakening. Over time the veins become

fragile. Under these conditions, massage might cause the vein to rupture, or release clots formed in the pools, into general circulation. Therefore, massage is locally contraindicated over superficial varicose veins and generally contraindicated for someone with a history of blood clots.

The mechanical action of kneading and other forms of petrissage also assist in venous return, much the same way muscle contraction does during exercise. Compression of the tissues increases local circulation and blood in the capillaries is moved along toward the larger veins.

Venostasis is a condition in which the normal flow of blood through a vein is slowed or halted. Lack of muscular activity can bring about venostasis, particularly in inactive or paralyzed limbs. Other causes for venostasis include varicose veins and pressure on the vessels from edema of the surrounding tissues. Massage given for this condition should first address the proximal aspects of an inactive limb before massage of the distal area. This ensures that the circulatory pathways are open enough to carry the venous flow from the distal area back toward the heart.

BLOOD PRESSURE

Researchers Barr and Taslitz found that blood pressure is temporarily decreased for about 40 minutes after a 1-hour massage session.[27] The decrease in pressure is thought to result from a greater capacity for blood in the capillaries due to local vasodilation and greater permeability of capillary walls. The more blood in the capillaries, the less there is in other vessels to cause pressure on vessel walls. Reduction in both systolic and diastolic pressure was duplicated in research by Cady and Jones.[28]

Also, as mentioned earlier, one of the long-term effects of eliciting the relaxation response regularly and learning to control stress is decreased blood pressure in individuals with hypertension. This saves wear and tear on the circulatory system and improves circulation overall.

RED BLOOD CELLS

Massage increases the number of circulating red blood cells, thereby increasing the oxygen-carrying capacity of the blood. Red blood cells (RBCs) stored in the liver and spleen are thought to be discharged during massage, as well as RBC in stagnant capillary beds returned to circulation.[29, 30]

Lymphatic System and Immunity

The lymphatic system is made up of a network of lymphatic vessels, a fluid called lymph, and small organs (i.e., lymph nodes) that contain a large number of lymphocytes. The lymphatic system functions to return fluids from body tissues to the blood; transports hormones, nutrients, and waste products from tissues into general circulation; and defends the body from infection and disease via white blood cells or lymphocytes. A more detailed account of the lymphatic system is given in Chapter 23, *Lymphatic Facilitation*.

LYMPH FLUID MOVEMENT

Lymph is a viscous fluid that moves slowly through the lymphatic vessels. Lymphatic pressure is naturally lower, and lymph fluid movement slower, than venous blood flow.

The movement of lymph through the capillaries, ducts, and nodes of the lymphatic system depends on outside sources, such as the contraction of muscles, action of the diaphragm, and pressure generated by filtration of fluid from the capillaries. Lack of mobility due to a sedentary lifestyle, confinement to a bed or a wheelchair, pain, or paralysis seriously interferes with flow of lymph fluid.

It has been known for some time that massage techniques, especially effleurage and petrissage, mechanically assist general lymphatic flow.[31, 32, 33] In addition, special lymphatic facilitation techniques have been developed to maximize the effects of moving lymph through superficial capillaries (Figure 6–10 ■). Manual lymph drainage (MLD) techniques along with other therapies are used effectively in the treatment of a condition called *lymphedema*.[34] Lymphatic facilitation techniques used to move lymph fluid during injury rehabilitation, for relieving allergy symptoms, and other health purposes are described in Chapter 23, *Lymphatic Facilitation*.

IMMUNITY

Immunity is defined as "the resistance to injuries and disease caused by specific foreign chemical compounds and pathogens."[35] It is a complex phenomenon in which the lymphatic system plays an important part.

Massage affects immunity by enhancing the immune response, which is designed to destroy or inactivate pathogens, abnormal cells, and foreign molecules such as toxins. By improving lymphatic flow, as previously described, massage facilitates the transport of lymphocytes that participate in the immune response. This is a direct mechanical result of massage techniques such as effleurage and petrissage, both of which help move body fluids.

Massage also appears to improve immunity through a number of other mechanisms. Recent studies suggest that massage may be associated with increased natural killer (NK) cells and increased CD4 cells, as well as decreased anxiety and cortisol levels. High cortisol levels inflict wear and tear on the body over time by inhibiting the production and release of white blood cells, blocking T and B cell

FIGURE 6–10
Lymphatic massage techniques improve the circulation of lymph fluid.

Source: Pearson Education, Inc./Segal Photography.

function, and interfering with the production of interleukins, which are important for communication among white blood cells.[36, 37, 38]

Respiratory System

The respiratory system includes the lungs and the passageways leading to the lungs (i.e., nose, nasal cavity and sinuses, trachea, bronchial tubes). It acts with the circulatory system to achieve an exchange of gases between the body and the environment. The respiratory system relies on the diaphragm and other skeletal muscles to produce breathing.

Massage enhances respiratory function by improving general blood circulation and encouraging relaxed diaphragmatic breathing. Massage can also address tension and shortening in skeletal muscles involved in respiration. To the extent that massage facilitates good posture, it helps achieve the structural alignment and rib cage expansion necessary for optimal vital capacity (i.e., the amount of air moved into or out of the lungs during a single respiratory cycle).

Digestive System

The digestive system consists of a muscular tube called the digestive tract (i.e., oral cavity, pharynx, esophagus, stomach, small intestine, large intestine, rectum, and anus) and accessory organs, including the salivary glands, gall bladder, liver, and pancreas. Functions of the digestive system include ingestion, mechanical processing, and chemical breakdown of food and drink, secretion of digestive enzymes, absorption of water and nutrients, and excretion of waste products.

Massage enhances digestion through eliciting the relaxation response, in which digestive activity is increased. One of the negative effects of stress accumulated over a long period of time is disruption of the normal digestive processes, which can cause indigestion. Relaxation massage as part of a stress reduction program helps prevent digestive maladies.

Abdominal massage has been used for decades to facilitate bowel movement in people suffering from constipation. The direct mechanical effects of massage move the contents of the large intestine and initiate reflex effects that stimulate peristaltic movement.[39] See Figure 6–11 ■. Abdominal techniques of infant massage assist bowel and gas movement and help relieve distress. Abdominal massage for adults is described in Chapter 14, *Full-Body Swedish Massage*, and for infants in Chapter 18, *Special Populations and Adaptations*.

Urinary System

The structures of the urinary system include the kidneys, ureters, urinary bladder, and the urethra. The primary function of the urinary system is removal of waste products from the blood and their excretion from the body. It also helps regulate blood volume and pressure, as well as blood composition.

Because massage enhances function of the cardiovascular system, it indirectly affects the urinary system, which filters the blood. Better circulation to the kidneys leads to improved blood filtration overall. In addition, one of the results of activation of the parasympathetic nervous system via relaxation massage is increased urinary production and bladder tension. It is not uncommon to have to use the toilet after receiving a relaxing massage.

— Large intestine
— Small intestine

FIGURE 6–11 Abdominal massage facilitates bowel movement.

Reproductive System

The male and female reproductive organs are not appropriate targets for therapeutic massage. They do, however, benefit from improved general cardiovascular function, as do all body systems. There is evidence that chronic stress can impair sexual function, so to the extent that massage promotes relaxation, it could be said to benefit the reproductive function.

There are specialized approaches to massage for pregnant women. Postgraduate training in pregnancy massage is valuable for massage therapists in general practice or those working in places such as spas and salons. Some massage therapists are trained to work with midwives and other health care practitioners during delivery. They often combine Swedish massage techniques with others such as shiatsu or, in some cases, folk-healing traditions. Chapter 18, *Special Populations and Adaptations*, describes pregnancy massage.

Women's breasts contain mammary glands and lymphatic vessels surrounded by pectoral fat pads and other connective tissues. A layer of loose connective tissue separates the mammary complex from underlying muscle. Breast massage is a specialized skill that helps promote well-breast health and is a complementary therapy for women undergoing treatment for breast cancer.[40] Breast massage requires informed consent from the client and may be beyond the legal scope of practice for some practitioners.

Occasionally in males, increased circulation to the groin area as a result of massage produces an erection. This does not necessarily indicate sexual arousal. With no sexual arousal, the erection will subside naturally. This is the situation in the vast majority of cases.

However, if there appears to be sexual arousal, it is advised to stop the session immediately, state your perception, and ask the client if your perception is correct. If you still believe that there is sexual arousal regardless of what the client says, or if you are uncomfortable, inform the client that the massage is over, and leave the massage room to allow the client to get dressed. The ethical issues with the client should be dealt with outside the immediate massage environment. See the discussion about the intervention model in Chapter 5, *Ethics and the Therapeutic Relationship*.

PHYSIOLOGICAL EFFECTS— ORGANISM LEVEL

The effects of massage at the organism level include phenomena that go beyond the effects on one or two organ systems. Growth and development in infants, stress reduction, pain reduction, and certain psychological benefits are instances of the whole person effects commonly encountered by massage therapists.

Growth and Development

Touch and movement have been found to be essential for the proper growth and development of infants and children. Holding, cuddling, rocking, stroking, and other forms of touching are all necessary for infants to thrive. There is also evidence that adequate pleasurable tactile experience in early life can influence the development of personality traits such as calmness, gentleness, and nonaggressiveness.[41, 42, 43, 44]

The importance of stimulation to the skin for proper growth and development cannot be overestimated. The skin develops from the same primitive cells as the brain and is a prime sensory organ. Stimulation of the tactile nerve endings in the skin provides information about the outside world and helps the brain organize its circuitry for proper development. This is also true for movement and information received through the kinesthetic sense. Thus "the use of touch and sensation to modify our experience of peripheral conditions exerts an active influence upon the organization of reflexes and body image deep within the central nervous system."[45]

As infants learn about the world around them through touch and movement, they also learn about themselves and their own bodies. Juhan expresses this idea with these words: "by rubbing up against the world, I define myself to myself."[46]

Massage is an excellent way to provide systematic and regular touching to growing infants. See Figure 6–12 ■. The massage of infants has been practiced widely all over the world and has been increasing in use in the United States as more caregivers become aware of its benefits. Chapter 18, *Special Populations and Adaptations*, describes infant massage in greater detail.

Pain Reduction

Pain reduction is one of the most frequently cited reasons that people get massage therapy.[47] Pain comes from many sources and is characterized by an unpleasant sensation of discomfort, distress, or suffering caused by injury, disease, or emotional upset. It occurs in varying degrees of intensity from mild to severe. *Analgesia,* or pain reduction, is one of the benefits of massage that follows from its ability to elicit the relaxation response, reduce anxiety, relieve muscle

FIGURE 6–12 Massage promotes proper growth and development of infants.

tension, and improve local circulation. Pain is a complex subject that involves many physical and emotional factors, which perhaps explains why massage (which has effects at many different levels) has been found effective for pain relief in so many cases. Massage is reported to be effective in reducing chronic, long-term, and diffuse pain. Subjects reported reduced pain immediately after sessions, as well as in follow-up interviews.[48, 49]

Massage has been used effectively to reduce pain caused by muscle tension. The pain associated with hypertonic muscles is related to *ischemia* or lack of blood supply caused by inhibited blood vessels. This condition is relieved by muscle relaxation that reestablishes normal blood flow in an area. Massage can also be used to interrupt the pain–spasm–pain cycle set off by muscle spasm. By relaxing the muscle and relieving the pain of the spasm, the cycle is broken, and healing can take place.[50, 51]

A neurological phenomenon called the *neural-gating mechanism* may also play a part in pain reduction. Massage is thought to activate this neural-gating mechanism in the spinal cord through increasing sensory stimulation. The theory is that by activating the fast, large nerve fibers that carry tactile information, transmissions from the slower pain-transmitting nerve fibers are blocked. The perception of pain may be reduced for minutes or hours through the additional sensory input created by massage techniques. Activation of the neural-gating mechanism has been suggested as an explanation for the temporary analgesia associated with deep friction massage in the treatment of injuries to tendons and ligaments.[52]

Myofascial trigger points (TrPs) are painful fibrous nodules that occur in muscle and connective tissue. They are known to cause pain at the site of the TrP, at satellite trigger points, and in muscles that lie within the reference zone of the TrP. Massage techniques of ischemic compression, muscle stripping, and stretching are often used in deactivating trigger points.[53] Trigger points along with muscle relaxation account for much of the pain relief from massage in cases of tension headache and low back pain. See Chapter 22, *Trigger Point Therapy*, for further discussion.

There is also evidence that massage induces the release of neurochemicals called endorphins and enkephalins. These substances modulate pain-impulse transmission in the central nervous system and induce relaxation and feelings of general well-being. They are the body's natural painkillers. The mechanism involved is not clearly understood and may be a combination of psychological, as well as physical, reactions to massage.[54]

Stress Reduction

Soothing massage is commonly recognized as an effective relaxation technique. It is one of several stress-management methods known to trigger the relaxation response. Other popular methods include meditation, guided imagery, progressive relaxation, abdominal breathing, hatha yoga, and biofeedback.

Back massage is especially effective for stress management, and its application for relaxation is described in more detail in Chapter 14, *Full-Body Swedish Massage*. Several studies have confirmed the benefits of back massage for reducing stress in hospitalized patients.[55, 56, 57] The value of back massage for stress reduction is directly related to its ability to activate the parasympathetic nervous system and elicit the physiological phenomenon called the *relaxation response*. Inducing the relaxation response counters the damaging effects of a chronic stress response by bringing balance to the body's systems.

Specific health benefits of the relaxation response include[58]

- Decreased oxygen consumption and metabolic rate, and less strain on energy resources

- Increased intensity and frequency of alpha brain waves associated with deep relaxation

- Reduced blood lactates, blood substances associated with anxiety

- Reduced levels of cortisol, norepinephrine, and epinephrine

- Significantly decreased blood pressure in individuals with hypertension

- Reduced heart rate and slower respiration

- Decreased muscle tension

- Increased blood flow to internal organs

- Decreased anxiety, fear, and phobias, and increased positive mental health

- Improved quality of sleep

During the relaxation response, a person feels totally relaxed and is in a pleasant semi-awake state of consciousness.

Full-body massage consisting predominantly of effleurage and petrissage, with fewer specific techniques that cause discomfort, is very effective in eliciting the relaxation response. The qualities of such a session could be described as light, smooth, and flowing. The relaxing effects of this type of session may be enhanced with certain types of music, soft lighting, warm room temperatures, and minimal talking.

PSYCHOLOGICAL EFFECTS

The psychological effects of massage (i.e., on the mind and emotions) are less well understood than the physical effects, although they are related to the physical effects in many ways. The most well-studied mental and emotional effects of massage include increased mental clarity, reduced anxiety, and feelings of general well-being. A phenomenon called *emotional release*, which is an interesting interface of body, mind, and emotions, may also occur during massage.

Mental Clarity

Two studies performed at the Touch Research Institute in Miami suggest that massage helps improve mental clarity (i.e., sharpening cognitive skills like solving problems, remembering information, or paying focused attention). In one study, 15-minute massage sessions were given to hospital personnel over a 5-week period during their lunch breaks. People reported feeling more relaxed, in better moods, and more alert after receiving massage. Similarly, students who received massage during finals week reported being more relaxed and less anxious and said that they remembered information better after an 8-minute massage session.[59]

In a job-stress study conducted in 1993, subjects received a 20-minute massage in a chair twice weekly for a month. They reported less fatigue and demonstrated greater clarity of thought, improved cognitive skills, and lower anxiety levels. See Figure 6–13 ■. EEG, alpha, beta, and theta waves were also altered in ways consistent with enhanced alertness.[60]

Massage is used with athletes in pre-event situations to help spark the alertness necessary for competition. For pre-event readiness, sports massage sessions are 15–20 minutes in duration, have an upbeat tempo and use techniques to increase circulation and joint mobility. Tapotement is frequently applied for stimulation.

In each of the cases mentioned, the massage sessions were relatively short—between 8 and 20 minutes. Increased mental alertness is most likely related to sensory stimulation and enhanced circulation to the brain. Improved mental clarity may also be the result of a calmer mind and activation of the sympathetic nervous system.

Reduced Anxiety and Depression

A consistent finding of research on massage is that it reduces anxiety significantly. Interestingly, this is true for both the receiver and the giver. This applies to the general public, as well as to those with chronic diseases and to those who are hospitalized for various reasons. Anxiety is measured through subjective self-reporting instruments, or by the more objective measure of cortisol levels in saliva and urine. Anxiety reduction would be an expected result of the relaxation response and action of the parasympathetic nervous system. It may also be related to the release of endorphins.[61, 62, 63, 64]

Character Armor and Emotional Release

Wilhelm Reich (1897–1957) introduced the concept of *character armor*, or muscular tension caused by suppression of emotions. For example, unexpressed anger often causes tension in the muscles of the back and arms that would have been used to strike out. Or unexpressed grief may result in shallow breathing and stiffening of muscles used in crying. In the process of relaxing the affected muscles, the suppressed emotions may be felt by the recipient. Massage practitioners sometimes encounter such armoring and should be prepared to help the patient or client understand the release of emotions that sometimes happens during a massage session.

During an emotional release, unexpressed emotions that are held in the receiver's body may come to the surface in various forms, such as tearfulness, anger, fear, grief, or laughter and joy. Although emotional release is a phenomenon familiar to many massage practitioners, relatively little is known about the mechanisms involved. It is possible

FIGURE 6–13 Short, upbeat massage sessions can improve mental alertness.

Source: Pearson Education, Inc./Segal Photography.

that during deep relaxation, a person's natural psychological defenses are lowered, allowing him or her to feel or express emotions held inside.

Since the unconscious mind is actively involved in controlling experience and emotional flow, thereby maintaining the status quo, alteration of a person's body–mind patterns can threaten or loosen unconscious control of feelings and memories. If this control weakens, then what is stored or blocked in the unconscious can surface to consciousness and may be expressed emotionally in the form we know as emotional release.[65]

Some forms of massage and bodywork specifically address the emotions, and practitioners are trained to deal with issues brought up during emotional release. Releasing unexpressed emotions can be an important step in a physical or psychological healing process.

Massage practitioners should be considerate of their clients during an emotional release and be good listeners, but at the same time be mindful of their own scope of practice. Clients should be referred to other health professionals as needed to resolve deep emotional problems.

Feelings of General Well-Being

Stated in positive terms, massage is shown to increase feelings of general well-being. This likely involves the same mechanisms as anxiety reduction, that is, relaxation response and release of endorphins. Tactile pleasure associated with relaxation massage and simple caring touch may also contribute to feelings of well-being.

It is interesting to note that prolonged exposure to pain and other stressors has been shown to deplete the stores of endorphins, leading to an increased perception of pain and despair. To the extent that massage helps to manage pain and stress, and to release endorphins, it may contribute to a more positive outlook.

Limbic System

The concept of the *limbic system* helps shed light on how the physical and emotional components of a person are related and how body memories are created. From a physiological perspective, the limbic system is defined as follows:

The limbic (LIM-bik) system includes several groups of neurons and tracts of white matter along the border (*limbus* means border) between the cerebrum and diencephalon. This system is concerned with (1) the sense of smell and (2) long-term memory storage. One part of the limbic system, the hippocampus, plays a vital role in learning and storage of long-term memories. . . . The limbic system also includes centers within the hypothalamus responsible for (1) emotional states, such as rage, fear, and sexual arousal, and, (2) the control of reflexes that can be consciously activated such as . . . movements associated with eating.[66]

Memory researchers have been able to trace the flow of information from touch receptors in the skin through the spinal cord and brain stem into different parts of the brain. This activates the limbic system to experience emotions related to touch and to create memories or images of tactile experiences.[67]

There is the possibility, therefore, that memories are activated, as well as created, by touch. This has a variety of important implications for practitioners. For example, if the recipient of massage has experienced caring touch primarily

CASE FOR STUDY

Jim Learns about the Benefits of Massage

Jim is in his mid-30s. He works on a computer most of the day and likes to play sports on the weekends. He is in good physical condition but is feeling tired and sore lately. His job is stressing him out, too. A friend has suggested that Jim add massage to his wellness routine. Jim says he needs to learn more about the good things massage would do for him.

Question:

What information about the effects of massage might convince Jim to make a massage appointment?

Things to consider:

- What are Jim's major needs, given what you know about him?
- Which effects at the tissue or organ system level might he be interested in?
- Do any organism levels or psychological effects seem relevant in this case?

Write a brief description of the effects of massage that might convince Jim that making an appointment would be to his benefit.

_____

_____

_____

in a sexual context, the touch of the practitioner might bring up feelings and memories that would be confusing and inappropriate during a session. Or a recipient who has been physically or sexually abused may have difficulty accepting healing touch without hardening against it. The structured touch of massage has been used to help in the healing and recovery process for those who have experienced physical and emotional trauma, including those diagnosed with post-traumatic stress disorder (PTSD).[68]

MECHANISMS OF MASSAGE

Several mechanisms have been identified to explain how the effects of massage are produced. Some of these theories are recognized within the Western biomedical model, whereas others are on the cutting edge of alternative and body–mind studies. The mechanisms presented here include mechanical, physiological, reflex, body–mind, and energetic. Table 6–5 ■ outlines the mechanisms commonly used to explain the effects of massage.

Some effects are produced by more than one mechanism. For example, changes in local blood circulation during and after massage are thought to occur through direct physical and mechanical effects on vessels; circulatory changes mediated by the local release of vasodilator chemicals (e.g., histamine); or circulatory changes elicited by reflex responses of the autonomic nervous system to tissue stimulation.[69]

Furthermore, a specific massage technique may produce a number of different effects. This is a good example of the holistic nature of human beings and the complexity of effects produced by something seemingly as simple as massage.

Mechanical Effects

Mechanical effects are the result of physical forces of massage, such as compression, stretching, shearing, broadening, and vibration of body tissues. These effects occur on the more gross level of physical structure. Examples of mechanical effects include enhanced venous return from deep effleurage; elongation of muscles by stretching; increased lymph flow from kneading and deep effleurage; and breaking tissue adhesions with deep transverse friction or myofascial massage.

Physiological Effects

Physiological effects refer to organic processes of the body. These effects involve biochemical processes at the cellular level, but may also occur at the tissue and organ system levels. Examples of physiological effects include the various results of the relaxation response produced by activating the parasympathetic nervous system; decrease in anxiety by facilitating the release of mood-enhancing hormones; and proper development and growth in infants assisted by the tactile stimulation that occurs during massage.

Reflex Effects

Reflex effects are functional changes mediated by the nervous system. Sensory receptors in the skin and proprioceptors in muscles are stimulated by massage and joint movements, thereby eliciting reflex effects. Some examples of reflex effects are muscle relaxation, enhanced mental clarity, and pain reduction.

A different type of reflex effect forms the theoretical basis for a type of bodywork called *reflexology*. In this largely unexplained phenomenon, pressing or massaging one part of the body (e.g., ears, hands, or feet) is believed to have a normalizing effect on an entirely different part of the body. It is not clear if the apparent effects occur through the nervous system or some other mechanism. Chapter 24, *Reflexology*, explains more about this bodywork approach.

Body–Mind Effects

Body–mind effects result from the interplay of body, mind, and emotions. This concept has a long tradition in natural healing, in most indigenous cultures, and in medical traditions of China and India. Western medical science is beginning to confirm demonstrable links between our physical bodies and our mental and emotional states. The science of psychoneuroimmunology (PNI) is an interdisciplinary

TABLE 6–5	Mechanisms to Explain the Effects of Massage
Mechanism	**Description and Examples**
Mechanical	The result of physical forces such as compression, stretching, shearing, broadening, and vibration of tissues; occurs on the gross level of physical structure *Examples*: Venous return, lymph flow, breaking adhesions
Physiological	Organic processes of the body on cellular, tissue, or organ system levels *Examples*: Activation of parasympathetic nervous system; release of mood-enhancing hormones
Reflex	Functional changes mediated by the nervous system; pressure or movement in one part of the body has an effect in another part, as in reflexology *Examples*: Muscle relaxation, increased mental clarity, pain reduction, normalizing system function
Body–mind	The result of the interplay of body, mind, and emotions in health and disease processes *Examples*: Relaxation response, anxiety reduction
Energetic	The result of balancing or improving the flow of energy within and around the body *Examples*: Removing energy restrictions, dispersing pooled energy, strengthening deficient energy

CRITICAL THINKING

Think about the many effects of massage on human beings at the organ system and organism levels (refer to Table 6–1). Analyze the primary mechanisms involved in creating these effects (refer to Table 6–5).

1. Are some effects elicited by more than one mechanism?
2. How are the mechanisms of different effects and massage techniques related?
3. Why is it important for massage therapists to understand the effects and mechanisms of massage?

approach that studies interactions between psychological processes and the body's nervous and immune systems.

The body–mind connection can be seen clearly in the relaxation response, a physiological process involving the parasympathetic nervous system. The relaxation response is elicited by practices such as meditation, which quiets the mind, or by the tactile stimulation of massage. Other examples of body–mind effects of massage include reduction in anxiety and release of unexpressed emotions held in the body.

Energetic Effects

Massage and bodywork have been described as balancing and improving the flow of energy, thus providing **energetic effects**. What this energy is and how it relates to the body are yet to be determined in terms of Western science; however, several ancient and more modern massage and bodywork approaches are based on concepts of energy. Examples of popular forms of energy-based bodywork are traditional Chinese medicine (TCM), Ayurveda from India, Therapeutic Touch adopted by many nurses, polarity therapy, and Reiki from Japan. Chapter 25, *Asian and Energy-Based Bodywork*, examines three approaches widely used by massage therapists.

There are a variety of theories about how energy flows in and around the body, and many practitioners and receivers report "feeling" energy. Energy work is currently outside the understanding and general acceptance of Western biomedicine, but it has persisted over time and is found to be useful by many people.

BENEFITS OF WELLNESS MASSAGE

When the effects of massage support general health and well-being or the ongoing healing process, there are benefits by definition. A wellness or general massage aims to normalize body tissues and to optimize function. Everyone can benefit from the health-promoting effects of a broad-spectrum wellness massage.

The main intention of this type of massage is to elicit the relaxation response, promote muscular relaxation, and enhance circulation of fluids, digestion, and elimination. The effects of general relaxation alone have an impact on many physiological and psychological aspects of health and well-being. Wellness massage also provides healthy touch, which is a basic human need.

The effects of wellness massage may be especially beneficial for people with special needs. These benefits are the natural effects of a general massage tailored for each unique individual. For example, athletes, pregnant women, infants, the elderly, the terminally ill, and clients with psychological problems or physical disabilities may find specific benefits derived from massage sessions planned to take into consideration their special needs. See Chapter 18, *Special Populations and Adaptations*, for more information on how the benefits of massage can improve the quality of life—both physiologically and psychologically—for all people.

CHAPTER HIGHLIGHTS

- *Effects of massage* refer to changes that occur in the body, mind, and emotions of the recipient during a massage session.
  - Effects of massage can be beneficial or detrimental, depending on the circumstances.
  - Effects are beneficial if they have a positive impact and lead toward healing and greater wellness.

- Massage is *indicated* if its effects are likely to be beneficial to a person with a specific medical condition.
- Massage is *contraindicated* if its effects are likely to be harmful to a person with a specific medical condition.

- Different massage techniques and different methods of application can produce very different physiological and psychological outcomes.
- Time and dose are important considerations when describing the effects of massage applications.
  - Short-term effects are changes that occur during a massage session and last for a few hours or a day afterward.
  - Long-term effects are changes that occur during a massage session and last for a longer period, such as a few days or weeks.
  - Single-dose effects occur after one massage application.
  - Multiple-dose effects occur over time from repeated massage applications.

- A holistic view of effects of massage looks at connections of body, mind, and emotions.
  - In touching the outermost part of the physical body, we are able to touch the innermost parts of our clients.
  - Massage is called a body-centered therapy because it works primarily through touch and movement to create its effects.

- Information about the physiological and psychological effects of massage comes from several different sources.
  - These sources include tradition, personal experience, and rational understanding of human anatomy and physiology.
  - Scientific research is conducted to examine theories about the effects of massage.

- Systematic reviews look at a number of different studies on a specific topic to discover consistent findings.
- Research literacy includes understanding the scientific method, locating and evaluating research articles, and gleaning practical information from research studies.
- Scientific research is based on observations about what actually happens, rather than taking the word of an authority or anecdotes from individuals.
  - Different types of research studies offer weaker or stronger evidence of cause and effect.
  - Comparing pre- and posttreatment measurements provides evidence that real change took place.
  - Research studies may have flaws that make their findings less valid.

- Research studies can be located in research databases found on the Internet.
- Peer-reviewed journals contain credible research reports that have been evaluated by experts in the field.

- Massage improves the overall health of cells and tissues of the body.
  - Massage can assist in the tissue repair process, especially in the regeneration and remodeling phases, but is contraindicated in the inflammatory phase.
  - Massage causes connective tissues to become more fluid and pliable and prevents some connective tissue abnormalities and dysfunction.

- Massage improves the overall function of organ systems.
  - *Integumentary system*—Oil applied during massage moisturizes the skin; massage stimulates sensory receptors; friction techniques assist in healthy scar formation.
  - *Skeletal system*—Massage promotes good joint mobility and flexibility and proper alignment.
  - *Muscular system*—Massage can reduce muscle stiffness and soreness after strenuous activity and relax hypertonic or tense muscles; massage alleviates some of the negative effects of underactivity and overactivity of the muscular system.
  - *Nervous and endocrine systems*—Massage works through the nervous system to increase body awareness, relax muscles, and reduce pain.
    - Massage helps trigger the release of stress, anxiety, and pain-reducing hormones, and of mood-enhancing hormones.
  - *Cardiovascular system*—Massage improves the function of the cardiovascular and lymphatic systems by helping to move fluids through the systems.
    - Massage produces hyperemia locally and increases blood volume in an area.
    - Mechanical action of deep effleurage enhances venous flow.
    - Massage can play a part in decreasing blood pressure and increasing the number of circulating red blood cells.
  - *Lymphatic system*—Massage can assist in movement of lymph fluid through the lymphatic system and enhances immunity.
  - *Respiratory system*—Massage enhances general circulation, relaxes muscles of respiration, and encourages deep diaphragmatic breathing.
  - *Digestive system*—Relaxation massage improves digestive system function, and abdominal massage is used to treat constipation.
  - *Reproductive system*—Although this system is not ordinarily a target for massage, massage can indirectly improve its function through improved circulation and general relaxation.
    - Massage can address the needs of pregnant women.

- Breast massage is a specialty used for well-breast health and as complementary treatment for breast cancer.
- Men can experience a nonsexual erection during massage due to increased circulation in the groin area.

- Massage can have a positive effect at the whole organism level.
  - Massage enhances growth and development of infants.
  - Massage has pain-reduction effects and can elicit the relaxation response.

- Psychological effects of massage include increased mental clarity, reduced anxiety, emotional release, and increased feelings of general well-being.

- Mechanisms through which the effects of massage are produced include mechanical, physiological, reflex, body–mind, and energetic.
- Everyone can benefit from the health-promoting effects of general or wellness massage.
- Special populations also benefit from wellness massage planned to take into consideration their special needs.

EXAM REVIEW

Key Terms

Match the following key terms to their descriptions. For additional study, look up the key terms in the Interactive Glossary, and note other terms that compare or contrast with them.

_____ **1.** Body–mind effects
_____ **2.** Effects of massage
_____ **3.** Energetic effects
_____ **4.** Hypothesis
_____ **5.** Long-term effects
_____ **6.** Mechanical effects
_____ **7.** Multiple-dose effects
_____ **8.** Peer-reviewed journals
_____ **9.** Physiological effects
_____ **10.** Reflex effects
_____ **11.** Research literacy
_____ **12.** Scientific method
_____ **13.** Short-term effects
_____ **14.** Single-dose effects

a. Changes that start during a massage session and last for a longer period of time, such as a few days or weeks

b. Effects that happen over time from repeated massage applications

c. Research publications that meet certain standards and that have been evaluated by experts in the field

d. Functional changes mediated by the nervous system such as muscle relaxation, enhanced mental clarity, and pain reduction

e. Organic processes of the body that occur at the biochemical, cellular, tissue, and organ system levels

f. Changes that occur during a massage session and may last for the time of the session and for a brief period afterward

g. Understanding the scientific method, locating and evaluating research articles, and gleaning practical information from research studies

h. Systematic way of testing theories through gathering and analyzing relevant information to see if it supports the theory in question

i. Effects that result from the interplay of body, mind, and emotions in health and disease

j. Changes that happen from one application of massage

k. Balancing and improving the flow of energy

l. An unproven theory about how something works or what will happen in a certain situation

m. Changes that occur in the body, mind, and emotions of the recipient as a result of soft tissue manipulation

n. The result of physical forces of massage, such as compression, stretching, shearing, broadening, and vibration of body tissues

Memory Workout

To test your memory of the main concepts in this chapter, complete the following sentences by circling the most correct answer from the two choices provided.

1. Massage promotes the overall health of tissues, primarily through increased blood and (lymph) (waste) circulation.
2. Research is the systematic examination of a phenomenon based on careful observation using (anecdotes) (measurements).
3. A systematic review of a number of different research studies looking at the same subject is called a (case study) (meta-analysis).
4. The capacity of research findings to be generalized to a larger group than the one that participated in the study is called (external) (internal) validity.
5. A quick overview of background, methods, results, conclusion, and keywords in a research report is found in the (abstract) (discussion).
6. During the remodeling phase of tissue repair, deep friction massage helps in healthy (scab) (scar) formation.
7. Joint movement techniques stimulate production of (synovial fluid) (lymph fluid).

8. Muscles that are tense and in a state of partial contraction are said to be (hypotonic) (hypertonic).
9. The (fight-or-flight) (relaxation) response occurs with activation of the parasympathetic nervous system, which has effects on skeletal muscles as well as several other organ systems.
10. A condition in which normal blood flow in the veins is slowed or halted is called (venous return) (venostasis).
11. Resistance to injuries and disease caused by foreign substances is called (immunity) (approximation).
12. There is evidence that massage can produce the release of neurochemicals called (analgesia) (endorphins) that induce relaxation and feelings of well-being.
13. Effects of massage that are the result of physical forces such as compression, stretching, and vibration of body tissues are called (physiological) (mechanical) effects.
14. Character (development) (armor) is a concept used to explain muscular tension caused by suppressed emotions.

Test Prep

The following multiple-choice questions will help to prepare you for future school and professional exams.

1. Changes that occur over time from repeated massage applications are called:
   a. Short-term effects
   b. Single-dose effects
   c. Multiple-dose effects
   d. Indications

2. Understanding the scientific method and locating and evaluating research articles are essential skills of:
   a. Research literacy
   b. Massage literacy
   c. Principle-based therapy
   d. Treatment planning

3. The type of research study that offers the strongest evidence of cause and effect is the:
   a. Case series
   b. Case study
   c. Randomized controlled trial
   d. Meta-analysis

4. Elements within the design or execution of a research study that make it more or less credible affect the study's:
   a. External validity
   b. Internal validity
   c. External reliability
   d. Statistical significance

5. Which section of a research report describes the research design in detail?
   a. Abstract
   b. Introduction
   c. Methods
   d. Discussion

6. The section of a research report that speculates on why the massage application worked or did not work as hypothesized is the:
   a. Introduction
   b. Methods
   c. Results
   d. Discussion

7. What is the primary mechanism of massage techniques that remove adhesions in fascial tissues?
   a. Reflex
   b. Body–mind
   c. Mechanical
   d. Energetic

8. Which of the following explains how massage promotes muscle relaxation?
   a. By evoking the relaxation response
   b. By providing an environment for recipients to consciously let go of tension
   c. By creating increased sensory input
   d. All of the above

9. Superficial friction produces an increase in local circulation in the skin and underlying connective tissue. This effect is called:
   a. Ischemia
   b. Hyperemia
   c. Hypertonicity
   d. Immunity

10. Which of the following massage techniques most effectively enhance venous circulation?
    a. Petrissage and deep effleurage
    b. Passive touch and direct pressure
    c. Deep and superficial friction
    d. Vibration and tapotement

11. A holistic view understands human beings as:
    a. Divided into body and mind
    b. Whole persons in body, mind, and spirit
    c. Separated into tissues and organ systems
    d. Body-centered beings with a mind

12. Which of the following statements about breast massage is *not* correct?
    a. Breast massage is a skill that requires specialized training.
    b. Breast massage is contraindicated for women undergoing treatment for breast cancer.
    c. Breast massage requires informed consent from the client.
    d. Breast massage may be beyond the legal scope of practice for some practitioners.

13. Massage techniques that promote better blood circulation are used to address a condition called:
    a. Ischemia
    b. Fibrosis
    c. Hyperemia
    d. Adhesion

14. Effects of massage that involve biochemical processes at the cellular, tissue, and organ system levels are called:
    a. Reflex
    b. Physiological
    c. Energetic
    d. Mechanical

15. What is the greatest benefit for infants of the tactile stimulation of regular massage?
    a. Better digestion
    b. Improved circulation
    c. Normal growth and development
    d. More relaxed muscles

Video Challenge

Watch this video, which can be found at MyHealthProfessionsLab.com, Chapter 6, and then answer the following questions.

Goal-Oriented Planning

1. How is knowledge of the effects of massage used in goal-oriented planning?

2. How might awareness of single-dose and multiple-dose effects influence a long-term plan for massage to treat a certain condition?

3. At what point in goal-oriented planning might you want to read research studies on the effects of massage?

Comprehension Exercises

The following short-answer questions test your knowledge and understanding of chapter topics and provide practice in written communication skills. Explain in two to four complete sentences.

1. Explain how massage reduces pain using the neural-gating mechanism theory.

2. Explain the origin of the connection between skin, brain, and nervous system.

3. Name the parts of a research report, and briefly describe the contents of each part.

For Greater Understanding

The following exercises are designed to take you from the realm of theory into the real world. They will help give you a deeper understanding of the subjects covered in this chapter. Action words are underlined to emphasize the variety of activities presented to address different learning styles and to encourage deeper thinking.

1. Write a brief personal health history for the past one or two years. Using the information in this chapter, identify any areas that might have benefited (or did benefit) from receiving massage. Discuss your conclusions with a study partner or group.

2. Choose one particular effect of massage to study in more depth. Search several sources for further information, including anatomy and physiology textbooks and research databases. Discuss your findings with a study partner or group.

3. Choose one research study to read, analyze, and evaluate. Present your findings and conclusions to a study partner or group.

MyHealthProfessionsLab™

MyHealthProfessionsLab.com is a premium online homework management system that includes a host of features to help you study. Registered users will find:

- Powerful tools that track and analyze your results—allowing you to create a personalized learning experience
- Videos, flashcards and other learning tools to help enrich your progress
- Streaming lesson presentations and self-paced learning modules
- A space where you and your instructors can view and manage your assignments

Clinical Applications of Massage

CHAPTER OUTLINE

Learning Outcomes

Key Terms

Clinical Massage Therapy

Evidence-Based Practice

Client-Centered Massage

Therapeutic Outcomes

Musculoskeletal Applications

Cardiovascular and Lymphatic
Applications

Respiratory Applications

Back Massage for Hospitalized
Patients

Massage for Cancer Patients

Pediatric Applications

Psychological Clinical Applications

Therapeutic Touch

Complement to Chiropractic Care

Case Reports

Chapter Highlights

Exam Review

LEARNING OUTCOMES

After studying this chapter, you will have information to:

1. Define clinical massage therapy.

2. Explain the nature of evidence-based practice.

3. Explain the theory of client-centered massage.

4. Discuss different clinical approaches to massage.

5. Describe the benefits of massage in treatment of various pathologies.

6. Explain how massage is used to complement chiropractic care.

7. Discuss the importance of case reports in developing massage therapy research.

KEY TERMS

Case reports

Client-centered massage

Clinical massage therapy

Direct therapeutic
outcomes

Evidence-based practice
(EBP)

Evidence funnel

Indirect therapeutic
outcomes

Palliative care

Principle-based therapy

Recipe-based massage

CLINICAL MASSAGE THERAPY

Massage has been used to treat injuries and illnesses since ancient times and is currently being integrated into a number of medical settings as an effective therapy. The term **clinical massage therapy** describes applications of massage for the treatment of pathological conditions.

Clinical massage therapy is not a technique or group of techniques. It includes Swedish massage as well as manual therapy approaches that address specific tissues and organ systems or enhance healing on a holistic level. It also encompasses forms of energy-based bodywork and manual therapies from non-Western health care such as traditional Chinese medicine. The number of private massage practices that specialize in clinical applications is growing, and health care professionals routinely refer patients for massage therapy for a variety of ailments. Medical settings that sometimes offer massage therapy include hospitals, rehabilitation facilities, sports medicine clinics, nursing and assisted-living homes, hospices, and medical spas. Massage therapists working in clinical settings must understand the operating procedures there and develop the required skills, such as charting and note-taking.

Clinical applications require massage therapists to have greater knowledge of human pathology, the effects of medications, factors that enhance healing, and indications for various massage applications. Also important to know are current standard and alternative treatments for the pathologies being addressed and possible contraindications for massage therapy. Books on pathology and clinical applications written specifically for massage therapists are useful resources that contain information describing common medical conditions and their treatments, as well as contraindications and recommendations for massage therapy. A selection of these books are listed in *Additional Resources* in Appendix E.

For clinical applications, it is essential to understand the effects that various massage techniques have and how to apply them for the greatest therapeutic benefit in each individual case. The growing interest in clinical massage therapy has led to an increased number of research studies about its efficacy in the treatment of a variety of pathologies. See Chapter 6, *Effects of Massage and Research Literacy*, for a general discussion about research and how to find and read research reports.

EVIDENCE-BASED PRACTICE

The original concept of **evidence-based practice (EBP)** was "the integration of best research evidence with clinical expertise and patient values."[1] In this model, best research evidence is clinically relevant research that can improve practice. It requires that clinical practitioners "learn to evaluate and bring evidence into the equation" when developing a treatment plan.[2] Figure 7–1 ■ shows the three foundations of evidence-based practice.

FIGURE 7–1 Foundations of evidence-based practice.

That broad viewpoint has sometimes been narrowed to focus only on experimental research as the "evidence" referred to. In the emerging integrative health care scene, those therapies that are supported by scientific research are more likely to be valued and used. As stated in the Foreword to *Touch Therapy*:

> One of the principal requirements of modern health care provision can be summed up by the term, "evidence-based." It is no longer sufficient for any therapeutic approach to simply rely on a long history of use, or popularity, or widespread availability, to justify its continued acceptance (especially if insurance reimbursement is anticipated).[3]

Evidence from scientific studies can more clearly substantiate the benefits of massage in treating certain diseases, as well as identify contraindications. Applications of clinical massage therapy will become safer and more effective long term as the result of research. However, this narrow view discounts both the practitioner's experience and judgment and the patient's involvement in the treatment.

Dividing research into levels of evidence, as described in the previous discussion of research literacy in Chapter 6, also has drawbacks because many of the lower levels, such as case studies, provide valuable practice-based information. (*Memory refresher*: The levels of evidence from low to high are case study, case series, experimental study with no control group, randomized control trial, and systematic review.) Replacing this evidence hierarchy with the concept of a nonhierarchical **evidence funnel** has been suggested.[4] In the evidence funnel model, all types of research as well as untested theories and expert opinions would be placed into a conduit leading to the practitioner, who would sort out relevant information and combine it with personal expertise and the patient's values, to come up with the best massage application in the situation. Some use the term *evidence-informed* to place the practitioner back at the center of decision making for clinical applications of massage.

CLIENT-CENTERED MASSAGE

When a massage treatment plan is based on the client's unique situation, needs, and goals, it is **client-centered massage**. This is in contrast to *formula* or **recipe-based massage**, in which every client receives exactly the same treatment (i.e., the same techniques applied in the same way) for a particular medical condition.

The concept of **principle-based therapy** proposed by Yates similarly puts the client at the center of treatment, but also accounts for the choice of massage techniques and application.[5] The foundation of principle-based therapy is the creation of an overall plan directed toward the achievement of specific treatment goals. This plan takes into consideration the pathology being treated, the condition of the client or patient, and most significantly, the therapeutic potential of different treatment methods. Principle-based therapy allows for variation:

> Appropriate treatment techniques and modalities are selected, integrated, and adapted as necessary to achieve specific effects and are modified according to the changing physiological and psychological state of the patient as treatment proceeds. Treatment is therefore patient-centered rather than technique-centered.[6]

Research helps sort out which massage techniques and approaches have the most therapeutic potential for specific clinical applications. Research is most useful for adding to our understanding of the applications of massage, not as a means for developing recipes for treatment. There is room for consideration of research, experience, and the client in the client-centered practice of clinical massage therapy. A summary of important concepts in clinical massage therapy appears in Table 7–1 ■.

TABLE 7–1	Important Concepts in Clinical Massage Therapy
Concept	**Explanation**
Clinical massage therapy	Applications of massage in the treatment of pathological conditions; sometimes referred to as *medical massage therapy*
Evidence-based practice	Massage applications based on research, clinical expertise, and client values
Client-centered massage	Treatment plan based on the client's unique situation, needs, and goals; opposite of recipe-based massage
Principle-based therapy	Directed toward achievement of specific treatment goals; takes into consideration the pathology, the client's condition, and the therapeutic potential of different treatment methods
Recipe-based massage	Treatment based on predetermined formula or protocol for a specific pathology or condition; opposite of client-centered massage

THERAPEUTIC OUTCOMES

The intended outcomes of clinical massage therapy fall into three major categories:

1. Direct therapeutic outcomes

2. Indirect therapeutic outcomes

3. Palliative care

It is important to be clear about the intended outcomes when planning in a clinical situation, in order to choose the most appropriate massage techniques and applications.

Direct therapeutic outcomes of clinical massage focus on the healing of a diagnosed medical condition, or easing of its symptoms. An example would be the use of deep transverse friction in treating repetitive strain injuries. Another is massage for healthy nervous system development and weight gain in preterm infants. Massage may be used to help manage chronic conditions such as asthma and autism. In these cases, massage may be the primary treatment approach, but is more often part of a multifaceted plan of care. This team approach to treatment is commonly found in integrative and alternative health care settings.

Indirect therapeutic outcomes of clinical massage focus on enhancing the effectiveness of a primary treatment, or creating a more favorable environment for healing. For example, massage is used to help reduce anxiety, thereby improving the body's immune response. Massage may also help alleviate some of the negative effects of a primary treatment, for example, massage used to reduce nausea associated with some cancer treatments. In these cases, massage may be considered to be complementary health care.

Palliative care is concerned with easing discomfort and improving the quality of life for those with chronic medical conditions or terminal illness. Palliative care is provided for hospitalized or institutionalized patients, as well as in some outpatient services such as home hospice. For example, massage has been suggested to help reduce the dehumanizing effects of nursing homes. It is also used in hospice care for a variety of outcomes, including positive physical, psychological, and social effects.

Although these categories are not mutually exclusive, they offer a way to sort out the intention behind clinical massage applications. They answer the question: What does massage contribute to the healing of this medical condition or to the well-being of this client/patient? A summary of these therapeutic outcomes in clinical massage therapy can be found in Table 7–2 ■.

The remainder of this chapter discusses some of the uses of massage in medical settings and some of the promising research that has been done on its clinical applications. It is just a sampling of the growing amount of information available and points to areas where the study of the clinical applications of massage has been strong.

CRITICAL THINKING

Locate a scientific research report about a clinical application of massage. Read, analyze, and evaluate the study reported. Read each section carefully to understand the researcher's approach to the study and the results. Refer to Table 6-3: Typical Sections of a Research Report and Table 6-4: Research Report Evaluation Worksheet.

1. What was the researcher trying to find out about massage? What was the hypothesis?
2. How did the researcher go about testing the hypothesis? What was the research method?
3. What did the research find out? What were the results?
4. What do the findings mean for clinical massage applications?

TABLE 7–2	Therapeutic Outcomes in Clinical Massage Therapy
Outcomes	Description
Direct therapeutic outcomes	Focus on the healing of a diagnosed medical condition, or easing of its symptoms; alternative or integrated health care.
Indirect therapeutic outcomes	Focus on enhancing the effectiveness of a primary treatment, or creating a more favorable environment for healing; complementary health care.
Palliative care	Focus on easing discomfort and improving the quality of life for those with chronic medical conditions or terminal illness; often provided for hospitalized or institutionalized patients.

MUSCULOSKELETAL APPLICATIONS

Massage is routinely incorporated into the rehabilitation of musculoskeletal injuries by physical therapists, athletic trainers, and massage therapists (Figure 7–2 ■). It is also used as a complement to chiropractic care as discussed later in this chapter.

Massage is particularly effective in relieving muscle tension, increasing flexibility and range of motion, promoting healthy connective tissue, and reducing muscular pain. These direct therapeutic effects on the muscular system are outlined in Chapter 6, *Effects of Massage and Research Literacy*. Because of these physiological effects, massage can be a valuable ingredient in the treatment of muscle injuries such as sprains, strains, and inflammation of tendons.[7]

Deep transverse friction has been especially effective in the treatment of repetitive strain injuries (RSI) such as tendinitis/tenosynovitis (i.e., inflammation of tendons and tendon sheaths) and bursitis (i.e., inflammation of the fluid sacs around joints).[8] Deep friction techniques increase local circulation, help separate adhesions, and have an analgesic or pain-reducing effect.[9]

Pain caused by hypertonic muscles can be relieved with massage. For example, chronic tension headaches caused by tense and shortened cervical muscles have been successfully treated using a combination of Swedish massage, myofascial release, and trigger point therapy.[10] Massage has also been effective in treating subacute chronic low back pain.[11, 12] These findings are particularly encouraging because tension headaches and low back pain afflict so many people in the modern world.

Myofascial massage and trigger point therapy include specialized techniques that target myofascial pain and dysfunction. See Chapter 21, *Myofascial Massage*, and Chapter 22, *Trigger Point Therapy*, for more detail on these approaches to normalizing muscle and related tissues.

Fibromyalgia Syndrome

Fibromyalgia syndrome (FMS) is a chronic condition characterized by widespread muscle pain and stiffness and tenderness at specific body sites. See Figure 7–3 ■. The pain and fatigue associated with FMS can be debilitating. Other common symptoms of FMS are disturbed sleep, chronic fatigue, inability to tolerate exercise, and impaired cognitive function. Severe headaches, irritable bowel syndrome, systemic lupus erythematosus, and emotional problems such as anxiety and depression often accompany FMS. Because the cause of FMS has not been established, it is classified as a syndrome rather than as a disease.[13]

Although there is no known cure for FMS, massage can address many of its symptoms. The general effects of massage that offer relief are reduction of stress and anxiety, more restful sleep, more positive outlook, improved circulation, and relief for sore and stiff muscles.[14, 15] One FMS study found that with massage there was an improvement in sleep and a decrease in substance P (SP), which is a neuropeptide associated with inflammation and pain.[16]

Research investigating the use of massage for treatment of FMS has had mixed results. Some reported no relief with massage, whereas others indicated some positive results. Experiments that showed positive outcomes with massage used connective tissue massage,[17] massage combined with exercise,[18] and manual lymph drainage and connective tissue massage.[19]

FIGURE 7-2

Massage is routinely incorporated into the rehabilitation of musculoskeletal injuries.

Source: Pearson Education, Inc./Segal Photography.

1. Low cervical: anterior aspects of the intertransverse spaces at C5–C7

2. Second rib: second costochondral junctions

3. Occiput: suboccipital muscle insertions

4. Trapezius: midpoint of the upper border

5. Supraspinatus: above the medial border of the scapular spine

6. Lateral epicondyle: 2 cm distal to the epicondyles

7. Gluteal: upper outer quadrants of buttocks

8. Greater trochanter: posterior to the trochanteric prominence

9. Knee: medial fat pad proximal to the joint line

FIGURE 7-3 Fibromyalgia tender point sites.

CARDIOVASCULAR AND LYMPHATIC APPLICATIONS

Relaxation massage may be beneficial in treating some cardiovascular pathologies, such as hypertension (high blood pressure) and cardiac arrhythmia.[20, 21, 22] It not only reduces heart rate and blood pressure, but also reduces anxiety, which helps give the patient a more positive outlook and improved feelings of well-being. These particular effects of massage are supported in a meta-analysis of massage research studies.[23]

A study by nurses found that back massage consisting of effleurage had a positive effect on the perception of relaxation and comfort reported by patients with acute myocardial infarction. Although they could not confirm improvement in the pathology, the massage had no apparent detrimental effects and did have positive palliative outcomes.[24]

In another study, patients hospitalized in a cardiovascular unit of a large medical center in New York City who received Therapeutic Touch had a significantly greater reduction in anxiety scores than those who received casual touch or no touch.[25] A fuller discussion of Therapeutic Touch can be found later in this chapter.

Edema and Lymphedema

Edema, or excess interstitial fluid in the tissues, is not a disease, but rather a condition of fluid buildup or swelling. It may be caused by injury, tissue damage, inflammation, or poor circulation. The edema itself can cause pain from increased fluid pressure and the buildup of toxins in the tissues. Applying massage safely in cases of edema requires knowledge of the reason for the condition because some types of swelling are contraindications for massage. For example, circulatory massage is contraindicated in cases of heart failure, kidney disease, and liver congestion.[26]

Traumatic edema occurs with minor muscular injuries such as strains and sprains. It is "localized swelling of tissue associated with soft tissue injury and/or the exertion of exercise, including the acute or chronic sprains, strains, and hematomas common to sports and exercise."[27] Lymphatic facilitation techniques can be used effectively for treatment of traumatic edema. See Chapter 23, *Lymphatic Facilitation*, for more information about manual lymphatic facilitation techniques.

Lymphedema is a specific type of edema caused by lymphatic system defect or damage. Primary lymphedema results from congenital or hereditary defects. Secondary lymphedema occurs when nodes or vessels are damaged by trauma, surgery, infection, radiation, or chemotherapy.[28] Manual lymphatic drainage (MLD) techniques have been developed as part of complete decongestive therapy to address lymphedema specifically.

The beneficial effects of manual lymph drainage for patients with chronic and postmastectomy lymphedema continues to be confirmed. Lymphatic massage in these cases is for management of the condition and must be received regularly for long-term benefit.[29, 30, 31, 32]

Immune Function

One of the basic positive effects of massage is improvement in immune function, as noted in Chapter 6, *Effects of Massage and Research Literacy*. One of the first major studies to link massage and improved immunity was conducted by the Touch Research Institute in 1996. In a group of HIV-positive men who received daily massage for a month, the majority had significant increase in the number and activity of natural killer (NK) cells. The men showed reduced anxiety and stress, lower cortisol levels, as well as increased serotonin levels during the month of massage.[33] A study of women with breast cancer found a similar increase in NK cells and lymphocytes after massage therapy.[34]

To the extent that massage helps reduce stress and thus improves immune function, it can be considered an important disease prevention measure. Health problems associated with compromised immunity include frequent infections, autoimmune disorders, and possibly, cancer.[35]

RESPIRATORY APPLICATIONS

Massage is used as a complementary therapy for people with respiratory conditions such as chronic bronchitis, emphysema, and asthma. The benefits of massage for these patients include anxiety reduction and relaxation that deepens breathing patterns, relaxation and lengthening of muscles tense from labored breathing, and reduced fatigue overall. Passive movement of the rib cage, as well as percussion on the back and chest, can help loosen mucus for more productive coughs.

Children with asthma have been the subjects of several recent research projects. In one study, children with asthma were found to have lower anxiety, improved attitude toward the asthma condition, and increased peak airflow after regular massage by their parents. Over a 1-month period, these children had fewer asthma attacks. The study suggested that daily massage may lead to improved airway tone, decreased airway irritability, and better control of asthma in children.[36]

In another study, patients with asthma, bronchitis, and emphysema received a form of bodywork called Trager Psychophysical Integration®, which consists of gentle, painless, passive movements. Focus was on the neck, abdomen, and chest wall. After treatment, improvement was found in forced vital capacity, respiratory rate, and chest expansion. Patients reported general relaxation and decrease in anxiety and tension.[37]

An increase in thoracic gas volume, peak flow, and forced vital capacity was found in four out of five chronic obstructive pulmonary disease (COPD) patients receiving a combination of massage and myofascial trigger point therapy. The trigger point techniques were specifically directed to improve the function of chronically hypertonic muscles involved in breathing.[38]

Note that the studies cited here used different massage therapy approaches to achieve their positive results. The overall objectives were to reduce stress, improve diaphragmatic breathing, and relax and lengthen the muscles of respiration. Studies help identify specific techniques that are effective for these outcomes.

BACK MASSAGE FOR HOSPITALIZED PATIENTS

The ability of massage to reduce anxiety, promote restful sleep, and manage pain accounts for much of its value as a complement to standard medical treatment in hospitals and skilled nursing facilities. Back massage in particular has been found useful in caring for patients hospitalized for a variety of conditions (Figure 7–4 ■). For example, back massage was found to be effective in promoting sleep in critically ill patients. It has been suggested as an alternative or adjunct to sleep medications in some cases.[39]

A randomized control study conducted in Veteran's Administration (VA) hospitals found back massage to be useful for patients who had just undergone major surgery. Patients who received 20 minutes of effleurage on the back daily experienced a short-term decrease in pain intensity and unpleasantness. They also had a faster rate of decrease of pain intensity and unpleasantness over the first 4 postoperative days than the control group, which did not receive massage.[40]

Back massage was also found to be an effective, noninvasive technique for promoting relaxation and improving communication with elderly, institutionalized patients. The nurses who conducted the study noted the potential of massage for reducing the common dehumanizing effects of institutional care.[41] Those results confirmed the results of a previous study by two nurses that looked at slow-stroke back rub for older adults.[42]

MASSAGE FOR CANCER PATIENTS

Massage was once listed as a general contraindication for cancer patients. It is now recognized as a valuable complementary therapy. Cancer patients who receive massage are reporting relief from a number of physical, mental, and emotional discomforts related to the disease and its treatment.[43]

General benefits of massage especially important to cancer patients include reduced stress and anxiety, improved sleep, improved immune system function, pain relief, and the comfort of caring touch.[44, 45, 46, 47]

Cancer patients who undergo surgery may benefit from the effects of massage related to faster recovery from anesthesia, faster wound healing, separation of adhesions around incisions, healthy scar formation, and reduction of edema and lymphedema. Massage has also been linked to reduced pain and less need for pain medication. Hospitalized patients find relief from muscle soreness caused by prolonged bed rest. Improved circulation from massage helps prevent pressure and bed sores.

In one study, nurses examined the effects of therapeutic massage on hospitalized cancer patients. Primary techniques used were effleurage, petrissage, and trigger point therapy. They found that massage therapy significantly reduced the patients' perceived levels of pain and anxiety while enhancing their feelings of relaxation. Objective physiological measures (i.e., heart rate, respiratory rate, and blood pressure) tended to decrease, providing further indication of relaxation.[48]

Massage has also been found to reduce some of the negative side effects of radiation and chemotherapy, such as fatigue, nausea, diarrhea, loss of appetite, and insomnia.[49] However, the timing of massage in relation to treatment can be important; for example, the patient may be overtaxed and

FIGURE 7–4
Massage is used as a complement to standard medical treatment in hospitals and skilled nursing facilities.

Source: Pearson Education, Inc./Segal Photography.

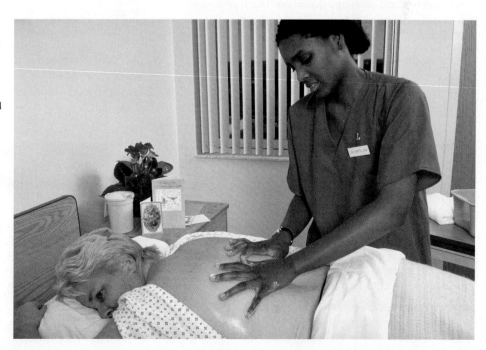

negative side effects worsened if massage is received too soon after a bout of chemotherapy.

The benefits of massage on the emotional level can be significant. Massage can help a cancer patient deal with depression and offer pleasant social interaction providing relief from isolation. It can help reestablish a positive body image and reclaim the body as an ally. It empowers patients to participate in their healing process and helps rebuild hope.[50, 51]

Breast massage is increasing in use as a clinical application for women who have experienced breast cancer. It is especially useful for postmastectomy patients, including for general wound healing, healthy scar formation, and treating lymphedema.[52, 53, 54, 55] The concern about massage causing metastasis, or that massage may spread cancer, is still real in some cases. For example, massage should be avoided completely around the site of a tumor or where a tumor has recently been removed. Massage practitioners should consult the patient's physician to assess the potential for harm from massage and to get advice on how to proceed safely.[56]

Evidence-based treatment guidelines for giving massage to cancer patients have been compiled by a nurse, Janice Post-White.[57] These guidelines will continue to evolve as further research becomes available.

- Massage is recommended as part of a multimodality treatment for cancer patients experiencing anxiety or pain.[58]

- Massage therapists treating patients with cancer should be trained in how and when to modify techniques.

- Avoid deep or intense pressure near cancer lesions or enlarged lymph nodes, radiation field sites, medical devices (such as indwelling intravenous catheters), and anatomic distortions (such as postoperative changes), or in patients with a bleeding tendency.[Ibid.]

- Adapt the massage technique, length, and depth according to the patient's age, symptoms, tolerance, and experience with previous massage. When in doubt, always choose a light touch.

- Assess and document effectiveness, outcomes, and any adverse reactions or responses.

- Offer massage or teach willing family members to give massage to spouses, children, siblings, and other family members.

PEDIATRIC APPLICATIONS

Massage is being used increasingly in the care of hospitalized children, from infants to adolescents. Many of the uses of massage in pediatric care are similar to uses for adults (e.g., rehabilitation and anxiety reduction). Massage has also been found to reduce sleep problems in infants generally.[59] A unique benefit for infants is the tactile stimulation provided by massage, which is essential for proper growth and development.

Much of the recent interest in massage for children has been generated by the work of Tiffany Field, PhD, who founded the Touch Research Institute (TRI) in 1991 at the University of Miami School of Medicine, Department of Pediatrics. The research being performed at TRI on a variety of pediatric conditions can be reviewed on their website (see Appendix E).

Preterm Infants

Building on research done in the 1970s, Field found that preterm infants who received tactile stimulation during their stays in transitional care nursery settings experienced greater weight gain, increased motor activity, more alertness, and improved performance on the Brazelton Neonatal Behavioral Assessment Scale. Tactile stimulation was applied by gentle stroking of the head and neck, across the shoulders, from upper back to the waist, from the thighs to the feet, and from the shoulders to the hands. Additional stimulation was provided by passive flexion/extension movements of the arms and legs.[60]

Subsequent research has shown that massage also benefits cocaine-exposed preterm infants. In addition to better weight gain, massaged infants showed significantly fewer postnatal complications and stress behaviors than the control infants did.[61]

PRACTICAL APPLICATION

Investigate the uses of massage in the treatment of a particular pathology. Look at a variety of resources to locate information, for example, pathology textbooks, books about massage and/or the pathology, research reports, massage therapists with relevant experience, and other credible sources.

1. Is massage used for its direct therapeutic outcomes? Indirect outcomes? Palliative care?

2. What specific techniques are applied for the desired outcomes?
3. Are there contraindications or cautions to be aware of?
4. How would you defend the use of massage as evidence-based therapy in the treatment of this pathology?

More recent studies support the effectiveness of massage therapy for preterm infants to increase weight gain.[62, 63] It has also been shown to shorten hospital stays and improve their quality of sleep.[64] A study that followed low-birth-weight infants for 2 years after they received massage therapy, found that they had higher scores on mental and psychomotor development indexes.[65]

Additional Pediatric Applications

A review of some of the research being done at TRI demonstrates the broad range of situations in which massage is found to be a useful treatment for children. Descriptions of the research related to the following results, and many other studies related to pediatrics, can be found on the TRI website.

- *Asthmatic children.* Twenty-minute massages given to asthmatic children by their mothers for 1 month resulted in decreased anxiety levels and improved mood for both children and parents; the children's cortisol levels decreased, and they had fewer asthma attacks and were able to breathe better.

- *Autistic children.* After 1 month of massage therapy, the autistic children were less touch sensitive, less distracted by sounds, more attentive in class, related more to their teachers, and received better scores on the Autism Behavior Checklist and on the Early Social Communications Scales.

- *Diabetic children.* A pilot study showed that as a result of massage given to diabetic children by their parents, both children and parents showed lower anxiety and less depressed mood levels; the children's insulin and food regulation scores improved, and blood glucose levels decreased to the normal range.

- *Depressed adolescent mothers.* After 10 massage sessions over a 5-week period, depressed adolescent mothers reported lower anxiety; showed behavioral and stress hormone changes, including decreases in anxious behavior, pulse rate, and salivary cortisol levels; and a decrease in urine cortisol levels, suggesting lower stress levels.

- *Infants of depressed adolescent mothers.* Full-term infants born to depressed adolescent mothers were given 15 minutes of massage twice a week for 6 weeks. These infants gained more weight; showed greater improvement on emotionality, sociability, and soothability temperament dimensions, and on face-to-face interaction ratings; and had greater decreases in urinary stress catecholamines/hormones (norepinephrine, epinephrine, cortisol) than the control infants who were simply rocked.

- *Children with posttraumatic stress disorder.* Children traumatized by Hurricane Andrew were massaged at their schools twice a week for 1 month. The massaged children had less depression, lower anxiety levels, and

lower cortisol (stress hormone) levels than children in the control group.

Although further research is needed to substantiate much of what has been found to date, massage appears to be a promising adjunct to treatment of children with a variety of disorders.[66]

REALITY CHECK

JERMAINE: I'm interested in working with clients in a substance abuse rehabilitation facility, but don't feel qualified right now. We learned a little in school, but not enough for me to feel confident. What can I do to gain the knowledge and skills needed for this career goal?

ANTONIA: Entry-level training usually does not go very deeply into any of the wide variety of clinical applications of massage. For your career goal, I'd suggest a multifaceted approach. First look for information on the subject in professional publications and in psychology books, and read it for background understanding. Be sure that material found on the Internet is from credible sources. (Chapter 8, *Endangerment Sites, Contraindications, Cautions*, has a discussion of resources for reliable information.) At the same time, search for relevant studies in medical research databases. Once you have this foundation, look for continuing education related to massage and substance abuse. Also try to interview a massage therapist working with this population. Locate a facility that fits your future employment goal, and find out if they hire massage therapists and what qualifications they are looking for. A volunteer or internship position at a rehab facility might be a good place to get some experience and training. Or you might work with outpatient clients to begin learning about their characteristics and needs. Rather than learning additional massage techniques, it probably will be more important to learn how to apply techniques you already know to achieve the goals of this population, to keep proper boundaries, and to avoid some of the pitfalls of working in this setting. By reading, searching, interviewing, and getting some experience, you will eventually feel confident and ready to find the position you seek.

ANTONIA

PSYCHOLOGICAL CLINICAL APPLICATIONS

Massage is sometimes used to address the psychological and emotional problems of patients receiving medical treatment. For example, several of the studies mentioned in this chapter found massage to be beneficial in the reduction of the anxiety of patients hospitalized for serious medical conditions.

Massage may also help in the treatment of patients with medical conditions significantly worsened by stress. For example, in one study, patients with chronic inflammatory bowel disease, ulcerative colitis, or Crohn's disease (ileitis) who received massage for relaxation had fewer episodes of pain and disability from the disease.[67]

Massage may also help patients hospitalized for psychiatric reasons. In a study of hospitalized depressed and adjustment-disorder children and adolescents, those who received massage were less depressed and anxious and had lower saliva cortisol levels (an indication of less depression) than patients who watched relaxation videotapes.[68]

Psychotherapy patients not hospitalized may also benefit from the effects of massage related to stress and anxiety reduction, improved body awareness, and the ability to receive pleasurable nonsexual touch. For example, some massage therapists work with psychotherapists in the treatment of survivors of sexual and physical abuse.[69] Massage has been found to be beneficial in helping these patients reconnect with their bodies, develop a more compassionate relationship with their physical being, and experience their bodies as a "source of groundedness and eventually of strength and even pleasure—good things instead of bad things."[70]

Reduction of depression and state anxiety were two of the effects of massage confirmed in a meta-analysis of massage research. A course of massage treatment for these conditions was estimated to provide benefits similar in magnitude to those of psychotherapy.[71]

THERAPEUTIC TOUCH

Therapeutic Touch (TT) is a form of manual therapy in which the energy field of the recipient is rebalanced, thus promoting health and healing. Although it does not fall directly into the category of soft tissue massage, it is performed by many massage practitioners and integrated into their work. It has found special acceptance by nurses, who find it effective in caring for patients.

Therapeutic Touch was developed by Dolores Krieger, PhD, RN, in the 1970s.[72] She explains the technique as one of centering; then placing the hands in the recipient's energy field to detect a break in energy flow, pressure, or dysrhythmias; then rebalancing or repatterning the energy field by sweeping hand movements a few inches above the skin. She explains what happens as a profound relaxation response that has a positive effect on the immune system, which allows self-healing to reassert itself.

Kreiger explains that Therapeutic Touch has been found to have more effect on some conditions than others. For example, it seems to have a positive effect in working with fluid and electrolyte imbalances, dysfunctions of the autonomic nervous system, lymphatic and circulatory dysfunctions, and musculoskeletal problems. She further explains that:

 CASE FOR STUDY

Chloe Applies Massage for PTSD

Chloe has a client who was diagnosed with posttraumatic stress disorder (PTSD). The client was referred for massage by her doctor, who thought that massage might be good to reduce stress and anxiety. Chloe does not know much about PTSD but has an appointment with the client in a few days.

Question:

How can Chloe find out about PTSD and massage to provide a safe environment for the client and apply massage most effectively?

Things to consider:

- Where can Chloe go to find out about PTSD and its treatment?
- How can Chloe find out if massage has been used successfully in the treatment of PTSD?

- What might the potential therapeutic outcomes be? The contraindications or cautions?
- What massage approaches or techniques are important to know for this clinical application?
- What are Chloe's professional boundaries related to scope of practice in this situation?

Put yourself in Chloe's shoes and prepare for this client with PTSD. From what you found out, what would be your general approach to the massage session? What cautions would you observe?

_____

_____

_____

Some collagen dysfunctions respond, such as rheumatoid arthritis, but lupus is resistant. Within the endocrine system, the thyroid, adrenals, and ovaries respond, but there is little success with the pituitary and variable success with the pancreas in treating diabetes. In psychiatric disorders, manic depressives and catatonics respond, but there has been little success with schizophrenics.[73]

Therapeutic Touch has been found to have potential in the treatment of tension headache pain and fibromyalgia syndrome pain.[74, 75] A large clinical study showed TT to be beneficial for hospitalized patients by promoting feelings of comfort, calming, and general well-being.[76]

Research and articles about Therapeutic Touch can be found in nursing journals such as *American Journal of Nursing, Nursing Research*, and *Holistic Nursing Practice*. Further information about Therapeutic Touch research is available from Nurse Healers–Professional Associates (NH–PA), which was established in 1977 under the leadership of Dolores Kreiger. The NH–PA is a voluntary, nonprofit cooperative whose international exchange network facilitates the exchange of research findings, teaching strategies, and developments in the clinical practice of Therapeutic Touch.

COMPLEMENT TO CHIROPRACTIC CARE

Chiropractic care is gaining recognition as an effective treatment for certain conditions, especially back pain. Massage is often given as a complement to chiropractic care to help prepare the body for chiropractic adjustments, to relieve tension and pain in muscles and related soft tissues, and to prevent future musculoskeletal misalignment.

The term *chiropractic adjustment* is used here to mean a technique in which bones and joints are manipulated to return the body to proper alignment. This often involves a forceful thrusting movement or manipulation, which is not within the scope of practice of massage. Such adjustments are performed on subluxations, a condition of misalignment in a joint, which often results in structural, nervous system, and chemical dysfunctions.

Local massage is sometimes used in preparation for an adjustment. Massage relieves muscle tension and warms up the soft tissues in the area, making joints more pliable and more easily adjusted. Massage may be given along with heat and ultrasound in this preparatory routine.

A general massage (30–60 minutes long) may also be good preparation for an adjustment. In addition to preparing the immediate area of concern, it helps induce general relaxation and accustoms the recipient to touch. The recipient may be more receptive to other hands-on treatment in such a relaxed state. Massage after an adjustment may help the muscles remain relaxed and prevent a tightening reaction to the treatment. Regular massage may help adjustments last longer by keeping muscles relaxed and lengthened.

Therapeutic massage may also be used to address some of the muscular problems that bring patients for adjustments. These include nerve constriction due to tight muscles, poor circulation, trigger points, damaged tissues, and the pain–spasm–pain cycle. Massage used with ice can help relieve muscles in spasm. Recent research shows massage to be an effective treatment for low back pain, which is a common reason people seek chiropractic care.[77, 78]

CASE REPORTS

A good way to learn the basics of clinical massage therapy research is to design a case study for one client with a particular condition, implement the treatment plan, and write a report on the experience. **Case reports** contain most of the elements of larger research projects, including background information (introduction and literature review), client description (subject), measurement of variables pre- and posttreatment, and discussion of results. Examples of case studies and useful information about writing case reports can be found on the Massage Therapy Foundation (MTF) website, including articles and webinars on various aspects of the process (see Appendix E).

Published case reports contribute to the growing body of knowledge about massage. They are a way to share with other practitioners the techniques and approaches that have been tried for a particular pathology and those that have worked or not worked in a specific case. They are also useful to researchers designing experimental studies, informing them about the results of various approaches used in real life situations.[79] MTF encourages massage therapists to write case reports by publishing them in the open access journal, *International Journal of Therapeutic Massage and Bodywork (IJTMB)*, and by conducting annual case report contests, one for students and one for practitioners.

CHAPTER HIGHLIGHTS

- Clinical massage therapy refers to applications of massage for the treatment of pathologies.
- Client-centered massage makes the client's unique situation, needs, and goals the focus of treatment planning.
  - This is in contrast to recipe-based massage, in which every client receives exactly the same treatment for a particular medical condition.
- Principle-based therapy takes into consideration the pathology being treated, the condition of the individual, and the therapeutic potential of different treatment methods.
- Approaches to clinical massage therapy are focused on its therapeutic outcomes.
  - Three major categories of outcomes are direct therapeutic outcomes, indirect therapeutic outcomes, and palliative care.
- Massage has been found effective in relieving many musculoskeletal conditions, such as repetitive strain injuries, tension headaches, low back pain, and symptoms of fibromyalgia.
- Massage is used in treatment of cardiovascular and lymphatic disorders such as hypertension, edema, and lymphedema.
- Massage improves immune function, which is important in the treatment of many diseases.
- Massage is a useful complementary therapy for people with respiratory conditions, such as chronic bronchitis, emphysema, and asthma.
  - Several different massage therapy approaches have been studied for their effects on people suffering from COPD.
- Back massage has been used effectively with hospitalized patients to reduce anxiety and pain and to improve communication.
- Benefits of massage for cancer patients include reduced stress and anxiety, faster recovery from surgery, and reduction of the side effects from cancer treatment.
  - Emotional benefits for cancer patients include help in dealing with depression, reestablishing a positive body image, and rebuilding hope.
- Massage has been used successfully in pediatric care for children with asthma, autism, diabetes, depression, and posttraumatic stress disorder. It helps preterm infants gain weight and develop more normally.
- Massage is an effective complement to treatment of conditions worsened by stress. It relieves the anxiety and stress of psychiatric patients.
- Therapeutic Touch is a form of manual therapy that rebalances the energy field of the patient.
  - It has been found effective in treatment of several pathological conditions and beneficial for the comfort and general well-being of hospitalized patients.
  - Nurses have been particularly involved in the development of Therapeutic Touch and its use with patients.
- Massage is an effective complement to chiropractic care.
  - It helps prepare the body for adjustment and addresses some of the muscular problems of chiropractic patients.
- A good way to learn about clinical massage research is to write a case report.
  - Case reports include introduction, literature review, client description, measurement of variables pre- and posttreatment, and discussion of results.
  - Case reports are useful for informing researchers designing experimental studies about how massage is being applied in real life situations.

EXAM REVIEW

Key Terms

To study the key terms listed at the beginning of this chapter, match the appropriate lettered meaning to each numbered key term listed below. For additional study, look up the key terms in the Interactive Glossary and note other terms that compare or contrast with them.

_____ 1. Case reports
_____ 2. Client-centered massage
_____ 3. Clinical massage therapy
_____ 4. Direct therapeutic outcomes
_____ 5. Evidence-based practice
_____ 6. Indirect therapeutic outcomes
_____ 7. Palliative care
_____ 8. Principle-based therapy
_____ 9. Recipe-based massage

a. Eases discomfort and improves the quality of life for those with chronic medical conditions or terminal illness
b. Enhance the effectiveness of a primary treatment, or create a more favorable environment for healing
c. Every client receives exactly the same treatment for a particular medical condition
d. The creation of an overall treatment plan directed toward the achievement of specific treatment goals
e. Focuses on the client's unique situation, needs, and goals as the basis for treatment planning
f. Written accounts of the use of massage for individual clients
g. Focus on the healing of a diagnosed medical condition, or easing of its symptoms
h. Applications of massage in the treatment of human pathologies
i. Use of massage applications that are supported by scientific research

Memory Workout

To test your memory of the main concepts in this chapter, complete the following sentences by circling the most correct answer from the two choices provided.

1. The term _(clinical) (client-centered)_ _massage therapy_ describes applications of massage in the treatment of human patholgies.
2. The growing interest in massage for _(rest and rejuvenation) (treatment of pathologies)_ has led to an increased number of research studies about its efficacy.
3. Having verifiable _(objective) (anecdotal)_ evidence for the effectiveness of therapies chosen for a treatment plan is the cornerstone of evidenced-based practice.
4. Massage that focuses on the client's unique situation, needs, and goals as the basis for treatment planning is called _(client-centered) (evidence-based)_.
5. Massage used to ease discomfort and to improve the quality of life for those with chronic medical conditions or terminal illness is referred to as _(indirect) (palliative)_ care.

6. Research studies are most useful for adding to our understanding of the applications of massage, _not_ as a means for developing _(protocols) (principles)_ for treatment.
7. Two important effects of massage on the cardiovascular system are _(reduced) (increased)_ heart rate and blood pressure.
8. The _(Touch Research Institute) (Massage Therapy Foundation)_ at the University of Miami conducts and publishes many research studies on clinical massage applications.
9. A form of manual therapy sometimes used by nurses in clinical settings in which the energy field of the recipient is rebalanced is Therapeutic _(Massage) (Touch)_.
10. One of the benefits of massage for cancer patients is reduction of the _(therapeutic effects) (side effects)_ of cancer treatment.

Test Prep

The following multiple-choice questions will help to prepare you for future school and professional exams.

1. A complete description of evidence-based practice includes:
   a. Scientific research
   b. Scientific research and experience
   c. Scientific research and old traditions
   d. Scientific research, experience and judgment, and client values

2. Client-centered massage is the *opposite* of:
   a. Principle-based therapy
   b. Recipe-based massage
   c. Evidence-based practice
   d. Research-based massage

3. The use of deep transverse friction in treating repetitive strain injuries is an example of:
   a. Palliative care
   b. Indirect therapeutic outcome
   c. Direct therapeutic outcome
   d. Therapeutic Touch

4. Massage given to patients in hospices is an example of:
   a. Direct therapeutic outcome
   b. Palliative care
   c. Acute care
   d. Intensive care

5. The effect of massage therapy for which there is the best evidence from scientific research is:
   a. Increased general circulation
   b. Relief from negative mood
   c. Reduction of trait anxiety
   d. General weight loss

6. In Therapeutic Touch, the energy field of the recipient is rebalanced or repatterned by sweeping hand movements performed:
   a. On the arms and legs
   b. A few inches above the skin
   c. Directly on the skin using light pressure
   d. On the back

7. A massage application found to be an effective, noninvasive technique for promoting relaxation and improving communication with elderly, institutionalized patients is:
   a. Abdominal massage
   b. Lymphatic drainage
   c. Deep transverse friction
   d. Back massage

8. Indirect therapeutic outcomes of massage:
   a. Create a favorable environment for healing
   b. Treat a pathology and ease its symptoms
   c. Address the comfort of the recipient
   d. Focus on cause and effect

9. In chiropractic care, a condition of misalignment in a joint, which often results in structural, nervous system, and chemical dysfunctions is called a(n):
   a. Mobilization
   b. Adjustment
   c. Subluxation
   d. Adhesion

10. The benefits of massage for patients with chronic inflammatory bowel disease, ulcerative colitis, and Crohn's disease are based on its ability to:
    a. Increase circulation
    b. Relieve stress
    c. Increase flexibility
    d. Increase body awareness

Video Challenge

Watch this video, which can be found at MyHealthProfessionsLab.com, Chapter 7, and then answer the following questions.

Documentation

1. What do massage therapists in the video say about the usefulness of documentation for clinical massage applications?

2. How do SOAP notes as described in the video support evidence-based clinical massage therapy?

3. How are the Subjective and Objective sections of SOAP notes as described in the video used in client-centered massage?

Comprehension Exercises

The following short answer questions test your knowledge and understanding of chapter topics and provide practice in written communication skills. Explain in two to four complete sentences.

1. Describe the additional knowledge and skills needed for clinical massage therapy applications.

2. Explain the benefits of massage for hospitalized patients for which there is evidence from research studies.

For Greater Understanding

The following exercises are designed to take you from the realm of theory into the real world. They will help give you a deeper understanding of the subjects covered in this chapter. Action words are underlined to emphasize the variety of activities presented to address different learning styles, and to encourage deeper thinking.

1. Choose a specific pathology to study. Locate information about contraindications and cautions related to the pathology. Identify implications for giving massage to a person with the pathology studied. Discuss with a study partner or group.

2. Interview someone who is receiving massage as treatment for a particular pathology. Ask the individual to identify the benefits he or she feels from receiving massage. Compare this with conventional wisdom and available research.

3. Interview a massage practitioner who specializes in clinical applications or the director of a clinical massage setting. Ask the person about the types of pathologies seen in his or her practice and the benefits patients receive from massage. Report to a study partner or group.

4. Design a case study, implement the plan, and write a case report describing the results. Give an oral presentation of the case and your findings to the class. Consider submitting the report to the Massage Therapy Foundation Student Case Report Contest.

MyHealthProfessionsLab™

MyHealthProfessionsLab.com is a premium online homework management system that includes a host of features to help you study. Registered users will find:

- Powerful tools that track and analyze your results—allowing you to create a personalized learning experience
- Videos, flashcards and other learning tools to help enrich your progress
- Streaming lesson presentations and self-paced learning modules
- A space where you and your instructors can view and manage your assignments

8 Endangerment Sites, Contraindications, Cautions

Pearson Education, Inc.

CHAPTER OUTLINE

Learning Outcomes

Key Terms

Do No Harm

Endangerment Sites

General Principles for Safety
  around Endangerment Sites

Contraindications

Principles for Contraindications
  and Cautions

Medications

Person-Centered Massage

Resources for Reliable Information

Chapter Highlights

Exam Review

LEARNING OUTCOMES

After studying this chapter, you will have information to:

1. Locate endangerment sites on the body.
2. Apply massage safely around endangerment sites.
3. Recognize contraindications and cautions for massage.
4. Distinguish between general and local contraindications for massage.

5. Adapt massage sessions for clients taking medications.
6. Demonstrate a person-centered approach to massage.
7. Locate information about endangerment sites and contraindications for massage in professional resources.

KEY TERMS

Cautions

Contraindications

Do no harm

Endangerment site

General contraindications

Health history

Local contraindications

Person centered

DO NO HARM

One of most basic principles of giving therapeutic massage is to **do no harm**. Guidelines for helping you make decisions about what to do and what to avoid to protect the health and safety of your clients are presented in this chapter. Topics addressed include endangerment sites, contraindications, cautions, medications, and useful resources for further information.

The variety of massage and bodywork approaches used today complicates the issue somewhat. These forms vary from deep tissue structural massage of the physical body to light touch affecting the energy within and around the physical body. An endangerment site or a contraindication in one form of manual therapy may be considered perfectly safe for a different form.

This chapter focuses on endangerment sites, contraindications, and cautions that are important when giving Swedish massage and forms that use similar techniques. This includes all techniques applied to the physical body that involve pressing, stroking, friction, kneading, tapping, vibrating, and joint movements. Chapters devoted to other types of massage and bodywork address contraindications and cautions for that particular approach.

Knowledge of anatomy, physiology, and pathology is essential to ensure the safety of persons receiving massage and bodywork. It is particularly important to know the location of major nerves, blood vessels, glands, and visceral organs. Endangerment sites, contraindications, and cautions are discussed in this chapter from the perspective of the health and medical sciences.

ENDANGERMENT SITES

Endangerment sites are areas of the body where delicate structures are less protected and, therefore, may be more easily damaged when receiving massage. Tissues and structures particularly vulnerable include blood vessels, nerves, lymph nodes, glands, eyes, and all the internal organs. Caution is required when performing massage on or around endangerment sites. The following sections identify the location of endangerment sites and describe cautions when working in those areas. See Figure 8–1 ■ for the general location of endangerment sites on the anterior and posterior body.

Head and Face

The head and face contain several relatively superficial structures that require caution when giving massage. These include arteries, lymph nodes, nerves (facial and trigeminal), salivary glands, and eyes. See Figure 8–2 ■. Practitioners should be aware of the underlying structures they are touching when applying massage techniques to the area and use only light to moderate pressure.

Arteries supplying blood to the face and head branch off from the carotid artery in the neck. The temporal artery goes up around the sides and top of the head and can be felt as a pulse at the temple. The facial artery travels through the nose and cheek area supplying blood to muscles and structures there. The facial nerve that regulates facial expression and the trigeminal nerve that transmits sensations spread across the cheek area in a similar fan-like pattern from the ear to the midline of the nose and to the mandible.

The path of the lymph vessels and nodes in the face runs under and along the jawline, up to the nose, and in front of and behind the ear. The node will feel hard or swollen and may be tender if a client is fighting an infection such as a sinus infection. Avoid direct pressure over the nodes if this seems to be the case. However, lymphatic drainage techniques, which are very light and superficial, may be applied to the area to facilitate lymph flow in the absence of other contraindications. For example, lymphatic massage might be beneficial for someone with seasonal allergies or general puffiness in the face.

Salivary glands are found in the soft tissue under the jaw (submandibular gland) and in front of the ear on the face (parotid gland). Superficial skin movement and the very light pressure of lymphatic massage is acceptable over these areas. However, deep pressure should be avoided and care taken when performing massage on the masseter muscle to prevent contact with the parotid gland.

Use caution when working around the eyes. Be careful not to slip and hit the eyeball by accident. Only the very lightest pressure is used when stroking the eyelid.

Anterior Neck

The anterior neck is the triangular area on the front of the neck defined by the sternocleidomastoid (SCM) and includes the sternal notch, which is the depression found on the superior aspect of the sternum. Delicate structures located in the anterior neck triangle are the carotid artery, jugular vein, vagus nerve, larynx, and thyroid gland. Deep pressure on any of these structures can be harmful. See Figures 8–3 ■ and 8–4 ■.

Pressure within the anterior triangle of the neck, including the depression formed by the sternal notch, should be avoided entirely in most forms of massage. The gentle superficial stroking during lymphatic massage and noncontact forms of energy work are possible exceptions to the no-touch rule.

Great care should be taken when performing neck massage on older adults due to the likelihood of atherosclerosis and the potential for dislodging a thrombus that could lead to stroke. Too much pressure from massage could also cause further damage to blood vessels in the area. Moderate pressure on the muscles of the posterior cervical triangle may be safe to apply with care.

Vertebral Column

The vertebral column protects the spinal cord of the central nervous system. The spinous processes of the cervical, thoracic, and lumbar vertebrae can be felt along the midline of

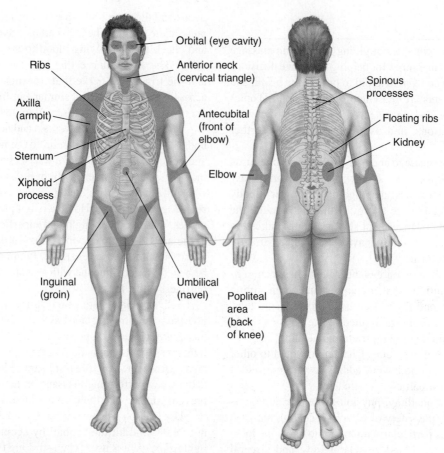

FIGURE 8–1 Endangerment sites—anterior and posterior views.

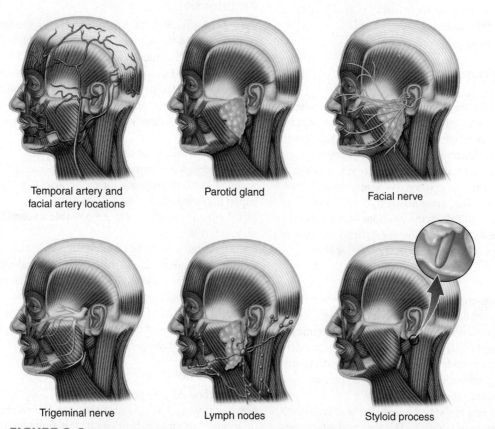

Temporal artery and
facial artery locations

Parotid gland

Facial nerve

Trigeminal nerve

Lymph nodes

Styloid process

FIGURE 8–2 Endangerment sites of the head and face. Use only light to moderate pressure on head and face.

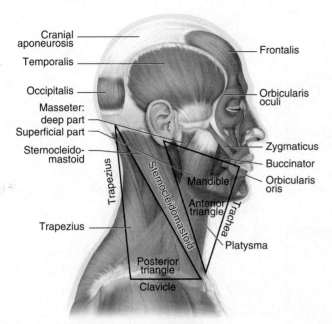

FIGURE 8–3
Anterior and posterior triangles of the neck. Avoid massage in anterior neck.

FIGURE 8–4
Anterior neck structures. Avoid massage in anterior neck.

the neck and back. See Figure 8–5 ■. Massage techniques that apply heavy pressure or that involve percussion should not be performed directly over the spinous processes.

Thoracic Cage

The thoracic cage consists of the ribs and sternum. The thoracic cage is relatively flexible to allow for breathing. Ribs 1–10 attach to the sternum with cartilage, whereas ribs 11–12 do not attach and are called floating ribs. The inferior tip of the sternum, called the *xiphoid process*, is a slender piece of bone that can break under pressure and be driven into the liver, causing severe damage. See Figure 8–6 ■.

Avoid heavy pressure or impact directly over the sternum, and especially on the xiphoid process. Forceful pressure over the rib cage should also be avoided, especially in older adults and those at risk for osteoporosis.

Shoulder and Axilla

Delicate circulatory and nerve structures are relatively exposed in the shoulder and axilla (i.e., armpit) area. These structures include the brachial artery, axillary artery and vein, cephalic vein, basilica vein, brachial plexus nerve complex, and axillary lymph nodes (Figure 8–7 ■). Deep specific pressure in this area should be approached with caution. Moderate broad pressure may be applied to the armpit, but deep specific pressure should be restricted to the surrounding musculature (e.g., pectoral and subscapularis muscles) and their attachments.

Elbow and Wrist

Two places around the elbow or cubital area require caution. One is the space just medial to the olecranon process, where the ulnar nerve is relatively exposed. This is the "funny bone" area that causes sharp pain when hit. Another sensitive place is the anterior fold of the elbow. This area is similar to the popliteal area found posterior to the knee. Vulnerable structures that pass through the elbow include the brachial vein and artery, median cubital vein, and median nerve. These structures are all close to the surface and unprotected by muscle. Moderate broad pressure may be applied to the area, but deep specific pressure should be restricted to the surrounding muscles and their attachments (e.g., forearm flexors and extensors).

The wrist, particularly the anterior wrist, is unprotected by muscular structures. Bones are close to the surface under the skin, as are blood vessels and nerves. The pulse can be felt in the radial brachial artery at the lateral (thumb side) inner wrist. Avoid deep pointed pressure in the area.

Torso

The torso contains the internal organs of the body. Massage therapists should be familiar with the location of the organs for certain massage applications, particularly abdominal massage. See Figure 8–8 ■. The umbilicus or "belly button" is a sensitive area superficial to the descending aorta and abdominal aorta. Avoid direct, pointed pressure to the umbilicus. See Chapter 18, *Special Populations and*

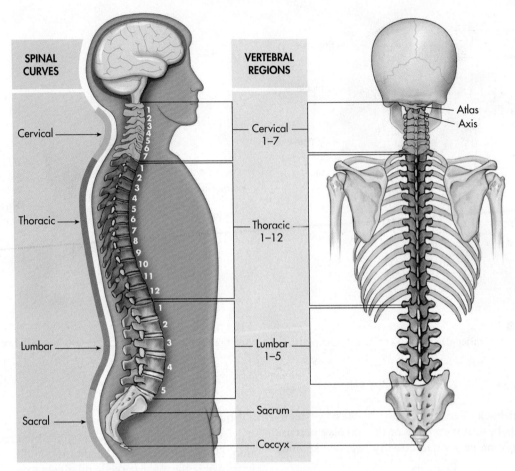

FIGURE 8–5 Vertebral column. Avoid heavy pressure directly over spinous processes.

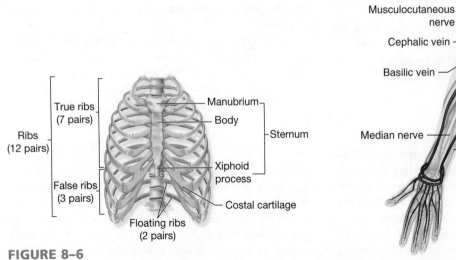

FIGURE 8–6

Thoracic cage. Avoid heavy pressure over the sternum and xiphoid process; caution over rib cage.

FIGURE 8–7 The anterior arm (shoulder, axilla, anticubital, and inner wrist areas). Approach deep pressure in these areas with caution.

Adaptations, for contraindications and cautions when giving massage to pregnant clients.

The kidneys are located on either side of the spine, generally at the level between the third lumbar and twelfth thoracic vertebrae. See Figure 8–9 ■. They are positioned behind the parietal peritoneum and against the deep muscles of the back. Superficial or deep stroking and pressing techniques may be applied carefully to the muscles of the back located in the kidney area. However, only light pressure should be used when performing percussion techniques over the kidneys.

Inguinal Area

The inguinal or groin area is located roughly where the thigh and the trunk meet on the anterior side of the body. The femoral nerve and major blood vessels to the lower extremities cross there (i.e., femoral artery, great saphenous and femoral veins). See Figure 8–10 ■. When the thigh is flexed, a depression is created in the area, exposing the more delicate structures. Great care should be taken when applying deep pressure into this area, for example, when addressing the iliopsoas muscle. This should be attempted by students only under supervision and by practitioners with adequate training.

Popliteal Area

The muscles of the posterior lower extremity cross the knee laterally and medially, leaving the center space relatively unprotected. This space is called the popliteal area. The popliteal artery and vein and the tibial nerve are located there. See Figure 8–11 ■. Broad flat hand strokes over this area may be safe, but avoid heavy specific pressure over the back of the knee joint. Follow the muscles around the popliteal area when massaging them.

Major Veins in Extremities

Major veins in the extremities are being included under endangerment sites because structural damage may occur to the valves within the veins if deep effleurage is applied improperly. Always apply deep flushing effleurage to the arms and legs from distal to proximal (i.e., toward the heart, and with the flow that opens the valves). See Figure 8–12 ■.

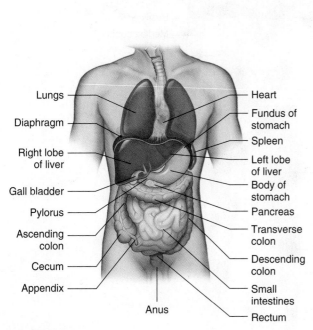

FIGURE 8–8
Abdominal organs. Proceed with caution during abdominal massage.

Lungs
Diaphragm
Right lobe of liver
Gall bladder
Pylorus
Ascending colon
Cecum
Appendix
Anus
Heart
Fundus of stomach
Spleen
Left lobe of liver
Body of stomach
Pancreas
Transverse colon
Descending colon
Small intestines
Rectum

FIGURE 8–9 Location of the kidneys—posterior view. Avoid heavy percussion over the kidneys.

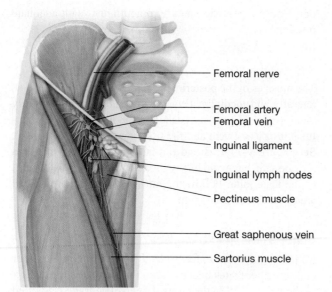

Femoral nerve

Femoral artery
Femoral vein

Inguinal ligament

Inguinal lymph nodes

Pectineus muscle

Great saphenous vein

Sartorius muscle

FIGURE 8–10 The inguinal area. Take great care when applying deep pressure in this region

Semitendinosus

Biceps femoris

Semimembranosus

Sciatic nerve

Popliteal vein
Popliteal artery
Tibial nerve
Small saphenous vein
Gastrocnemius

Common peroneal nerve

FIGURE 8–11 The popliteal area. Avoid heavy pressure over the back of the knee joint.

FIGURE 8–12

Major veins of the body. Apply deep flushing effleurage to the arms and legs from distal to proximal, or toward the heart.

External jugular vein
Internal jugular vein

Superior vena cava

Hepatic portal vein

Superior mesenteric vein
Inferior vena cava
Ulnar vein
Radial vein
Common iliac vein
External iliac vein
Internal iliac vein

Digital veins

Femoral vein
Great saphenous vein

Popliteal vein

Posterior tibial vein

Anterior tibial vein

Fibular vein

Subclavian vein
Right and left brachiocephalic veins

Cephalic vein
Brachial vein

Basilic vein

Median cubital vein

Renal vein

GENERAL PRINCIPLES FOR SAFETY AROUND ENDANGERMENT SITES

Here are some general principles to keep in mind to protect the receiver's body from structural damage during massage. Remember, your first responsibility is to do no harm.

1. Always adjust the pressure applied to match the part of the body, the condition of the tissues, and the recipient's comfort. Any part of the body can be damaged if too much pressure is used.

2. Avoid heavy pressure anyplace where nerves, blood vessels, or lymph vessels are close to the surface or are unprotected by muscle or bone.

3. Be careful around joints where delicate structures are less protected by skeletal muscle.

4. If you feel a pulse, it means that you are on a major artery. Move to a different place immediately.

5. If the receiver feels searing, burning, shooting, electrical sensations, "pins and needles," or numbness, you may be pressing on a nerve. Move to a different place immediately.

6. Any abnormal structure is a potential endangerment site. Get information about structural abnormalities, and proceed with caution when you are sure it is safe to do so.

7. Always work with awareness, and when in doubt, do not take a chance that might lead to injury.

CONTRAINDICATIONS

Contraindications are conditions or situations that make the receiving of massage inadvisable because of the harm it might do. In the treatment model, a contraindication is any symptom or condition that renders a particular medication, procedure, or treatment unwise given the circumstances. For **general contraindications**, avoid massage altogether. For regional or **local contraindications**, avoid only the specific area of the body affected.

Cautions are situations of potential danger that require thoughtful consideration and possible modifications of technique application. Cautions may or may not involve pathology.

Be alert to possible contraindications and cautions for every client. A **health history** taken during the initial visit provides information about previous conditions or health issues to be aware of. Chapter 9, *Medical Terminology, Goal-Oriented Planning, Documentation,* discusses in greater detail the health history and intake interview. See samples of intake, health history, and note forms on MyHealthProfessionsLab .com. Check with regular clients at every session to see if their health status has changed in significant ways, especially if they are known to have conditions that are contraindications or for which special cautions apply.

Knowledge of normal anatomy and physiology, as well as the nature of common pathologies, is important for massage practitioners. Such knowledge may help prevent a well-meaning practitioner from causing harm. Those performing clinical applications need to be especially well versed in the pathologies that they are treating.

Be sure to fully understand the origin of any symptom of disease reported by a client. This information will help in the selection of appropriate techniques. It will also be useful in positioning clients to best support their health and comfort. If a client reports having a condition or disease that you are not familiar with, use your professional resources (as described in a later section of this chapter) to get more information before proceeding with the massage session.

Some general principles can be used to help determine whether receiving massage might be harmful. Some of the more common conditions and situations encountered in a massage practice are listed in the next section.

PRINCIPLES FOR CONTRAINDICATIONS AND CAUTIONS

1. *Severe Distress.* Do not perform massage when the recipient is experiencing severe distress.
   For example:
   - Feels physically ill or nauseated
   - Is in severe pain
   - Has a fever
   - Has been seriously injured recently

2. *Acute Inflammation.* Do not perform massage in the presence of acute inflammation. Signs of inflammation are redness, heat, swelling, and pain. Any diagnosed condition that ends in "-itis" is either a general or local contraindication.
   For example:
   - *Appendicitis.* Massage will spread inflammation throughout abdomen; avoid massage entirely.
   - *Rheumatoid arthritis.* Avoid massage over acutely inflamed joints (local contraindication); use caution even when subacute; avoid traction of joints and spine.
   - *Phlebitis.* Inflammation of a vein; completely avoid site of disease, usually the legs.
   - *Locally inflamed tissues.* Signs are redness, heat, swelling, and pain; avoid the surrounding area; on limbs, only work proximal to the affected area.

3. *Loss of Structural Integrity.* Understand the physician's recommendations and the relevant anatomy and physiology in cases where there is a loss of integrity in an area.
   For example:
   - *Over recent surgery.* Only those specifically trained to work with scar tissue should attempt this work.

REALITY CHECK

ROB

WENDY: The other day I was giving a massage and noticed that the client didn't have any toenails. It hadn't come up in the intake interview, and I was a little surprised. I didn't know what to say, but also didn't want to hurt her when massaging her feet. What can you do in a case like that?

ROB: Remember that many people have structural abnormalities that they have lived with for a long time and might forget to mention. If your demeanor is professional and you don't act embarrassed or overly concerned, it will put the client at ease in talking about the situation. Be matter of fact and say something like, "I notice that you don't have any toenails. Is there anything I need to know when massaging your feet? Are your toes tender?" This might be enough to get the person to talk to you about the situation. Then you can determine if any contraindications or cautions apply. The important thing is to acknowledge the situation, get the information you need to make good decisions, and document the condition on his or her health history after the session.

• **Around burns.** Avoid any pressure over or around recent burns.
• **Recent fractures.** With the client's permission, request information from his or her physician about the phase of healing of the fracture. Recent fractures or unset broken bones are contraindications for massage. See Figure 8–13 ■. Use caution around plates and screws used to hold bones together. Avoid pressure to injured soft tissues. Lymphatic facilitation may be helpful to reduce related swelling.

• **Artificial joint replacements.** Follow recommended restrictions in range of motion for artificial joint replacements. Take care in positioning the client comfortably after replacement of knee, hip, or shoulder joints. Avoid positions that put pressure directly on joint replacements.

4. **Skin Conditions.** Do not touch areas of the skin where there is a pathological condition that is contagious or that may be worsened or spread by applying pressure or rubbing.
For example:

• **Acne vulgaris.** Avoid massage over acne lesions. Acne is a localized bacterial infection of the sebaceous glands in the face, neck, or upper back. Acne lesions include pimples, cysts, blackheads (open comedones), and whiteheads (closed comedones). See Figure 8–14 ■.
• **Rashes.** Avoid touching on or near contagious skin rashes. A rash is a general term for red spots on the skin. Inquire about the cause of the rash. Avoid massage altogether if the rash is caused by a systemic disease (e.g., Lyme disease or lupus).
• **Cellulitis.** is a streptococcal infection of cells in the skin and is a general contraindication for massage. The infected area becomes red, tender, and swollen.
• **Dermatitis.** is an umbrella term for a skin inflammation and is most often reserved for noninfectious problems. Dermatitis caused by contact with poison ivy is a local contraindication for massage.
• **Boils.** Avoid touch on or near a boil. This is a localized staphylococcus infection of the skin.
• **Athlete's foot.** Avoid touch on or near fungal infections such as athlete's foot.
• **Ringworm.** Avoid touch on or near fungal infections such as ringworm. See Figure 8–15 ■.
• **Herpes simplex (e.g., cold sores).** Avoid massage altogether during an acute outbreak of herpes. See Figure 8–16 ■. Avoid massage locally during the scabbing phase.
• **Impetigo.** Avoid massage until lesions have completely healed. This is a highly contagious bacterial infection.
• **Hives.** Avoid massage altogether in the acute phase of hives and locally in the subacute stage. Hives (urticaria) are areas of redness, itching, heat,

Femur, AP view, comminuted fracture

Tibia, simple, transverse fracture

Greenstick fracture

Pott's fracture—dislocation

Compression fracture

Epiphyseal plate fracture

Colles' fracture

FIGURE 8–13 Types of fractures. Massage is contraindicated near fractures in early stages of healing.

and swelling that occur in reaction to an allergy or emotional distress. See Figure 8–17 ■. Common allergens that can result in hives are certain foods, pet dander, dust and mold, and certain materials such as latex.

- **Skin cancer.** Cancerous skin lesions should be diagnosed by a doctor. If diagnosed as nonmalignant, a cancerous lesion is a local contraindication for massage. If it is diagnosed as metastasizing, massage may be generally contraindicated. The signs of malignant melanoma are a mole that changes size and color, bleeds and itches, and has an irregular border. Alert the client if you notice a suspicious-looking skin growth. Suggest that he or she get it examined by a doctor. Figures 8–18 ■ and 8–19 ■ show different types of skin cancers.

FIGURE 8–14 Acne. Avoid massage over acne.
Source: Ocskay Bence/Fotolia.

FIGURE 8–17 Hives is a general contraindication in the acute phase and a local contraindication in the subacute phase.
Source: Rob Byron/Shutterstock.

FIGURE 8–15 Ringworm is a local contraindication for massage.
Source: Centers for Disease Control and Prevention.

FIGURE 8–18 Basal cell carcinoma is a local contraindication for massage.
Source: Vizual Studio/Shutterstock.

FIGURE 8–16 Herpes is a local contraindication during active phase.
Source: Centers for Disease Control and Prevention.

FIGURE 8–19 Melanoma is a local contraindication for massage.
Source: Centers for Disease Control and Prevention.

- *Allergies.* Clients with skin allergies may react negatively to certain oils or lotions used during massage. Check with recipient for substances to avoid, and be alert to skin reactions during the session.
- *Other skin disorders.* Some skin disorders such as benign moles (Figure 8–20 ■) and psoriasis (Figure 8–21 ■) are not contraindications for massage.

5. *Decreased Sensation.* Use extreme care in amount of pressure used when the client has decreased sensation, which may be caused by stroke, diabetes, spinal cord injury, or medication. Recipients cannot give accurate feedback regarding pressure and may also have abnormal vasomotor response to the massage.

6. *Increased Sensitivity to Touch.* Massage only to recipient's tolerance or comfort when there is increased sensitivity to touch. Clients who are ticklish

FIGURE 8–20 A common mole (nevus) is not a contraindication for massage.

Source: Schankz/Fotolia.

FIGURE 8–21 Psoriasis is a local contraindication for massage only during an acute outbreak.

Source: Quayside/Fotolia.

or who have ticklish areas (e.g., feet) generally find light superficial stroking unpleasant and annoying. They may respond well to deeper, slower pressure, or to percussion techniques on the ticklish area.

7. *Cardiovascular Disorders.* For clients with cardiovascular system disorders, research the condition carefully, and with the client's permission, consult with his or her physician if the condition is advanced. Be aware of medications the client is taking and their potential as contraindications for massage.
For example:

- *High blood pressure.* For clients with borderline or mild high blood pressure, relaxation massage may be beneficial. For those with high blood pressure accompanied by other cardiovascular or kidney disease, avoid massage that increases general blood circulation. Other forms of bodywork may be safe to apply if they do not significantly increase blood flow. Abdominal massage is contraindicated.
- *Low blood pressure.* Someone with low blood pressure may be more susceptible to fainting after receiving massage either on a table or a massage chair. Orthostatic hypotension is a condition that causes light-headedness or fainting when changing from lying down or semireclining to standing up. Be sure that these clients get up slowly from a horizontal or semireclining position.
- *Cardiac arrhythmias or carotid bruit.* Avoid lateral and anterior neck.
- *Severe atherosclerosis.* Massage only with physician's permission and then only very superficially. Avoid heavy pressure with clients on anticoagulant medication. See Figure 8–22 ■.
- *Severe varicose veins.* Tissues can be easily damaged, and there may be a tendency to clotting; avoid massage of the area. See Figure 8–23 ■.
- *Stroke.* Avoid circulatory massage, especially massage of neck. Blood thinners are usually prescribed after stroke, so use light pressure with all soft tissue manipulation.

8. *Spreading Disease by Circulation.* Do not perform circulatory massage when there is a pathological condition that might be spread through the lymph or cardiovascular systems.
For example:

- *Blood poisoning (lymphangitis).* Inflammation of the lymphatic vessels; appears as streaks of red on the skin.
- *Swollen glands (i.e., lymph nodes).* The immune system may be attempting to filter out bacteria or other pathogens, and draining them may cause an infection to spread.

9. *Bleeding and Bruising.* Do not perform massage near an area where there is bleeding or bruising.

FIGURE 8–22 Arteriosclerosis is a local contraindication for massage of the lateral neck.

FIGURE 8–23 Severe varicose veins are a local contraindication for massage.

For example:

- *Bruise.* Avoid pressure to immediate area in the acute stage, and use gentle pressure around the area after healing has begun. Bruises can be classified as hematoma (i.e., bleeding and pooling of blood between muscle sheaths) and ecchymosis (i.e., more superficial blood leakage).
- *Whiplash or other acute trauma.* Any situation in which there is tearing of tissue and where there may be bleeding into the tissue during the first 24–48 hours after the trauma; avoid massage in area, and if severe trauma avoid massage totally (see Principle #1 earlier).

10. *Edema.* Be sure of the cause of edema before proceeding with massage. Edema from inflammation due to bacterial or viral infection, pitted edema indicating tissue fragility, lymphatic obstruction due to parasites, and edema due to deep vein thrombosis are all contraindications for massage. In cases of general edema caused by cardiac, liver, or kidney disease, avoid massage altogether. Traumatic edema resulting from musculoskeletal injury may be treated with specialized lymphatic facilitation techniques.

11. *Compromised Immunity.* Take added sanitary precautions when working with clients who are ill or elderly. Be especially careful with personal and environmental hygiene when a client's immune function is depressed (e.g., after organ transplant when immune system is depressed with medication, with AIDS/HIV, or chronic fatigue syndrome).

12. *Osteoporosis.* Avoid deep pressure and vigorous joint movements with a client with diagnosed osteoporosis, someone whom you suspect to have the disease, or someone in a high-risk category. Osteoporosis is a disease in which bones become fragile, brittle, and fracture easily. The high-risk category includes small, sedentary postmenopausal women; frail older adults; or someone with hyperkyphosis or "dowager's hump." See Figure 8–24 ■.

13. *Cancer.* Massage may be contraindicated for a client with cancer in certain circumstances. Cancer is characterized by uncontrollable growth in abnormal cells forming malignant tumors. Although cancer has been removed as a general category from the list of contraindications for massage, caution is still advised. With the client's permission, consult his or her health care provider before giving massage to a cancer patient. Patients undergoing treatment for cancer often find symptomatic relief from massage. Cautions related to wounds, burns, nausea, compromised immunity, and weakness may apply.

    Massage therapists are advised to educate themselves about giving massage to people who have had or now have cancer. Physicians may not know or

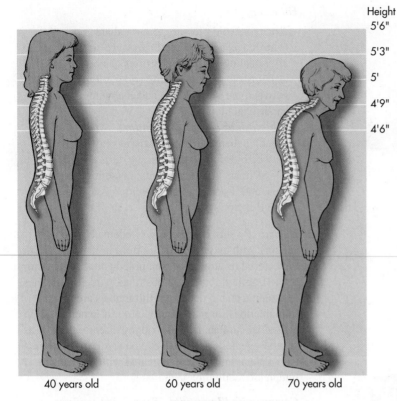

Height
5'6"
5'3"
5'
4'9"
4'6"

FIGURE 8–24 Spinal changes caused by osteoporosis. Use light pressure and gentle stretches only with frail or postmenopausal women.

40 years old   60 years old   70 years old

understand the different types of massage and their effects. They may also not be aware of current research about massage and cancer. See Chapter 7, *Clinical Applications of Massage*, for further discussion of massage and cancer, and for general treatment guidelines.

14. ***Personal Appliances.*** Avoid contact with personal appliances or aids that clients may be wearing. See Chapter 18, *Special Populations and Adaptations*, for a discussion of clients with medical appliances. *For example:*

• ***Contact Lenses.*** If a client is wearing contact lenses, take special care when working around the eyes to avoid pressure on the lenses and to avoid dislodging or moving the lenses. Make sure there is no pressure on the eyes when the client is prone and using a face cradle. Taking the contact lenses out during massage is preferable.

• ***Hearing Aid.*** If a client wears a hearing aid, be careful not to dislodge it while massaging around the ears. If it is turned on, massage on the head or around the ears may make a lot of noise for the client and be annoying. Be sure that these clients can see you if you talk to them.

MEDICATIONS

Medications are used by an increasing number of people for a variety of ailments. This includes prescription drugs, as well as over-the-counter drugs. Some medications are for short-term use, for example, common cold medications and painkillers

(analgesics) such as aspirin; and some are for long-term use, for example, heart medications or antidepressants. Massage practitioners need to be aware of what medications their clients are taking and understand the implications for massage therapy. Box 8–1 ■ lists some of the most common considerations for massage and medications. It summarizes some important points to keep in mind when working with clients taking medication. If in doubt, check with clients and their health care providers about potential for harm and how to avoid it.

A client's medications may affect the scheduling of massage sessions, the length of sessions, and techniques used and their application. They may also influence client behavior. Types of medications that require caution include, but are not limited to, those that:

• Alter sensation (e.g., numbing, increase sensitivity)

• Affect the blood and circulation (e.g., prevent clotting, regulate blood sugar level)

• Compromise tissue integrity (e.g., corticosteroids)

• Alter mood (e.g., depressants, antidepressants)

Table 8–1 ■ presents a pharmacology overview, listing a sampling of different classes of drugs, their functions, and generic and brand names. Additional information about common medications can be found in published pharmacology guides and on the Internet. Books that look specifically at medications and massage are also available. Be aware that new medications are continually being developed, and information about a particular drug's safety may change at any time.

Massage is generally contraindicated for persons under the influence of alcohol or recreational drugs. These drugs

BOX 8–1 Guidelines for Massage and Medications

Scheduling of Sessions

- Massage **after** the client's scheduled dosage if the medication is needed for condition stability (i.e., to ensure maximum bioavailability of the medication). For example, with insulin-dependent diabetics, chronic pain clients, epileptic patients.
- Massage **before** or **shortly after** the client's scheduled dosage if medication decreases the client's perception of pain and his or her ability to give accurate feedback. For example, clients taking drugs such as nonsteroidal anti-inflammatories, narcotic analgesics, and central nervous system depressants.

Session Length

- **Shorten the session** if the medication significantly depletes the energy level of the client, causing abnormal fatigue. For example, clients taking hypertension medications, antianxiety drugs, and many antidepressants.
- **Shorten the session** if the medication significantly decreases the emotional stability of the client, causing him or her to feel emotionally volatile or easily overwhelmed. For example, clients taking corticosteroids (long term) or medications that have side effects that cause mood fluctuations, anxiety, or depression.

Selection of Massage Techniques

- **For drugs that alter clotting mechanisms** (e.g., anticoagulants, platelet inhibitors, and aspirin and other nonsteroidal anti-inflammatory drugs): Avoid high-pressure techniques such as muscle stripping, deep kneading, ischemic compression, and cross-fiber friction.
- **For drugs that alter protective responses** (e.g., centrally acting muscle relaxants, narcotic analgesics, antianxiety drugs): Avoid deep massage, tense–relax stretching, and any technique that requires accurate client feedback for safe application.
- **For drugs that compromise tissue integrity** (e.g., corticosteroids, long-term use or injected directly into joints or tissue): Avoid deep pressure techniques, heavy tapotement, forced stretching, skin rolling and wringing.
- **For drugs that mask pain responses** (e.g., anti-inflammatory drugs, analgesics): Rely less on client feedback and more on observation and palpation to determine appropriate pressure and technique applications. Err on the side of caution.
- **For drugs that alter a client's cooperativeness or make him or her less communicative** (e.g., narcotic analgesics and antianxiety medications): Take time to ask questions as needed for accurate health histories and ongoing feedback during massage.

Source: Adapted from Persad, R. S. (2001). *Massage Therapy & Medications: General Treatment Principles.* Toronto, ON: Curties-Overzet Publications.

TABLE 8–1 Pharmacology Overview

Classification	Action	Generic and *Brand* Names
ACE inhibitor drugs	Cause vasodilation and decrease blood pressure	benazepril, *Lotensin* captopril, *Capoten*
Analgesics	Treat minor to moderate pain	salicylates, *Bayer Aspirin, Ecotrin* acetaminophen, *Tylenol* ibuprofen, *Advil* naproxen, *Aleve*
Androgen therapy	Replaces male hormones	testosterone, *Androderm, AndroGel* testosterone cypionate, *Andro-Cyp, Depo-Testosterone*
Anesthetics—local	Applied to the skin to deaden pain	lidocaine, *Lidoderm, Xylocaine* procaine, *Novocain*
Anesthetics—general	Produce a loss of consciousness or sensation	propofol, *Diprivan* fospropofol, *Lusendra*
Anorexiants	Treat obesity by suppressing appetite	benzphetamine, *Didrex* phentermine, *Adi-pex-P, Suprenza*
Antacids	Neutralize stomach acids	calcium carbonate, *Tums* aluminum hydroxide and magnesium hydroxide, *Maalox, Mylanta*
Antibiotic ointments	Kill bacteria causing skin infections	bacitracin, neomycin, *Neosporin ointment*

(continued)

TABLE 8–1	(continued)	
Classification	Action	Generic and *Brand* Names
Antibiotics for the respiratory system	Kill bacteria causing infections	amoxicillin, *Amoxil* ciprofloxacin, *Cipro* ampicillin
Antibiotics for the urinary system	Treat bacterial infections of the urinary tract	ciprofloxacin, *Cipro* nitrfurantoin, *Macrobid*
Anticoagulants	Prevent blood clot formation by "thinning" the blood	heparin, *Hep-Lock* warfarin sodium, *Coumadin*, *Warfarin*
Anticonvulsants	Prevent seizures by reducing the excitability of neurons	carbamazepine, *Tegretol* lacosamide, *Vimpat*
Antidiarrheals	Control diarrhea	loperamide, *Imodium* diphenoxylate, *Lomotil* kaolin/pectin, *Kaopectate*
Antiemetics	Treat nausea, vomiting, and motion sickness	prochlorperazine, *Compazine* promethazine, *Phenergan*
Antifungals	Kill fungi infecting the skin	miconazole, *Monistat* clotrimazole, *Lotrimin*
Antihemorrhagics	Prevent or stop hemorrhaging	aminocaproic acid, *Amicar* vitamin K
Antihistamines	Block the effects of histamine released by the body during an allergic reaction	cetirizine, *Zyrtec* diphenhydramine, *Benadryl* fexofenadine, *Allegra* loratadine, *Claritan*
Antilipidemics	Reduce amount of cholesterol and lipids in the blood to treat hyperlipidemia	atorvastatin, *Lipitor* simvastatin, *Zocor*
Antiparasitics	Kill lice or mites	lindane, *Kwell* permethrin, *Nix*
Antiplatelet agents	Prolong bleeding time by interfering with the action of platelets; used to prevent heart attacks and strokes	clopidogrel, *Plavix* ticlopidine, *Ticlid*
Antiprostatic agents	Treat early stages of benign prostatic hypertrophy	finasteride, *Proscar* dutasteride, *Avodart*
Antipruritics	Reduce itching	diphenhydramine, *Benadryl* benzocaine, *Anbesol, Orajel*
Antiseptics	Kill bacteria in cuts or wounds of the skin	isopropyl alcohol hydrogen peroxide
Antispasmodics	Prevent or reduce bladder muscle spasms	oxybutynin, *Ditropan* neostigmine, *Prostigmin*
Antithyroid agents	Block production of thyroid hormones in people with hypersecretion disorders	methimazole, *Tapazole* propylthiouracil, *Propyl-Thyracil*
Antitussives	Relieve the urge to cough	hydrocodon, *Hycodan* dextromethorphan, *Vicks Formula 44*
Antivirals	Treat herpes simplex infection	valacyclovir, *Valtrex* famcyclovir, *Famvir* acyclovir, *Zovirax*
Beta-blockers	Lower the heart rate to treat hypertension and angina pectoris	metoprolol, *Lopressor* propranolol, *Inderal*

Classification	Action	Generic and *Brand* Names
Bone resorption inhibitors	Reduce the resorption of bone in conditions such as osteoporosis	denosumab, *Prolia* ibandronate, *Boniva*
Bronchodilators	Treat asthma by relaxing muscle spasms in bronchial tubes	albuterol, *Proventil, Ventolin* salmeterol, *Serevent* theophylline, *Theo-24*
Calcium channel blockers	Cause the heart to beat less often and less forcefully to treat hypertension, angina pectoris, and congestive heart failure	diltiazem, *Cardizem* nifedipine, *Procardia*
Cardiotonics	Lower blood pressure by increasing urine production, which reduces blood volume	furosemide, *Lasix*
Corticosteroid creams	Anti-inflammatory creams applied topically	hydrocortisone, *Cortaid* triamcinolone, *Kenalog*
Corticosteroids	Anti-inflammatories used in conditions such as rheumatoid arthritis or other autoimmune diseases	prednisone methylprednisolone, *Medrol* dexamethasone, *Decadron*
Corticosteroids for the respiratory tract	Reduce inflammation and swelling	fluticasone, *Flonase* mometasone, *Nasonex* triamcinolone, *Azmacort*
Decongestants	Reduce congestion in the respiratory system	oxymetazoline, *Afrin, Dristan, Sinex* pseudoephedrine, *Drixoral, Sudafed*
Diuretics	Increase the volume of urine produced by the kidneys	furosemide, *Lasix* spironolactone, *Aldactone*
Dopaminergic drugs	Treat Parkinson's disease by replacing the dopamine that is lacking or increasing the strength of the dopamine that is present	levodopa L-dopa, *Laradopa* levodopa/carbidopa, *Sinemet*
Emetics	Induce vomiting	ipecac syrup
Expectorants	Improve the ability to cough up mucus from the respiratory tract	guaifenesin, *Robitussin, Mucinex*
Fertility drugs	Stimulate ovulation	clomiphene, *Clomid, Milophene*
H_2-receptor antagonists	Treat peptic ulcers and gastroesophageal reflux disease (GERD) by blocking H_2-receptors, which results in a low acid level in the stomach	ranitidine, *Zantac* cimetidine, *Tagament* famotidine, *Pepcid* esomeprazole, *Nexium*
Hematinics	Increases the amount of hemoglobin in the blood	epoetin alfa, *Procrit* darbepoetin alfa, *ARANESP*
Hormone therapy (HT)	Replaces estrogen in the postmenopausal woman	conjugated estrogens, *Cenestin, Premarin*
Human growth hormone therapy	Stimulates skeletal growth	somatropin, *Genotropin, Nutropin*
Hypnotics	Promote sleep	secobarbital, *Seconal* alprazolam, *Xanax* zolpidem, *Ambien*
Immunosuppressants	Prevent rejection of a transplanted organ by blocking certain actions of the immune system	mycophenolate mofetil, *CellCept* cyclosporine, *Neoral*
Insulin	Replaces insulin in type 1 diabetics or to treat type 2 diabetics	human insulin, *Humulin R* Insulin lispro, *Humalog*
Laxatives	Treat constipation by stimulating a bowel movement	senosides, *Senokot* psyllium, *Metamucil*

(continued)

TABLE 8–1 *(continued)*		
Classification	Action	Generic and *Brand* Names
Mucolytics	Liquefy mucus so it is easier to cough up and clear from respiratory tract	*N*-acetyl-cysteine, *Mucomyst* guaifenesin, *Mucinex*
Narcotic analgesics	Used to treat severe pain; can be habit forming	morphine, *MS Contin* pxycodone, *OxyContin* meperidine, *Demerol*
Nonsteroidal anti-inflammatory drugs (NSAIDs)	Anti-inflammatory and mild pain relief for conditions such as arthritis	ibuprofen, *Advil, Motrin* naxoproxen, *Aleve, Naprosyn* salicylates, *Bayer Aspirin*
Oral contraceptive pills	Prevent conception by blocking ovulation	estrogen-progestin combination, *Ortho-Cept, Lo/Ovral, Yaz, Zovia*
Oral hypoglycemic agents	Cause a decrease in blood sugar	metformin, *Glucophage* glipizide, *Glucotrol*
Oxytocin	Begins or improves uterine contractions during labor and delivery	oxytocin, *Pitocin*
Protease inhibitors	Stop viruses from reproducing by inhibiting the enzyme protease	indinavir, *Crixivan* saquinavir mesylate, *Invirase*
Proton pump inhibitors	Block the stomach's ability to secrete acid	esomeprazole, *Nexium* omeprazole, *Prilosec*
Reverse transcriptase inhibitor drugs	Stop viruses from reproducing by inhibiting the enzyme reverse transcriptase	lamivudine, *Epivir* zidovudine, *Retrovir*
Sedatives	Produce a relaxing or calming effect	amobarbital, *Amytal* butabarbital, *Butisol*
Skeletal muscle relaxants	Relax skeletal muscles to reduce muscle spasms	cyclobenzaprine, *Flexeril* carisoprodol, *Soma*
Thrombolytics	Dissolve existing blood clots	clopidogrel, *Plavix* alteplase, *Activase*
Thyroid replacement hormones	Replace thyroid hormones for people with hypothyroidism or who have had their thyroid glands surgically removed	levothyroxine, *Levoxyl, Synthroid* liothyronine, *Cytomel*
Vasoconstrictors	Raise blood pressure by contracting smooth muscle in walls of blood vessels	norepinephrine, *Levophed, Noradrenaline*
Vasodilators	Increase circulation to an ischemic area and reduces blood pressure by relaxing smooth muscle in artery walls	nitroglycerine, *Nitro-Dur* amyl nitrate
Vasopressin	Controls diabetes insipidus and promotes reabsorption of water in the kidney tubules	desmopressin acetate, *DDAVP, Stimate* conivaptan, *Vaprisol*

have the potential to alter sensation, affect mood, lessen the ability to give accurate feedback, and, in many cases, reduce good judgment. Giving massage therapy to a person "high" or in an altered state of consciousness is potentially dangerous for him or her and also for the massage practitioner.

PERSON-CENTERED MASSAGE

It is easy to lose sight of the person when there is pathology involved. From the wellness perspective, massage is best thought of as **person centered** rather than *pathology*

centered. In other words, practitioners may give massage to people with pathologies, but the people are more than their pathologies. In fact, practitioners often find themselves working around pathologies.

This may be the case when a person has a condition for which deep or vigorous massage is contraindicated. A light massage may be appropriate to add an element of care, comfort, and stress reduction as a complement to standard medical care. For example, there would be few cases in which stroking the hand or head of a seriously ill person is contraindicated.

Most of the contraindications and cautions discussed in this chapter are based on common sense, given some

CASE FOR STUDY

Kayla Adapts Her Routine Massage

Kayla gave a health history interview to a new client who came for a relaxation massage. She discovered that the client has skin allergies, ticklish feet, varicose veins in her legs, and periodic fainting. Several years ago the client broke her elbow in a fall and has a metal plate in her forearm. She has no major or chronic illnesses to report.

Question:

What precautions would Kayla take to ensure the health, safety, and comfort of her client during the massage session?

Things to consider:

● Is anything the client mentioned a general contraindication for massage?
● Does any of the health information point to local contraindications?
● Are any cautions around certain body areas warranted?

Write a brief description of what Kayla can do to provide for the safety and comfort of this client during the massage session.

_____

_____

_____

knowledge of anatomy, physiology, and pathology. If the giver of massage is motivated by sincere concern, gentle in giving massage, and receptive and responsive to feedback from the recipient, the experience will most likely be a healthy one for both people. Even in the hands of a child, massage given with love and sensitivity can be supportive and helpful.

RESOURCES FOR RELIABLE INFORMATION

The health history given at the client's first visit will often reveal health and medical conditions that deserve the massage therapist's attention. Even regular clients may develop new health issues over the years, changing some aspects of their massage sessions, for example, the type of lotion, or positioning, or areas of caution. Massage therapists should always be on the lookout for general and local contraindications and situations that require caution. Although your initial training and continuing education may give you knowledge of many conditions and the implications for massage, it is important to have reliable resources to look up information on health concerns that arise in the course of massage sessions.

People commonly get information they need from the Internet. Although this can be convenient and fast, the information is not always reliable. Just searching for a specific term (e.g., psoriasis or Coumadin) will generate hundreds of websites to click on, the first listed often being paid advertising. As a massage professional, it is good to have a few trustworthy websites in your "favorites" or "bookmarks" for easy access. Examples are: PubMed Health (http://www .ncbi.nlm.nih.gov/pubmedhealth); WebMd (http://www .webmd.com); MedicineNet (http://www.medicinenet.com);

and Mayo Clinic (http://www.mayoclinic.com). These sites have useful information about diseases and their symptoms, as well as common medications and their possible side effects.

Massage therapists also need *massage-specific* information related to contraindications and cautions and will find it helpful to keep personal professional libraries with reference books. These libraries should include some basic resources for information about conditions and pathologies commonly encountered in massage practices.

A basic professional library for massage practitioners might include a good anatomy and physiology text, an atlas of human anatomy, a pathology text, a medical dictionary, and a recently published pharmacology guide. Pathology and pharmacology books written especially for massage therapists are available and are valuable references that include special considerations for massage, including contraindications and cautions.

Practitioners working with special populations should have applicable references for basic information. There are books available on massage with specific populations (e.g., pregnant women, infants and children, older adults, cancer patients). Organizations for special populations may also have websites for information, for example, the American Heart Association and the American Cancer Society. Nonprofit groups have ".org" in their web addresses and may provide more unbiased information than commercial sites.

One of the best resources for information may be the recipient him- or herself. Recipients are often very knowledgeable about their own pathologies, especially if they have lived with a chronic condition for some time. The recipient's health care providers may also serve as valuable resources when there is any doubt as to the safety of an individual receiving massage.

PRACTICAL APPLICATION

Interview one of your practice clients using one of the health history forms that can be found at MyHealthProfessionsLab.com. Look over the information, and identify contraindications and cautions relevant to this person receiving massage therapy.

1. Does he or she have a chronic illness or recent injury?
2. Are there structural anomalies?
3. Is the individual taking medications regularly or occasionally?

CRITICAL THINKING

Think about the contraindications and cautions identified in the Practical Application exercise for this chapter. Apply the *Principles for Safety around Endangerment Sites* and the *Principles for Contraindications and Cautions* to this case.

1. Are there specific techniques that you would avoid?
2. Are there certain areas of the body that require caution?
3. How might medications the client is taking affect your approach or choice of techniques?

CHAPTER HIGHLIGHTS

- One of the most basic principles of giving therapeutic massage is to do no harm.
- Awareness of endangerment sites, contraindications, and cautions ensure the health and safety of clients.
- Endangerment sites are areas of the body where delicate structures are less protected and therefore more easily damaged when receiving massage.
  - Endangerment sites include the head and face, anterior neck, vertebral column, thoracic cage, shoulder and axilla, elbow, wrist, torso, umbilicus, kidney area, inguinal area, popliteal area, eyes, and the major veins in the extremities.
- General principles for performing massage related to endangerment sites include caution around delicate or abnormal anatomical structures, adjusting pressure to avoid damage, and always working with awareness.
- Contraindications are conditions that make receiving massage inadvisable because of the harm it might do.
  - For general contraindications, massage should be avoided altogether.
  - For local or regional contraindications, only the specific area of the body affected should be avoided.
- Cautions are areas of potential danger that require thoughtful consideration and possible modifications of technique application.
- Contraindications and cautions for massage include:
  - Severe distress, acute inflammation, skin problems, osteoporosis, decreased or increased sensation, and compromised immunity.

- Bleeding and bruising, some types of edema, cardiovascular disorders, diseases spread by circulation, and loss of structural integrity.
- Contact lenses, hearing aids, and other personal appliances.
- Medications including prescription and over-the-counter drugs that clients are taking must be considered.
  - Medications may affect the scheduling of massage sessions, the length of sessions, techniques used and their application, or the client's behavior.
  - Types of medications that require caution include those that alter sensation, affect the blood and circulation, compromise tissue integrity, or alter mood.
  - Persons under the influence of alcohol or recreational drugs should not receive massage because such substances alter sensation, affect mood, and reduce good judgment.
- From the wellness perspective, massage is person centered, not pathology centered.
- Massage therapists should be able to find reliable information about contraindications and cautions.
  - Websites used for information should have unbiased and reliable information.
  - Personal professional libraries include books and other resources for information about pathologies and related contraindications and cautions for massage.

EXAM REVIEW

Key Terms

To study the key terms listed at the beginning of this chapter, match the appropriate lettered meaning to each numbered key term listed. For additional study, look up the key terms in the Interactive Glossary, and note other terms that compare or contrast with them.

_____ 1. Cautions
_____ 2. Contraindications
_____ 3. Do no harm
_____ 4. Endangerment site
_____ 5. General contraindications
_____ 6. Health history
_____ 7. Local contraindications
_____ 8. Person centered

a. One of the most basic principles of giving therapeutic massage
b. For these, avoid only the specific area of the body affected
c. For these, avoid massage altogether
d. Provides information about previous medical conditions or health issues to be aware of
e. Focuses on the client rather than his or her pathologies
f. Situations of potential danger that require thoughtful consideration and possible modifications of technique application
g. Areas of the body where delicate structures are less protected and, therefore, may be more easily damaged when receiving massage
h. Conditions or situations that make the receiving of massage inadvisable because of the harm it might do

Memory Workout

To test your memory of the main concepts in this chapter, complete the following sentences by circling the most correct answer from the two choices provided.

1. Endangerment sites are areas of the body where delicate anatomical structures are (encased) (exposed) and, therefore, may be more easily damaged when receiving massage.
2. Always apply deep effleurage on the limbs from (distal to proximal) (medial to lateral) to avoid damage to the valves in the large veins.
3. Always adjust the amount of (pressure) (oil) you use to match the condition of the tissues being manipulated.
4. Avoid massage altogether for (general) (regional) contraindications.

5. A client health history should be taken to identify possible (preferences) (contraindications) for massage.
6. Acute inflammation is a general or local contraindication for massage, for example, almost any condition that ends in (-osis) (-itis).
7. Bruising is a (local) (mild) contraindication.
8. A client's compromised (immunity) (integrity) calls for extra care in personal and environmental hygiene.
9. If a medication significantly depletes a client's energy level, it may be advisable to (lengthen) (shorten) a massage session.
10. From a wellness perspective, massage is best thought of as (pathology centered) (person centered).

Test Prep

The following multiple-choice questions will help to prepare you for future school and professional exams.

1. Which region of the neck should be avoided during massage?
   a. Posterior
   b. Anterior triangle
   c. Lateral aspect
   d. Suboccipital

2. Forceful or heavy pressure techniques are generally contraindicated if a client has:
   a. Skin allergies
   b. Contact lenses
   c. Osteoporosis
   d. Low blood pressure

3. If you feel a pulse, it means that you are touching a(n):
   a. Nerve
   b. Artery
   c. Vein
   d. Lymph node

4. If the receiver feels a shooting or electrical sensation, you have probably hit a(n):
   a. Nerve
   b. Artery
   c. Tendon
   d. Ligament

5. For massage, skin acne is a:
   a. General contraindication
   b. Local contraindication
   c. Local indication
   d. Nonconsideration

6. Clients with diabetes usually have this condition in the feet:
   a. Warts
   b. Fallen arches
   c. Decreased sensation
   d. Increased sensation

7. If a client's medication decreases his or her sensitivity to pain, it is best to conduct the massage:
   a. Before the scheduled dosage
   b. After the scheduled dosage
   c. Not at all (contraindicated)
   d. Anytime

8. A primary concern related to long-term use of corticosteroids (e.g., for allergies or chronic inflammation) is that it tends to:
   a. Make a person less talkative
   b. Deplete energy
   c. Compromise tissue integrity
   d. Reduce blood clotting mechanisms

9. For a frail or seriously ill person, in addition to choosing less-vigorous massage techniques, you might also:
   a. Make the session shorter
   b. Make the session longer
   c. Include a lot of joint movements
   d. Reduce the amount of lotion used

10. Which of the following precautions applies specifically to clients with low blood pressure?
    a. Avoid percussion techniques
    b. Get up slowly from a horizontal position
    c. Avoid massage of the feet
    d. Shorten the session

Video Challenge

Watch this video, which can be found at MyHealthProfessionsLab.com, Chapter 8, and then answer the following questions.

Goal-Oriented Planning

1. In what step of planning a massage session might a contraindication to massage be discovered?

2. How is knowledge of contraindications used in planning massage sessions?

Comprehension Exercises

The following short-answer questions test your knowledge and understanding of chapter topics and provide practice in written communication skills. Explain in two to four complete sentences.

1. Describe massage techniques that would be contraindicated and those that are safe to apply over the back of the knee or popliteal area.

2. Identify four types of medications that create conditions requiring caution for the application of massage techniques.

3. Explain why massage is contraindicated for a person under the influence of alcohol or recreational drugs.

For Greater Understanding

The following exercises are designed to take you from the realm of theory into the real world. They will help give you a deeper understanding of the subjects covered in this chapter. Action words are underlined to emphasize the variety of activities presented to address different learning styles and to encourage deeper thinking.

1. On yourself, or working with a study partner, <u>explore</u> the surface anatomy of the major endangerment sites. Carefully and safely <u>feel</u> the structure of the area and <u>visualize</u> the tissues and anatomical structures underneath the skin. <u>Imagine</u> how deep specific structures are to the surface and how exposed they are to pressure. <u>Use</u> an anatomy book or atlas as an aid to visualization.

2. <u>Interview</u> a massage practitioner who specializes in clinical applications or the director of a clinical massage setting. <u>Ask</u> the person about the types of pathologies he or she sees in his or her practice and the cautions taken in working with those clients. <u>Report</u> to a study partner or group.

3. <u>Interview</u> a person taking one or more medications. <u>List</u> the medications he or she takes and the related pathology for which the individual is being treated. <u>Identify</u> modifications you would make in a massage session with this person. <u>Discuss</u> your session plan with a study partner or group.

MyHealthProfessionsLab™

MyHealthProfessionsLab.com is a premium online homework management system that includes a host of features to help you study. Registered users will find:

- Powerful tools that track and analyze your results—allowing you to create a personalized learning experience
- Videos, flashcards and other learning tools to help enrich your progress
- Streaming lesson presentations and self-paced learning modules
- A space where you and your instructors can view and manage your assignments

9 Medical Terminology, Goal-Oriented Planning, Documentation

Pearson Education, Inc.

CHAPTER OUTLINE

Learning Outcomes

Key Terms

Medical Terminology

The Importance of Planning

Steps in Goal-Oriented Planning

Long-Term Planning

Individual Session Planning

Treatment Planning

Collecting Subjective Information

Collecting Objective Information

Importance of Documentation

SOAP Note Overview

Writing SOAP Notes

Simplified Documentation

Designing a System of Documentation

Legal and Ethical Issues

Chapter Highlights

Exam Review

LEARNING OUTCOMES

After studying this chapter, you will have information to:

1. Use medical terminology in treatment planning and documentation.

2. Use the six-step process for planning goal-oriented massage sessions.

3. Develop long-term, individual session, and treatment plans for meeting clients' goals.

4. Perform intake interviews to gather client information for planning.

5. Use basic evaluation tools to collect objective information for planning.

6. Describe four types of SOAP notes.

7. Write SOAP notes clearly, concisely, and correctly.

8. Write simplified session notes.

9. Design a documentation system for a massage practice.

10. Identify legal and ethical issues related to documentation.

KEY TERMS

Assessment

Clinical reasoning

Continuing session notes

Discharge notes

Documentation

Goal-oriented planning

HIPAA privacy rules

Intake notes

Long-term planning

Progress notes

SOAP notes

Treatment planning

MEDICAL TERMINOLOGY

Medical terminology is the shared language of health professionals. Standard medical terms enable clear communication, precise descriptions, and common understanding. Knowledge of common terms is useful when taking health histories, determining contraindications and cautions, planning treatments, and writing session notes. An overview of medical terminology is provided here in preparation for goal-oriented planning and documentation discussed later in the chapter.

Understanding medical terminology and becoming proficient in using it correctly begins with learning the word parts, or components, that form the terms. These word parts are prefixes, word roots/combining forms, and suffixes. For instance, the prefix *mal-* (bad) and the word root *format* (a shaping) plus the suffix *–ion* (process) produces the term *malformation*, meaning the process of being deformed or badly shaped.

Once you learn the word parts, you have a logical system for interpreting what an unfamiliar term means and for speaking and writing in a language used by others in the health professions. The most efficient way of understanding a medical term is to read the term from the end of the word (suffix) back to the beginning (prefix) and then look at the word root. For example, the term *pericarditis* can be translated as inflammation (*-itis*) surrounding (*peri-*) the heart (*cardi/o*).

Prefixes

A prefix is added to the front of a word root/combining form to alter or modify its meaning or to give additional information, such as the location of an organ, the number of parts, or the frequency of an action. For example, the prefix *bi-* means two, and the term *bilateral* means having two sides. The prefix *dys-* means difficult, and the term *dyspnea* means difficult breathing. Not all medical terms have prefixes. Table 9–1 ▪ lists common prefixes.

TABLE 9–1 Common Prefixes

Prefix	Meaning	Example (Pronunciation)	Definition
a-	Without, away from	Aphasia (ah FAY zee ah)	Without speech
an-	Without	Anoxia (ah NOK see ah)	Without oxygen
ante-	Before, in front of	Antepartum (AN tee par tum)	Before birth
anti-	Against	Antibiotic (AN tee BYE ott ik)	Against life
auto-	Self	Autograft (AW toe graft)	A graft from one's own body
bi-	Two	Bilateral (by LAT er uhl)	Two sides
brady-	Slow	Bradycardia (brad ee KAR dee ah)	Slow heartbeat
circum-	Around	Circumduction (sir kum DUK shun)	Joint movement around a circle
contra-	Against, opposite	Contraindicated (kon truh IN duh kayt ed)	Not indicated
di-	Two	Diplegic (dih PLEJ ik)	Paralysis of two extremities
dia-	Through	Dialysis (dye AHL ah siss)	Procedure that removes uric acid from circulating blood
dis-	Separate, away from	Distal (DISS tal)	Pertaining to away from a point of reference
dys-	Bad, abnormal	Dysplasia (diss PLAY zee ah)	Abnormal tissue development

(continued)

TABLE 9–1 (*continued*)

Prefix	Meaning	Example (Pronunciation)	Definition
ecto-	Outer, outside	Ectoderm (ek toe derm)	Outer layer of cells
endo-	Within, inner	Endoderm (ehn doe derm)	Inner layer of cells
eu-	Good, normal	Eupnea (yoop NEE ah)	Normal breathing
ex-	Out, away from	Extension (ex TEN shun)	Move away from
hemi-	Half	Hemiplegia (hem ee PLEE jee ah)	Paralysis of one side or half of the body
hetero-	Different	Heterograft (HET er oh graft)	A graft from another person's body
homeo-	Same, similar	Homeostasis (ho mee oh STAY siss)	State of equilibrium in the body
hydro-	Water	Hydrotherapy (high droh THER ah pee)	Water treatment
hyper-	Over, above	Hypertrophy (high PER troh fee)	Overdevelopment
hypo-	Under, below	Hypotension (HIGH poh ten shun)	Chronic low blood pressure
in-	In, into, not	Insomnia (in SAHM nee ah)	Condition of not being able to sleep
inter-	Among, between	Intervertebral (in ter VER teh bral)	Between the vertebrae
intra-	Within, inside	Intramuscular (in trah MUS kue lar)	Within a muscle
macro-	Large	Macrocephalic (MAK roh SEH falik)	Having a large head
meta-	Beyond, over, between	Metacarpals (met ah KAR pals)	Pertaining to the bones beyond the wrist
micro-	Small	Microcephaly (MY kroh SEFF ah lee)	Having a small head
mono-	One	Monoplegia (mon oh PLEE jee ah)	Paralysis of one extremity
multi-	Many	Multipara (mull tee PAR ah)	More than one birth
neo-	New	Neonate (NEE oh nate)	Newborn
pan-	All	Pansinusitis (PAN sigh nuss EYE tiss)	Inflammation of all paranasal sinuses
para-	Beside, beyond, near	Paraspinal (pair ah SPY nahl)	Alongside the spine
per-	Through	Percutaneous (per kyoo TAY nee uss)	Through the skin
peri-	Around	Pericardial (pair ih KAR dee al)	Around the heart

Prefix	Meaning	Example (Pronunciation)	Definition
poly-	Many	Polyuria (POLL ee YOO ree ah)	Large amounts of urine
post-	After	Postprandial (post PRAN dee al)	More than 2 hours after a meal
pre-	Before, in front of	Prefrontal (pree FRUN tahl)	In front of the frontal bones
quad-	Four	Quadriplegia (kwahd rih PLEE jee ah)	Paralysis of all four extremities
retro-	Backward, behind	Retrograde (REH troh grayd)	Movement in a backward direction
semi-	Partial, half	Semiconscious (sem ee KON shus)	Partially conscious
sub-	Below, under	Subcutaneous (sub kyoo TAY nee us)	Under the skin
super-	Above, upper, excess	Superficial (soo per FISH uhl)	Pertaining to the surface
supra-	Above	Supraspinatus (soo prah SPY nayt us)	Muscle above the spine of the scapula
tachy-	Rapid, fast	Tachycardia (tak ee KAR dee ah)	Fast heartbeat
trans-	Through, across	Transdermal (trans DERM al)	Through the skin
tri-	Three	Triceps (TRI seps)	Muscle with three heads
ultra-	Beyond, excess	Ultrasound (ULL trah sound)	Beyond sound
uni-	One	Unilateral (yoo nih LAT er uhl)	One side

Word Roots/Combining Forms

The main part of the word is the word root, which provides the general meaning of the word. For instance, *cardi* means heart, as in the term *cardiac*, and tells us which body system is being discussed. *Cis* means to cut, as in the term *incision*, and tells us the action being taken. Sometimes more than one word root can form a term. For instance, *osteoarthritis* is formed from two word roots, *oste* meaning *bone*, and *arthr* meaning *joints*. Adding the suffix *–itis*, which means *inflammation*, gives us the meaning of the term: inflammation of bone at the joints.

The combining form is simply the word root combined with a vowel, which makes it easier to pronounce long medical terms. Most often this is the vowel *o* used between two word roots (oste/o arthr -itis) or between a word root and a suffix (cardi/o -logy). Table 9–2 ▪ lists common word roots and their combining vowel.

Suffixes

A component added to the end of a word, a suffix adds additional meaning to the term, such as condition, disease, or procedure. Every medical term has a suffix. Generally it is added to a word root; however, it can also be added to a prefix without a word root. For example, the term *prognosis*, which means the prediction of the course of disease and recovery, is formed from the prefix *pro-*, meaning *before*, and the suffix *–gnosis*, meaning *knowledge*. If a suffix begins with a vowel, the combining vowel of the word root is dropped. Table 9–3 ▪ lists common suffixes.

Singular and Plural Endings

Forming the singular and plural versions of many medical terms follows the rules of the originating languages of the terms, which are Greek and Latin. For example, the heart has a left atrium and a right atrium. When we speak of two,

TABLE 9–2 Common Root Words and Combining Forms

Root Word/ Combining Form	Meaning	Example (Pronunciation)	Definition
abdomin/o	Abdomen	Abdominopelvic (ab DOM ih no PELL vik)	Abdominal and pelvic regions of the body
aden/o	Gland	Adenopathy (add eh NOP a thee)	Gland disease
arteri/o	Artery	Arteritis (ar tuh RITE us)	Inflammation of an artery
arthr/o	Joint	Arthroplasty (AHR throh PLASS tee)	Surgical repair of a joint
carcin/o	Cancer	Carcinoma (kar sih NOH ma)	Cancerous tumor
cardi/o	Heart	Cardiopulmonary (KAR dee oh PULL mon air ee)	Pertaining to the heart and lungs
cephal/o	Head	Cephalic (seh FAL ik)	Pertaining to the head
chem/o	Chemical	Chemotherapy (KEE moh THAIR ah pee)	Treatment with chemicals
cis/o	To cut	Incision (in SIH zhun)	Process of cutting into
cost/o	Rib	Intercostals (in ter KOHST uls)	Pertaining to between the ribs
crani/o	Skull	Craniotomy (KRAY nee ot uh mee)	Incision into the skull
dermat/o	Skin	Dermatology (DER mah TAHL oh jee)	Study of the skin
enter/o	Small intestines	Enteric (en TER ik)	Pertaining to the small intestines
gastr/o	Stomach	Gastric (GAS trik)	Pertaining to the stomach
gynec/o	Female	Gynecology (GYE neh KOLL oh jee)	Study of females
hemat/o	Blood	Hematology (HEE mah TOLL oh jee)	Study of the blood
hydr/o	Water	Hydrotherapy (high droh THER ah pee)	Treatment with water
immun/o	Immune	Immunology (IM yoo NOLL oh jee)	Study of immunity
laryng/o	Voice box	Laryngeal (LAIR in jee uhl)	Pertaining to the voice box
mamm/o	Mammary gland, breast	Mammography (mam OG rah fee)	Process of obtaining images of the breast
my/o	Muscle	Myoma (MY oh ma)	Tumor containing muscle tissue
nephr/o	Kidney	Nephrology (neh FROLL oh jee)	Study of the kidneys
neur/o	Nerve	Neural (NOOR uhl)	Pertaining to a nerve

Root Word/ Combining Form	Meaning	Example (Pronunciation)	Definition
ophthalm/o	Eye	Ophthalmic (off THAL mik)	Pertaining to the eye
oste/o	Bone	Osteoporosis (oss tee oh peh ROH siss)	Condition that results in reduction of bone mass
ot/o	Ear	Otic (OH tik)	Pertaining to the ear
path/o	Disease	Pathology (path OLL oh jee)	Study of disease
ped/o	Foot, child	Pedal (PED uhl)	Pertaining to the foot
phleb/o	Vein	Phlebitis (fleh BYE tiss)	Inflammation of the vein
psych/o	Mind	Psychology (sigh KOLL oh jee)	Study of the mind
pulmon/o	Lung	Pulmonary (PULL mon air ee)	Pertaining to the lungs
rhin/o	Nose	Rhinoplasty (RYE noh plass tee)	Surgical repair of the nose
therm/o	Heat	Thermotherapy (therm oh THAIR ah pee)	Treatment with heat
thorac/o	Chest	Thoracic (THOR ah sik)	Pertaining to the chest
ur/o	Urine, urinary tract	Urology (yoo ROHL oh jee)	Study of the urinary tract
ven/i, ven/o	Vein	Venipuncture (VEN ih punk cher)	To pierce a vein with a needle
vertebr/o	Spine, vertebra	Vertebral (VER teh bral)	Pertaining to a vertebra

TABLE 9–3 Common Suffixes

Suffix	Meaning	Example (Pronunciation)	Definition
-algia	Pain	Neuralgia (noo RAL jee ah)	Nerve pain
-cele	Hernia, protrusion	Cystocele (SISS toh seel)	Protrusion of the bladder into the vagina
-cise	Cut	Excise (EX size)	To cut out
-cyte	Cell	Hemocyte (HEE moh site)	Blood cell
-dynia	Pain	Cardiodynia (kar dee oh DIN ee ah)	Heart pain
-ectomy	Surgical removal	Appendectomy (app ehn DEK toh mee)	Surgical removal of the appendix

(continued)

TABLE 9–3 *(continued)*

Suffix	Meaning	Example (Pronunciation)	Definition
-genesis	Produces, generates	Osteogenesis (OSS tee oh JEN uh siss)	Producing bone
-genic	Producing	Carcinogenic (kar SIH na jen ik)	Producing cancer
-gram	To record	Electrocardiogram (ee lek troh KAR dee ah gram)	Record of heart's activity
-graph	Instrument for recording	Electrocardiograph (ee lek troh KAR dee ah graf)	Instrument for recording the heart's electrical activity
-ia	State, condition	Hemiplegia (hem ee PLEE jee ah)	Condition of being half paralyzed
-ism	State of	Hypothyroidism (HIGH poh THIGH royd izm)	State of low thyroid
-itis	Inflammation	Cellulitis (sell you LYE tiss)	Inflammation of cells
-logist	One who studies	Cardiologist (kar dee AHL oh jist)	One who studies the heart
-logy	Study of	Cardiology (kar dee AHL oh jee)	Study of the heart
-lysis	Destruction	Osteolysis (OSS tee oh LYE siss)	Bone destruction
-megaly	Enlargement, large	Cardiomegaly (kar dee oh MEG ah lee)	Enlarged heart
-meter	Process of measuring	Audiometer (aw dee AH meh ter)	Instrument to measure hearing
-ology	Study of	Hematology (HEE mah TALL oh jee)	Study of the blood
-oma	Tumor, mass	Carcinoma (kar sih NOH ma)	Cancerous tumor
-osis	Abnormal condition	Lordosis (lor DOH siss)	Abnormal curvature of the lumbar spine
-ostomy	Surgically create an opening	Colostomy (koh LOSS toh mee)	Surgically create an opening for the colon through the abdominal wall
-pathy	Disease	Myopathy (my OHP ah thee)	Muscle disease
-penia	Lack of, deficiency	Osteopenia (OSS tee oh PEEN ee ah)	Lack of bone
-plasia	Development, growth	Dysplasia (dis PLAY zee ah)	Abnormal development
-plasty	Surgical repair	Dermatoplasty (DER mah toh PLASS tee)	Surgical repair of the skin
-rrhage	Excessive, abnormal flow	Hemorrhage (HEM er aj)	Excessive bleeding
-rrhea	Discharge, flow	Rhinorrhea (rye noh REE ah)	Discharge from the nose
-sclerosis	Hardening	Arteriosclerosis (ahr tee ree oh skleh ROH siss)	Hardening of an artery

Suffix	Meaning	Example (Pronunciation)	Definition
-scopy	Process of viewing or examining	Otoscopy (oh TOSS koh pee)	Viewing the ear through an otoscope
-stenosis	Narrowing	Angiostenosis (an jee oh sten OH siss)	Narrowing of a vessel
-therapy	Treatment	Hydrotherapy (high droh THER ah pee)	Treatment with water
-thermy	Heat	Hydrothermy (high droh THERM ee)	Treatment using heated water
-trophy	Development, nourishment	Hypertrophy (high PER troh fee)	Excessive development

however, we say *atria*, not *atriums*. Other words, such as *virus*, form their plurals using English rules, making the plural of virus *viruses*. Table 9–4 ■ illustrates how to form the singular and plural endings of some common medical terms.

Abbreviations and Symbols

Abbreviations and symbols are commonly used in medical records to save time and space. They can be confusing, however, and incorrect use of an abbreviation can cause serious problems in documents and records. If unsure, it is better to spell out the word rather than use an abbreviation or symbol. Never make up your own abbreviations or symbols. See Table 9–5 ■ for a list of common abbreviations and symbols that massage therapy professionals will find helpful. For greater ease of use, highlight terms used most often in your practice, and keep the list handy when you are writing or reading notes. Consult a medical dictionary for a complete list of medical abbreviations and symbols.

TABLE 9–4	Common Singular and Plural Endings	

Words Ending In	Singular	Plural
-a	Vertebra	Vertebrae
-ax	Thorax	Thoraces
-ex or -ix	Appendix	Appendices
-is	Metastasis	Metastases
-ma	Sarcoma	Sarcomata
-nx	Phalanx	Phalanges
-on	Ganglion	Ganglia
-us	Nucleus	Nuclei
-um	Ovum	Ova
-y	Biopsy	Biopsies

TABLE 9–5	Common Abbreviations and Symbols Used by Massage Therapists

Abbreviation/Symbol	Meaning
General	
ASAP	As soon as possible
@	At
Cl, CL	Client
CI, contra	Contraindication
DOB	Date of birth
Dx	Diagnosis
DKA	Did not keep appointment
Hx	History
HW	Homework
LTG	Long-term goal
MT	Massage therapist
MTx	Massage therapy session
meds	Medications
N/A	Not applicable
Ø	NO, none
#	Number
Rx	Prescription
rec	Recommendation
rpt	Reported
STG	Short-term goal
Sx	Symptoms
X	Times, repetitions
Tx	Treatment, therapy
unk	Unknown
w/	With
w/o	Without

(continued)

TABLE 9–5 (continued)

Abbreviation/Symbol	Meaning
Descriptions, Symptoms	
Abn	Abnormal
ADL	Activities of daily living
adh, *X*	Adhesion
post	After
&, +	And
~	Approximate
BA	Backache
pre	Before
Δ	Change
c/o	Complains of
CSTx	Continue same treatment
crep	Crepitus
DOI	Date of injury
↓	Decrease, down
DDD	Degenerative disk disease
DJD	Degenerative joint disease
ed	Edema
/	Elevation
=	Equals, is
xs	Excessive
FT	Fibrous tissue
HA	Headache
HOH	Hearing impaired (hard of hearing)
HBP	High blood pressure, hypertension
tens, ≡ HT	Hypertonic, tense muscle
→	Leading to, resulting in
↔	Lengthened, longer than normal
L	Light, low, mild
LBP	Low back pain
mob	Mobility
mod	Moderate
N	Normal
≈	Numbness, tingling
•	Pain
P & B	Pain and burning
POM	Pain on motion
1°	Primary
2°	Secondary, due to
sev	Severe
>-<	Shortened, shorter than normal
SD	Sleep disturbance

Abbreviation/Symbol	Meaning
STI	Soft tissue injury
SP, ≈	Spasm, cramping
st	Stiffness
INFLAM, ⇔	Inflammation
TeP, ∞	Tender point
TP, TrP, ς	Trigger point
↑	Up, increase
VGH	Very good health
Massage and Related Techniques	
AAS	Active assisted stretching
AROM	Active range of motion
ACU	Acupuncture, acupressure
aroma	Aromatherapy
CP	Cold packs
CTM	Connective tissue massage
CST	Craniosacral therapy
XFF	Cross fiber friction
DT	Deep tissue
DP	Direct pressure
eff	Effleurage
EW	Energy work
Ex	Exercise (active movement)
Fx	Friction
FBM	Full-body massage
FBRM	Full-body relaxation massage
HP	Hot packs
hydro	Hydrotherapy
ICES	Ice, compression, elevation, support
MLD	Manual lymph drainage
M	Massage
MET	Muscle energy technique
MFR	Myofascial release
NMT	Neuromuscular therapy
palp	Palpation
PB	Paraffin bath
PROM	Passive range of motion
pet	Petrissage
PR	Positional release
PNF	Proprioceptive neuromuscular facilitation
RI	Reciprocal inhibition
reflex	Reflexology
SFT	Soft tissue mobilization
SCS	Strain, counterstrain
str	Stretching

Abbreviation/Symbol	Meaning
SwM	Swedish massage
T&R	Tense and relax
Anatomical Terms	
abs	Abdominals
ACL	Anterior cruciate ligament
ASIS	Anterior superior iliac spine
C, C1-7	Cervical, cervical vertebrae
CT	Connective tissue
delt	Deltoid
ES	Erector spinae
gastroc	Gastrocnemius
gluts	Gluteal muscles
hams	Hamstrings
ITB, IT band	Iliotibial band
lats	Latissimus dorsi
lev scap	Levator scapulae
LB	Low back
L, L1-5	Lumbar, lumbar vertebrae
mm	Muscles
pecs	Pectoralis muscles
PSIS	Posterior superior iliac spine
QL	Quadratus lumborum
quads	Quadriceps femoris
rhomb	Rhomboid muscles
scal	Scalene muscles
ST	Soft tissue
SCM	Sternocleidomastoid muscles
SI	Sacroilia
T, T1-12	Thoracic, thoracic vertebrae
TFL	Tensor fascia latae
TMJ	Temporomandibular joint
traps	Trapezius muscles
Locations, Directions, Movement	
abd	Abduction
add	Adduction
ant	Anterior
BL, B	Bilateral, both
circ	Circumduction
dep	Depression (e.g., scapula)
DF	Dorsiflexion
ele	Elevation
ever	Eversion
ext	Extension
ext	External
flex	Flexion

Abbreviation/Symbol	Meaning
int	Internal
inv	Inversion
lat	Lateral
lat flex	Lateral flexion
L	Left
med	Medial
PF	Plantar flexion
post	Posterior
pro	Pronation
prox	Proximal
ROM	Range of motion
AROM	Active range of motion
PROM	Passive range of motion
RROM	Resisted range of motion
rot	Rotation
R	Right
SB	Sidebending
sup	Supination
WNL	Within normal limits

THE IMPORTANCE OF PLANNING

Every massage session needs a plan. This is true whether you are giving a set massage routine to a healthy client, or designing a session to meet specific client goals. Session planning is the logical process of thinking through the massage. It includes collecting relevant information, assessing the situation and setting goals, choosing massage applications, performing the massage, and evaluating results.

The thoroughness of the session planning process varies with the situation. At a minimum, a short verbal or written intake to screen for contraindications may be sufficient before giving a standard massage routine. This is a common situation when offering sample massage at a health fair, postevent massage at a sports event, or signature massage to one-time clients at a destination spa. Planning in those cases is done quickly. Modifications to the routine are made during the session from client feedback. The *plan* in that case involves performing the standard massage and making changes necessary for the safety, comfort, and satisfaction of the client.

Goal-Oriented Planning

Goal-oriented planning focuses on meeting specific client needs, rather than giving a standardized massage routine. Planning to achieve client goals provides a focal point for organizing massage sessions and choosing appropriate techniques. It increases both practitioner and client awareness of positive results and improves satisfaction of regular clients. Goal-oriented planning is an intellectual process

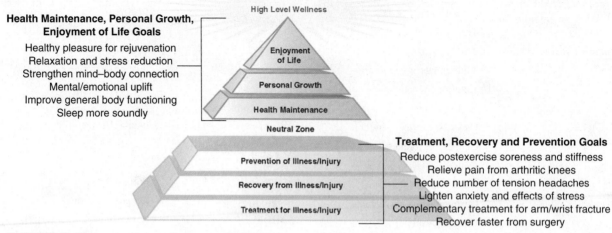

FIGURE 9–1 Sample client goals from the Wellness Massage Pyramid.

that provides a foundation for the artful and intuitive side of massage.

Clients come for massage for a reason. It is either to improve feelings of well-being, rejuvenate the mind/body, relax, reduce pain, improve mobility, alleviate symptoms of a disease, or some other specific desire. Goal-oriented planning can be applied to the entire Wellness Massage Pyramid (WMP). Figure 9–1 ■ shows the WMP and lists some of the many goals clients have related to massage therapy. The more aware you are of your clients' goals, the better you can serve them.

Clinical reasoning, the cognitive process used in goal-oriented planning, is essentially a problem-solving exercise. The client presents you with a problem to be solved (e.g., stress, muscle tension, pain), and you devise a plan using massage therapy to solve the problem. The goal-oriented planning process presented later uses a basic problem-solving approach.

In massage therapy, three variations of goal-oriented planning are long-range planning, individual session planning, and treatment planning. The steps in the process are the same, but are applied differently for the different circumstances.

STEPS IN GOAL-ORIENTED PLANNING

Goal-oriented planning involves six steps with a feedback loop for making adjustments. The general process is outlined in Box 9–1 ■.

Planning is presented here as *steps*, which implies a linear process. In practice however, the thinking involved is not entirely linear. For example, subjective and objective information is gathered continuously as you listen to and observe your client before, during, and after a massage session. Information acquired during a massage from palpation or client feedback may signal a need to modify

your session goals or massage application. Goal-oriented massage sessions are works in progress with adjustments as part of the process. Talking about the process as *steps* simply provides an orderly way to grasp the basic concepts and stay focused on the goals.

Taking time for goal-oriented planning is important. However, in most cases it does not need to be lengthy. For most wellness applications, a 5- to 10-minute interview in the initial massage session will suffice, followed by brief check-ins before subsequent sessions to review goals for

---

BOX 9–1   Six-Step Process for Goal-Oriented Planning

Step 1   Gather information from the client. Obtain subjective information from the client via written forms and verbal interviews.

Step 2   Collect information through observation and measurement. Compile objective information through practitioner observations, tests, and measurements.

Step 3   Assess the situation and set goals. Analyze the subjective and objective information obtained, make your conclusions, and determine client goals.

Step 4   Develop a plan to reach goals. Design a long-term program to achieve client goals. If it is an individual session, choose massage applications to achieve the day's goals.

Step 5   Implement your plan. Perform the massage therapy application.

Step 6   Evaluate the results. Analyze the outcomes of a series of sessions, or of one specific session.

Adjust goals and/or plans based on new information and results.

Document the process in session notes (SOAP notes).

the day. Treatment of injuries and the use of massage as complementary to medical treatment require more planning and discussion with the client. More time is taken for tests, measurements, and assessment in the initial session and progress evaluation sessions for those clients. Many massage therapists schedule an extra 30 minutes for new client intake and interview.

LONG-TERM PLANNING

Long-term planning is typically part of the initial massage session with a new client. It is focused on gathering subjective and objective information to get a big picture of the situation, determining overall client goals, and planning a series of massage sessions to reach those goals. The term *long term* is used here to mean more than one session, or the interval between an initial session and a progress session to check the extent to which goals have been reached. The interval might be anywhere from 1–8 weeks. The steps in long-term planning are summarized in Appendix C, *Goal-Oriented Planning*.

Step 1 Subjective information is gathered from the client intake form, health history form, and initial client interview.

Step 2 Objective information is collected from observing things such as the client's posture, movement, expression, and stress level. Tests are conducted, and measurements are taken related to the client's stated goals, complaints, written referral, or prescription for massage. Tools for information

gathering are described in more detail later in the chapter. Their purpose is to collect enough information to assess the situation and identify reachable goals.

Step 3 In Step 3 you assess the situation and establish long-term goals. Wellness goals that can be addressed with massage are identified, as well as problems for which massage is indicated. Also part of assessing the situation is identifying contraindications for massage and cautions to take into consideration later in planning. It may be determined at this point that the client should be referred for medical diagnosis before proceeding with massage.

For clients who receive regular massage as part of their general wellness plan, setting goals depends on what is happening in their lives at the time. They may go through a particularly stressful time, or participate in a seasonal activity like gardening or skiing. They may sustain injuries or get a new job with different physical requirements. Check in with regular clients on an ongoing basis for a continuous updating of long-term goals or goals for a particular session.

An important aspect of Step 3 is prioritizing goals with the client. This helps you determine what to focus on the most without losing sight of the bigger picture. It also brings the client into the process as he or she participates consciously in planning with you. Remember that it is the client's massage, and it is his or her goals that direct the sessions.

Step 4 With the results of Steps 1–3 in mind, an action plan is developed to achieve the client goals. For a long-term plan, this means suggesting the frequency and length of massage

---

 ## CASE FOR STUDY

Solana and Long-Term Planning

Solana has decided to add regular massage to her overall wellness lifestyle. She contacts a massage therapist recommended by a friend and schedules her first massage. She is not sure what to expect but believes that massage will be beneficial for her.

The massage therapist has Solana fill out intake and health history forms. Solana reports that she is taking medication for allergies, but otherwise has no major medical conditions. She broke her left arm a few years ago, but it has healed. She is also adjusting her diet for healthier eating and plans to exercise more.

The massage therapist observes that Solana has some limitation in motion in the upper extremities around the past fracture. She checks with Solana about her sensitivity to certain massage oils and lotions. They briefly discuss the potential health benefits of massage and Solana's expectations. They agree to focus on stress reduction and relief of tension in the left arm and shoulder for the next few sessions.

Solana plans to come for massage every other week. Before each session, the massage therapist checks on the effects the massage sessions are having. Additional goals are expected to

be set as the client learns more about massage and expands her ideas about how it can help her achieve her wellness goals.

The massage therapist will apply Swedish massage techniques, adding trigger point therapy and stretching to the shoulders and arms, for the first few sessions. She writes intake information, observations, assessment, and the long-range plan in the session notes for the day. After 2 months, the massage therapist will evaluate progress toward the original goals and modify them as needed as the therapeutic relationship develops over time.

Questions for planning:

- What subjective information did Solana provide?

  _____

- What objective information was gathered by the massage therapist?

  _____

- What were the agreed-upon goals for massage therapy?

  _____

- What was the resulting long-range plan?

  _____

sessions. For example, to reduce chronic stress, the plan may be for the client to receive a 1-hour massage weekly at the end of the workweek. Or during a competitive season, the plan may be for an athlete to get a weekly maintenance massage with an additional recovery massage the day after an event. Or to facilitate rehabilitation of soft tissue injury such as a sprain, a half-hour massage twice a week for 3 weeks may be the plan.

The action plan includes selecting a general approach, such as relaxation massage sessions, trigger point therapy, myofascial massage, passive joint movements, or some combination. Perhaps polarity therapy, or shiatsu/acupressure, lymphatic facilitation, or some other form of bodywork is called for. Massage therapists survey their repertory of techniques and methods to see which ones are most likely to effectively address client goals. Obviously, the larger your repertoire, the more choices you have. Also, the more knowledgeable you are about the effects of different techniques and approaches, the better able you will be to choose an approach to help clients reach their goals. If a client is seeking treatment for a health issue, this would be a good time to see if any scientific research is available concerning the effectiveness of massage for the condition.

Home care is another important aspect of Step 4. Note that massage therapists do not *prescribe* activities for their clients, which is outside their scope of practice. But they can suggest different additional activities to be done on the clients' own time at home that may help them achieve their goals more quickly or effectively. Common home-care activities include self-massage techniques, hot and cold applications, stretching, active exercises, and relaxation techniques.

Step 5 Implementing a long-term plan entails reviewing the plan with the client and making appointments. Being an educator is part of being a massage therapist as you teach your clients how to do their home-care activities.

Step 6 Long-term planning involves taking time to evaluate the results of a series of massage sessions and answering the question, "How well are the client's goals being met?" This is done in special progress sessions for well-defined goals, or on a less formal basis in presession interviews with the client, or with observations made during sessions.

The important point is to keep goals in mind and be aware of positive results toward those goals as time passes. You will thus gain from your experiences and become a better massage therapist than if you just give massage sessions without paying attention to the results. Your clients benefit from achieving their goals, and you benefit as you learn from your experiences.

Loop After the evaluation of results, the process loops to one or more of the steps described earlier as more information is gathered, and goals and plans are updated. Goal-oriented planning is less a linear process and more of a looping spiral.

Long-term plans are documented in notes that go into client files. These notes are essentially a recap of the steps in the planning process. Sections later in this chapter explain in detail what goes into the notes and how to write them.

A client who comes for massage to achieve a specific goal (e.g., to reduce tension headaches) may stop appointments once that goal is met. Many clients, however, benefit from regular massage to achieve high-level wellness or address a chronic health problem. Working with a client over time is a continuous process of assessing the situation and modifying your approach accordingly.

INDIVIDUAL SESSION PLANNING

Each individual massage session is a step toward achieving long-term client goals. Some basic questions to ask are, "Where are we today, and what can we do in this session to move closer to the long-term goals?" The goal-oriented planning process for individual massage sessions is summarized in Appendix C, *Goal-Oriented Planning*.

Step 1 Before a client arrives, it is useful to do a quick review of previous session notes, and, in some cases, his or her intake and health history forms. Reacquaint yourself with the long-term goals and the results of the last session. From that point of orientation, you greet your client and perform a brief presession interview. In that interview, you ask the client about any changes in health status or medications and any progress or regression related to his or her goals since the last massage session.

Step 2 As you greet and interview your client, observe general posture, facial expression, voice quality, and other outward indicators of his or her state of being. Either before or during the session when the client is on the massage table, use brief tests and measurements to collect objective information (e.g., assessing flexibility during a stretch, tissue quality while performing massage techniques, or ability to relax and let go of tension).

Step 3 Prior to beginning the massage, assess the current situation and prioritize the day's goals with the client. Determine any contraindications and cautions to be taken into consideration in this session. This may include long-standing conditions or temporary conditions, such as a recently acquired bruise or aspirin taken an hour before for a minor headache. Agree on goals for the session, and briefly review your general plan for the day with the client.

Step 4 While assessing the situation in Step 3, begin formulating your plan for the day. This is a good example of the steps in the planning process as overlapping and blending, rather than being discrete sequential steps. The goals for the session will lead logically to an appropriate session organization and choice of techniques. While the client is undressing and getting onto the table, you can go

CRITICAL THINKING

Explore the truth of the statement: "Every massage session needs a plan." Consider these questions:

1. What purpose does planning serve?
2. Can you give a massage without a plan?

3. How detailed does a plan for massage need to be?
4. When is a more detailed plan appropriate? When is an abbreviated plan a better choice?

---

over the plan in your mind, start your notes for the day, or prepare adjunct modalities such as hot packs.

Step 5 Begin the massage with the action plan in mind. For example, you begin at a certain place on the body using techniques chosen to achieve specific client goals. During the session, you might see reactions or results that either support the approach planned or signal a need to modify the plan. As you become aware of additional subjective and objective information, you will modify the original action plan for best results.

Step 6 Evaluating progress during a massage session is an essential part of the implementation phase as explained in Step 5. A postsession evaluation is also important. When you are saying good-bye to the client, you can make general observations and conduct a brief postsession interview. Questions should be open-ended and designed to elicit information useful to evaluating the outcomes of the massage; for example, "How is your arm feeling now?" or "Are you feeling more relaxed?"

Each session is documented in notes that go into client files. The SOAP note format described later in this chapter is well suited for capturing the goal-oriented planning process. The notes from the last session become a point of departure for planning the next time the client comes for massage.

TREATMENT PLANNING

Treatment planning is a form of goal-oriented planning in which the goal is alleviation of symptoms, or facilitation of healing of a pathological condition. It is used for medical, clinical, and orthopedic massage applications and the treatment and recovery levels of the Wellness Massage Pyramid (see Figure 9–1). A treatment plan is sometimes called a *plan of care*. See Appendix C, *Goal-Oriented Planning*.

Treatment planning requires a greater knowledge of pathology and massage research, as well as more advanced assessment and manual skills than other massage applications. Massage therapists who treat structural problems learn advanced musculoskeletal anatomy, biomechanics, and kinesiology, the study of human movement.

The terms *clinical massage*, *medical massage*, and *orthopedic massage* are sometimes used to describe advanced specialties within the broader field of massage therapy that focus on treatment. These terms do not refer to a unique set of techniques, but rather to the application of massage in a treatment planning process.

One major difference between treatment planning and other types of goal-oriented planning is in Step 3, that is, assessment of the situation. In medical settings, assessment typically means identifying or diagnosing a pathological condition. Because massage therapists do not diagnose, **assessment** is more about measuring function or loss of function (e.g., range of motion) or evaluating the condition of tissues (e.g., fibrosis and adhesions). It may be determining how massage can alleviate symptoms such as pain or facilitate healing. Clients often come to massage therapists seeking complementary care for a condition already medically diagnosed and under treatment by other health care professionals.

Yates sums up the critical competencies for developing treatment plans for medical conditions. First is the "ability to accurately *assess* the cause of the patient's presenting complaint in order to select and plan appropriate treatment." Second is the "capacity to *recognize* conditions for which some therapeutic approaches are contraindicated and to modify treatment accordingly." And third is "mastery of a sufficient variety of soft tissue techniques and other modalities to be able to safely and effectively *perform* the most appropriate form of treatment."[1]

Another difference in treatment planning is the end point of treatment. Medical settings that take their lead from health insurance companies often define the point of discharge or end of treatment as reaching the neutral point. The neutral point is the point at which symptoms are relieved (e.g., pain), normal function is restored, or signs of illness become undetectable. It may also be the point at which no further improvement is expected. However, in the wellness model, the neutral point is the jumping off place toward high-level wellness.

Collecting subjective and objective information from the client is the foundation of the goal-oriented planning process. These essential steps are explained in greater detail in the following sections.

CASE FOR STUDY

Alex and Individual-Session Planning

Alex signs up for a massage at the health club about once a month. He believes that regular massage helps him relax and relieves the aches and pains from his sports activities. Alex has been getting massage at the club for about 2 years. He sees whichever massage therapist is available at the time he wants to schedule the session.

While the massage therapist is waiting for Alex to arrive, he quickly reviews Alex's health history. He also looks at past session notes, especially from the last four massage sessions. He is looking for contraindications, past injuries, recent goals for sessions, and notes about results.

When Alex arrives, the massage therapist screens for changes in health status and current medications and asks about Alex's specific goals for the session. Alex reports that his legs and feet are a little stiff, and that he has some bruises on his legs from a hiking trip the past weekend. Alex is looking for general relaxation, reduced stiffness, and overall rejuvenation.

The massage therapist plans a full-body basic maintenance sports massage session. He will spend a little extra time on the legs and feet, but will avoid deep pressure over bruised areas. The session will include effleurage and kneading techniques, trigger point therapy, and myofascial massage as needed. Joint mobilizing and stretching, especially in the lower extremities, will be done. Problems found through palpation and range-of-motion evaluation will be noted and addressed if there is time. The massage therapist writes observations, techniques applied, and results in the individual session notes.

Questions for planning:

● What subjective information did Alex provide?

_____

● What objective information was gathered by the massage therapist?

_____

● What were the agreed-upon goals for massage therapy?

_____

● What was the resulting session plan?

_____

COLLECTING SUBJECTIVE INFORMATION

Intake is the process of gathering relevant information from a new client. This is considered to be subjective information. Intake forms are usually filled out by the client without direct help from the massage therapist. They contain general information about the client (e.g., name, address, phone, occupation); identification of the primary health care provider, and insurance company, if relevant; and the reason for the initial visit.

Intake forms also explain the nature and scope of the massage practice and fees and policies (e.g., fees, payment, and cancellation policy). Intake forms usually include a privacy statement explaining confidentiality policies and consent for care.

Give a copy of this form to the client to take home for reference, and keep a signed copy for his or her client file. A basic intake form for massage therapy can be found at MyHealthProfessionsLab.com.

Health/Medical History

A general health history is also filled out by the client as part of the intake process. The purpose of the health history is to learn more about the client's health and medical history, as well as to identify potential contraindications and cautions for massage. In treatment planning, information about medical conditions, diagnoses from health care providers, and treatment goals help massage therapists plan sessions specifically to address the condition for which massage is sought and indicated.

A sample health history form for general wellness applications, and a different form for more medically oriented situations, can be found at MyHealthProfessionsLab.com The medically oriented form has more detail about past and current injuries, surgeries, diseases, and medications.

There are situations when intake forms and health histories are impractical or unnecessary, for example, for a short massage at a health fair, trade show, or sports event. In these cases, a minimum amount of information is necessary to provide a safe massage session. Some basic screening questions to ask are

- Have you ever had massage before? (If no, provide more explanation and instructions.)

- Have you been ill recently?

- Do you have any skin conditions, injuries, or bruises I should avoid?

- Have you taken any medication today that affects your blood pressure or circulation?

- Have you taken any pain relievers today?

- If a woman: Are you pregnant?

- Is there any area that is especially tense that you'd like me to spend more time on?

The main purpose of these screening questions is to identify specific areas to focus on and contraindications or places to avoid massaging. A short consent statement and liability

CASE FOR STUDY

Angela and Treatment Planning

Angela comes for massage complaining of frequent tension headaches. In the client intake interview, she reports having headaches at least 3 times a week. She mentions that her neck is stiff. The massage therapist notices that she has trouble turning her head from side to side. Angela takes aspirin, but that is becoming less effective. The headaches are more likely to occur in the afternoon after she works at her desk for a long period of time.

She has not been in an accident lately and has no other signs of contraindications for massage. Her doctor has ruled out any underlying medical conditions that might cause frequent headaches and prescribed moist heat and a pain reducer to alleviate the headache pain.

It appears to be a typical case of chronic tension headache with no contraindications for massage. After discussion, the massage therapist and Angela both agree that the goal for massage will be to reduce the intensity and frequency of the headaches. The plan is for Angela to come for massage twice a week for 2 weeks and perform home care of self-massage and stretching, as well as hot applications. She will also begin using a headset for the telephone and reposition her computer screen to achieve better neck alignment when working.

The general approach for massage sessions will be to focus on the shoulder, neck, and head muscles most often associated with tension headaches. General relaxation will be included for the beneficial effects of the relaxation response. Techniques will be drawn from Swedish massage, trigger point therapy, and myofascial massage.

The plan is to reassess the situation after 2 weeks to see if there are fewer or less severe headaches. Before and after each session, the massage therapist asks Angela to rate her headache pain on a scale from 1 to 10 (1 = no pain; 10 = severe pain). She also notes days when headaches occurred and how severe they were.

As her headaches subside, Angela reduces her sessions to once a week and then to twice a month. Regular massage and home care activities help keep shoulders and neck muscles relaxed and reduce the number of headaches and their intensity.

Questions for planning:

- What subjective information did Angela provide?

  _____

- What objective information was gathered by the massage therapist?

  _____

- What were the agreed-upon goals for massage therapy?

  _____

- What was the resulting treatment plan?

  _____

---

release form should also be signed before giving even a short massage. A sample intake list for massage events can be found at MyHealthProfessionsLab.com.

Intake Interview

After the client fills out the intake and health history forms, the massage therapist conducts a short intake interview. The purpose of the interview is to clarify items on the forms and fill in any gaps of information. For example, if a client says that he or she was in a car accident last week, you would want to ask further questions about medical treatment received, injuries sustained, or lingering aftereffects. This is also the opportunity to confirm the client's top priorities for massage and collect more specific information about problems the person may be having.

INTERVIEW SKILLS

Interview skills include a variety of methods for eliciting useful information from clients. These communication skills are important from the time you screen potential clients on the phone, to intake interviews with new clients, to taking health histories, and conducting pre- and postsession interviews.

Listening skills are essential to interviews, as are different methods for framing client answers. Some basic client interview methods are asking open-ended and multiple-choice questions and using rating scales and body charts.

Open-Ended Questions Open-ended questions steer clients to specific topics, but leave space for them to answer in their own words. Rather than dictating the form of response, the massage therapist listens to what the client has to say in answer to a simple question. Responses to open-ended questions often give clues for further questions. Examples of general open-ended questions used in presession interviews appear in the following list.

- How are you feeling today?

- How has your shoulder been feeling since the last massage?

- How were your legs during the marathon last weekend?

- How has your stress level related to that work situation been?

- How were you able to rearrange your workstation so you aren't straining your neck so much?

- What are your goals for the massage today?

Multiple-Choice Questions Multiple-choice questions give clients a choice of descriptors, which helps them to be more specific and helps you to better assess the situation they are trying to describe. It gives them choices that they might not have thought of themselves, but that have meaning to you. Some useful descriptors for common complaints appear in the following list.

- Is the sensation you feel numbness, tingling, or pain?

- Would you describe your pain as sharp, diffuse, dull, aching, or throbbing?

- Would you describe the pain as: mild, moderate, or severe?

- Would you describe movement at your shoulder as free, fluid, stiff, or restricted?

- Are your headaches seldom, occasional, frequent, or almost constant?

Rating Scales Rating scales offer a rough measurement of things from the client's subjective view. Ratings use numbers to measure the degree or level of the client's experience of some factor related to their goals. Ratings give an indication of the client's experience of his or her condition and can be used to measure progress or regression from the client's perspective.

A scale from 1 to 10 is familiar to most clients, with 1 indicating the best scenario and 10 indicating the worst scenario for the item being rated. Following are examples of rating stress level, pain, and function.

- On a scale of 1 to 10—1 being pleasantly relaxed and 10 being totally stressed—how would you rate your level of stress today?

- On a scale of 1 to 10—1 being pain free and 10 being extreme pain—how would you rate how your back feels today?

- On a scale from 1 to 10—1 being easy and 10 being extremely limited—how would you rate your ability to walk up stairs today?

Body Charts These forms show diagrams of the human figure (e.g., front, back, and side views) that are marked by the client to locate problem areas and indicate the nature of a complaint. They offer the client a visual and kinesthetic (as opposed to verbal) way to give subjective information. Body charts can be used in the initial interview, as well as before individual massage sessions.

Clients mark with a pen the exact spots of concern on an outline of a body. Symbols can be used to locate painful areas, recent injuries, or bruises. Symbols can also be used to indicate different feelings in the area, for example, tension, numbness, tingling, and pain.

A body chart marked by the client is similar to the body chart filled in as part of the massage therapist's written SOAP notes (refer to Figure 9–10). Documentation should clearly indicate whether the client or the massage therapist is the source of information on the chart.

INTERVIEW GUIDELINES

In addition to framing relevant questions, conducting good interviews includes knowing how to create an openness to response, when to lead the questioning, what to avoid, and when to stop.

Clients feel more open to giving responses if they understand the reason for your questions. Explain why you are asking questions in the interview. For example, while setting up an appointment for a first-time client, say something like: "I'm going to ask you a few questions to see if massage therapy would help you reach your goals, and if so, to plan your first session." Before taking a health history explain: "I need a little more information about your health and any medications you are taking to plan the massage session."

Speak clearly and use body language that encourages answering. For example, look directly at the client and listen for the answer, rather than shuffling papers or looking around the room.

Give clients time to respond if you want thoughtful and accurate answers to questions. Do not rush the client's answers, and pause for 5–10 seconds before repeating the question or asking further questions. Elderly clients may need more time to respond. Remember that silence gives clients the space they need to collect their thoughts.

Some clients may need more direction, especially if you are relying on open-ended questions. Switch to multiple-choice questions, rating scales, or body charts for clients who have trouble expressing themselves verbally.

Ways to take more of a lead in questioning include asking for clarification of a statement, keeping clients on the topic if they are digressing, and helping them to get to the point. Ask clients to clarify conflicting statements. Ask for a final statement of agreement in important matters such as billing policies, informed consent, or goals of a massage session. For example, say, "Do we agree on those two primary goals for this session?"

Avoid creating an atmosphere in which clients feel like they're being interrogated, for example, by not smiling, or asking rapid-fire questions, or questioning their answers. Avoid being judgmental or dismissing their answers as unimportant. Do not deny their experiences.

Avoid questions not directly relevant to their massage therapy sessions. For example, it would be inappropriate to have a person coming to you for a relaxation massage go through an extensive medical history interview.

A good rule of thumb is to make interviews just long enough to get the essential information for planning a safe and effective massage session—no longer. Clients are coming for massage, which is a hands-on experience. Unnecessary questions take away from that valuable session time. A summary of interview guidelines is shown in Box 9–2 ■.

BOX 9–2 Summary of Interview Guidelines

When conducting client interviews, follow these guidelines:

1. Create an inviting and open atmosphere.
2. Explain to the client *why* you are asking questions.
3. Look directly at the client when asking a question.
4. Give clients time to think and speak.
5. Use affirmative listening for encouragement.
6. Use active listening to clarify what was said.
7. Lead back a client who is digressing.
8. Ask for clarification of conflicting statements.
9. Use open-ended questions to hear the client's own words.
10. Use multiple-choice, rating, or body charts to frame answers.
11. Ask only relevant questions.
12. Stop when you know enough.

Avoid:

1. Creating an atmosphere of interrogation
2. Asking rapid-fire questions
3. Speaking too fast
4. Being judgmental
5. Dismissing answers
6. Denying the client's experience
7. Posing unnecessary questions

COLLECTING OBJECTIVE INFORMATION

Objective methods of collecting information include the massage therapist's own observations, evaluations, and measurements. These methods do not rely on a client's subjective view, but come from the practitioner's objective or outside perspective.

The type of information collected varies according to the client's reason for seeking massage or to his or her initial complaint. Initial sessions and progress evaluation sessions will contain more evaluation than ongoing sessions. Methods for collecting objective information include making general observations about the client, palpation of the client's tissues, range-of-motion evaluation, posture analysis, biomechanics analysis, and gait analysis.

Be mindful that there is a difference between what you observe and your interpretation of those observations. For example, you might observe that a client is moving slowly and stiffly. It will take further investigation to assess why this might be the case. The cause might be any number of things, such as osteoarthritis, low mood, habitual movement pattern, a recent accident, or the marathon the individual ran the day before.

Be careful that you do not jump to conclusions or diagnose, that is, put the name of a pathology or medical condition to what you observe. Massage therapist are limited in their interpretations by their level of training. Beginning massage therapists have less knowledge to make interpretations than those with more training and experience. This means that you should sharpen your skills at observation, while understanding your limitations at interpretation of what you see.

General Observations

Observation is a basic tool for evaluation of the client's condition. Massage therapists use their senses to *observe* clients, that is, with their eyes, ears, noses, and hands. Some general observations and examples of descriptors are listed here.

- Skin: dry patches, blotches or red spots, acne, unusual marks or moles, rashes, bruises, wounds, scars

- Movement quality: slow, stiff, fluid, controlled, unstable, guarded

- Facial expression: smile, frown, nervous tick, furrowed brow, blank, serene

- Level of communication: nonstop talking, talkative, quiet, nonresponsive, silent

- Voice quality: loud, soft, weak, raspy, high pitched, low pitched

- Breathing: relaxed, diaphragmatic, chest breathing, labored, rapid, sighing, congested, wheezing, coughing

- Mental clarity: sharp, alert, fuzzy, vacant, distracted, forgetful, sleepy

- Emotional state: relaxed, agitated, nervous, angry, worried, anxious

For session notes, general descriptors are more useful if accompanied by specific or detailed descriptions of behaviors. For example, "The client seemed nervous and was tapping her pencil through the whole interview" is more informative than "The client seemed nervous." Another example, "The client's breathing was relaxed, from the diaphragm, and even" tells more than "The client seemed relaxed." Note that the simpler descriptions (e.g., nervous and relaxed) are actually interpretations of more specific behaviors that you observed.

Be as specific as you can in your notes. You may find out later that your interpretation of what you observed was incorrect. It is useful to be able to refer back to the original observation when reinterpreting or reviewing a situation. Although you observe many things about the client during the course of a massage, notes written about the session are limited to information used in planning and evaluating the current or future massage sessions. Session notes are discussed in more detail later in the chapter.

Palpation

Palpation is the act of sensing information about the client through touch. Palpation is about the *feel* of tissues and of movement at joints. Palpation has been described as "an art and skill which involves (1) locating a structure, (2) becoming aware of its characteristics, and (3) assessing its quality or condition so you can determine how to treat it."[2] A fourth aspect of palpation is to detect changes in quality or condition of tissues as a result of massage.

Palpatory sensitivity can only be developed through hands-on practice, aided by describing in words what is felt. Chaitow observed that "We need to unleash a torrent of descriptive words for what we feel when we palpate" and "to obtain a thesaurus and to look up as many words as possible to describe accurately the subtle variations in what is being palpated."[3] The physical skill of sensing qualities and the verbal skill of describing them accurately together make up palpatory literacy.

The first step in palpatory literacy for massage therapists is to be able to locate specific structures, that is, to feel where anatomical structures are located on the body. This is usually learned in anatomy class with a hands-on lab. Focus is on muscles, bones, joints, and related tissues and structures. This is useful knowledge for any type of massage therapy.

As palpation skills develop, you become more aware of differences in tissue temperature, texture, and firmness. You sense the ease of movement in healthy tissue and joints.

You are then able to detect abnormal tissue conditions. Descriptors for abnormal tissues include *spongy, hard, grainy, stringy, taut, taut bands, nodules, thick, congested, dehydrated,* and *adhering.* When assessing fascia, you feel for restrictions to movement or sticking. Abnormal joint movements may be described as *stiff, clicking, shortened, grinding,* or *bound.*

Certain forms of massage therapy key into the body's rhythms that can be felt in the tissues. Body rhythms include circulatory rhythm or pulse, respiratory rhythm or breathing, and craniosacral rhythm in the circulation of cerebrospinal fluid. Practitioners of Chinese medicine read the subtle radial pulse and detect the health of each organ and flow of energy, or *chi,* in the body.

Some forms of energy-based bodywork rely on detection of the body's energy field and the flow of energy in and around the body. These include polarity therapy, reiki, and therapeutic touch.

Developing palpation skill takes time and attention. Biel offers three principles of palpation.[4]

1. Move slowly. Haste only interferes with sensation.

2. Avoid using excessive pressure. Less is truly more.

3. Be consciously aware of what you are feeling. In other words, be present.

The more focused hands-on time you log, the better your palpation skills will be. Palpation skills develop throughout your entire career as a massage therapist. Examples of useful terms to describe palpation findings are listed in Box 9–3 ■.

Range of Motion Evaluation

Objective information about the general condition and degree of flexibility at a specific joint can be obtained by a range of motion evaluation. This is done by active or passive

---

BOX 9–3 Descriptors for Documenting Palpation Findings

Words used to describe palpation findings are presented here in relative terms. Although most of these terms have inexact definitions, they are useful in describing general palpation findings.

Skin

> hot / warm / cold
> dry / damp / oily
> hairless / hairy
> smooth / rough
> loose / taut
> thin / thick
> elastic / mobile
> scarred

Soft Tissues (General)

> spongy / firm
> hard / tough / pliable / soft
> dehydrated / puffy / swollen
> congested
> grainy / smooth

Muscles and Tendons

> hypertonic / hypotonic
> hard / firm / pliable
> taut / taut bands / lax
> knotty / smooth
> ropey or ropelike
> stringy
> spasm / relaxed

Fascia

> adhering / sticking / moving freely
> restricted / unrestricted

Joint Movement

> stiff / easy / free
> clicking / hitches / glitches
> crepetations
> grinding / grating
> stuck / bound / freely moving

Pulses

> strong / weak
> fast / slow
> even / uneven
> regular / irregular

Energy

> stagnant / blocked / free flowing
> pooled
> fluid
> excess / deficient

---

movement of the joint through its range, while observing any restrictions or shortening and any discomfort experienced by the client. Figure 9–2 ■ shows normal range of motion at the shoulder and hip joints.

A. Flexion and extension of the shoulders.

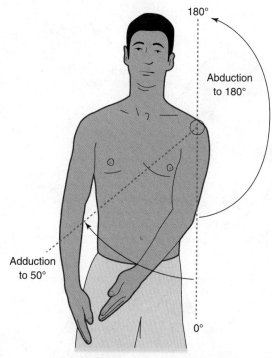

B. Abduction and adduction of the shoulder.

C. Flexion and extension of the elbow.

D. Flexion of the hip with straight knee.

FIGURE 9–2 Range of motion at the shoulder and hip joints.

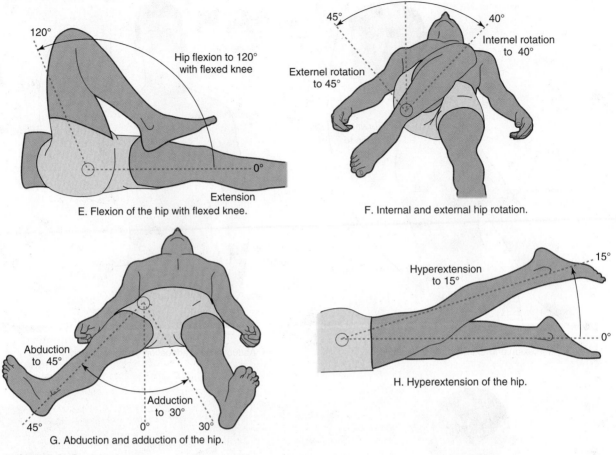

E. Flexion of the hip with flexed knee.

F. Internal and external hip rotation.

G. Abduction and adduction of the hip.

H. Hyperextension of the hip.

FIGURE 9–2 continued

For evaluating active range of motion (AROM) at a joint, first demonstrate the movement you want the client to perform. Ask him or her to move slowly and steadily. Observe the client's ease of movement and any limitations or weakness. The client may report pain or discomfort verbally or by facial expression. Compare movement on both sides of the body. Document any deviation from normal, pain-free movement in your session notes.

Three simple (AROM) tests for the shoulder are the Apley Scratch Test and two tests for internal rotation and adduction.[5] See Figure 9–3 ■. Tests like these are simple for clients to perform and offer quick, objective evaluations.

For evaluating passive range of motion (PROM) at a joint, have the client relax the muscles surrounding the joint while you move the joint through its range or apply a mild stretch. A passive stretch offers a good estimate of the degree of motion at a joint. For upper and lower extremities, compare the degree of flexibility on both the right and left sides. Note any restrictions in movement, differences in left and right sides, or discomfort experienced by the client. Document any positive findings, that is, any deviations from normal, pain-free movement at the joint.

You can also measure the range of motion quantitatively using an instrument called a goniometer, which is similar to a protractor used in geometry to measure angles

(Figure 9–4 ■). There are specific protocols for measuring range of motion with this instrument that take some practice to master and are used primarily for medical applications.

Range of motion evaluation offers clues to potential muscle and tendon problems (AROM), or problems with ligaments and joint structures (PROM). Swelling, discoloration, or severe pain with passive joint movement signals that massage is contraindicated in the area. For any suspected joint injury, the client should see a health care provider for a diagnosis of his or her condition.

On the other hand, restricted range of motion may simply be a sign of tense, shortened muscles that can benefit from increased circulation in the area, muscle relaxation, and lengthening of muscles fibers. Joint movements are discussed in greater detail, along with examples of mobilizing techniques and stretches for the neck and upper and lower extremities, in Chapter 13, *Joint Movements*.

Posture Analysis

Posture, or body alignment, can tell a lot about a client's physical and emotional state and reveals habitual patterns that can cause problems in the musculature. Standing, sitting, and sleeping posture are three basic points of reference for evaluating a client who complains about back, neck, and

FIGURE 9–3 Active range of motion (AROM) tests for the shoulder. A, Apley Scratch Test. B and C, Internal rotation and adduction tests.

shoulder tension or pain. Evaluation of the body's structural alignment is called *posture analysis.*

Important guidelines for good posture include standing straight and tall while avoiding locking the knees. The weight of the body should be mostly over the balls of the feet, not back on the heels. The head should be in alignment on top of the neck and spine and the chin not pushed forward. To keep the head level, the chin can be tucked slightly. The arms hang naturally down at the sides of the body. The shoulders are relaxed.

Standing posture analysis can be as simple as asking a client to stand for a moment and observing his or her alignment. This can be done with the client clothed, shoes off, standing comfortably with feet slightly apart, and arms hanging at the sides. View the client from the front, back,

and sides. Look for uneven height in shoulders or hips, leaning, head and chin forward, stooping, head tilted to one side, twisting, one arm hanging lower than the other, and any other deviation from good body alignment. A vertical point of reference such as a door frame can be used to identify leaning or other asymmetry.

Wall grid charts are useful for formal postural analysis and essential for structurally focused massage therapists. Grid charts have both vertical and horizontal lines to measure more accurately any deviations from balanced posture. Photos taken of clients standing in front of grid charts are useful for the initial analysis, client education about posture, and evaluation of progress toward goals of improving posture. Body charts that show boney landmarks are useful for visual charting of posture deviations. Reference points for assessment of standing posture are shown in Figure 9–5 ■.

Sitting posture analysis is especially important for clients who work at desks or tables and complain of neck and shoulder tightness or pain. Some guidelines for good sitting posture are that the back is supported by the back of the chair, and the knees are aligned evenly with the hips, or slightly higher. Both feet are flat on the floor, or on a foot support. Slouching or sitting forward should be avoided, and the head should be aligned over the shoulders with the chin tucked slightly, as in good standing posture. If working at a desk, the arms should be flexed at a 75- to 90-degree angle, with shoulders squared and relaxed. Stretching breaks should be taken to avoid sitting in one position too long. Aligned sitting posture is shown in Figure 9–6 ■.

A client's sleeping posture may also cause problems. Subjective information about sleeping habits may reveal a source of muscular aggravation. Firm mattresses are generally better than soft ones for proper back support. Sleeping on the side or back offers better alignment than sleeping on the stomach, which can strain the neck and lower back. Pillows should help keep the natural curvature of the neck and not cause hyperextension or flexion. While the client is supine on the massage

FIGURE 9–4 Using a goniometer to measure joint ROM.

Source: Pearson Education, Inc.

Posture Analysis Front View
Midsagittal and Horizontal Planes

EYES →

ACROMION PROCESS

12th RIB
ILIAC CRESTS →

GREATER TROCHANTER

TIBIAL TUBEROSITIES →

MEDIAL MALLEOLUS →

Posture Analysis Side View
Coronal Planes

EAR →

HEAD OF HUMERUS →

0°
10°

GREATER TROCHANTER →

FEMORAL LATERAL CONDYLE →

LATERAL MALLEOLUS →

FIGURE 9–5 Reference points for posture analysis.

table, you can demonstrate using a neck roll for added support and the use of a pillow under the knees to relieve pressure on the lower back. You can also show proper use of pillows for good alignment while in the side-lying position.

Biomechanical Analysis

Biomechanics is the study of movement in living organisms. It takes into account principles of motion and the structure and function of the human body, especially the muscle and skeletal systems. Whereas posture analysis looks at the body at rest, biomechanics looks at the body in motion. It is a branch of kinesiology and an important aspect of sports medicine.

Biomechanical analysis of your own movements while performing massage is an important aspect of your training. It can help you avoid injuries from poor body mechanics and serve as a starting point for understanding your clients' body mechanics. Good body mechanics for massage therapists are described in greater detail in Chapter 11, *Body Mechanics, Table Skills, Application Guidelines,* and various aspects of self-care are discussed in Chapter 4, *Physical Skills, Fitness, Self-Care for the Massage Therapist.*

Knowledge of biomechanics is essential for massage therapists who work with athletes, dancers, musicians, artists, craftspeople, and others who use their bodies in their daily activities. Massage therapists who specialize in musculoskeletal complaints or structural bodywork should also be well versed in analyzing how the body moves, and how it applies and absorbs force.

Biomechanical analysis is the examination of common movements, such as lifting, and job-related movements, such as using a computer keyboard, and can help massage therapists identify points of stress and strain on their clients' bodies. This is especially helpful in providing objective information about clients with overuse injuries.

Biomechanical analysis not only points to specific structures affected by a movement (e.g., muscles, tendons, joints, ligaments), but also can suggest ways of correcting movement patterns that may be causing a client musculoskeletal problems.

FIGURE 9–6 Good alignment for sitting posture.

Source: Pearson Education, Inc.

FIGURE 9–7 Good body mechanics for lifting heavy objects.

Source: Pearson Education, Inc.

Lifting a heavy object with good alignment is shown in Figure 9–7 ■. Notice that the knees bend to reach the object, with the back bending as little as possible. In proper alignment, the leg muscles do the lifting and not the lower back or arm muscles. Keep the weight of the object as close as possible to your center of gravity. Poor alignment when lifting puts strain on the lower back.

Advise your clients to carry heavy objects close to the body and switch arms frequently if carrying something in one hand, such as a suitcase. Balance equal weight on both sides if possible when carrying more than one object. When carrying a backpack, avoid leaning forward and rounding the shoulders. If unable to keep good alignment, consider using a pack or case with wheels.

Gait Analysis

Gait analysis looks at biomechanics while walking or running. Gait analysis starts when your client walks into the room, and you begin to observe his or her movement pattern.

For further analysis, watch the client walk away from you and toward you. Figure 9–8 ■ shows the phases of walking.

The phases of walking for each foot include a stance phase (heel strike, flat foot, push off, and acceleration), and a swing phase (toe-off, midswing, and deceleration). While one foot is in the stance phase, the other foot is in the swing phase. Points to look for in walking are base width (2–4 inches from heel to heel), vertical movement of the center of gravity, knee flexion, lateral shifting, length of step, and pelvis rotation.

Deviations from normal include slow gait, limping, shuffling, twisting at the waist, dragging the feet, waddling (lateral movement), wide base, lurching. Compensations may also be made for arthritic or fused joints in the feet or legs. Some of the common causes of walking gait deviations are listed in Table 9–6 ■. More detailed analysis of gait is found in biomechanics, clinical massage, and orthopedic massage texts.[6]

Orthopedic Tests

A number of orthopedic tests are available to assess pathology in musculoskeletal structures, movement and locomotor disorders, and sources of soft-tissue pain and dysfunction. These tests are also utilized by other professionals, such as physical therapists, athletic trainers, and orthopedic doctors.

Orthopedic or clinical massage is an advanced specialty for massage therapists who focus on the use of massage to treat orthopedic conditions. Details about orthopedic massage and assessment skills are outside the scope of this foundations book, but can be found in other texts (see Appendix E, *References and Additional Resources*).

Massage therapists who apply these tests do so in the context of their scope of practice. They do not diagnose pathologies. The purpose of massage therapists using orthopedic tests is for observation of function, ruling out conditions and injuries that may be contraindications for massage, and for decisions about referrals to doctors for medical diagnosis.

Heel strike	Foot flat	Midstance	Heeloff	Pushoff	Early swing	Midswing	Late swing
	Right leg stance phase				Right leg swing phase		
Double support 10%	Single support 40%			Double support 10%	Single support 40%		

FIGURE 9–8 Phases of the normal walking gait.

TABLE 9–6	Common Causes of Walking Gait Deviations
Gait Deviation	**Common Causes**
Slow walk	Old age, neurological disorder, joint disease, or injury
Limping	Injury to foot or leg, short leg
Shuffling	Weak quadriceps, Parkinson's disease, neurological disorder
Twisting	Arms crossing midline during walk
Dragging	Tibialis anterior weakness (also called drop foot, toe scraping)
Waddling	Pain in lower back, hips, lower extremities
Wide base	Unsteadiness, dizziness, general weakness, vision problems
Lurching	Weakness in gluteal muscles

IMPORTANCE OF DOCUMENTATION

Documentation is the process of writing massage session records for future reference. It is also called note-taking or charting. Session notes are kept on paper or in electronic form in client files.

Notes can be considered legal documents when used for insurance reporting, or may be subpoenaed as evidence in legal cases. Notes are official client health records. Massage therapy practices that store and transmit client information electronically are subject to **HIPAA privacy rules**. HIPAA stands for the Health Insurance Portability and Accountability Act, which was passed by the U.S. Congress in 1996 to protect the privacy of medical records. (Find more information about HIPAA in Chapter 27, *Private Practice and Finances*).

Notes are also very practical. Notes assist the massage therapist in remembering what happened the last time a client came for massage and may show meaningful patterns over time. If two or more massage therapists share clients, they can review each other's notes while planning an upcoming session. Notes demonstrate the care taken to ensure a client's safety and well-being. Well-written SOAP notes also reflect a logical or clinical reasoning process by presenting information in an organized way and keeping the focus on goals for the massage sessions.

Documentation is not an extra chore or optional task. It is an important part of every massage session. Time can be set aside either between sessions or at the end of every day for completing client records.

Each massage practice or business creates its own system of keeping client notes. It is common for all regular clients to have personal files with an official record of their massage sessions. The systems of note-taking explained in this chapter contain the essential elements of documentation that can be adapted for your own or a specific employer's requirements. The goal-oriented SOAP note format and simplified formats for note-taking are presented in the remainder of the chapter.

SOAP NOTE OVERVIEW

SOAP notes have become a standard for charting massage sessions. *SOAP* refers to the format used to write the notes and is an acronym for *subjective, objective, assessment,* and *plan.* The SOAP format helps sort information into meaningful categories and provides a standard outline for reports. SOAP notes are written in a kind of shorthand using standard abbreviations. SOAP notes capture the relevant information in a goal-oriented session plan. The SOAP format also serves as a guideline for planning sessions from the beginning. If you understand the planning process well, SOAP notes will be easier to write.

The SOAP format records the elements of logical and clinical reasoning. You start with *subjective (S)* and *objective*

 PRACTICAL APPLICATION

Use the goal-oriented planning process to plan a 1-hour individual massage session with a practice client. Implement the plan. Afterward, write down your experience with each step. Ask yourself the following questions:

1. How long did it take to gather enough subjective and objective information to determine client goals for the session?

2. During the session, did you learn any information that caused you to modify the original plan?

3. Do you think that the approach and techniques you used helped achieve the goals for the session?

4. Did the practice client report results consistent with the goals you agreed on before the session? Did he or she report results that you did not anticipate?

REALITY CHECK

BARBARA

CHRISSY: How do you find the time to document massage sessions? I allow 30 minutes between sessions, and by the time one client leaves and the other arrives, I have no time.

BARBARA: There are some ways to make the time you need to document your massage sessions properly. For example, at the beginning of the day I pull all of the files for the clients I will see that day, and put them in a secure but accessible place. Then I write some notes about the previous client while the next client is getting undressed. Even if I can't complete the notes, I jot down some things I want to be sure to document later. Then I schedule in 30–40 minutes at the end of the day to finish my notes, return the files, and clean up the space. I've found that it takes less time to write notes now that I've had more practice, and I don't consider the day finished until the documentation is completed.

(O) information about the client, come to an *assessment (A)* of the situation (either the nature of a condition and/or goals for sessions), create a general *plan (P)* for achieving the goals and a plan for each massage session. The initial session plan is followed in continuing sessions, and progress is evaluated regularly.

Even if you see a client for only one session, or have limited time for interviews, the session organizing and logical reasoning reflected in SOAP notes help you to aim the session at meeting client needs instead of giving exactly the same 1-hour massage routine to everyone. Even if the record forms or charts you use have only blank lines for recording session notes, you can use the SOAP format to better organize your thoughts about the client and the session.

Four types of notes are commonly reported on SOAP charts. These are intake notes, continuing session notes, progress notes, and discharge notes. The four types of notes reflect different stages in planning massage sessions. **Intake notes** are comprehensive and include the client's stated reason for massage or specific complaint, related subjective and objective information, agreed-upon long-term goals, and a general plan. **Continuing session notes** are briefer and record the session-by-session history of a client's visits. **Progress notes** are for special sessions that reevaluate a client's progress related to his or her long-term goals. Progress notes contain more assessment information than regular session notes and may identify new goals and plans. **Discharge**

notes are a final summary of the client's progress and any comments about the course of treatment.

SOAP Note Format

Although originally designed for medical record keeping, the general format for SOAP notes can be adopted for non-medical settings. The SOAP format is useful in settings such as health clubs, spas, and private offices. However, the detail required and abbreviations used in different settings may vary. Insurance companies may require that certain terms be used in SOAP notes to qualify for reimbursement.

Massage therapists working in the same office or with the same clients should use standard abbreviations so they can read each other's notes. The elements in notes are generally the same; however, a specific type of information may appear in different sections in different systems. Follow the format established and used in your current location.

Some massage therapists have adopted a variation called a *SOTAP note*. The *T* stands for *treatment*, and provides a separate section in the note for recording the massage and related techniques used in the session. In the SOAP format, the *T* description is often included in the *P* or *plan* section of the note.

SOAP Note Content

S stands for *subjective* and refers to subjective information reported by clients. It includes things like what clients say about their reasons for getting massage, how they feel overall, where they feel pain or tension, stresses in their lives, and recent accidents, illnesses, or other changes in health status. For continuing session notes, the *S* section summarizes complaints on the day of the session and any changes clients perceive from their last sessions to their current ones.

O stands for *objective* and refers to what the practitioner observes about the client. Objective information provides clues about the client's state of well-being. It includes observations (e.g., facial expression, general posture, or skin conditions); qualitative measurement from palpation of soft tissues or movement at joints; or results of standardized tests (quantitative measurement) for range of motion, muscle strength, posture, or specific muscle injuries.

A stands for assessment, and in medical charting, it is the practitioner's conclusions from the subjective and objective record. It is the assessment of the situation. For example, in an initial visit, a doctor may conclude that a patient has an arthritis flare-up that is causing a swollen, painful knee. That is the diagnosis that goes into the *A* section of the note. Because diagnosis is *not* in the scope of practice of massage therapists, the *A* section can be used for other information.

A good use of the *A* section, from a wellness perspective, is to identify long-term goals for the client. Goals follow from an assessment of the client's needs (based on subjective and objective information) and ideally are agreed on by the practitioner and client. This provides a basis from which to plan sessions that meet defined goals.

Examples of goals include reducing chronic muscle tension in the forearm, improving flexibility in the hip joint, or alleviating chronic stress or anxiety. Goals could be higher up the Wellness Massage Pyramid (see Figure 9–1), for example, maintaining overall health, or body–mind–spirit rejuvenation. Another use suggested for the *A* section is to "summarize the patient's functional ability: limitations, previous ability, and current situation; and to set goals that, when accomplished, demonstrate functional progress."[7]

For health care professionals whose scope of practice includes diagnosis of pathologies, the *A* section is fairly straightforward. *A* is used to record the diagnosis and prognosis of a medical condition as a prelude to writing a treatment plan. For wellness practitioners, the goals identified in the *A* section might fall anywhere within the full scope of the Wellness Massage Pyramid from treatment to health maintenance to life enjoyment.

P stands for plan and refers to the strategy for meeting the goals in the *A* section. It includes the plan as carried out for the current session, as well as long-term, general plans.

In addition, *P* includes a description of the immediate massage application, including the length of the session, techniques used, and parts of the body massaged. Record specific work in more detail, such as when addressing neck and shoulder tension within the context of a general wellness massage.

In medical settings, *P* is the treatment plan for the diagnosed pathology. In massage therapy, the long-term plan might include the number and frequency of massage sessions to meet the goals; details about the massage and related therapies to be used; home care such as self-massage, relaxation exercises, or stretching; and a reevaluation date.

For regular massage clients in nonmedical settings, the *A* and *P* sections can be revisited regularly to provide continuous focus on client needs and goal-oriented massage sessions. Although the goals of the regular sessions may change over time and may be special in any one session, meeting long-term client needs is the foundation of a successful practice. The more conscious you are of your clients' needs, the better you will be able to serve them. A summary of the SOAP note content appears in Table 9–7 ■.

WRITING SOAP NOTES

SOAP notes are written in a sort of shorthand using brief descriptions, abbreviations, and symbols. They tell a lot with few words, like text messaging on cell phones. With some practice, they can be written quickly using little space. However, they must be readable and able to be transcribed by others. Notes that cannot be read are not very useful. Common abbreviations and symbols used in SOAP notes are listed in Table 9–5.

Notes do not contain complete sentences. They are typically strings of descriptions separated by commas and semicolons, or bulleted lists.

Notes contain anatomical terms for locations, adjectives, symptoms, measurements, and ratings. They might report quotes from the client such as "can't get to sleep at night," or "trouble turning my head when driving." Some examples of SOAP note entries are found in Figure 9–9 ■.

SOAP charts that include diagrams of the body are useful to manual therapists. They show front, back, and side views. Symbols can be used to locate problem areas visually and indicate the general symptoms felt there, such as pain, numbness, inflammation, adhesions, or shortening. Postural deviations can also be noted. Elsewhere on the form there is space for the narrative SOAP notes. Figure 9–10 ■ is an example of a SOAP chart with body diagrams.

Entries are descriptions, *not* diagnoses, unless reporting a diagnosis made by a health care provider. In that case, the note would read something like, "client reported a diagnosis by his physician of arthritis in the R knee." A client's self-diagnosis should be reported as just that; for example, "client complained of arthritis in knees—not diagnosed by physician." The massage therapist's note might read, "R knee infl and P," meaning, "right knee inflamed and painful." This is a subtle but important point and must be observed to stay within the scope of practice of massage therapy.

If you or a client will be filling out health insurance claim forms for massage sessions, use terminology in your notes that will be recognized by the insurance company, and learn current medical codes that apply. This is important because medical codes are used to process claims, and your records might be subpoenaed to support a client's insurance claim. Massage therapy covered may include hot and cold packs, massage, and manual therapy.

The medical codes change periodically, so if you do insurance billing, check with your state licensing or other appropriate agency for which codes are currently legally acceptable for massage therapy. Be aware that code numbers for physical and occupational therapy may be different from code numbers for massage therapy. Chapter 27, *Private Practice and Finances*, discusses insurance issues as they pertain to massage therapy in more detail.

Guidelines for Writing SOAP Notes

The following guidelines summarize standard procedures for writing SOAP notes. They approach SOAP notes as legal documents and reflect some of the same standards used for legal contracts and accounting. With a little practice, these procedures can become second nature.

- Write legibly in blue or black ink.

- Write in concise, clear language using standard abbreviations and symbols; no need for complete sentences.

- Do not use so many symbols or abbreviations that the meaning of the note is lost; abbreviations make the most sense in context.

- Aim for spending only 5–10 minutes writing each SOAP note. Writing concise, useful, readable notes comes with practice.

TABLE 9–7	Summary of SOAP Note Content	
SOAP Note Section		**Content Possibilities**
S	Subjective	Client's stated reason for massage
		Initial and subsequent complaints
		Health history information
		Report of medications taken
		Report of recent illness or injury
		Description of symptoms (e.g., pain, trouble sleeping)
		Report of functional limitations (e.g., walking, sitting)
		Qualitative description (e.g., tension, pain, numbness, stress)
		Quantitative rating (e.g., tension, pain, numbness, stress)
		Diagnosis from health care provider
O	Objective	Visual observations (e.g., posture, skin color, facial expression)
		Palpation (e.g., tissue quality, joint movement quality)
		Range-of-motion measurement
		Posture analysis
		Gait analysis
		Orthopedic tests of function
A	Assessment	Summary of conditions or limitations
		Identification of contraindications and cautions
		General goals for a series of massage sessions
		Goals for a specific massage session
P	Plan	General plan to achieve goals
		• Number of sessions and frequency of massage
		• Use of adjunct modalities (e.g., hot/cold packs)
		• Homework (e.g., stretching, relaxation exercises)
		Plan for specific massage session
		• Time spent on each body area
		• Techniques used
		• Adjunct modalities used
		• Results

Logical/clinical reasoning behind SOAP notes: *Subjective* information from the client and *objective* information gathered by the massage therapist are used in an *assessment* of the situation to set goals for the massage sessions, followed by the development of *plans* to achieve those goals.

- Start your note right after the last note entered so that it will always be in chronological order, and difficult for notes to be altered or added to.

- Date the note clearly at the beginning or in the space provided on the form.

- Print your name and initial or sign your note at the end.

- If you make a mistake, draw a single line through the mistake, and write "error" next to or above the area, and initial and date it. This makes it clear what was originally written and who altered the record and when. Never scribble over a note or use correction fluid over a mistake.

- Be objective, impersonal, and respectful in your notes.

- Stick to descriptions of symptoms and conditions (e.g., swollen, red, warm, painful), and do not make statements that could be mistaken for a medical diagnosis (e.g., tendinitis).

- Do not write anything that is personal, slanderous, or that you would not want the client to read. Clients have a legal and ethical right to see what is in their official records.

- Keep client records for at least 7 years, even if the client has stopped coming to you for massage. The records may be needed for legal or insurance purposes.

- Follow HIPAA Privacy Rules for storage and access to client records when applicable.

Intake SOAP Note – Example 1

S: CL 1° reason for M = stress ↓; 2° c/o is mild LBP with st in legs; Hx of LB ≈ 2 weeks ago; ↓ with use of CP and rest; CL walks and gardens for Ex; does mod lifting in job; previous M = 0.

O: CL walks slowly w/st and mildly bent over; mm in LB felt ≡; flexibility in hams = poor; Mild ed in ST around knees; mm in shoulders and neck ≡ and short.

A: 1° LTG = stress ↓; 2° LTG = ↓ st in LB, legs, shoulders, neck.

P: GP = FBRM 1 X per wk w/M for ↓≡ in mm in extremities and LB; HW of str in legs and back & gen relax Ex; CP if spasm in LB returns.

Continuing Session SOAP Note – Example 2

S: CL c/o ↑ stress at job from ↑ in workload; ↑ in # HA from ↑ ≡ in shoulders and neck; sev bruise on R lower arm; rpt ↑ mob in lower legs after str last M.

O: CL face looked ↑ tired; rubbed his neck; bruise on R lower arm ~ inch in diameter + dark color.

A: 1° goal = gen relax & ↓ ≡ in shoulders and neck; 2° = flex in hips and legs; bruise on R arm = local contra.

P: 1 hr M + NMT; 40 min on upper body + 20 min on hips & legs; DP to TrP in traps and neck mm + str; deep eff, pet & str to legs; used neck roll; enjoyed relax music; rpt feeling ↑ relax overall after M; HW: HP on shoulders and neck 2X day & str at night.

Continuing Session SOAP Note – Example 3

S: CL rpt feeling ↑ depression this wk; not heard from son in days; SD; yesterday in house all day & 0 visit w/ friends; skin dry; c/o cramp forearm mm.

O: Looked tired & sad; CL rated energy very L; skin dry; forearm mm ≡ on palp; held fist.

A: 1° goal ↑ feeling well-being & ↑ energy; 2° lube skin & ↓ forearm mm ≡.

P: 1 hr FBRM w/mod pace & eff + gentle pet; 15 min M forearms and hands; music upbeat; oil & lotion to FB w/ more in dry areas; HW: relax Ex and str for forearms; CL ↑ talk and alter post Tx.

FIGURE 9–9

Examples of SOAP Note entries.

SIMPLIFIED DOCUMENTATION

There are circumstances in which documentation of a massage can be minimized, and postsession notes can be shortened or dispensed with altogether. However, at the very least, it is a good idea to keep a record of who received massage and to have clients sign a legal release form.

At venues such as health fairs, trade shows, sports events, and outreach events where people are receiving short, standard massage routines and will not be seen by the practitioner again, no postsession notes are necessary. An example of a form used at outreach events where massage recipients sign their names after reading a statement at the top is found at MyHealthProfessionsLab.com.

A simplified form can also be used for walk-in clients at a street venue, at a stand within a store or mall, or in public places such as airports. In those cases, adequate documentation might consist of a short intake form with a general statement about the massage to be given, a few questions asking for information about major contraindications, and the client's signature granting permission for the massage. This provides a record of who received massage and evidence that they knew what to expect. See Figure 9–11 ■. This type of form works well with one-time clients.

A simplified note system is adequate when a standard routine is given and then modified for a client's safety and/ or preferences. It might also be appropriate at a spa or health club where clients come for massage periodically, but have no long-term goals in mind. Figure 9–12 ■ shows an example of a short note form with space for more than one date on a page for use with regular or periodic clients in a nonmedical setting.

FIGURE 9–10
Example of SOAP chart with body diagram.

SOAP NOTE CHART
CONTINUING MASSAGE SESSION

Practitioner's Name _____ Date _____

Client's Name _____

S: Reason for massage, complaints, reports

O: Observations, qualitative/quantitative measurements

A: Primary and secondary goals for the session; contraindications

P: Duration of massage; areas addressed; techniques used; results; suggested home care

Practitioner Signature _____ Date _____

Symbols:

Primary 1°	Secondary 2°	Change Δ	Increase ↑	Decrease ↓	Tension ≡
Adhesion *X*	Pain **P**	Numbness ∿∿	Inflammation ✳	TrP ⊗	

The short form contains some of the elements of a SOAP chart (e.g., subjective and objective information), but the *A* section is unnecessary, and a *C* section for general comments is added. The *P* section documents the length of the session, the general approach used (e.g., relaxation with attention to back and neck) and significant modifications made to address contraindications and cautions. If a client comes for a more goal-oriented massage, a regular SOAP chart can be used to document that session.

As with all documentation, it is recommended that even shortened and simplified records be kept for a period of 7 years. Legible and understandable entries are a must.

DESIGNING A SYSTEM OF DOCUMENTATION

Consider several factors when designing a note-taking system for your own practice. You may develop a few different forms for different circumstances. For example, if you have

SHORT INTAKE and NOTE FORM

Client _____ Date _____

Address _____ Phone _____

Massage Therapist _____

Please answer the following questions to ensure a comfortable and safe massage session:

1. What is your primary goal for this massage?
   ☐ Relaxation, stress reduction
   ☐ Relieve muscle tension, specify area: _____
   ☐ General health and wellbeing
   ☐ Other, please specify _____

2. Have you had any illness, accidents, or injury recently? ☐ No ☐ Yes

   If so, please explain briefly _____
   _____

3. Are you experiencing any of the following today? Check all that apply.

   ☐ pain or soreness   ☐ numbness or tingling   ☐ dizziness
   ☐ stiffness   ☐ swelling   ☐ nausea

4. Do you have any allergies, especially to oils or lotions? ☐ No ☐ Yes

   If so, please explain briefly _____
   _____

5. For women – Are you pregnant? ☐ No ☐ Yes ☐ Maybe

6. Have you taken any medications today? ☐ No ☐ Yes

   If so, please list _____

I have answered the above questions to the best of my ability. I acknowledge that massage therapy does not include medical diagnosis and that I should see an appropriate health care provider to diagnose and treat medical problems. I give my consent for the massage session.

_____ Date _____
Signature

Plan:

Comments:

FIGURE 9–11

Example of simplified note for one-time client.

an office, do house calls, and work trade shows, you may want to use three different forms. Or if you have an office and offer routine massage as well as medical treatment, you may use two different forms.

As a general rule, use SOAP notes for goal-oriented or treatment sessions. A simplified form can be used for routine massage, or for one-time, walk-in clients. For a trade show or health fair, a signature list following a short statement might be adequate. See MyHealthProfessionsLab.com for samples of different forms.

If you process claims for insurance reimbursement, be sure to document the services performed in the claims.

Design your note forms to include all the information required by the insurance companies you deal with. Electronic note systems may be more efficient in these cases.

If you keep hard copy or paper records, make a separate file for each regular client. File folders with fasteners are useful for keeping papers in order. In a file with two fasteners, general information (e.g., intake form, signed privacy and policy statement, health history, referral letter) can be kept on one side, and individual session notes on the other side.

Records for one-time clients can be kept in alphabetical order in a group file. If they become regular clients,

FIGURE 9–12

Example of simplified note for a nonmedical setting.

SHORT NOTE CHART

Client's Name _____

Date _____ Practitioner's Name _____

S: Comments, complaints, reports, recent illness or injury, medications

O: Visual observations, palpation

P: Length of session, routine given, significant modifications

C: General comments

MT Initials _____

Date _____ Practitioner's Name _____

S: Comments, complaints, reports, recent illness or injury, medications

O: Visual observations, palpation

P: Length of session, routine given, significant modifications

C: General comments

MT Initials _____

Date _____ Practitioner's Name/Initials _____

S: Comments, complaints, reports, recent illness or injury, medications

O: Visual observations, palpation

P: Length of session, routine given, significant modifications

C: General comments

MT Initials _____

you can make an individual file for them. Signature lists from events can have their own file in chronological order. The important thing is to have a system that allows you to locate records easily and one that works for your type of practice.

LEGAL AND ETHICAL ISSUES

Legal and ethical issues related to documentation and note-taking revolve around scope of practice, accuracy, honesty, confidentiality, and respect for the client. Because diagnosis is not in the scope of practice of massage therapists, no diagnoses by them should appear in session notes. References to others' diagnoses need to be clearly identified, for example, "condition as diagnosed by client's physician," or "client self-diagnosis," or "self-reported." This is a legal as well as an ethical matter.

Write session notes to accurately reflect what happened in the session. Writing notes as soon as possible after a session increases the likelihood of complete and accurate documentation. Record only those procedures that were performed in the session. Defrauding an insurance company is unlawful and unethical.

Keep session notes in a secure place such as a locked cabinet, and do not leave them lying around for others to see. Follow all HIPAA rules related to privacy of health records where applicable. Share the contents of clients' files only with their permission. See Chapter 27, *Private Practice and Finances*, for more information about HIPAA confidentiality rules.

Write notes using respectful and professional language. Omit opinions and personal comments about clients that are unrelated to their massage session. Remember that clients have a right to look at their notes, and others may someday have access to the notes as well. Your notes are a reflection of your level of professionalism.

PRACTICAL APPLICATION

Obtain a blank copy of the documentation form used in student clinic at your school. Examine the form to see how it is formatted and what information is requested for each massage session. Use the form to document practice sessions in preparation for your student clinic experience. Answering the following questions will help you with student clinic documentation.

1. What level of detail will be required at student clinic?
2. Is there a chart of standard abbreviations used in student clinic?
3. Does the clinic have specific guidelines related to completing documentation, for example, what information goes in each section and how each entry should be signed?

CRITICAL THINKING

Obtain examples of three or four different note-taking forms used by massage therapists. Compare, contrast, and analyze the forms to determine which forms might be appropriate for different settings (e.g., spa, health club, clinic, private practice, outreach event). Redesign the forms to improve their appearance or usefulness. Consider the following:

1. Is the form complete? Is all important information included?
2. Is it easy to use? Is the format logical?
3. Is the form useful for the intended setting?
4. Does the spacing allow for writing entries?

CASE FOR STUDY

Jennifer and Simplified Documentation at the Salon

Jennifer, a massage therapist with a small practice within a community beauty salon, uses a simplified format for documentation of massage sessions given there. She has informed clients that the massage offered in the salon is primarily for relaxation and rejuvenation and refers clients to other massage therapists for more clinical massage applications. The form she developed has three sections to document each massage session.

- The *H* section is for recording relevant health information including contraindications.
- The *MT* section is for a description of the massage therapy application for the day.
- The *C* section is for comments, including noteworthy events and results.

Jennifer can fit notes for four sessions with a client on one page and has learned to be concise in her documentation.

Session with Isabel

Isabel came in for her regular massage and in the brief presession interview reported that she had been to the doctor in the past week for a skin rash on her leg. The doctor thought it might be an allergic reaction and prescribed some oral medication and some anti-itch crème. Isabel was stressed out from a family situation and was looking forward to relaxing. Jennifer gave her the relaxation massage as usual, but switched to a hypoallergenic lotion. She spent more time on the neck and shoulders, where Isabel had reported tension, and avoided massage around the rash. Isabel was a little more talkative than usual, and Jennifer tried to help her focus on her breathing and letting go of tension. She played special relaxation music for a calming atmosphere. Jennifer sensed that Isabel was distracted, but did seem a little more relaxed at the end of the session. Isabel thanked Jennifer and reported feeling less anxious.

Write notes for this session using Jennifer's system of documentation.

H _____

MT _____

C _____

Date _____ Time _____

CHAPTER HIGHLIGHTS

- Medical terminology is the shared language of health professionals.
- Medical terms typically consist of a prefix, a root word, and a suffix.
- Session planning is the logical process of thinking through the massage from beginning to end.
- Goal-oriented planning focuses on achieving specific client goals, as reflected in the Wellness Massage Pyramid.
- Clinical reasoning is the cognitive process used in goal-oriented planning and is essentially a problem-solving exercise.
- The six steps in goal-oriented planning are (1) collecting subjective information from the client; (2) collecting objective information through observation, tests, and measurements; (3) assessing the situation and setting client goals; (4) devising a plan to achieve client goals; (5) implementing the plan; and (6) evaluating the results. The plan is revised as needed based on the results obtained.
- Three basic variations of goal-oriented planning are long-range planning, individual session planning, and treatment planning.
  - Long-range planning is done in the initial session and in progress evaluation sessions.
  - Individual session planning is done before each massage session.
  - Treatment planning is done when the goal is the alleviation of symptoms or facilitating healing of a pathological condition.
  - Each of the variations uses the six-step session planning process, modified for its specific application.
- Intake is the process of gathering relevant information from a new client.
- Intake involves the client filling out an intake form and a health history form and the therapist conducting a new client interview.
  - A health history provides information to identify contraindications and as background for planning sessions.
  - When providing routine massage at an outreach event, the intake process can be shortened to a few relevant questions and signing a consent form.
- Objective methods of collecting information include the massage therapist's own general observations, palpation, range-of-motion evaluation, posture analysis, biomechanical analysis, gait analysis, and orthopedic tests.

- Subjective and objective information gathered in Steps 1 and 2 of the session planning process is used in Step 3 to assess the situation and prioritize client goals.
- Documentation is the process of writing massage session records for future reference; also called note-taking or charting.
- Session notes are kept on paper or in electronic form in client files.
- Notes are legal documents, are used for insurance reporting, and may be subpoenaed as evidence in legal cases.
- Notes are official client health records, and electronic records may be protected by HIPAA Privacy Rules.
- Notes are practical as an aid to memory and in planning sessions. Writing notes is an important part of completing a massage session.
- SOAP notes have become a standard for charting goal-oriented massage sessions.
- The SOAP format reflects a logical or clinical reasoning process.
  - Four types of SOAP notes are initial, continuing, progress, and discharge notes.
  - Massage therapists working in the same office should use standard abbreviations and symbols and follow the format required by their employer.
- SOAP is an acronym for subjective, objective, assessment, and plan.
  - The *S* or subjective section contains information provided by the client.
  - The *O* or objective section contains observations, tests, and measurements made by the massage therapist.
  - The *A* or assessment section identifies the goals for the massage session and any contraindications.
  - The *P* or plan section lays out the steps planned to achieve identified goals.
- SOAP notes are written using brief descriptions, abbreviations, and symbols.
  - Notes are strings of descriptions separated by commas or semicolons, or are bulleted lists.
  - Diagrams of the body are useful in writing notes.
  - Entries are descriptions and not diagnoses of conditions.
- SOAP notes are written legibly in clear, concise language in blue or black ink. They conform to standards for legal documents related to making and initialing changes and are dated and initialed at the end.

○ Personal comments about clients should not be written.
○ Clients have the right to see their files.
○ Files are kept for at least 7 years.

● Simplified note formats may be used when routine massages are given, and with one-time, walk-in clients.
○ Documentation can include at a minimum a short intake form asking about contraindications, a description of the massage to be given, a date, and a signature from the client giving permission for the session.

● Massage therapists design systems of documentation and note-taking appropriate for the type of practice they have.
○ Therapists can design their own charting forms or use premade forms.
○ A separate file is created for each regular client.

● Legal and ethical issues related to documentation revolve around scope of practice, accuracy, honesty, confidentiality, and respect for clients.
● Client files should be kept secure and shared only with the client's permission.
○ The way you keep your files is a reflection of your level of professionalism.

EXAM REVIEW

Key Terms

To study the key terms listed at the beginning of this chapter, match the appropriate lettered meaning to each numbered key term listed. For additional study, look up the key terms in the Interactive Glossary, and note other terms that compare or contrast with them.

_____ 1. Assessment
_____ 2. Clinical reasoning
_____ 3. Continuing session notes
_____ 4. Discharge notes
_____ 5. Documentation
_____ 6. Goal-oriented planning
_____ 7. HIPAA privacy rules
_____ 8. Intake notes
_____ 9. Long-term planning
_____ 10. Progress notes
_____ 11. SOAP notes
_____ 12. Treatment planning

a. General process of planning massage sessions to meet client needs and goals
b. Notes related to the initial massage session with a client
c. Planning a series of massage sessions over time to reach specific goals
d. Step in goal-oriented planning in which the situation is analyzed and goals are prioritized
e. Common format used for documenting massage
f. Notes that evaluate achievement related to long-term goals
g. Record the session-by-session history of a client's visits
h. Process of planning massage sessions in which the goal is alleviation of symptoms or facilitation of healing of a pathological condition
i. Cognitive process used in goal-oriented planning
j. Protects the privacy of medical records
k. Process of writing massage session records for future reference; also called note-taking or charting
l. Final summary of the client's progress and any comments about the course of treatment

Memory Workout

To test your memory of the main concepts in this chapter, complete the following sentences by circling the most correct answer from the two choices provided.

1. Session planning is the (logical) (intuitive) process of thinking through a massage session.
2. Before (ending) (beginning) a massage session with a regular client, ask about any recent changes in his or her health status or medications.
3. The goal of treatment planning is the facilitation of healing of a (kinesiological) (pathological) condition.
4. The main purpose of a short intake interview before giving massage at outreach events is to identify possible (contraindications) (indications).
5. Rating scales offer a rough measurement of things from the client's (objective) (subjective) view.
6. Palpation is the act of sensing information about a client through (vision) (touch) and through the (look) (feel) of tissues.

7. In good standing posture, the head is in alignment over the shoulders, and the chin is slightly (tucked) (forward).
8. In proper lifting mechanics, power comes from the (shoulder) (leg) muscles.
9. Documentation is the process of writing detailed (records) (plans) of massage sessions for future reference.
10. The *O* in SOAP notes stands for (other) (objective).
11. SOTAP is a variation of the SOAP note, and the *T* stands for (theory) (treatment).
12. Body charts are good visual aids for collecting (objective) (subjective) information from clients.
13. Initial or sign your note at the (beginning) (end) of an entry.
14. Records for one-time clients can be kept in (alphabetical) (chronological) order in a group file.
15. Signature lists from events can have their own file in (alphabetical) (chronological) order.

Test Prep

The following multiple-choice questions will help to prepare you for future school and professional exams.

1. Which of the following is a method of collecting subjective information from clients?
   a. Range-of-motion evaluation
   b. Gait analysis
   c. Health history forms
   d. Palpation of tissues

2. Suggesting activities to be done outside the massage session on the client's own time is correctly referred to as:
   a. A prescription
   b. Home care
   c. Contraindication
   d. An assignment

3. The goal-oriented planning process is best described as:
   a. Rigid and linear
   b. Logical but disorderly
   c. Linear and disorderly
   d. Looping spiral

4. Which of the following is *not* within the massage therapist's scope of practice?
   a. Measuring function or loss of function
   b. Assessing the condition of tissues
   c. Diagnosing a medical condition
   d. All of the above

5. At what point in a massage session does the massage therapist clarify the client's top goals for the massage?
   a. Presession interview
   b. Postsession interview
   c. Midpoint in the session
   d. When writing postsession notes

6. Which type of interview question steers clients to specific topics, but leaves space for them to answer in their own words?
   a. Open-ended question
   b. Multiple-choice question
   c. Rating scale
   d. Body chart

7. Which of the following tends to reduce the ability to feel or palpate the condition of tissues?
   a. Moving slowly
   b. Being focused and present
   c. Using heavy pressure
   d. Putting descriptive words to what your feel

8. In good sitting posture, the knees should be aligned with the hips or slightly:
   a. Lower
   b. Higher
   c. Turned in
   d. Turned out

9. The *S* section of a SOAP note contains:
   a. A transcription of the client's words from the intake interview
   b. A summary of subjective information from the client
   c. A summary of measurements taken during the intake interview
   d. A summary of the session plan

10. In the PSOAP variation of SOAP notes, the first *P* contains:
    a. Possible contraindications
    b. Plans developed in a prior session
    c. Permission to send records to the insurance company
    d. Prescription or diagnosis from a primary health care provider

11. In which section of SOAP notes for an individual massage session are the results of the day's massage typically recorded?
    a. S
    b. O
    c. A
    d. P

12. Once you have mastered writing SOAP notes, about how much time would you expect to spend after each massage session writing an entry?
    a. 1–2 minutes
    b. 5–10 minutes
    c. 25–30 minutes
    d. 45–50 minutes

13. Which of the following instructions for correcting a mistake made in SOAP notes is *not* acceptable?
    a. White-out or erase the mistake
    b. Put a single line through the mistake
    c. Write "error" above or next to the area
    d. Initial the correction

14. What is the recommended number of years that client records are kept?
    a. 1
    b. 3
    c. 5
    d. 7

15. The most acceptable place to store client records securely in a massage office is:
    a. In a locked file cabinet
    b. In a desk drawer
    c. In a box in the closet
    d. On a shelf behind the desk

Video Challenge

Watch these videos, which can be found at MyHealthProfessionsLab.com, Chapter 9, and then answer the following questions.

Goal-Oriented Planning

1. Match the scenes in this video segment with the steps in the goal-oriented planning process. Which step does each scene illustrate?
2. Identify scenes in the video where massage therapists are collecting subjective data from clients. During which parts of massage sessions does subjective data collection occur?
3. For each scene in the video showing sitting posture, point out aspects of good alignment, as well as deviations that may result in muscle tension and pain.

4. Review scenes from the video explaining good standing alignment. What are important instructions for assessing a client's standing alignment?
5. List the different occupations illustrated in the video in the section on biomechanics. Identify potential musculoskeletal problems clients in these occupations might develop.

Documentation

6. List the many practical uses for session notes mentioned in the video.
7. Identify where the massage therapist gets the information contained in each section of the SOAP note as explained in the video.

Comprehension Exercises

The following short-answer questions test your knowledge and understanding of chapter topics and provide practice in written communication skills. Explain in two to four complete sentences.

1. List the six steps in the goal-oriented planning process. Give an example of using the process for planning an individual massage session.
2. Explain why goal-oriented planning is a work in progress rather than a strictly linear process? At what point in the massage might goals or plans be adjusted? Based on what information?

3. Describe good standing posture. List some anatomical markers for evaluating proper alignment when viewed from the front and from the side.
4. What is the difference between a *diagnosis* and a *description* of a complaint by a client? Which is within the scope of practice of massage therapists? Give an example.

For Greater Understanding

The following exercises are designed to take you from the realm of theory into the real world. They will help give you a deeper understanding of the subjects covered in this chapter. Action words are underlined to emphasize the variety of activities presented to address different learning styles and to encourage deeper thinking.

1. <u>Interview</u> a family member or friend after he or she has filled out a health history form. <u>Lead</u> the person in a discussion of the potential benefits of massage in helping to improve his or her overall wellness using the Wellness Massage Pyramid. <u>Help</u> the individual determine his or her top three goals for getting massage in the future.

2. <u>Perform</u> a posture, biomechanical, or gait analysis of a classmate's movements. <u>Describe</u> what you observe, and <u>offer</u> instructions for more balanced alignment or biomechanically sound movement.

3. <u>Analyze</u> a list of ten medical terms chosen by a study partner. Identify the prefix, suffix, and root word, then <u>translate</u> the term into English. Alternatively, translate English expressions for certain conditions (e.g., lack of bone, nerve pain) into correct medical terminology (e.g., osteopenia, neuralgia). Study partners take turns quizzing each other.

4. <u>Write</u> a sample SOAP description in complete sentences without abbreviations or symbols. <u>Give</u> that description to a study partner, and <u>ask</u> him or her to <u>translate</u> the longer descriptions using the SOAP shorthand format. Now <u>give</u> the abbreviated SOAP notes to a third study partner, and see if he or she can <u>translate</u> the note correctly back into longhand.

MyHealthProfessionsLab™

MyHealthProfessionsLab.com is a premium online homework management system that includes a host of features to help you study. Registered users will find:

- Powerful tools that track and analyze your results—allowing you to create a personalized learning experience
- Videos, flashcards and other learning tools to help enrich your progress
- Streaming lesson presentations and self-paced learning modules
- A space where you and your instructors can view and manage your assignments

Pearson Education, Inc.

10 Hygiene, Equipment, Environment

CHAPTER OUTLINE

Learning Outcomes

Key Terms

Introduction

Personal Hygiene and Hand
   Washing

Massage Equipment

Supplies for Massage

Topical Substances

Physical Environment for Massage

Infection Control

Chapter Highlights

Exam Review

LEARNING OUTCOMES

After studying this chapter, you will have information to:

1. Practice good personal hygiene.

2. Wash hands thoroughly for massage therapy.

3. Evaluate massage tables and chairs in relation to practice needs.

4. Set up and care for massage tables and chairs properly.

5. Describe the variety of bolsters and pillows used in massage.

6. Describe the uses of sheets, blankets, and towels in massage.

7. Choose topical substances for their specific effects.

8. Keep equipment and supplies clean and sanitary.

9. Create a comfortable, sanitary, and safe environment for clients.

10. Follow infection control procedures to prevent the spread of serious diseases.

KEY TERMS

Bolsters

Equipment

Hygiene

Hygienic hand washing

Massage chairs

MRSA

Portable massage table

Sanitation

Topical substance

Universal precautions

INTRODUCTION

Preparation for massage therapy includes consideration of hygiene, equipment, and environment. Hygiene is especially important when people are in close contact, such as when giving and receiving massage. Habits of personal and environmental hygiene are established from day one in massage training programs as you learn to keep yourself, your equipment, and your space clean.

Practicing massage therapy also requires knowledge of basic equipment and supplies. Massage tables and chairs provide the platform for massage applications and are essential tools of the profession. Additional basic tools are various accessories such as linens and bolsters and the oils and lotions typically used in Swedish massage. Hydrotherapy equipment is described in Chapter 17, *Hydrotherapy and Temperature Therapies.*

Practicing massage techniques outside school and experience in student clinic provide opportunities for learning to create a suitable environment for massage therapy. The goal is to provide for the comfort and safety of clients, as well as to organize a space conducive to relaxation and healing. Hygiene, equipment, and environment are interrelated aspects of preparation for massage and the foundation for hands-on applications.

PERSONAL HYGIENE AND HAND WASHING

Massage practitioners have a responsibility to follow good hygiene and sanitation practices that make the client comfortable and that prevent the spread of disease. Although the original meaning of the words *hygiene* and *sanitation* referred generally to practices that promote good health, they are primarily used today to refer to cleanliness and removing disease-causing organisms. In this textbook, **hygiene** will be used in relation to personal cleanliness, whereas **sanitation** will be used when referring to cleaning equipment, supplies, and the massage space.

Personal Hygiene

The close physical contact inherent in massage therapy calls for excellent personal hygiene. Massage therapists must look neat and smell clean to inspire the confidence and trust of clients. This applies to clothes as well as to the body, and especially to the hands. Professional appearance, grooming, and personal hygiene are discussed in greater detail in Chapter 3, *Professional and Personal Development.*

In addition to looking clean and neat, avoid offensive odors. This includes odors from the body and clothes, including strong perfumes and colognes. Some practitioners bathe or change shirts during the day to stay fresh. After a spicy meal, or just a long day, consider using a breath freshener. Smokers should be particularly aware to eliminate odors on their clothes, hands, and breath.

The hands are the primary means for giving massage. The following hand-care guidelines for the practitioner help to make the massage a more pleasant experience for the recipient.

- Keep fingernails clipped short and below the level of the fingertips. If you hold your hands up with the palms facing you, you should not be able to see the fingernails.

- Use lotion to keep the hands soft and moisturized. Smooth out rough spots and calluses that might feel scratchy to a receiver.

- Avoid wearing rings and bracelets. They can distract and possibly scratch the receiver, and harbor germs.

- Wash hands thoroughly before and after each session to prevent the spread of disease. Remove odors from hands.

- Keep hands warm and dry before touching a client. They can be warmed beneath a heat lamp, by hot water, or by rubbing them together briskly. Use a towel to dry hands thoroughly after washing them. Cornstarch or powder may be used to absorb moisture and keep hands dry.

Without good hygiene and sanitation, pathogens can be passed from practitioner to client or from client to client in various ways. One of the most basic personal hygiene measures for massage therapists is hand washing.

Hand Washing

The most effective method for preventing the transfer of pathogens during massage is **hygienic hand washing**. Massage practitioners wash their hands before and after each session. They may also wash during a session, for example, before touching the face after massaging the feet. A thorough hand-washing procedure includes nine steps, which are illustrated in Practice Sequence 10–1, *Hygienic Hand Washing.*

REALITY CHECK

MARIA

RACHELLE: My hands are getting irritated from all of the hand washing that goes with doing massage. And my cuticles are raw from using a nail brush. How can I keep my hands in better shape while practicing good hygiene?

MARIA: Try always using soap with a skin conditioner like aloe in it. You might also find a brand that is used by nurses or other health care professionals. They wash their hands even more than massage therapists and have products formulated for their needs. I use a nail brush with soft natural bristles. It is less abrasive than a synthetic brush. Dry your hands thoroughly, too. And at the end of the day, use a good hand cream to restore and protect the skin.

PRACTICE SEQUENCE 10–1

Hygienic Hand Washing

1

Figure 10–1 Adjust the water coming from the faucet so that the temperature is comfortable. Water too hot can damage your skin and is not necessary for cleaning. Water must be running to wash away pathogens.

2

Figure 10–2 Wet the forearms and hands from elbow to fingertips. Keep the hands lower than the elbows. Water flows off the fingertips.

3

Figure 10–3 Scrub the nails with a nail brush to loosen oil and dirt. Clean under the nails.

4

Figure 10–4 Create a soapy lather with the hands and spread the soap up to the elbows. Liquid soap is preferred. If using a bar of soap, be sure to rinse it after each use. Cover the entire skin surface, including the finger and thumb webs.

Figure 10–5 Rub for at least 15 seconds. Particles and pathogens become suspended in the soapy lather and are washed away.

Figure 10–6 Rinse the soap off completely from fingertips to elbows. Water flows off the forearms near the elbows.

Figure 10–7 Dry hands and forearms thoroughly with clean paper towels to prevent chapping.

Figure 10–8 Use the same paper towels to turn off the faucet.

Figure 10–9 If before a massage, use the same paper towels to operate door handles and then discard in the massage room.

After you perform the Practice Sequence, evaluate how well you did by filling out Performance Evaluation Form 10-1, *Hygienic Hand Washing*. The form can be found in Appendix D, *Performance Evaluation Forms*, and at MyHealthProfessionsLab.com.

Figures source: Pearson Education, Inc./Segal Photography.

FIGURE 10–10 Use a rubber finger cot to cover an open wound on a finger.

Source: Pearson Education, Inc./Segal Photography.

FIGURE 10–11 Use rubber gloves (latex or nonlatex) to cover hands as needed to protect against contamination in certain settings.

Source: Pearson Education, Inc./Segal Photography.

If washing with soap and water is not feasible, commercial hand sanitizers are an option. These gel-like substances typically contain ethyl alcohol to kill common pathogens. Choose a brand with a moisturizer included to prevent skin damage with frequent use. Be sure to follow directions.

If you have cuts or scrapes on your hands or forearms, cover them before touching a client. Use either rubber gloves or finger cots. A finger cot is adequate if the exposure is just on one finger. See Figure 10–10 ■. Many people are allergic to latex, so if you have a skin reaction to it, use a nonlatex alternative. Also ask clients if they are allergic to latex, and use nonlatex alternatives if they are. If you have a skin abrasion on the forearm, avoid use of the forearm when applying techniques.

Other situations in which glove protection might be appropriate is when a client has a potentially contagious condition, or in the presence of blood or other body fluids. This may be necessary in some hospital and clinical settings and sometimes at sports events. Be sure that there are no contraindications for massage present before giving massage with rubber gloves on. See Figure 10–11 ■.

MASSAGE EQUIPMENT

Equipment refers to items that are relatively costly and that last for several years. Massage tables and massage chairs are the biggest equipment investments that beginning massage therapists make. Considering them as investments makes sense because wise choices now will pay rich dividends in both the short and long terms. The aim is to select good-quality massage tables and massage chairs to meet your needs in the foreseeable future.

You will begin learning about massage equipment as you set up, use, and take down massage tables and chairs in class. This presents a great opportunity to practice using and caring for equipment properly.

Massage Tables

Massage tables are specially designed for the needs of massage practitioners and may be stationary or portable. Massage tables are adjustable for height. Most have a removable, adjustable face cradle. Tables vary in length, width, and type of padding and covering. A typical portable massage table and adjustable face cradle are shown in Figure 10–12 ■.

The most appropriate table for a particular situation depends on the type of practice and the setting. For example, in settings where tables are rarely moved, stationary tables may be best for their stability. However, if the table will be carried from place to place, or set up and taken down frequently, then a **portable massage table** would be a better choice. A hinged tabletop is another option that allows easy positioning of clients in a semireclining position. This may be important when working with special populations or if specializing in a type of bodywork such as reflexology.

Table width, length, and height are also important considerations. Table widths vary from 27–32 inches or wider. Narrower tables are lighter weight, but may be less comfortable for larger clients. Wider tables are heavier to carry, but accommodate bigger people and have more space for positioning the side-lying client. If you are short, maintaining good body mechanics while reaching over a wider table may be a challenge, but in that case you can use a step stool if you need more extension.

Standard table length is 73 inches long, which fits people up to about 6 feet tall. Taller clients can be accommodated in various ways, including using special table extenders. A typical size massage table for Swedish massage is 29–31 inches wide and 73 inches long.

Massage tables are adjustable for height. Massage therapists can then set up their tables at a height that allows for good body mechanics. Shorter massage therapists generally

FIGURE 10–12 Adjustable massage table with face cradle.

need lower tables, and taller people need higher tables. Proper table height might also vary depending on the size of the client, special client positioning (e.g., side-lying), or type of massage being given. Proper table height is the height that allows for massage applications without bending too much at the waist or neck. Massage tables typically have a height range of 8–10 inches, for example, a standard table is adjustable to 24–34 inches in height. Shorter massage therapists can get tables that start out lower (e.g., range of 18–26 inches), and taller massage therapists need tables that start out higher (e.g., range of 26–36 inches).

Stationary tables with electric lifts allow massage therapists to easily change the height of the table before or even during a massage session. The table can be lowered to accommodate the client getting onto the table and then raised to the appropriate height when starting the massage. The table height can also be changed during a session when massaging different parts of the body, or for a special massage application. The electric lift table is a good choice for an office practice.

For sports massage, a narrower table is often preferred. Some shiatsu practitioners get up on the table for better leverage, and so a wider, stronger table is more desirable. There are special tables for pregnant clients and tables with hinged tops that allow for a semireclining position.

A massage table is an important purchase for a student or recent graduate. To research a variety of tables, it is advisable to visit a massage supplies showroom, attend a trade show or convention, or check table manufacturers' websites. Avoid massage tables sold for personal, not professional, use. These lower-grade tables are not made to stand up to the use of a massage therapy practice. A good-quality professional-grade massage table is a wise investment. A checklist of considerations for choosing a massage table is presented in Table 10–1 ■.

Massage Chairs

Massage chairs are specially designed to provide maximum comfort for people receiving massage in a seated position while fully clothed. Chairs typically have a seat,

TABLE 10–1   Checklist for Choosing a Massage Table

1. Type of Massage or Bodywork	☐ Swedish ☐ Deep tissue ☐ Sports massage ☐ Special populations ☐ Other _____
2. General Type of Table	☐ Portable ☐ Stationary ☐ Hinged tabletop for semireclining
3. Table Width	☐ Standard (29–31 inches) ☐ Narrow (28 inches or less) ☐ Wide (32 inches or more)
4. Table Length	☐ Standard (72–73 inches) ☐ Short (68–70 inches) ☐ Long (over 73 inches)
5. Table Height	☐ Standard (24–34 inches) ☐ Short (18–26 or 22–30 inches) ☐ Tall (26–36 inches)
6. Tabletop Features	☐ Thick foam layer ☐ Thin foam layer ☐ Smooth vinyl cover ☐ Suede vinyl cover ☐ Other cover _____ ☐ Dark color ☐ Light color
7. Table Legs	☐ Wood ☐ Metal ☐ Height adjustment on legs ☐ Leg-stabilizing mechanism ☐ Special height needs ☐ Electric lift

(continued)

TABLE 10–1	*(continued)*	
8. Weight of Table	☐ Light weight (25–28 lbs)	
	☐ Medium weight (29–34 lbs)	
	☐ Heavy weight (35+ lbs)	
9. Table Strength*	☐ Strong enough for client	
	☐ Strong enough for client plus massage therapist	
	*Standard maximum operating capacity: 300–600 lbs	
10. Special Features Needed	☐ _____	
	☐ _____	
	☐ _____	
11. Additional Factors	☐ Ease of setup and takedown	
	☐ Ease of care and durability of table cover	
	☐ Cost	

knee rests, armrest, chest cushion, and face cradle. A typical massage chair is shown in Figure 10–13 ■. This type of massage chair was introduced in the 1980s, and chairs are continually undergoing improvement in design.

Things to consider when choosing among different massage chair models are ease of setup, takedown, and carrying from place to place. Massage chairs are designed to be used for on-site massage, that is, taken to a location such as a workplace, store, or community event. Look at the chair when it is folded up, and try carrying it. Find out how much the massage chair weighs. Check to see if it has wheels. Set the chair up and then take it down a few times to see how easy or difficult it is.

Consider stability. Get onto the chair yourself to see how stable it feels. Is it easy to get onto and out of? Have someone else get on the chair while you apply a few massage techniques. Does the chair move a lot or feel like it will tip over easily? A wider base helps prevent tipping from side-to-side, which is a client safety consideration.

Be aware of the range of clients the chair can accommodate. Chairs have a maximum weight allowance, for example, 300–600 pounds. How tall or short clients are can also make a difference. A typical chair can seat clients from 4 feet 6 inches to 6 feet 6 inches tall. Shorter or taller clients may have difficulty being positioned properly. Never place

A   **B**

FIGURE 10–13 A. Adjustable massage chair. B. Recipient positioned in massage chair.

CRITICAL THINKING

Determine the ideal massage table for you at this time. Complete a features and cost comparison of massage table models from different companies. Pick one brand and model that seems best for you and your start-up practice after graduation.

1. Use the chart in Table 10–1 to identify important features of your ideal table.

2. Look at different massage tables in person or on company websites, and pick out options for tables that have the features you want.
3. Determine the cost of your ideal table, and think about how you will go about financing its purchase.

---

a client in a massage chair if you suspect the chair is not designed to handle his or her weight.

Look for adjustments in the face cradle, chest pad, armrest, and kneeler. Different massage chair models might also have special adjustments for client positioning variations. Some have seat and kneeler adjustments that allow clients to sit on the chair "backward" for different massage applications. Before purchasing a massage chair, investigate different models to find the features that you want.

Equipment Setup and Care

Massage tables and chairs will remain in good condition longer with proper use and care. Follow the manufacturer's guidelines for basic care of equipment.

To set up a typical portable massage table, place it on the floor on its side with the handles up. Unlatch the closures and swing the table open to about 60 degrees. Remove the face cradle if it is stored inside. Then straighten out the legs and open the table completely. If there are two people, one stands at each end and they lift the table together, turning it onto its feet. If there is one person setting up the table, he or she can stand in the middle or at an end and pull the table onto its feet, while bracing a table leg.

Once the table is set up, check to make sure the legs are straight and supporting cables or braces are in place properly. The table can then be adjusted for height and the face cradle slid into place. Never sit on a portable massage table directly over the hinge in the middle. This weakens the table over time. Periodically check to make sure that nuts and bolts are tightened securely because they can come loose from the movement of massage. See Figure 10–14 ■.

Massage chair designs differ greatly, and so there is no standard method of setup. Check the manufacturer's guidelines for instructions. Be sure that all attachments are in place properly. Get into the chair to check to make sure that it is stable. Tighten nuts and bolts as needed.

There are many choices of upholstery for massage tables. Some are softer and some harder. Some are suedelike and some smooth. Check the manufacturer's instructions for care of the upholstery on your equipment. Generally avoid cleaning with harsh chemicals that can dry out and damage the fabric. Depending on the type of massage or bodywork you practice, you may need to clean your table every day or week. Some recommend wiping the face cradle cushion

after each client, even when a face cradle cover is used. Using a padded or plastic barrier under the bottom drape can save wear and tear on upholstery. See Figure 10–15 ■.

Massage chairs should be wiped down after each client, especially the face cradle and armrests. Use a disinfectant to kill germs that could spread disease. Face cradle covers help keep sweat and makeup off the upholstery. See Figure 10–16 ■.

Alternatives to Tables and Chairs

Whenever possible, use equipment specially designed for massage. However, sometimes practitioners have to improvise in less-than-ideal situations. For example, massage is sometimes given to people in wheelchairs, to the bedridden elderly or ill, to workers at their desks, or even at poolside at a swim meet. In these circumstances, care should be taken to ensure the safety and comfort of the receiver while providing for good body mechanics for the practitioner.

SUPPLIES FOR MASSAGE

In addition to a massage table, some basic supplies are needed for massage therapy. Bolsters and pillows, draping materials, and topical substances such as oil and lotions are essential for most massage applications.

Bolsters and Pillows

Bolsters and pillows are used to position the client for comfort and safety. Body support may be provided in different positions as needed under the knees, neck, ankles, shoulders, and wrists (Figure 10–17 ■). Positioning clients correctly is addressed in Chapter 11, *Body Mechanics, Table Skills, General Guidelines*.

Bolsters are long narrow pillows or cushions used to support or prop clients into position for massage. Massage bolsters are typically as wide as a standard table, and come in round, half-round, and quarter-round shapes. Small bolsters are useful for neck support. Soft wedges of various sizes and shapes are made for positioning different parts of the body. Some whole-body support systems are available for pregnant and other special-needs clients.

Bolsters are usually covered with the same upholstery materials used on massage table tops. If a bolster touches a

FIGURE 10–14 A. Open portable massage table on its side. B. Straighten out legs completely and check that leg supports are locked. C. Turn table upright. D. Adjust table height.

Source: Pearson Education, Inc./Segal Photography.

FIGURE 10–15 Use a rubber or padded barrier to save wear and tear on the tabletop.

Source: Pearson Education, Inc./Segal Photography.

FIGURE 10–16 Use face cradle covers to prevent the client's skin from touching the face cradle upholstery.

Source: Pearson Education, Inc./Segal Photography.

CASE FOR STUDY

Jayden and Buying a Massage Chair

Jayden has been given the opportunity to become an independent contractor providing on-site chair massage for the employees of a large corporation located close to his home-based massage therapy practice. However, Jayden will need to purchase a massage chair before he can begin this new venture. He has discovered that there are many chairs available from which to choose and is concerned about finding the best-quality chair within his budget.

Question:

What are the criteria Jayden needs to bear in mind as he shops for a massage chair?

Things to consider:

- Is the chair sturdy but lightweight enough for him to set up and move around easily?

- Will the armrests hold up to the deep compression and friction techniques commonly used on the arms?
- Is the chair easy to adjust? What adjustments can be made?
- Are there any hinges or other metal components that could scratch or pinch the skin of either the therapist or client?
- Does the chair come with a warranty?

Investigate massage chairs by visiting manufacturers' showrooms or websites or studying their catalogs. Has another massage therapist made a recommendation? Which chair would you choose if you were Jayden? Why?

_____

_____

_____

client's skin during massage, wash it afterward. Bolsters can also be covered or placed under the bottom drape for protection.

Standard bed pillows are sometimes useful for positioning clients, especially for those in the side-lying position. Be sure that pillows are washable. Pillows should be covered with liners and pillow cases, with cases changed after each client.

Sheets, Blankets, and Towels

Sheets are the most common draping material for Swedish massage. See Figure 10–18 ■. The mechanics of draping with sheets are described in Chapter 11, _Body Mechanics, Table Skills, General Guidelines_. Single bed sheets can be used on most massage tables, or sheets specially made for massage tables can be purchased. Sheets come in different fabrics with most made of cotton or cotton blends. Flannel sheets are sometimes used for warmth. Stock at least enough sets of sheets for the number of clients seen daily. Having extra sheets reduces the number of trips to the laundry.

Blankets are good to have when a client gets cold and can be placed over the top drape. Blankets sized for massage tables can be bought or made. Blankets that hang over the sides of the table too much are difficult to handle when

draping and undraping arms and legs. Bulky and heavy blankets may feel uncomfortable to clients. Many find fleece and flannel blankets ideal for massage. In most circumstances, blankets that do not touch a client's skin may be used on other clients without washing first. In hospital or clinical settings, blankets would not be shared.

Having a variety of sizes of terry cloth or Turkish towels available is very practical. See Figure 10–19 ■. Towels are serviceable for draping women's breasts and can be rolled up for use as bolsters. They are employed for temperature therapy applications such as applying hot packs and cold packs. They are used to wipe off excess oil and lotion and for cleaning up spills. A large towel can be laid over a top drape instead of a blanket for increased warmth.

FIGURE 10–17 Bolsters and pillows are essential for most massage applications.

Source: Pearson Education, Inc./Segal Photography.

FIGURE 10–18 Sheets are the most commonly used draping material.

Source: Pearson Education, Inc./Segal Photography.

FIGURE 10–19 Towels have many uses during a massage therapy session.

Source: Pearson Education, Inc./Segal Photography.

FIGURE 10–20 Topical substances, such as liniments, oils, lotions, and creams, enhance the effects or minimize skin friction during the application of many massage techniques.

Source: Pearson Education, Inc./Segal Photography.

Sheets must be changed after every client. Used sheets and towels should be placed in a covered or closed container, preferably away from the massage table. Never let·a sheet or towel used on one client touch another client.

Wash sheets and towels as needed. An alternative to using a home washer and dryer is to take sheets and towels to a commercial self-service laundry. That way, you save wear and tear on your own machines and may be able to wash more sheets and towels in one load. Some businesses will do the laundry for you for a fee. Massage therapists sometimes contract with linen services to supply their sheets and towels. The service then takes care of laundering and delivers clean sheets as needed. This is a business decision that usually involves signing a contract, so it should be entered into thoughtfully. Figure the time and cost of washing sheets and towels as part of the expense of your massage practice.

TOPICAL SUBSTANCES

Many forms of massage and bodywork use some kind of **topical substance** to enhance their effects or to minimize skin friction during the application of techniques. Topical substances are classified as liniments, oils, lotions, creams, or combinations of these. See Figure 10–20 ■.

Uses of Different Topical Substances

Liniments have been used for centuries for sore and stiff muscles and for sprains and bruises. They are particularly popular with athletes. A liniment is a liquid or semiliquid preparation for rubbing on or applying to the skin for therapeutic purposes. Liniments are typically counterirritants that produce a slight skin irritation to relieve symptoms of inflammation. They contain ingredients such as camphor, menthol, and turpentine. Herbal preparations might contain rosemary, wild marjoram, or cayenne pepper. Because they contain irritants, rubbing with them too vigorously may cause blistering. If liniments are used, they are usually rubbed onto the skin after massage of an area.

Oil serves as a lubricant to minimize uncomfortable skin friction during sliding and kneading techniques. Certain vegetable oils may also add moisture and nutrients to the skin. Commonly used vegetable oils include almond, olive, and grape seed. Vegetable oils for massage should be cold pressed; they are not the same as oils used for cooking. Mineral oils are sometimes used and generally wash out of sheets more easily than vegetable oils. Vegetable oils trapped in sheets can spoil and turn rancid, causing sheets to have an unpleasant odor. However, some consider vegetable oils healthier for both the giver and the receiver of massage.

Jojoba (pronounced ho-ho-ba) is an oil-like substance made from seeds of the jojoba plant found in the North American desert. Native Americans used jojoba for skin and hair care. Many massage practitioners use jojoba either by itself or in combination with lotions because it is hypoallergenic, healthy for skin, and washes out of sheets easily.

Practitioners choose their oils based on a number of factors. These include properties such as the "feel" of the oil (e.g., thick or thin), inherent nutrients, and scent. Unscented oils are available. High-quality oils developed specially for massage can be purchased from suppliers.

Lotions are semiliquid substances containing agents for moisturizing the skin or for therapeutic purposes such as reducing itching or local pain. Lotions are readily absorbed into the skin, unlike oils, which tend to stay on top of the skin longer. Lotions are good for situations in which lubrication is desired for a warm-up phase, but more friction is desired later in the session. Those who don't like the feel of oil on their skin may prefer lotions. Lotions also tend to be more water soluble than oils and are, therefore, more easily washed out of sheets.

Practitioners experiment with different topical substances and concoct combinations of substances to get the properties that best enhance their work. They frequently mix different oils or mix lotions and oils.

Some substances are more likely to cause allergic reactions. Also, some skin types are more easily irritated.

During the intake interview, always ask clients about any skin allergies they might have or adverse reactions to particular scents. People going back to work after massage may desire an unscented substance. Men usually prefer different scents than women. Care should be taken in choosing a topical substance for each unique client or patient situation.

Sanitation and Topical Substances

A few simple practices can prevent cross-contamination from oils, lotions, and creams used in massage. First, wipe off bottles and jars after each session, and any topical substances spilled or dripped on surfaces in the massage room.

Use oil bottles with closeable spouts, and keep them closed between uses. Pumps are available for dispensing lotion.

Do not dip your fingers into a jar to remove creams. Instead, take out what you intend to use with a little spatula and place it on a small plate or piece of paper. Wash the tool after each use or use disposable spatulas. Use the separated supply of cream for the massage, and discard any excess afterward. The original jar then remains uncontaminated. "Double-dipping" can result in cross-contamination from one client to another.

Wash topical substances out of sheets and towels thoroughly. Some topical substance blends are formulated to be more easily washed out of sheets. Organic oils and lotions left in cloth can turn rancid over time, leaving a disagreeable odor. Once this happens, it is advisable to get rid of the sheets and buy new ones.

PHYSICAL ENVIRONMENT FOR MASSAGE

Regardless of the specific setting, certain environmental factors will help maximize the benefits of massage. Important factors to consider include the configuration of the room, floor, wall, and window coverings, lighting and color, temperature and air quality, music or tranquil sounds, and dressing arrangements.

Room Setup

The room in which massage is given must be large enough to accommodate the necessary furniture and equipment, plus the client and the massage therapist. At a minimum, a massage room contains a massage table and sitting stool on wheels, with adequate space for movement around the table. A step

stool can help short or less mobile clients get onto the table. A nearby tabletop or countertop holds oils and lotions, small hand tools, hot packs, and other objects used during massage. A cabinet or closet is useful to store linens, lotions, and other supplies. Soiled linens are kept in a separate covered container. A chair and clothes rack for clients' belongings round out the furnishings in a well-equipped massage room.

Provide convenient dressing arrangements and a private space for clients to disrobe. If there is only one table in the room, then the practitioner may simply leave the room while the recipient is disrobing. A privacy screen or curtain can be used if needed. In situations where there is more than one table in the room, such as in a training room or clinic, gowns may be provided for clients to use when walking from the dressing area to the massage table. Robes are often provided for this purpose at spas.

It is considered a breach of professional boundaries for clients to be seen naked as they prepare for massage. Exceptions are in cases where the person receiving massage needs assistance undressing or dressing, such as with the elderly or disabled. Even in these cases, care should be taken to preserve the modesty of the recipient as much as possible.

Floors, Walls, and Windows

Floors in massage rooms should be able to be washed and disinfected regularly. Wood and tile floors are most easily washed, but can be cold for the client. Area rugs can add warmth, but look for those with rubber backing to avoid slipping when people walk on them. Carpet is the hardest floor covering to keep clean and is liable to stain if oil or lotion is spilled on it. Some local health ordinances may require a specific type of flooring for massage establishments.

Windows in a massage room allow for fresh air and natural sunlight. Be sure that curtains, shades, or blinds provide adequate privacy at all times.

Walls in a massage room may be decorated with artwork, and provide a place to hang certificates or anatomy charts. A small wall mirror is useful for clients to check their hair or makeup after massage. Place mirrors so that they do not reflect clients on the table during the massage. A typical massage room is shown in Figure 10–21 ■.

Keep a regular maintenance schedule for removing dust and dirt and cleaning surfaces in massage rooms. Using an electric air cleaner with a filter can help keep dust to a

PRACTICAL APPLICATION

Experiment with various topical substances to become familiar with their different qualities and potential uses for massage therapy. Sample various liniments, oils, lotions, and creams. Use each one in a massage application, and evaluate how it performs and how it compares to others.

1. What are the ingredients in each topical substance?
2. What are the advantages of each for different massage applications? Disadvantages?
3. Do you like some better than others? Why?

FIGURE 10–21
A typical massage room has adequate space for equipment and pleasant decorations.

Source: Istock/Diane Diederich.

minimum. Daily cleaning is a must, with more thorough cleaning on a weekly or monthly schedule.

Lighting and Color

Lighting is another important consideration. Soft and indirect lighting is more restful than harsh and direct lighting. Overhead lighting may shine in the receiver's eyes when he or she is supine on a table, as will the sun if doing massage in an outdoor setting such as at a spa or an athletic event. In places where overhead lighting cannot be controlled, you may provide the receiver with a light shield for the eyes when he or she is supine.

Temperature, Humidity, and Fresh Air

Keep the massage room temperature and humidity at a comfortable level. A good temperature is around 75°F when the receiver is partially or fully unclothed under a drape. A comfortable humidity range is 45%–50%. Lower humidity can cause drying of the skin and difficulty breathing, and damage equipment and furniture.

Clients often get cold during massage as they relax. Ways to help keep them warm include an electric mattress pad underneath the bottom sheet, a heat lamp overhead, or a blanket on top. Turning up the heat in the room is a less desirable solution because the practitioner may then get overheated while working.

Well-ventilated rooms keep air quality fresh and pleasant. This may be a challenge in some places such as hospitals or beauty salons where strong odors are present. Eliminate allergens such as pollen and animal hair as much as possible. Electric air cleaners may be used, and in the summer, air conditioners can help keep air fresh. Wash filters as needed. However, if using an air conditioner, be sure that the room does not get too cold for the client.

Music and Sound

Sound can help create a peaceful and healing environment or a stimulating one. Music elicits certain emotions and is often used to create a particular effect. In general, popular and vocal music should be avoided if the intent is to relax. Use of popular music may also confuse the professional relationship because it is normally heard in social situations. Numerous music recordings are available that are specifically designed for relaxation, some explicitly for massage. Some massage therapists keep special playlists in digital form on an iPod or MP3 player for their massage sessions.

Sometimes it is desirable to have a background of more stimulating music, for example, when the receiver must go back to work immediately or for an athlete receiving massage just before an event. Music that is stimulating, while not stressful or frenetic, is appropriate in these situations. The receiver's taste in music should be taken into consideration and a variety of choices made available.

For some people, silence, or a fish tank bubbling in the background, is most restful. Fish tanks are known to have a relaxing effect on most people. There are also machines that produce "white noise" to mask annoying outside noises.

Safety

The safety of clients is the responsibility of massage therapists. Be aware of potential hazards in the massage environment and minimize them. Make sure that all equipment and furniture is stable and in good repair. Provide adequate lighting. Remove objects that clients might fall over or slip on. Make sure that wall hangings are secure and that room dividers or screens will not fall over. Watch out for sharp edges on furniture, walls, doors, and other places that can cause harm. If something spills, wipe it up immediately to prevent falls.

FIGURE 10.22 Wash all surfaces in a massage room daily, including the massage table.

Source: Pearson Education, Inc./Segal Photography.

There is a special responsibility with clients who are disabled or elderly. Help them onto and off of the massage table as necessary to prevent falls.

Although "slip-and-fall" insurance protects you legally when accidents occur, you may be considered liable for injuries if you are deemed to have been negligent in your duty to provide a safe environment.

Maintenance Schedule

Overall cleanliness and neatness of the space where massage is given is essential. Not only does this provide a sanitary environment for the recipient, but also it helps create a calm, peaceful, and cheerful atmosphere. Neatly arrange oil bottles and wipe them clean. Stack and store clean linens. Place used sheets and towels in a closed container, and keep them out of sight. Clean floors, vacuum carpets, and dust furniture regularly. Set time aside at the beginning and end of the day to care for the space. See Figure 10–22 ■. A checklist of daily maintenance tasks is provided in Box 10–1 ■.

There may be local health department regulations concerning sanitation in places where massage is provided. Requirements sometimes include washable floors, floors disinfected regularly, sheets and towels stored away, and other rules.

BOX 10–1	**Massage Room Daily Maintenance Checklist**

✓ Clean all furniture surfaces (e.g., tabletops, chairs).
✓ Wipe off oil and lotion bottles.
✓ Clean massage table upholstery.
✓ Stack and store clean linens out of sight.
✓ Remove dirty linens and store in closed container.
✓ Empty wastebaskets.
✓ Clean or vacuum floors.

INFECTION CONTROL

The hygiene and sanitation measures discussed throughout this chapter help prevent infections from disease-causing organisms in the massage environment. This applies to the massage school setting, as well as to a future massage practice. Infections can spread in school as students practice massage on one another and also in student clinic. Infection control measures are important from the first day in massage school.

Two final topics related to infection control focus on less common situations, but important ones nonetheless because of their potential seriousness. These are universal precautions and MRSA.

Universal Precautions

The aim of **universal precautions**, sometimes called *standard* or *sanitary precautions*, is to prevent the transmission of serious communicable diseases. Among these are HIV, hepatitis B, and other blood- and fluid-borne pathogens. Although massage therapists are generally at low risk for coming into contact with blood and body fluids, it is prudent to know the standard precautions related to sanitation. Massage therapists who work in skilled nursing facilities, hospitals, hospice, or

---

CASE FOR STUDY

Alina and Sanitation on the Road

Alina has a number of home-visit clients in her massage therapy practice. That means she must carry whatever she needs for massage to the client's home in her car. She has become more concerned recently about hygiene and sanitation and wants to establish a more thorough cleaning and maintenance plan.

Question:

What might the elements of a thorough hygiene and sanitation plan look like for a home-visit massage practice?

Things to consider:

- What personal hygiene measures must be set up for a home visit?

- How might Alina plan for carrying clean linens? Removing used linens? Avoiding contamination of topical substances?
- What are some potential areas of difficulty for sanitation during a home visit session?
- What cleaning products might she need to have on hand, and how might she carry them around?
- How might she best care for and sanitize her equipment?

Write a brief description of a hygiene and sanitation plan for Alina's home-visit massage practice.

_____

_____

_____

with the elderly or with athletes at competitive events have a special need to know about universal precautions.

Universal precautions apply to body fluids such as blood, semen and vaginal/cervical secretions, urine, feces, and vomit. They do not apply to nasal secretions, saliva, sweat, tears, and sputum, unless they contain visible blood. The risk of transmission of serious diseases from these latter substances is extremely low or negligible. Basic sanitary precautions are as follows:

1. Use protective barriers such as latex or nonlatex gloves to prevent contact with body fluids to which universal precautions apply. When removing gloves that have touched such fluids, hold them at the wrist and turn them inside out. This keeps the fluids from contact with the outside.

2. If your skin comes in contact with body fluids to which universal precautions apply, wash the area with a bleach solution of 1 part bleach to 10 parts water, or comparable disinfecting solution (Figure 10–23 ■).

3. If other surfaces, such as the massage table or chair, are exposed to contamination, immediately wash the surface with the bleach solution described. Wear protective gloves when washing the surface.

4. If sheets or towels come into contact with body fluids for which universal precautions apply, place them into a plastic bag separate from other laundry. Wear protective gloves. Wash the sheets or towels in a disinfecting solution.

MRSA

MRSA stands for *methicillin-resistant Staphylococcus aureus*, which is a drug-resistant bacterial infection typically found on the skin but which can occur elsewhere in the body. MRSA (pronounced *mersa*) has become a serious problem in hospitals, schools, athletic facilities, and other places where people come in close contact or may share personal items such as towels and razors. If detected and treated early, MRSA is less difficult to control.

MSRA is a staph infection that is spread by direct contact with another person's infection or by contact with items

10 parts water

1 part bleach

FIGURE 10–23 A good disinfecting solution you can make yourself consists of 1 part bleach to 10 parts water.

that have touched an infection. MSRA appears as a bump or infection on the skin that is red, swollen, warm, painful, and with pus or other drainage. It is sometimes accompanied by a fever. If MRSA is suspected, cover the area and see a health care professional immediately. If you detect a suspicious bump or infection on a client, avoid touching the area and ask the client about the condition. Remember that fever is a general contraindication for massage. If you detect a suspicious skin condition while in school, tell a teacher or administrator immediately so that he or she can follow up to prevent potential infection in the school.

For further information on infection control visit the U.S. Department of Health and Human Services, Centers for Disease Control and Prevention (CDC) website (http://www.cdc.gov).

CHAPTER HIGHLIGHTS

- A massage therapist's good personal hygiene helps the client feel comfortable with him or her and prevents the spread of disease.
- Massage practitioners wash their hands thoroughly (hygienic hand washing) before and after each session to prevent the spread of pathogens.
- When choosing a massage table, consider the type of massage or bodywork for which it will be used and the setting.

- Evaluate the massage table for type (stationary or portable), height, width, length, padding, upholstery, weight, strength (operating capacity), and ease of set up and take down.
- Special massage tables with hinged tops for semi-reclining positioning or other special features are available.

- ○ Choose a professional-grade massage table, and check out table models at showrooms, at trade shows or conventions, or on table manufacturers' websites.

- Massage chairs are specially designed to provide maximum comfort while receiving massage in a seated position while fully clothed.
  - ○ Massage chairs have a seat, knee rests, armrest, chest cushion, and face cradle.
  - ○ When choosing a massage chair, consider its overall design, ease of setup and carrying, weight, stability, adjustments, and special features.

- Follow manufacturer's instructions for proper care of massage tables and chairs.
  - ○ Clean upholstery regularly, but avoid using harsh chemicals.
  - ○ Set up tables and chairs carefully to avoid damage to them.
  - ○ Do not sit directly in the center of a portable massage table over the hinge.
  - ○ Check nuts, bolts, and other hardware regularly and tighten or fix as needed.

- Sheets, blankets, and towels are supplies needed by massage therapists.
  - ○ Sheets are typically used for draping and should be easily washable.
  - ○ Blankets are used for added warmth.
  - ○ Various size towels are useful in massage therapy for draping, bolstering, wiping off oil, cleaning up spills, hot and cold applications, and other uses.

- Many forms of massage and bodywork use some kind of topical substance (liniments, oils, lotions, creams, or combinations of these) to enhance their effects or to minimize skin friction during the application of techniques.
  - ○ Sanitation measures related to topical substances help prevent cross-contamination and the spread of disease.
  - ○ Wipe off bottles and jars after each session.
  - ○ Use oil bottles with closeable spouts, and keep them closed between uses.
  - ○ Use pump jars for dispensing lotion.
  - ○ Do not dip your fingers into a jar to remove creams; instead, take out what you intend to use with a little spatula, and place it on a small plate or piece of paper.

- Important factors to consider in creating the physical environment for massage include the configuration of the room, floor, wall, and window coverings, lighting and color, temperature and air quality, music or tranquil sounds, and dressing arrangements.
- Temperature, ventilation, lighting, and sound in a room can help set the tone for massage.
- Eliminate safety hazards in the massage environment such as slip-and-fall hazards.
- Set up a regular maintenance schedule for dusting, washing equipment, and cleaning floors and furniture in your massage room.
- Universal precautions are procedures for preventing contamination from certain body fluids that can carry serious diseases such as HIV and hepatitis B.
  - ○ Body fluids for which universal precautions apply include blood, semen, vaginal/cervical secretions, urine, feces, and vomit.
  - ○ Body fluids with extremely low or negligible potential for spreading serious disease include nasal secretions, saliva, sweat, tears, and sputum.
  - ○ Wear latex or nonlatex gloves in the presence of body fluids for which universal precautions apply.
  - ○ Wash contaminated surfaces with a bleach solution of 1 part bleach to 10 parts water, or comparable disinfectant.
  - ○ Isolate and dispose of contaminated items (gloves, sheets, towels) properly.

- MRSA stands for methicillin-resistant *Staphylococcus aureus*, which is a drug-resistant bacterial infection typically found on the skin but that can occur elsewhere in the body.
  - ○ Signs of MRSA are a skin bump or infection that is red, warm, swollen, painful, with pus or other drainage, and may be accompanied by fever.
  - ○ MRSA is spread by direct contact with an infected area or contact with an item that has had direct contact with the infection.
  - ○ If MRSA is suspected, cover the area and have the client see a health care professional immediately.

- Good personal hygiene, environmental sanitation, and infection control are serious matters in the massage school environment to promote the health and safety of students, teachers, and clinic clients.

EXAM REVIEW

Key Terms

Match the following key terms to their descriptions. For additional study, look up the key terms in the Interactive Glossary, and note other terms that compare or contrast with them.

_____ **1.** Bolsters
_____ **2.** Equipment
_____ **3.** Hygiene
_____ **4.** Hygienic hand washing
_____ **5.** Massage chairs
_____ **6.** MRSA
_____ **7.** Portable massage table
_____ **8.** Sanitation
_____ **9.** Topical substance
_____ **10.** Universal precautions

a. Drug-resistant bacterial infection typically found on the skin
b. Hinged table that can be carried from place to place and set up and taken down easily
c. Personal cleanliness
d. Removing disease-causing organisms
e. Liniments, oils, lotions, and creams
f. Long narrow pillows or cushions used to support or prop clients
g. Procedures to prevent the transmission of serious communicable diseases
h. Most effective method for preventing the transfer of pathogens during massage
i. Designed to provide maximum comfort for people receiving massage in a seated position
j. Massage tables and massage chairs

Memory Workout

To test your memory of the main concepts in this chapter, complete the following sentences by circling the most correct answer from the two choices provided.

1. The words *hygiene* and *sanitation* refer to procedures that prevent the spread of (disease) (dust).
2. For hygienic hand washing, the water must be (hot) (running) to wash away pathogens.
3. If you have a cut or scrape on your finger, cover it with a (Band-Aid) (finger cot) before touching a client.
4. Keep fingernails clipped short (below) (above) the level of the fingertips.
5. It is a wise investment to buy a (professional-) (personal-) grade massage table.

6. Long narrow pillows used to support or prop clients into position for massage are called (cushions) (bolsters).
7. Used sheets and towels should be placed in a (plastic) (closed) container.
8. Because (lotions) (liniments) contain irritants, rubbing with them too vigorously may cause blistering.
9. Floors in massage room should be able to be washed and (sanitized) (refinished) regularly.
10. The aim of (universal) (therapeutic) precautions is to prevent the transmission of serious communicable diseases.

Test Prep

The following multiple-choice questions will help to prepare you for future school and professional exams.

1. Which of the following statements about hand washing before and after massage is *not* correct?
a. Water must be running to wash away pathogens.
b. Water should be as hot as possible to kill germs.
c. Hands are rubbed for at least 15 seconds.
d. Dry hands thoroughly to prevent chapping.

2. When rinsing off soap in hygienic hand washing, the arm is held at an angle so that water flows from:
a. Wrist to fingers
b. Elbow to fingers
c. Fingers to wrist
d. Fingers to elbow

3. A typical size massage table for Swedish massage is:
   a. 30 inches wide and 73 inches long
   b. 28 inches wide and 80 inches long
   c. 35 inches wide and 70 inches long
   d. 40 inches wide and 75 inches long

4. The width of the base of a massage chair helps determine its:
   a. Agility
   b. Adjustability
   c. Stability
   d. Portability

5. A topical substance that reduces friction during massage and that is readily absorbed into the skin is:
   a. Liniment
   b. Lotion
   c. Oil
   d. Cornstarch

6. Camphor, menthol, rosemary, and cayenne pepper are ingredients commonly found in:
   a. Liniments
   b. Aromatherapy oils
   c. Infant massage lotions
   d. Natural cleaning solutions

7. Comfortable temperature and humidity for a massage room is about:
   a. 55°F and 20% humidity
   b. 68°F and 30% humidity
   c. 75°F and 45% humidity
   d. 82°F and 75% humidity

8. The ideal lighting for a massage room is:
   a. Overhead and direct
   b. Soft and indirect
   c. Bright and direct
   d. Dark

9. Which of the following is *not* a good sanitary practice for handling topical substances?
   a. Using a pump to dispense lotion
   b. Wiping oil bottles clean after each massage
   c. Wiping up spills as soon as they happen
   d. Dipping your fingers into a jar to remove creams

10. Exposure to which of the following body fluid requires use of universal sanitary precautions?
    a. Tears
    b. Blood
    c. Sputum
    d. Sweat

11. The disinfecting solution used as a universal precaution is:
    a. 1 part bleach to 10 parts water
    b. 10 parts bleach to 1 part water
    c. 1 part bleach to 1 part water
    d. 100% bleach

12. MRSA is:
    a. A disinfectant cleaning solution
    b. A blood-borne disease-causing agent
    c. A drug-resistant staph infection
    d. A universal precaution procedure

Video Challenge

Watch this video, which can be found at MyHealthProfessionsLab.com, Chapter 10, and then answer the following questions.

Hygienic Hand Washing

1. How did the person in the video begin the hygienic hand washing procedure?

2. How would you describe the method of cleaning the fingernails shown in the video?

3. How did the person in the video turn off the water faucet?

Comprehension Exercises

The following short-answer questions test your knowledge and understanding of chapter topics and provide practice in written communication skills. Explain in two to four complete sentences.

1. Describe the steps in hygienic hand washing. How is this different from ordinary hand washing?

2. Describe the important features of a portable massage table. What are the dimensions of a standard massage table for Swedish massage?

3. Explain universal precautions. What body fluids are of concern? How would you handle sheets that were contaminated?

For Greater Understanding

The following exercises are designed to take you from the realm of theory into the real world. They will help give you a deeper understanding of the subjects covered in this chapter. Action words are underlined to emphasize the variety of activities presented to address different learning styles and to encourage deeper thinking.

1. Evaluate different models of massage chairs. Note special features of each, and do a comparison of different models.

2. Take an inventory of your own massage therapy equipment and supplies. Note your method of storage and transport. Develop a maintenance plan for keeping them neater, cleaner, and more sanitary.

3. Visit a spa, health club, or other facility that offers massage therapy. Note the massage room setup, windows, walls, floors, lighting, sound, and air quality. Ask about hygiene and sanitary procedures. Evaluate your findings, and identify ways you might change that environment to make it more comfortable and safe for clients.

MyHealthProfessionsLab™

MyHealthProfessionsLab.com is a premium online homework management system that includes a host of features to help you study. Registered users will find:

- Powerful tools that track and analyze your results—allowing you to create a personalized learning experience
- Videos, flashcards and other learning tools to help enrich your progress
- Streaming lesson presentations and self-paced learning modules
- A space where you and your instructors can view and manage your assignments

Body Mechanics, Table Skills, General Guidelines

Pearson Education, Inc.

CHAPTER OUTLINE

Learning Outcomes

Key Terms

Principles of Hand and Body Mechanics

Preventing Injury and Overuse

Hand Mechanics for Different Techniques

Body Mechanics for Table Massage

Body Mechanics for Seated/Chair Massage

Table Skills

Positioning

Draping

General Guidelines for Massage

Chapter Highlights

Exam Review

LEARNING OUTCOMES

After studying this chapter, you will have information to:

1. Practice good body mechanics and self-care.
2. Describe proper body mechanics for table massage.
3. Describe proper body mechanics for seated massage.
4. Use good hand mechanics for different massage applications.
5. Vary hand positions during massage to lessen strain.
6. Assist clients onto and off of the table as needed.
7. Position clients for safety, comfort, and accessibility.
8. Perform draping techniques skillfully.
9. Analyze massage application elements.

KEY TERMS

Body mechanics

Bow and arrow stance

Bracing

Draping

Hand mechanics

Horse riding stance

Neutral position

Positioning

Specificity

Stacking the joints

Table skills

Tenting

PRINCIPLES OF HAND AND BODY MECHANICS

Practicing good body and hand mechanics is essential for your well-being and longevity as a massage therapist. **Body mechanics** refers to the overall alignment and use of the body while performing massage. Good body mechanics minimize shoulder, neck, and back problems, as well as injuries to the arms and hands. Good **hand mechanics** minimize strain on the fingers, thumb, and wrist.

A major concern for those performing massage on a regular basis is avoiding strain and overuse injuries. To prevent injuries, special attention must be paid to the care of the hands and wrists and to practicing good body mechanics.

PREVENTING INJURY AND OVERUSE

Avoiding undue strain and overuse injuries is accomplished in a number of ways. Being in good physical condition and using good hand and body mechanics are essential. See Chapter 4, *Physical Skills, Fitness, Self-Care for the Massage Therapist*, for information on physical fitness.

Common upper-body injuries for massage practitioners include repetitive strain injuries such as tendinitis and nerve impingement syndromes such as carpal tunnel and thoracic outlet. In addition to strengthening and stretching exercises, self-massage and hydrotherapy can head off injuries due to the wear and tear of giving massage (Figure 11–1 ■).

The beginning of a massage session can serve as a warm-up for the practitioner. It is like an athlete doing warm-ups before a competition. Begin the session slowly, and gradually increase pressure and pace. This benefits both the giver and receiver and eases both into the massage.

Using a variety of techniques in a session helps minimize repeated strain on a particular joint or body area. Some massage techniques are less strenuous than others, for example, light effleurage and passive touch. More strenuous techniques, such as compression and kneading, can be alternated with less stressful ones to provide a resting phase to a session. At the end of a session, the hands may feel hot or "charged" with energy. Running cold water over the wrists and hands after washing aids in recovery.

The number of massage sessions performed in 1 day and throughout the week is also important to take into consideration. The number that can be performed without leading to injury depends on several factors. These include the type of massage given, the practitioner's physical fitness, and the quality of his or her body mechanics. Practitioners starting out in their careers must build strength and stamina to meet the physical stress on their bodies. A sudden increase in the number of sessions given per week can lead to strain, pain, and possible injury.

The following are guidelines for scheduling sessions per week. They project the number of massage sessions that can be given safely by most practitioners.

FIGURE 11–1 Self-massage of the forearm helps reduce the effects of stress on muscles used for massage.
Source: Pearson Education, Inc./Segal Photography.

Schedule no more than:

- Five 1-hour sessions in 1 day, if you work 4 days per week
- Four 1-hour sessions in 1 day, if you work 5 days per week
- Twenty hours of massage per week total

In addition:

- Take 15- to 30-minute breaks between sessions.
- Take an additional 15- to 30-minute break after three consecutive 1-hour sessions.
- Do no more than four 1-hour sessions in 1 day if the type of massage is strenuous.

Hand and Wrist Care

The hands are the primary means for giving massage. Conditioning exercises for the hands, wrists, forearms, and shoulders can help prevent overuse injuries. These include both strengthening and stretching exercises. Different exercise devices can be used to build strength in the small muscles of the hand. See Figure 11–2 ■. Simple strengthening exercises for the hands include squeezing a rubber ball and extending the fingers against resistance using a rubber band. Conditioning is especially important when learning massage and before embarking

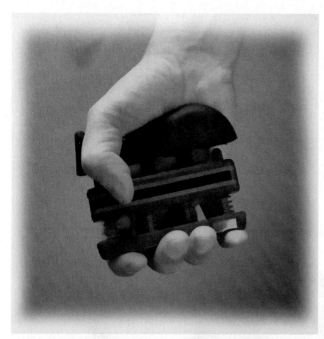

FIGURE 11–2 Hand exercise devices build strength for injury prevention.

Source: Pearson Education, Inc./Segal Photography.

on a full-time practice. Self-massage of the hands and wrists are also beneficial for conditioning and to relieve fatigue.

HAND MECHANICS FOR DIFFERENT TECHNIQUES

Good hand mechanics emphasize joint alignment and efficient movement. Proper alignment reduces stress on hand and wrist joints, and efficient movement prevents muscle fatigue.

The thumb is especially vulnerable during high-pressure techniques such as direct pressure, trigger point therapy, and acupressure. A principle called **stacking the joints** can help protect the thumbs from damage. According to this principle, the bones of the thumb and wrist are lined up so that pressure passes in a straight line through the bones, as demonstrated in Figure 11–3A ■. This avoids pressure applied at an angle to or across the joint, which causes strain on joint structures and tissues. Applying pressure with the thumb abducted is especially harmful (Figure 11–3B ■).

Other parts of the hand can be used to apply techniques, and to avoid strain on the thumb and fingers. A close look at the structure of the hand reveals a variety of points and flat surfaces that may be useful. For example, the point formed at the knuckle of the middle phalangeal joint of the middle finger can be used to apply direct pressure. The flat surface on the back of the fingers of a loose fist or of curled fingers can be used for broad sliding and friction techniques. Hand position variations are demonstrated in Figure 11–4 ■.

Keep the wrist in a **neutral position** (i.e., neither flexed nor extended) as much as possible when applying massage techniques (see Figure 11–5 ■). For compression techniques, avoid hyperextension of the wrist. To reinforce one hand with the other during compression techniques, place the top hand directly over the metacarpals of the bottom hand as demonstrated in Figure 11–6A ■. Do not hold onto the bent wrist (Figure 11–6B ■), or hyperextend the wrists (Figure 11–6C ■).

The elbow and forearm can be very useful for applying heavier pressure to large muscles. For example, the forearm can be used to apply broad effleurage to the thighs or back muscles as demonstrated in Figure 11–7 ■.

A

B

FIGURE 11–3 Stacking the joints. A. Correct thumb–wrist alignment for applying direct pressure. B. Incorrect position with thumb abducted will cause injury to the joints.

Source: Pearson Education, Inc./Segal Photography.

C

FIGURE 11–4 Different hand positions and working surfaces for massage applications on large muscles. A. Flat surface between second and third finger joints. B. Point of second joint of the middle finger. C. Loose fist.

Source: Pearson Education, Inc./Segal Photography.

BODY MECHANICS FOR TABLE MASSAGE

Good body mechanics help minimize shoulder and back problems. A key element is adjusting the table height to fit you properly. A table too high or too low can lead to poor body mechanics and put undue strain on your body. To determine the correct table height for you, stand facing the table with your hands at your sides as shown in

FIGURE 11–5 Wrist in neutral position while performing effleurage.

Source: Pearson Education, Inc./Segal Photography.

Figure 11–8 ■. Adjust the legs so that your knuckles touch the tabletop. Notice your alignment when applying massage at this table height. Further adjust the table height up or down as needed to keep good alignment of the back and neck. For example, when working on large clients you can lower the table somewhat to avoid raising your shoulders when applying pressure downward.

To keep proper back alignment during a massage session, bend the knees to lower your body. Avoid bending the back excessively or dropping the head as depicted in Figure 11–9 ■. This puts strain on the upper back and neck muscles. Bend forward from the waist, not from the upper back, to extend your reach, for example, when applying a long effleurage stroke to the leg.

Tai chi stances are effective for keeping good alignment when giving massage. They also position you to use body leverage to apply pressure via weight transfer from leg to leg. This allows you to apply maximum force with the least amount of effort. These stances emphasize keeping the back in upright alignment while using the legs to generate power. Two stances especially useful for massage practitioners are the forward-leaning or **bow and arrow stance**, and the side–side or **horse riding stance**.

FIGURE 11–6 Correct wrist position while performing compression. A. Correct wrist position for compression techniques. B. Incorrect position with pressure directly on the wrist with the other hand will cause wrist injury. C. Incorrect position with wrist hyperextended will cause wrist injury.

Source: Pearson Education, Inc./Segal Photography.

FIGURE 11–7 Use of forearm for performing effleurage on the hamstring muscles.

Source: Pearson Education, Inc./Segal Photography.

FIGURE 11–8 Determining a good table height. Stand facing the table with your hands at your sides. Adjust the table legs so that your knuckles touch the tabletop.

Source: Pearson Education, Inc./Segal Photography.

FIGURE 11–9 Incorrect body alignment with back bent and head forward.

Source: Pearson Education, Inc./Segal Photography.

The bow and arrow stance is used when facing the head or foot of the table as demonstrated in Figure 11–10A ■. Both feet face the direction of movement. Notice that the legs are bent to lower the body, and the leg closest to the table is behind and turned out slightly (Figure 11–10B ■). The torso is upright. Power can be generated by shifting the weight from the back leg to the front leg while keeping the back in alignment.

The horse riding stance is used when facing the table directly. Both feet face the table with head and back in alignment (Figure 11–11A ■). The knees are bent equally to lower the body into position, and the feet are turned out slightly (Figure 11–11B ■). Weight is shifted from side to side as techniques are applied.

A   B

FIGURE 11–10 Good body mechanics when facing the head or foot of the table. A. Head and back in alignment. B. Legs and feet in bow and arrow stance.

Source: Pearson Education, Inc./Segal Photography.

A   B

FIGURE 11–11 Good body mechanics when facing the table directly. A. Head and back in alignment. B. Legs and feet in horse riding stance.

Source: Pearson Education, Inc./Segal Photography.

A   **B**

FIGURE 11–12 Good body mechanics for sitting on chair while performing massage. A. Sit with back and head in alignment. B. Sit near edge of chair with feet flat on floor.

Source: Pearson Education, Inc./Segal Photography.

Sitting on a chair or stool is common when massaging the receiver's head, hands, or feet. This helps minimize strain on the body. Sit near the edge of the seat with the feet flat on the floor and upper body upright as shown in Figure 11–12 ■. Adjust the height of the chair to allow you to keep your wrists in a neutral position.

BODY MECHANICS FOR SEATED/CHAIR MASSAGE

The principles of good hand and body mechanics are the same whether the client is lying on a massage table or seated in a chair. Keeping the back upright and neck in good alignment are essential. Avoid hyperextending the wrists and applying pressure with the thumb abducted. Bend the knees, not the back, to lower the body.

With the client more or less vertical in the chair, you will experience some differences in body mechanics compared to working on a person who is horizontal on a table. You must be able to reach up to the head, as well as down to the hands. The bow and arrow stance and horse stance described in the preceding section are ideal for such changes in level. Using a wider stance and bending the knees more lowers the body. Shortening the stance and straightening the legs raises the body. You can rise up on your toes for brief periods to gain more height. Avoid raising the shoulders when reaching upward.

 CASE FOR STUDY

Nadia and Preventing Overuse Injuries

Nadia is finishing massage school in a few months and plans to begin a job at a spa when she graduates. She has recently begun to get pains in her hands and wrists and has a lot of tension in her upper back after giving massage in class.

Question:

What can Nadia do to minimize the negative effects she is feeling from giving massage?

Things to consider:

● What aspects of body and hand mechanics might be causing her problems?
● What fitness exercises can she do to condition her body and especially her hands?
● How can she build up to a job doing massage full-time?

What advice would you give Nadia as she prepares for her job at the spa?

_____

_____

FIGURE 11–13 Good hand and body mechanics when applying thumb pressure to the back.

Source: Pearson Education, Inc./Segal Photography.

FIGURE 11–14 Use of the forearm to apply pressure to points on the upper trapezius muscle.

Source: Pearson Education, Inc./Segal Photography.

Pressing into the recipient's back calls for more forward motion, rather than downward. Shift your weight forward, pushing from the rear leg to generate power. Joints are stacked from the shoulder through the elbow, wrist, and thumb when applying thumb pressure to the back, as shown in Figure 11–13 ∎.

Applying pressure down onto the upper trapezius muscle can be done with the forearm. Lean your body weight into the forearm by sinking at the knees. The point of the elbow can be used with sensitivity to apply pressure to specific points. See Figure 11–14 ∎.

Massage of the arms and hands requires lowering your body significantly. Options for keeping good alignment include sinking the knees farther in the bow and arrow stance, or kneeling on one or both knees. See Figure 11–15 ∎. If a chair or stool is accessible, massage of the arms and hands can be given from a sitting position.

With practice, keeping good body alignment becomes second nature. It may take a little experimentation at first to discover the most effective body mechanics for seated massage.

FIGURE 11–15 Kneeling on one knee to keep good alignment when massaging the arms and hands.

Source: Pearson Education, Inc./Segal Photography.

PRACTICAL APPLICATION

Experiment with different ways to apply effleurage or sliding techniques to various areas on a practice client. Focus on ease of application and avoiding strain on your body.

1. How do you maintain good overall body alignment when applying sliding techniques?
2. How do you apply effleurage to a long leg or arm without leaning forward too much?

3. What are different hand positions and surfaces you can use for different areas, for example, effleurage on the arm, shoulder, foot, neck, or face?
4. Repeat the experiment with different massage techniques such as kneading and compression.

TABLE SKILLS

Table skills include a variety of actions required to position and drape a client properly on a massage table. The goals of table skills include the safety and comfort of the receiver and accessibility of different parts of the body for massage applications.

Assistance Getting Onto and Off of the Table

Occasionally clients need assistance getting onto the massage table before the session, and off the table afterward. These include people with disabilities, the elderly, and pregnant women. Ask the client if he or she wants assistance, but take responsibility for helping anyone you believe needs assistance to be safe.

Keep a step stool available for use by clients. Make sure that it is stable and has a nonslip surface. If you are tall, and your table is set relatively high, shorter people may need a boost from a step stool to get onto the table safely. See Figure 11–16 ■. If you work in a place with a hydraulic table, you can set the table low for clients to get onto and raise it to the proper height for you before the session starts.

Different clients need different degrees of assistance. In some cases, you might only need to stand close by to assist if necessary. Stand close enough to be able to react effectively if a client loses balance or cannot complete the movement he or she is attempting. In other cases, you might have to hold onto the client's arm, and/or put your arm around his or her shoulder while guiding the person onto or off the table.

For weak or frail individuals, a higher degree of assistance may be called for. In these cases, you can help clients to a sitting position on the side of the table, and then support

FIGURE 11–16 Step stool can help clients get onto and off of a high table.

Source: Pearson Education, Inc./Segal Photography.

their backs and heads as they lie down. They may also need help getting their legs up onto the table.

The reverse works well for getting off the table. Stand to the side of the table and put one arm around the client's shoulder, and the other under his or her knees (Figure 11–17 ■). As he or she attempts to sit up, offer as much assistance as necessary. Keep the drape covering the client during this process. Have him or her sit on the side of the table for a moment, especially if dizzy. Hold onto the client while he or she steps onto the stool and floor.

FIGURE 11–17
Assistance in getting off the massage table.

Source: Pearson Education, Inc./Segal Photography.

Maintain clients' modesty while you are helping them. In some cases, it might be too difficult for clients to take off all their clothes for massage. They can be assisted onto the table fully clothed and then remove shoes and as much clothing as desired. Drape appropriately for modesty and warmth.

Assistance Turning Over

Clients may need assistance in turning from a supine to prone position or vice versa. A skill called **tenting** keeps clients from getting rolled up in the drape. To create a tent, pin one side of the sheet against the table with your leg or hip. Then lift the sheet so that the client can turn over underneath the drape. Have him or her turn away from you. The client should be out of your sight and the sight of anyone else in the room, while turning over. See Figure 11–18 ■.

If clients have trouble turning over by themselves, you might consider using the semireclining, side-lying, or seated positions instead of supine and prone. This may be preferable for certain special populations such as the elderly and people with disabilities.

POSITIONING

Placing the receiver in a comfortable and safe position on the table, called **positioning**, is essential for effective application of massage. The recipient's position can also allow easier access to particular muscles or regions of the body.

The receiver should not have to exert muscular effort to stay in position or to hold draping in place. Various size bolsters, pillows, or rolled towels are used to support body areas and position receivers properly. See Chapter 10, *Hygiene, Equipment, Environment*, for more information about bolsters and pillows.

FIGURE 11–18 Creating a tent for turning from prone to supine or vice versa. Pin one side of the sheet against the table with the leg or hip, and lift the sheet so that the recipient can turn over underneath the sheet.

Source: Pearson Education, Inc./Segal Photography.

FIGURE 11–19 Supine position. Placement of bolsters under the knees and neck.

Source: Pearson Education, Inc./Segal Photography.

Supine

In the supine or faceup position, a bolster placed under the knees takes pressure off the lower back. A neck roll is sometimes used for support in the cervical area. This can be a small bolster or rolled-up towel. See Figure 11–19 ■.

If the table is wide enough, clients' arms can lie alongside them on the table. If the table is narrow, clients can rest their hands on their abdomen. Attachable side extenders are available to widen a table temporarily at the arms if needed. Sometimes clients' arms do not lie flat on the table due to their structure or muscular tightness. In those cases, small bolsters or rolled towels can be placed under the wrists or hands for support.

Prone

In the prone or facedown position, support is placed under the ankles to take pressure off them. Small pillows may be placed under the shoulders for people with large chests. See Figure 11–20 ■. Positioning women with large breasts is discussed in Chapter 18, *Special Populations and Adaptations*.

Face Cradle Adjustment

When a client is lying prone, using an adjustable face cradle provides the most options for positioning. Note that some face cradles are not adjustable and extend straight out from the table. This limits positioning and is less desirable for professional massage.

FIGURE 11–20 Prone position. Placement of bolsters under ankles and shoulders, head supported by face cradle.

Source: Pearson Education, Inc./Segal Photography.

Most modern face cradles have two adjustments. One adjustment elevates and lowers the entire face cradle, and the other controls the angle. First adjust the face cradle height so that the head is in proper alignment with the spine, and then adjust the angle so that the face is tilted slightly downward. This opens the shoulder and neck region for better access. Avoid hyperextending or flexing the neck too much when adjusting the face cradle. Figure 11–21 ■. Always ask clients if the adjustment is comfortable for them. Practice adjusting the face cradle with different body types to learn to perform this essential table skill quickly and effectively. See Figure 11–22 ■.

Side-Lying and Semireclining

For the side-lying position, have the client straighten out his or her lower leg on the table and bend the upper leg at the hip and knee. Place one or two pillows under the upper leg for support. Ideally, from the knee down the upper leg ends up parallel to the table, which keeps the pelvis and spine in

FIGURE 11–21 Face cradle adjustment for comfort of receiver.

Source: Pearson Education, Inc./Segal Photography.

good alignment. Place another pillow under the upper arm. Some clients like to hug the pillow with both arms, whereas others prefer to place the lower arm on the table near the head. A pillow or bolster supports the head and keeps the

A

B

C

FIGURE 11–22 Positioning the face cradle. A. Neck in proper alignment. B. Avoid hyperextension. C. Avoid too much flexion.

Source: Pearson Education, Inc./Segal Photography.

FIGURE 11–23 Side-lying position. Placement of bolsters under the superior leg, arm, and head.

Source: Pearson Education, Inc./Segal Photography.

neck in good alignment. The face cradle pad can be used for this purpose. See Figure 11–23 ▪.

For the semireclining position, the client is sitting up at a 30- to 60-degree angle. A backrest is created either by adjusting a special hinged table or by propping the recipient up with a wedge-shaped bolster. A long round or quarter-round bolster is placed under the knees to prevent hyperextension. The arms lie alongside the body or may be placed on the abdomen. A pillow is used under the head if needed for comfort. See Figure 11–24 ▪.

Seated

Seated massage is given with the client positioned in a special massage chair or in a regular chair adapted for the purpose. Special massage chairs offer the best options for receiving massage in the seated positionand are described in detail in Chapter 10, *Hygiene, Equipment, Environment*.

Positioning in regular chairs is less than ideal but necessary in some cases. The use of regular household or folding chairs typically occurs in special circumstances. Examples are massage at a health fair, in offices at employee desks, with athletes at events, or at institutions such as senior centers.

If a massage chair is unavailable, choose a sturdy regular chair with a low back and comfortable seat. Clients should be able to place their feet flat on the floor. If the feet do not touch the floor, place a support under them so that the thighs are level. The rest of the positioning depends on the massage application.

One option for foot massage is to sit opposite the client and place his or her foot on your thigh. Place a towel on your leg to protect it from any lotion used. Change the protection for each client. For giving arm and hand massage, use

FIGURE 11–24 Semireclining position. Back supported and placement of bolster under the knees.

Source: Pearson Education, Inc./Segal Photography.

FIGURE 11–25 Bracing the head while applying pressure to the neck.

Source: Pearson Education, Inc./Segal Photography.

an arm chair with a pillow over the chair arm for support. Place a protective covering over the pillow and change it for each client.

Head, neck, and shoulder massage can be given with the recipient in a regular chair with some consideration for bracing. Pressure applied against the posterior neck and back muscles tends to push the client forward. **Bracing** refers to offering a counterresistance to prevent the movement of the body in the opposite direction. You can apply massage with one hand while bracing the client's head with the other hand to resist the push forward when massaging the neck (Figure 11–25 ▪).

Better yet, have clients lean against a table or desk. They can place their forearms on the table and let their heads rest on them. For added comfort, they can place a pillow in front of them and lean on that (Figure 11–26 ▪). Some tabletop massage equipment provides a chest brace and face cradle for use with regular chairs at desks (Figure 11–27 ▪). Remember the basic principles, and use your creativity to provide stability, accessibility, and comfort for massage in regular chairs.

DRAPING

Covering the body during massage, or **draping**, serves to protect the receiver's privacy, maintains clear professional boundaries, and keeps the receiver warm. Skill in draping helps the client feel safe and allows for maximum relaxation. Choose draping material that is substantial enough to provide a sense of privacy and modesty. The use of thin sheets or small, narrow towels can leave the recipient feeling exposed, self-conscious, and uncomfortable.

When clients remove their clothing and are draped for massage, some general guidelines apply. The genitals and women's breasts should be draped at all times. Mutual

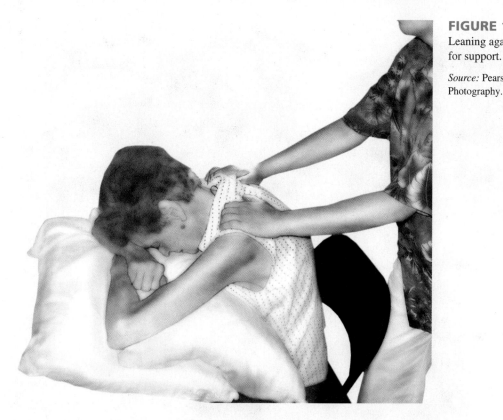

FIGURE 11–26
Leaning against a table with a pillow for support.

Source: Pearson Education, Inc./Segal Photography.

consent or familiarity between practitioner and receiver are not good reasons to ignore this guideline. An exception might be during breast massage, but only after special training in breast massage for the practitioner and with informed consent from the client. Draping can be adjusted to allow

FIGURE 11–27 Portable tabletop equipment that provides support for recipients receiving massage.

Source: Pearson Education, Inc./Segal Photography.

access to areas close to the genitals or breasts (e.g., attachments to the adductors or pectoralis major muscle), while maintaining clear professional boundaries. This should be done only with informed consent.

Draping with a sheet provides maximum coverage. The part to be massaged is uncovered and then recovered during the session. Skillful tucking will enhance the security of the drape and prevent inadvertently exposing the receiver. Figure 11–28 ■ demonstrates undraping the arm prior to massage.

Preserve the client's modesty when undraping the leg. Lift the leg at the knee and then pull the drape underneath the thigh. Tuck the drape securely at the hip. The genitals, perineum, and gluteal cleft are covered at all times. Figure 11–29 ■ shows draping and undraping of the leg in a supine position, and Figure 11–30 ■ demonstrates undraping and securing the drape for the leg in a prone position.

Prior to massage of a woman's abdomen, the breasts are draped with a towel. This is done with informed consent. To begin, a towel is placed over the breasts on top of the sheet. Either you or the client can hold the towel in place as you pull the sheet down to the waist, exposing the abdomen. The towel remains covering the breasts. Tuck the sheet around the recipient's hips. Figure 11–31 ■ demonstrates proper draping for a woman's breasts.

Large towels may also be used for draping. The same general guidelines for modesty apply whatever type of drape is used.

In some situations, receivers do not remove their clothes, and draping is unnecessary. For example, receivers

A

B

C

FIGURE 11–28 Draping for massage of arm. A. Hold arm to side and tuck drape at ribs. B. Lift arm across chest and tuck sheet underneath the shoulder. C. Place the arm on table ready for massage.

Source: Pearson Education, Inc./Segal Photography.

usually remain clothed during pre- and postevent sports massage, chair massage, and some shiatsu and other energy-balancing sessions.

GENERAL GUIDELINES FOR MASSAGE

There are a number of general performance elements to keep in mind when applying massage techniques. Important elements include the length of sessions, amount of lubricant to use, sequence of techniques and routines, specificity and direction, and pressure, rhythm, and pacing.

Length of Sessions

Session lengths vary depending on the goals of the massage and the setting in which it is given. For example, massage sessions for general health purposes typically last from 30–90 minutes. The most common length is 60 minutes. Seated massage given in the workplace may last from 15–20 minutes. Athletes may receive preevent massage for 15 minutes; however, maintenance or recovery massage may last for 30–60 minutes. Massage that is part of a larger therapy session (e.g., physical therapy) may last for as little as 5–10 minutes. Guidelines for session lengths for different types of massage are suggested in later chapters.

 CRITICAL THINKING

Think about the different positioning options for table massage. Analyze supine, prone, side-lying, and semireclining positions in terms of the client's alignment and the support needed.

1. In each position, what stresses are put on the joints when a client lies on a massage table without support?

2. What shape and size bolster gives the best support for each area of stress?

3. Why does each client's size and unique structure need to be taken into consideration? Give examples.

FIGURE 11–29 Draping for massage of leg in supine position. A. Lift the leg with one hand, and with the other hand pull the drape underneath the thigh. B. Pull the drape snugly around the thigh. C. Tuck top of drape under the hip.

Source: Pearson Education, Inc./Segal Photography.

FIGURE 11–30 Draping for massage of leg in prone position. Pull the drape underneath the thigh. A. Uncover the buttocks muscles without exposing the gluteal cleft. B. Tuck the end of the drape under the hip.

Source: Pearson Education, Inc./Segal Photography.

A

B

C

D

FIGURE 11–31 Draping for a woman's chest. A. Place a towel over the sheet on the upper chest. B. Hold the towel in place while you pull the sheet down to expose the abdomen. C. Tuck the towel securely at the sides. D. The towel remains in place while you massage the chest or abdomen.

Source: Pearson Education, Inc./Segal Photography.

Amount of Lubricant

A good general guideline is to use the least amount of lubricant needed to apply the massage techniques effectively. Too much oil or lotion prevents firm contact and causes slipping and sliding over the surface of the skin. Specific techniques applied to small areas, such as deep friction, use little or no lubricant. Too little lubricant can cause skin irritation, especially for people with fair or thin skin and those with a lot of body hair. Look at and feel the skin mindfully to determine its physical characteristics before deciding what type and how much lubricant to use for the massage.

You may apply more oil or lotion when warming an area with effleurage and petrissage techniques, and then wipe it off for more specific applications. Or you may finish an area by applying additional lotion as a moisturizer if the recipient has dry skin. This will be especially appreciated during dry weather.

The face is an area where little, if any, lubricant is usually needed. Also take care not to get oil or lotion in the client's hair when massaging the neck. Recipients can wear surgical or shower caps to keep lubricants out of their hair.

PRACTICAL APPLICATION

Practice draping for a recipient in different positions; for example, supine, prone, side-lying, and semireclining. Aim for skillful, secure, and effective draping.

1. Can you uncover and recover different parts of the body with ease?
2. Can you drape a woman properly for abdominal massage?
3. Do recipients feel that their modesty is preserved?

REALITY CHECK

LUTHER

LEE: I feel really awkward when I drape a client. The sheets seem bulky, and it is worse when there is also a blanket. And the drape seems to come loose a lot, especially when I am massaging the legs. I keep having to tuck and retuck, which is disruptive to the flow of the massage. What can I do to make draping easier?

LUTHER: Draping is an art in itself. It takes determination, practice, and the right draping materials to do the job smoothly. Make it a priority to become a draping expert early in your training, and good draping will come naturally after a while. First consider the size of your drape. If it is too large, it will hang over the sides of the table too much and will be difficult to handle. You can get sheets made specifically for massage tables or use standard twin-size sheets. Use lightweight blankets such as fleece to minimize bulk, and consider cutting them to hang only about 8 inches over the sides and foot of the table. Don't rush through draping. Take time to tuck securely the first time. Through watching experienced massage therapists in person and on videos, you will see some of the draping tricks developed through the years. Practice and develop your own draping methods. Take pride in learning this skill as much as your massage techniques, and over time draping will not seem like such a chore.

Lubricants absorb into the skin during massage, and the excess can be wiped off afterward. This avoids getting oily substances on the clothes. Some substances stain clothes, and certain scents may be difficult to wash out of fabrics. Rubbing the skin with a dry towel will remove most lotions and oils. Rubbing alcohol can be applied to the skin when more thorough cleaning is desired.

Sequence of Techniques and Routines

Different massage techniques are blended into sequences to create desired effects. Superficial warming techniques precede and follow deeper or more specific technique applications. Smooth transitions between techniques give a skillful feel to a session.

Routines are organized sequences of techniques performed in almost the same way every time. A routine may also refer to a systematic sequence of body regions addressed during the session, for example, starting on the back with the recipient prone and ending on the head with the recipient supine. Practice Sequence 14–1, *Full-Body Swedish Massage*, describes a full-body massage routine that can be used as a model for practice.

Experienced massage practitioners usually establish a routine way of approaching their massage sessions. They vary parts of the routine depending on the needs and desires of the receiver. Routines are useful to establish a smooth pattern or flow for a session. They are also an effective way to learn new massage approaches. Several Practice Sequences or routines for different massage applications appear throughout the remaining chapters.

Specificity and Direction

Many massage techniques are applied over large regions in sweeping movements. For example, the long, sliding strokes of effleurage are often used as a warming technique for large areas such as the back or the entire arm. And muscle groups are often kneaded and stretched, as opposed to individual muscles. This more general way of applying techniques is appropriate for effects such as warming an area, eliciting the relaxation response, relaxing muscle groups, or increasing general circulation. Transition and finishing techniques also usually cover larger areas.

There is greater **specificity** if techniques are focused on smaller areas or specific structures. For example, applying direct pressure with the thumb to a trigger point or deep transverse friction on a tendon are more specific applications. Working with specificity requires thorough knowledge of anatomical structures and good palpation skills.

The direction of technique application may be expressed in terms of general anatomical terminology (e.g., proximal, distal, medial, lateral, superior, inferior). See Figure 11–32 ■. An age-old dictum in massage is to apply deep effleurage to the limbs moving fluids from distal to proximal, or toward the heart. Lighter sliding movements using superficial pressure may be performed proximal to distal as when applying nerve strokes.

Direction also may be described in relation to a specific anatomical structure, for example, toward the muscle attachment. Or it could be said to be along the length of the muscle fibers as in stripping, or across the fibers as in cross-fiber friction. Massage approaches described in later chapters use the concepts of sequence, direction, and specificity to clarify their applications.

Pressure, Rhythm, and Pacing

Pressure, rhythm, and pacing describe different qualities of applying massage techniques. These qualities vary with the desired effect of the application of a single technique, a technique combination, or an entire session.

FIGURE 11–32
Anatomical terms for location and direction.

Source: Pearson Education, Inc./Richard Logan.

Pressure Pressure is related to the force used in applying techniques and to the degree of compaction of tissues that results. The amount of pressure used in any one situation depends on the intended effect and on the tolerance or preference of the recipient. Generally speaking, when applying pressure to an area, it should start out light and then proceed to deeper pressure if desired. This allows tissues to warm up and become accustomed to the pressure. Tissues usually soften as pressure is applied gradually. Removing pressure slowly also allows tissues to adjust to the lightening of pressure over time. Pressure too light may cause tickling, whereas too deep too fast may elicit a tensing response. Either effect is undesirable during massage.

Rhythm Rhythm refers to a recurring pattern of movement with a specific cadence, beat, or accent. The rhythm of massage may be described as smooth, regular, or in some cases, uneven. Rhythm is important for establishing the flow of a session. Working with specificity may slow or stop a regular rhythm, as when stopping to press a tender point. A smooth, flowing, regular rhythm tends to elicit the relaxation response. An uneven rhythm can be stimulating or sometimes distracting. A general rule is to avoid breaking contact with the skin once a session has begun, or to break and resume contact gently, not abruptly.

Playing music during massage sessions can help establish and keep a certain rhythm. Over time, massage practitioners tend to develop their own rhythm for working.

Pacing Pacing refers to the speed of the massage movements. Generally, a slower pace is more relaxing, whereas a faster pace is more stimulating. Relaxation massage tends to be slower, whereas preevent sports massage is faster paced. Applying techniques too slowly and a lack of variation can actually seem boring to a recipient. Choose a pace that accomplishes the intended goals of the session.

The art of massage is the skillful blending of all of these performance elements. Massage practitioners apply techniques with these elements in mind to create healthy, satisfying experiences for their clients. Table 11–1 ■ summarizes the performance elements in the art of massage.

TABLE 11–1	Performance Elements in the Art of Massage
Performance Element	**Description**
Length of Session	Number of minutes from start to finish of a session; general massage: 30–90 minutes, 60 minutes most common; seated massage: 15–20 minutes
Amount of Lubricant	Quantity of lubricant needed to apply massage effectively; use least amount necessary
Sequence of Techniques	Order of techniques applied for desired effects; blended to achieve session goals
Routine	Organized sequences of techniques and order of body regions addressed; modified to address needs of the client
Specificity	Degree of focus on a specific area or anatomical structure; warm area with techniques applied broadly before performing specific applications
Direction	Path of massage application in terms of relationship to the body: proximal, distal, medial, lateral, superior, inferior
Pressure	Force used in applying techniques; prepare area with lighter broader applications before using deeper pressure; modify pressure as needed for the individual client.
Rhythm	Specific cadence, beat, or accent in the application: smooth, regular, uneven
Pacing	Speed of application: slow, moderate, fast; slower more relaxing, faster more stimulating

CHAPTER HIGHLIGHTS

- Good body mechanics minimize shoulder, neck, and back problems, as well as injuries to the arms and hands.
- Good hand mechanics minimize strain on the fingers, thumb, and wrist.
- Using a variety of techniques in a session helps minimize repeated strain on a particular joint or body area.
- Practitioners starting out on their careers must build strength and stamina to meet the physical stress on their bodies.
- Twenty hours of massage per week can be given safely by most practitioners; no more than 4–5 hours per day.
- Take 15- to 20-minute breaks between sessions, and at least a 30-minute break after three consecutive 1-hour sessions.
- Keep the hands and wrists in good alignment while applying massage techniques for minimal strain and injury.
- Stack the joints so that the bones of the thumb and wrist line up, and pressure passes in a straight line through the bones when applying direct pressure.
- Avoid pressure applied at an angle to or across the joint.
- Keep the wrist in a neutral position (i.e., neither flexed nor extended) as much as possible when applying massage techniques.
- To determine the correct table height for you, stand facing the table with your hands at your sides and adjust the legs so that your knuckles touch the tabletop.

- To keep proper back alignment during a massage session, bend the knees to lower your body, and avoid bending the back excessively or dropping the head.
- Use the bow and arrow stance when facing the head or foot of the table and the horse riding stance when facing the table directly.
  - Keep the back in upright alignment while using the legs to generate power by shifting the weight from one leg to the other.
- When sitting on a stool to give massage, sit on the edge of the seat with the feet flat on the floor.
- Body mechanics are adapted for applying massage with the client in a seated position.
  - With the recipient vertical, pressing into his or her back calls for more forward motion, rather than downward, which can be achieved by shifting your weight forward and pushing from the rear leg to generate power.
  - Massage of the arms and hands of a seated client requires lowering your body significantly to maintain good alignment.
- Positioning involves placing the receiver in a comfortable and safe position on the massage table; use bolsters, pillows, and rolled towels for positioning.
- Draping the body during massage serves to protect the receiver's modesty, provide clear professional boundaries, and keep the receiver warm; genitals and women's breasts are draped at all times.

- Massage sessions for general health purposes typically last from 30–90 minutes, with the most common length being 60 minutes.
- Use the least amount of lubricant needed to apply the massage techniques effectively and to prevent skin irritation.
- Massage routines are organized sequences of techniques performed in almost the same way every time.
- Superficial warming techniques precede and follow deep specific technique applications.
- The direction of technique application may be expressed in terms of general anatomical terminology (e.g., proximal, distal, medial, lateral, superior, inferior).
- Pressure, rhythm, and pacing describe different qualities of applying massage techniques.
  - Pressure is related to the force used in applying techniques and to the degree of compaction of tissues that results.
  - Rhythm refers to a recurring pattern of movement with a specific cadence, beat, or accent.
  - Pacing refers to the speed of the massage movements.
- The art of massage is the skillful blending of all application elements.
  - Application elements include the length of the session, the sequence of techniques, and the specificity and direction of applications.
  - Greater specificity means working on a smaller area or specific structure.
  - The rhythm and pacing of massage sessions establish their flow.

EXAM REVIEW

Key Terms

Match the following key terms to their descriptions. For additional study, look up the key terms in the Interactive Glossary, and note other terms that compare or contrast with them.

_____ 1. Body mechanics
_____ 2. Bow and arrow stance
_____ 3. Bracing
_____ 4. Draping
_____ 5. Hand mechanics
_____ 6. Horse riding stance
_____ 7. Neutral position
_____ 8. Positioning
_____ 9. Specificity
_____ 10. Stacking the joints
_____ 11. Table skills
_____ 12. Tenting

a. Minimize strain on the fingers, thumb, and wrist
b. Neither flexed nor extended
c. Placing the receiver in a comfortable and safe position on the table
d. Overall alignment and use of the body while performing massage
e. Keeps clients from getting rolled up in the drape
f. Actions required to position and drape a client properly on a massage table
g. Avoids pressure applied at an angle to or across the joint
h. Forward-leaning stance used when facing the head or foot of the table
i. Tai chi side to side stance
j. Offering a counterresistance to prevent the movement of the body in the opposite direction
k. Covering the body during massage
l. Techniques focused on smaller area

Memory Workout

To test your memory of the main concepts in this chapter, complete the following sentences by circling the most correct answer from the two choices provided.

1. The maximum number of massage hours per week that can be safely given by most massage therapists is (30) (20).
2. When joints are lined up so that pressure passes through them rather than across them, it is called (stacking) (extending) the joints.
3. When reinforcing one hand with the other during compression techniques, the top hand is placed over the (metacarpals) (wrist) of the other hand.
4. The wrist is kept in a(n) (extended) (neutral) position as much as possible when applying massage techniques to prevent strain.
5. The (bow and arrow) (horse riding) stance is used when facing the massage table directly.
6. Actions required to position and drape a client properly on a massage table are called (table) (mechanical) skills.
7. Ask the client to turn over (away from) (toward) you when tenting to avoid getting wrapped up in the sheet.
8. Tilting the face cradle slightly (downward) (upward) opens the shoulder and neck region for better access.
9. A recurring pattern of movement with a specific cadence, beat, or accent is referred to as (pacing) (rhythm).
10. The (science) (art) of massage is the skillful blending of performance elements.

Test Prep

The following multiple-choice questions will help to prepare you for future school and professional exams.

1. Which of the following is *avoided* when applying direct pressure with the thumb?
   a. Stacking the joints
   b. Adduction
   c. Abduction
   d. Alignment with the wrist

2. In the bow and arrow stance, the body is lowered by:
   a. Widening the stance and bending the knees
   b. Narrowing the stance and straightening the knees
   c. Bending at the waist
   d. Bending the knees and the neck

3. Which of the following is the best option for lowering the body for massage applications to the forearms and hands of a person positioned in a massage chair?
   a. Kneeling on one or both knees
   b. Bending at the waist
   c. Taking an extra wide stance
   d. Bending forward and reaching down

4. Broad pressure to the upper trapezius muscle of a person positioned in a massage chair is best applied with your:
   a. Forearm
   b. Fingertips
   c. Palms
   d. Thumb

5. Where are bolsters typically placed to support a client in the supine position on a massage table?
   a. Neck and lower back
   b. Neck and knees
   c. Shoulders and feet
   d. Upper back and knees

6. When sitting on a stool to give massage, position yourself:
   a. Near the back with the ankles crossed
   b. Near the back with the feet flat on the floor
   c. Near the edge with the ankles crossed
   d. Near the edge with feet flat on the floor

7. When lying supine, if a client's arms do not lie flat on the table due to his or her structure or muscular tightness, support can be provided with a small bolster placed under the:
   a. Shoulder or upper arm
   b. Elbow
   c. Wrist or hand
   d. Fingertips

8. In the side-lying position, the upper leg is best supported so that it is:
   a. Perpendicular to the table
   b. Parallel to the table
   c. At a 45-degree angle to the table
   d. Touching the table

9. A good guideline for the use of lubricant for massage applications is:
   a. Use a lot of oil to provide maximum slide
   b. Use liberally for specific techniques such as deep friction
   c. Use no lubricant for people with a lot of body hair
   d. Use the least amount needed to apply techniques effectively

10. Pressure applied too deeply too fast during massage usually causes:
    a. Tension and pain
    b. Tickling
    c. Relaxation
    d. Sliding

Video Challenge

Watch these videos, which can be found at MyHealthProfessionsLab.com, Chapter 11, and then answer the following questions.

Body Mechanics

1. What principles of good body mechanics did you see demonstrated in this video segment?

Positioning and Draping

2. How many bolsters were used, and where were they placed for the side-lying position?
3. How did the massage therapist's draping technique show a sense of respect for the client?

Comprehension Exercises

The following short-answer questions test your knowledge and understanding of chapter topics and provide practice in written communication skills. Explain in two to four complete sentences.

1. Explain the principles of good hand mechanics for reducing stress on the thumb and wrist.

2. Describe the challenges to good practitioner body mechanics when applying massage techniques with the recipient in a more vertical position.
3. Describe proper draping for abdominal massage for women.

For Greater Understanding

The following exercises are designed to take you from the realm of theory into the real world. They will help give you a deeper understanding of the subjects covered in this chapter. Action words are underlined to emphasize the variety of activities presented to address different learning styles and to encourage deeper thinking.

1. Make a video of yourself performing massage for about 10 minutes. Analyze your performance for good hand and wrist care and general body mechanics. Get feedback from observers. Repeat your video performance, making corrections.

2. Observe someone giving a massage, and analyze the performance elements you see. Look at the technique sequence, direction, specificity, pressure, pacing, and rhythm. Explain how these elements put together in a specific application exemplify the art of massage.

3. Experiment with using different amounts of lubricant for a variety of massage applications. Notice how the skin in different areas of the body absorbs the oil or lotion and what effect that has on different technique applications.

MyHealthProfessionsLab™

MyHealthProfessionsLab.com is a premium online homework management system that includes a host of features to help you study. Registered users will find:

- Powerful tools that track and analyze your results—allowing you to create a personalized learning experience
- Videos, flashcards and other learning tools to help enrich your progress
- Streaming lesson presentations and self-paced learning modules
- A space where you and your instructors can view and manage your assignments

PART

3

Tappan's Guide to Healing Massage

Chapter 12

Swedish Massage Techniques

Chapter 13

Joint Movements

Chapter 14

Full-Body Swedish Massage

Chapter 15

Regional Massage Applications—Upper Body

Chapter 16

Regional Massage Applications—Lower Body

Chapter 17

Hydrotherapy and Temperature Therapies

CHAPTER

12 Swedish Massage Techniques

Pearson Education, Inc.

CHAPTER OUTLINE

Learning Outcomes

Key Terms

Swedish Massage Overview

Swedish Massage Techniques

Effleurage

Petrissage

Friction

Tapotement

Vibration

Touch without Movement

Chapter Highlights

Exam Review

LEARNING OUTCOMES

After studying this chapter, you will have information to:

1. Describe the Swedish massage technique categories.

2. Apply Swedish massage techniques for specific effects.

3. Use Swedish massage techniques appropriately within a session.

4. Perform variations of basic massage techniques.

5. Vary rhythm, pacing, and pressure of massage techniques for different effects.

KEY TERMS

Cyriax friction

Direct pressure

Effleurage

Friction

Passive touch

Petrissage

Tapotement

Touch without movement

Vibration

Swedish massage

SWEDISH MASSAGE OVERVIEW

Swedish massage is the basis of most massage therapy performed in North America and Europe today. It is the most common form of massage found in spas, health clubs, and private practice. It is the foundation for therapeutic applications within the professions of massage therapy, physical therapy, athletic training, and nursing.

The beginning of Swedish massage can be traced to the latter nineteenth century. It is the legacy of people like Pehr Henrik Ling (Swedish movements), Johann Mezger (classic European massage), John Harvey Kellogg (massage in natural healing), Mary McMillan (massage in physical therapy), and many others. Swedish massage has been popular in North America for over 100 years. A more detailed view of the history of Swedish massage can be found in Chapter 2, *The History of Massage as a Vocation*.

The effects, benefits, and indications for Swedish massage are understood in terms of the sciences of anatomy, physiology, and kinesiology, and Western beliefs about health and disease. This is in contrast to Chinese medicine, Ayurveda (from India), and other traditional healing systems. The techniques of Swedish massage are effective for improving circulation of blood and lymph, relaxing muscles, improving joint mobility, inducing general relaxation, and promoting healthy skin. See Chapter 6, *Effects of Massage and Research Literacy*, and Chapter 7, *Clinical Applications of Massage*, for more thorough discussions of the science of massage.

SWEDISH MASSAGE TECHNIQUES

Swedish massage techniques fall into seven general categories:

- Effleurage
- Petrissage
- Friction
- Tapotement
- Vibration
- Touch without movement
- Joint movements

This is the same broad classification of techniques used by Kellogg in the late nineteenth century to describe the "procedures of massage."[1] This chapter describes the techniques of soft tissue manipulation, whereas joint movements are described in Chapter 13, *Joint Movements*. The categories of Swedish massage are useful for thinking about how techniques are performed, their physiological effects, and common uses.

Keep in mind that there are an endless number of variations of massage techniques, and the ones presented in this text merely represent a few of the many possibilities. Successful massage therapists develop manual skill in applying a wide variety of technique variations. This gives them more options for accomplishing session goals, as well as providing a more pleasurable and interesting experience for clients. Swedish massage techniques and variations are summarized in Table 12–1 ■.

TABLE 12–1	Swedish Massage Techniques and Variations*	
Technique	Description	Variations
Effleurage	Slide over skin; long smooth strokes	Basic sliding effleurage Stripping Shingles effleurage Bilateral tree stroking Three-count stroking Horizontal stoking Mennell's superficial stroking Nerve strokes Knuckling
Petrissage	Lift, wring, squeeze, press, or roll soft tissues	Basic two-handed kneading One-handed kneading Circular two-handed petrissage Fingers-to-thumb petrissage Skin lifting Compression Rolling
Friction	Rub one surface over another repeatedly	
Superficial friction	Rub hand on skin briskly	Warming friction with palms Warming knuckle friction Warming sawing friction
Deep friction	Shift, broaden, and separate tissues	Cross fiber, parallel, circular Cyriax friction (deep transverse)

(continued)

TABLE 12–1 *(continued)*

Technique	Description	Variations
Tapotement	Percussion with rapid, stimulating movements	Hacking Rapping Cupping Clapping Slapping Tapping Quacking Squishes
Vibration	Oscillating, quivering, or trembling movements	Fine vibration with electric device Deep vibration Light effleurage with vibration Shaking (muscle movement) Jostling (joint movement)
Touch without Movement	Touch without visible movement	Passive touch Direct static pressure Ischemic compression

*A selection of the endless number of variations of basic Swedish massage techniques.

Always perform techniques taking into consideration endangerment sites, contraindications, and cautions, as described in Chapter 8, *Endangerment Sites, Contraindications, Cautions*, and using good hand and body mechanics, as presented in Chapter 11, *Body Mechanics, Table Skills, General Guidelines*.

EFFLEURAGE

Effleurage techniques slide or glide over the skin in a smooth, continuous motion. Pressure may be light to moderate, as when applying oil or warming an area, or may be deep, as when facilitating venous return in heavily muscled areas. Experienced practitioners can perform effleurage in many different ways to suit the body area and to evoke specific effects.

Effleurage is perhaps the most versatile of the Swedish techniques and is used most frequently. For example, effleurage is usually used to begin a session, especially when oil or lotion is applied. It accustoms the receiver to the touch of the practitioner. It is used as a connecting or transition technique. Effleurage is often performed as a break from more specific techniques, to move gracefully from one area to another, to conclude work on an area, or to end the session.

While performing effleurage, a practitioner skilled in palpation can assess the general condition of the soft tissues and the firmness and shape of the musculature. Sensitive fingers may find areas of tension or holding. In some cases where there is pain, effleurage may be the only technique employed.

Effleurage can affect the recipient's body and mind in a variety of ways. The qualities of pressure, pacing, and rhythm may be varied for different effects. For example,

when effleurage is performed with moderate pressure slowly and smoothly on the back, it may stimulate the parasympathetic nervous system and evoke the relaxation response. It enhances venous return in the limbs when performed with moderate to deep pressure moving distal to proximal. Deep effleurage may also provide a passive stretch to a muscle group.

Variations of Effleurage

Basic Sliding Effleurage Basic sliding effleurage is performed with the palms and fingers of the hands, thumbs, fists, or forearms. When using the palms and fingers, mold the hands to the surface of the body. This provides full contact, as shown in basic effleurage of the leg in Figure 12–1 ■. The thumbs may be used in small places

FIGURE 12–1 Basic sliding effleurage using the palms of the hands provides full contact with the leg.

Source: Pearson Education, Inc./Segal Photography.

FIGURE 12–2 Basic sliding effleurage using the thumb gets into the small spaces between the metatarsals of the foot.

Source: Pearson Education, Inc./Segal Photography.

like between the metatarsals of the foot, as in Figure 12–2 ■. More pressure may be applied using the forearms or fists in broad places like the back and hamstrings, as seen in Figure 12–3 ■.

Stripping Stripping is a type of effleurage performed with deep pressure along the length of the muscle fibers, typically done with the thumb. See Figure 12–4 ■. It is commonly performed on the long muscles in the arms and legs, and on the cervical muscles. Stripping is specific to a particular muscle and usually follows the muscle to its site of attachment. If the muscle is wider than the thumb, stripping is performed in parallel lines to cover the entire muscle. Stripping separates and lengthens muscle fibers. It is a useful technique to apply after direct pressure to trigger points.

Shingles Effleurage Shingles effleurage refers to alternate stroking, first one hand then the other in continuous motion, with the strokes overlaying each other like shingles on a

FIGURE 12–3 Basic sliding effleurage using the forearm applies broad, deep pressure to an area.

Source: Pearson Education, Inc./Segal Photography.

FIGURE 12–4 Stripping is performed with deep pressure along the length of a muscle to its attachment. Parallel strips are applied to cover the entire muscle width.

Source: Pearson Education, Inc./Segal Photography.

roof. Fingers and palms make firm contact with the skin. One hand always remains in touch with the tissues as the other hand is lifted. This gives the feeling of unbroken contact. Shingles effleurage is commonly applied to the back with hands parallel to the spine and to the direction of movement as shown in Figure 12–5 ■.

A

B

FIGURE 12–5 Shingles effleurage with hands parallel to the spine and to the direction of movement.

Source: Pearson Education, Inc./Segal Photography.

Bilateral Tree Stroking Bilateral tree stroking traces a pattern reminiscent of branches growing out from both sides of the trunk of a tree. It is usually performed on the back, starting with the hands on either side of the spine and moving laterally across the shoulders or around the sides as far as you can reach. This movement is repeated as you progress to cover the entire back. Fingers and palms make secure contact with the skin. It may be performed standing at the head and progressing from the shoulders toward the hips as shown in Figure 12–6 ■. It may also be done standing at the side moving from hips to shoulders.

Three-Count Stroking of the Trapezius Three-count stroking of the trapezius is performed in three movements, alternating hands with each stroke. Count 1 begins at the origin of the lower trapezius and moves toward its insertion in the shoulder. Count 2 begins just as the first stroke concludes, moving from the origin of the middle trapezius toward the insertion. As soon as the first hand has completed its

FIGURE 12–6 Bilateral tree stroking across the back.
Source: Pearson Education, Inc./Segal Photography.

slide over the lower trapezius, it lifts and crosses over to the origin of the upper trapezius to begin count 3. Count 3 moves laterally to the insertion to complete the sequence. Figure 12–7 ■ shows how the stroke is performed with the

A   B   C

FIGURE 12–7 Three-count stroking of the trapezius.
Source: Pearson Education, Inc./Segal Photography.

practitioner standing on the opposite side. Maintain firm contact with the skin through the entire stroke. The three-count sequence is repeated several times. This particular method of stroking the whole trapezius is rhythmic and relaxing when done well. It must be timed so that despite the lost touch as each hand is raised, the receiver feels unbroken contact.

Horizontal Stroking Horizontal stroking is usually applied to broad, rounded areas like the thigh, abdomen, or lower back. The movement is across the width of the body part, rather than over the length. Horizontal stroking may be considered a hybrid form of effleurage and petrissage because, in addition to sliding, there may be a lifting and pressing motion. Some call this technique *wringing*, as in wringing out a towel.

To perform horizontal stroking on the lower back, stand facing the table at the side of the receiver near the waist. Place your hands lightly on the receiver's back, one hand on each side with the fingers of both hands pointing away from you, as shown in Figure 12–8 ■. Slide both hands toward the spine using firm pressure, and then continue the movement all the way to the other side. One hand will move forward and one hand backward, crossing at the spine. The motion is then reversed without changing the position of the hands. As the hands slide from side to side, they execute a lifting and pushing together of the soft tissues. No pressure should be placed over the spinous processes of the vertebrae as the hands pass over them. Greatest pressure comes with the lift and push together of the tissues as the hands move upward and inward to meet and cross over.

Mennell's Superficial Stroking Mennell's superficial stroking is a light effleurage technique usually performed

FIGURE 12–9 Mennell's superficial stroking over the arm.

on a limb, moving in one direction only—either distal to proximal or proximal to distal—but never in both directions. Use enough pressure to comfortably engage the skin, but not the deeper tissues. To perform it on the arm with the recipient prone, slide your hand from the recipient's wrist to the shoulder while maintaining full contact. See Figure 12–9 ■. Return to the starting position through the air just over the skin surface. Take the same time to perform both the forward and the return movements. Repeat the stroke in a controlled, even rhythm. This should be a gentle, relaxing application.

Nerve Strokes Nerve strokes are another very light effleurage movement. They are performed with the fingertips gently brushing the skin, or they may be done on top of the drape. Nerve strokes can go in any direction and are often used when finishing a section of the body or when ending the session. Be careful not to tickle the client. A few seconds of nerve strokes are usually enough to create a relaxing effect.

Knuckling Knuckling is an effleurage variation in which the pressure is first applied with the back of the fingers in a loose fist, gradually turning the fist over as it slides over the skin, and finishing with the palm of the hand. See Figure 12–10 ■. Knuckling is further described in an early massage textbook:

> Gradually bring the hand from plantar (flexion) to dorsal (hyperextension) flexion. Pressure is not continuous, but swells up and down, starting lightly and becoming stronger, then decreasing again in pressure. The hand must not adhere to the part but should glide over it lightly. Knuckling should only be used where there is enough room for the hand to be applied.[2]

FIGURE 12–8 Horizontal stroking across the lower back.

Source: Pearson Education, Inc./Segal Photography.

A   B

C

FIGURE 12–10 Knuckling effleurage (knuckle to palm) performed on the back.

Source: Pearson Education, Inc./Segal Photography.

PETRISSAGE

Petrissage techniques lift, wring, or squeeze soft tissues in a kneading motion, or press or roll the tissues under or between the hands. Petrissage may be performed with one or two hands, depending on the size of the muscle or muscle group. There is minimal sliding over the skin except perhaps in moving from one area to another when using lubricant. The motions of petrissage serve to "milk" a muscle of accumulated metabolic waste products, increase local circulation, and assist venous return. Petrissage may also help separate muscle fibers and evoke muscle relaxation.

Before performing petrissage, prepare and warm the area, usually with effleurage. Use only a small amount of oil or lotion when warming up the area because too

much lubricant will make it difficult to grasp the tissues during petrissage. If you are working without lubricant, light compressions may be used to prepare the tissues involved.

Avoid pinching or bruising the tissues when applying petrissage techniques, and do not work too long in one area. Adjust the amount of pressure used to match the overall condition of the recipient. Muscular and physically strong clients may enjoy harder pressure, whereas smaller or frail individuals will tolerate less force. Get feedback to adjust pressure to the client's comfort level.

Variations of Petrissage

Basic Two-Handed Kneading Basic two-handed kneading is performed by lifting, squeezing, and then releasing the soft tissues in a rhythmical motion. Hands can either alternate

FIGURE 12–11 Basic two-handed kneading. Tissues are lifted with the whole hand in firm contact.

Source: Pearson Education, Inc./Segal Photography.

FIGURE 12–12 One-handed kneading. Tissues are lifted with the whole hand in firm contact.

Source: Pearson Education, Inc./Segal Photography.

left and right or lift the tissues at the same time. In basic kneading, tissues are lifted with the whole hand in firm contact as shown in Figure 12–11 ■, rather than with just the fingertips. The movement is a lifting away from the underlying bone. Two-handed kneading works well on the larger muscles of the arms, shoulders, and legs.

One-Handed Kneading One-handed kneading may be used on smaller limbs, for example, arms and children's legs. Place your hand around the part, picking up the muscle mass using the whole hand. The kneading movement may be described as circular—grasping the tissues on the up motion and relaxing the hand on the down motion without losing contact. As with two-handed kneading, the rhythm should be slow and regular. Progression to a new position should follow three or four repetitions in the same place. In general, the movements should be performed distal to proximal, and effleurage may be interspersed with petrissage or may follow it, to enhance venous return.

The biceps is a good place to practice one-handed kneading. Grasp the biceps with one hand as shown in Figure 12–12 ■. Let the muscle belly fit firmly into the palm of the hand while the thumb and fingers apply pressure and lift as they begin the kneading motion.

Alternating One-Handed Kneading Alternating one-handed kneading may be used to work flexors and extensors at the same time. For example, on the upper arm, grasp the biceps with one hand and the triceps with the other hand. Alternate lifting and squeezing first the biceps and then the triceps using an even rhythm. See Figure 12–13 ■. Perform this technique rapidly for a more stimulating effect.

Circular Two-Handed Petrissage Circular two-handed petrissage is best performed on broad, flat areas like the

back. This technique may be applied to one side of the spine after warming the area using deep effleurage. Stand facing the receiver from the side and near the hips and be ready to move along toward the head while performing the technique. Place both hands firmly on one side of the receiver's back, with the hand nearest the hips ready to start the movement over the upper portion of the gluteals. Each hand will describe a clockwise circle, timed so that when the hands pass each other, the soft tissues are picked

FIGURE 12–13 Alternating one-handed kneading. Alternate lifting and squeezing biceps and triceps in an even rhythm.

Source: Pearson Education, Inc./Segal Photography.

FIGURE 12–14 Circular two-handed petrissage. Tissues are picked up between the hands as they pass each other.

Source: Pearson Education, Inc./Segal Photography.

FIGURE 12–15 Fingers-to-thumb petrissage. The soft tissues are pressed between the thumb of one hand and the fingers of the other hand.

Source: Pearson Education, Inc./Segal Photography.

up and pressed between the hands. The hands lie flat as they shape themselves to the contours of the back. Pick up tissues between the hands (not *with* the hands) as they pass each other, as shown in Figure 12–14 ■. After one or two repetitions of this technique in one place, slide the lower hand up to where the upper hand has just been working, while the upper hand slides to a new position closer to the head. Eventually, the technique progresses from lower back to upper back, ending over the shoulders. Circular petrissage can also be applied to the forehead using the thumbs.

Fingers-to-Thumb Petrissage Fingers-to-thumb petrissage is a useful way to manipulate the superficial tissues. In this technique, the skin and underlying tissues are pressed between the thumb of one hand and the first two fingers of the other hand, causing the tissue between them to lift. Variations include fingers-to-fingers and loose fists-to-fingers petrissage. Another variation is to form a "V" with the index finger and thumb of one hand and use it to lift and press the enclosed tissues against the opposite thumb. At the same time, the thumb is moving toward, and pressing the tissues against, the fingers of the opposite hand. See Figure 12–15 ■. The technique is applied from place to place over an area with an even rhythm and moderate pace.

Skin Lifting Skin lifting is a technique in which the skin and subcutaneous tissue are picked up between the thumb and the first two fingers and gently pulled away from the deeper tissues. Figure 12–16 ■ shows skin lifting on the back. Once the skin is pulled away, the thumbs may push forward, lifting the tissues in a smooth, continuous motion causing a rolling effect. Skin rolling, a basic myofascial massage technique, stretches the underlying fascia and increases superficial circulation. It is often applied to the back, but may be used on almost any part of the body.

Compression In compression techniques, tissues are pressed or rolled against underlying tissues and bone in a rhythmic motion. The effects are similar to other petrissage techniques, as the tissues are compressed under the hands. Figure 12–17 ■ shows compression using the palm of one hand, while the other hand provides additional force from above. Note that the heel of the top hand is placed so that it does not put pressure on the wrist of the bottom hand. The compressing force is applied through the palms, as you lean into the movement with your body weight. Avoid using just your arms and shoulders to perform compression techniques. Review the principles of good hand and body mechanics for compression in Chapter 11, *Body Mechanics, Table Skills, General Guidelines.* A variation for massaging the large muscles of the buttocks is compression with a loose fist. Rhythmic compression is

FIGURE 12–16 Skin lifting. Superficial tissues are picked up and gently pulled away from deeper tissues.

Source: Pearson Education, Inc./Segal Photography.

FIGURE 12–17 Compression using reinforced palm. The heel of the top hand is placed to avoid putting pressure on the wrist of the bottom hand.

Source: Pearson Education, Inc./Segal Photography.

often used in postevent sports massage because it is easily applied over clothes.

Rolling Rolling is a form of petrissage performed on the limbs. Grasp the limb lightly on opposite sides between the palms of the hands. The muscles of the limb are compressed against each other as the hands press in and perform an alternating back-and-forth motion. Rolling progresses from proximal to distal. In addition to compressing tissues, rolling causes movement in the shoulder or hip joint. See Figure 12–18 ■. The larger your

hands are in proportion to the limb, the easier rolling is to perform.

FRICTION

Friction is performed by rubbing one surface over another repeatedly. For example, the hand is used to rub the skin for superficial warming, as in a traditional rubdown. The resistance to the motion provided by the surfaces creates heat and stimulates the skin.

Friction may also be created between the skin and deeper tissues. In deep friction, the practitioner's fingers do not move over the skin, but instead move the skin over the tissues underneath. Deep friction addresses one small area at a time and adds specificity to the massage by affecting specific structures, such as a particular section of a muscle or tendon. Cross-fiber, parallel, and circular friction are the basic forms of deep friction.

Variations of Friction

Superficial Warming Friction In superficial warming friction, the palm or some other part of the practitioner's hand is rubbed briskly over the skin. This generates heat and stimulates superficial circulation. Variations of warming friction use different parts of the hands to create the friction. Greater pressure may be applied to affect deeper tissues such as when using the knuckles (Figure 12–19 ■) and in *sawing,* also called *ulnar friction* (Figure 12–20 ■). Warming friction is best done dry or with little lubricant because oil or lotion reduces the amount of resistance between the two surfaces and thus reduces the amount of friction. It can be applied over clothing, for example, during sports massage or seated massage.

FIGURE 12–18 Rolling on the arm. Hands on opposite sides of the arm compress and roll the soft tissues and create movement in the surrounding joints.

Source: Pearson Education, Inc./Segal Photography.

FIGURE 12–19 Warming friction using the knuckles. The first two knuckles move back and forth on the skin to create friction in the area to be warmed.

Source: Pearson Education, Inc./Segal Photography.

FIGURE 12–20 Warming friction created with a sawing motion (i.e., ulnar friction). The ulnar sides of the hands move back and forth on the skin to create friction in the area to be warmed.

Source: Pearson Education, Inc./Segal Photography.

FIGURE 12–21 Deep circular friction around the knee with the fingertips.

Source: Pearson Education, Inc./Segal Photography.

Deep Friction Deep friction is used to create movement between the deeper tissues and helps keep them from adhering to one another. For example, tissues of the musculoskeletal system are designed for smooth and efficient movement and should slide over each other without sticking. With lack of movement, stress, or trauma to an area, muscle fibers may stick together or tendons stick to tissues with which they come in contact. Deep friction can help keep tissues separated and functioning smoothly.

Deep friction may also be used to create movement in tissues around joints such as the ankle and knee, reach into small spaces like the suboccipital region, or be used in areas that lack muscle bulk such as on the head. Areas that don't lend themselves well to petrissage (e.g., at tendonous attachments) may be massaged with deep friction. See Figure 12–21 ∎.

Deep friction may be performed in a cross-fiber, parallel, or circular motion. *Cross-fiber friction* refers to deep friction applied across the direction of the fibers, whereas *parallel friction* is applied in the same direction as the fibers. *Circular friction* is performed using circular movements, which move the underlying tissues in many directions. Figure 12–22 ∎ shows cross-fiber friction being applied to the paraspinal muscles.

Deep friction is performed with the tips of the fingers, the thumb, or the heel of the hand, depending on the size of the surface to be covered. For example, small tendons in places such as the wrist or around the ankle may be frictioned with the fingertips. In Figure 12–23 ∎, circular friction is applied with the heel of the hand to free up the broad iliotibial band on the side of the leg.

Before deep friction is applied, warm the area thoroughly using effleurage and petrissage. The lubricant used in the warming-up phase may have to be wiped off before performing friction, to allow the hands to move the skin without sliding over it. Deep friction is a three-dimensional

technique. Practitioners must be keenly aware of the depth at which they are working and the depth of the tissues they wish to affect. If the tissues are just beneath the skin, then lighter pressure is called for. If the tissues are deep or under other tissues then you must "work through" the more superficial tissues. It is helpful to visualize the tissues in superficial to deep layers. You will develop palpation skills that allow you to feel through the layers of tissue. Take care when applying deep pressure. Do not try to "muscle through" more superficial tissues, but instead soften them layer by layer. This process takes patience and sensitivity.

FIGURE 12–22 Cross-fiber friction to the paraspinal muscles. Friction is created by moving the more superficial muscle and connective tissues over the deeper tissues underneath.

Source: Pearson Education, Inc./Segal Photography.

FIGURE 12–23 Circular friction to the broad iliotibial band. The heel of the hand is used to create friction between the skin and the underlying tendon and between the tendon and underlying muscles.

Source: Pearson Education, Inc./Segal Photography.

Friction Used in Rehabilitation

Deep transverse friction or **Cyriax friction** is a specific type of cross-fiber friction that is applied directly to the site of a lesion. It is used to facilitate healthy scar formation at an injury site. The mechanical action across tissues causes broadening and separation of fibers. Cyriax friction is "specifically intended to disrupt and break down existing and forming adhesions in muscles, tendons and ligaments using compression and motion."[3] Deep transverse friction encourages a more parallel fiber arrangement of scar tissue and fewer cross-connections that limit movement. See Figure 12–24 ■.

Deep transverse friction is reserved for subacute and chronic musculoskeletal injuries, (e.g., repetitive strain injuries) and in the remodeling stage of tissue healing. It is contraindicated for acute injuries in the inflammatory and regeneration stages.

FIGURE 12–24 Deep transverse friction (i.e., Cyriax friction) on an ankle ligament.

Source: Pearson Education, Inc./Segal Photography.

Cyriax popularized the use of deep transverse friction in injury rehabilitation.[4] He specified the following principles for treating muscle and tendon lesions:

- The fingers and skin move together to affect deep tissues.
- The effect of friction is most important, not the amount of pressure used.
- The movement must be over the precise site of the lesion.
- The tissue must be in the appropriate tension.
- Do 6–12 sessions of 5–10 minutes each on alternate days. (*Note*: This application is for subacute and chronic conditions only. Begin with 1–5 minutes, and gradually increase the time per session, depending on the tolerance of the recipient and the tissue condition.)

Cyriax also recommended 10–20 minutes of effleurage and gentle friction to prepare the tissues before applying deep friction. This warms the area and makes connective tissues more pliable.

In addition to promoting healthy scar formation, circular and cross-fiber friction around an injury site can help keep normal tissues from adhering to the scarred area. Such adhering of tissues may cause chronic pain or inflammation. This is especially important where there is a large wound, such as after surgery.

TAPOTEMENT

Tapotement consists of a series of brisk percussive movements following each other in rapid, alternating fashion. Tapotement, also called *percussion*, has a stimulating effect and is pleasant to receive if performed skillfully. The most common forms of tapotement are hacking, rapping, cupping, clapping, slapping, tapping, and pincement.

The movement of tapotement is light, rapid, and rhythmic. The hands should "bounce off" the surface as they make contact, lightening the impact. The recipients should not feel like they are taking a beating, but should feel pleasantly stimulated. The percussive sound itself can be pleasing and can add to the therapeutic effect. Different hand positions create different sounds, and different parts of the body sound different when struck. Quacking and squishes described later are nontraditional forms of tapotement that make distinctive, interesting sounds.

Tapotement takes a certain rhythmic ability and much practice to master. The effort to learn it, though, is well worthwhile for the diversity it can bring to your work. Experiment with varying rhythms and hand positions for different effects.

Tapotement is often used in finishing either a section of the body, a side of the body, or the session itself. Because it can be stimulating if received for a short period of time, tapotement is useful in situations in which the receiver must be alert when leaving the session. For example, it may be used if the receiver must drive directly after a session or go back to work. Athletes benefit from tapotement before a competition. Some people simply like the tingling and alive feeling that tapotement can provide.

When applying tapotement, the amount of force to use and the degree of stiffness of the hands depends on the area receiving the technique. Heavily muscular areas like the back and thighs can withstand more force, whereas more delicate areas like the head need a light touch. When performing tapotement over a broad area, as in ending a session on the back of a body, the amount of force used will vary as you move from one section to another.

Variations of Tapotement

Hacking Hacking is performed with the hands facing each other, thumbs up. The striking surface is the ulnar surface of the hand and sometimes the sides of the third, fourth, and fifth fingertips. See Figure 12–25 ■. The wrists, hands, and fingers should be held loosely during the rapid percussion movement. Alternate hitting with the left and right hands. Performed correctly, the effect of hacking is one of pleasant stinging and stimulation.

To practice hacking, shake your hands letting the wrists, hands, and fingers relax and flap up and down. No attempt should be made to hold the fingers together or the hands and wrists in any particular position. If relaxation is complete, you will notice that the hands fall into a neutral plane of motion that neither supinates nor pronates the forearms. Move the hands rapidly, alternating one up and one down, keeping the wrists and hands relaxed. Practice on the back moving from the hips to the shoulders, and then back to the hips again. Never hit hard over the kidneys.

Rapping Rapping, a similar movement to hacking, may be performed using lightly closed and loosely held fists. The fists may be held palms down as in rapping on a door, as shown in Figure 12–26 ■. In side-rapping (sometimes called *beating*), the striking surface is the ulnar side of the fist. Keep

FIGURE 12–26 Rapping. Tapotement performed with the knuckles of a loosely closed fist, as if rapping lightly on a door.
Source: Pearson Education, Inc./Segal Photography.

the force of the blows light and "rebounding" in effect rather than jarring.

Cupping and Clapping Cupping and clapping are applied with the same rhythmic, rapidly alternating force. For both techniques, cup the hand so that the thumb and fingers are slightly flexed and the palmar surface contracted. The thumb is held tightly against the first finger. For cupping, strike the body surface with the outside rim of the cupped hand, keeping the palm contracted, as shown in Figure 12–27 ■. There will be a hollow sound. A slight vacuum is created with each blow, which may loosen broad, flat areas of fascial adhesion. Cupping is also used for loosening congestion in the respiratory system.

FIGURE 12–25 Hacking. Tapotement performed with the ulnar side of relaxed hands.
Source: Pearson Education, Inc./Segal Photography.

FIGURE 12–27 Cupping. Tapotement performed with the outside rim of a cupped hand.
Source: Pearson Education, Inc./Segal Photography.

FIGURE 12–28 Tapping. Tapotement performed with the fingertips of a relaxed hand.

Source: Pearson Education, Inc./Segal Photography.

FIGURE 12–29 Pincement. Tapotement performed by gently picking up superficial tissues between the thumb and the first two fingers with a light rapid movement.

Source: Pearson Education, Inc./Segal Photography.

Let the palm contact the body surface for *clapping*. This produces a less hollow sound and provides a broader contact surface.

Slapping Slapping is performed with an open hand, the fingers held lightly together. Strike gently and briskly with the palmar surface of the fingers, rather than with the whole hand.

Tapping Tapping is done with the ends of the fingers. Sharp, light taps are applied with the padding of the fingers. See Figure 12–28 ■. Light tapping can be applied to the head.

Pincement Pincement is a rapid, gentle movement in which superficial tissues are picked up between the thumb and the first two fingers. It might be described as "plucking."

A rhythm is established alternating left and right hands. See Figure 12–29 ■.

Quacking Quacking is performed with the palms together and fingers loosely apart. The striking surface is the lateral edges of the tips of the fourth and fifth (little) fingers, as shown in Figure 12–30 ■. As the fingers hit the bony surface, they come together, making a quacking sound.

Squishes Squishes are applied with the hands loosely folded, making an air pocket between the palms. The striking surface is the back of one of the hands. As the back of the hand hits, the palms push out the air between them, creating a "squishing" sound.

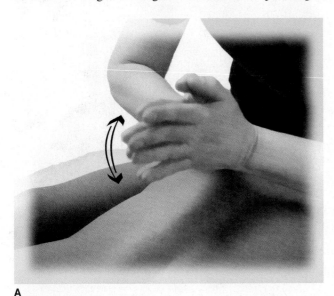

A
B

FIGURE 12–30

Quacking. Tapotement performed with the hands together and fingers loosely apart. Fingers come together as the little finger strikes, making a "quacking" sound.

Source: Pearson Education, Inc./Segal Photography.

REALITY CHECK

DENISE

KIM: When I practice massage techniques, my wrists and fingers don't bend the way my teachers' or the massage therapists in the video bend. And I can't get my hands around larger arms and legs in the same way. Is there anything I can do to make my hands perform more like the professionals I see demonstrating techniques?

DENISE: Everyone's hands are different, so don't expect to perform massage techniques exactly like someone else. Look at the structure of your hands compared to the teachers' or your practice partners. Compare the overall size, the length of the fingers, and the ratio of palm to fingers. See how far your hands can spread and the amount of abduction possible at the thumb. Check out how far your finger and thumb joints extend. Techniques often need to be modified depending on the size and structure of your hand, and the size of the person to whom you are giving massage. Trying to force your hands to move in ways they are not designed for can cause damage. So within the principles of good hand mechanics, experiment with ways to modify the techniques you see demonstrated so that they make sense for your hands.

VIBRATION

Vibration may be described as an oscillating, quivering, or trembling motion, or movement back and forth or up and down performed quickly and repeatedly. The vibration may be fine and applied to a small area with the fingertips. Or it may be coarse and involve shaking a muscle belly back and forth.

Vibration over the abdomen is sometimes used to stimulate the organs of digestion and elimination. Coarse vibration, in the form of jostling, may be used to help a recipient become aware of holding tension, to bring greater circulation to a muscle, and to help it relax. Fine vibration techniques impart an oscillating motion to the soft tissues and have an overall stimulating effect. Applied to a specific muscle for several seconds, fine vibration can also help the muscle relax.

Electronic vibration devices are useful for imparting fine vibration to tense muscles. The motion of vibration can be sustained for a longer period of time with a machine than if performed by hand. There are many types of handheld electronic

vibration instruments. Some impart a coarser vibration, others a finer oscillation. One type of device straps to the back of the hand and causes vibration in the fingers. This allows the practitioner to stay in direct contact with the receiver and perform another technique such as light effleurage or friction. A still finer vibration may be created by sound waves. There are devices that impart a lower frequency wave than ultrasound and are within the scope of practice of most practitioners.

Variations of Vibration

Deep Vibration A deep vibration or trembling motion is imparted through the fingertips, but generated by the forearm. To practice deep vibration, place one hand on a muscle with the fingertips slightly apart. The trembling movement comes from the whole forearm, through the elbow, and the wrist and finger joints are kept in a fixed position. The elbow should be slightly flexed. This vibrating motion should be more in and out than side to side. The fingers remain in contact with the same spot during the vibration and are then lifted off the skin and placed on a new spot. Heavy pressure should be avoided. Deep vibration on the abdomen is shown in Figure 12–31 ■.

Light Effleurage with Vibration Light effleurage with vibration may be used for a soothing effect. Apply the effleurage technique, adding a slight back and forth motion with the fingertips. In areas that are hypersensitive or painful, use gentle contact between the hand and the skin for an overall calming effect.

Shaking Shaking is a coarse form of vibration that can assist muscular relaxation. For example, a muscle such as the biceps or gastrocnemius may be grasped with one hand and shaken gently back and forth. Figure 12–32 ■ shows shaking of the muscles of the leg.

FIGURE 12–31 Deep vibration applied with fingertips to the abdomen.

Source: Pearson Education, Inc./Segal Photography.

FIGURE 12–33 Jostling. A form of coarse vibration that includes mobilizing joints.

Source: Pearson Education, Inc./Segal Photography.

FIGURE 12–32 Shaking. A form of coarse vibration to a muscle or muscle group.

Source: Pearson Education, Inc./Segal Photography.

Jostling In jostling the upper leg, two hands are used, one on each side of the leg. In this case, the muscle movement is back and forth from hand to hand, as shown in Figure 12–33 ■. It is helpful at times to jostle the entire limb gently to mobilize the surrounding joints and encourage relaxation and "letting go" of the whole area.

TOUCH WITHOUT MOVEMENT

Touch without movement is a unique massage technique category. It is defined by touch with the hands, but without any visible movement. Touch without movement is not casual or social touch, but is skilled touch with intention. Kellogg cautions that this is not ordinary touch, but "touch applied with intelligence, with control, with a purpose; and simple as it is, is capable of producing decided physiological effects."[5]

Passive Touch

Passive touch is simply laying the fingers, one hand, or both hands lightly on the body. Passive touch may impart heat to an area, have a calming influence on the nervous system, or as some believe, help balance energy. Historically, the effects of passive touch have been attributed to "hypnotic" or "electrical" effects, "magnetism," and "subtle qualities of manner, a peculiar softness of the hand, or other personal quality not easy to describe."[6] The use of passive touch to balance energy is more fully developed in systems of massage outside classic Western systems.

Passive touch is often used to begin or end a session, or before turning over. It is used effectively for its calming effects when applied to the feet or to the head, as shown in Figures 12–34 ■ and 12–35 ■.

FIGURE 12–34 Passive touch by holding the head lightly.

Source: Pearson Education, Inc./Segal Photography.

FIGURE 12–35 Passive touch by holding the feet lightly.

Source: Pearson Education, Inc./Segal Photography.

CASE FOR STUDY

Hector Chooses Techniques to Address George's Goals

Hector's client, George, wants a massage to reduce stress, enhance general circulation, and address occasional constipation. George has had stiffness in his arm and leg joints lately and wonders if massage can help keep those joints loose and moving freely. George also enjoys the mental alertness he feels after massage.

Question:

What massage techniques might Hector incorporate into the massage session to meet George's goals?

Things to consider:

- Which technique variations directly address each of George's goals for his massage?
- When in the session might Hector address each goal?
- Are some techniques more appropriate to apply at the beginning of the session? At the end? Somewhere in the middle?

Write a brief description of the techniques Hector can include in George's massage session and when they might be most effectively applied.

_____

_____

_____

Direct Pressure

Direct pressure, also called _direct static pressure_, may be applied with a thumb, finger, knuckle, or elbow. Tissues are compressed using light to heavy pressure. Once tissues are compressed, the technique is held for 5–30 seconds, depending on the intent. There is no movement after the initial compression.

Although this text categorizes direct pressure as touch without movement, it might also be considered _static friction_, or a form of compression. _Ischemic compression_, a form of direct pressure applied with enough force to cause blanching, causes vasodilation on release of pressure, thus increasing local circulation. Ischemic compression is used to treat trigger points, as described in Chapter 22, _Trigger Point Therapy_.

Pressure is applied slowly and carefully to avoid bruising or damaging tissues. Direct pressure is often preceded by warming the area with effleurage or rhythmic compressions and followed with effleurage to "smooth out" the area or transition to another place. Figures 12–36 ■ and 12–37 ■ show two different uses for direct pressure.

Direct static pressure to various points is known to relieve pain, diminish congestion, and help muscles relax. Theories about how it works have evolved over the years and include the concepts of zone therapy, motor points, stress points, reflex points, trigger points, and acupressure points. The intentions of practitioners using direct static pressure may differ, and the amount of pressure used, location of areas pressed, and duration of pressure may also vary.

FIGURE 12–36 Direct pressure to suboccipital muscles. Fingers press up into the cervical muscle attachments along the occipital ridge.

Source: Pearson Education, Inc./Segal Photography.

FIGURE 12–37 Ischemic compression (i.e., direct pressure) to a trigger point in the trapezius muscle.

Source: Pearson Education, Inc./Segal Photography.

PRACTICAL APPLICATION

Verbally describe Swedish massage technique variations as you perform them. Explain to the recipient or to an observer what you are doing and why.

1. How are you moving your hands on the receiver's body?
2. How do you describe the manipulation of soft tissues?
3. What effects are you having as you apply different techniques?

CRITICAL THINKING

Think about the different categories of Swedish massage techniques. Compare the categories, noting their essential differences and any similarities.

1. What makes each technique category clearly different from the rest?
2. Does every technique variation fit neatly into only one of the categories?
3. Can you accurately categorize massage techniques that you observe in person or on a video of a massage session?

CHAPTER HIGHLIGHTS

- Swedish massage is the most common form of massage found in North America and is used for a variety of wellness and therapeutic applications.
- Swedish massage is the legacy of historical figures such as Pehr Ling of Sweden, Johann Mezger of Amsterdam, J. Harvey Kellogg of the United States, and Mary McMillan of the United States and Britain.
- Swedish massage is understood in terms of the sciences of anatomy, physiology, and kinesiology, and Western notions about health and disease.
  - It is recognized as valuable for improving circulation, relaxing muscles, improving joint mobility, inducing general relaxation, and promoting healthy skin.
- Swedish massage techniques fall into seven broad categories: effleurage, petrissage, friction, tapotement, vibration, touch without movement, and joint movements.
- Effleurage techniques slide or glide over the skin with a smooth, continuous motion.
  - Effleurage is used to begin a session, apply lubricant, accustom the receiver to touch, connect or transition from one body region to another, assess the condition of tissues, and conclude work on an area.

- The pressure, rhythm, and pace of effleurage is varied for different effects.
- Variations include basic sliding effleurage, stripping, shingles effleurage, bilateral tree stroking, three-count stroking of the trapezius, horizontal stroking, Mennell's superficial stroking, nerve strokes, and knuckling.

- Petrissage techniques lift, wring, or squeeze soft tissues in a kneading motion, or press or roll the tissues under or between the hands.
  - Petrissage is used to increase local circulation, "milk" tissues of accumulated waste products, assist venous return, separate muscle fibers, and evoke muscular relaxation.
  - Variations include basic two-handed kneading, one-handed kneading, alternating one-handed kneading, circular two-handed petrissage, alternating fingers-to-thumb petrissage, skin rolling, compression, and rolling.

- Friction is performed by rubbing one surface over another repeatedly.
  - Superficial friction is used for warming tissues and is performed by rubbing the palms briskly over the skin.

○ Deep friction is used to separate tissues, break adhesions, form healthy scar tissue, or create movement in less-muscled areas, such as around joints and over the head.

○ Deep friction is performed in cross-fiber, parallel, or circular motions.

○ Cyriax friction is a form of deep cross-fiber friction used in injury rehabilitation.

● Tapotement consists of a series of brisk percussive movements following each other in rapid, alternating fashion.

○ Tapotement is used for stimulation and as a finishing technique.

○ Variations include hacking, rapping, cupping, clapping, slapping, tapping, pincement, quacking, and squishes.

● Vibration is an oscillating, quivering, or trembling motion, or movement back and forth or up and down performed quickly and repeatedly.

○ Deep vibration is applied with the fingertips or with an electric vibrator.

○ Coarse vibration is applied with the whole hand over a larger area and includes light effleurage with vibration, shaking, and jostling.

● Touch without movement is defined by touch with the hands, but without any visible movement.

○ Touch without movement is used to impart heat, have a calming effect, or balance energy.

○ Variations include passive touch and holding.

○ Direct pressure (e.g., ischemic compression) is applied to points for a number of effects, including relieving pain, diminishing congestion, relaxing muscles, and stimulating points according to zone therapy, motor points, stress points, reflex points, trigger points, or acupoint theories.

EXAM REVIEW

Key Terms

Match the following key terms to their descriptions. For additional study, look up the key terms in the Interactive Glossary, and note other terms that compare or contrast with them.

_____ 1. Cyriax friction
_____ 2. Direct pressure
_____ 3. Effleurage
_____ 4. Friction
_____ 5. Passive touch
_____ 6. Petrissage
_____ 7. Tapotement
_____ 8. Touch without movement
_____ 9. Vibration
_____ 10. Swedish massage

a. Lift, wring, squeeze soft tissues
b. Stimulating percussion
c. Contact with no visible movement
d. Oscillating, quivering, trembling
e. Legacy of Pehr Ling and Johann Mezger
f. Thumb pressure into soft tissues
g. Deep friction for rehabilitation
h. Rubbing one surface over another repeatedly
i. Long, smooth sliding stroke
j. Laying hand lightly on the body

Memory Workout

To test your memory of the main concepts in this chapter, complete the following sentences by circling the most correct answer from the two choices provided.

1. Classic Swedish massage includes (five) (seven) technique categories.
2. (Effleurage) (Friction) techniques slide over the skin with a smooth, continuous motion.
3. (Pacing) (Pressure) used during petrissage should avoid bruising the tissues.
4. (Superficial) (Subcutaneous) friction generates heat on the skin by brisk rubbing over the skin surface and is done best with little or no lubricant.
5. (Fine) (Deep) friction is applied in parallel fiber, cross-fiber, or circular movements.
6. Tapotement consists of a series of brisk (percussive) (sliding) movements following each other in light, rapid, rhythmic, alternating fashion.
7. Variations of tapotement are achieved by altering (hand position) (force used).
8. Deep vibration or trembling motion is imparted by the fingertips, but generated by (forearm) (shoulder).
9. Sound can be a pleasant aspect of the technique of (petrissage) (tapotement).
10. Sliding along the length of the muscle fibers using deep pressure with the thumb is called (shingles) (stripping).
11. Fingertips gently brush over the drape to finish a session with (nerve strokes) (rolling).
12. A rhythmic petrissage technique applied over clothing and often used in sports massage is (compression) (knuckling).

Test Prep

The following multiple-choice questions will help prepare you for future school and professional exams.

1. The variation of effleurage that is applied with deep pressure along the length of the muscle fibers, often with the thumb, is:
   a. Basic sliding effleurage
   b. Stripping
   c. Shingles effleurage
   d. Bilateral tree stroking

2. Horizontal stroking applied to broad, rounded areas like the thigh and lower back can be considered a hybrid form of:
   a. Basic stroking and vibration
   b. Petrissage and friction
   c. Vibration and tapotement
   d. Effleurage and petrissage

3. If your intention were to increase superficial circulation *and* remove fascial adhesions in the skin on the recipient's back, your best choice of technique would be:
   a. Basic effleurage
   b. Skin rolling
   c. Tapping
   d. Deep vibration

4. The form of tapotement that makes a hollow sound, creates a slight vacuum when applied, and is used on the back and chest for treating respiratory congestion is:
   a. Hacking
   b. Pincement
   c. Rapping
   d. Cupping

5. For ending a session with a calming technique that is also thought to help balance energy in the body, the best choice would be:
   a. Passive touch
   b. Ischemic compression
   c. Fine vibration
   d. Quacking

6. The best technique for moving soft tissues around boney joints like the knee, ankle, and wrist is:
   a. Mennell's superficial stroking
   b. Knuckling
   c. Fingertip friction
   d. Passive touch

7. A form of touch without movement that has also been referred to as *static friction* is:
   a. Deep friction
   b. Direct pressure
   c. Pincement
   d. One-handed kneading

8. In deep transverse or Cyriax friction:
   a. Fingers slide over the skin to stretch deeper tissues.
   b. Fingers and skin move together over deeper tissues.
   c. Friction on the skin increases superficial circulation.
   d. Fingertips move in circular motion around a tender spot.

9. How is full, firm contact best achieved when applying effleurage techniques with the hands?
   a. Hands mold to the surface of the body.
   b. Hands are held stiffly, and only the palms touch the body.
   c. Hands are relaxed, and only fingertips touch the body.
   d. Fingers are spread and rake the skin.

10. Before applying deep massage techniques, tissues in the area should be thoroughly:
    a. Cooled off
    b. Warmed up
    c. Frictioned
    d. Lubricated

Video Challenge

Watch the Swedish Massage Techniques videos, which can be found at MyHealthProfessionsLab.com, Chapter 12, and then answer the following questions.

1. In the video, various types of petrissage are demonstrated on different parts of the body. Why were specific body areas chosen for these petrissage demonstrations?

2. Notice that variations of the tapotement technique make different sounds. Can you describe the different sounds made by these tapotement variations?

3. What do you notice about the color of the receiver's skin in the area of technique application for effleurage, petrissage, and friction? Why does this change in color occur?

Comprehension Exercises

The following short-answer questions test your knowledge and understanding of chapter topics and provide practice in written communication skills. Explain in two to four complete sentences.

1. Describe superficial and deep friction. Why are both of these techniques considered friction? How are they different?

2. What are the possible effects of passive touch? How is it typically used in a massage session?

3. Describe the use of lubricant when applying Swedish massage techniques. How does the optimal amount of lubricant differ among different techniques? Give an example.

For Greater Understanding

The following exercises are designed to take you from the realm of theory into practical applications. They will help give you a deeper understanding of the techniques covered in this chapter. Action words are underlined to emphasize the variety of activities presented to address different learning styles and to encourage deeper thinking.

1. Make a video of yourself performing each massage technique variation. Watching the video, analyze your hand and body mechanics. Perform the techniques again, correcting mechanics. (Alternative: substitute an observer for the videotape.)

2. After developing skill in the techniques illustrated in the book, experiment with your own technique variations. Explain to a practice partner what effects you are trying to accomplish, and why you think your variation would be effective for that purpose.

3. Watch a video of a full-body Swedish massage (or portion of a session) and identify the techniques observed. Describe how the techniques are used in the session (e.g., warming, transition, ending), and their different potential effects (e.g., circulatory, muscle relaxation, general relaxation). (Alternative: substitute a live massage session for the video.)

4. Receive a massage and pay attention to the feel of the different techniques; name them in your mind as they are applied. Notice how they are used by the practitioner.

MyHealthProfessionsLab™

MyHealthProfessionsLab.com is a premium online homework management system that includes a host of features to help you study. Registered users will find:

- Powerful tools that track and analyze your results—allowing you to create a personalized learning experience
- Videos, flashcards and other learning tools to help enrich your progress
- Streaming lesson presentations and self-paced learning modules
- A space where you and your instructors can view and manage your assignments

CHAPTER 13 Joint Movements

CHAPTER OUTLINE

Learning Outcomes

Key Terms

Overview of Joint Movements

Methods of Stretching

Safety

General Guidelines for Joint
  Movement Techniques

Regional Applications of Joint
  Movements

Chapter Highlights

Exam Review

LEARNING OUTCOMES

After studying this chapter, you will have information to:

1. Distinguish between active and passive movements.

2. Compare joint mobilizing techniques and stretching.

3. Describe four different stretching methods.

4. Explain the therapeutic benefits of joint movements.

5. Describe the structure of joints in different areas of the body.

6. Apply mobilizing techniques to different joints in the body.

7. Apply stretching techniques in different areas of the body.

8. Follow the general guidelines for applying joint movements.

KEY TERMS

Active assisted stretch

Active movements

Assisted movements

Contract–relax–stretch (CRS)

Mobilizing techniques

Passive movements

Reciprocal inhibition

Resisted movements

Simple static stretch

Stretching

290

OVERVIEW OF JOINT MOVEMENTS

Swedish massage includes both soft tissue manipulation and joint movement techniques. This combination can be traced back to the original system of Swedish medical gymnastics developed by Pehr Henrik Ling, which included both types of movements.[1] Joint movements are an integral part of Swedish massage sessions that complement soft tissue techniques and produce unique therapeutic effects. Skeletal system anatomy including the location of major joints can be found on the inside back cover of this textbook.

Categories of Movements

Movements of the body can be categorized generally as either active or passive. **Active movements** are initiated and powered by the individual him- or herself. **Passive movements** refer to movements initiated and controlled by another person, while the recipient remains totally relaxed and receptive.

Movements can be further divided into free, assisted, and resisted. *Free active movements* are performed voluntarily without assistance from anyone else and are also called *exercises*. In **assisted movements**, a person initiates the movement, while another person helps him or her complete it. In **resisted movements**, a person initiates the movement, while a second person offers resistance, thereby challenging the muscles used. Resisted movements are sometimes used in rehabilitation to restore strength to a muscle. Assisted and resisted movements also can be used in stretching techniques.

Joint Movement Techniques

In massage therapy, joint movements are used for a variety of therapeutic goals. Joint movement techniques can be categorized as joint mobilizing and stretching techniques. A comparison of the two types of joint movement techniques is made in Table 13–1 ■. A third category, joint manipulations or adjustments, is important to know about, but is outside the scope of massage therapy.

Mobilizing techniques, or *free passive joint movements*, used in massage therapy are nonspecific movements applied within the normal range of motion. Nonspecific means that the movements are not applied in a precise manner (as in a chiropractic adjustment), but are applied to facilitate movement at the joint generally. Joint mobilizing techniques can be further described as having a *smooth* and *loose* quality.

These nonspecific joint movements warm the surrounding soft tissues and elicit muscle relaxation. They stimulate proprioceptors in the surrounding area, which develops kinesthetic awareness. These techniques loosen up motion at the joints involved and stimulate the production of synovial fluid. Recipients can learn to let go of tension and unconscious holding patterns during passive joint movements.

Some contemporary systems of bodywork, such as Trager Psychophysical Integration®, use joint mobilizing techniques to affect the nervous system. Mobilizing techniques that are free and easy help reeducate muscles and integrate function within the nervous system.

Stretching is a type of joint movement applied to the limit of a joint's normal range in a specific direction. Stretching elongates the muscles and connective tissues that cross the joint. It is used to increase flexibility at the joint and for muscle relaxation. Stretching techniques typically target a specific muscle or muscle group. Different methods of stretching are discussed later in the chapter.

Joint movements add a kinetic dimension to massage sessions and provide diversity of technique. They are useful for increasing flexibility and improving posture and body alignment. Athletes find joint movements particularly beneficial for improving performance, preventing injuries, and enhancing rehabilitation.

Joint manipulations or adjustments (sometimes called chiropractic adjustments) are not within the scope of massage therapy. By joint manipulations and adjustments, we mean techniques that take a joint beyond its normal range of motion. They are direct attempts to realign a misaligned joint, or free a frozen joint, usually using a thrusting movement. They should be performed only by those trained to do so within their legal scope of practice. "Cracking" necks and backs and "popping" toes are potentially dangerous and are not within the scope of standard Swedish massage.

TABLE 13–1	Comparison of Joint Mobilizing and Stretching Techniques	
	Joint Mobilizing Techniques	Stretching Techniques
Definition	Nonspecific passive movements of joints within their normal range of motion	Joint movements performed to the limit of the normal range in a specific direction.
Movement qualities	Free, smooth, loose	Slow, sustained, controlled (static stretching)
Effects	Warms associated soft tissues; stimulates proprioceptors; elicits muscle relaxation; stimulates production of synovial fluid	Elongates targeted muscles and associated connective tissue; elicits muscle relaxation
Benefits	Freer movement of joints; increases kinesthetic awareness; decreases muscle tension	Greater flexibility; decreases muscle tension and stiffness
Example	Wagging the arm (Figure 13–5)	Cervical stretch (Figure 13–4)

This chapter focuses on joint movement techniques that fall under the categories of nonspecific joint mobilizing and stretching. These movements can be incorporated into a general massage session or used for achieving specific therapeutic goals.

METHODS OF STRETCHING

Four basic methods of stretching are the following:

1. Simple static stretch
2. Contract–relax–stretch (CRS)
3. CRS using reciprocal inhibition
4. Active assisted stretch

With practice, these methods of stretching can be easily integrated into a massage session.

A **simple static stretch** is a type of passive stretch characterized by slow, sustained, and even application. Avoid sudden, forceful, or bouncing movements when applying static stretches.

To apply a simple static stretch, move the body part to be stretched into position and hold at the comfortable limit of range of motion. The limit is determined by feeling for the point of resistance from the tissues involved. The receiver is passive during the entire stretch. Use feedback from the recipient for safety. The recipient should feel the stretch, but not feel pain. Hold for 10–15 seconds, and then try to increase the stretch. The muscles will often relax after a short time, allowing further stretch (30 seconds overall).

Stretches can be facilitated with techniques that utilize muscle physiology. In **contract–relax–stretch (CRS)** techniques, the practitioner gets into position to apply the stretch, but first asks the client to contract the muscle to be stretched against a resistance (resisted movement). Immediately following the targeted muscle's relaxation, the stretch is applied.

When CRS incorporating **reciprocal inhibition** is used, the practitioner gets into position to apply the stretch, but first asks the client to contract the target muscle's antagonist against a resistance. The target muscle relaxes as its antagonist contracts. Immediately following the antagonist's relaxation, the stretch is applied.

Applying the stretch during the recipient's exhalation can enhance the stretch. The body is more relaxed during exhalation than during inhalation, and holding the breath causes tension in the musculature and restricts movement. So it is better to stretch a muscle on the exhalation. Once you and the recipient are in position to apply a stretch, ask him or her to "take a deep breath and then let it out slowly." During the exhalation, apply the stretch.

For an **active assisted stretch**, the practitioner gets into position to apply the stretch and then directs the recipient to actively move the body part in the desired direction. The practitioner then assists the stretch, providing additional force in the direction of the movement. Have the recipient breathe normally during the active stretch; however, move more deeply into the stretch on an exhale.

The four methods of stretching are summarized in Table 13–2 ■.

SAFETY

Knowledge of the joint structure and surrounding soft tissues is essential for the safe and effective application of joint movements. Anatomical structure determines the type and degree of movement possible at the joint. Review of musculoskeletal anatomy and kinesiology related to joints is useful before attempting to perform joint movement techniques. Six types of synovial joints are shown in Figure 13–1 ■.

Normal range of motion refers to the degree of movement typically found at a particular joint. Normal range of motion is a point of comparison for assessing the degree of flexibility of a joint in a specific person, and how it might vary from the norm. Knowing the limitations of movement at each joint also decreases the likelihood of inadvertently damaging a joint or the surrounding tissues and increases safety for the recipient. Evaluating range of motion is described in Chapter 9, *Medical Terminology, Goal-Oriented Planning, Documentation*, and Figure 9–2 shows normal range of motion at the shoulder and hip joints.

Palpation skills are important for learning how joints move. Practitioners can learn much about the condition of the joint and surrounding tissues from the kinesthetic feel of its movement. Sensations such as "drag" and "end feel"

 PRACTICAL APPLICATION

Visualize the anatomical structure of the joints as you practice mobilizing and stretching techniques. Compare the picture in your mind and in your textbooks to what you palpate with your hands.

1. How is the movement of the joint related to its bony structure and to associated muscles and other soft tissues?

2. What limitations does the structure place on the movement of the joint?
3. Does this particular joint show deviation from what is considered normal? How do you modify your technique to account for such deviations?

TABLE 13–2   Methods of Stretching

Method	Description	Example Using Quadriceps Stretch (see Figure 13–25)
Simple static stretch	• Position targeted muscle • Apply static stretch • Recipient is passive	Relax the entire leg before the stretch
Contract–relax–stretch (CRS)	• Position targeted muscle • Contract targeted muscle against resistance • Relax targeted muscle • Apply static stretch	Resistance to quadriceps contraction applied before the stretch
CRS using reciprocal inhibition	• Position targeted muscle • Contract antagonist against resistance • Relax antagonist • Apply static stretch	Resistance to hamstrings contraction applied before the stretch
Active assisted stretch	• Position targeted muscle • Client actively performs the stretch • Practitioner assists by applying additional force in the desired direction	Assistance for the stretch is applied by the practitioner

FIGURE 13–1
Six types of synovial joints.

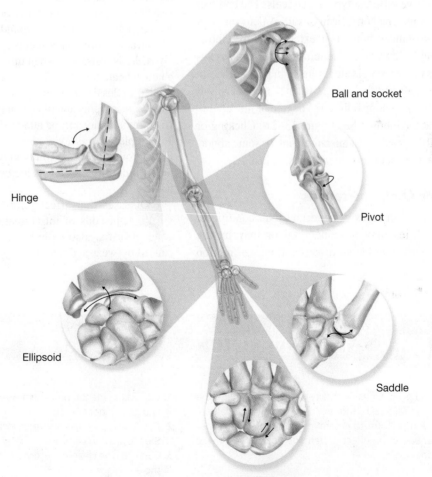

Ball and socket

Hinge

Pivot

Ellipsoid

Saddle

Plane (gliding)

Hard-end feel   Firm-end feel   Soft-end feel

FIGURE 13–2 Three types of "end feel" in normal joints.

offer clues to restrictions to normal range of motion, areas of tightness, patterns of holding, and the limits of stretches. *Drag* refers to resistance felt as the soft tissues around a joint are stretched, and *end feel* refers to the quality of restriction as the limit of the range of motion is reached. Different types of joints have different typical end feels. The end feel at healthy joints may be bony, firm, or soft. A bony end feel occurs when bone meets bone, as in extension of the elbow. A firm end feel follows when the joint capsule and associated ligaments reach their elastic limits, as in plantar flexion at the ankle. A soft end feel results when surrounding soft tissues (muscle and tendons) limit the degree of movement, as in flexion at the elbow.[2] See Figure 13–2 ■. Clicking or grinding in a joint may signal misalignment, or some abnormality or pathology such as osteoarthritis.

Cautions and Contraindications

Caution is advised in cases of abnormal joint conditions. Joint abnormalities may be congenital or may be the result of accidents, injuries, or diseases. Range of motion at an abnormal joint may be limited, or the joint may be hypermobile and unstable. Remember that massage and joint movements are contraindicated when acute inflammation is present.

Past trauma to a joint can cause unusual conditions in the area. These include shortening or loss of muscle tissue, scarring in connective tissues, or abnormal joint structure. Recent soft tissue injuries around a joint can leave swelling and inflammation that affect the joint itself.

Care is warranted when moving joints in the vicinity of a newly healed fracture. Even if the break was distant from a joint, muscles that cross the joint may be affected. Hardware, such as metal pins and plates, may have been used to treat a fracture and may still be attached, thus limiting movement. Joint replacements are becoming more common, and movement around artificial joints may be restricted. Hip, knee, and shoulder replacements are especially common in older adults.

Diseases that affect joints directly can cause pain, swelling, periods of inflammation, and loss of mobility. Osteoarthritis, also called degenerative joint disease, is caused by wear and tear of the joint structures. Bursitis, or

CRITICAL THINKING

Think about the variations on static stretching that utilize the principles of contract–relax and reciprocal inhibition. Evaluate each stretch you perform to determine if one of these variations might enhance the effect. Determine how to best make the application.

1. Can you name the primary muscle targeted with the stretch and its antagonist?
2. Can you apply adequate resistance to the muscle you want the recipient to contract?
3. Can you give clear instructions to the recipient to perform the technique correctly?

inflammation of the fluid sacks in synovial joints, results in pain and limited mobility. Osteoporosis, or loss of bone tissue, leaves bones thin, brittle, and prone to injury. These and other joint pathologies have implications for applications of joint movements and massage.

Take the time to learn about joint conditions presented by clients, and note them in their health history files. Additional information can be obtained from a recipient's medical records or from his or her physician. Make the effort to learn more about unfamiliar conditions by consulting anatomical and medical references.[3] Greater knowledge helps to ensure a safe application of joint movements.

GENERAL GUIDELINES FOR JOINT MOVEMENT TECHNIQUES

The following is a summary of the general guidelines for performing joint mobilizing and stretching techniques:

- Check for contraindications before applying joint movements.
- Adapt techniques for structural abnormalities.
- Stay within the normal range of motion of the joint.
- Stay within the comfort range of the recipient.
- Warm surrounding soft tissues before stretching.
- Apply joint mobilizing techniques with smooth, free, loose quality.
- Apply stretching techniques with slow, sustained, even motion.
- Apply a stretch as the recipient exhales.
- Use contract–relax and reciprocal inhibition to enhance a stretch.
- Use client feedback to determine the limit of a stretch.

REGIONAL APPLICATIONS OF JOINT MOVEMENTS

The following sections discuss applications of joint movements to the neck, shoulder girdle, elbow, wrist, hand, chest, hip, knee, ankle, and foot.

Neck

Structure and Movement The *neck* is a general term for the region between the head and the trunk. It includes the seven cervical vertebrae and the surrounding soft tissues. The cervicals are the smallest, most delicate vertebrae and are designed to allow for a lot of movement but not bear a lot of weight. They are arranged vertically with an anterior convex curve.

The musculature in the neck region is complex, with deeper, smaller muscles entirely within the neck, and larger and more superficial muscles attaching superior and inferior. The bony and muscular structures allow a variety of movements, including flexion, extension, hyperextension, lateral flexion, protraction, retraction, and rotation.

Mobilizing Techniques Mobilizing techniques for the neck are performed when the recipient is lying supine. The mobilizing movement occurs between the cervical vertebrae and in the suboccipital region. All the following examples may be performed with the practitioner seated at the head of the recipient. It is useful to have an adjustable stool or chair on wheels so that you can get in good position, for both leverage and good body mechanics.

Simple mobilizing movements of the neck may be performed by lifting the head slightly off the table and moving the neck into lateral flexion, rotation, forward flexion, or hyperextension. Be sure to have a firm grip on the head. You may have to remind the recipient to relax because it takes great trust to let someone hold and move your head. You may also assure the individual that you will not "crack" his or her neck, and that such manipulations are not part of this type of joint movement. Keep the movements small at first and gradually increase the range of motion as the recipient allows.

Finger push-ups may be used to produce gentle movement between the cervical vertebrae. First warm up the neck muscles with effleurage and circular friction along each side. Straighten the neck so that the recipient is directly facing up. Simply place the fingers at the base of the neck on either side, palms up, and push up with the fingers, applying direct pressure. Move your hands about an inch at a time along the neck, pressing up at each spot as you move along. You will feel movement between the vertebrae and notice movement at the head. Variations of finger push-ups include alternating pressing from side to side. The rhythm would be to press right, press left, move along; press right, press left, move along; repeating the sequence along the neck, moving toward the head.

The *suboccipital release* is a variation of the finger push-up applied in the suboccipital region. Place your hands, palms up, under the recipient's head, with fingers along the suboccipitals, similar to Figure 12–36. Lift the head with the hands, and then lower the wrists to the table, while leaving the head balanced on the fingertips. Usually within 5–10 seconds, the neck muscles relax, the suboccipital tissues release, and the head hyperextends. You will notice the recipient's head falling back, and your fingers will be deep into the suboccipital space. This pressure usually feels good to the recipient. Finish by gently pulling on the occiput to return the neck to a neutral position with its natural curve.

A *wave movement* may be created in the neck by simply applying deep effleurage on both sides at the same time, moving from the base to the suboccipital region. You exaggerate the natural curve of the neck by pressing up as you slide along. The neck will return to its normal curve as you finish the movement. (See Figure 14–68.) At the end of the movement, give a gentle pull on the occiput to straighten any hyperextension remaining from the movement. The wave is a good technique to use to detect tension in the neck. The wavelike motion will not occur if the recipient is unconsciously holding tension in the neck or if the neck muscles are shortened and tight.

Stretches Massage and simple mobilizing techniques are used to warm up the neck thoroughly before applying stretches. The following stretches may be performed when the recipient is lying supine on a table.

A stretch in *lateral flexion* helps lengthen the muscles on the sides of the neck. Place the head in position to one side at a point where you feel the tissues just starting to stretch. The head placement, either faceup or turned to the side, will determine which muscles are stretched most. Place one hand on the shoulder and the other on the side of the head. You can create a gentle stretch of tissues by pushing the head and shoulders in opposite directions, as shown in Figure 13–3 ■. Guide the recipient to exhale as you apply the stretch. The head will move to a position of greater lateral flexion as the upper trapezius relaxes and lengthens. Repeat on the other side.

Range of *rotation* may be enhanced with a simple stretch. Position the head faceup so that the neck is straight. Then rotate the head to one side, keeping the neck vertically aligned. Gently push the head into greater rotation, stretching the neck muscles. Repeat on the other side.

Position the head faceup to stretch the neck in *forward flexion*. Lift the head with one hand, and with the other hand, reach under the head and across to the tip of the shoulder. The head rests on the forearm. Reach under that arm with the free hand and place it on the other shoulder. The head should be cradled safely at the place where the forearms cross, as shown in Figure 13–4 ■. Slowly stretch the neck into forward flexion. Stand during this movement for best leverage.

FIGURE 13–4 Cross-arm stretch of cervical muscles with neck in forward flexion.

Source: Pearson Education, Inc./Segal Photography.

The *cross-arm stretch* may also be performed with the head rotated. This will stretch neck muscles at a different angle. After forward flexion, return to the starting position, and turn the head to one side. Repeat the forward flexion to each side with the head in rotation. For safety, get feedback from the client to be sure that the stretch is pain free.

REALITY CHECK

KELLY

TAMIKA: I'm not sure how to integrate joint movements to a Swedish massage. I thought I would simply be stroking and kneading muscles. How will I know when to add mobilizing and stretching?

KELLY: There's no fixed rule for when to add joint movements. There are some techniques I include in my general approach, mainly free movements of the arms and shoulders, and legs and hips. If I sense that a client is holding tension, I'll add some mobilizing in the area to help them let go and relax. Other than that I include joint movements when I think it will support the goals for the session. For example, I notice that some clients have shortened posterior neck muscles, possibly from driving or looking at computer screens for long periods of time. I'll add stretches for the neck to help bring it into better alignment and to ease tension in the area. Once you become skilled in applying joint movements, you will intuitively integrate them with soft tissue skills to address individual client needs as you become aware of them.

FIGURE 13–3 Stretch of trapezius and cervical muscles with neck in lateral flexion.

Source: Pearson Education, Inc./Segal Photography.

Shoulder Girdle

Structure and Movement The shoulder girdle is a complex region that can be defined in different ways. For our purposes, the shoulder girdle will be defined as including the glenohumeral, acromioclavicular, and scapulocostal joints. The glenohumeral joint is classified as a ball-and-socket joint and the acromioclavicular joint as diarthrodial or capable of free movement. The scapulocostal juncture may be described as a gliding joint of the scapula over the rib cage, with associated muscles, connective tissue, and bursa.

The shoulder girdle is the most mobile area of the body. Movements possible in the shoulder girdle include the upper arm movements of flexion, extension, hyperextension, abduction, adduction, rotation, and horizontal flexion. Movements of the scapulae themselves include elevation, depression, upward and downward rotation and tilt, and retraction and protraction. The entire shoulder girdle is structured to accomplish circumduction.

Mobilizing Techniques Mobilizing movements of the shoulder girdle can be performed with the recipient in supine, prone, side-lying, or seated position. Motion in the shoulder joints can be accomplished indirectly by movement of the arm or by movement of the scapula.

To mobilize the shoulder girdle with the recipient in the supine position, take hold of the hand and lift and wag the arm, as shown in Figure 13–5 ■. While *wagging* the arm, there will also be movement at the wrist and elbow. *Shaking* is performed by creating a slight traction of the arm toward the feet, holding onto the hand, and leaning back, as shown in Figure 13–6 ■. Loosely shake the arm up and down. Movement will be felt at the wrist, elbow, and shoulder.

The *passive shoulder roll* may be used for mobilizing the shoulder. Hold onto the upper arm with one hand close to the glenohumeral joint and the other hand at the tip of the

FIGURE 13–6 Shaking: an arm and shoulder mobilizing technique.

Source: Pearson Education, Inc./Segal Photography.

shoulder. Simply move the shoulder through the full range of motion possible in the supine position. The quality of movement should be smooth, free, and loose. This same technique is effective in the prone, side-lying, and seated positions. Figure 13–7 ■ shows the passive shoulder roll with the recipient supine.

With the recipient prone, *scapula mobilizing* may be accomplished using pressure applied at the top of the shoulder. Position the recipient's arm on the table with elbow bent and hand near the waist. Then place your hand on top of the shoulder near the tip and press lightly toward the feet. The scapula will move and lift if the attached muscles are relaxed, as shown in Figure 13–8 ■. Don't force the movement, but encourage relaxation by gentle motions and reminding the recipient to let go of tension in the area. Once the medial border lifts, you may apply effleurage to massage the muscles that attach there.

Stretches Use massage and mobilizing technique to warm up the shoulder girdle before stretching. Shoulder girdle stretches are effective in the supine, prone, and side-lying

FIGURE 13–5 Wagging: an arm and shoulder mobilizing technique.

Source: Pearson Education, Inc./Segal Photography.

FIGURE 13–7 Passive shoulder roll: mobilizing technique for the shoulder with recipient in supine position.

Source: Pearson Education, Inc./Segal Photography.

FIGURE 13–8 Scapula mobilizing technique: move and lift the scapula by pulling back at the shoulder.

Source: Pearson Education, Inc./Segal Photography.

positions. The muscles of the shoulder girdle are stretched primarily with movements of the upper arm.

In the supine position, a stretch in *horizontal flexion* may be performed by moving the arm over the chest. This elongates the muscles that attach to the medial border of the scapula, including the rhomboids, as well as the posterior shoulder muscles. Hold onto the recipient's lower arm near the wrist with one hand, while the other hand reaches under to the medial border of the scapula. Stretch the arm over the chest, and enhance the stretch by gently pulling back on the scapula at the same time. See Figure 13–9 ■.

A very pleasant stretch may be applied with the recipient's arms extended overhead. This *overhead stretch* may be performed one arm at a time or both arms at the same time. For a two-arm stretch, simply place the arms overhead,

FIGURE 13–10 Overhead stretch for the shoulder muscles. Lean back to create the stretch using your body weight.

Source: Pearson Education, Inc./Segal Photography.

grasping the forearms near the wrists. Lean back to create the stretch at the shoulder, as shown in Figure 13–10 ■. This technique stretches all the muscles of the shoulder girdle, including the latissimus dorsi and pectoral muscles.

A similar stretch may be applied with the recipient seated in a massage chair. Grasp the forearm with both hands and move the arm overhead to a position in line with the angle of the body. You should be facing in the same direction as the recipient. Lift the arm upward, and give it a gentle shake, as shown in Figure 20–10.

Elbow

Structure and Movement The elbow is formed by the junction of the distal end of the humerus and the proximal ends of the radius and the ulna. Movements of the humeroulnar joint are limited to flexion and extension. The bony structure of the joint further limits the range of motion in extension. What we think of as the point of the elbow is the olecranon process of the ulna. The movements of pronation and supination of the forearm (palm down and palm up) occur as the head of the radius rotates over the surfaces of the capitulum of the humerus and the radial notch of the ulna. At the same time, the distal ends of the radius and ulna glide over one another.

Mobilizing Techniques Movements at the elbow are limited by the structure of the joint. *Wagging* of the arm as described previously offers some mobilization at the elbow. You may also *pronate and supinate* the forearm by holding the hand and turning it alternately palm up and palm down.

To perform a simple mobilizing technique at the elbow called *circling the forearm,* bend the arm at the elbow so that it is perpendicular to the table. Hold the arm just below the wrist. Trace a circle with the hand creating movement at the elbow, as shown in Figure 13–11 ■.

Stretches Stretches of muscles that cross the elbow are accomplished largely by stretching the whole arm as in the *overhead stretch* of the shoulder described earlier. If the biceps muscles are shortened, the stretch is created by simply straightening out the arm at the elbow.

FIGURE 13–9 Stretching the shoulder muscles with arm in horizontal flexion.

Source: Pearson Education, Inc./Segal Photography.

FIGURE 13–11 Circling the forearm to create movement at the elbow.

Source: Pearson Education, Inc./Segal Photography.

Wrist

Structure and Movement The wrist joint is formed by the union of the slightly concave surface of the proximal row of carpal bones with the distal end of the radius and the midcarpal joint. What people commonly call the "wrist bone" is actually the distal end of the ulna. Movements possible at this juncture include flexion, extension, hyperextension, radial and ulnar deviation (side-to-side movement), and circumduction.

Mobilizing Techniques Mobilizing the wrist is best performed with the recipient supine. The soft tissues in the wrist area may be warmed up with small effleurage movements with the thumbs prior to mobilizing and stretching. A useful starting position for basic mobilizing techniques and stretching is achieved by clasping the recipient's hand with your own, palms facing and fingers interwoven. The recipient's elbow is bent and may be resting on the table. In the hand-clasp position, you may move the hand through its entire range of motion at the wrist, including flexion, extension, hyperextension, side-to-side in radial and ulnar deviation, and circumduction. Keep the passive movement well within the possible range of motion.

A light, quick mobilizing technique may be performed at the wrist with a *waving* movement. Face the head of the table and hold the forearm just proximal to the recipient's wrist (palm down) with both of your hands, the thumbs on top and index fingers below. Use the remaining fingers to cause the hand to wave, by pressing up against the heel of the hand quickly and repeatedly, letting gravity help it fall between times. Movement at the wrist also occurs during less specific mobilizations, including wagging the arm, shown previously in Figure 13–5, and supination and pronation of the forearm.

Stretches *Flexion* and *hyperextension* are the major stretches performed at the wrist. Figure 13–12 ■ shows stretching the flexors of the forearm by hyperextending the wrist. Press down gently on the palm side of the fingers to create the stretch. Now flex the wrist by pressing down on the back side of the hand to create a stretch of the extensors

FIGURE 13–12 Stretching the flexor muscles of the forearm by hyperextending the wrist.

Source: Pearson Education, Inc./Segal Photography.

of the forearm, as shown in Figure 13–13 ■. During these stretches, be careful to approach the limit of motion slowly.

Hand

Structure and Movement Joints within the hand and distal to the wrist include the metacarpophalangeal juncture (i.e., knuckles) and the small joints between phalanges. The second through fifth fingers each have three phalanges with two joints, whereas the thumb has just two phalanges

FIGURE 13–13 Stretching the extensor muscles of the forearm by flexing the wrist.

Source: Pearson Education, Inc./Segal Photography.

with one joint. The joint between the carpal and metacarpal of the thumb is designed to allow freer movement than similar junctures of the carpals and metacarpals. Movement may also occur between metacarpals. Movements of the fingers include flexion, extension, abduction, and adduction. The hand as a whole is capable of holding and grasping objects.

Mobilizing Techniques Perform mobilizing techniques of the hand joints very carefully, matching the force used to the size and strength of the hand you are working with. Warm the muscles in the recipient's hands with effleurage and light frictions before performing mobilizing techniques and stretches.

Mobilizing the knuckles one at a time may be achieved making *figure-8s*. Hold the recipient's hand with one of your hands, his or her fingers pointing toward you, palm down. With your other hand, grasp the fifth (little) finger firmly near the knuckle and move in a small figure-8 pattern two or three times, mobilizing the joint. See Figure 13–14 ■. Repeat for each knuckle joint. A similar, but lighter, mobilizing of the knuckles may be achieved by grasping the fingers more distally. Perform the figure-8s as described.

You can mobilize the soft tissues between the meta-carpals with a *scissoring* motion. With the recipient's palm down, take hold of the knuckles of the fifth and fourth fingers, as shown in Figure 13–15 ■. Simply move one knuckle up and the other down at the same time, alternating in a scissoring motion. Repeat along all of the knuckles.

Stretches There are a few simple stretches for the joints of the hand. Perform them slowly and with care. The fingers can be *hyperextended* at the knuckles. Interlace your fingers with the recipient's, palm to palm, placing the tips of your fingers just below the recipient's knuckles. Gently press between the metacarpals, bending the fingers into hyperextension. This movement may also cause the metacarpals to spread out, stretching the tissues between them.

Taking the whole hand into *hyperextension* can stretch all the flexor muscles (*flexion*) within the hand and the wrist flexors in the forearm. Hold the forearm with one hand and

FIGURE 13–15 Scissoring motion to create movement between the metacarpals of the hand.

Source: Pearson Education, Inc./Segal Photography.

with the other hand, press back on the phalanges, causing hyperextension at the knuckles and at the wrist. Gently stretch the tissues of the hand and the forearm. See Figure 13–12.

Chest

Structure and Movement The *chest* is a common term for the area on the front and sides of the upper body generally defined by the ribs, sternum, and clavicle. It is the part of the thorax accessible when lying supine. The entire thorax, including the chest, expands and contracts with the inhalation and exhalation of breathing. The pectoral muscles are located on the chest.

Mobilizing Techniques The rib cage may be mobilized by *gentle rocking* from the side. Stand facing the side of the table in line with the rib cage. Put one hand on top of the other and place them on the rib cage, as shown in Figure 13–16 ■. Gently rock the rib cage by repeatedly pushing and then letting up the pressure in a rhythmic manner. Move around on the rib cage to mobilize different areas. You will feel the elastic quality of the rib cage as it springs back after you push.

FIGURE 13–14 Figure-8s at the knuckles of the hand.

Source: Pearson Education, Inc./Segal Photography.

FIGURE 13–16 Placement of hands for mobilizing the rib cage from one side.

Source: Pearson Education, Inc./Segal Photography.

FIGURE 13–17 Placement of hands for mobilizing the rib cage from side to side.

Source: Pearson Education, Inc./Segal Photography.

FIGURE 13–18 Rocking the leg to create rotation in the hip joint.

Source: Pearson Education, Inc./Segal Photography.

If you can reach far enough with your arms, you can cause movement in the chest from both sides. Facing the head of the table, reach over with one hand to the far side of the chest, fingers pointing down toward the table. Place the other hand on the near side, fingers pointing up. See Figure 13–17 ■. Gently rock the rib cage by alternately pulling with the far hand and pushing with the near hand. Establish a smooth rhythm to encourage relaxation of the surrounding musculature.

Stretches There are no highly movable joints on the chest itself. However, the pectoral muscles of the shoulder girdle attach there. Use the *overhead stretch* of the arms, as shown in Figure 13–10, to lengthen the pectorals.

Hip

Structure and Movement The hip joint is a typical ball-and-socket joint formed by the articulation of the head of the femur with the deep cup-shaped acetabulum of the pelvis. The large muscles that move the hip joint are located primarily on the thigh and the buttocks. The iliopsoas is a strong hip flexor that attaches to the lumbar vertebrae and inner surface of the ilium and the lesser trochanter of the femur. Movements possible at the hip joint include flexion, extension, hyperextension,

abduction, adduction, diagonal abduction and adduction, outward and inward rotation, and circumduction.

Mobilizing Techniques Most hip movements are performed with the recipient in the supine position. Mobilizing techniques are an excellent way to affect the deeper muscles that move the hip.

With the recipient supine, remove the bolster from under the knees. The legs should be straight and slightly apart. Stand facing the thigh at the side of the table. Gently *rock the leg* into rotation by placing the hands palms down on the top of the thigh and pressing down and away. See Figure 13–18 ■. The leg will usually rotate back, especially if the gluteals are tight. The foot will wag from side to side if performed properly. Repeat with a rhythmic rocking motion.

To achieve *passive movement through the full range of motion* of the hip, bend the leg, placing the foot in one hand and using the other hand for support at the knee. See Figure 13–19 ■. Let the knee trace a circle as the hip flexes, adducts diagonally, extends, abducts diagonally, and goes round again in circumduction. The movement should be smooth and controlled.

A   B

FIGURE 13–19 Moving the hip through its full range of motion.

Source: Pearson Education, Inc./Segal Photography.

FIGURE 13–20 Stretching the gluteals by bringing knee to chest.

Source: Pearson Education, Inc./Segal Photography.

Stretches The muscles that move the hip can be stretched in many directions. The following are a few simple yet useful stretches for the hip joint.

A stretch for the gluteals may be applied with the hip in flexion by pressing the knee toward the chest in the supine position (*knee to chest flexion*). See Figure 13–20 ■. The hamstrings may be stretched with the leg straight and in flexion (*straight leg flexion*), as shown in Figure 13–21 ■. To enhance the stretch and involve all the gluteal and leg muscles, dorsiflex the foot while you bring the leg into flexion as close to perpendicular as possible.

Diagonal adduction of the thigh while lying supine will also stretch the gluteals. Bring the knee toward the chest, and then let it cross the body diagonally, as shown

FIGURE 13–22 Stretching the muscles of the hip and lower back with diagonal adduction of the bent leg.
Source: Pearson Education, Inc./Segal Photography.

in Figure 13–22 ■. The recipient's shoulders remain flat on the table, while the spine rotates and the hip muscles stretch. This is also a good stretch for the lower back.

The flexors may be stretched from the prone or side-lying position. With the recipient prone, stand at the side of the table facing the head. Bend the leg at the knee and grasp the thigh from underneath; the lower leg can rest against your shoulder. Lift the knee off the table, putting the hip into hyperextension. You may anchor the hip with the other hand. This stretch takes some strength and is most easily performed if the recipient is smaller than you are.

The stretch into *straight leg hyperextension* can be more easily performed with the recipient in side-lying position. Stand behind the recipient facing the table at the hip. Cradle the upper leg with one arm while you stabilize the trunk with the other. Pull the upper leg back into hyperextension, as shown in Figure 13–23 ■. Because you are pulling the leg back, instead of lifting it up, this technique is more efficient and takes less strength. It primarily stretches the quadriceps and iliopsoas muscles.

FIGURE 13–21 Stretching the hamstrings with straight leg flexion.

Source: Pearson Education, Inc./Segal Photography.

FIGURE 13–23 Stretching the hip flexors with the recipient side-lying.
Source: Pearson Education, Inc./Segal Photography.

Knee

Structure and Movement The knee is classified as a hinge joint and is formed by the articulation of the distal end of the femur with the proximal end of the tibia. A large sesamoid bone embedded in the connective tissues that cross the joint forms the knee cap or patella. The major movements of the knee joint are flexion and extension. Some minor inward and outward rotation of the tibia is possible when the knee is flexed in a non-weight-bearing situation.

Mobilizing Techniques The knee joint is best mobilized with the recipient in the prone position. For a simple mobilizing technique, stand facing the side of the table at the knee. Pick up the leg near the ankle with both hands, so that the lower leg is perpendicular to the table. Lift the leg slightly off the table and *wag* it back and forth. This also mobilizes the hip joint. See Figure 13–24 ■.

Another simple mobilization at the knee involves tossing the lower leg back and forth from hand to hand. This *leg toss* technique helps the recipient learn to relax and let go of tension in the legs. After the leg toss, you may perform a different knee mobilization by *circling the lower leg*. Place one hand on the thigh to steady it and grasp the lower leg near the ankle with the other hand. Make small circles with the lower leg. Stay well within the small range of this circular motion.

Stretches A few of the stretches for the hip joint, performed with a straight leg, also stretch muscles that cross the knee. See Figure 13–21. An additional stretch (*heel to buttocks*) for the knee extensors can be created with the recipient in the prone position by bringing the heel of the foot toward the buttocks. See Figure 13–25 ■. Table 13–2 describes four different methods of applying this stretch.

FIGURE 13–25 Stretching the quadriceps by bringing the heel of the foot toward the buttocks.
Source: Pearson Education, Inc./Segal Photography.

Ankle

Structure and Movement The ankle is a hinge joint formed by the junction of the talus with the malleoli of the tibia and fibula. The structure is bound together with many ligaments for stability. The tendons of the muscles of the lower leg that attach to the foot all pass over the ankle. They are bound neatly at the ankle by a band of connective tissue called the retinaculum. Movements possible at the ankle include dorsiflexion (flexion), plantar flexion (extension), pronation (eversion and abduction), and supination (inversion and adduction).

Mobilizing Techniques When the recipient is prone, the ankle may be accessed by lifting the lower leg so that the foot comes off the table. For mobilizing with *dorsiflexion,* stand at the feet facing the end of the table. Lift one leg and place both hands on the foot, thumbs on the bottom of the foot. Lean into the foot with the thumbs in the arch, moving the foot into dorsiflexion, as shown in Figure 13–26 ■. Repeat the mobilization several times in a rhythmic manner, changing the location of the thumbs to affect different spots on the foot.

FIGURE 13–24 Wagging the leg with recipient prone.
Source: Pearson Education, Inc./Segal Photography.

FIGURE 13–26 Dorsiflexion of the foot with direct pressure to bottom of foot with the thumbs.
Source: Pearson Education, Inc./Segal Photography.

With the lower leg lifted so that it is perpendicular to the table, the ankle can be put through a *full range of motion through passive movement*. Grasp the bottom of the foot from above and move the ankle through dorsiflexion, pronation, plantar flexion, and supination in a circular movement. This is also an excellent position from which to apply simple dorsiflexion and plantar flexion.

With the recipient supine, the ankle can be put through *side-to-side mobilizing* by placing the heels of the hands on the foot just under the malleoli of the tibia and fibula (ankle bones) and alternately pressing one side and then the other. The movement is rapid and causes the heel of the foot to move from side to side at the articulation of the talus and malleoli of the tibia and fibula. (See Figure 14–36.)

Stretches Stretches at the ankle are primarily performed in *dorsiflexion* and *plantar flexion* and may easily be done with the recipient prone or supine. Stretches may be applied from any of the positions mentioned for mobilizations. Simply move the foot into dorsiflexion or plantar flexion and take it to the limit of range of motion. Figure 13–27 ■ shows the ankle and foot stretching in plantar flexion. This movement helps elongate the foot flexors located on the front of the lower leg and may be felt across the top of the foot.

Foot

Structure and Movement The foot may be described as an elastic arched structure made up of 26 bones and designed for support and propulsion. A foot has seven tarsal bones (i.e., calcaneus, talus, navicular, cuboid, and three cuneiforms), five metatarsals, and 14 phalanges. There is a longitudinal arch, which extends from the heel to the heads of the five metatarsals, and a transverse arch, which extends side to side and is formed by the anterior tarsal bones and the metatarsals. The intertarsal joints are irregular joints and allow slight gliding movements, and the interphalangeal joints of the toes are hinge joints that allow for flexion and extension.

Mobilizing Techniques Mobilizing techniques for the feet are similar to those for the hands. They are best performed with the recipient supine. The soft tissues in the feet may be warmed up with small sliding effleurage movements with the thumbs or fingers, and compressions with the fist on the bottom of the foot.

Hold the foot steady with one hand and with your other hand, grasp the fifth (little) toe firmly near the knuckle and move in a small *figure-8* pattern two or three times, mobilizing the joint. Repeat for each knuckle joint. See Figure 13–28 ■. You can mobilize the tissues between the metatarsals with a *scissoring* motion. Take hold of the knuckles of the fifth and fourth toes. Simply move one knuckle up and the other down at the same time, alternating in a scissoring motion. Repeat for all the metatarsals.

Sometimes the toes curl under due to shortening of the toe flexors that are located on the bottom of the feet. The toes can be mobilized into extension using *effleurage* along the underside of the toes. This is usually performed with the thumbs. Do not "pop" or pull on the toes forcefully to straighten them. This is uncomfortable and may cause injury.

Stretches There are a few stretches for the intrinsic tissues of the foot itself. As described earlier, you can plantar flex the foot from either the prone or supine positions, stretching the tissues on the top of the foot, including the extensor muscles. The toes alone may easily be stretched back at the ball of the foot or pressed forward for a stretch (*hyperextension*).

FIGURE 13–27 Stretching the flexors of the foot in plantarflexion, recipient prone. Lower leg perpendicular to the table.

Source: Pearson Education, Inc./Segal Photography.

FIGURE 13–28 Figure-8s on the toes mobilize joints of the foot.

Source: Pearson Education, Inc./Segal Photography.

FIGURE 13–29 Create space between metatarsals by pulling sides of foot away from each other.

Source: Pearson Education, Inc./Segal Photography.

The foot may be spread stretching the spaces between the metatarsals and the muscles that run across them. Simply grasp both sides of the foot and pull in opposite directions, *widening the foot at the metatarsals* and stretching related tissues, as shown in Figure 13–29 ■.

Because the foot is a small part of the body with many joints, it can be massaged thoroughly rather quickly combining soft tissue techniques with mobilizations and stretches. Joint movements help recipients regain a sense of their feet as having moving parts and help sharpen their kinesthetic sense. This is important, especially for those who live in cultures where shoes are worn all day.

Table 13–3 ■ provides a quick, at-a-glance overview of joint movement techniques described in this chapter. Remember that these are just a sample of the possible joint mobilizing and stretching techniques. Others will appear in the practice sequences in the remaining chapters.

TABLE 13–3	**At-a-Glance Joint Movement Techniques**	
Region	**Mobilizing Techniques**	**Stretches**
Neck	Finger push-ups	Cross-arm stretch
	Meltdown	Forward flexion
	Simple mobilizing movements	Lateral flexion
	Wavelike movement	Rotation
Shoulder Girdle	Passive shoulder roll	Horizontal flexion
	Scapula mobilizing (prone)	Overhead stretch
	Shaking	
	Wagging	
Elbow	Circling the forearm	Overhead stretch
	Pronation and supination	
	Wagging	
Wrist	Passive movement through full range of motion	Hyperextension
	Waving	Flexion
Hand	Figure-8s	Flexion
	Passive movements of all joints	Hyperextension of fingers and wrist
	Scissoring	
Chest	Gentle rocking of rib cage	Overhead stretch
Hip	Passive movement through full range of motion	Diagonal adduction with flexed knee
	Rhythmic rocking of straight leg	Knee to chest flexion
		Straight leg flexion
		Straight leg hyperextension—prone and side-lying
Knee	Circling the lower leg	Heel to buttocks
	Leg toss	
	Wagging	
Ankle	Dorsiflexing foot with thumb pressure	Dorsiflexion
	Passive movement through full range of motion	Plantar flexion
	Side-to-side mobilizing	
Foot	Figure-8s of toes	Fingers interlocked between toes
	Scissoring metatarsals	Foot widening at metatarsals
	Straightening toes with effleurage	Hyperextension of toes

CASE FOR STUDY

Claudelle Applies Joint Movements to Improve Roger's Walk

Claudelle has a client named Roger who complains of stiffness in his legs and feet. Roger sits for long periods of time at work, and when he stands up has a hard time getting moving smoothly. He can barely touch his toes anymore with his legs straight and has tripped a few times from not picking up his toes high enough as he walks. Other people have commented that he seems to be limping a little.

Question:

How can Claudelle incorporate joint movements into Roger's massage sessions to help improve his walking?

Things to consider:

- Does Roger have any recent injuries to his lower limbs or other contraindications for joint movements?
- Does Roger have good flexibility in his legs at the ankles, knees, and hips?
- Are there specific leg muscles that seem tight or shortened?

Write a brief description of which joint mobilizations and stretches to include in Roger's next massage session. Assume that there are no contraindications.

_____

_____

_____

CHAPTER HIGHLIGHTS

- Joint movement techniques are part of Swedish massage.
  - Joint movements within the scope of massage therapy are nonspecific joint mobilizing and stretching techniques.
  - Joint manipulations or adjustments that involve thrusting movements are not within the scope of massage therapy.
- Movements of the body may be generally categorized as active and passive.
  - Active movements are initiated and powered by the person him- or herself.
  - During passive movements, the client remains totally relaxed and receptive while the practitioner initiates and controls the movement.
- Movements may be free, assisted, or resisted.
  - In free active movements, a person is unaided during the movement.
  - In assisted movements, a person initiates the motion and is assisted by another person in completing it.
  - In resisted movements, a person initiates the motion, and another person offers resistance to it.
- Joint mobilizing techniques are nonspecific passive movements performed within the normal range of joint motion.
  - Qualities are smooth, free, and loose.
  - Purposes are to warm surrounding tissues, elicit muscle relaxation, stimulate proprioceptors, free up motion, and stimulate production of synovial fluid.

- Stretching is a type of joint movement that is performed to the limit of the range of motion in a specific direction.
  - Stretching elongates muscles and connective tissue and elicits muscle relaxation.
- Four basic stretching methods are used in massage therapy.
  - A simple static stretch is a slow, smooth, and even stretch application, holding the end point for up to 30 seconds.
  - Contract–relax–stretch (CRS) involves contracting the targeted muscle before a stretch.
  - CRS with reciprocal inhibition involves contracting the antagonist of the targeted muscle before a stretch.
  - Active assisted stretch involves the recipient initiating the stretch and the practitioner assisting by applying additional force in the desired direction.
- Practical knowledge of the structure and the movement possible at each joint is essential to ensure the safety of the recipient during joint movements.
- Joint movements add a kinetic dimension to a massage session and provide diversity of technique.
- General guidelines for performing joint mobilizations and stretching techniques include
  - Check for contraindications before applying joint movements.
  - Adapt techniques for structural abnormalities.

o Stay within the normal range of motion of the joint.
o Stay within the comfort range of the recipient.
o Warm surrounding soft tissues before stretching.
o Apply joint mobilizing techniques with smooth, free, loose quality.
o Apply stretching techniques with slow, sustained, even motion.
o Apply a stretch as the recipient exhales.

o Use contract-relax and reciprocal inhibition to enhance a stretch.
o Use client feedback to determine the limit of a stretch.

- The areas of the body for which joint movement techniques are effective include the neck, shoulder girdle, elbows, wrists, hands, chest, hips, knees, ankles, and feet.

EXAM REVIEW

Key Terms

Match the following key terms to their descriptions. For additional study, look up the key terms in the Interactive Glossary, and note other terms that compare or contrast with them.

_____ **1.** Active assisted stretch
_____ **2.** Active movement
_____ **3.** Assisted movement
_____ **4.** Contract–relax–stretch
_____ **5.** Mobilizing techniques
_____ **6.** Passive movements
_____ **7.** Reciprocal inhibition
_____ **8.** Resisted movements
_____ **9.** Simple static stretch
_____ **10.** Stretching

a. Nonspecific passive joint movement technique
b. Movement that meets with resistance supplied by the practitioner
c. Movements initiated and controlled by another person
d. The practitioner helps a client complete a movement
e. Client initiates the stretch and practitioner helps stretch further
f. Techniques used to increase flexibility at the joints and for muscle relaxation
g. Unassisted voluntary movement; exercise
h. Target muscle relaxes as its antagonist contracts
i. Stretch applied to a muscle immediately after its contraction
j. Type of passive stretch characterized by slow, sustained, and even application

Memory Workout

To test your memory of the main concepts in this chapter, complete the following sentences by circling the most correct answer from the two choices provided.

1. In (resisted) (assisted) movements, the client initiates the movement, while the practitioner helps complete it.
2. Joint manipulations intended to realign misaligned joints by sudden thrusting movements (are) (are not) within the scope of massage therapy.
3. Stay within the (extended) (normal) range of motion of the joint when performing joint movement techniques.
4. Joint mobilizing techniques can be characterized as (smooth, loose) (controlled, precise).
5. When using reciprocal inhibition to enhance a stretch, the (agonist) (antagonist) of the targeted muscle is contracted prior to the stretch.

6. Use client (feedback) (height) to determine the limits of a stretch.
7. Joint abnormalities may be (congenital) (constitutional) or may be the result of accidents, injuries, or diseases.
8. Sense of restriction as the limit of the range of motion at a joint is reached is called (end feel) (inhibition).
9. The recipient is totally passive during a simple (resisted) (static) stretch.
10. Apply a stretch as the recipient (inhales) (exhales).
11. Muscles should be (strengthened) (warmed) before applying stretching techniques.
12. Neck stretches are best applied when the client is (supine) (side-lying).

Test Prep

The following multiple-choice questions will help to prepare you for future school and professional exams.

1. Movements performed entirely by a person without assistance from anyone else are called:
   a. Passive resisted
   b. Free active
   c. Active assisted
   d. Free resisted

2. Which of the following joint movements is not within the scope of massage therapy?
   a. Figure-8s of the toes
   b. Extension of the arm overhead
   c. Thrusting on the back
   d. Flexion of the ankle

3. A simple, static stretch is a type of stretch characterized by:
   a. Slow, sustained, and even application
   b. Sudden, forceful movements
   c. Bouncing
   d. Both a and c

4. A contraindication for joint movement techniques is:
   a. Muscle soreness
   b. Muscle shortening
   c. Acute inflammation
   d. Osteoarthritis

5. Time the stretch to the client's:
   a. Holding his or her breath
   b. Inhale
   c. Exhale
   d. Either b or c

6. For the contract–relax–stretch technique, the client contracts the:
   a. Target muscle just before the stretch
   b. Target muscle right after the stretch
   c. Antagonist to the target muscle just before the stretch
   d. Antagonist to the target muscle right after the stretch

7. Mobilizing techniques for the cervical vertebrae are best applied with the client:
   a. Sitting
   b. Side-lying
   c. Prone
   d. Supine

8. Which of the following techniques creates free movement in the shoulder, elbow, and wrist?
   a. Horizontal flexion of the arm
   b. Wagging the arm
   c. Stretching the arm overhead
   d. Passive shoulder roll

9. Which is the best indication that a stretch is at its safe limit?
   a. When the practitioner feels a little resistance in the tissues
   b. When the skin in the area turns color
   c. When the practitioner hears a snap
   d. When the client tells the practitioner the limit has been reached

10. Care around hypermobile joints is advised because they may be prone to:
    a. Dislocation
    b. Adhesions
    c. Swelling
    d. Hyperextension

Video Challenge

Watch this video, which can be found at MyHealthProfessionslLab.com, Chapter 13, and then answer the following questions.

Joint Movements
1. What are the three guidelines mentioned in the video for joint mobilizations?

2. Describe the technique shown in the video for mobilizing the shoulder with the client in the supine position.
3. What are the four guidelines mentioned in the video for stretching techniques?

Comprehension Exercises

The following short-answer questions test your knowledge and understanding of chapter topics and provide practice in written communication skills. Explain in two to four complete sentences.

1. Contrast joint mobilizing and stretching techniques.
2. Explain how the principle of reciprocal inhibition can enhance a static stretch.

3. Describe two techniques for mobilizing the shoulder joint when the client is supine.

For Greater Understanding

The following exercises are designed to take you from the realm of theory into practical applications. They will help give you a deeper understanding of the techniques covered in this chapter. Action words are underlined to emphasize the variety of activities presented to address different learning styles and to encourage deeper thinking.

1. For each of the stretches covered in the chapter, name the muscles involved and locate their attachments on a skeleton. If possible, perform the joint movements on the skeleton and observe how the bones move in relation to each other.

2. One person performs mobilizing techniques on a joint, while another observes. The observer verbally describes the hand and body position of the person performing the technique and evaluates the giver's body mechanics.

3. In a group of three, one person talks another through performing a particular stretch on a receiver lying on the massage table. He or she describes step-by-step how the technique is performed. Include static, contract–relax–stretch, CRS with reciprocal inhibition, and active assisted stretching.

4. Videotape your application of mobilizing and stretching techniques. Watching the video, analyze your body mechanics. Perform the technique again, correcting body mechanics.

MyHealthProfessionsLab™

MyHealthProfessionsLab.com is a premium online homework management system that includes a host of features to help you study. Registered users will find:

- Powerful tools that track and analyze your results—allowing you to create a personalized learning experience
- Videos, flashcards and other learning tools to help enrich your progress
- Streaming lesson presentations and self-paced learning modules
- A space where you and your instructors can view and manage your assignments

14 Full-Body Swedish Massage

Pearson Education, Inc.

CHAPTER OUTLINE

Learning Outcomes

Key Terms

Overview

Guidelines for Full-Body Swedish Massage

Full-Body Swedish Massage Practice Sequence

Chapter Highlights

Exam Review

LEARNING OUTCOMES

After studying this chapter, you will have information to:

1. Describe a full-body Swedish massage session.

2. Organize a massage session from body region to body region.

3. Apply techniques in appropriate order within each body region.

4. Choose opening, warm-up, transition, and finishing techniques appropriately.

5. Apply the principles of continuity, rhythm, pacing, specificity, and pressure.

6. Perform a 1-hour full-body Swedish massage for health promotion.

KEY TERMS

Continuity

Finishing techniques

Flow

Full-body Swedish massage

Opening technique

Pacing

Pressure

Rhythm

Specificity

Transition techniques

Warming technique

OVERVIEW

A **full-body Swedish massage** addresses all regions of the body. It usually includes techniques from all seven of the basic Swedish massage technique categories. Oil, lotion, or other lubricant is typically used to enhance sliding over the skin and to prevent chafing. Full-body Swedish massage sessions last from 30–90 minutes, with the 50 or 60 minute formats being the most common.

Performed from a wellness perspective, these sessions focus on general health and well-being, as well as meeting the specific therapeutic needs of the recipient. The goals for health promotion include improving circulation, relaxing the muscles, improving joint mobility, inducing the relaxation response, promoting healthy skin, and creating a general sense of well-being.

GUIDELINES FOR FULL-BODY SWEDISH MASSAGE

Although each practitioner combines and blends various massage techniques in different ways, there are some general guidelines for giving a full-body Swedish massage. These guidelines address draping, sequence of body parts, order of techniques, continuity, rhythm, pacing, specificity, and pressure. Table 14–1 ■ summarizes the guidelines for performing full-body Swedish massage.

TABLE 14–1	Summary of the Elements of a Swedish Massage Session
Goals	General health promotion
	Improved circulation, relaxed muscles, improved joint mobility, relaxation response, healthy skin, sense of well-being
	Therapeutic needs (e.g., reduce muscle stiffness and soreness, relieve trigger points, injury recovery)
Length of Time	30–90 minutes (typically 50 or 60 minutes)
Draping	Full sheet or large towel
	Body regions uncovered for massage and then recovered
	Genitals and women's breasts covered at all times
Sequence of Body Regions *Starting point* *Direction* *(e.g., clockwise)* *Ending point*	Starting prone:
	Start on back
	Buttocks, legs
	Turn to supine
	Legs/feet, arms/shoulders, chest, abdomen
	End with neck, head, and face
	Starting supine:
	Start on head and face
	Neck, arms/shoulders, chest, abdomen, legs/feet
	Turn to prone
	Legs, buttocks
	End with back
Order of Techniques on a Specific Body Region	Opening technique (e.g., effleurage to apply oil or compressions)
	Warming techniques (e.g., effleurage or compressions)
	Combination of techniques
	For general health (e.g., effleurage, petrissage, superficial warming friction, joint movements)
	Specific therapeutic goals (e.g., deep friction, vibration, direct pressure)
	Transition techniques (e.g., effleurage, tapotement, compression)
	Finishing techniques (e.g., effleurage, tapotement, compression)
Continuity	Sense of continuous touch throughout the session
	Avoid abrupt removal of touch
Flow	Orderly sequence and smooth transitions
	Skillful draping
Rhythm	Smooth and even rhythm
Pacing	Moderate speed
Specificity	Attention to specific muscle or small area
	Shorter length session = less specificity in full-body massage
Pressure	Medium to light pressure, heavier pressure by request
	Vary according to part of body massaged and condition of tissues
	Get feedback about pressure at the beginning of the session and after moving to a different area

Draping

Draping is done with a sheet or large towel, and body parts are skillfully uncovered and recovered as needed. Genitals are covered at all times. Women's breasts are always covered, except when breast massage is performed by a practitioner with special training and then only with informed consent of the recipient. Breast massage is not yet common in the United States and, therefore, will not be included in the general full-body routine described in this chapter.

Sequence of Body Regions

In a full-body session, the practitioner massages each region of the body (e.g., back, arms, and legs) in a particular sequence. The sequence usually includes supine and prone positions and has a starting point, direction (e.g., clockwise), and an ending point. This establishes organization and a routine way of working.

Recipients lie prone or supine for the first part of the massage, and then turn over for the second part. Whether they start prone or supine is a matter of preference for the practitioner and the recipient. Sometimes the side-lying or semireclining positions are used, for example, with special populations.

There are no hard-and-fast rules for sequence, but it should facilitate a smooth flow from one region of the body to the next. Some advocate moving clockwise around the table. The following are two suggestions for sequences in a full-body Swedish massage session.

- If a session starts with the recipient in the prone position, a commonly used sequence of body sections would be the back, buttocks, and legs. The neck and feet are sometimes addressed prone, but are more easily accessed supine. Then turn over to the supine position with a sequence moving from legs and feet, shoulders, arms and hands, chest and abdomen, neck, and ending with the head and face.

- If the session starts with the recipient in the supine position, a commonly used sequence of body sections would be head and face, neck and shoulders, arms and hands, chest and abdomen, legs and feet. Then turn over to the prone position with a sequence moving from buttocks to legs and ending on the back.

One advantage to starting in the prone position is that it may feel safer to someone new to massage. Another advantage is that back massage generally triggers the relaxation response sooner, so relaxes the client more quickly. It also allows those who need to be more alert at the end of the session to finish faceup. An advantage of starting in the supine position is that the practitioner can massage the head, face, and neck right away, which may be appreciated by recipients who do a lot of desk or computer work.

Order of Techniques

The general order of techniques for each region of the body is similar. Once a part is undraped, opening and warming techniques are applied. These are followed by a combination of techniques for general health promotion, as well as techniques for specific therapeutic effects. Finishing and transition techniques complete work on the region. Vary techniques throughout the application. Too much repetition of one technique can be monotonous and boring for the client.

The most common **opening technique** and **warming technique** for each area to be massaged is effleurage. It is used to apply oil or lotion, to warm the area, and to facilitate circulation. It is applied first using lighter and then deeper pressure. Effleurage on the limbs should always be performed moving distal to proximal, unless the pressure used is very light. Compressions may also serve as an opening or warming technique.

The opening is followed by a combination of techniques to improve circulation, relax muscles, improve joint mobility, and other health promotion goals. Technique combinations at this stage usually include effleurage, petrissage, warming friction, and joint movements. Deep friction, vibration, and direct pressure are applied as appropriate for more specific applications. Finish massage of the area with effleurage, tapotement, and/or compression.

Transition techniques serve to provide continuity and flow from one section to another. For example, when moving from massage of the upper leg to the lower leg, a few effleurage strokes to the entire leg help tie the regions together kinesthetically for the recipient.

When ending work on a specific part of the body, the prone or supine side, or the entire session, some thought should be given to finishing techniques. **Finishing techniques** may be used to reconnect parts of the body that have been worked on more specifically or to further sedate or stimulate the recipient. Effleurage, tapotement, and compression are typical finishing techniques that can create a sense of wholeness, connectedness, and completeness. Light effleurage, sometimes called nerve strokes, is more soothing, whereas tapotement is more stimulating. Passive touch in the form of simple holding at the head or feet is calming and is sometimes used to end a session.

Continuity and Flow

A skillful full-body massage has a sense of continuity and flow. **Continuity** is achieved by creating a sense of continuous contact throughout the session from the initial touch to the finishing touches. Establishment or removal of touch is never abrupt. This does not mean that you may never take your hands off a recipient during a session, but that doing so is kept to a minimum and is done as imperceptibly as possible.

A sense of **flow** is achieved through an orderly sequence and smooth transitions from one part of the body to the next. Skill in draping, including uncovering and recovering, can add to the sense of smooth transitions.

Rhythm, Pacing, Specificity, Pressure

The **rhythm** of a classic Swedish massage session may be described as smooth and even and the **pacing** as moderate in speed. Trying to perform a full-body session in half an hour will necessitate a faster pace with less attention to detail. A session focusing on general relaxation will be slower paced and usually minimize or eliminate such stimulating techniques as tapotement.

Specificity is required for attention to a specific muscle or small area. If the recipient requests more attention to certain parts of the body, such as the back and neck, then those areas would receive more time and specific techniques, and the rest of the body would receive less specific massage. Every area should be addressed in a full-body massage, even if the techniques used are broadly applied for a brief time. Avoid the pitfall of spending so much time in one area, such as the back, that no time is left for other parts of the body. Even a few effleurage strokes or light compressions will feel more satisfactory to a client than leaving an area untouched.

The amount of **pressure** used for full-body massage varies from medium to light, although some clients may like deeper pressure. Vary the pressure used according to the part of the body massaged. For example, use lighter pressure on the face and medium to deep pressure on more muscular areas. Ask for feedback about pressure near the beginning of the session to get a sense of the client's preference and after moving to a new region.

FULL-BODY SWEDISH MASSAGE PRACTICE SEQUENCE

There is no one best way to perform a full-body Swedish massage. Practitioners usually develop their own styles and routine ways of performing a massage session. Routines generally involve a regular starting point and opening techniques, a specific sequence of body regions, a certain order of techniques in each body region, and a regular way of ending the session. These routines typically change with further training and experience and are modified to meet the needs of the recipient on the table. Today's eclectic practitioners may use a full-body Swedish massage routine as a starting point and then integrate contemporary techniques as appropriate to accomplish the therapeutic goals of the session.

Some spas and salons offer what they call a *signature massage,* which is a massage routine that is given uniformly by all massage therapists in the establishment. This provides some standardization, and customers know what to expect.

REALITY CHECK

ESTEBAN

JENNIFER: I think I'm using too much pressure in my full-body massage. I can feel my practice clients tensing up, and sometimes they tell me to "lighten up." I don't realize I'm hurting them until they say something to me. I'm just really strong. How can I learn to develop a better sense of the pressure I'm using?

ESTEBAN: Varying pressure according to the situation is part of the art of massage. Work with a practice partner to learn to vary the pressure you are applying. It doesn't matter how strong you are, you can learn to control how much pressure you use. And remember that individual preferences regarding pressure vary a lot. Some people have lower tolerance for pressure for reasons that are not always apparent. That's why it's good to start with what you think is medium pressure (less than your heaviest pressure), and ask for feedback. You can go lighter or deeper from there. Also look for nonverbal signs earlier. Be prepared to go as light or heavy as clients want within reasonable limits.

Establishments train their employees to perform their signature massages.

The following Practice Sequence is an example of a 1-hour full-body routine that may be used to practice the basic Swedish massage techniques on different parts of the body. By having a routine as a framework, the learner is free to focus on specific skills, including good body mechanics, draping, specific techniques, smooth transitions, continuity, rhythm, and pacing.

It is impossible to describe every single movement of a routine in writing. Use the Practice Sequence offered here as a framework, but feel free to add variations of techniques as you become more attuned to the work. Experiment with what feels right to you. To lengthen the routine, you may repeat techniques or insert additional techniques as appropriate.

PRACTICE SEQUENCE 14–1

Full-Body Swedish Massage | 1-hour massage

Preliminary Instructions
• Before leaving the client alone to undress in private, request that he or she be covered with the drape and lying facedown on the table when you return. Explain how the face cradle works.
• Before the session starts, adjust the position of the face cradle and place a bolster under the ankles.

Recipient prone
Region: Back (15 minutes)

1

Figure 14–1 Uncover the back down to the waist. Stand at the head to apply lubricant to the back using long effleurage strokes. Cover the entire back and sides using light to moderate pressure.

2

Figure 14–2 Without losing contact, move to the recipient's right side. Stand at the hip and face the head. Apply shingles effleurage along the right side of the spine with fingers pointing toward the head. Use moderate to deep pressure. Repeat 3–4 times.

3

Figure 14–3 Apply deep circular friction with the fingertips to the erector muscles on the right side, moving from the sacrum to the neck. To apply deeper pressure, use both hands, placing one hand on top of the other. Circle away from the spine. Repeat twice.

4

Figure 14–4 Apply deep effleurage with the thumbs between the iliac crest and the last three ribs. Keep the thumbs in proper alignment. Repeat this technique in two or three strips, moving out laterally from the spine. Alternative (not shown): Warming friction using the knuckles may be substituted as easier on the hands. Less lubricant is used so that friction can be created.

5

Figure 14–5 Reconnect the lower back with the shoulder with a few deep effleurage strokes. Then place one hand over the other to apply greater pressure for a circular movement around the shoulder. Repeat 3–4 times.

6

Figure 14–6 Starting at the waist, apply circular two-handed petrissage over the entire right side. Keep hands flat with full contact on the back surface. Both hands move clockwise. Lift superficial soft tissues as hands pass each other.
Alternative (not shown): Use skin rolling if the skin does not lift easily and appears to be adhering to soft tissues underneath. It can be applied to the entire back or in specific areas of adhering.

7

Figure 14–7 Knead the upper trapezius with one or two hands. Lift, squeeze, and release the soft tissues in a rhythmical motion.

Apply kneading across the shoulder and up the neck. Get feedback from client about the amount of pressure you are using.

8

Figure 14–8 Walk around the head of the table to the left side and reach across to perform three-count stroking to the right shoulder (trapezius). Cover the lower, middle, and upper trapezius. Keep flat, firm contact that conforms to the body contour. Repeat 3–4 times.

Note: Perform from same side if it is too difficult to reach across the table.

9

Figure 14–9 Reconnect the lower and upper back with horizontal stroking from lower back to shoulders. Keep flat, firm contact that conforms to the body contour. Repeat twice. Repeat Steps 2–9 on the left side.

10

Figure 14–10 When both sides of the back have been massaged, redrape the back. With light to moderate force, use rapping or some other form of tapotement as a finishing technique for the entire back.

Region: Lower Limbs and Buttocks (10 minutes)

Figure 14–11 Undrape the left leg up to the waist, being careful not to expose the gluteal cleft. Tuck the drape securely under the hip and at the waist. When massaging the legs and buttocks, your hands should never touch or come unreasonably close to the genital area.

Figure 14–12 Stand at the side of the table facing the head. Apply lubricant with effleurage from ankle to hip following the curves of the leg and using moderate pressure. Contact the sides and posterior surfaces. The inside hand will slide onto the back of the leg about halfway up the thigh and follow the outside hand around the buttocks and hip. Hands return together to the ankle with a light sliding motion.

Figure 14–13 Apply deep circular effleurage to the buttocks muscles as a warming technique. Place one hand on top of the other for reinforcement. Follow the contour of the area moving medial to lateral and around the hip.

Figure 14–14 Apply compressions over the entire buttocks region with the fist using moderate to heavy pressure. Include the attachments along the iliac crest. Finish with circular effleurage, using either the hand-over-hand position or the fist. Transition with 2–3 long effleurage strokes to the entire leg.

15

Figure 14–15 Apply effleurage to hamstring muscles with fists from just above the popliteal fossa to the superior attachments of the hamstring muscles. Alternative: Use the forearm to apply the effleurage for more pressure.

16

Figure 14–16 Continuing with one fist, perform effleurage along the iliotibial band and the tensor fascia lata muscle moving from the hip to the knee. This broad band of fascia and muscle can accept moderate to deep pressure.

17

Figure 14–17 Place one hand on the medial and one on the lateral thigh to begin horizontal stroking. Slide hands up and around the thigh, exchanging positions with a smooth sliding and lifting motion. Apply from the knee to just below the attachments of the adductors. Be mindful of professional boundaries when touching the inside of the leg.

18

Figure 14–18 Two-handed kneading on the upper leg. Apply kneading to medial, posterior, and lateral muscles of the thigh.

Figure 14–19 Basic effleurage distal to proximal as a transition technique. Apply first to the upper thigh and then to the entire leg.

Figure 14–20 Two-handed kneading to lower leg muscles. Knead the belly of the calf muscles using two hands alternating in an even rhythm.

Figure 14–21 Basic sliding effleurage to the lower leg. Apply from heel of foot to knee. Conform hands to contour of leg for full contact.

Figure 14–22 Finishing techniques to entire leg. Start with basic effleurage from ankle to hip. Redrape the leg. Finish with a few nerve strokes from the buttocks to the ankle.

Repeat Steps 11–22 on the right side. Afterward, continue with Step 23.

23

Figure 14–23 Finishing techniques for the back of the body. With the recipient fully draped, gently rock the body from side to side, from back to hips to legs for about 5 seconds. Perform 2–3 light effleurage stokes from shoulders to feet over the drape as a connecting maneuver, and to signal the end of the massage on the back side of the body.

24

Figure 14–24 Turning over technique: Use tenting to assist the recipient turning to supine position. Anchor the drape with your leg against the side of the table and hold the other side of the drape up slightly. Have the recipient roll away from you to prevent him or her from getting wrapped up in the sheet. Lower the drape.

Note: The recipient should have been out of your sight as he or she turned over under the tent. If there is more than one session going on in the room, be sure that you do not expose the recipient to others.

Recipient supine
Region: Lower limbs (10 minutes)

25

Figure 14–25 Undrape the right leg. Tuck the drape securely under the thigh.

26

Figure 14–26 Apply lubricant to the entire right limb using basic sliding effleurage. Apply moderate pressure distal to proximal, and slide back with light touch. Hands conform to the contour of the leg for maximal contact. Lighten pressure over knee. Cover anterior, medial, and lateral aspects of the limb.

Figure 14–27 Apply deep effleurage to the thigh from knee to superior thigh. Cover anterior, medial, and lateral aspects of the thigh. Use flat hands or loose fists to apply pressure.

Figure 14–28 Apply two-handed kneading to quadriceps, adductor, and abductor muscles of the thigh.

Figure 14–29 Jostle the thigh, tossing from side to side, hand to hand. Causes loose, free movement in the hip and knee joints.

Figure 14–30 Place one hand on the medial and one on the lateral thigh to begin horizontal stroking. Slide hands up and around the thigh, exchanging positions with a smooth sliding and lifting motion. Apply from the knee to the superior thigh. Be mindful of professional boundaries when touching the inside of the leg.

31

Figure 14–31 Effleurage to transition to lower leg—distal to proximal. Apply effleurage with moderate pressure to thigh first, and then to entire limb from ankle to thigh. Follow with effleurage from ankle to knee.

32

Figure 14–32 Apply circular friction around the knee with the heels of the hands moving the skin over soft tissues underneath. Stay to sides of the kneecap.

33

Figure 14–33 Use thumbs to apply stripping effleurage to the muscle just lateral to the shin bone (tibialis anterior). Apply from ankle to the attachments near the lateral condyle of the tibia. Complete 2–4 strips, depending on the size of the muscle.

34

Figure 14–34 Direct thumb pressure along the tibialis anterior. Start at proximal end, moving about 1 inch at a time to distal end. Keep thumb and wrist in good alignment. Use moderate to heavy pressure. Transition with effleurage over lower limb.

Figure 14–35 Circular friction around the ankle with the fingertips. Applying pressure with the fingertips, move the skin around the ankle over underlying soft tissues. Follow the contour of the ankle bones.

Figure 14–36 Mobilize the ankle using the heels of the hands. Place the heels of the hands just under the ankle bones. Shift the hands back and forth causing movement side to side in the ankle. Action is free and loose.

Figure 14–37 Squeeze the foot lightly from heel to toes. Fingers of hands on top with thumbs around the sides and underneath. Apply slight pressure to the sides to spread the metatarsals.

38

Figure 14–38 Effleurage between the metatarsals using the thumb or fingers. Slide between the metatarsals one-by-one from the toes to the ankle.

39

Figure 14–39 Slide along the bottom of the foot with the fist. Apply from the ball of the foot to the heel. Use moderate to deep pressure. Other hand supports the foot from the dorsal side.

40

Figure 14–40 Slapping tapotement on the bottom of the foot. Slap lightly 4–5 times.

41

Figure 14–41 Effleurage to the entire limb with moderate pressure, followed by nerve strokes as a finishing technique. Apply effleurage distal to proximal, and then redrape the leg. Apply nerve strokes proximal to distal over the drape to finish.

Repeat Steps 25–41 on the left leg. Afterward, continue with Step 42.

Figure 14–42 Transition from the lower to the upper limbs with compression over the drape. Apply compression with palms over the leg and then up the arm to the shoulder as a connecting and transition technique.

Region: Arms, Shoulders, Chest (10 minutes)

Figure 14–43 Uncover the left arm and shoulder. Apply oil or lotion to the arm with effleurage from hand to shoulder, including the deltoid muscle.

Figure 14–44 Alternating one-hand kneading to the upper arm. Squeeze the biceps side, then the triceps side, alternating in a rhythmical motion. Cover the entire upper arm from the shoulder to the elbow.

Figure 14–45 Passive shoulder roll. Place one hand on the anterior and the other on the posterior shoulder. Circle the shoulder clockwise, then counterclockwise twice in each direction.

46

Figure 14–46 Effleurage to transition to forearm—distal to proximal. Apply effleurage with moderate pressure to upper arm first, and then to entire arm from wrist to shoulder. Follow with deep effleurage from wrist to elbow.

47

Figure 14–47 One hand kneads the forearm muscles, while the other hand stabilizes the arm at the wrist.

48

Figure 14–48 Apply stripping effleurage with the thumb to the flexor and extensor muscles of the forearm. Apply from the wrist to their attachments near the elbow.

Figure 14–49 Warm wrist and hand. Palm down, hold the hand on the little finger and thumb sides, then gently squeeze the hand while broadening the palm and separating the metacarpals. Apply effleurage with the thumbs to back of the wrist, and then between metacarpals. Turn the palm up to apply effleurage to the palm of the hand.

Figure 14–50 Mobilize the joints in the hand. Follow with figure-8s at the knuckles and scissoring the metacarpals.

Figure 14–51 Lightly squeeze along each finger applying pressure first near the knuckle and then moving along the finger to the tip.

Figure 14–52 Effleurage to entire arm to reconnect and transition to the chest. Apply effleurage with moderate pressure from hand to shoulder 2–3 times.

53

Figure 14–53 Effleurage to pectoral muscles using fist. Lift the arm, holding just below the wrist. Apply effleurage over the pectoral muscles with a loose fist, moving lateral to medial and stopping at the breast tissue.

54

Figure 14–54 Effleurage over sternum. Apply with the palm of the hand between breast tissue. Omit this technique if a woman recipient has large breasts or if she might feel it is an invasion of her personal boundaries. Ask permission if in doubt.

55

Figure 14–55 Effleurage to the entire area with moderate pressure as a finishing technique. Apply effleurage distal to proximal, and then redrape the arm and shoulder.

Repeat Steps 43–55 on the right arm. Afterward, continue with Step 56.

Region: Abdomen (5 minutes)

Preliminary Considerations:
• Ask permission to massage the abdomen if the recipient is new to massage or new to you.
• Explain to women that the breasts will be draped.
• Avoid if recipient has eaten in the last hour.
• People experiencing constipation or gas in the bowels may be sensitive to pressure. Get feedback about their comfort.

Figure 14–56 Drape recipient for abdominal massage. Tuck drape along sides for secure anchoring. Do not expose the pubic area. (Cover women's breasts before pulling the sheet to the iliac crest exposing the abdomen. See Figure 11–31.)

Figure 14–57 Circular clockwise pattern. Gently lay a hand on the abdomen to establish contact. Apply effleurage with one hand while the other rests on top. Move in a large circle along the bottom of the ribs and around the outline of the pelvis. Check with the recipient to make sure the pressure is comfortable.

Figure 14–58 Vibration to the abdomen with the fingertips. Apply vibration from spot to spot in a clockwise pattern. Stop if the recipient reports feeling pain.

Figure 14–59 Petrissage with a flat hand. Apply compression across the abdomen in a wavelike motion. Push in first with the heel of the hand and then roll onto the fingertips, repeating the wave with rhythmic movement.

Figure 14–60 Horizontal stroking of the abdomen. Place a hand on either side of the waist, fingers pointing away from you. Slide and lift the hands to the other side simultaneously. Hands cross in the middle. Repeat 3–4 times.

Figure 14–61 Passive touch in center of abdomen as finishing technique. Place a hand gently in the center of the abdomen, and rest there for a moment. Remove your hand, and recover the recipient to the shoulders with the larger drape. (If the recipient is a woman, the breast drape may remain in place for warmth or may be removed at this time.)

Region: Neck and Shoulders (5 minutes)

Figure 14–62 Mobilize shoulders with "cat paw" technique. Place a hand on each shoulder to establish contact. Mobilize the shoulders by alternating pushing one side and then the other with a slow rhythmical motion. Perform from a sitting position or a low horse riding stance at the head of the table.

Figure 14–63 Apply oil or lotion with effleurage to both sides of the neck. With recipient faceup, apply oil or lotion with both hands (one on each side of the neck) sliding along the upper trapezius from the shoulder tips to the occipital ridge.

Note: Steps 64–67 are all applied to one side of the neck at a time before proceeding with Step 68.

Figure 14–64 Effleurage with loose fist to left side of neck. Turn the head slightly to the right side, exposing the left side of the neck. Perform effleurage with the fist on the upper trapezius from the occipital ridge to the shoulder. Creates a mild stretch in the upper trapezius.

Figure 14–65 Apply circular friction to the left side of the neck along cervical muscles with the fingertips of your left hand. Start at the base of the neck moving up along the cervical muscles to the suboccipital region. Use moderate pressure to warm the deeper muscles.

Figure 14–66 Stripping effleurage along cervical muscles. Using the fingertips or a knuckle to apply deep effleurage to the posterior cervical muscles from the suboccipital region to the base of the neck. Feel the stretching and broadening of the cervical muscles.

67

Figure 14–67 Effleurage as a finishing and transition technique. Finish the left side with effleurage moving back and forth from the tip of the shoulder to the suboccipital region. Use palm of hand or fist. Return the head to face upward.

Repeat Steps 64–67 on the right side. Afterward, continue with Step 68.

68

Figure 14–68 Wavelike neck mobilization. Place the hands palms up at the base of the neck, one on either side of the spine, with fingertips pressing up on the cervical muscles. Draw the fingers toward the occiput, maintaining pressure upward. The cervical vertebrae will rise and fall as the fingers pass underneath. If the muscles are relaxed, this will create a wavelike motion in the neck.

69

Figure 14–69 Finish with effleurage and passive touch. Apply effleurage to both sides simultaneously, starting at the tips of the shoulders and drawing the hands toward the base of the neck and up to the occipital ridge. Repeat twice.

70

Figure 14–70 Cradle the head briefly in both hands to end this section.

Region: Face and Head (5 minutes).

Preliminary Considerations:
• Ask permission to massage the face, especially if the recipient is wearing makeup.
• Do not use oil on the face and use lotion only if the skin is dry.

Figure 14–71 Apply effleurage to face with palms. Place the hands gently on the face with fingertips at the jaw. Draw the hands toward the temples using the full palm-side of the hands. Repeat 2–3 times.

Figure 14–72 Circular friction to jaw muscles and temples. Apply circular friction with the fingertips over the masseter and then the temporalis muscles.

Figure 14–73 Effleurage to forehead. Use the thumbs to stroke the muscles of the forehead, applying effleurage medial to lateral. Repeat 2–3 times.

74

Figure 14–74 Circular petrissage to forehead. Use the thumbs moving in counterclockwise circles. The movement is timed so that the tissues are lifted and pressed as the thumbs move past one another.

75

Figure 14–75 Stroke alongside the nose and under the cheekbones. Use the thumbs to slide down the sides of the nose, ending in the indentation at the inferior end. Continue under the cheekbones, moving bilaterally. Repeat twice.

76

Figure 14–76 Press up under the cheekbones. Use light to moderate pressure to press into the soft tissues up against the underside of the cheekbones.

77

Figure 14–77 Loosen the scalp by applying circular friction to the sides, back, and top of head (over entire hair area). The fingers and scalp move together over a spot before moving to the next spot. Do not slide over the skin or hair.

Figure 14–78 Cradle the head briefly in both hands to end this section. Hold for a few seconds until you can feel the recipient completely relax.

Figure 14–79 Finish the entire session with brushing over front of the body. Apply brushing movements with fingertips from head and shoulder areas to toes. Sweep along the sides to avoid the genital area. Hold feet gently and tell the recipient that the session has ended.

 After you perform the Practice Sequence, evaluate how well you did by filling out Performance Evaluation Form 14–1, Full-Body Swedish Massage. The form can be found in Appendix D, *Performance Evaluation Forms* and at MyHealthProfessionsLab.com.

Figures source: Pearson Education, Inc./Segal Photography.

PRACTICAL APPLICATION

Use the Practice Sequence presented in this chapter to develop skill in combining techniques for a full-body Swedish massage session. With practice, you will be able to complete a full-body session in 50–60 minutes.

1. Can you complete the routine for each separate region in the time allotted?
2. Are your transitions smooth?
3. Can you maintain awareness of the recipient's comfort and safety while practicing?

CRITICAL THINKING

Think about the sequence of techniques used in the Practice Sequence and the flow of the entire session. Analyze one region closely and describe how you might alter or add to it to make it more effective.

1. How might you transition from one technique to the next to create better continuity or flow?
2. How might you create more specificity?
3. How much can you add and still stay within the time allotted in the 60-minute session?

CHAPTER HIGHLIGHTS

- A typical full-body Swedish massage lasts 50 or 60 minutes and includes massage of the back, legs, abdomen, chest, arms, neck, and head.
- Wellness massage sessions focus on general health and well-being, as well as meeting the therapeutic needs of the recipient.
- Practitioners develop their own styles and routine ways of performing a massage session.
- The recipient is typically unclothed and draped with a sheet for modesty.
- The seven basic Swedish massage techniques are blended into a sequence to create a routine.
- The sequence usually includes both supine and prone positions and has a starting point, a direction (e.g., clockwise), and an ending point.
- Oil or lotion is used to enhance movement over the skin and to prevent chafing.
- The order of techniques for each part of the body includes opening and warming techniques such as effleurage or compressions, followed by technique combinations for general health and specific therapeutic effects.
- Massage of a particular area is concluded with finishing techniques to reconnect, smooth out, and gradually lighten touch.
  - Finishing techniques typically include light effleurage, tapotement, or passive touch, such as holding.
- A full-body massage has a sense of continuity and flow.
  - Touch is established at the beginning of a session and maintained continuously throughout, with minimal interruption.
  - A sense of flow is achieved through an orderly sequence and smooth transitions from one part of the body to the next.
- The rhythm of a full-body massage is smooth and even, and the pacing is moderate in speed.
- Specificity is required when giving attention to small areas or applying techniques for specific therapeutic purposes.
- Pressure varies according to the part of body receiving massage and the preference of the client; usually medium to light, but deeper on request.
- Eclectic practitioners may use Swedish massage as a starting point and then integrate other massage forms as appropriate to meet the client's needs.

EXAM REVIEW

Key Terms

Match the following key terms to their descriptions. For additional study, look up the key terms in the Interactive Glossary, and note other terms that compare or contrast with them.

_____ 1. Continuity
_____ 2. Finishing techniques
_____ 3. Flow
_____ 4. Swedish massage
_____ 5. Opening technique
_____ 6. Pacing
_____ 7. Pressure
_____ 8. Rhythm
_____ 9. Specificity
_____ 10. Transition techniques
_____ 11. Warming technique

a. Type of massage developed in Europe and North America
b. Attention to a specific muscle or small area
c. The speed of a massage session
d. Techniques that provide a sense of continuity when moving from one section of the body to another
e. Element of full-body massage described as smooth and even
f. Sense of continuous touch throughout a massage session
g. Sense of fluid movement or smoothness in a massage session
h. Technique used to prepare and warm tissues for massage
i. Techniques to create a sense of wholeness and completion
j. Technique used to begin a massage
k. Force used in applying massage

Memory Workout

To test your memory of the main concepts in this chapter, complete the following sentences by circling the most correct answer from the two choices provided.

1. A typical full-body massage lasts for (60) (120) minutes.
2. Practitioners blend massage techniques into logical sequences or (routines) (treatments).
3. Recipients are usually draped with a (towel) (sheet).
4. The (genitals) (buttocks) should always be covered.
5. A massage (sequence) (technique) has a beginning, a middle, and an end point.
6. Advantages of starting prone are that it often feels (safer) (lighter) to those new to massage.
7. Massage of each region of the body begins with (warming) (transition) techniques.
8. Establishment or removal of touch should never be (made) (abrupt).
9. The (shorter) (longer) the session, the less specificity is possible on any one region.
10. Routines are (lengthened) (modified) to meet the needs of the recipient on the table.

Test Prep

The following multiple-choice questions will help to prepare you for future school and professional exams.

1. Which of the following is an appropriate goal for a Swedish massage session?
   a. Improve circulation
   b. General relaxation
   c. Reduce muscle soreness
   d. Any of the above

2. When is it considered ethical to uncover a client completely during a massage?
   a. Only if he or she requests it
   b. Only if it is hot in the room
   c. Only if the drape interferes with technique application
   d. Never

3. Which of the following is the most versatile transition technique?
   a. Effleurage
   b. Petrissage
   c. Friction
   d. Vibration

4. Which of the following statements about the continuity of touch during a full-body massage session is *most* correct?
   a. Once a session has begun, never remove your hands from the body until the session is finished.
   b. Reestablish touch quickly if you remove your hands from the body during a session.
   c. Establishment or removal of touch during a session should not be abrupt.
   d. Continuity of touch during a session is not important to its flow.

5. Which of the following would be the *least* appropriate place to begin a full-body Swedish massage session?
   a. Face and head
   b. Back
   c. Abdomen
   d. Feet

6. Which of the following is the best choice for a finishing technique for a massage session if the recipient needs to be alert and ready to go back to work afterward?
   a. Nerve strokes over the drape from head to feet
   b. Holding the feet with passive touch
   c. Light tapotement from shoulders to feet
   d. Holding the head with passive touch

7. A massage session focusing on general relaxation would be:
   a. Faster paced with stimulating techniques
   b. Slower paced and avoiding stimulating techniques
   c. Medium paced with deep specific techniques
   d. Slower paced with deep specific techniques

8. When draping for abdominal massage to a woman:
   a. Simply pull the large drape down to the waist and tuck securely
   b. Use a separate drape to cover the breasts, then pull the large drape down to the waist and tuck securely
   c. Always apply abdominal massage through the drape
   d. Any of the above

9. Experienced massage therapists usually develop:
   a. A routine way of approaching their massage sessions
   b. A specific set routine that they use for all clients
   c. Separate routines for each client
   d. A routine for women and a different routine for men

10. If a portion of a massage session is focused on a particular anatomical structure or a small area, it is referred to as working with:
    a. Continuity
    b. Flow
    c. Specificity
    d. Generality

Video Challenge

Watch the Full-Body Swedish Massage videos, which can be found at MyHealthProfessionsLab.com, Chapter 14, and then answer the following questions.

1. In the full-body session demonstrated in the videos, in what order are the body regions massaged?

2. How are transitions made from one region to another in the full-body session?

3. What is the intent of each massage technique used in the full-body session? Analyze the applications in one or more body regions.

Comprehension Exercises

The following short-answer questions test your knowledge and understanding of chapter topics and provide practice in written communication skills. Explain in two to four complete sentences.

1. What is the purpose of applying finishing techniques at the end of a full-body Swedish massage session? Give two examples of different ways to end a massage session.

2. Discuss the decision to begin a massage session with the recipient prone or supine. What are the factors to consider? What are the advantages of each starting position?

3. Explain the health benefits of full-body Swedish massage. How are those benefits achieved?

For Greater Understanding

The following exercises are designed to take you from the realm of theory into the real world. They will help give you a deeper understanding of the subjects covered in this chapter. Action words are underlined to emphasize the variety of activities presented to address different learning styles and to encourage deeper thinking.

1. Receive two professional massages from the same person. Compare and contrast the two experiences. Did you notice a routine way of working, favorite techniques, and other similarities? Were there differences in the two sessions? If yes, what were they, and why do you think there were differences?

2. Receive a 60-minute full-body massage and, at a later time, a 30-minute full-body massage from the same practitioner. Analyze how the practitioner shortened the second session. How did the two experiences compare?

3. Watch a video of a full-body Swedish massage routine. Analyze the elements of the routine with particular attention to the techniques chosen and the continuity and flow. Discuss with a study partner or group.

MyHealthProfessionsLab™

MyHealthProfessionsLab.com is a premium online homework management system that includes a host of features to help you study. Registered users will find:

- Powerful tools that track and analyze your results—allowing you to create a personalized learning experience
- Videos, flashcards and other learning tools to help enrich your progress
- Streaming lesson presentations and self-paced learning modules
- A space where you and your instructors can view and manage your assignments

Regional Massage Applications—Upper Body

Pearson Education, Inc.

CHAPTER OUTLINE

Learning Outcomes

Key Terms

Regional Massage

Head and Face

Neck

Back

Upper Extremities

Chest and Abdomen

Chapter Highlights

Exam Review

LEARNING OUTCOMES

After studying this chapter, you will have information to:

1. Apply massage to upper body regions with greater specificity.

2. Describe upper body regions in terms of their human meaning.

3. Describe the general anatomy of upper body regions.

4. Appreciate the interconnections among body regions.

5. Perform massage Practice Sequences for various upper body regions.

KEY TERMS

Human meaning

Interconnections

Regional massage

Specificity

Upper body regions

REGIONAL MASSAGE

Often in massage sessions more time and attention is given to a particular region of the body, for example, to the back, neck, or feet. Information on a health history form or a referral from a health care provider could prompt more focus on a particular body region. In some cases, a client's request or the practitioner's assessment may lead to the added attention. Massage focused on a particular area of the body is sometimes called **regional massage**.

Extended massage sessions on smaller body areas provide an opportunity for greater **specificity**. This requires a shift of attention from simply applying techniques to the surface of the body toward awareness of specific anatomical structures being affected.

Massage applications and Practice Sequences for various upper regions of the body are described in this chapter. The face and head, neck, back, shoulders, upper extremities, chest, and abdomen are the **upper body regions** represented. A discussion of the meaning of each region in human terms is followed by its muscular anatomy, applications of massage, and a Practice Sequence for the region. Skeletal anatomy for the various regions is described in Chapter 13, *Joint Movements*. The applications presented can be integrated into the full-body Swedish massage described in Chapter 14, *Full-Body Swedish Massage*.

Interconnections and Meaning

The body is typically addressed region by region during a massage session. However, the body's **interconnections** should always be kept in mind. Although the following massage applications focus on different regions of the upper body, a body is not so easily divided in reality. It has wholeness and integrity.

For example, structurally the upper trapezius is in the cervical region, whereas the whole trapezius extends down the spine through the thoracic region. In addition, individual structures and whole regions are connected through a continuous wrapping of fascial tissues. Fluid circulates through vessels, and energy flows through channels that extend from head to feet. The effects of massage in a certain area will necessarily flow into the surrounding regions and sometimes to the entire body. Observations about interconnections will be made throughout this chapter and in Chapter 16, *Regional Massage Applications—Lower Body*.

Another consideration when addressing different regions of the body is that they have special significance in human terms. Body regions have **human meaning** determined by what they allow us to do and to be in this world, and their social and emotional associations. A body region may have special meaning in a particular person's life (e.g., a musician's hands or runner's legs). Keep in mind that you are not just massaging body parts such as shoulders or neck, but that you are in relationships with human beings. As you interact with clients, be aware that you are touching unique individuals.

Regional Practice Sequences

The Practice Sequences in this chapter and in Chapter 16 build on the more general Swedish massage described in Chapter 14. They expand on the treatment of each upper- and lower-body region and add techniques to address anatomical structures with more specificity. Some knowledge of musculoskeletal anatomy and skill in palpation are assumed.

Practice Sequences provide a starting point for focusing on specific regions. You are encouraged to build on these routines as you learn more advanced massage techniques. Greater knowledge of muscles and connective tissues will suggest additional ways to address normalizing soft tissues in these regions. Although the Practice Sequences are useful for generating ideas for massage, eventually you will adapt your approach to address the tissues you are actually touching during a session.

Practice Sequences follow the basic progression from general to specific to general. They include warming of the area, followed by attention to specific structures, then connecting and finishing techniques. When performing a Practice Sequence, you may find that it feels right to add some transition or other techniques to enhance the flow of the session.

HEAD AND FACE

Much of human consciousness is focused in the head and face. The head is the center for thinking and processing information. Our senses of sight, hearing, taste, and smell

PRACTICAL APPLICATION

Close your eyes and briefly scan your body mentally. Think about the significance of each region to you personally. Then sketch your body on a piece of paper using different colors to represent different regions. Explain your drawing to a study partner or group.

1. Which regions have special significance to you?
2. How did your choice of color reflect your feelings toward each region?
3. How might the personal meaning of a body region affect how you experience touch and massage there?

CRITICAL THINKING

Think about the interconnections within the upper body. Examine how massage of one upper region might affect other regions, and how this might impact massage applications.

1. What structural and functional interconnections are there in the upper extremities?

2. How might an abdominal massage affect the rest of the body?

3. Why are the head, neck, and shoulders frequently addressed together?

are housed here. The structures for bringing food into our bodies are here. We communicate with others through the structures of speech, and our faces convey our feelings and emotional states through facial expression. The muscles of the face are part of the process of thinking, as seen in furrowed brows and frowns of concentration. Relaxing the muscles of the head and face helps bring clarity of mind and release of mental and emotional stress.

Anatomy of the Head and Face

The musculature of the face and head is complex and includes muscles of expression, mastication, and movement. The muscles of expression in the face are embedded in the cutaneous tissue and move the skin itself. These muscles are relatively thin and more delicate than skeletal muscles. Common facial movements and some of the major muscles involved are listed in Table 15–1 ■.

There is an old adage that says "It takes more muscles to frown than to smile, so why overwork?" This saying appears to be true. It is estimated that it takes 41 muscles to frown and only 17 to smile. Wiggling the ears is accomplished using small muscles just above and behind the ears, the auricularis superior and posterior.

Some muscles on the head are skeletal muscles that create movement at joints, such as the masseter moving the mandible. The temporalis muscle also helps elevate the mandible and aids in mastication. The major muscles of the head and face are shown in Figure 15–1 ■.

The head is connected skeletally to the spine and muscularly to the cervical muscles. Tension in the head musculature can spread down to the neck area. Conversely, tension and trigger points in the cervical muscles can refer into the head. Head, neck, and shoulders are interconnected functionally and are often treated as a unit.

Applications of Massage for the Head and Face

Massage can help release tensions in the face and head acquired in daily living. This may be an area of tension for people whose jobs involve a lot of thinking or require extensive use of the eyes. Reading, writing, looking at a computer monitor, and doing activities that require fine hand–eye coordination, such as needlework or drawing, put strain on the muscles of the face, especially around the eyes. People who wear eyeglasses may feel strain from the weight of the glasses on the nose and ears.

Emotional distress may also lead to tension in the face and head. Worry and anxiety can result in tension in the forehead and temporal area. Habitual clenching of the jaw can cause tension in the masseter and temporalis muscles and lead to temporomandibular joint (TMJ) pain syndrome. Although crying can lead to a healthy release of emotions, it can also create strain around the eyes. Holding back emotions, and holding back tears, are accomplished by tension in the face, throat, and diaphragm.

The muscles of the face and head may also be affected by certain pathologies, such as stroke and Bell's palsy, a temporary paralysis of the face due to damage of the seventh cranial nerve. With appropriate precautions, face and head massage can help during recovery from these conditions.

TABLE 15–1	Facial Movements and Muscles
Facial Movement	**Major Muscles Involved**
Raising the eyebrows (surprise)	Frontalis
Pulling eyebrows downward and medially (frown)	Corrugator procerus
Closing the eyes (squint)	Orbicularis occuli
Flaring the nostrils	Dilator naris
Pulling corners of the mouth downward (frown)	Depressor anguli oris, platysma
Closing and protruding the lips (kiss)	Mentalis, orbicularis oris
Drawing corners of the mouth outward (smile)	Risorus, zygomaticus

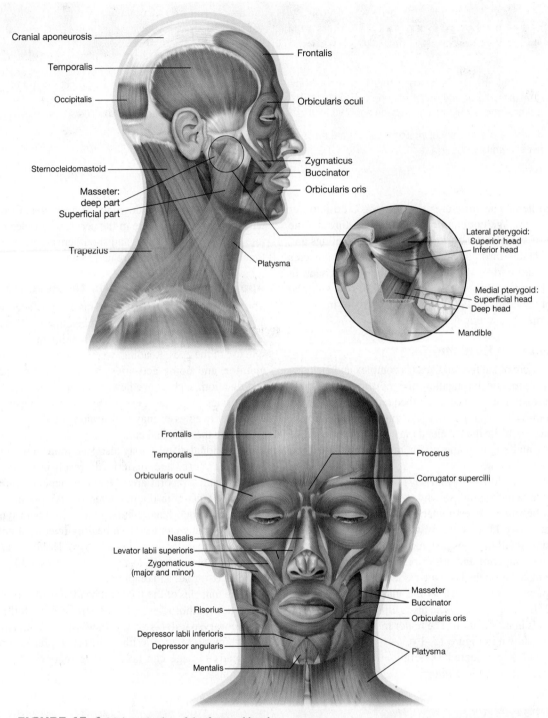

FIGURE 15–1 Major muscles of the face and head.

Massage techniques applied to the head and face address specific areas and muscles located there. There are several areas important in a head and face massage.

Eyebrow Area The tissues in the eyebrow area become tense in people who squint, are sensitive to light, or use their eyes a lot in their work (e.g., computer work, reading, or activities that require fine hand–eye coordination). Congestion in this area often accompanies tension headache. The corrugator muscle, which draws the eyebrow downward and medially, is located there.

Eyelids Gentle rubbing over the eyelids and around the eye orbit is similar to the common gesture of rubbing the eyes when tired. This action massages orbicularis oculi, the sphincter muscle of the eyelids.

Bridge of the Nose People who wear glasses often rub or squeeze the tissues between the eyebrows at the bridge of the nose to relieve pressure where the glasses sit. The procerus, a small muscle located there, draws the medial angles of the eyebrows downward and produces transverse wrinkles over the bridge of the nose. Those with sinus congestion may also feel tenderness in the external tissues of the upper nose area.

Cheekbones Pressure to the zygomatic or cheekbone area will sometimes help relieve sinus congestion.

Mouth and Jaw A number of muscles around the mouth and jaw create movement for eating, speaking, and expression. For example, chewing, sipping, whispering, singing, smiling, frowning, and sneering all involve muscles around the mouth and jaw. Muscles that aid in mastication include the masseter, pterygoid muscles, and temporalis.

Ears The ears are made of soft cartilage and have many curves and folds. People who wear glasses, clip-on earrings, or any type of heavy earrings usually enjoy massage to the ears. Take care around hearing aids.

Scalp The skin that covers the head (the scalp) moves freely on most people. Mobilizing the scalp has similar effects to skin rolling, which frees the underlying fascia and increases superficial circulation. Because circulation to hair follicles is increased, this helps promote healthy hair. Stress can lead to tension in the muscles of the head and a less mobile scalp. Tension in these muscles can contribute to tension headaches.

PRACTICE SEQUENCE 15–1

Head and Face Massage
10–15 minutes
Recipient supine

Preliminary Instructions
• Stand or sit at the head of the table during the application.
• Do not use oil or lotion on the face.
• Use light to moderate pressure.
• Avoid pressure over the eyes if a recipient is wearing contact lenses.

Figure 15–2 Apply effleurage to the face using palms. Stroke bilaterally from chin to temples, lifting facial tissues gently.

Figure 15–3 Apply effleurage to forehead with thumbs. Stroke from middle of forehead to the temples. Begin just above the eyebrows and repeat in rows as necessary to cover the entire forehead.

3

Figure 15–4 Apply gentle circular friction to the temple area.

4

Figure 15–5 Gently squeeze the tissues along the eyebrow line between your thumb and forefinger. Begin at the nose and move from place to place along the eyebrow line laterally to the outside edge of the eye orbit.

5

Figure 15–6 Apply effleurage over eyelids. Using very light pressure, stroke the closed eyelids with your thumbs medial to lateral. Stroke a few times to cover the entire lid.

6

Figure 15–7 Thumb slides along the nose. Slide a thumb over the procerus muscle, then use both thumbs to slide along the outline of the nose from the eyes to the depression at the base.

Figure 15–8 Apply direct pressure under the zygomatic arch. Moving laterally, gently press up and under the zygomatic arch with the index and third fingers. The area will be tender if the sinuses are congested.

A

B

Figure 15–9 Thumb slides above and below the mouth. (A) Use the thumbs to stroke above the upper lip and then (B) under the lower lip. Knead the tissues on the chin and along the jawline with the thumb and first two fingers.

Figure 15–10 Apply circular friction with the fingertips over the masseter muscle.

10

Figure 15–11 Rub the ears between your thumbs and index fingers. Follow the curves to rub the entire ear, including the ear lobes. As you approach the outer edges of the ear while rubbing, give a gentle pull.

11

Figure 15–12 Apply circular friction to the area of the head around the base of the ears.

12

Figure 15–13 Use friction to mobilize the entire scalp. Place the fingers on the scalp, and move the skin over the underlying muscle and bone. As the skin moves, the fingers stay in place on the skin surface.

13

Figure 15–14 Apply circular friction to muscles on the head using moderate pressure to the frontalis and temporalis muscles and the attachment of the suboccipital muscles on the occipital ridge.

14

Figure 15–15 Press the sides of the head with the palms. Fingertips meet on the forehead and palms lay along the sides of the head. Use the full hand to press with moderate pressure. Slowly release the pressure.

15

Figure 15–16 Apply passive touch over the eyes and cheeks to finish. Place the hands, using very light pressure, on the face with palms over the eyes. Similar to the self-comforting gesture of holding your face in your hands.

After you perform the Practice Sequence, evaluate how well you did by filling out Performance Evaluation Form 15–1, Head and Face Massage. The form can be found in Appendix D: *Performance Evaluation Forms*, and at MyHealthProfessionsLab.com.

Figures source: Pearson Education, Inc./Segal Photography.

NECK

The cervical or neck region is *pivotal* in many senses of the word. It links the head with the torso and houses the delicate spinal cord. Nerves and blood vessels going to the brain pass through the neck. It contains the muscles that hold the head in position during upright posture and movement in different planes. It is the pivot point for the head and provides the structure and musculature that allows us to access sensation as we turn our heads to look, listen, smell, and taste.

For some people, the neck and throat are areas to be protected from touch by others. People who have experienced choking, near suffocation or drowning, neck trauma, or who fear such occurrences may respond negatively to touching

the neck. Protective responses may include tightening the shoulder and neck muscles, raising the shoulders, lowering the chin, covering the throat with the hands, or even pulling the practitioner's hands from the neck. Talk to clients about any protective reactions you sense. Ask for their permission to touch the neck region. Alerting them before you touch the neck may put them more at ease.

Anatomy of the Neck

The neck is defined by the seven cervical vertebrae that connect the skull to the thoracic region. At this upper level of the spine, the spinal cord is thick and contains most of the nerves that connect the brain to the rest of the body. That is why a broken neck that damages the spinal cord at this level can lead to severe paralysis. The major muscles in the neck include

- Upper trapezius
- Splenius capitis and cervicis
- Semispinalis capitis and cervicis
- Longissimus capitis
- Levator scapulae
- Sternocleidomastoid (SCM)

The deeper smaller muscles in the neck are

- Suboccipitals (rectus capitis posterior major and minor, oblique capitis superior and inferior)
- Multifidi
- Rotatores

The more superficial muscles are larger and thicker, and the deeper ones are smaller and thinner.

Note that some of the muscles of the neck attach to the thoracic spine. See Figure 15–17 ■. When applying passive forward flexion of the neck, you can sometimes feel a resistance at the lower attachments of the cervical muscles. The deep suboccipital muscles are shown in Figure 15–18 ■.

CAUTIONS

Endangerment sites in the cervical region include the anterior neck triangle and throat and the arteries and veins that supply the brain. The carotid artery and jugular vein are located on the sides of the neck. These areas should be avoided, especially in older adults or anyone with a history of atherosclerosis (i.e., hardening of the arteries).

Applications of Massage for the Neck

Poor posture and body mechanics can lead to excessive tension in the neck. The head-forward posture and poor sitting posture at workstations are two common sources of chronic neck tension. A cold draft on the back of the neck or sleeping in a cramped position can sometimes cause neck stiffness. Long airplane or automobile rides can also leave neck muscles painful and stiff.

Stressful life situations may aggravate cervical tension and may literally be a "pain in the neck." A major cause of tension headache is hypertonicity, or excessive tension, of the cervical muscles, which refer pain into the head. Trigger point work on the cervical and upper back muscles may be integrated into a Swedish massage session for effective relief of a tension headache. Massage can also help in recovery from injuries in the neck region, such as whiplash and torticollis, sometimes called *wryneck*, which is a twisting of the neck to one side due to muscle spasms.

Massage techniques applied to the cervical area address specific muscles. When working in the cervical area, attention is given first to relaxing the superficial muscles, which allows better access to the deeper muscles. The area is thoroughly warmed up before deeper techniques are applied.

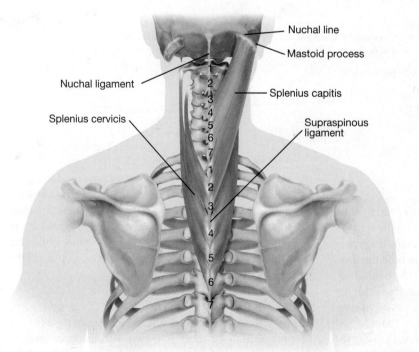

Nuchal line

Mastoid process

Nuchal ligament

Splenius capitis

Splenius cervicis

Supraspinous ligament

FIGURE 15–17

Deep muscles of the posterior neck; splenius capitis and cervicis attachments.

FIGURE 15–18
Suboccipital muscles.

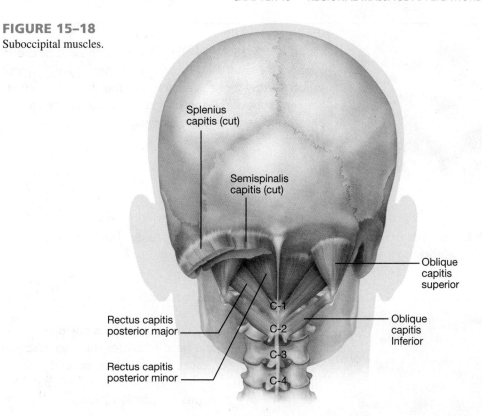

Splenius
capitis (cut)

Semispinalis
capitis (cut)

Oblique
capitis
superior

Rectus capitis
posterior major

Oblique
capitis
Inferior

Rectus capitis
posterior minor

C-1
C-2
C-3
C-4

PRACTICE SEQUENCE 15–2

Massage of the Neck Region

15–20 minutes
Recipient supine

Preliminary Instructions
• Stand or sit at the head of the table during the application.
• Use good hand mechanics, especially when using the thumb to apply techniques.
• Do not apply pressure within the anterior triangle.

Figure 15–19 Apply oil or lotion across shoulders and to posterior neck. Turn the head to one side to access the area. Apply lubricant from the tip of the shoulder to the occiput. Repeat on the other side.

1

2

Figure 15–20 Apply effleurage to both sides of the upper trapezius using loose fists. When moving laterally, apply slightly more pressure near the shoulder. When moving superiorly, apply slightly more pressure to the posterior neck to cause elongation of the muscles at the points of attachment.

Apply Steps 3–9 to one side of the body first, then repeat on the other side. Turn the head as needed to access the area.

3

Figure 15–21 Apply direct pressure along upper trapezius, turning the head to access the area. Use your thumb to apply pressure every inch or so along the upper trapezius from the shoulder to the occiput. Hold tender or trigger points for about 20 seconds.

4

Figure 15–22 Holding the head with one hand, apply effleurage to upper trapezius on one side using the fist. When moving laterally, apply slightly more pressure near the shoulder. When moving superiorly, apply slightly more pressure to the posterior neck to cause elongation of the muscles at the points of attachment.

5

Figure 15–23 Still holding the head with one hand, apply effleurage to scalene muscles with fingertips, from superior to inferior.

Figure 15–24 Continue holding the head with one hand, and apply effleurage superior to inferior along the sternocleidomastoid muscle (SCM) with the fingertips. Avoid pressure over the carotid artery.

Figure 15–25 Stretch the cervical muscles with neck in lateral flexion. Place one hand on the shoulder and the other hand on the head. Slowly apply pressure to elongate the cervical muscles.

Figure 15–26 Apply circular friction and direct pressure to suboccipital muscles one side at a time. Turn head to access suboccipitals on one side. Apply direct pressure to tender points.

Figure 15–27 Mobilize neck in wavelike motion. Return the head to a neutral position facing upward. Apply pressure up bilaterally while sliding fingertips from the base of the neck to the occiput. Pull back at the occiput to elongate the cervical muscles.

Figure 15–28 Cross-arm stretch with head in forward flexion. With your arms crossed, place one hand on each shoulder. Let the head rest on your arms as you gently lift it to elongate the cervical muscles.

Figure 15–29 Traction the neck by placing the head, in neutral position facing upward, in one hand. Place the other hand lightly on the forehead. Pull gently to traction the cervical region.

Figure 15–30 Cradle the head to finish. Rest the head on the table. Place your fingers on the sides of the head just behind the ears with thumbs over the temporal area. Hold for 10–15 seconds.

After you perform the Practice Sequence, evaluate how well you did by filling out Performance Evaluation Form 15–2, Massage of the Neck Region. The form can be found in Appendix D: *Performance Evaluation Forms*, and at MyHealthProfessionsLab.com.

Figures source: Pearson Education, Inc./Segal Photography.

BACK

"Spend more time on my back" is a frequent request from clients. The back is the core area for maintaining upright posture and the place of attachment for muscles that move the arms and legs. It is a heavily muscled area that works hard and is prone to tension, aches, and stiffness. Poor body mechanics when sitting, lifting, playing sports, or during physical activities such as gardening can cause backache.

The expression "carrying the weight of the world on your shoulders" describes the physical sensation of stress and worry. A bent-over posture evokes the image of weakness, discouragement, and defeat. An upright, aligned back presents the image of strength, self-confidence, and vigor.

Anatomy of the Back

For purposes of massage, the back can be thought of in three sections: upper back, mid-back, and low back. The upper back includes the musculature attached to the thoracic vertebrae, whereas the low back is defined by the lumbar vertebrae. The area between the shoulder blades is sometimes referred to as the mid-back. The entire back is interconnected through a complex musculature and fascial tissues.

It is important for massage practitioners to develop a three-dimensional concept of the back. This includes the recognition that the back is the posterior portion of the torso, which also has sides. The back is thick with layers from large, broad superficial muscles to the tiny, deep muscles of the spine. See Figure 15–31 ■. The scapulae, or shoulder blades, located on the upper back are an integral part of the shoulder girdle. They glide over the posterior ribs and have numerous muscular attachments, which generate the free movement of the shoulder complex. Practitioners work at various depths of penetration during massage of the back.

The large superficial muscles of the back include

- Trapezius

- Latissimus dorsi

Spinal muscles include

- Erector spinae (iliocostalis, longissimus, spinalis)

- Deep posterior spinal muscles: multifidi, rotatores, interspinales, intertransversarii, and levatores costarum

- Semispinalis thoracis

Muscles surrounding the scapulae include

- Subscapularis

- Upper trapezius

- Posterior deltoid

- Supraspinatus

- Infraspinatus

- Serratus anterior

- Teres major and minor

- Levator scapulae

- Rhomboids on the medial border

FIGURE 15–31
Major back and shoulder muscles.

Levator scapulae
Rhomoid
Trapezius
Spine of scapula
Deltoid (cut)
Teres major
Deltoid
Triceps brachii
Latissimus dorsi
Serratus anterior
Serratus poster

The lower back includes

- Quadratus lumborum, with attachments on the last rib, the transverse processes of the upper four lumbar vertebrae, and the iliac crest

Applications of Massage for the Back

Soothing back massage is associated with the qualities of nurturing, sympathy, and deep relaxation. Perhaps because the nerves of the parasympathetic nervous system exit the posterior vertebrae, the relaxation response is easily triggered during massage of the back. Back massage is often used to help people go to sleep.

Deep massage of the back muscles can help release tension held there and relieves the stiffness and soreness that accompanies heavy physical labor. Joint movements improve the mobility of the shoulder blades, increasing movement in the shoulder girdle. Tension in the upper trapezius can refer pain into the head, and massage of the shoulders and neck can help relieve tension headache.

Back Massage for Relaxation If the purpose of back massage is general relaxation, either avoid specific painful work on the back altogether, or spend at least 5–7 minutes after painful work on lighter, soothing techniques. Use long, flowing effleurage strokes with oil, maintaining full contact with the palm of the hand throughout the stroking.

Use moderate to slow continuous motion. The movement should feel "seamless."

Vary the pattern to avoid boredom. Mix up vertical, circular, and horizontal patterns of effleurage. Some petrissage of the shoulder may be integrated for variety. Avoid tapotement, and finish either with nerve strokes or passive touch over the scapulae.

Sedating Effleurage of the Back Back massage is sometimes used in hospitals and nursing homes for those having trouble falling asleep. Sedating effleurage may be performed without oil or lotion. It is very effective for evoking the relaxation response and promoting sleep. The movement consists of long, gliding strokes directly over the spine that begin at the base of the skull and go all the way to the coccyx. Hands alternate. As one hand is about to complete its motion near the coccyx, the other hand begins the next stroke starting at the base of the skull. This gives the recipient the feeling of continuous contact, with one hand beginning the next stroke before the other hand finishes. Keep the motion going for 1 or 2 minutes to help the recipient relax completely. Pressure must be light but firm and the rhythm monotonous. Pressure that is too light might stimulate rather than sedate. A tingling sensation may be felt in the arms and legs as relaxation occurs. If this technique is applied for more than 2 or 3 minutes, it tends to stimulate rather than relax, so it should not be continued for too long.

PRACTICE SEQUENCE 15–3

Upper Back and Shoulder Massage
15–20 minutes
Recipient prone

Preliminary Instructions
- Avoid heavy pressure over the spinous processes.
- Avoid abducting thumb when applying techniques.

1

Figure 15–32 Standing at the head of the table, apply oil or lotion to the entire back and shoulders with bilateral stroking. Slide hands from shoulders to hips using palms to spread lubricant to the back and sides.

Perform Steps 2–9 on one side of the back and then the other before going on.

Figure 15–33 Standing at the side and facing the head, apply shingles effleurage to paraspinal muscles of the upper back. Gradually deepen pressure of strokes.

Figure 15–34 Standing at the side and facing the head, apply deep circular effleurage over shoulder area using palms. Place one hand on top of the other to apply added pressure through the palm. Circle from the spine over the shoulder, and return to starting position to repeat several times. Follow the curve of the shoulder.

Figure 15–35 Using the same hand position as in Step 3, apply circular friction along paraspinal muscles of the upper back using fingertips. Make small circles along side of spine (clockwise on right side, counterclockwise on left side) and move spot to spot from lower to upper back.

Figure 15–36 Knuckle friction between and over the shoulder blades. Superficial friction between shoulder blade and spine, transverse to the rhomboid muscles. Friction over the shoulder blade.

6

Figure 15–37 Standing at the side of the table facing the head, mobilize the scapula by pressing along medial border. Outside hand is on the shoulder, inside hand along the medial border of the scapula. Pull back on the shoulder lifting the scapula, and press under medial border at the same time.

7

Figure 15–38 Using one or two hands, knead the upper trapezius.

8

Figure 15–39 Standing at the head of the table, apply effleurage to upper trapezius from neck to shoulder using a loose fist. Stroke from base of neck to shoulder to elongate the area.

9

Figure 15–40 Apply direct thumb pressure into points along the upper trapezius from base of neck to shoulder. Hold for 2–3 seconds each.

Repeat shingles effleurage (Step 2) to side of back as finishing technique. Repeat Steps 2–9 on the other side of back.

Figure 15–41 Apply two-hand petrissage over the entire upper back. Place palms flat on back next to each other. Circle in opposite directions, and lift skin between the hands as they pass each other.

Figure 15–42 Finish with bilateral stroking to the entire back. Stand at head of the table with fingers pointing toward spine. Slide hands from shoulders to hips using palms. On return, point fingers toward the table, and spread hands to "rake" between ribs on sides.

After you perform the Practice Sequence, evaluate how well you did by filling out Performance Evaluation Form 15–3, Upper Back and Shoulder Massage. The form can be found in Appendix D: *Performance Evaluation Forms*, and at MyHealthProfessionsLab.com.

Figures source: Pearson Education, Inc./Segal Photography.

PRACTICE SEQUENCE 15–4

Low Back Massage | 10–15 minutes
Recipient prone

Preliminary Instructions
• Area of focus is between the last rib and the iliac crest of the pelvis.
• Avoid abducting thumb when applying techniques.

Figure 15–43 Standing at the head of the table, apply oil or lotion to the entire back with bilateral stroking. Slide hands from shoulders to hips using palms to spread lubricant to the back and sides. Slide thumbs along paraspinal muscles, increasing pressure to warm tissues.
Source: Pearson Education, Inc./Segal Photography.

Perform Steps 2–5 on one side of back and then repeat on the other side.

Figure 15–44 Standing at the side, apply circular friction along paraspinal muscles of the low back using fingertips. Make small circles along side of spine (clockwise on right side, counterclockwise on left side). Move spot to spot from iliac crest to last rib.

Figure 15–45 Slide thumbs along spine in strips (thumb stripping) to paraspinal and quadratus lumborum muscles in lower back. Move both inferior to superior and superior to inferior.

Figure 15–46 Apply direct pressure to points on low back. Press into paraspinal muscles from the side. Move spot to spot from below the last rib to the iliac crest. Hold 2–3 seconds each.

Repeat Step 3 along paraspinal muscles in low back.

Figure 15–47 Lift sides of waist with deep effleurage strokes from the side. Move to opposite side and reach over to apply lifting effleurage to waist area just massaged.

Repeat Steps 2–5 on other side of low back.

Figure 15–48 Finish with bilateral stroking to the entire back. Stand at head of the table with fingers pointing toward spine. Slide hands from shoulders to hips using palms. On return, point fingers toward the table, and spread hands to "rake" between ribs on sides.

After you perform the Practice Sequence, evaluate how well you did by filling out Performance Evaluation Form 15–4, Low Back Massage. The form can be found in Appendix D: *Performance Evaluation Forms*, and at MyHealthProfessionsLab.com.

Figures source: Pearson Education, Inc./Segal Photography.

 CASE FOR STUDY

Dan's Request for Extra Time on the Back

Dan receives regular massage at a local spa. He painted his living room over the weekend and complained to his massage therapist that his back was tense and stiff from the work. He requested that more time be spent treating his back in this session.

Question:

How will Dan's request affect the plan of his usual 1-hour full-body massage?

Things to consider:

- How much time should the massage therapist spend on Dan's back?
- How might the massage therapist locate specific muscles or areas to focus on?
- How might the rest of the body receive some attention also?

Describe your approach to Dan's request:

_____

_____

_____

UPPER EXTREMITIES

Upright posture is thought to be an adaptation in the evolution of human beings to free us to use our hands for grasping and manipulating objects. Everyday activities such as cooking and eating, personal grooming, cleaning the house, and gardening are performed using the arms and hands. Hobbies and sports and most work activities also depend on the upper extremities.

The upper extremities are also important in communication. Many of us use our hands to augment verbal expression. The hearing impaired use their hands for sign language. To be friendly or affectionate we shake hands, give pats on the back, and hug. Loss of the use of the arms or hands can be personally and socially devastating.

Anatomy of the Upper Extremities

For purposes of massage, the upper extremities may be thought of in four sections, that is, the shoulders, upper arms, forearms, and hands. The shoulders may be addressed as part of the upper back during massage because the shoulder blades are located there. Functionally, however, the shoulder blades are part of the shoulder girdle and designed to facilitate use of the arms and hands. The rotator cuff muscles are a special muscle group involved in shoulder movement. See Figure 15–49 ■. The joints of the upper extremities include the complex shoulder girdle, elbows, wrists, and several small joints in the hands.

The muscles that move the shoulder include

- Pectoralis major and minor
- Deltoid
- Subscapularis
- Supraspinatus

- Infraspinatis
- Teres major and minor
- Serratus anterior
- Levator scapulae
- Rhomboid major and minor
- Trapezius

Latissimus dorsi is located on the back, but functions primarily to move the upper arm.

Muscles of the upper arm and forearm include

- Biceps brachii
- Triceps brachii
- Brachialis
- Pronator teres, pronator quadratus, supinator (smaller muscles of pronation and supination)
- Anconeus
- Coracobrachialis
- Brachioradialis

The anterior forearm also contains the wrist flexors and palmaris longus, whereas the posterior forearm contains the wrist extensors. See Figure 15–50 ■. There are many small muscles intrinsic to the hand, which move the fingers and thumbs.

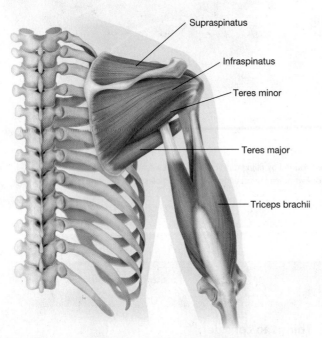

FIGURE 15–49 Rotator cuff muscles of the shoulder.

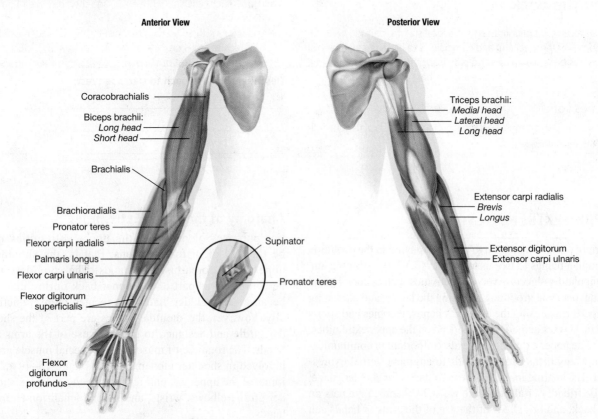

FIGURE 15–50 Major muscles of the arm.

Applications of Massage for the Upper Extremities

Massage and joint movements can help maintain shoulder flexibility. They can also improve mobility lost by poor posture, overuse, aging, or injury.

People who perform repetitive movements with the arms and hands often experience tightness and soreness in the upper extremities. Hand and arm massage is beneficial for them as well as those who do manual labor. The hands can be massaged and mobilized to help retain their function in old age.

The muscles of the forearms create movement at the wrist and the hands. Certain occupations and activities tend to stress these muscles and produce chronic tension in them.

This is common among computer users, artists, craftspeople, and musicians. Video games and text messaging may also create strain in the muscles and joints of the hand and wrist.

Tennis elbow and golfer's elbow are repetitive strain injuries (RSIs) that involve tendinitis at the elbow and tenderness in the forearm. These RSIs may also result from activities requiring similar movements of the arms. Regular, specific massage of the hands and forearms can help prevent overuse injuries in this area. A complete prevention program would also include regular resting time, stretching, self-massage, and proper biomechanical performance of the movements. Massage therapists themselves are prone to such overuse in the upper extremities.

PRACTICE SEQUENCE 15–5

Massage of the Upper Extremities

20–30 minutes
Recipient supine

Preliminary Instructions

• For complete attention to the upper extremities, perform Practice Sequence 15–3, Upper Back and Shoulder Massage, before or after this one.
• Secure drape to prevent exposure of women's breasts.
• Use bolster under wrist or forearm.

Figure 15–51 Apply oil or lotion to the entire arm from distal to proximal, including around the shoulder.

Figure 15–52 Wag the arm to mobilize the joints of the upper extremities. Grasp the hand and lift the arm off the table. Wag back and forth to effect movement in the wrist, elbow, and shoulder joints.

3

Figure 15–53 Stretch shoulder in horizontal flexion by grasping at the forearm and reaching the entire arm across the body. With your other hand on medial border of the scapula, assist the stretch.

4

Figure 15–54 Apply effleurage to pectoral muscles with fist, moving along pectoral muscles from shoulder to inferior attachments, stretching the soft tissues. Avoid heavy pressure over breast tissue. Afterward replace the arm at the side.

5

Figure 15–55 Place your hands on both sides of the upper arm, and squeeze along the anterior and posterior muscles from armpit to elbow.

6

Figure 15–56 Apply transverse friction to tendons at the shoulder with thumb or fingertips. Add stripping effleurage along length of tender tendons.

Figure 15–57 Apply deep effleurage to triceps. Position arm with elbow pointing upward to access the triceps muscles. Stabilize with one hand while the other applies the effleurage. Replace the arm on the table.

Figure 15–58 Squeeze forearm by placing your hands on both sides of the forearm and squeeze from elbow to wrist.

Figure 15–59 Stripping along flexor and extensor muscles with your thumb from attachments at wrist to elbow.

10

Figure 15–60 Apply friction to tendons at the elbow with thumb or fingers. Add stripping effleurage along length of tender tendons.

11

Figure 15–61 Apply draining stroke to forearm. Hold forearm off of the table with one hand. With the other hand, slide from wrist to elbow while applying pressure around the forearm tissues. Apply first to lateral side of the arm, then the medial side.

12

Figure 15–62 Use your thumbs to apply circular friction over the wrist bones, with recipient's palm down.

13

Figure 15–63 Hold hand around thumb and little finger and apply broadening strokes across the metacarpals. Press up on palm with fingers.

Figure 15–64 Apply thumb slides between metacarpals from knuckles to wrist.

Figure 15–65 Turn the hand over and apply broadening effleurage across the palm. The thumbs fan out from the center of the palm to the sides. Separate metacarpals with the movement.

Figure 15–66 Mobilize knuckles with figure-8s. Turn the hand so palm faces the table. Grasp the proximal phalange just above the knuckle between your thumb and index finger. Mobilize the joint with a figure-8 movement.

Figure 15–67 Squeeze along the length of each finger from web to nail. First along top/bottom and then along the sides. Include over the nail and along its sides.

18

Figure 15–68 Stretch the flexor muscles with hyperextension at the wrist. Hold the forearm vertical with one hand. Use the other hand to apply pressure to stretch wrist flexor muscles. The recipient's palm is up.

19

Figure 15–69 Stretch the extensor muscles with flexion at the wrist. Reposition the palm to face the table. Apply pressure on the back of the hand to stretch the wrist extensor muscles.

20

Figure 15–70 With the arm placed on the table, apply effleurage over the entire upper limb as a reconnecting and finishing technique.

Repeat Steps 1–20 on the other arm.

After you perform the Practice Sequence, evaluate how well you did by filling out Performance Evaluation Form 15–5, Massage of the Upper Extremities. The form can be found in Appendix D: *Performance Evaluation Forms*, and at MyHealthProfessionsLab.com.

Figures source: Pearson Education, Inc./Segal Photography.

CHEST AND ABDOMEN

The anterior torso includes the chest and the abdomen. Although these areas may be addressed separately during massage, they are considered together here as the front of the torso. The internal organs of the chest and abdominal cavities are more exposed in the anterior torso, as opposed to the back of the body. And the entire torso is connected for certain functions such as respiration and trunk flexion movements.

The expansion and contraction of the chest for breathing is evidence of life itself. Because it is the location of women's breasts, the chest is associated with both nurturing and sexual appeal. The chest is also identified with strength and power, particularly in men, as when the pectoral muscles are more developed.

In the United States, women's breasts are kept covered in public and, therefore, should be draped to maintain modesty and proper professional boundaries. Practitioners can access the pectoral and intercostal muscles of women working around or over a drape. Massage of the breast tissue itself is becoming more common as both a general health measure and for certain clinical applications. Breast massage should be performed only after special training and with informed consent from the recipient. Breast massage can be a valuable complementary therapy in the treatment of breast cancer. In such cases, it would be part of an overall plan of care.

The abdomen is a relatively vulnerable area extending from the diaphragm to the pubis. It contains the *viscera,* or internal organs, of digestion, elimination, and reproduction. It lacks the bony protection afforded the lungs and heart in the chest. The abdomen is contained and supported principally by the abdominal muscles. It is the soft belly exposed in humans because of our upright posture.

The word *visceral* has come to mean deeply felt, instinctive, or having to do with elemental emotions. This area is sensitive for many people and should be approached with care.

Anatomy of the Chest and Abdomen

The chest or thorax is defined by the rib cage, sternum, and muscles of the shoulder girdle that attach to them. The prominent muscles of the chest are pectoralis major and minor. See Figure 15–71 ■. Muscles located on the chest with the primary function of respiration include the diaphragm (separates the chest from the abdomen) and the intercostals.

The breast structure sits over the muscles of the chest wall. It is a specialized gland structure that evolved as an appendage of the skin. The female breast is made up of fat tissue and mammary glands and ducts with supporting connective tissue. Breast tissue lies beyond the obvious contour of the breast, and extends inferior and laterally on the chest. When working on women with large breasts, it may be difficult to reach the muscles underneath.

The abdomen lies between the chest and the pelvis. The abdominal cavity contains the stomach, liver, spleen, pancreas, small and large intestines, kidneys, bladder, reproductive organs in females, and other visceral organs. The

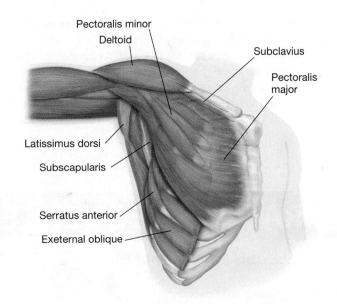

FIGURE 15–71 Major muscles of the chest.

abdominal muscles surrounding and supporting the viscera include the rectus abdominus and internal and external obliques. See Figure 15–72 ■.

Applications of Massage for the Chest and Abdomen

Poor posture, long periods of sitting at a desk, and carrying objects in the arms can all lead to shortening of the muscles of the chest and abdomen. A chronic slumped posture can inhibit the functions of the visceral organs, lead to back and neck tension and fatigue, and restrict breathing. Massage can help stretch and lengthen shortened anterior muscles that are the result of and contribute to chronic slumped posture and rounded shoulders. Along with proper strengthening exercises for the back and abdominal muscles, massage can help people maintain good postural alignment.

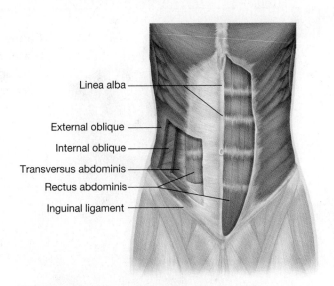

FIGURE 15–72 Major muscles of the abdomen.

The chest cavity expands to accommodate expansion of the lungs during inhalation. Therefore, any muscular restriction in the area can adversely affect breathing. The major muscles of respiration are the diaphragm and intercostals. Forced inhalation and exhalation also involve the abdominal muscles and muscles that move the rib cage, such as pectoralis minor, serratus anterior, scalenes, and sternocleidomastoid. Massage can help maintain the muscles of respiration in optimal condition and relieve tension caused by poor posture or stress.

Breast massage is a specialized technique performed as a wellness measure for female breast health. It is also used to address discomforts associated with the menstrual cycle, pregnancy, and nursing.[1]

PRACTICE SEQUENCE 15–6

Chest and Abdominal Massage

15–20 minutes
Recipient supine

Preliminary Instructions
- Cover women's breasts securely with an adequate drape.
- During abdominal massage, cover genitals completely and avoid exposing pubic hair.
- Avoid deep pressure directly over breast tissue.
- Apply techniques to the abdomen only in a *clockwise* direction.
- Use informed consent for massage of chest for women and massage of abdomen for men and women.

Figure 15–73 Standing at the head of the table, apply oil or lotion to chest area. Spread lubricant fanning out over the upper chest from clavicles to sides of the torso.

Figure 15–74 Apply effleurage to upper chest bilaterally over pectoral muscles and sternum. Medium pressure superior to inferior, and light pressure back to starting point.

Figure 15–75 Use fingertips to apply friction to muscle attachments along inferior length of the clavicle.

Figure 15–76 Apply effleurage and direct pressure on attachments of pectoralis minor. Lift one arm off the table to access the pectoral muscles. Use the fingertips of your hand to apply broadening effleurage along the pectoralis minor. Finish with more broadening effleurage. Repeat on other side.

Figure 15–77 Stretch anterior tissues by pressing down on shoulders. Stand at the head of the table. Place the heels of your hands on the shoulders over the anterior deltoid muscle. Apply bilaterally downward.

Figure 15–78 Mobilize chest and shoulders with *cat paw* movement. Move your hands just superior to their position in Step 5. Alternate pressing shoulders toward the feet, left then right, in a gentle rhythmic movement.

7

Figure 15–79 Mobilize the rib cage. Redrape to cover the chest, and stand to one side of the table. Place your hands on each side of the rib cage. Rock the rib cage from side to side in a gentle rhythmic movement.

8

Figure 15–80 Adjust drape for abdominal massage, and stand at the side of the table facing the head. Place hands on the rib cage bilaterally, and rake between the ribs superior to inferior.

9

A

B

Figure 15–81 (A) Thumb slide along diaphragm, and lift around the waist. Place thumbs just under the rib cage, and slide along the muscle attachments there from medial to lateral. Do not press on the xiphoid process of the sternum. (B) After each slide, lift up the tissues around the waist.

10

Figure 15–82 Effleurage clockwise to abdomen. Place palm over palm, and apply effleurage in a circle around the abdomen. Fingertips trace along the rib cage and pelvis. Avoid touching the pubic hair.

Figure 15–83 Apply vibration clockwise around abdomen with fingertips to points in a circle over the colon.

Figure 15–84 With your fingertips, using medium pressure, trace the colon over the abdomen. Move in clockwise direction.

Figure 15–85 Apply petrissage to center of abdomen. Place hands palm over palm in center of the abdomen. Create an undulating movement by (A) pressing with the heel of the hands and then (B) rolling onto the fingertips in repeated rhythmical motion.

A

B

Figure 15–86 Apply light effleurage around abdomen in a large circle with the palm of a flat hand.

Figure 15–87 Apply passive touch over abdomen to finish. Slow the circle stroke you performed in Step 14, and let the hands rest on the center of the abdomen for a few seconds. Gradually lift the hands from the skin, and redrape the abdomen.

After you perform the Practice Sequence, evaluate how well you did by filling out Performance Evaluation Form 15–6, Chest and Abdominal Massage. The form can be found in Appendix D: *Performance Evaluation Forms*, and at MyHealthProfessionsLab.com.

Figures source: Pearson Education, Inc./Segal Photography.

CHAPTER HIGHLIGHTS

- More time and attention is sometimes given to a particular region of the body during a massage session.
  - This could result from a request from the client, the practitioner's own judgment, information on a health history form, or referral from a health care provider.
- Even though the body is massaged region by region during a session, its interconnections should always be kept in mind.
- Different body regions also have significance or human meaning to an individual person.
- The body regions addressed in regional massage of the upper body are the head and face, neck, back, upper extremities, and chest and abdomen.
- Knowledge of each region in terms of its human meaning, anatomy, cautions, and relevant massage applications is essential for meeting the recipient's needs.

- Practice Sequences for regional massage build on the more general massage described as full-body massage.
  - Regional massage addresses anatomical structures with more specificity.
  - Students are encouraged to build on Practice Sequences with more advanced massage techniques and with greater knowledge of muscles and connective tissues in these regions.
  - Although the Practice Sequences are useful for generating ideas for massage, adapt your approach to address the tissues you are actually touching.
  - Practice Sequences follow the basic progression from general to specific to general; they include warming of the area, followed by attention to specific structures, and connecting and finishing techniques.

- When actually performing the Practice Sequences, add techniques to enhance the flow of the session.

- The head and face region is the center for thinking and communication.
  - The senses of sight, hearing, taste, and smell are housed there.
  - Massage can release tension caused by job-related activities, by emotional distress, and by pathologies that affect the facial muscles.

- The neck region links the head and torso and contains the muscles that hold the head upright.
  - Muscle tension in the neck may result from poor posture, stress, or injury.
  - Endangerment sites in the region include the anterior neck and arteries and veins to the brain.

- The back region is the core area for maintaining upright posture and the place of attachment for arms and legs.
  - Soothing back massage helps elicit the relaxation response.
  - Tension in the back may result from heavy labor, sports, poor posture, or stress.

- The upper extremities allow humans to use the hands and manipulate objects.
  - They are important for everyday and work activities and for communication.
  - Problems in the upper extremities can result from repetitive motion, poor posture, old age, or injury.
  - Mobility of the shoulder girdle can be enhanced with massage.

- The chest and abdomen are connected for certain functions such as respiration, digestion, and trunk flexion movements.
  - The chest is the location of pectoral muscles and breasts and is associated with both nurturing and sexual appeal in women and with strength in men.
  - The abdomen is a relatively vulnerable region containing the viscera or internal organs.
  - Applications of massage in the chest region include addressing poor posture, rounded shoulders, and enhancing respiration.
  - Massage techniques performed on the abdomen help stimulate movement of the contents of the lower digestive tract; massage only in *clockwise* direction.

EXAM REVIEW

Key Terms

Match the following key terms to their descriptions. For additional study, look up the key terms in the Interactive Glossary, and note other terms that compare or contrast with them.

_____ 1. Human meaning
_____ 2. Interconnections
_____ 3. Regional massage
_____ 4. Specificity
_____ 5. Upper body regions

a. Attention to anatomical structure
b. Massage to large body areas
c. Association of body area with self
d. Above the waist
e. Links between regions

Memory Workout

To test your memory of the main concepts in this chapter, complete the following sentences by circling the most correct answer from the two choices provided.

1. Even though the body is massaged region by region during a session, its (interconnectedness) (meaning) should always be kept in mind.
2. As you interact with a client, be aware that you are not just touching a body, you are touching a(n) (anatomical structure) (human being).
3. Much of human consciousness is focused in the (heart) (head).
4. Clients often have a (protective) (welcome) response to massage near the neck and throat.
5. When performing effleurage over the eyelids, keep pressure (firm) (light).
6. Tension headaches can often be relieved with massage of the (back) (neck).
7. It is important for practitioners to develop a (two-) (three-) dimensional concept of the body.
8. Flaring the nostrils is accomplished with the (orbicularis oris) (dilator naris) muscle.
9. When giving neck massage to a client in the supine position, the practitioner is typically (kneeling) (sitting) to maintain good body mechanics.
10. In the United States, women's breasts are kept covered in public and should therefore be (exposed) (draped) during massage.

Test Prep

The following multiple-choice questions will help to prepare you for future school and professional exams.

1. Extended massage sessions on smaller body areas provide an opportunity for greater:
   a. Generality
   b. Specificity
   c. Range of motion
   d. Pacing

2. Although the Practice Sequences are useful for generating ideas for massage, eventually you would alter them to:
   a. Make them easier
   b. Make them shorter
   c. Address the tissues you are actually touching
   d. Include everything you learn

3. This old adage appears to be true:
   a. It takes more muscles to smile than to frown
   b. It takes more muscles to frown than to smile
   c. Frowning causes wrinkles
   d. Don't frown—your face may freeze that way

4. If a client seems protective of the neck region, try to put him or her more at ease by:
   a. Asking for permission before you touch the area
   b. Ignoring any protective actions as if nothing were wrong
   c. Touching the area quickly before he or she can react
   d. Touching the area softly, hoping that he or she will not notice

5. Although they are in the upper back region, the scapulae are functionally part of the:
   a. Torso
   b. Lower back
   c. Pelvic girdle
   d. Shoulder girdle

6. Long gliding strokes directly over the spine that start at the base of the skull and go all the way to the coccyx, if applied repeatedly over a short period of time, tend to have a(n):
   a. Stimulating effect
   b. Sedating effect
   c. Annoying effect
   d. No particular effect

7. If the main purpose of a back massage is general relaxation, the following strategy would be the *most* effective:
   a. Include specific deep massage techniques for muscle tightness and end with tapotement.
   b. Apply about 10 minutes of nerve strokes and brushing.
   c. Address specific muscle tension as needed and end with several minutes of lighter, soothing techniques.
   d. Spend the majority of time on joint movements.

8. Passive stretches for the neck muscles are best applied with the client:
   a. Sitting
   b. Side-lying
   c. Prone
   d. Supine

9. The pectoral muscles and intercostals of women may be properly accessed by:
   a. Undraping the chest to the waist
   b. Undraping one breast at a time
   c. Working around a drape
   d. None of the above

10. The direction of abdominal massage is always:
    a. Clockwise
    b. Counterclockwise
    c. Superior to inferior
    d. Lateral to medial

Video Challenge

Watch the Regional Applications of Massage—Upper Body videos, which can be found at MyHealthProfessionsLab .com, Chapter 15, and then answer the following questions.

1. How does the massage therapist in the video maintain good body mechanics while applying massage to the face, head, and neck?

2. What does the massage therapist in the video do to avoid endangerment sites in the neck?
3. In the massage of the upper extremities, which specific techniques are used to create more specificity in the application?

Comprehension Exercises

The following short-answer questions test your knowledge and understanding of chapter topics and provide practice in written communication skills. Explain in two to four complete sentences.

1. Explain why more time and attention might be given to a particular region of the body during a massage session.

2. Explain why the recipient's personal meaning for a particular body region is an important consideration for massage of that region.
3. Give examples of how massage of the forearm can be applied with greater specificity than in a general massage of the region.

For Greater Understanding

The following exercises are designed to take you from the realm of theory into the real world. They will help give you a deeper understanding of the subjects covered in this chapter. Action words are underlined to emphasize the variety of activities presented to address different learning styles and to encourage deeper thinking.

1. Interview someone who has received massage recently. Ask if massage of any particular body region was uncomfortable for him or her, and if so, ask for an explanation. Discuss with a study partner or group.

2. Interview someone who has received massage recently. Ask the person to identify his or her favorite part of the massage and to explain the choice. Discuss your findings with a study partner or group.

3. Receive a massage from a professional practitioner. Request special attention to the back and neck. Note how the massage therapist addresses the request and his or her approach to massage of the region. Report your experience to a study partner or group.

4. Create a 30-minute massage for an upper body region. Include warming, therapeutic combinations, and transition and finishing techniques. Demonstrate your sequence, noting how you achieved specificity, avoided monotony, and made transitions.

MyHealthProfessionsLab™

MyHealthProfessionsLab.com is a premium online homework management system that includes a host of features to help you study. Registered users will find:

- Powerful tools that track and analyze your results—allowing you to create a personalized learning experience
- Videos, flashcards and other learning tools to help enrich your progress
- Streaming lesson presentations and self-paced learning modules
- A space where you and your instructors can view and manage your assignments

16 Regional Massage Applications—Lower Body

Pearson Education, Inc.

CHAPTER OUTLINE

Learning Outcomes

Key Terms

Regional Massage of the Lower Body

Hips and Buttocks

Lower Extremities

Chapter Highlights

Exam Review

LEARNING OUTCOMES

After studying this chapter, you will have information to:

1. Apply massage to lower body regions with greater specificity.

2. Describe lower body regions in terms of their human meaning.

3. Describe the general anatomy of lower body regions.

4. Appreciate the interconnections among body regions.

5. Perform massage Practice Sequences for various lower body regions.

KEY TERMS

Bipedal locomotion

Lower body regions

Mobility restrictions

Palpatory sensitivity

Specificity

REGIONAL MASSAGE OF THE LOWER BODY

In this chapter, we turn our attention to regional massage of the lower body. **Lower body regions** are typically defined for massage as hips and buttocks, upper and lower legs, and feet. Keep in mind that these regions are connected to each other structurally and functionally, as well as being connected to the upper body.

Each lower body region is addressed here with greater **specificity** than in a full-body massage. More attention is paid to specific anatomical structures, and sequences include techniques that allow for greater specificity, such as deep friction. Some knowledge of the musculoskeletal anatomy of the lower body and skill in palpation are assumed.

As discussed in Chapter 15, *Regional Massage Applications—Upper Body*, the Practice Sequences in this chapter are designed to be a starting point for focusing on specific regions. Build on these routines as you learn more advanced massage techniques and acquire greater knowledge of muscles and connective tissues. You are encouraged to adapt your approach to address the tissues you are actually touching.

Practice Sequences follow the basic progression from general to specific to general. They include warming of the area, followed by attention to specific structures, then connecting and finishing techniques. When performing a Practice Sequence, you may find that it feels right to add some transition or other techniques to enhance the flow of the session.

HIPS AND BUTTOCKS

The large muscles of the hips and buttocks region help support the entire body and provide the power for locomotion. They are the most important and the most stressed muscles in many sports. They are also the perch points for sitting.

The hips and buttocks are associated with sexual appeal. They may also be a source of poor self-image and embarrassment, particularly in women. For those physically or sexually abused as children, it is often a region of remembered pain and suffering. Practitioners should take great care when working in this region to create a feeling of safety and modesty.

Anatomy of the Hips and Buttocks

The more superficial muscles of the hip region are the large gluteal muscles (maximus, medius, minimus), which run superior to inferior. See Figure 16–1 ■. The smaller, deeper hip rotators include the:

- Piriformis

- Gemellus superior and inferior

- Quadratus femoris

- Obturator internus and externus

These deeper muscles run more medial to lateral, as shown in Figure 16–2 ■. They are sometimes referred to as "the deep six."

Gluteus maximus (cut)

Gluteus medius

Gluteus medius

Gluteus minimus

Gluteus medius removed (origin attachement)

Gluteus medius

Gluteus maximus

Iliotibial tract

FIGURE 16–1 Gluteal muscles of the hip region.

Gluteus minimus

Piriformis

Gemellus superior

Gelmellus inferior

Quadratus femoris

Obturator internus

Cut obturator internus

Obturator externus

Cut quadratus femoris

FIGURE 16–2 Deep hip rotator muscles.

Applications of Massage for the Hips and Buttocks

Sports and fitness participants are often stiff and sore in the hip area from the strain of physical activity. On the other hand, those who are more sedentary may also experience stiffness from lack of movement. This includes people who work on computers and sit at their desks for many hours at a time. Tight buttock muscles can impinge on the sciatic nerve and cause leg pain. Soft tissue manipulation and joint movements improve circulation to the area, relax muscles, and improve mobility at the hip joint. Older adults may especially benefit from improved hip mobility and, therefore, improved locomotion.

Some practitioners massage the buttocks as part of a back routine, whereas others include the buttocks in a lower limb sequence. Because most of the attachments of the buttocks muscles are on the ilium and femur and create movement in the thigh, the buttocks are often addressed when massaging the lower limbs.

Use of the Elbow and Forearm Because you must work through the large superficial muscles to reach the smaller deeper muscles, it is useful to use the elbow or forearm to apply some techniques to the buttocks. You can apply more pressure and avoid straining the hands. However, take care not to use too much pressure, especially around the sciatic nerve outlet in the buttocks. **Palpatory sensitivity** will allow you to feel the condition of the tissues as you would with your hands. The elbow or forearm is not used

to "muscle through" the tissues, but to apply more pressure skillfully.

The elbow or forearm may be used for broad strokes, and the point of the elbow (olecranon process) may be used for more specific techniques, such as direct pressure to a particular spot. The elbow or forearm may be used to apply effleurage, direct pressure, and circular or transverse friction.

Use of the Fist A closed hand or fist is useful for applying deep pressure for compressions, effleurage, and circular friction over the large muscles of the buttocks. A loose or open fist is preferred because a tight fist can feel hard and insensitive to the recipient. One advantage of this technique over using the palms is that the wrist can be kept straight, thus avoiding potential wrist damage when applying deep pressure. Figure 11–4 shows different hand positions for applying massage techniques to large muscles such as those in the hips and buttocks region.

Joint Mobilizing and Stretching A thorough treatment of the muscles of the buttocks includes both massage and joint movements. Joint mobilizing techniques and stretching help condition the deep rotators of the hip joint, which are difficult to reach directly with massage. Although massage of the buttocks is necessarily performed with the recipient prone, most joint movements are done supine. If one of the major goals of the session addresses mobility in the hips, it may be useful to begin prone to warm up the muscles and finish supine for the joint movements.

PRACTICE SEQUENCE 16–1

Hip and Buttocks Massage

20 minutes
Recipient prone and supine

Preliminary Instructions
• Secure the drape around the leg, and do not expose the gluteal cleft.
• Use sensitivity when applying pressure with the fist, knuckles, and elbow.
• To begin, recipient is prone.

Figure 16–3 Apply oil or lotion to the entire leg and hip. Slide palms from lower leg to buttocks. Inside hand slides laterally around the hip before returning down the leg.

Figure 16–4 Deep effleurage to buttocks muscles using reinforced palm. Place one hand over the other to apply pressure to the gluteal muscles. Fingertips trace the muscle attachments along the iliac crest and around the hip joint.

Figure 16–5 Rhythmic compression to gluteal muscles using the fist. Press into the large gluteal muscles moving from one spot to another in moderate pace.

4

Figure 16–6 Circular friction to gluteal muscle attachments using the fist. Use the knuckles or the middle phalangeal surface to apply circular friction to attachments of gluteal muscles along the sacrum and iliac crest.

5

Figure 16–7 Direct pressure to deep rotator muscles using the elbow. Use the elbow tip to apply pressure moving from one spot to another along the rotator muscles.

6

Figure 16–8 Effleurage along deep rotator muscles using the knuckles. Slide knuckles from sacrum to hip, tracing the deep rotator muscles.

7

Figure 16–9 Deep friction around the hip joint using the knuckles. Use the knuckle of the middle finger to apply circular friction around the head of the femur at the hip joint.

8

Figure 16–10 Effleurage to buttocks muscles using reinforced palm. Place one hand over the other to apply pressure and slide over the entire gluteal and hip area as a finishing technique.

9

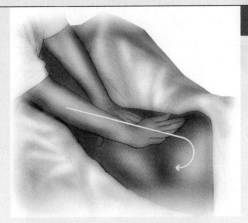

Figure 16–11 Effleurage with palms to reconnect the hip area to the leg. Slide the palms from foot to around the hip a few times as a connecting technique.

Redrape the leg and repeat Steps 1–9 on the other side. After both sides have been massaged, assist the recipient in turning over.

Preliminary Instructions
• Secure the drape around the leg, and do not expose the genital area during joint movements.
• Recipient is supine.

10

Figure 16–12 Facing the table, place one hand on the thigh and the other on the lower leg. Gently rock the leg medially several times for passive rotation of hip joint. Let it come back into position naturally.

11

Figure 16–13 Passive movement of the hip through its full range. With one hand just above the knee and the other hand on the foot, flex the knee and hip, and then take the leg through its full range: lateral, neutral, and medial.

12

Figure 16–14 Stretch the hip in flexion. With one hand just above the knee and the other hand on the foot, gently push the knee directly toward the chest to stretch the hip region.

13

Figure 16–15 Stretch the hip in lateral flexion. Bring the knee toward the chest. Place one hand on the shoulder to prevent movement and the other hand on the knee. Gently push the knee medially to stretch the deep rotator muscles.

14

Figure 16–16 Effleurage to leg and around hip joint. Slide palms over the front of the leg as a connecting and finishing movement. Outside hand slides over the hip joint. Rock the leg from side to side gently as hands return to the ankle.

After you perform the Practice Sequence, evaluate how well you did by filling out Performance Evaluation Form 16–1, Hip and Buttocks Massage. The form can be found in Appendix D: *Performance Evaluation Forms*, and at MyHealthProfessionsLab.com.

Figures source: Pearson Education, Inc./Segal Photography.

LOWER EXTREMITIES

The lower extremities, the legs and feet, are the principal means of locomotion for humans. They afford us a great degree of independence as we can get from one place to another employing **bipedal locomotion**. Loss or diminished use of the legs through disease, injury, or old age results in greater dependence and loss of freedom. Having a "spring in your step" is a sign of vitality and positive outlook. Athletes depend on their legs to play their sports, and walking has become a popular fitness activity.

In Western cultures, shoes are worn for protection and also to confine the feet. It feels good to free the feet and kick off your shoes after wearing them all day. Going barefoot or wearing sandals is a sign of leisure and relaxation. It has been said that if your feet hurt, you hurt all over. Foot massage is commonly valued as a pleasurable treat.

Anatomy of the Lower Extremities

For purposes of massage, the lower extremities may be thought of in three sections: thighs, lower legs, and feet. In the prone position, the buttocks are often included with the lower extremities. There are three large joints in the lower extremities—hip, knee, and ankle—and several small joints within the feet.

Thigh The major muscles of the anterior thigh include

- Quadriceps (rectus femoris, vastus intermedius, vastus lateralis, vastus medialis)
- Sartorius

Muscles found on the medial thigh include the adductors:

- Adductor brevis
- Adductor longus

- Adductor magnus
- Gracilis
- Pectineus

High on the lateral thigh is

- Tensor fasciae latae

The posterior thigh includes the hamstrings:

- Biceps femoris
- Semimembranosus
- Semitendinosus

The iliopsoas muscle group acts on the hip joint, but, for the purposes of massage, is palpated in the abdomen. Those muscles are

- Psoas
- Iliacus

The muscle chart on the inside front cover of this book shows the more superficial leg muscles. The deeper adductor muscles are illustrated in Figure 16–17 ■.

Lower Leg The muscles of the lower leg act largely on the ankle joint and include

- Anterior muscles (tibialis anterior, peroneus tertius, and the flexors)
- Lateral muscles (peroneus longus and brevis)
- Posterior muscles (gastrocnemius, soleus, tibialis posterior, and the extensors)

The superficial and deeper muscles of the posterior lower leg are shown in Figure 16–18 ■.

FIGURE 16–17 Adductor muscles of the medial thigh.

Feet There are many small muscles intrinsic to the feet, most of which are on the plantar side or the bottom. See Figure 16–19 ■. The plantar muscles include a superficial layer:

- Abductor hallucis
- Flexor digitorum brevis
- Abductor digiti minimi

a middle layer:

- Lumbricales
- Quadratus

and a deep layer:

- Adductor hallucis
- Interossei plantares
- Flexor hallucis brevis

The plantar aponeurosis is a superficial strong fibrous band of fascia that runs from the heel to the ball of the foot and binds the longitudinal arch. It is the central part of a broad band of fascia that covers the muscles on the plantar side of the foot. The dorsal surface of the foot is fairly bony. The extensor digitorum brevis and the dorsal interossei are accessible there to massage.

FIGURE 16–18
Muscles of the posterior lower leg.

Superficial layer

- Abductor digiti minimi
- Flexor digitorum brevis
- Abductor hallucis

Second layer

- Lumbricals
- Quadratus plantae

Third layer

- Flexor digiti minimi brevis
- Adductor hallucis
- Flexor hallucis brevis

Deepest layer

- Plantar interossei

FIGURE 16–19 Intrinsic muscles of the foot.

CAUTIONS

Major endangerment sites in the lower extremities include the popliteal fossa located behind the knee, and the inguinal area or groin. Care should be taken not to apply heavy pressure in these areas. However, attachments of muscles may be followed to or around the area. Avoid deep pressure over varicose veins, which are common in older adults. Do not massage the legs if blood clotting or phlebitis is present. Avoid irritating bunions found at the base of the great toe. Watch for athlete's foot and other fungal infections that may be spread through touch. Avoid massaging feet with active infections.

Applications of Massage for the Lower Extremities

People who stand long hours in their jobs often experience stress and pain in the legs and feet. Women especially tend to wear shoes with little support and often wear high heels, which puts the feet and legs in a strained position. Those who sit a lot typically have problems with loss of strength, muscle shortening, and poor circulation in their legs. With age there is loss of strength, flexibility, and agility, and the leg muscles are more frequently stiff and sore. Massage and stretching can help the legs and feet feel and function better by improving circulation, joint mobility, and muscle relaxation.

A thorough foot massage can make you feel good all over. It touches all the small intrinsic muscles of the feet, as well as attachments of muscles of the lower leg, and mobilizes the many joints found there. It relaxes the muscles, improves circulation, and restores feeling to a part of the body encased in shoes most of the time. Special lubricants are available for the feet that contain cooling substances such as peppermint and menthol.

Leg and foot massage is especially beneficial for athletes. Runners and joggers enhance training and help prevent injuries with proper care of the lower extremities.

ENHANCING MOBILITY IN THE LOWER EXTREMITIES

Mobility restrictions in the lower extremities may occur for a number of reasons. Overuse and shortening of muscles in athletes and physical workers, lack of use or aging, recuperation from an extended illness or injury, or a sedentary lifestyle can all contribute to stiff joints and lack of fluid movement in the lower limbs.

For best results, all the muscles of the hips, thighs, lower legs, and feet are thoroughly massaged with effleurage and petrissage and conditioned with stretching. The major tendons are frictioned near their points of attachment. Joints are taken through their full range of motion. Direct pressure along muscles and tendons helps relax them.

CRITICAL THINKING

Think about the structural and functional connections in the lower body. Describe interconnections among the hips, buttocks, legs, and feet.

1. Which muscles cross joints into different regions?
2. What common movements involve more than one region?
3. How are interconnections acknowledged during massage?

PRACTICE SEQUENCE 16–2

Thigh and Lower Leg Massage

20–30 minutes
Recipient supine and prone

Preliminary Instructions
• Secure the drape properly; do not expose the genital area.
• Place a small bolster under the knees to prevent hyperextension.
• Avoid heavy pressure directly over the knee.
• Get informed consent to massage high on the thigh.
• To begin, recipient is supine.

1

Figure 16–20 Apply oil or lotion to the entire leg with effleurage. Use light to medium pressure to warm superficial tissues.

Figure 16–21 Warming effleurage to thigh muscles. Use reinforced palm over palm method to apply deeper pressure from knee to superior muscle attachments. Follow contour of the leg.

Figure 16–22 Petrissage to adductor and quadriceps muscles. Knead, lift, and squeeze muscle bellies.

Figure 16–23 Effleurage to adductor muscles. Bend the knee and open the leg to access adductor muscles. Resecure drape. Slide over adductor muscles with fingertips using medium pressure.

Figure 16–24 Straighten the leg and effleurage to quadriceps with forearm. Apply in three parallel strokes from above knee to superior attachments.

Figure 16–25 Effleurage to iliotibial band with palm. Apply with heel of the hand from superior attachment to attachment at knee.

Figure 16–26 Horizontal stroking to thigh from superior to inferior. Lift tissues as hands cross over top of thigh.

Figure 16–27 Circular friction over attachments at knee. Apply with fingertips or palms.

Figure 16–28 Broadening effleurage to lower leg. Place heels of the hands together over tibia (no pressure over the bone). Slide heels around the leg and toward the table, stretching soft tissues. Move along lower leg, knee to ankle. Repeat twice.

Figure 16–29 Squeeze posterior leg muscles. Apply along muscles from knee to ankle. Use same hand position as in Step 9. Fingers squeeze muscles against heels of the hands.

Figure 16–30 Knuckle friction to tibialis anterior. Apply superficial friction along lateral side of tibia from ankle to superior attachment of tibialis anterior.

Figure 16–31 Apply circular friction around ankles with fingertips.

Finish with abbreviated foot massage sequence (see Practice Sequence 16–3, Foot Massage, which follows). Perform Steps 1–12 plus foot massage on the other extremity, then assist the client in turning over to prone position.

Preliminary Instructions
• Secure the drape properly; expose the buttocks muscles if including the hip area; do not expose the gluteal cleft.
• Place small bolster under the ankles.
• Recipient is prone.

13

Figure 16–32 Apply oil or lotion to the entire leg. Include hip if performing massage to hip region as part of massage of lower extremities.

14

Figure 16–33 Longitudinal and horizontal effleurage to the thigh. Apply with medium pressure to warm tissues.

15

Figure 16–34 Petrissage adductor muscles.

16

Figure 16–35 Deep effleurage with forearm to hamstring muscles. Apply from above knee to superior attachments.

Figure 16–36 Stretch quadriceps, pushing the heel to the buttocks.

Figure 16–37 Effleurage (A) and petrissage (B) to lower leg.

A

B

Figure 16–38 Thumb slides to Achilles tendon.

20

Figure 16–39 Mobilize the ankle with dorsiflexion.

21

Figure 16–40 Slide fist over foot bottom.

22

Figure 16–41 Finish with effleurage from ankles to hips.

 After you perform the Practice Sequence, evaluate how well you did by filling out Performance Evaluation Form 16–2, Thigh and Lower Leg Massage. The form can be found in Appendix D: *Performance Evaluation Forms*, and at MyHealthProfessionsLab.com.

Figures source: Pearson Education, Inc./Segal Photography.

PRACTICAL APPLICATION

Develop a lower body massage sequence that primarily uses compression and joint movements and is applied over clothing such as sweat pants. Focus on muscle relaxation and mobility.

1. Where do you start? What is the progression from region to region?
2. Which mobilizing techniques and stretches do you apply?
3. Can you complete the sequence on both legs in 30 minutes?

PRACTICE SEQUENCE 16–3

Foot Massage   15–20 minutes
Recipient supine

Preliminary Instructions
• Foot massage can be applied with the practitioner sitting on a stool.
• Check the condition of the skin and joints in the feet for contraindications and cautions before beginning.
• Do not pull or bend the toes forcefully.

Figure 16–42 Apply lubricant to the foot and ankle, plantar and dorsal surfaces, and to each toe separately.

Figure 16–43 Mobilize the ankle using the heels of the hands. Place a palm on either side of the ankle just below the malleolus. Move the hands back and forth alternately to create movement.

3

Figure 16–44 Sliding effleurage with a thumb between metatarsals on the dorsal foot surface. Slide from web to tarsal bones.

4

Figure 16–45 Mobilize the space between metatarsals with a scissoring action. Hold the toe "knuckles" of adjoining toes to apply the scissoring action one space at a time.

5

Figure 16–46 Mobilize each metatarsal–phalangeal joint with figure-8s. Hold the tarsal just below the "knuckle" to perform the figure-8s on each toe.

6

Figure 16–47 Gently squeeze along the length of each toe. Move proximal to distal. Squeeze top and bottom first, and then along the sides, one toe at a time.

7

Figure 16–48 If toes are curled, straighten them with effleurage along the length of each toe. Use thumb on top and index finger underneath. Apply more pressure on the underside to stretch the tissues.

8

Figure 16–49 Effleurage to the foot bottom using the fist. Hold the dorsal surface of the foot with one hand while the other slides from toes to heel. Shape the foot around the fist, stretching the top of the foot and accentuating the longitudinal and transverse arches.

9

Figure 16–50 Circular friction with knuckles to various spots on the foot bottom. Concentrate on places with thicker soft tissues.

10

Figure 16–51 Transverse friction to the plantar aponeurosis with the thumb. Brace the foot with one hand while the other applies the deep friction.

11

Figure 16–52 Separate the metatarsals. Create space between the metatarsals by holding onto the sides of the foot and pulling the hands away from each other.

12

Figure 16–53 Slap the foot bottom with the back of the hand. Rapid, light slaps create a stimulating sensation.

After you perform the Practice Sequence, evaluate how well you did by filling out Performance Evaluation Form 16–3, Foot Massage. The form can be found in Appendix D: *Performance Evaluation Forms*, and at MyHealthProfessionsLab.com.

Figures source: Pearson Education, Inc./Segal Photography.

 CASE FOR STUDY

Jody and the Client with Ticklish Feet

Jody has a client with very ticklish feet. At first he told Jody to skip his feet during massage. But the client now has a job where he stands all day and wants massage for relief of his sore legs and feet.

Question:

What can Jody do to avoid tickling the client's feet, and yet provide a thorough foot massage?

Things to consider:

- Where are his feet ticklish? What causes the ticklish reaction?
- Is he ticklish if touched through his socks?
- What massage techniques are least likely to cause tickling?

Describe three approaches Jody can try to avoid tickling while giving foot massage to this client:

_____

_____

_____

CHAPTER HIGHLIGHTS

- Lower body regions addressed during massage include the hips and buttocks, upper and lower legs, and feet.
  - These regions are interconnected and also connected to upper body regions both structurally and functionally.

- Practice sequences for the lower body provide a basic routine for addressing the regions.
  - More advanced massage techniques may be incorporated as learned.
  - Greater specificity may be achieved as greater knowledge of muscles and connective tissues is acquired.
  - Adapt your approach to address the tissues you are actually touching.

- The hips and buttocks support the entire body and provide the power for locomotion.
  - They can be a source of sexual appeal, as well as embarrassment.
  - They are often massaged in conjunction with the lower extremities.
  - Draping while massaging this region should provide for safety and modesty.

- The lower extremities, the legs and feet, are the principal means of bipedal locomotion.
  - Stress and pain in the legs and feet may be the result of injury, old age, sports, or job requirements.
  - Foot massage involves massage of intrinsic muscles of the feet and attachments of leg muscles, and mobilizing of joints.
  - Mobility in lower extremities can be enhanced with massage of the hips, thighs, lower legs, and feet.

EXAM REVIEW

Key Terms

Match the following key terms to their descriptions. For additional study, look up the key terms in the Interactive Glossary, and note other terms that compare or contrast with them.

_____ **1.** Bipedal locomotion
_____ **2.** Lower body regions
_____ **3.** Mobility restrictions
_____ **4.** Palpatory sensitivity
_____ **5.** Specificity

a. Difficulty moving from place to place
b. Below the waist
c. Massage of individual muscle
d. Allows detection of deeper tissues
e. Walking upright on two feet

Memory Workout

To test your memory of the main concepts in this chapter, complete the following sentences by circling the most correct answer from the two choices provided.

1. Lower body regions are connected structurally and (specifically) (functionally).
2. When working with greater specificity, more attention is paid to (broad areas) (distinct structures).
3. The ability to feel the condition of tissues being massaged requires (palpatory) (emotional) sensitivity.
4. When massaging the hips and buttocks take care to create a feeling of safety and (relaxation) (modesty).
5. The large muscles of the hips and buttocks region provide power for (locomotion) (assisted motion).
6. The lower extremities are generally massaged in (two) (three) sections.
7. A major endangerment site in the lower extremities is the popliteal fossa located behind the (ankle) (knee).
8. Special lubricants are available for the feet that contain (cooling) (warming) substances such as camphor and menthol.
9. Before massaging high on the recipient's thigh, get his or her informed (assessment) (consent).
10. If there are varicose veins in the legs, apply only (deep specific) (broad light) techniques to the area.

Test Prep

The following multiple-choice questions will help to prepare you for future school and professional exams.

1. To condition the deep rotators of the hip joint, which are difficult to reach directly with massage, practitioners can apply:
   a. Lotion with menthol
   b. Joint movements
   c. Effleurage techniques
   d. Passive touch

2. When draping for massage of the hips and buttocks region:
   a. Pull the drape down on both sides and secure at the upper thighs
   b. Undrape one side at a time, avoiding exposure of the gluteal cleft
   c. Never expose the buttocks themselves
   d. Either a or b

3. Passive stretches for the hips and buttocks muscles are best applied with the client:
   a. Sitting
   b. Side-lying
   c. Prone
   d. Supine

4. If a recipient has mild varicose veins on his or her legs, it is generally safe to use the following over the area:
   a. Deep thumb stripping
   b. Vigorous kneading
   c. Light effleurage with palms
   d. Any of the above

5. Because of their function for locomotion, the buttocks muscles are typically massaged as part of the:
   a. Lower extremities
   b. Back
   c. Abdomen
   d. Feet

6. During foot massage, the space between metatarsals is best mobilized using:
   a. Figure-8s
   b. Scissoring action
   c. Flexion
   d. Circumduction

7. The main purpose of using the forearm to apply massage to the large hips and buttocks muscles is to:
   a. Avoid straining the hands
   b. Muscle through the dense tissues
   c. Apply more pressure skillfully
   d. Both a and c

8. The first step in any massage sequence is to:
   a. Address individual muscles specifically
   b. Apply finishing techniques
   c. Apply deep pressure for stimulation
   d. Warm the tissues

9. When the recipient is prone, pushing the heel to the buttocks primarily stretches the:
   a. Hamstrings muscles
   b. Quadriceps muscles
   c. Tensor fascia latae
   d. Gracilis

10. Most of the small muscles intrinsic to the feet are palpated on the:
    a. Dorsal side
    b. Plantar side
    c. Medial side
    d. Lateral side

Video Challenge

Watch the Regional Applications of Massage—Lower Body videos, which can be found at MyHealthProfessionsLab.com, Chapter 16, and then answer the following questions.

1. How does the massage therapist in the video drape the client for massage of the hips and buttocks?

2. What massage technique variations are shown in the video demonstrations for the lower extremities? Note how the massage therapist's hands are used.

3. Which techniques used in the video demonstration of massage of the feet add specificity to the application?

Comprehension Exercises

The following short-answer questions test your knowledge and understanding of chapter topics and provide practice in written communication skills. Explain in two to four complete sentences.

1. Describe alternatives to using the palm of the hand for applying massage to large muscles of the body, such as the buttocks muscles.

For Greater Understanding

The following exercises are designed to take you from the realm of theory into the real world. They will help give you a deeper understanding of the subjects covered in this chapter. Action words are underlined to emphasize the variety of activities presented to address different learning styles and to encourage deeper thinking.

1. Receive a massage from a professional practitioner, and request special attention to the legs. Note how the massage therapist addresses the request and his or her approach to massage of the region. Report your experience to a study partner or group.

2. Practice the foot massage sequence on three different people. Note structural differences in their feet and the ways that you adapted the massage to accommodate for their individuality. Report your experience to a study partner or group.

2. Explain how the use of deep friction offers greater specificity in massage of the lower extremities. Give an example.

3. Give massage of the buttocks and legs to two different practice clients. Get informed consent before massaging the buttocks area. Note the reaction of the recipient to massage of this region. Notice how you felt massaging the buttocks muscles and each recipient's personal reaction. Discuss with a study partner or group.

4. Create a 30-minute massage for a lower body region. Include warming, therapeutic combinations, and transition and finishing techniques. Demonstrate your sequence, noting how you achieved specificity, avoided monotony, and made transitions.

MyHealthProfessionsLab™

MyHealthProfessionsLab.com is a premium online homework management system that includes a host of features to help you study. Registered users will find:

- Powerful tools that track and analyze your results—allowing you to create a personalized learning experience
- Videos, flashcards and other learning tools to help enrich your progress
- Streaming lesson presentations and self-paced learning modules
- A space where you and your instructors can view and manage your assignments

17 Hydrotherapy and Temperature Therapies

Pearson Education, Inc.

CHAPTER OUTLINE

Learning Outcomes

Key Terms

Introduction

History of Hydrotherapy

Healing Properties of Water

Hydrotherapy Facilities

Hot Applications

Cold Applications

Chapter Highlights

Exam Review

LEARNING OUTCOMES

After studying this chapter, you will have information to:

1. Discuss the history of hydrotherapy.

2. Describe the healing properties of water.

3. Describe hydrotherapy facilities found in spas and health clubs.

4. Compare degree ranges for different temperature therapy modalities.

5. Recognize contraindications for hydrotherapy and temperature therapy.

6. Use hydrotherapy facilities effectively and safely.

7. Apply thermotherapy and cryotherapy effectively and safely.

8. Use hot packs within the scope of massage therapy.

9. Use cold packs within the scope of massage therapy.

10. Apply ice massage for therapeutic benefit.

KEY TERMS

Cold packs	Hunting reaction	Sauna	Thermotherapy
Cryotherapy	Hydrotherapy	Steam rooms	Whirlpool bath
Hot packs	Ice massage	Temperature therapy	

INTRODUCTION

Hydrotherapy is the use of water in health and healing practices. The trio of water, massage, and exercise is a natural combination found all over the globe in bathhouses, spas, and health clubs. The word *spa* is an acronym for the Latin *salus per aquam* meaning "health from water." A more general term for therapeutic applications of hot and cold, whether or not water is involved, is **temperature therapy**.

This chapter explores some of the more common hydrotherapy methods and hot and cold applications within the scope of massage therapy. For more in-depth information on the use of physical agents overall and within the context of rehabilitation, refer to specialty textbooks listed for this chapter in Appendix E, *References and Additional Resources*.

HISTORY OF HYDROTHERAPY

The use of water for bathing, relaxation, and recreation is universal. From time immemorial, humans have enjoyed mineral and hot springs for their soothing and cleansing effects. Native Americans are said to have frequented natural springs for their healing properties. Later, in places such as Saratoga Springs, New York; Hot Springs, Arkansas; and Calistoga, California, resorts were built where the hot and cold mineral waters were taken internally as well as used for bathing. At spas today, hot and bubbling mineral waters are collected in pools for bathers seeking relaxation and healing.

Archaeologists studying the ancient Maya and Aztec civilizations have found the ruins of sweat baths throughout Central America. The oldest of the sweat baths date from about 1350 BCE. These structures, called *temezcalli,* are described in the first written history of Mexico by Friar Diego Duran in 1567. Most were small buildings with low ceilings and small entranceways and held about 10 people. Steam was created by pouring water over hot rocks. Herbs were used with the steam for their healing effects. Sweating was thought to purify the body and cure illnesses. Mayan sweat baths are the antecedents of today's *temescal* or sweat houses still found in Central America.

In North America, the sweat lodge ceremony is one of the most important traditional practices of Native Americans. In the past, sweat lodges were circular domed structures constructed from animal skins stretched over frames made of tree branches, but today sweat lodges take many forms. In this ritual for spiritual cleansing, stones are heated in a central fire pit and added in increments to increase the heat in the lodge. Water is added to the stones to increase steam, and herbs (sage, copal, lavender) are placed on the stones for therapeutic purposes. Native American spiritual objects and rituals are typically part of the traditional sweat lodge ceremony.

The sauna was developed centuries ago in Finland. The sauna is typically a wood-lined room or shed heated to a high temperature by hot rocks. Water is poured on the rocks periodically to add some moisture to the room. After sitting and sweating in these superheated rooms, hardy Finns would jump into cold rivers and snow banks to cool off. It is a practice that many believe builds stamina, energy, and strength.

Today's spa and health club facilities such as whirlpool baths, showers, and steam rooms can be traced in Western civilization directly to the ancient Greek gymnasia and Roman baths. Turkish baths, based on the Roman prototype, became popular in Europe and the United States in the latter nineteenth century. Baths were also popular in ancient Asia, particularly India, China, Korea, and Japan. Massage and bodywork was and still is an integral part of the bathhouse experience.

The Water Cure

The healing effects of water applications were known in ancient Greece. The famous Greek physician Hippocrates (c. 460 BCE) used compresses, sponging, bathing, and drinking water in his treatments.

Water therapies of various kinds were among the natural healing methods that blossomed in the 1800s. Vincent Priessnitz (1799–1851), a farmer in the Austro-Hungarian Empire, was well known for the methods of water therapy he developed and made popular. Priessnitz created an entire system of baths, compresses, and other hot and cold applications to treat various diseases.

Sebastian Kneipp (1821–1897) from Bavaria is perhaps the most famous water cure practitioner of his era. Kneipp was a priest who built on Priessnitz's water-based therapies and his own knowledge of herbal remedies, becoming the foremost authority on the subject. His book, *My Water Cure,* first written in 1889, was translated into many languages through the years. People flocked to him from all over Europe to be cured of a variety of ailments.

European spas, which cater to people seeking healing as well as relaxation, adopted the methods of Priessnitz and Kneipp. An example of a Kneipp treatment given at the Biltz Sanitarium in Weisbaden, Germany, in 1898 is shown in Figure 17–1 ■. The great spas at Baden-Baden and Weisbaden in Germany, Montecatini Terme in Italy, and Evian-les-Bains in France, as well as many smaller hydrotherapy establishments, carry on the tradition of the water cure.

The idea of the natural healing resort was imported to the United States in places such as J. Harvey Kellogg's Battle Creek Sanitarium in Michigan. Kellogg wrote *Home Handbook of Domestic Hygiene and Rational Medicine* in 1880, which covered hydrotherapy, electrotherapy, and Swedish remedial gymnastics. His book *Rational Hydrotherapy,* written in1900, described 200 water treatments.

Hydrotherapy versus Hydropathy

Sir John Floyer, a physician in Lichfield, England, wrote a treatise in 1702 titled *The History of Cold Bathing to the Ancient and Modern.* Later that century, Dr. Currie of

FIGURE 17–1 Kneipp treatment: Upper affusion with hose at the Biltz Sanitarium in Weisbaden, Germany, 1898.

Liverpool, England, wrote *Medical Reports on the Effects of Water, Both Warm and Cold, as a Remedy in Fevers and Other Diseases* (1797). The use of water as a therapeutic agent was well established within the developing field of biomedicine by the eighteenth century.

Almost a century later in Vienna, Wilhelm Winternitz (1835–1917) experimented with various forms of external water applications to treat a variety of diseases. He used the shower, spray, alternating hot and cold baths, along with manipulations and massage. He varied the temperature of the water and the force with which it was applied and measured the results. Winternitz brought hydrotherapy into the domain of science.

Mineral water hospitals were opened in England as early as 1738 in Bath, 1824 in Harrogate, 1836 in Droitwich, and 1858 in Buxton. Physicians managed the larger spas, but had competition from lay natural healers whom they considered quacks. The medical-versus-lay healer split widened, although each side adopted methods of the other.

By the 1890s, the use of water as a therapeutic agent had two main branches and two terms to describe it. At places such as Nauheim, Germany, and Bath and Malvern in England, where the medical influence was strong, the term used was *hydrotherapy,* a rational system of baths, exercises, and electricity. The term *hydropathy* was reserved for "barefoot back-to-nature cults masterminded by lay philosophers" practiced at continental mountain resorts.[1]

Methods of natural healing and those of modern biomedicine were diverging into separate paths by the turn of the nineteenth century. Biomedicine opted largely for treatments with drugs and surgery. The old hydropathy became the province of naturopaths and other natural healers. Hydrotherapy retained its association with massage and movement therapies.

Members of the Chartered Society of Trained Masseuses (later Physiotherapy) in England treated injured servicemen during World War I (1914–1918) with hydrotherapy, massage, and related therapies. This idea was imported to North America at about the same time, and the profession of physical therapy, as it is known in the United States, was born. Physical therapists continue to research the therapeutic uses of water and temperature as a science.

HEALING PROPERTIES OF WATER

Water is relaxing to look at in rivers, lakes, and ponds, and to listen to by the seashore, at a waterfall, or in a desktop water fountain. Flowing water feels pleasurable on the skin.

Taken internally and experienced externally, water is the basis of many natural healing methods. The therapeutic use of water taken internally is outside the scope of massage therapy, aside from encouraging clients to drink water to stay hydrated.

External applications of water in various forms and immersion in water, however, have an association with massage that goes back to ancient times. Hydrotherapy and temperature therapy may be roughly divided into *thermo, neutro,* and *cryo.* **Thermotherapy** involves methods above normal body temperature. Neutrotherapy uses methods at about body temperature. **Cryotherapy** involves methods below body temperature. Table 17–1 ■ outlines the sensations associated with these temperature ranges. Note that descriptions such as hot, tepid, and cold are based on personal perception of temperature on the skin. These perceptions are subjective and vary from person to person.

TABLE 17–1	Temperature Sensations for Thermo-, Neutro-, and Cryo-Hydrotherapy		
Type	**Description**	**Fahrenheit**	**Celsius***
Thermo	Very hot	111° to 120°	44° to 49°
	Hot	101° to 110°	38° to 43°
	Warm	96° to 100°	36° to 38°
Neutro	Neutral	91° to 95°	33° to 35°
Cryo	Tepid	80° to 90°	27° to 32°
	Cool	70° to 79°	21° to 26°
	Cold	55° to 69°	13° to 21°
	Very cold	31° to 54°	1° to 12°
	Freezing	32° and below	0° and below

*Temperature conversion Fahrenheit (°F) to Celsius (°C):
°F = °C × 9/5 + 32.

Source: Data from Miller, E. (1996). Day Spa Techniques. Albany, NY: Milady Publishers; Belanger, A. (2002). Evidenced-Based Guide to Therapeutic Physical Agents. Philadelphia, PA: Lippincott Williams & Wilkins.

Methods within the scope of massage therapy include types of hydrotherapy used for health promotion, such as those found in health clubs and spas. It also includes therapeutic uses of hot and cold applications in the forms of hot and cold packs and ice. The general temperature ranges for these methods are listed in Table 17–2 ■.

Healing properties of water are related to its use in cleansing the body and its ability to raise and lower the core body temperature or the temperature of specific body tissues. Water can assume different forms—liquid, steam, and ice—each with its own contribution to healing. Water pressure from a shower, hose, or water jets is also used for a type of massage of the soft tissues.

HYDROTHERAPY FACILITIES

Typical spa and health club settings offer whirlpool baths, showers, steam rooms, and/or saunas in addition to massage services. Hot tubs and Esalen massage have been part of the California scene since the 1970s. Massage practitioners should know something about these facilities to be able to give clients guidance and to suggest their safe and effective use in relation to massage.

The benefits of warm to hot forms of hydrotherapy include raising the body temperature, producing sweating, cleansing skin pores, increasing superficial circulation, muscular relaxation, and general relaxation. These are best used before receiving massage.

The benefits of cool to cold forms of hydrotherapy include lowering body temperature, closing skin pores,

decreasing superficial circulation, and general invigoration or stimulation. The cold shower is the most common form of cryo-hydrotherapy in the spa setting. Cold showers, or a contrasting hot to cold shower, are best taken after massage. See Table 17–3 ■ for major effects of hot and cold hydrotherapy.

A **whirlpool bath** consists of a water-filled tub that has air or water jets causing movement or churning of the water. Private whirlpool bathtubs are deep enough so that a person can lie down. Whirlpool baths within the context of physiotherapy may be smaller to accommodate an arm or a leg and are made of stainless steel.

The temperature of the water in a whirlpool bath is generally hot, but may vary considerably depending on the purpose of the bath and the health of the patron. The recommended water temperature for relaxation ranges from about 95°F to 105°F (35°C to 41°C).

The healing effects of the whirlpool bath stem from the water heat and the pressure of the water coming out of the jets and hitting the body. The churning of the water helps sustain the heat of the water on the skin and stimulates the touch receptors of the skin.

Communal whirlpool baths may be found in spas, health clubs, and bathhouses. In these baths, people sit on benches and are immersed in hot water with just their shoulders and heads above the water line. Whirlpool jets cause the water to churn and swirl. A hot tub is a variation made with wood

TABLE 17–2	Degree Ranges for Hydrotherapy and Temperature Therapy Methods from Cold to Hot Applications
Method	**Temperature Range**
Ice	23° to 32°F (25° to 0°C)
Cold pack	33° to 50°F (1° to 10°C)
Cold water	50° to 80°F (10° to 27°C)
Bath—cool/cold	70° to 80°F (21° to 27°C)
Whirlpool bath—warm	95° to 104°F (35° to 40°C)
Whirlpool bath—hot	105° to 110°F (41° to 43°C)
Steam room*	105° to 130°F (41° to 54°C)
Sauna**	160° to 180°F (71° to 82°C)
Hot pack—wet	165° 2 170°F (74° to 77°C)

*Wet heat with 100% humidity
**Dry heat with 6–8% humidity

Source: Data from Miller, E. (1996). Day Spa Techniques. Albany, NY: Milady Publishers; Belanger, A. (2002). Evidenced-Based Guide To Therapeutic Physical Agents. Philadelphia, PA: Lippincott Williams & Wilkins.

TABLE 17–3	General Effects of Hydro-therapy* Comparing Thermo-Hydrotherapy and Cryo-Hydrotherapy	
Thermo-hydrotherapy	**Cryo-Hydrotherapy**
• Increase core body temperature	• Decrease core body temperature
• Increase pulse rate	• Decrease pulse rate
• Decrease blood pressure	• Increase blood pressure
• Increase respiratory rate	• Decrease respiratory rate
• Decrease muscle tone	• Increase muscle tone
• Induce sweating	• Induce shivering
• Relaxing/sedative effect	• Invigorating/stimulating effect
	• Reduce inflammation
	• Decrease pain

*Hydrotherapy refers here to methods that are applied to the whole body, such as whirlpool, shower, steam room, and sauna.

Note: The actual effects of specific hydrotherapy methods depend on the health of the client, the actual temperature of the water or room, and the length of time a person is exposed to the heat or cold.

Source: Data from Body Systemic Effects Generally Associated with Cryo-, Thermo-, and Neutro-Hydrotherapy, in Belanger, A. (2002). Evidenced-Based Guide to Therapeutic Physical Agents. Philadelphia, PA: Lippincott Williams & Wilkins.

slats and a rubber or plastic liner and may or may not have whirlpool jets. The safety guidelines for whirlpool baths and hot tubs are the same.

Showers are created by water streaming out of showerheads mounted on the wall. Showers may have no added pressure, falling like rain, or may have added pressure or pulsing pressure. Showers may be hot or cold. Hot showers have a similar effect as whirlpool baths, that is, relaxation and increased superficial circulation.

Cold showers are stimulating and help reduce general body heat. They may be taken as a cool down after thermo-hydrotherapy or exercise. Variations of the showers found in spas include the Swiss shower in which showerheads surround the bather at different levels from head to toe. In a Scotch shower, the patron is sprayed alternately with hot and cold water, which is thought to stimulate circulation. The Vichy shower is given with the patron lying down on a table with water showering down from about 4 feet above (see Figure 19–1). The Vichy shower can be varied with pulsating water, with alternating hot and cold water, or with a salt or shampoo scrub. An attendant controls the water pressure and temperature from a panel.

Steam rooms are typically spaces tiled from floor to ceiling with benches for sitting. Steam comes out from jets in the walls and fills the space with wet heat from 105°F to 130°F (41°C to 54°C) with 100% humidity. Patrons in the steam room inhale the steam, which helps clear sinuses and relieve respiratory congestion. Steam also raises the body temperature and causes sweating. It is a relaxing, cleansing experience.

A variation of the stream room is the steam cabinet. The patron sits on a stool in an enclosed box with his or her head sticking out. Steam is pumped into the box, raising core body temperature and causing sweating. Because the head is out of the box, the steam is not inhaled. A cold shower following a steam room or steam cabinet experience can help wash off sweat and bring body temperature down to normal.

When raising the core body temperature is contraindicated or undesirable, facial steam may be beneficial. Facial steam devices focus steam to the face and are used in skin care, as well as to improve respiration.

Taking a **sauna** involves sitting in a room with dry heat from 160°F to 180°F (71°C to 82°C) with 6% to 8% humidity. The sauna is typically a wood-lined room heated without steam, and the air is very dry. Patrons sit on wooden benches. Occasionally, water may be poured over hot rocks to produce steam, adding some moisture to the air. A cold shower or a plunge into a swimming pool or lake (or snowbank) after sitting in a sauna is stimulating, closes the skin pores, and helps reduce body temperature back to normal.

Contraindications for thermo-hydrotherapy are listed in Box 17–1 ■. The most serious contraindications are related to heart, circulatory, and other systemic diseases. People with skin rashes should also avoid the increase in superficial circulation that results from immersing in hot water. Of

---

BOX 17–1   Contraindications for Thermo-Hydrotherapy

- High or low blood pressure
- Heart or circulatory problems
- Pregnancy
- Systemic diseases such as hepatitis
- Seizures
- Multiple sclerosis
- Infection or inflammatory condition
- Vascular problems associated with phlebitis, varicose veins, diabetes
- Skin rashes
- Allergies to water additives
- Contagious conditions
- Some cancers and cancer treatments

Certain medications may make hydrotherapy unsafe for a client. These include drugs that:

- Alter how blood vessels react to hot and cold
- Change skin sensitivity to hot and cold
- Alter the body's temperature control or cooling mechanism

Note: These contraindications apply to hydrotherapy methods that raise the core body temperature. In some cases, using water with lower temperature and/or limiting the time in the hot water or steam may make their use safer.

Source: Data From Miller, E. (1996). Day Spa Techniques. Albany, NY: Milady Publishers; Persad, R. S. (2001). Massage Therapy And Medications. Toronto, On: Curties-Overzet Publications; Belanger, A. (2002). Evidenced-Based Guide To Therapeutic Physical Agents. Philadelphia, PA: Lippincott Williams & Wilkins.

---

course, people using public facilities should be careful not to spread contagious disease of any kind.

Although it is possible to overdo cryo-hydrotherapy causing adverse reactions, it is more common for people to stay too long in the heat of the thermo-hydrotherapy baths and rooms. First-time bathers should only stay 5 to 15 minutes in hot water, whereas healthy, experienced bathers may stay up to 30 minutes. People who are weak or over 60 years old should limit their exposure to hot baths and steam to 5 to 15 minutes.

If a client reports feeling lightheaded or dizzy, is nauseous, or develops a headache, he or she probably stayed immersed too long in hot water or steam. Take measures to reduce the body temperature gradually, such as sitting or lying in a neutral temperature environment and sipping tepid to cool water. If symptoms persist or get worse, consider medical evaluation. Guidelines for safe use of thermo-hydrotherapy facilities are summarized in Box 17–2 ■.

The most commonly used methods of temperature therapy within the scope of massage therapy are hot packs, ice, cold packs, and ice massage. The focus of the following section is on local applications of temperature therapy.

BOX 17–2	Guidelines for Safe Use of Thermo-Hydrotherapy Facilities: Whirlpool, Shower, Steam Room, and Sauna

1. Check to make sure that no contraindications are present before using thermo-facilities (see Box 17–1).
2. Wait for at least 1 hour after eating before using thermo-facilities.
3. Avoid alcohol before or during use of thermo-facilities.
4. Wear sandals or shoes with nonslip bottoms to avoid slipping and falling.
5. Check temperature of the water or room (steam and sauna) for therapeutic range (see Table 17–2) and for individual tolerance.
6. Limit use according to experience in thermo-facilities and factors such as general health and age. In general, for those less experienced, less healthy, weaker, or over age 60, limit use to 15 minutes; otherwise 15 to 30 minutes is appropriate.
7. Drink plenty of water during and after thermo-hydrotherapy to replace loss through sweating.
8. Always have someone to call for help if needed.
9. Monitor how you feel, and if weak, dizzy, or nauseous get out of the water or room. Lie or sit down in a cooler place, and replace fluids by sipping a cool drink of water.
10. If reaction to heat is severe or lasts a long time, consider seeking medical evaluation.

Note: Use of thermo-hydrotherapy facilities *before massage* is beneficial for initiating general relaxation, muscle relaxation, and increased superficial circulation and connective tissue pliability. Use of the thermo-hydrotherapy facilities *after massage* may continue the benefits described. Be sure to drink water to replenish fluids, and wash off oil and lotion thoroughly before entering thermo-facilities. Lubricants can contaminate water and leave slippery films on benches and floors.

HOT APPLICATIONS

Heat applied locally to muscles and related soft tissues not only feels good, but also helps muscles relax, increases local circulation, and makes connective tissues more pliable. Sore, stiff muscles benefit from the increased circulation and heat.

Raising tissue temperature to between 104°F and 113°F (40°C to 45°C) increases cell metabolism and blood flow for various therapeutic results. Lower temperatures have little therapeutic effect, and higher temperatures will damage cells.[2]

Although heat is applied locally, use of hot packs can raise core body temperature. In that case, contraindications for thermo-hydrotherapy also apply. See Box 17–1. Local contraindications for the use of hot packs include burns, wounds, swelling, inflammation, and skin conditions (e.g., rashes) that could be made worse by heat. Check the area visually and/or by palpation for evidence of contraindications before deciding to use hot packs.

Hot Packs and Massage

The application of **hot packs** prior to massage can help begin muscle relaxation, enhance circulation locally, and prepare the area for deeper massage techniques. After massage of an area, hot packs can enhance muscle relaxation and prolong increased local circulation.

Heat sources include moist hot packs or dry hot packs or pads. Moist hot packs are more penetrating. A rubber hot water bottle is an inexpensive yet effective heat source. Some newer types of hot packs heated in microwave ovens can be good heat sources and are generally easy to use. They can be applied over warm, damp cloths to create moist heat.

Typical moist hot packs come in various sizes and shapes and are heated in hot water. Hydrocollator units are metal containers with electrical heating elements used to keep the water within a constant range: 158°F to 168°F (51°C to 54°C). Hot packs are suspended in the hot water to a therapeutic temperature and then applied to the client.

Always check how the hot pack feels on your own skin (e.g., at the wrist) prior to applying it to a client. Packs that have been sitting in the hydrocollator for a long time (i.e., over 60 minutes) will be hotter than packs that are rotated in and out often, or that have been heating for only a few minutes.

Take care not to burn the client's skin. This is accomplished by placing towels between the hot pack and the skin. Ask the client for feedback every 5 to 7 minutes about how the pack feels (i.e., if it feels too hot). A visual and tactile check is also a good idea. Clients taking medications that reduce skin sensation, or alter the reaction of blood vessels to heat, or reduce their body heat control mechanisms, are not good candidates for hot packs. See Box 17–3 ▪ for guidelines for the use of moist hot packs with massage. Practice Sequence 17–1 shows a hot application on the upper back.

CRITICAL THINKING

Experiment with three different heat sources or hot packs for thermotherapy applications. Compare their ease of application, safety considerations, and overall effectiveness.

1. What materials is each heat source or hot pack made from?
2. How do you get the application to the desired temperature? Is additional equipment required?
3. What are the most cost-effective methods for different therapeutic goals?

REALITY CHECK

KELLY

TAMIKA: I'd like to use heat applications for clients, especially in the winter, but it takes so many towels. I end up having to do a lot of extra laundry. Do you have any suggestions for alternatives?

KELLY: Hot packs heated in hydrocollators are very wet, so you have to use several towels to protect the client's skin from burning. This type of wet heat is best in clinical situations. But if your goal is to provide warmth, comfort, and some muscle relaxation, other heat sources that can be applied over the drape may be adequate. This type of hot pack is generally filled with therapeutic beads, gel, aromatic herbs, or rice and is typically heated in a microwave oven, so is more convenient for nonclinical settings. Some hot pack fillings also generate some moisture when heated, but not so much that towels are needed.

BOX 17–3 Summary of Guidelines for Safe Use of Moist Hot Packs Before and During Massage

1. Be clear about your goals for using hot packs in association with massage.
2. Check to make sure that no contraindications are present and that the client is not taking medications that reduce sensation or alter circulation.
3. Get informed consent from the client to apply hot packs.
4. Instruct the client on the need for feedback about how the hot pack feels to him or her, especially if it feels too hot.
5. Check the hot pack to make sure it is the correct temperature. Touch it to your own skin (e.g., wrist) to judge if it is hot enough or too hot, and how many layers of towels to use.
6. Apply layers of towels between the client's skin and the hot pack to help avoid burns. Use more layers for more sensitive skin and for clients over 60 years old.
7. Apply a towel over the hot pack to help keep heat from escaping.
8. Ask for feedback from the client every 5 to 7 minutes or more if needed. Heat of tissues increases the longer the hot pack is applied.
9. Add additional towels beneath the hot pack if the client complains of too much heat.
10. Remove hot pack immediately if you judge potential for damage to skin or if client is having negative reaction to heat (e.g., dizziness, nausea).
11. Maximum time for hot pack use on a local area is about 20 minutes.

PRACTICE SEQUENCE 17–1

Hot Application on Upper Back
15 minutes
Recipient prone

Preliminary Instructions
• Prepare heat source ahead of time.
• Check for contraindications for heat applications.
• Get informed consent for the hot application.
• Get frequent feedback about heat intensity from recipient.

1

Figure 17–2 Prepare upper back for hot application. Undrape upper back. Check tissues visually and through palpation.

Figure 17–3 Check heat source for temperature. Evaluate the amount of heat given off from the source using your own sense of touch. Use your judgment on how thick a heat barrier to start with.

Figure 17–4 Place sheet or towel over area to be heated. Use sufficient heat barrier for the heat source used. Use at least one depth of towel under moist heat source.

Figure 17–5 Apply the heat source, and ask for immediate feedback on the heat intensity felt by the recipient. Heat should not cause pain, but feel soothing. Add or subtract heat barriers as needed to protect the skin.

Figure 17–6 Instruct recipient on giving you feedback immediately if heat becomes too intense. Remind the person that the effects of heat can build over time.

Figure 17–7 Cover heat source to slow cooling by placing a towel over it.

Figure 17–8 Get feedback every 5 to 7 minutes about heat intensity. Add or subtract heat barriers to maintain therapeutic effect. Massage other areas while heat is on upper back.

Figure 17–9 Remove the heat source, and check the skin for redness. Massage the area, and notice muscle relaxation that has occurred.

After you perform this practice sequence, evaluate how well you did by filling out Performance Evaluation Form 17–1, Hot Application on Upper Back. The form can be found in Appendix D, *Performance Evaluation Forms*, and at MyHealthProfessionsLab.com.

Figures source: Pearson Education, Inc./Segal Photography.

COLD APPLICATIONS

Cryotherapy, which is cold applied locally to muscles and related soft tissues, causes vasoconstriction and decreased local circulation. There is also decrease in cell metabolism, nerve conduction velocity, pain, muscle spindle activity, and spasm in the cold area. After about 20 to 30 minutes of continuous application, cold-induced vasodilation is thought to occur. This may lead to increased circulation, but it is doubtful that circulation rises to a baseline of what it was before the cold was applied. Cold applied locally can also lower core body temperature over time.

The **hunting reaction**, also called the *hunting response* or *Lewis reaction*, occurs when the temperature of tissues is reduced for 12 to 15 minutes or more, or when the temperature is lowered to 50°F (10°C). The hunting reaction consists of alternating periods of vasodilation and vasoconstriction in the tissues affected. It is a protective mechanism designed to prevent tissue damage or frostbite.[3] Local cold applications are usually set at about 15 minutes to avoid triggering the hunting reaction.

Cold applications after trauma or injury can decrease secondary cell and tissue damage. Cold helps prevent the worsening of a soft tissue injury by causing vasoconstriction. This limits internal and external bleeding. It also reduces acute inflammation and swelling.

First aid for a strain or sprain, or a blow to soft tissues, includes immediate application of cold, preferably ice cold. This limits hemorrhaging, swelling, and secondary cell hypoxia or damage. If a limb is involved, the RICES first aid principle applies (i.e., rest, ice, compression, elevation, and stabilization).

Cryotherapy is used most often with massage in settings where clients are likely to have soft tissue injury or pain. These include sports medicine and rehabilitation settings and chiropractic offices. However, any client may have had a recent injury or have muscle spasms, so knowledge of the use of cold applications can be useful. Contraindications to local cold applications include circulatory insufficiency, such as with Raynaud's disease and diabetes, allergic reaction to cold, cold sensitivity, and low core body temperature or chilling. Clients with multiple sclerosis or asthma may not react well to cold. Take special care with clients taking medications that reduce skin sensation, alter the reaction of blood vessels to heat and cold, or reduce their body temperature control mechanisms. See Box 17–4 ▪ for a summary of contraindications for cryo-hydrotherapy and cold applications.

The person receiving the cold application will normally feel the following stages: (1) a sensation of cold, (2) tingling or itching, (3) pain, aching, or burning, and (4) numbing or analgesia. It is good to inform the client about what he or she will feel because some of the sensations can be uncomfortable. Be careful not to apply very cold applications for too long (1-hour maximum) to avoid tissue damage and frostbite. Guidelines for cold applications are summarized in Box 17–5 ▪.

BOX 17–4 | **Contraindications for Cryo-Hydrotherapy and Cold Applications**

- Circulatory insufficiency or vasospastic disorders (e.g., Raynaud's disease, diabetes)
- Cardiac disorder
- Allergy to cold
- Cold hypersensitivity or chilling
- Multiple sclerosis
- Asthma
- Fibromyalgia
- Rheumatoid arthritis
- Osteoarthritis
- Some cancers and cancer treatments
- Infection
- Depression
- Pregnancy

Certain medications may make hydrotherapy unsafe for a client. These include drugs that:

- Alter how blood vessels react to hot and cold
- Change skin sensitivity to hot and cold
- Alter the body's temperature control or cooling mechanisms

Note: These contraindications and cautions apply to cryo-hydrotherapy methods that lower the core body temperature.
Source: Data from Knight, K. L. (1995). Cryotherapy in Sports Injury Management. Champaign, IL: Human Kinetics; Belanger, A. (2002). Evidenced-Based Guide To Therapeutic Physical Agents. Philadelphia, PA: Lippincott Williams & Wilkins; Persad, R .S. (2001). Massage Therapy And Medications. Toronto, ON: Curties-Overzet Publications.

BOX 17–5 | **Summary of Guidelines for Safe Use of Cold and Ice Packs before and during Massage**

1. Be clear about your goals for using cold applications in association with massage.
2. Check to make sure that no contraindications are present and that the client is not taking medications that reduce sensation or alter circulation.
3. Get informed consent from the client to apply cold packs.
4. Instruct the client on the need for feedback about how the cold application feels to him or her.
5. Inform the client of the stages of sensation to expect with cold applications, i.e., (1) cold sensation, (2) tingling or itching, (3) aching or burning, and (4) numbness or analgesia.
6. Apply the cold or ice pack directly to the desired area.
7. Take care when applying a cold-gel pack directly to the skin under a compression bandage because it may cause frostbite over time.
8. Use the RICES principle if the injury is to a limb: rest, ice, compression, elevation, stabilization.
9. Ask for feedback on the cold application every 5 to 7 minutes.
10. Remove the cold pack immediately if it causes an adverse reaction (e.g., skin rash, chilling).
11. Maximum time for continuous cold application is 1 hour; 15 minutes is usually sufficient in the context of a massage session.

Cold Packs and Massage

Cold packs of various kinds are commercially available. They are usually made of materials that hold cold over a period of time and stay pliable even when near freezing. They have coverings for comfortable contact with skin.

Ice packs are made with ice cubes or crushed ice inside plastic bags that can be sealed. A disadvantage of ice is that it melts over time, and plastic bags can leak water. Ice, water below 32°F (0°C), is also hard to the touch and may be less comfortable over injuries. However, ice is readily available and generally stays cold longer than cold packs.

Ice can be replaced in bags as needed to hold a freezing temperature.

Cold packs are used as adjuncts to massage to reduce muscle spasm or muscle pain, or if a client has swelling from a recent injury such as a sprained ankle. Cold may be applied to reduce spasm and pain so that the area can be massaged. It can also be used instead of massage if massage would further aggravate the injury or spasm. Cold or ice may be applied to a specific area during massage of other parts of the body. Practice Sequence 17–2 illustrates a cold application for the knee.

PRACTICE SEQUENCE 17–2

Cold Application for Knee | 15 minutes
Recipient supine

Preliminary Instructions
• Use a cold source that will conform to the shape of the knee.
• Check for contraindications for the cold application.
• Get informed consent for the cold application.
• Get frequent feedback about cold intensity from recipient.

1

Figure 17–10 Prepare knee for cold application. Undrape the leg. Check tissues visually and through palpation, and notice any swelling.

2

Figure 17–11 Place a towel or sheet over knee area. Use a thin barrier to protect skin from cold source.

Figure 17–12 Instruct recipient on stages of feeling cold. Tell the recipient to let you know right away if cold becomes too intense.

Figure 17–13 Apply the cold source, and ask for immediate feedback. Conform the cold source to the shape of the knee covering the kneecap and lateral areas.

Figure 17–14 Cover and secure the cold source in place. Wrap the cold source using a towel or elastic bandage to keep it in place. Let the cold source remain in place for about 12 minutes.

Figure 17–15 Get feedback every 5 to 7 minutes about cold intensity. Massage other areas while cold source is on the knee.

7

Figure 17–16 Remove cold source, and check the knee for changes. Notice skin color and changes in swelling around the knee.

After you perform this practice sequence, evaluate how well you did by filling out Performance Evaluation Form 17–2, Cold Application for Knee. The form can be found in Appendix D, *Performance Evaluation Forms*, and at MyHealthProfessionLab.com.

Figures source: Pearson Education, Inc./Segal Photography.

Ice Massage

Ice massage involves rubbing ice directly on the skin using an ice cube or ice cup. Ice cups are made by filling paper cups with water and putting them in the freezer to harden. The paper is peeled back to expose the ice with some paper left on for holding the cup.

Ice massage is performed in a circular motion over a small area for about 5 to 10 minutes, until the area becomes numb. Ice massage may be used to numb an area before performing deep transverse friction such as in a case of tendinitis. It allows the therapist to work deep enough without causing severe pain. Ice is also used after this treatment to continue to numb the area. Ice massage for the elbow is demonstrated in Practice Sequence 17–3.

PRACTICE SEQUENCE 17–3

Ice Massage for Elbow

10 minutes
Recipient supine

Preliminary Instructions
• Prepare ice in paper cups ahead of time.
• Check for contraindications for ice massage in the elbow area.
• Get informed consent for the ice massage.
• Get frequent feedback about cold intensity from recipient.

1

Figure 17–17 Position the forearm for ice massage of the tendons around the elbow. Rest the forearm comfortably on a towel. Palm is down. Instruct recipient on stages of feeling cold, and to let you know right away if the cold becomes too intense.

Figure 17–18 Massage extensor muscles and apply transverse friction over tendons. Knead and press into forearm muscles just distal to the elbow to locate tense muscles and tender points. Apply transverse friction to tendons in the area for about 1 minute.

Figure 17–19 Circular movement of ice over lateral area just distal to the elbow. Use medium pressure to apply ice massage to the skin over the extensor tendons. Move ice in circular motion the entire time. Continue ice massage for 10 minutes.

Figure 17–20 Apply superficial friction with the towel to warm and dry the area.

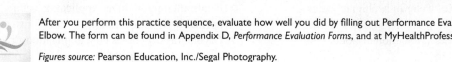

After you perform this practice sequence, evaluate how well you did by filling out Performance Evaluation Form 17–3, Ice Massage for Elbow. The form can be found in Appendix D, *Performance Evaluation Forms*, and at MyHealthProfessionsLab.com.

Figures source: Pearson Education, Inc./Segal Photography.

CASE FOR STUDY

Rod and Temperature Therapy Home Care

Rod is a client in his fifties who exercises regularly. He is usually stiff and tight in his shoulders when he comes for massage. His massage therapist thinks that temperature therapy applied between massage sessions can benefit Rod.

Question:

What temperature therapy methods might Rod's massage therapist suggest for home care?

Things to consider:

- Would thermotherapy or cryotherapy be most effective to reduce stiffness and tightness?
- What questions would help identify contraindications?
- What temperature therapy methods would be readily available to Rod at home?
- What safety considerations should the massage therapist caution Rod about?

Your Recommendation to Rod for Home Care:

_____

_____

_____

_____

 PRACTICAL APPLICATION

Perform the ice massage practice sequence on a practice client. Interview him or her to find a site that may benefit from the application and to identify any contraindications.

1. Did the practice client feel the four stages of sensation for cold applications?
2. How long did it take to cause numbness?
3. What changes did you notice in tissues receiving the ice massage?

CHAPTER HIGHLIGHTS

- Hydrotherapy is the use of water in health and healing practices.
- Temperature therapy is the application of hot or cold for therapeutic effects.
- The history of hydrotherapy can be traced to ancient times in all parts of the globe.
  - Native American traditions include the use of sweat baths and the sweat lodge ceremony.
  - Western traditions of hydrotherapy include the work of Priessnitz, Kneipp, Winternitz, Kellogg, and the Chartered Society of Trained Masseuses in England.
- Temperature therapy can be roughly divided into thermotherapy, neutrotherapy, and cryotherapy based on the temperature of the application.
  - Thermotherapy involves heat applications higher than normal body temperature.

  - Neutrotherapy involves applications at about normal body temperature.
  - Cryotherapy involves cold applications lower than normal body temperature.

- Water is used in temperature therapy in the form of liquid, steam, or ice.
- Water pressure from shower, hose, or water jets can serve as a type of massage of the soft tissues.
- Hot forms of hydrotherapy include whirlpool baths, showers, steam rooms, and sauna.
  - Effects of hot hydrotherapy include raising the body temperature, producing sweating, cleansing skin pores, increasing superficial circulation, and general relaxation.
  - Hot hydrotherapies are best used before a massage session.
  - Guidelines should be observed for safe use of these therapies.

- Heat applied locally to muscles and related soft tissues feels good, helps muscles relax, increases local circulation, and makes tissues more pliable.
  - Moist hot packs are typically used for thermotherapy.
  - Measures to avoid burning the client's skin include using towels as a safety barrier and limiting the time the hot pack is applied.
- Cold applications or cryotherapy causes vasoconstriction and decreased local circulation, cell metabolism, nerve conduction, and reduced pain and spasm.

- The hunting reaction occurs after 12 to15 minutes of cold application and involves alternating vasodilation and vasoconstriction in the affected tissues.
  - Cold applications are used in first aid for trauma and injury.
  - Cryotherapy methods include cold and ice packs and ice massage.
- Contraindications and safety guidelines for all forms of hydrotherapy and thermal therapies should be observed to avoid harm to the client.

EXAM REVIEW

Key Terms

To study the key terms listed at the beginning of this chapter, match the appropriate lettered meaning to each numbered key term listed below. For additional study, look up the key terms in the Interactive Glossary, and note other terms that compare or contrast with them.

_____ **1.** Cold packs
_____ **2.** Cryotherapy
_____ **3.** Hot pack
_____ **4.** Hunting reaction
_____ **5.** Hydrotherapy
_____ **6.** Ice massage
_____ **7.** Sauna
_____ **8.** Steam rooms
_____ **9.** Temperature therapy
_____ **10.** Thermotherapy
_____ **11.** Whirlpool bath

a. Application prior to massage can help begin muscle relaxation, enhance circulation locally
b. Facility that clears sinuses, relieves respiratory congestion, raises body temperature, and causes sweating
c. Cyclic periods of vasodilation and vasoconstriction caused by cold applications
d. Involves applications above normal body temperature
e. Involves applications below body temperature
f. Therapeutic applications of hot and cold
g. Healing effects stem from the water heat and the pressure of the water coming out of the jets and hitting the body
h. Made of materials that hold cold over a period of time and stay pliable even when near freezing
i. Used to numb a small area, allowing the therapist to work deep enough without causing severe pain
j. The use of water in health and healing practices
k. Wood-lined room with dry heat and low humidity

Memory Workout

To test your memory of the main concepts in this chapter, complete the following sentences by circling the most correct answer from the two choices provided.

1. Hydrotherapy is the use of (heat) (water) in health and healing practices.
2. Therapeutic use of hot and cold applications is called (temperature) (physical) therapy.
3. Sebastian (Kneipp) (Kellogg) from Bavaria further developed therapeutic use of water adding his knowledge of herbs (c. 1880).
4. Therapeutic use of water taken (internally) (externally) is outside the scope of massage therapy except for encouraging clients to drink plenty of clean pure water.
5. The (Vichy) (whirlpool) bath consists of a water tub with water jets that cause water movement or churning.
6. To prevent burns, towels are placed between the hot pack and the (top drape) (client's skin).
7. Increasing the temperature of tissues increases cell (division) (metabolism) and blood flow locally.
8. Cold applied locally causes (decreased) (increased) local circulation.
9. Cold applied to tissues after trauma (decreases) (increases) secondary cell or tissue damage.
10. Get (written consent) (informed consent) from clients before giving hot or cold applications along with a massage session.

Test Prep

The following multiple-choice questions will help to prepare you for future school and professional exams.

1. Temperature therapy that is below the body's normal temperature is called:
   a. Thermotherapy
   b. Neutrotherapy
   c. Cryotherapy
   d. Vichy therapy

2. The humidity in a steam room is typically:
   a. 10%
   b. 40%
   c. 60%
   d. 100%

3. A sauna provides:
   a. Dry heat
   b. Wet heat
   c. Cold plunge
   d. Steam heat

4. It is best to replenish fluids during and after using a steam room or sauna by:
   a. Drinking plenty of water
   b. Drinking an alcoholic beverage
   c. Draping a wet towel over your head
   d. Soaking your feet in a tub of water

5. The temperature sensation for an application at 31° degrees Fahrenheit (1°C) is:
   a. Tepid
   b. Warm
   c. Neutral
   d. Very cold

6. Exercise caution when giving hot or cold applications to clients taking medications that:
   a. Reduce sensation
   b. Alter circulation
   c. Affect temperature regulation
   d. All of the above

7. Which of the following is *not* an effect of thermo-hydrotherapy?
   a. Increased pulse rate
   b. Increased core body temperature
   c. Increased muscle tone
   d. Sweating

8. For a person with high blood pressure, using a steam room is:
   a. Highly beneficial
   b. Contraindicated
   c. Therapeutic
   d. Advised

9. First aid for an ankle sprain would include a:
   a. Hot moist pack
   b. Hot dry pack
   c. Cold pack
   d. Hot whirlpool treatment

10. The third stage of sensation during an ice application is:
    a. Burning or aching
    b. Tingling or itching
    c. Cold
    d. Numbness

Video Challenge

Watch these videos, which can be found at MyHealthProfessionsLab.com, Chapter 17, and then answer the following questions.

Hot Application on Upper Back

1. In the video demonstration of a hot application, what precautions did the massage therapist take to avoid burning the client?

Cold Application for Knee

2. How did the massage therapist in the video secure the cold pack to the recipient's knee? Why?

Ice Massage for Elbow

3. In the ice massage demonstration on the video, why did the massage therapist keep the ice moving in a circle?

Comprehension Exercises

The following short-answer questions test your knowledge and understanding of chapter topics and provide practice in written communication skills. Explain in two to four complete sentences.

1. Explain how to use thermo-hydrotherapy facilities in relation to a massage session.

2. Describe how you would ensure the comfort and safety of your client during hot and cold applications.
3. Describe the application of ice massage.

For Greater Understanding

The following exercises are designed to take you from the realm of theory into the real world. They will help give you a deeper understanding of the subjects covered in this chapter. Action words are underlined to emphasize the variety of activities presented to address different learning styles and to encourage deeper thinking.

1. Visit a spa or health club with hydrotherapy facilities. Observe how other people use the facilities. Was there anything you thought they needed instruction about, for example, contraindications or how best to enjoy the experience? Were there any signs or people to instruct patrons on how to use the facilities?

2. Immerse your foot or hand into a bucket of ice water. Notice the phases of sensation you experience. Say them out loud to a study partner as you experience them. (Variation: Apply a cold pack instead.)

3. Visit a training room with a certified athletic trainer. Observe how the trainer uses hydrotherapy and thermal therapy in treatment of athletes. Report your observations to a study partner or group.

MyHealthProfessionsLab™

MyHealthProfessionsLab.com is a premium online homework management system that includes a host of features to help you study. Registered users will find:

- Powerful tools that track and analyze your results—allowing you to create a personalized learning experience
- Videos, flashcards and other learning tools to help enrich your progress
- Streaming lesson presentations and self-paced learning modules
- A space where you and your instructors can view and manage your assignments

Chapter 18
Special Populations and
Adaptations

Chapter 19
Spa Treatments

Chapter 20
Seated Massage

PART

4

Tappan's Guide to Special Applications

Pearson Education, Inc.

CHAPTER

18 Special Populations and Adaptations

CHAPTER OUTLINE

Learning Outcomes

Key Terms

Introduction

Athletes

Pregnant Women

Infants

The Elderly

The Terminally Ill

Impairments and Disabilities

Amputees and Prostheses

Internal and External Medical Devices

Rewards and Challenges

Chapter Highlights

Exam Review

LEARNING OUTCOMES

After studying this chapter, you will have information to:

1. Plan massage sessions to meet the needs of athletes.
2. Provide massage safely to healthy women with low-risk pregnancies.
3. Massage infants for optimal growth and development.
4. Provide safe and effective massage to the elderly.
5. Plan massage to address the needs of the terminally ill and dying.
6. Adapt massage sessions for people with visual, hearing, and mobility impairments.

7. Accommodate large and small clients.
8. Accommodate clients with amputations and prosthetic limbs.
9. Provide massage safely to clients with internal and external medical devices.
10. Recognize the rewards and challenges of serving special populations.

KEY TERMS

Adaptations	High-risk pregnancies	Obesity	Physiological age
Colostomy bag	Infant massage	Palliative care	Special population
Disability	Mobility	Physical impairment	Sports massage

INTRODUCTION

A **special population** is a group of people with some distinctive life circumstance that sets them apart from a normal adult population. They include athletes, pregnant women, infants, the elderly, and people with various physical impairments and diseases. Whatever it is that makes a special population "special" can influence their goals for massage and may require adaptations to the session for safety or comfort. Contraindications might be different for members of a special population, and so more information about their individual situations is needed in planning massage sessions.

There is a difference between massage for special populations and clinical applications of massage. Clinical applications are distinguished by their focus on helping the client heal from or manage a specific pathology or injury and are provided in clinical settings. On the other hand, special populations are encountered in all settings, and individuals may be interested in massage for reasons that have nothing to do with their "special" circumstances.

Do not assume that someone with a medical condition is coming for massage to treat that condition. He or she may just want to relax or may be getting massage to enhance his or her general well-being. Always check with new clients about their goals for the massage. You may end up working around a special circumstance rather than addressing it directly.

Adaptations are adjustments or changes to the way things are normally done to meet the unique needs of an individual. Typical adaptations involve communication, positioning, and assistance with dressing and getting on and off the massage table. In some cases, it means giving a massage with the client in a bed or chair rather than on the massage table. For others, it requires eliminating or modifying massage applications for safety.

Attitude is important in working with special populations and clients with special needs. Remember that your job is to provide massage for their benefit. Be nonjudgmental and accepting of all clients as human beings. Be sensitive to their feelings about their situation. Be patient and work at the pace necessary for their comfort. Be flexible and open to making modifications. Above all, exercise good judgment and err on the side of doing no harm.

This chapter focuses on special populations commonly seen in massage practices. Massage therapists working in settings open to the general public must be ready to plan massage sessions for whomever walks in the door. Common sense, experience, and a little knowledge can aid in making the massage session safe and comfortable for these special clients.

ATHLETES

Massage has been used since ancient times in the training of athletes and to complement physical activity. This age-old tradition is carried on today in a specialization called **sports massage**. Physically active people in the modern world benefit from sports massage in much the same way

their ancestors did throughout history. Chapter 2, *The History of Massage as a Vocation*, contains a brief historical account of sports massage in ancient and modern times.

Athletes approach their sports and fitness activities in different ways—personal challenge, recreation, health practice, way of life, or possibly a career. Sports massage is a massage application specifically designed to meet the needs of this special population. It is not a set of unique manual techniques, but the application of a variety of techniques aimed at keeping active people healthy and in top form for participation in their sports or fitness activities.

There are five major applications of sports massage.

1. *Recovery* applications enhance physical and mental recovery from strenuous physical activity.

2. *Remedial* applications improve debilitating conditions such as muscle tension and soreness.

3. *Rehabilitation* applications facilitate healing after a disabling injury.

4. *Maintenance* massage is an all-purpose application for recovery, treating debilitating conditions, and overall health and well-being.

5. *Event* applications help athletes to prepare for competition and to recover afterward.

Techniques and Knowledge

Sports massage as practiced in the United States today primarily uses Swedish massage techniques to meet session goals. For example, effleurage and petrissage are applied with lubricant to increase circulation and for general and specific muscle relaxation. Compressions are typically used to increase circulation in situations where athletes are clothed (e.g., at events). See Figure 18–1 ■. Percussion techniques are mentally stimulating prior to events or practice sessions. Deep transverse friction treats debilitating conditions such as tendinitis and is used in

FIGURE 18–1 Compression used to increase circulation when the athlete is clothed.

Source: Pearson Education, Inc./Segal Photography.

rehabilitation after injuries. Contemporary forms of bodywork such as myofascial massage, lymphatic facilitation, and trigger point therapy are integrated into sports massage sessions as needed to accomplish therapeutic goals.

Sports massage specialists have well-developed palpation skills and knowledge of musculoskeletal anatomy and kinesiology. Understanding the biomechanics of a client's sport or fitness activity is useful in planning sessions and locating areas of stress. Familiarity with common sports injuries and their treatment is essential to remedial and rehabilitation applications. Massage therapists working with athletes should be well versed in their special needs and be able to plan massage sessions accordingly.

Recovery

A typical recovery massage addresses the tight, stiff, and sore muscles that accompany strenuous exercise and facilitates healing minor tissue damage. Recovery is a major component of postevent and maintenance sports massage. Focus is on areas stressed in recent activity. Recovery massage targets improved circulation, muscular relaxation, flexibility, and overall stress reduction. Effleurage, petrissage, and rhythmic compressions are the principle techniques used to enhance general circulation. Broadening techniques promote separation of muscle fibers that may be adhering from the stress of strenuous muscle activity. Stretches help muscles relax and lengthen, and jostling and rocking are good techniques to encourage muscles to let go and relax. See Figure 18–2 ■. Useful adjunct therapies for recovery include a hot shower, whirlpool, sauna, and steam room.

Remedial Massage and Rehabilitation

The most common remedial and rehabilitation sports massage applications address muscle tension and spasms, poor range of motion, trigger points, edema, tendinosis, tendinitis, tenosynovitis, strains, sprains, and general overwork and stress. Deep friction techniques are used for development of healthy scar tissue and freeing adhesions in connective

FIGURE 18–2 Joint movements of the lower leg for recovery after strenuous exercise.

Source: Pearson Education, Inc./Segal Photography.

tissues. Sports massage therapists may team with athletic trainers or physical therapists for rehabilitation applications.

Maintenance

A maintenance sports massage session is an all-purpose massage received regularly to address an athlete's needs at the time. Maintenance sessions last for 60 to 90 minutes. The intent is to keep the athlete in optimal condition as he or she trains. The foundation for the massage is recovery with remedial massage for problems as needed. Specific goals include the following:

• Reduce muscle tension and spasm

• Stretch, broaden, and free adhesions in connective tissue in high-stress areas

• Improve overall flexibility and range of motion

• Decrease the impact of delayed-onset muscle soreness and low-grade strains associated with intense training schedules

Injury prevention and anxiety reduction are added benefits from regular massage, and keeping an upbeat outlook is important for an athlete during a competitive season.

Events

Massage given at athletic events is designated as preevent, interevent, and postevent.

Preevent A preevent massage prepares athletes physically and mentally for an upcoming competition and may be considered part of their warm-up. Preevent massage is typically 15 to 20 minutes in duration, has an upbeat tempo, avoids causing discomfort, and concentrates on muscle groups to be used in the performance. Most athletes benefit from a stimulating session to increase their focus and alertness. Athletes are clothed for preevent massage. Preevent applications commonly include

• Compressions

• Direct pressure on stress points

• Friction techniques

• Lifting and broadening

• Percussion, jostling

• Joint movement and warm-up

Interevent An interevent massage is given between events at competitions such as track and swim meets. These sessions are short (10 to 15 minutes), avoid discomfort, and focus on recovery of muscles stressed in the event. It also readies the athletes for the next performance. It is a combination preevent and postevent application.

Postevent The primary goal of postevent sports massage is physical and psychological recovery. These sessions are short (10 to 15 minutes) if given soon after the event

CRITICAL THINKING

Think about the needs of athletes directly before and after competitive events and in between events. Compare and contrast their needs in each situation, and analyze how massage sessions might be used to address those needs.

1. What are the goals of massage in each situation?
2. Which massage techniques are effective in meeting those goals?
3. Which massage applications are best avoided in each situation?

and longer (30 to 90 minutes) if given over an hour after the event. The athlete should be cooled down, have taken adequate fluids, and be breathing normally before receiving massage. Pressure is generally lighter than maintenance massage, and the pace is moderate to slow. Special attention is given to muscles used in the past event. Techniques known to increase circulation and promote muscular and general relaxation are emphasized. These include

- Compression
- Kneading

- Jostling
- Joint movements
- Stretching

If the postevent massage takes place close to the time of the event, the practitioner may also identify and assess injuries received during the competition. The athlete may need first aid and/or be referred to other members of the health care team at the event. Practice Sequence 18–1 demonstrates a postevent sports massage for a walk/run event utilizing common sports massage techniques.

PRACTICE SEQUENCE 18–1

Postevent Sports Massage for Run/Walk Event

15 minutes
Begin with recipient supine

Preliminary Instructions
- Be sure the recipient has replaced fluids and cooled down before giving massage.
- Ask how he or she is feeling, and identify any contraindications for massage.
- Ask the person to remove his or her shoes.
- Apply techniques using light pressure then deeper pressure according to the athlete's needs.
- Do not use oil or lotion.

Figure 18–3 Establish contact by rocking the leg inward and outward in rotation. Hands move along the entire length of the leg. Look for movement at the hip joint. Compress tissues as you apply pressure.

2

A

B

Figure 18–4 To broaden and lift the quadriceps muscles, place the heels of the hands together directly on top of the quadriceps muscles. (A) With fingers pointing to the table, slide the hands apart as you press into the muscle. (B) Then lift the tissues as the hands return to the starting point. Repeat four times.

3

A

B

Figure 18–5 Alternate kneading and shaking the thigh muscles. (A) Perform two-handed kneading over the lateral, posterior, and medial musculature. (B) Periodically shake or "fluff up" the muscles with hands on either side of the thigh.

4

Figure 18–6 Apply knee to chest stretch for posterior hip and leg muscles. Facing the table directly, place one hand on the bottom of the foot and the other hand at the knee. Lift the leg and press the bent knee toward the chest.

Figure 18–7 Apply circular friction with the heels of the hands to tendons that cross the knee. Place heels of your hands on the sides of the knee, fingers pointing toward the head. Make circular movements using enough pressure to move the superficial tissues over the tissues underneath.

Figure 18–8 Knead the calf muscles with both hands. Place the foot flat on the table, knee bent. Reach behind from the front, and squeeze the calf muscles with the fingertips. Heels of the hands press on anterior muscles of the lower leg.

Figure 18–9 Mobilize the ankle. Place the heels of the hands just below the ankle bones, with fingers pointing up the leg. Move the hands back and forth alternately, causing free movement in the ankle joint.

Figure 18–10 Compression and broadening of foot. Place heels of your hands on top of the foot with fingers underneath. Squeeze the foot, broadening the structure along the longitudinal arch. Use the fist to apply compression to the foot bottom.

9

Figure 18–11 Apply scissoring between metatarsals and figure-8s on toe joints to mobilize the foot.

10

Figure 18–12 Use full palms to apply light sliding strokes from foot to hip. This connects and finishes massage of the leg. Repeat Steps 1–10 on the other leg.

Position the recipient prone with his or her feet hanging off the end of the table. Do not use a face cradle. Perform Steps 11–18 on both legs before proceeding to Step 19.

11

Figure 18–13 Stretch quadriceps muscles by bringing the heel of the foot to the buttocks. Hold the stretch for about 20 seconds.

12

Figure 18–14 Compression to gluteal muscles using the fists.

Figure 18–15 Compression along hamstring muscles using the fists. Alternating fists, press along the posterior and lateral musculature, moving from the knee to upper attachments on the ischial tuberosity of the hip.

Figure 18–16 Perform horizontal stroking of the thigh by facing the table and placing hands on the thigh with fingers pointing to the medial side. Lift tissues as the hands slide past each other as they move alternately medial to lateral and back again.

Figure 18–17 Shake the calf muscles. Pick up the calf muscles with one hand, and shake them back and forth.

Figure 18–18 Apply stroking from ankle to knee, using both palms to slide along the calf muscles. If hands will not slide easily, squeeze the calf with both hands, moving along from ankle to knee.

Figure 18–19 Dorsiflex the foot, applying direct pressure to the bottom. Standing at the end of the table, pick up the athlete's foot and press your thumbs into the bottom, causing dorsiflexion at the ankle. Repeat 3–4 times.

18

Figure 18–20 Apply light stroking with the palms from hip to ankles as a connecting and finishing technique. Repeat Steps 11–18 on the other leg.

19

Figure 18–21 Apply palm compressions using both hands over the entire back and shoulder musculature.

20

Figure 18–22 Use palms and fingers to brush off along the back of the body from shoulders to feet with long sweeping movements to finish massage. End by brushing off the feet.

After you perform the Practice Sequence, evaluate how well you did by filling out Performance Evaluation Form 18–1, Postevent Sports Massage for Run/Walk Event. The form can be found in Appendix D: *Performance Evaluation Forms*, and at MyHealthProfessionsLab.com.

Figures source: Pearson Education, Inc./Segal Photography.

PRACTICAL APPLICATION

Develop a postevent massage sequence that focuses on the upper extremities. Use the lower body Practice Sequence 18–1 as a general model. Practice the sequence until you can perform it effectively in 15 minutes.

1. What sports emphasize the upper extremities?
2. Which muscles are stressed most in those sports?

3. Which massage applications are most effective for recovery and relaxation of those areas?

_____

_____

_____

CASE FOR STUDY

Mike Helps Carl Prepare for a Triathlon

Carl is preparing for a triathlon (swimming, cycling, running) that is 1 month away. He has been experiencing some physical wear and tear from training, so he has asked Mike, a massage therapist, to help him prepare. Carl has some general soreness and feels that his shoulder and leg muscles are particularly tense. Muscle attachments at the knee are tender to the touch.

Question:

What sports massage applications will benefit Carl the most? What might Mike's recommendations be for the frequency and focus of sports massage?

Things to consider:

- What are Carl's needs leading up to event day and afterward?
- What would maintenance sessions focus on? Do any remedial applications apply?
- How might sessions be spaced out in time?

Using a blank 2-month calendar, write a schedule for maintenance, preevent, and postevent sports massage for Carl. Assume that time and money are not a problem. List the primary goals of Carl's sports massage sessions.

_____

_____

_____

PREGNANT WOMEN

Providing beneficial and safe massage to pregnant women requires some knowledge of pregnancy itself and of related contraindications and cautions. Massage sessions for healthy women with normal pregnancies involve adaptations for comfort and safety. Particularly important are skills in alternative positioning and draping and massage applications that focus on common problems of pregnant women.

Massage addresses many of the discomforts experienced by women during the 9-month pregnancy period. Benefits of massage during this time include less fatigue and more energy, less back and leg pain, headache relief, better sleep, and stress reduction. Many women experience improved mood and less anxiety and depression after massage. Pregnant women undergo a dramatic change in size, weight, and shape over a relatively short period of time. In a typical pregnancy posture, a woman's head is forward, chest back, belly forward, and lower back curved (Figure 18–23 ■). Massage can ease some of the stresses on the body experienced over the 9-month pregnancy period.[1]

Contraindications

Giving massage to women with high-risk pregnancies should only be done by massage therapists with specialized advanced training or avoided altogether if contraindicated. Therefore, it is important to identify high-risk situations and screen for warning signs of possible medical problems.

High-risk pregnancies are those in which the mother or fetus is at higher than normal risk for complications or negative developments. The following conditions are considered high-risk pregnancies:

- Mother's age (under 15 or over 35)
- Mother extremely underweight or overweight
- Mother with chronic illness (e.g., diabetes, heart disease)
- Mother with history of pelvic inflammatory disease (PID), endometriosis, or sexually transmitted disease (STD)
- History of miscarriage or preterm delivery
- More than five previous pregnancies—completed or not
- Twins, triplets, or other multiples

FIGURE 18–23 Typical pregnancy posture.

- Fetal abnormalities

- Serious complications: gestational diabetes, pregnancy-induced hypertension (PIH), pre-eclampsia, eclampsia, ectopic pregnancy (fertilized egg implants outside the uterus)

Screen for warning signs for contraindications before every massage session. Do not give massage if a pregnant client has any of the following signs:

- Morning sickness, nausea, vomiting

- Vaginal bleeding or discharge

- Fever

- Decrease in fetal movement in past 24 hours

- Diarrhea

- Abdominal pain

- Excessive swelling in the arms or legs

Some signs that require immediate medical attention are

- Chest discomfort or pain

- Pain in one or both arms, back, neck, jaw, or stomach

- Labored breathing

- Breaking into a cold sweat

- Nausea, lightheadedness, dizziness

- Seizure, convulsions, loss of consciousness

- Pitting edema (pressure leaves indentation in tissues)

- Swelling in the hands or face

Uterine contractions may indicate that the birth process has begun. If they continue, stop the massage, and advise the client to contact her health provider immediately.

Of course, all the normal contraindications and cautions apply to pregnant women. Find out what medications a client is taking. Ask if there have been any new or adverse reactions to them recently. Modify massage applications accordingly, especially for medications that affect circulation or sensation.

Pregnancy Massage Application

Once you identify that a pregnancy is normal, you can proceed with the massage with some adaptations. Considerations focus on the safety of the mother and the fetus and may call for restrictions on massage applications. Some restrictions are for the entire pregnancy, others are in certain trimesters. The position of the fetus in late pregnancy results in stresses on muscles and joints, internal organs, and major blood vessels along the spine(Figure 18–24 ■).

CREATING A COMFORTABLE ENVIRONMENT

The environment for pregnancy massage should be comfortable and relaxing. Keep the space well ventilated and with fresh air if possible. The temperature can be cooler

Lung
Heart
Diaphragm
Liver
Vena cava
Stomach
Small intestine
Aorta
Uterus
Cervix
Bladder
Vagina
Rectum

FIGURE 18–24 Position of the fetus in late pregnancy results in stresses on the mother's body.

than usual for massage, between 68°F to 72°F. Avoid strong scents in the air. Play music relaxing to the client.

An accessible bathroom is a must. Suggest that the client urinate just before beginning a massage session. Be prepared to stop the session and help the client off of the table to go to the bathroom and then to get back on again. Having a robe handy is practical for this purpose.

A step stool is useful for getting up onto the table. Be present if needed to assist the recipient and help her get into a comfortable position. A woman may require more assistance with this in the later stages of pregnancy.

Provide a glass of water for the client. Keep tissues and extra towels in reach.

POSITIONING OPTIONS

The primary purpose of positioning is to make the pregnant woman comfortable and safe during massage applications. In addition, positioning itself can be effective in reducing stress in the client's back and legs. The preferred positions for pregnancy massage are semireclining, side-lying, and seated. Although the supine and prone positions may be tolerated very early in the pregnancy, some experts recommend avoiding them altogether.

A general rule of thumb for positioning pregnant women is to fill in any spaces you find with bolsters, pillows, or rolled-up towels. The recipient should feel secure and supported all around.

Some massage tables and bolstering systems are designed specifically for pregnant women. These have both positive and negative features and are beyond the scope of this text. Focus here is on adaptations that can be made for pregnant women when using standard massage tables and bolstering with pillows. However, whenever a semireclining position is called for, a dense foam slanted wedge bolster provides a more stable base than standard pillows.

Semireclining Semireclining position, or half-sitting, is a good alternative to lying supine. With a slanted wedge providing a base, bolsters and pillows may be used to prop the recipient into a half-sitting position. Additional bolsters may be used to prop up the legs. A towel rolled up and placed under the right hip will shift weight slightly to the left, taking pressure off major blood vessels. Some massage tables have an adjustment to convert a flat tabletop into one with an inclined back support. A disadvantage of semireclining is limited access to the back of the body.

Side-Lying The side-lying position offers better access to more of the body. It does, however, require turning over to reach both left and right sides. If turning over is a problem, especially later in pregnancy, ask the client to lie on the side most comfortable for her.

In the side-lying position, the client's back and buttocks are near the edge of the table. This allows room for the arms, legs, and bolsters on the tabletop. The top leg is bent. Pillows are placed under the head, the top arm and leg, and around the belly if needed for support. Prop up the leg so that the hip, knee, and ankle are in a horizontal line (Figure 18–25 ■).

Seated The seated position can also be useful. The client sits on a chair placed at the side of the table and leans forward into pillows for support. The arms are crossed and placed on the pillows with the forehead resting on them (see Figure 11–26). This provides bracing for massage on the back. The client can sit up straight for massage of the arms and hands. A hospital gown or other clothing opened in the back provides draping and access to the back of the body.

Changing position during a massage session might also make sense. If a client becomes uncomfortable after some time in a particular position, change to a different position. If massaging a client in semireclining position, consider ending in the seated position with massage of the back. For safety, assist the client as needed when changing position, especially later in pregnancy.

TABLE HEIGHT

Adjust the table height to allow for your good body mechanics with the client in different positions. When the client is semireclining, a lower table height allows easier access to the head and shoulders. When the client is side-lying, a higher table height is sometimes better because techniques are applied more horizontally, rather than downward vertically. If you expect to specialize in pregnancy massage or work with other special populations, a mechanically adjustable table would be good to have.

CAUTIONS AND ADAPTATIONS

Unscented oils and lotions are the safest choice for pregnant women. Avoid heavily scented products. Some essential oils that promote relaxation, such as lavender and chamomile, may be used if the client is not adversely sensitive to smells. See Chapter 19, *Spa Treatments*, for more information about using essential oils on pregnant women.

Deep abdominal massage is contraindicated throughout pregnancy and in the weeks after delivery. In the second and third trimesters, gentle effleurage, passive touch, and some forms of energy bodywork may be performed safely on the abdomen. Use a broad flat hand to apply light effleurage in a clockwise direction over the enlarged abdomen.

Avoid aggressive or heavy pressure techniques applied to connective tissues. These include ligaments, tendons, and fascial tissues that are all affected by the hormone relaxin, which softens ligaments in the body in preparation for birth and can result in unstable joints. Stretching techniques are generally contraindicated.

Watch for excessive edema and varicose veins in the legs. Pregnant women are at higher risk for blood clots due to changes in blood chemistry during this time. Blood flow to and from the legs is restricted during pregnancy, especially in the third trimester. This creates a prime environment for blood clots.

Massage to the legs may be contraindicated if circulation is excessively poor, if the mother has been inactive or on bed rest by doctor's orders, or if she has varicose veins. Some advise avoiding massage to the legs altogether (except possibly the feet) during the third trimester.

FIGURE 18–25 Side-lying position and bolstering for pregnancy massage.

CASE FOR STUDY

Alissa and Pregnancy Massage

Alissa is a 30-year-old woman who just found out that she is pregnant. She has been getting massage regularly at the spa for the past 2 years. She is physically fit overall and would like to continue with massage during her pregnancy.

Question:

What does her massage therapist need to know to give Alissa a massage safely?

Things to consider:

- Is this a high-risk pregnancy?
- Are there any signs and symptoms indicating contraindications for massage?
- Is Alissa open to alterations in her massage sessions to accommodate her pregnancy?

Develop a brief questionnaire for interviewing Alissa to determine if massage is safe for her at this point.

_____

_____

_____

Advise pregnant clients to refrain from eating a meal for about 2 hours before a massage if possible. This is especially important later in the pregnancy.

Traditional Chinese medicine (TCM) prohibits certain techniques during pregnancy. Among these are pressure to acupoints LI-4 Tiger's Mouth in the web of the thumb, Sp-6 Yin Intersection above the inside ankle, Bl-60 Kunlun Mountain on lateral ankle, and GB-21 Shoulder Well on the shoulders. If there is worry about miscarriage, also avoid pressure on the Yin Channels on the inside of the lower legs. See Chapter 25, *Asian and Energy-Based Bodywork*, for locations of energy channels and acupoints.

TRIMESTER CONSIDERATIONS

The first and third trimesters are the most tenuous for the fetus. In the first trimester, the attachments to the mother are just becoming established. In the third trimester, the fetus and mother are preparing for eventual detachment and delivery. The fragility of these times calls for special attention and care.

First Trimester In the first trimester use only gentle relaxation massage techniques. Avoid pressure over the abdomen, sacrum, and low back. Stroking and kneading of the buttocks, legs, shoulders, and arms help relieve general tension. Head, face, and neck massage are also relaxing and pleasurable. Omit joint movements and stretching techniques, especially in the lower body. To be most

conservative, avoid pressure to LI-14 and Sp-6 acupoints and stimulation of the area on the feet between the ankle and the heel.

Second Trimester In a normal pregnancy, the second trimester is the safest and easiest part. Most women experience less nausea in this period. However, connective tissues continue to loosen, and prohibitions on joint movements and stretching still apply. Use positioning to help relax muscles that have begun to tighten and possibly spasm. Gentle stroking of the abdomen is permissible at this point. Attention to lower back muscles and along the muscle attachments on the iliac crest with circular friction and fingertip kneading can help relieve tightness there.

Third Trimester In the third trimester, discomfort increases as the fetus gains weight and the mother's body prepares for delivery. Massage sessions focus on comfort and relaxation. Watch for signs of poor circulation, swelling, and varicose veins in the legs. Omit massage of the legs if the client has been inactive and/or signs of poor circulation are evident. Refer the client to her health care provider if you notice pitting edema. Assist the client on and off the table and as needed for undressing and dressing.

Massage techniques can be adapted for the side-lying position. Practice Sequence 18–2 demonstrates techniques and applications for pregnant women in the side-lying position.

PRACTICE SEQUENCE 18–2

Pregnancy Massage in Side-Lying Position

Leg, back, and arm: 30 minutes
Recipient in side-lying position

Preliminary Considerations
• Adjust table height higher than normal.
• Screen for current health status and contraindications.
• Supplies: pillows for bolstering, sheet for draping, unscented oil or lotion.
• Secure drape for modesty.
• Find the best place to stand to maintain good body mechanics; move around the table as necessary.

Figure 18–26 Assist recipient into side-lying position. Woman sits on edge of table holding drape to cover her front and then lies down on her side; place pillows to support the head, arms, legs, and belly as needed; arrange and secure the drape for modesty.

Figure 18–27 Undrape top leg and apply warming effleurage to lateral leg, hip, and foot in distal to proximal direction. Secure drape between legs; apply oil or lotion to lateral leg, hip, and foot.

Figure 18–28 Knead accessible leg and hip muscles; alternate with effleurage. Avoid massage of the medial side of the thigh.

Figure 18–29 Knead accessible lower leg muscles; alternate with effleurage.

5

Figure 18–30 Massage the feet. Finish with light connecting strokes over the entire leg. Redrape the leg.

6

Figure 18–31 Secure drape under hip and top arm, and undrape back; stand in back at waist facing head. Apply warming effleurage to back and shoulders using both hands.

7

Figure 18–32 Apply circular friction along paraspinal muscles. Stand at waist facing head; use fingertips of outside hand to apply circular friction from hips to shoulders on one side and then the other. Use deeper pressure on tense spots.

8

Figure 18–33 Apply one-handed kneading of shoulder and neck muscles; end with flat palm circular superficial effleurage over entire back. Redrape the back.

9

Figure 18–34 Apply effleurage and petrissage on top arm. Stand in front of recipient and hold her hand with one hand while the other hand applies effleurage to the arm from wrist to shoulder; squeeze around arm from shoulder to hand. End with effleurage up the arm; redrape the arm.

10

Figure 18–35 Apply passive touch on the shoulder and hip. Stand in back and place one hand on the shoulder and the other on the hip. Hold for 5–10 seconds.

Assist recipient in turning over and repeat Steps 2–10 on the other side.

After you perform the Practice Sequence, evaluate how well you did by filling out Performance Evaluation Form 18–2, Pregnancy Massage. The form can be found in Appendix D: *Performance Evaluation Forms*, and at MyHealthProfessionsLab.com.

Figures source: Pearson Education, Inc./Segal Photography.

Labor, Delivery, and Recovery

Midwives, childbirth assistants, doulas, and others in the delivery room may use massage during labor and delivery as desired by the mother. This may be as simple as gentle stroking to reduce anxiety or circular strokes to the sacrum to relieve discomfort. Massage has been shown to reduce anxiety and labor pain and, for some women, to decrease the length of labor and need for medication.[2]

There are also certain acupressure points that may be pressed to relieve labor pain. These include the Shoulder Well (GB-21) on the trapezius; Sacral Points (GB-27–34); Hoku or Joining the Valley (LI-4) in the web of the thumb; Bigger Stream (K-3) near the Achilles tendon; and Reaching Inside (B-67) on the little toe.[3]

Massage may be helpful for recovery from the birth process. Traditional Swedish massage relaxes stressed and sore muscles and soothes nerves. Joint movements should remain limited for a few weeks as hormones return to prepregnancy state. Acupressure points to press

for postpartum recovery include Sea of Energy (CV-6) just below the navel; Inner Gate (P-6) inside the forearm just above the wrist; Sea of Vitality (B-23 and B-47) across the back at waist level; Womb and Vitals (B-48) lateral to the sacrum; Three Mile Point (St-36) just below the kneecap lateral to the shin bone; and Bigger Rushing (Lv-3) on top of the foot between the big toe and the second toe.[4]

After an appropriate amount of healing has taken place, women who have delivered their babies by cesarean section (C-section) may benefit from abdominal massage and massage around and on the scar itself. Deep transverse friction can help prevent adhesions and promote mobile scar tissue as in any wound-healing situation.

Contraindications in late pregnancy related to blood clots in the legs continue for 8 to 10 weeks postpartum. In addition, the side-lying position may continue to be the most comfortable position for a new mother even after delivery, especially if she is breast-feeding the baby.

PRACTICAL APPLICATION

Practice positioning practice partners in semireclining, side-lying, and seated position as if they were pregnant. Try out different approaches to massage applications appropriate for pregnancy massage.

1. How many bolsters do you need, and where are they placed for greatest security and comfort?
2. What is the best table height for each positioning alternative, taking into consideration your body mechanics?
3. How are massage applications adapted for different client positions?

Women with Infants and Toddlers

Women with infants and toddlers have a new set of stresses from the demands of motherhood. Massage affords an opportunity to take time out and relax. It may also address the stress on the upper back, neck, and arms from picking up, holding, and nursing their growing babies. Nursing mothers may find breast massage useful for relieving the discomforts of nursing. Specialized training is required before attempting breast massage.

INFANTS

Infant massage given by parents and other caregivers is an excellent way to provide the kinesthetic and tactile stimulation essential for the healthy growth and development of infants. A significant body of evidence confirms that massage not only contributes to the healthy development of normal babies, but also is effective in promoting recovery of preterm, cocaine-exposed, HIV-exposed, and other high-risk infants.[5]

Infant massage has other benefits, including helping babies release tension and learn to relax. It promotes bonding with parents, aids digestion and elimination, improves sleep, and eases growing pains. Massage helps calm colicky babies. In addition, touching and handling her baby promotes the mother's milk production by stimulating the secretion of the hormone prolactin. Massage can also provide fathers with an opportunity to touch and interact with their babies in a way that is satisfying and also builds confidence in handling small children.

Massage practitioners may include training in infant massage in their services to pregnant clients and their families before or after delivery. Dolls may be used to introduce massage techniques before the baby is delivered.

Infant Massage Application

Infant massage is about interacting socially as much as it is about applying massage techniques. Caregivers maintain eye contact and talk or sing to the child throughout the massage. Massage can be a time of playful interaction that enhances the infant's emotional, social, and physical development.

Be sure the space for infant massage is safe, secure, and warm. Minimize distractions such as noise and bright lights. Turn off the television and radio. Have all supplies in reach. Use unscented natural oil or lotion. Place a towel under the infant for the massage.

It is important that the massage giver be relaxed and comfortable throughout the session. Givers may sit on the floor with legs extended and back straight, perhaps supported against a wall or piece of furniture. The infant is placed supine on or between the giver's legs or prone across the legs. If the infant is on a bed or table, be sure that he or she cannot fall off. Infants can be very active during massage.

Infant massage is a simple, gentle, yet firm application of stroking, pressing, squeezing, and movement of the limbs. Use enough pressure to engage the tissues and avoid a light tickling touch. Infant massage is less specific than massage for adults. The idea is to provide pleasurable stimulation through touch and movement.

Practice Sequence 18–3, Infant Massage, includes basic techniques for the entire body, including stroking with the fingertips, thumb, and palm; gentle squeezing and milking; and circular fingertip friction. Two simple movements exercise the shoulder, hip, and leg joints. Bringing the baby's knees to the abdomen slowly and with repetition promotes good digestion and relieves constipation. Infant massage can be practiced on a doll to learn the basic progression and techniques.

 CRITICAL THINKING

Think about the nature of infants. Relate this to infant massage applications.

1. How do infants move when awake? Will they lie still for massage?

2. Is eye contact important for bonding? Do infants close their eyes for massage?

3. Are infants ever stressed? Can they relax with massage?

PRACTICE SEQUENCE 18–3

Infant Massage | 15–20 minutes

Preliminary Considerations
• Set up a secure and comfortable space.
• Make sure the room is warm.
• Minimize distractions.
• Have all supplies in reach.
• Use natural unscented oil or lotion.

1

Figure 18–36 Place the infant faceup on a soft surface, such as a towel, and remove his or her clothing. With one hand on each side, apply fingertip circles over the head. Do not use oil or lotion. Make eye contact and smile.

2

Figure 18–37 Slide thumbs over forehead and down sides of nose. (A) Using no oil or lotion, place thumbs in middle of forehead and slide out to the temples 2–3 times. (B) Slide down the sides of the nose.

A

B

3

Figure 18–38 Using the palm, apply oil with butterfly strokes across the chest. Alternate hands and move across the chest and up and around the opposite shoulder.

4

Figure 18–39 Gently squeeze/milk the arm with twisting motion. With oil or lotion on hands, use gentle but firm pressure, moving shoulder to wrist.

5

Figure 18–40 Apply thumb strokes on palm of hand and fingers. Hold the baby's hand palm up and use thumbs to stroke from wrist to fingers.

6

Figure 18–41 Using oil or lotion on your hands, squeeze/milk leg with twisting motion from ankle to thigh. Pressure is gentle but firm.

Figure 18–42 Apply thumb strokes on foot bottom and toes. Hold the baby's foot bottom-up and use thumbs to stroke from heel to toe.

Figure 18–43 Using oil or lotion, apply circular strokes on abdomen with fingertips. Move in a clockwise direction using firm pressure.

Figure 18–44 Hold baby's hands and (A) cross arms over chest and then (B) open out to the sides. Repeat several times.

A

B

Figure 18–45 Hold baby's feet and bend legs, moving knees into the abdomen/chest and then straighten. Repeat several times.

Figure 18–46 Turn baby over, placing him or her sideways across your legs if on floor or across pillow.

Figure 18–47 Apply circular fingertip friction on back, moving along spinal muscles from hip to shoulder and over shoulders.

Figure 18–48 Scoop from (A) shoulders to (B) heels. Hold feet in one hand; with other hand use the palm to apply long, broad strokes.

Figure 18–49 Turn the baby over and end with passive touch on the head. Gently hold the baby's head and look into his or her eyes and smile.

After you perform the Practice Sequence, evaluate how well you did by filling out Performance Evaluation Form 18–3, Infant Massage. The form can be found in Appendix D: *Performance Evaluation Forms*, and at MyHealthProfessionsLab.com.

Figures source: Pearson Education, Inc./Segal Photography.

THE ELDERLY

The elderly, defined roughly as people 70 years and older, are a rapidly growing special population. Massage has many benefits for elders, including helping them keep the strength and flexibility needed to do activities of daily living (ADLs) that contribute to maintaining independence. ADLs include things such as getting in and out of a chair, dressing and undressing, climbing stairs, and getting into and out of a bathtub. Another physical benefit is improved digestion and elimination.

Massage helps ease the pain of loss, frustration, and fear about the future. Loss of work, home, spouse, family, friends, independence, and financial security can result in anxiety and worry. The caring touch and relaxing benefits of massage help ease these emotional pains.

Massage also provides an avenue for social interaction, especially for elders in nursing homes, assisted living facilities, or homebound. The personal interaction with the practitioner helps reduce feelings of social isolation, and the inherent touch of massage provides a special connection to others.

Some of the common problem conditions experienced by the elderly that massage can help alleviate are insomnia, loss of appetite, constipation, immobility, poor circulation, and decreased immune system functioning. Massage can address skin problems such as loss of elasticity and dryness, pressure sores, and physical discomfort and pain. Massage reduces chronic stress, chronic depression, and feelings of being alone and useless.[6]

Some of the research about elders and massage in clinical settings is reviewed in Chapter 7, *Clinical Applications of Massage*. Studies have shown massage to be beneficial to those hospitalized for a number of conditions, including heart disease, cancer, and psychiatric problems. The benefits of back massage to institutionalized elderly included relaxation, improved communication, and a reduction in the common dehumanizing effects of institutional care.

There is promising research on massage for the agitated elderly in institutions and for those with Alzheimer's disease and dementia. Several studies have found reduction in certain agitated behaviors with regular 10-minute massage. Massage performed in the studies can be characterized as using light pressure, even rhythm, and slow strokes.[7]

Physiological Age

Elders are perhaps the most distinctive population to work with. Individuals in this age group are more different from each other than those in other age groups. By the time people have reached 70-plus years of age, they exhibit the accumulated effects of a lifetime of good and poor health habits, diseases and injuries, and life experiences. They are more likely to have chronic health problems and to be taking medications. Care should be taken in learning about each individual and in planning his or her massage sessions.

It is useful to think about older adults in terms of physiological age, rather than chronological age. **Physiological age** describes a person's health status relative to the norm in different age groups. For example, a 60-year-old person in good physical condition could be described as having the body of a normal 50-year-old.

People age at different rates depending on their genetic makeup, lifelong health habits, and unique life events. Traumatic events such as car accidents, work accidents, and sports injuries take their toll over time. Diseases experienced earlier in life may have effects later. An example is the incidence of post–polio syndrome affecting people 40 to 50 years after the acute phase of the disease. Negative factors can often be offset with healthy habits such as good nutrition and regular exercise.

Elders may be thought of as falling into one of three categories:

1. Robust

2. Age appropriate

3. Frail

Robust Elders These individuals show few outward signs of impaired health, look younger than their chronologic age, and are mentally sharp and physically active. Robust elders can generally be treated like the typical middle-aged recipient of massage. Information obtained on a health questionnaire can help you identify any areas of caution that are not obvious.

Age-Appropriate Elders People who show some of the typical signs of aging are considered age appropriate. Age-appropriate elders will have some problems associated with aging. Information from a health questionnaire is useful to identify contraindications and areas of caution. Use pillows and bolsters to ensure maximum comfort and the least stress on joints. Limit the prone position to 15 to 20 minutes. After the session, help the recipient sit up or at least stay near the massage table until he or she is sitting up. Leave the room only when you are sure that the recipient is not lightheaded and can get off the table safely.

Frail Elders Frail elders look and feel fragile to the touch and need special care. Check with their physicians before massaging the very frail. Frail elders will probably need assistance getting onto and off the table (see Figure 11–17). You might find it necessary to massage them in a regular chair or on their beds. Limit the session to 15 to 20 minutes until you know that they can handle longer sessions. Watch them carefully in the prone position on the table to be sure that they can lie there comfortably. Be extra gentle in lifting frail elders, avoiding pulling on their arms to help them up. Cradle their bodies to help them change position.

Positioning Options for the Elderly

Lying supine and prone as usual for full-body massage is a good option for most robust and many age-appropriate elders, although the prone position would normally be limited to a maximum of 20 minutes. The side-lying position puts stress on the hip and shoulder on the table, and is a less-desirable option in most cases.

Better positioning options for many age-appropriate and most frail elderly clients is either the seated (Figure 18–50 ■) or the semireclining positions (Figure 18–51 ■). These positions allow more social interaction between the elderly person and the massage therapist, including eye contact. They are also good options for clients with breathing difficulties and diminish the problem many elderly have with dizziness when changing from a horizontal to a more vertical

Figure 18–50 Seated position for massage for the elderly.

Source: Pearson Education, Inc./Segal Photography.

FIGURE 18–51 Semireclining position for massage for the elderly.
Source: Pearson Education, Inc./Segal Photography.

position, for example, when standing up after being supine for a time.

Guidelines for Massage of Older Adults

There are no special massage techniques that slow the aging process. However, there are certain points to keep in mind when working with older adults and especially with the elderly.

Do include the following in a massage session for healthy aging:

- Techniques to improve circulation in the extremities. Effleurage moving distal to proximal enhances venous return, and relaxing the muscles with kneading and jostling improves local circulation.

- Kneading, compression, and other petrissage movements that help keep muscle and connective tissue pliable and elastic.

- Joint movements and stretches of the lower extremities for improved mobility and flexibility. Spend time on the feet to relieve soreness, improve circulation, and mobilize joints. Mobilizing the legs and feet can help increase kinesthetic awareness, and thereby improve movements such as walking and climbing stairs.

- Movements and stretches for the shoulders to help maintain some important daily living functions, such as getting dressed and undressed and reaching for

things overhead. The hands may benefit from special attention to help them to stay mobile and sensitive.

- Passive motion and stretches for the cervical muscles to help maintain normal range of motion in the head and neck. With declining peripheral vision, the ability to turn the head to see things in the environment is important. This is essential for the safety of elders who drive motor vehicles.

- Techniques that focus on lengthening the front of the body, especially abdominal and pectoral muscles, to help maintain an erect posture. Exercises are also needed to keep postural muscles strong and to avoid a bent-over or collapsed condition later in life.

- Abdominal massage for the viscera, which may be important for sedentary elders to improve digestion and elimination. Use gentle but firm pressure, always going clockwise during circular movements (Figure 18–52 ■).

- Back massage is relaxing and comforting. It can be done even from a semireclining position if the client leans forward to allow access.

FIGURE 18–52 Abdominal massage can improve digestion and relieve constipation.
Source: Pearson Education, Inc./Segal Photography.

CRITICAL THINKING

Think about the physiological effects of aging and the cautions for giving massage to older adults. Analyze how screening interviews with older adults might be different from those with people in their 20s or 30s.

1. What contraindications might you look for specifically?
2. What medications might you expect older people to be taking?
3. What information about their joints would be good to know?

Cautions and Adaptations

Some problem conditions are more common in older adults and warrant special awareness. Massage is rarely contraindicated totally, but certain cautions apply with the conditions discussed next. It is important to take a thorough health history to identify the conditions that are contraindicated or for which cautions are warranted. Always consult the person's physician when in doubt about a condition or disease mentioned by a recipient of massage.

- Massage may be contraindicated with certain medications. If you work regularly with older adults and elders, it would be wise to have a reference book that explains the effects and possible side effects of common medications. Books written specifically about massage and medications are useful additions to a professional library. See Table 8–1 for at-a-glance information about medications. Check with the recipient's physician if in doubt about the advisability of him or her receiving massage while taking a certain medication.

- Elders typically have thin and delicate skin and bruise more easily than younger people. Some take anticoagulant medication as stroke prevention, which also makes them more prone to bruising. Pressure used in massage should be gentle to moderate, depending on the recipient's general condition. Use enough oil or lotion to prevent skin tearing.

- Watch for varicose veins in the legs, and do not perform deep effleurage or strong kneading over them. Light effleurage and jostling movements are better for circulation in this case. Elevating the legs slightly when the recipient is supine will help venous return during the massage.

- Deep vein thrombosis (DVT) and thrombophlebitis are two serious contraindications that may affect legs of elderly people. With these conditions, the legs will sometimes show typical signs of inflammation, that is, redness, heat, swelling, pain. There may be a cordlike hardness or a deep aching in the calf, or pitting edema in the skin. However, there may not be any signs of the underlying condition. Avoid massage of the legs if DVT is suspected.

- Older adults and elders may have diagnosed or undiagnosed atherosclerosis, or hardening of the arteries. This is especially dangerous in the cerebral arteries, which pass through the neck. Avoid deep work in the lateral neck area. Avoid movements that put the neck in hyperextension or increase the cervical curve because this position may further occlude blood vessels to the head and cause fainting.

- Use caution and consult a physician if an individual has bilateral ankle edema, as it could be due to disease of the cardiovascular or renal systems, and massage may be contraindicated.

- Use great care in performing mobilizing techniques and stretches around artificial joints. In the elderly, joint replacements are particularly common in the hip, knee, and shoulder. After a hip replacement, avoid movements involving abduction and circumduction in that joint. Consult the recipient's health care provider for instructions. Extreme care should be taken in the case of any joint replacement because of the potential instability of the joint or decreased range of motion due to scar tissue.

- In the case of cancer patients, always check with the physician before performing massage. Observe appropriate cautions with those receiving chemotherapy or radiation cancer treatments.

- Older adults and elders tend to have problems in their joints, including osteo- and rheumatoid arthritis. Massage of the area should be avoided if the joint is inflamed. When there is no inflammation, massage of the surrounding muscles is indicated to help relieve stress on the joint. Holding and warming arthritic and sore joints can be soothing. Heat is contraindicated if there is swelling.

- Because massage is commonly done directly on the skin, practitioners may detect possible skin cancers of which recipients are unaware. Basal and squamous cell carcinoma (see Figure 8–18) and malignant melanoma (see Figure 8–19) usually appear on sun-exposed areas of the body, including the face, arms, and chest. Malignant melanoma may develop at the site of a mole. Report any lesion or suspicious-looking skin condition to the recipient, or to the caregiver in the case of frail elders. Suggest that it be checked by a general physician or dermatologist. Do not massage directly over the site.

Massage in Semireclining Position

The semireclining position has several advantages for elderly massage recipients. It is usually easier for the elderly to get into and out of a chair, or onto and off of a low table. They are sitting up and so avoid potential problems associated with the prone position and turning over. They also avoid dizziness and instability commonly experienced when standing up after lying down for a period of time. None of these may be a problem for the robust elderly, but may be important for a frail elder or for octogenarians and older.

Disadvantages are related to access to different areas of the recipient's body. The lower back is difficult to reach, and the buttocks are largely inaccessible. Abdominal massage may also be more difficult than when a recipient is lying down. If abdominal massage is a high priority, then reclining at a greater angle will provide needed access to the mid region.

There are several options for equipment to facilitate a semireclining position. A recliner chair may be used or a regular chair with a footstool. Other options include massage tables with hinged tops, adjustable tables, or chairs used for spa treatments. The semireclining position can also be adapted for recipients in hospital beds.

Position fine-tuning is made by adjustments of the equipment and by using pillows and rolled towels. The back and head should be adequately supported and the knees flexed slightly. Arm rests on the chair, or support provided by bolsters or pillows, allow for relaxation of the upper body.

CASE FOR STUDY

Frank Puts Spring in Kristina's Step

Kristina just turned 80 years old. She gardens and walks short distances for exercise. She has noticed increasing difficulty walking and climbing stairs. Her legs feel stiff and heavy. Her sense of balance is getting worse. She has come to Frank, a massage therapist, to see if massage can help her get around better.

Question:

How might Frank plan a massage session to improve Kristina's mobility?

Things to consider:

- What types of massage techniques would best address Kristina's goals?
- What contraindications would it be good to screen for?
- What might Frank expect to find as he assesses Kristina's hips, legs, and feet?

Write a brief description of Frank's first massage session with Kristina. Describe how goals are set and cautions determined. List techniques likely to be included.

_____

_____

_____

Keeping good hand and body mechanics when massaging a semireclining recipient requires awareness and some creativity. The basic principles remain the same. Keep your neck and back in upright alignment. Move your body into position for applying techniques properly rather than putting the hand in an awkward position. Applying techniques to the lower body can be done from a sitting posture. Stand for massage of the upper body.

The height of the equipment (table or chair) is lower than for standard massage. This allows you to reach the recipient's head, neck, and shoulders without having to reach up or lift your shoulders. The following Practice Sequence adapts massage for clients in a semireclining position.

PRACTICE SEQUENCE 18–4

Massage for the Elderly in a Semireclining Position | 30 minutes

Preliminary Instructions

- Recipient removes as much clothing as practical and desirable.
- Help the recipient onto the table or chair.
- Drape for modesty and warmth.
- Place bolsters or pillows for comfort, support, and accessibility.
- Screen for contraindications and cautions. Note medications being taken.
- Sit at the recipient's feet to begin.

Figure 18–53 Apply compression and light effleurage techniques to the foot and ankle to warm the area.

1

2

Figure 18–54 Mobilize joints of the feet and ankle. Apply scissoring to metatarsals and figure-8s to toes. Dorsi- and plantar flex the ankle, and move side-to-side using the heels of the hands.

3

Figure 18–55 Apply lotion to the foot, lower leg, and thigh if accessible. Apply strokes from distal to proximal.

4

Figure 18–56 Knead lower leg muscles by bending the knee until the foot is flat on the supporting surface. Reach behind from the front, and squeeze the calf muscles with the fingertips. Heels of the hands press on anterior muscles of the lower leg.

Figure 18–57 Apply compression and kneading to thigh muscles. Address the entire thigh: anterior, posterior, medial, and lateral.

Figure 18–58 Rock the leg to create movement at the hip joint. Apply passive movements to mobilize knee and hip joints. Bend knee toward chest for a stretch. Move the leg in a circle to mobilize the hip. Slowly straighten the leg out. Redrape the leg.

Repeat Steps 1–6 on other leg.

Figure 18–59 Apply lotion to the arm from hand to shoulder. Use moderate pressure. Feel the quality of the tissues.

Figure 18–60 Use two hands to squeeze both sides of the arm at the same time. Apply from shoulder to wrist. Repeat twice.

9

Figure 18–61 Apply thumb strokes to the back of the hand (knuckle to wrist).

10

Figure 18–62 Turn the hand over and stroke the palm (wrist to finger web).

11

Figure 18–63 Mobilize hand and wrist joints. Apply scissoring to knuckles and figure-8s to fingers. Holding the hand, move the wrist through its range of motion.

Figure 18–64 Apply long effleurage stroke to entire arm—hand to shoulder. Brush off from shoulder to hand to finish.

Repeat Steps 7–12 on the other arm.

Figure 18–65 Stand behind and use two hands to knead both sides of upper trapezius.

Figure 18–66 Use one hand to knead posterior neck muscles. Place the other hand on the recipient's forehead to brace against forward pressure.

15

Figure 18–67 Use fingertips to apply deep friction to mobilize the scalp. Apply with one hand and brace with the other hand as necessary.

16

Figure 18–68 Reach from behind to apply circular friction to the temples on both sides.

17

Figure 18–69 Apply superficial friction to the upper and lower back. Stand to one side. Ask the recipient to lean forward so that the back is accessible. Apply superficial friction in circular motion to entire back. Brace against forward pressure at chest with other hand if necessary.

18

Figure 18–70 Apply light tapotement on the head. Tapping lightly with the fingertips works well for this purpose.

19

Figure 18–71 Brush off front to finish. Long brushing strokes from head to feet to finish.

Help the recipient slowly get up from the table or chair.

After you perform the Practice Sequence, evaluate how well you did by filling out Performance Evaluation Form 18–4, Massage for the Elderly in a Semireclining Position. The form can be found in Appendix D: *Performance Evaluation Forms*, and at MyHealthProfessionsLab.com.

Figures source: Pearson Education, Inc./Segal Photography.

PRACTICAL APPLICATION

Perform Practice Sequence 18–4 with the recipient in the semi-reclining position. Add massage techniques that address specific needs, for example, upper body tension.

1. Which techniques are most easily adapted for the semireclining position?

2. Are there variations of the semireclining position that provide better access to different areas of the body?

3. How do you maintain good body mechanics when giving massage to a semireclining recipient?

THE TERMINALLY ILL

Massage is used to bring caring and comforting touch to the terminally ill and dying. It is a valuable complementary therapy in hospital, hospice, and home care. Simple massage techniques may be used by health practitioners and taught to nonprofessional caregivers to aid those seriously ill or approaching the end of their lives.

From the wellness perspective, even those with terminal illnesses or nearing death continue to strive for optimal well-being in their unique life circumstances. Although massage will not cure or save someone from imminent death, it can help improve physical function and ease some of the pain and anxiety felt. **Palliative care** refers to measures that improve the quality of life for people with terminal illness. It has been observed that "attentive nurturing touch can be a significant therapeutic factor in treating despondency in the aging and/or the ill because of its multiple psycho-social, mental, emotional, and physical benefits."[8] Nurturing touch provides food for the soul, as well as for the body and mind.

General relaxation, improved circulation of blood and lymph, reduced muscular tension, and skin stimulation are effects of massage with benefits for everyone. These effects are relevant to the special needs of those who have been physically inactive or bedridden for a long period of time. Massage helps alleviate problems with insomnia, digestion, constipation, difficulty in breathing, and skin degeneration. It can help prevent bedsores.

People who are terminally ill and dying experience emotional distress for a number of reasons. They may feel isolation, grief from the loss of freedom and friends, fear of abandonment, fear of the disease or aging, or fear of dying. Depression is common among the seriously ill and elderly and may be caused or deepened by touch deprivation. Touch is essential nourishment for optimal well-being at all stages of life.

Gentle relaxation massage is known to reduce anxiety, provide a sense of connection, and generate feelings of general well-being. Massage may also facilitate a release of pent-up feelings, frustrations, sadness, and emotional energy. Pain that is aggravated by stress may be lessened with relaxing massage.

Near the end of life, massage can provide comforting touch and communicate care and love in a nonverbal way. The quality of touch for the dying should be gentle and the techniques simple, such as stroking and holding. When death is near, smooth, soothing touch is used as a form of comfort and a means of nonverbal communication. Some technical skills are needed to avoid causing pain or damaging delicate tissues.

In hospice and home-care situations, family members and other caregivers can be taught simple ways of giving massage to the dying person. This has benefits for both parties; it offers caregivers something active to do with their loved one and provides a means of connection even for those who may not be able to speak.

Adaptations for the Terminally Ill

A medical profile of the recipient is essential in working with the seriously ill and dying to protect both the recipient and you. As with any other massage, identify contraindications and areas of caution before proceeding with a session. It may also be useful to understand the symptoms expected as a specific disease or condition progresses.

Specific techniques are less important than other essential skills when working with this special population. Intuition and sensitivity to others are important qualities for giving massage to the terminally ill and dying. "If you develop the ability to 'see' an individual rather than just looking at a body, and if you reach out to that individual with a caring and open heart . . . out of your real and pure contact with the individual, you will intuitively know what to do and how to proceed."[9]

Other recommended characteristics and abilities include being touch oriented, able to adapt, open-hearted, able to focus energy, willing to face death, and able to focus on the individual. Important skills include

- Sensitive massage

- Active holding

- Listening and feedback

- Visualization and guided fantasy

- Guided meditation

- Shared breathing

- Communicating with the dying

Although some of these skills seem outside the normal scope of a massage practitioner, they are useful in working with this special population.

In planning massage sessions for the terminally ill or dying, there are no specific procedures to follow or ironclad rules to memorize. Each individual will be different in how he or she experiences dying and in how massage might be of benefit. However, there are some general guidelines to keep in mind.

In general, massage sessions with the dying should be softer, gentler, and shorter than a regular massage session. A person may only be able to benefit from 10 to 20 minutes of contact. Techniques may vary from simple hand-holding to full-body massage. Massage may be given with the receiver lying on a standard massage table, sitting in a chair or wheelchair, or lying in bed. Patients may be in hospital beds with tubes or IVs in their bodies. Massage practitioners in these situations need to be versatile and able to adapt to the circumstances. Listening and feedback skills are important because communication may be a great need for someone facing death. The key is to be caring, supportive, and accepting.

Hand and arm massage is a useful approach for getting to know a new patient or client. The hands are a familiar place of contact with other people. The hands are easily accessible, are relatively safe to massage, and benefit from the application of lotion. Having the hands touched is comforting in itself and affords the opportunity for eye contact while talking. Hand and arm massage is also easy for volunteers in nursing homes and hospices to learn. Practice Sequence 18–5 demonstrates a gentle hand and arm massage for palliative care of the terminally ill.

PRACTICE SEQUENCE 18–5

Gentle Hand and Arm Massage
20 minutes
Recipient seated

Preliminary Instructions
- Ask the person if he or she would like a massage today and for permission to begin.
- Identify any contraindications or cautions that apply. Check for open sores, bruises, and other skin problems.
- Use a lotion that is unscented and hypoallergenic.
- Position the recipient comfortably with the arm supported.
- Keep good eye contact throughout the massage.
- Use gentle but firm contact, and vary according to the recipient's needs. Many of the following techniques are the same as for healthy recipients. It is the way they are applied and the quality of touch that makes the difference.

Figure 18–72 Apply lotion to the entire hand and arm, moving up the arm from hand to shoulder. Use moderate pressure. Feel the quality of the tissues.

Figure 18–73 Alternate kneading and sliding on the upper arm. Knead the upper arm muscles with a hand on each side of the arm. Apply sliding strokes periodically toward the shoulder.

Figure 18–74 Alternate kneading and sliding on the forearm. Knead the forearm muscles with one hand. Apply sliding strokes periodically toward the elbow. Stabilize the arm with the other hand. Transition to step 4, using a few long, light sliding strokes from wrist to shoulder.

Figure 18–75 Gently press and roll the arm between your two hands, lightly mobilizing the shoulder and elbow joints. Hands move back and forth opposite each other to produce a rotational movement. If the person is especially frail, gently squeeze or simply hold places along the arm.

5

A

B

Figure 18–76
(A) Gently squeeze the whole hand between your fingers and palms. (B) Next squeeze each finger separately between your thumb and index finger. Apply from little finger to thumb.

6

Figure 18–77 Apply light circular friction over the wrist using your thumbs. Observe the skin moving over the wrist bones.

7

Figure 18–78 Joint movement of the fingers. Apply scissoring at the knuckles and figure-8s to the fingers to mobilize joints in the hand. Notice the degree of movement in the joints. Movements are extremely gentle and slow.

Figure 18–79 Perform thumb slides on the back of hand and palm. Slide your thumb between the metacarpals on the back of the hand, moving wrist to knuckles. Repeat thumb slides over the palm.

Figure 18–80 Gently squeeze along the length of the arm with both hands, moving down the arm from shoulder to wrist.

Figure 18–81 Finish by holding the hand briefly.

Repeat Steps 1–10 on the other arm.

After you perform the Practice Sequence, evaluate how well you did by filling out Performance Evaluation Form 18–5, Gentle Hand and Arm Massage. The form can be found in Appendix D: *Performance Evaluation Forms*, and at MyHealthProfessionsLab.com.

Figures source: Pearson Education, Inc./Segal Photography.

CRITICAL THINKING

Think about the various abilities needed in giving massage to the terminally ill and dying. Identify the important social and communication skills involved. Analyze how these skills are used best in a massage session.

1. Why might listening be more important than talking?
2. Why is being nonjudgmental essential?
3. What form does compassion take?

Self-Care

Working with the terminally ill and dying can be physically and emotionally challenging. It is important to practice conscious self-care to help maintain your own well-being.

The actual massage techniques used with the seriously ill or elderly tend to be simple and light and easy on the practitioner's hands. However, maintaining good body mechanics may be difficult when working with people in chairs or in beds. The general principles of good mechanics apply here also, and you need to find ways to keep your back straight and spine and neck in good alignment.

If the recipient has a communicable disease, proper precautions and hygiene should be observed. Although seemingly awkward, either latex or another type of glove should be worn if necessary for protection.

Maintaining emotional well-being involves a variety of factors. It helps to have confronted your own issues and fears around illness and death to a point of acceptance. Conscious awareness of how you feel when you are with someone seriously ill or nearing death can help you work through those feelings later with a friend, coworker, or supervisor.

IMPAIRMENTS AND DISABILITIES

Physical impairments commonly encountered in massage practices include visual, hearing, speech, size, and mobility challenges. These range from mild impairments such as needing a cane while walking to more severe circumstances such as being confined to a wheelchair. The difference between an impairment and disability is a matter of degree. Impairment becomes a **disability** when it severely limits a person's ability to perform daily life activities.

The Americans with Disabilities Act (ADA) is a U.S. federal civil rights law that prohibits the exclusion of people with disabilities from everyday activities. It went into effect in 1992 and applies to businesses of all sizes. It requires reasonable accommodation to make buildings and services accessible to all. How this applies legally to an individual business is a matter of interpretation, but the principle is clear and ethically sound. Massage therapists have a responsibility to accommodate all their clients, making reasonable adaptations when possible and safe to do so.

Visual Impairment

Many people wear glasses or contact lenses to correct mild vision problems. Clients wearing glasses will usually remember to take them off before getting on the massage table. If not, take the glasses from the client, and put them in a safe place until the session is over. Ask clients wearing contact lenses to remove them for the massage. If that is not convenient, take care that pressure is not applied to the eyes, especially when lying prone and using a face cradle.

Clients with more severe vision loss require more attention. During their first appointment, assess the situation. Ask them to explain their impairment, and discuss with them the level of assistance they need. Individuals vary on how well they can navigate on their own.

Having a magnifying glass on hand for reading would allow some people to fill out the health history without further assistance. Or a health history interview might be best. At the first visit, verbally describe the office and massage room as you walk them through the space, so that they can become familiar with it. Remove clutter from the floor space to prevent tripping. Show clients where to put their clothes and where the massage table is from that point. Ask if they would like further assistance, and if so, help them as requested.

CASE FOR STUDY

Keisha Prepares to Give Massage to a Client at the End of Life

Keisha's longtime client is coming close to the end of her life, ending a battle with inoperable cancer. The client has asked Keisha to provide her massage while she is in hospice care. Keisha agrees to do this and has scheduled her first session.

Question:

How does Keisha prepare for this first session, and how can she adapt her massage for this new situation?

Things to consider:

- Who, besides the client, would Keisha contact to integrate her service with other caregivers?
- How might Keisha find out more about possible contraindications and cautions for massage with this client?
- What about the physical setting would it be helpful for Keisha to know?
- What emotional challenges might Keisha face in this situation?

Write a possible scenario for Keisha's preparation for this massage session.

_____

_____

_____

There are a few general guidelines when working with the visually impaired.

- Let them know verbally when you are in the room.

- Position yourself in front and to their left when taking them through a space. They may or may not choose to touch your right arm for guidance.

- Describe your surroundings, and indicate where things are using clock face numbers. For example, a chair you can use for dressing is at 11 o'clock about 6 feet ahead.

- Do not interact with a client's service dog without his or her permission (Figure 18–82 ■). Discuss with the client where the best place would be for the dog to lie down during the massage.

Hearing Impairment

Hearing loss is common in older adults but can occur at any age. Suspect poor hearing if a client frequently asks you to repeat what you said, asks you to speak louder (if you had been speaking in a normal tone), or seems to be reading your lips. Simply speak more slowly, a little louder, and enunciate clearly. Do not exaggerate your lip movements. Face the client when you speak so that he or she can see your facial expression and read your lips. Maintain good eye contact. Eliminate background noise as much as possible.

Do not shout at someone wearing a hearing aid. If a client wears a hearing aid, ask if he or she would like to remove it during massage. Hearing aids pick up and magnify sounds in the room. If the client does remove the hearing aid, be aware that you will have to speak much louder, or

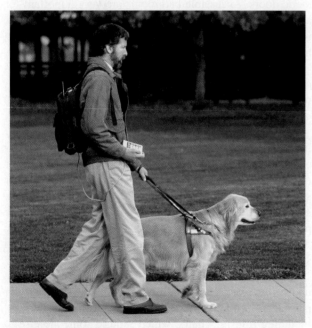

FIGURE 18–82 Do not interact with a service dog unless you have permission from its owner.

Source: Pearson Education, Inc./Segal Photography.

communication will have to be nonverbal. You will need to get his or her attention through touch and move within his or her line of sight so you can make eye contact and your face can be seen. If the hearing aid stays in, keep massage around the head and ears to a minimum because moving the hearing aid can cause annoying feedback.

If you work with a deaf client regularly, consider learning some sign language for common situations. Useful signs would be for hello, ready to start, turn over, finished, and questions about pressure, pain, and other feedback.

Speech Impairment

A person's difficulty communicating verbally can result from a variety of causes. Perhaps he or she has a physical abnormality that affects anatomical structures involved in speech, has had a stroke or head injury, or has a condition such as dementia. Some medications cause slurred speech. People deaf from birth have never heard speech and so may be difficult to understand. And although it is not a physical impairment per se, people speaking English as a second language may have heavy accents, mispronounce words, or use poor grammar, and therefore be hard to understand.

Whatever the cause of poor verbal expression, a little patience and attention will help you communicate adequately with clients. Ask clients to repeat anything you don't understand. Repeat back what you think they mean so that they can confirm it. Listen attentively, and remove background noise that can interfere with your own hearing. Watch their facial expressions and body language.

Distinguish between those who are fully capable mentally (e.g., has a physical impediment to speech) and those whose mental alertness may be clouded by diminished brain function or medication. The former case is a simpler matter of finding a way to communicate, whereas the latter case may require additional considerations.

Size Issues—Large and Small

Massage equipment is designed to accommodate a range of client sizes within normal limits. Tables are typically 6 feet long, are 28–32 inches wide, and can safely hold up to about 300 pounds. When clients fall outside this range, accommodations for their safety and general benefit are in order.

HEIGHT

Clients over 6 feet tall may extend past the foot of the table when they are supine. Extending the feet over the edge of the table a few inches is usually not uncomfortable. With some table models, you might be able to adjust the face cradle so that the client can use it comfortably as a table extender. The back of the head rests on the cradle with the client faceup, possibly covering or replacing the crescent with a pillow. Consider purchasing a specially made table extender for the foot of the table if you have a tall regular client. This is less of an issue when the client is prone because several inches are gained when using a face cradle.

People short in stature include those affected by one of the many medical conditions know as dwarfism. This special population has a support group called the Little People of America, who provide services and information for adapting to the larger world. "Little people" may need a foot stool to be able to get onto the massage table more easily. They frequently have orthopedic problems in the back and legs that can benefit from massage.

LARGE BREASTS

Women with large breasts can be made more comfortable lying prone by using some support. Rolled up towels or small pillows may be positioned to fill in the space above and below the breasts to spread out the weight on the chest area. The face cradle is elevated to maintain a comfortable curvature in the neck. Ready-made bolstering systems for women with large breasts are available from different table manufacturers.

Accessing the muscles under breast tissue can be a challenge, especially for women with large breasts. Remember that breast tissue extends from the front of the chest laterally to under the arm pit. If you need to massage the muscles in that area, perhaps the best strategy is to have the client take a side-lying position, so that gravity pulls the breast toward the table. You can hold the upper arm out of the way while you massage the exposed muscle with the other hand.

OBESITY

Having a body mass index of 30 or above is the definition of **obesity**. This calculation is based on height, weight, and an estimate of lean body mass. BMI is discussed in more detail in Chapter 4, *Physical Skills, Fitness, Self-Care for the Massage Therapist*. Obese clients have an excess accumulation of fat tissue in their bodies. It has been estimated that over 25% of people in the United States fit this definition, although estimates vary from region to region.

Extremely obese clients typically have mobility problems caused by increased weight and girth. Fitness exercises become more difficult, so inactivity may be a problem. They are likely to have related health issues such as joint pain, diabetes, and heart disease.

Depending on the size of the client, positioning on the massage table may pose challenges. Be sure to know the weight limit for your individual table model. You may need side extenders to accommodate larger girth. Lowering the table in these cases might facilitate better body mechanics for you as you work. Use adequate draping. Giving massage on a floor mat might be a better option for some clients.

It is important to maintain a nonjudgmental and caring attitude. Honor the clients' right to respect and their possible embarrassment about their physical condition. Do not lecture them about the health dangers of being overweight. This is insensitive and outside the scope of massage therapy. Make the necessary accommodations, and help them reach their wellness goals for the massage session.

Obesity does pose some unique challenges. A factor to consider is the nature of adipose tissue. It has a high proportion of blood capillaries, so it bruises easily. Palpating anatomical structures deep to the adipose tissue may be difficult. Specific structures that are usually palpable may be inaccessible. Asking a client to flex a particular muscle can help locate it. However, avoid applying deep pressure that can cause pain and bruising, and use the palms to apply broad strokes.

Carrying excess weight can distort posture and stress the musculature. Relaxation that accompanies massage and the mechanical action of stroking can help relieve some of that stress. In addition, massage reduces anxiety and increases an overall feeling of well-being. It can be a valuable adjunct to any medical weight-loss program. People who have experienced significant weight loss may have skin folds that hang loosely. Do not apply deep pressure to these folds, and avoid pinching the skin when applying techniques to adjacent tissues.

Weight loss surgery is becoming more commonplace and the types of these procedures continue to multiply. Some of the more common forms are gastric bypass, gastric band, and sleeve gastrectomy. If a client has had such a surgery, ask what type of surgery he or she received and become familiar with typical complications related to that procedure. Avoid abdominal massage with any client who has had weight loss surgery that alters the digestive system.

Mobility Challenges

Mobility refers to the ability to go from place to place independently. A person's mobility may be temporarily challenged by injury or illness, or he or she may have a permanent disability that affects mobility.

Accessibility to buildings and offices within buildings is improved with ramps, elevators, wide doors, and automatic doors. Accessible bathrooms are very important for a business like a massage practice. Getting into buildings, moving around in an office space, and getting on and off a massage table are typical mobility issues.

It is relatively easy to accommodate people using canes or crutches. Typically they can negotiate a few stairs and can walk from room to room. Ask if they need assistance, and watch for challenges they may be facing.

Walkers are usually associated with a higher level of impairment (Figure 18–83 ■). People typically use walkers because of general weakness, problems with balance, or chronic dizziness. Use of the walker may be temporary after surgery, injury, or illness. Or it may be more permanent, such as with the elderly. Those who use walkers in public places may get around fine at home or in small spaces. They will almost certainly need assistance getting on and off a standard massage table.

Wheelchair use indicates a more severe disability. The underlying reason for wheelchair use may be temporary or permanent. There are also different types of wheelchairs, including transfer chairs, which require someone else to push, standard models for self-wheeling, and motorized chairs. People who are paralyzed or extremely weak may be strapped into the chair.

FIGURE 18–83 People using walkers typically have a high level of mobility impairment.

Source: Pearson Education, Inc./Segal Photography.

In terms of mobility, know about your building's accommodations for outside access and inside maneuverability. Locate the handicapped accessible bathroom. If possible, meet the client at the building entrance to offer assistance, especially at the first appointment.

There are some general guidelines for working with people in wheelchairs. First, respect their autonomy, and do not push a wheelchair without permission. Ask what type of assistance they need because many have the ability to move into and out of the chair on their own. Do not assume the person is helpless, and be sensitive to his or her desire to live as independently as possible. But be ready to help when necessary.

Interview the client to learn the exact cause of his or her disability, which likely involves cautions and possibly contraindications for some massage applications. Sit or kneel so that you are at eye level for the interview to make good eye contact.

You and the client may decide that receiving massage in the wheelchair is the best plan. You can wheel the chair to the massage table and use pillows for support as the client rests his or her head and shoulders on the table. Then proceed with seated massage, observing appropriate precautions as needed related to the client's health problems.

AMPUTEES AND PROSTHESES

An amputee is a person who has lost one or more arms or legs. People lose limbs for a variety of reasons, such as car and workplace accidents or diseases like diabetes. And an increasing number of returning veterans have lost arms or legs in recent wars. Soldiers, who may have died of their injuries in the past, are returning home and getting rehabilitation services that include technologically advanced prosthetic devices.

Providing massage therapy in the context of treatment for a recent amputee recovering from surgery requires advanced training. However, clients who have lost limbs in the past may come for massage in any setting.

In the intake interview, get information about the limb loss. Ask how long ago it happened. Ask about the cause of the loss, which may uncover contraindications or cautions to be taken, and will help in session planning. If what remains of the limb, commonly called the *stump*, is to receive massage, find out more about the structure. For example, is there anything unusual about the muscles and bones involved? Ask if the stump is numb or sensitive to touch or pressure. The client will probably be able to tell you what will feel uncomfortable and what may feel good to the area. Ask if the client has any goals in mind related to the site of the amputation. Massage can be utilized to promote healthy scar tissue on the stump to facilitate better prosthetic fit and wearing tolerance.

Ask if the client needs assistance in any way, for example, undressing or getting onto the table. Depending on the extent of the loss, the client may be very self-sufficient or may need assistance.

A client with an amputation may experience what is called phantom limb sensation, or phantom limb pain. That is experiencing sensation or pain in a limb that does not physically exist. The missing limb may feel shorter or distorted. The pain is occasional, and the incidence of the sensation usually diminishes over time. This is a neurological

PRACTICAL APPLICATION

Role-play massage sessions for clients with various physical impairments and disabilities.

1. Ask appropriate screening questions in the intake interview.

2. Determine what assistance the client may need to prepare for the massage.

3. Position the client appropriately and practice a massage application you might use to meet his or her unique needs.

REALITY CHECK

LUTHER

SONIA: I feel totally inadequate to give massage to someone with special needs. I'm afraid I might say something inappropriate or hurt him or her. Can't I just take appointments from normal people?

LUTHER: I understand how you feel, but we don't always know ahead of time about our clients. And who's to say what normal is? I find that if I am open, honest, and respectful, and err on the side of caution, I do all right. The first time I had a client with a prosthetic leg, I wasn't sure what to do. I just stayed calm and asked her to tell me about her condition. I admitted that I had never massaged someone like her before and would need some direction about what to do and not to do. She had come in for relaxation massage and wasn't looking for anything related to her stump. When she left I did some research about amputees and was more informed the next time she came for an appointment. I've learned a lot through my career and take continuing education on different special populations when I can. You build confidence through experience.

FIGURE 18–84 Amputee and his prosthetic limb.

Source: Pearson Education, Inc./Segal Photography.

Pacemakers and Defibrillators

Artificial pacemakers and defibrillators are implanted under the skin in the upper chest with wires attaching to the heart itself. These devices keep the heart beating at a regular rhythm. Avoid massage in the immediate vicinity of an internal or external medical device. Also avoid movements that disturb the device. Use gentle massage techniques in areas that are sensitive around the site of a device.

Colostomy Bag

A colostomy is a surgery in which the colon is attached directly to the anterior abdominal wall, leaving an opening on the abdomen called a *stoma*. Feces leave the colon through the stoma and are collected in a **colostomy bag** attached to the outside of the body (Figure 18–85 ■). An ileostomy is similar except that the small intestine is attached to an opening in the abdominal wall. Clients with colostomies lower in the tract can often regulate their bowels. Colostomies and ileostomies may be temporary or permanent depending on the medical situation.

If a client has a colostomy or ileostomy, recommend that he or she not eat for about 2 hours prior to the appointment. Also suggest that he or she empty the bag before the session begins. Do not use lubricant around the stoma or bag opening to avoid weakening the adhesive that keeps the bag in place.

Use the side-lying position instead of prone to avoid pressure on the stoma. A protective pad under the bag area is a prudent step in case of accidental leakage. If a bag leaks or become detached, assist the client as needed to stabilize the situation. Use proper hygienic procedures, and use disposable glove and towels to sanitize any surface that becomes soiled. Keep a calm professional demeanor to minimize embarrassment to the client.

condition, and the overall calming effects of massage may help diminish phantom sensations.

Prostheses are artificial appliances that replace missing body parts (Figure 18–84 ■). The technology of these mechanical and electronic devices, especially those for the upper and lower extremities, can be quite advanced. Clients may or may not want to remove their prosthetic devices for massage. If they wear their devices, ask what precautions to take to avoid damaging them. If the device is removed, look for chafing, irritation, or skin lesions around the area of attachment. Avoid inflamed areas and breaks in the skin.

INTERNAL AND EXTERNAL MEDICAL DEVICES

Medical devices may be positioned inside or outside the body either temporarily or permanently. For example, hospital patients may have temporary urinary catheters or intravenous drips in place during their stays. A more permanent situation might be a heart disease patient with an implanted venous catheter or stent that keeps a blood vessel open.

FIGURE 18–85 Colostomy bag attached to the abdomen.

Source: Pearson Education, Inc./Segal Photography.

REWARDS AND CHALLENGES

This chapter touched on just some of the many special populations that massage therapists encounter in their careers. Serving special populations can be rewarding and challenging at the same time. It reminds us that each individual is unique and provides the opportunity to practice patience and compassion. It offers an appreciation of the many difficult circumstances life can present. Serving special populations can be mentally stimulating as we learn about different human conditions and plan massage sessions to meet client goals. It challenges us to stretch our minds and hearts and to learn new skills as we adapt to different situations.

Some massage therapists choose to specialize in a specific population as a special interest or marketing niche. Continuing education offers the opportunity to learn more about individual populations in greater depth.

CHAPTER HIGHLIGHTS

- A special population is a group of people with some distinctive life circumstance that sets them apart from a normal adult population.
  - This special circumstance can influence their goals for massage, may require adaptations to the session for safety or comfort, and may present contraindications.

- Clinical applications focus on treatment for a specific pathology or injury, whereas special populations may be interested in massage for reasons having nothing to do with their "special" circumstances.
- When working with special populations, maintain an open, nonjudgmental, sensitive, and patient attitude.
- Five major applications of sports massage are recovery, remedial, rehabilitation, maintenance, and event.
  - Maintenance massage is an all-purpose massage received regularly that includes recovery and remedial applications.
  - Preevent massage is upbeat and prepares an athlete for competition; postevent massage focuses on recovery.

- Massage can be given safely to healthy women with low-risk pregnancies.
  - Warning signs for contraindications include abdominal pain, discharge, swelling, fever, nausea, and pitting edema.
  - Abdominal massage and joint movements are contraindicated throughout a pregnancy and for several weeks after delivery; other contraindications and cautions apply during different trimesters.

  - Use the side-lying or semireclining positions for pregnancy massage.

- Infant massage provides tactile and kinesthetic stimulation for healthy growth and development.
  - Infant massage is a simple, gentle yet firm application of stroking, pressing, squeezing, and movement of the limbs.

- Massage helps the elderly keep the strength and flexibility needed to do activities of daily living (ADLs) and provides pleasurable social interaction.
  - Think of elders in terms of physiological age rather than chronological age.
  - Include massage techniques to improve circulation, promote relaxation, and improve mobility.

- Massage brings caring and comforting touch to the terminally ill and dying and is a valuable complementary therapy in hospital, hospice, and home care.
  - Near the end of life, massage can provide comforting touch and communicate care and love in a nonverbal way.
  - Massage sessions with the dying should be softer, gentler, and shorter than a regular massage session.

- Physical impairments commonly encountered in massage practices include visual, hearing, speech, and mobility challenges.
- When clients fall outside a normal size range, accommodations for their safety and general benefit are in order.
  - Excessively obese clients may be better positioned on a floor mat for massage.

- Assist clients with amputated limbs as needed, and watch for irritated or chafed skin at the site of attachment of prosthetic devices.
- Avoid sites around internal and external medical devices.
  - Position clients with colostomy bags in the side-lying position, and be prepared for hygienic cleanup if a bag leaks.

- Working with special populations challenges us to stretch our minds and learn new skills as we adapt to different situations.

EXAM REVIEW

Key Terms

To study the key terms listed at the beginning of this chapter, match the appropriate lettered meaning to each numbered key term listed. For additional study, look up the key terms in the Interactive Glossary, and note other terms that compare or contrast with them.

_____ **1.** Adaptations
_____ **2.** Colostomy bag
_____ **3.** Disability
_____ **4.** High-risk pregnancies
_____ **5.** Infant massage
_____ **6.** Mobility
_____ **7.** Obesity
_____ **8.** Physical impairment
_____ **9.** Physiological age
_____ **10.** Special population
_____ **11.** Sports massage

a. Distinctive life circumstance that sets them apart from the norm
b. A person's age relative to his or her health status
c. Adjustments to the way things are normally done to meet the unique individual needs
d. Visual, hearing, speech, size, and mobility challenges
e. The mother or fetus is at higher than normal risk for complications or negative developments
f. An application specifically designed to meet the needs of athletes
g. External medical device
h. Provides kinesthetic and tactile stimulation for healthy growth and development
i. Unhealthy accumulation of fat tissue
j. An impairment that severely limits a person's ability to perform daily life activities
k. The ability to go from place to place independently

Memory Workout

To test your memory of the main concepts in this chapter, complete the following sentences by circling the most correct answer from the two choices provided.

1. Preevent sports massage applications are typically (upbeat and stimulating) (calming and mild).
2. Use (unscented) (fragrant) oils and lotions when giving massage to pregnant women.
3. The pressure used for infant massage is gentle but (deep) (firm).
4. (Age appropriate) (Robust) elders show few outward signs of impaired health.
5. Programs designed to provide high-quality palliative care to the dying are called (nursing homes) (hospice).
6. Perhaps the most important skill for people giving massage to the dying is their ability to (listen) (speak with authority).

7. When guiding a visually impaired person through a space, position yourself in front and to their (left) (right).
8. A person who comes for massage using a walker for balance, will (almost certainly) (not necessarily) need assistance getting onto and off a standard massage table.
9. When giving massage to an extremely obese client, consider (raising) (lowering) your massage table to facilitate better body mechanics for you as you work.
10. If a client has a colostomy or ileostomy, recommend that he or she not eat for about two hours (after) (prior to) the massage appointment.

Test Prep

The following multiple-choice questions will help to prepare you for future school and professional exams.

1. Improving a debilitating condition such as muscle soreness and tension is the goal of what sports massage application?
   a. Preevent
   b. Postevent
   c. Remedial
   d. Rehabilitation

2. If a pregnant woman has been on bed rest by a doctor's orders, massage of the legs is:
   a. Beneficial
   b. Contraindicated
   c. Indicated
   d. Welcomed by the recipient

3. In a normal pregnancy, which trimester is the safest and easiest part?
   a. First
   b. Second
   c. Third
   d. No significant difference

4. The following technique promotes bowel movement in infants:
   a. Foot massage
   b. Milking the legs
   c. Bringing the knees to the chest repeatedly
   d. Back massage

5. To avoid tearing or bruising skin that has thinned over time, it is advisable to use:
   a. Less pressure
   b. More pressure
   c. Generous amount of lotion or oil
   d. Both a and c

6. Which of the following is most important when giving massage to the terminally ill?
   a. Critical thinking
   b. Technical skill
   c. Using a wide variety of techniques
   d. Intuition and sensitivity

7. When speaking to someone with a hearing impairment do not:
   a. Speak more slowly
   b. Exaggerate your lip movements
   c. Speak a little louder
   d. Face the person directly

8. To better access chest muscles in women with large breasts, have them lie in this position.
   a. Side-lying
   b. Supine
   c. Prone
   d. Seated

9. When someone comes for massage in a wheelchair, the best approach is to:
   a. Give assistance before being asked to
   b. Assume they are helpless
   c. Ask about what assistance they might need
   d. Assume they have developed skills for complete independence

10. Pacemakers are medical devices that are typically:
    a. Hung externally on the chest
    b. Hung externally on the abdomen
    c. Implanted into the abdomen
    d. Implanted in the chest

Video Challenge

Watch these videos, which can be found at MyHealthProfessionsLab.com, Chapter 18, and then answer the following questions.

Postevent Sports Massage

1. In the postevent sports massage video, what did you notice about positioning that is different from standard relaxation massage? Why do you think it is done this way?

Pregnancy Massage

2. What massage techniques are shown in the video for addressing tight muscles in the low back of a pregnant woman?

Infant Massage

3. In the video showing infant massage, what techniques are used to massage the arms and legs? How does this differ from massage of the average adult?

Massage for the Elderly

4. In the video showing massage of an elderly person, how was he positioned and draped? What challenges did this present to the massage therapist in terms of the massage application and of maintaining good body mechanics?

Gentle Hand and Arm Massage

5. What qualities of touch can you see in the massage application demonstrated in the video? In what other ways does the massage therapist convey caring?

Comprehension Exercises

The following short-answer questions test your knowledge and understanding of chapter topics and provide practice in written communication skills. Explain in two to four complete sentences.

1. Explain some of the restrictions on massage applications for pregnant women. Relate those restrictions to the physiology of pregnancy.

2. Describe how skin changes as we age. What precautions should be taken during massage to avoid damage to the skin of an elderly recipient?

3. What questions would you include in an intake interview with a man who is wearing a prosthetic device on his leg? How might his answers impact session plans?

For Greater Understanding

The following exercises are designed to take you from the realm of theory into the real world. They will help give you a deeper understanding of the subjects covered in this chapter. Action words are underlined to emphasize the variety of activities presented to address different learning styles and to encourage deeper thinking.

1. Observe treatment of athletes at a sports medicine rehabilitation center. Note the roles of physical therapists, athletic trainers, and massage therapists in the setting. How are the roles different? How are they similar? How did different therapists use massage? What adjunct therapies were offered?

2. Observe people of a variety of ages in a public place such as a park or shopping mall. Note differences in the way they move, their posture, and other visible characteristics. Compare and contrast children, young adults, older adults, and the elderly. Describe any physical impairments you observe.

3. Interview a health professional who is working or who has worked with the terminally ill or dying. Ask the individual about the type of setting and his or her personal challenges working in that environment. What were the patients' greatest needs? Inquire about the role of massage, if any, where he or she worked, and the potential benefits of massage for this special population. Discuss your findings with a study partner or group.

MyHealthProfessionsLab™

MyHealthProfessionsLab.com is a premium online homework management system that includes a host of features to help you study. Registered users will find:

- Powerful tools that track and analyze your results—allowing you to create a personalized learning experience
- Videos, flashcards and other learning tools to help enrich your progress
- Streaming lesson presentations and self-paced learning modules
- A space where you and your instructors can view and manage your assignments

Spa Treatments

Ann L. Mihina
Sandra K. Anderson

CHAPTER

19

Pearson Education, Inc.

CHAPTER OUTLINE

Learning Outcomes

Key Terms

Overview

Equipment and Supplies

Helping Clients Choose Spa
   Treatments

Exfoliation

Body Wraps

Aromatherapy

Stone Massage

Chapter Highlights

Exam Review

LEARNING OUTCOMES

After studying this chapter, you will have information to:

1. Describe equipment and supplies needed for spa treatments.

2. Explain the sanitation practices necessary for a spa practice.

3. Help clients choose spa treatments for themselves.

4. Describe exfoliation and its benefits.

5. Explain full-body and quick prep dry brushing.

6. Describe how to perform scrubs.

7. Explain chemical, enzyme, and dissolving exfoliations.

8. Describe how to perform body wraps.

9. List the features of 10 foundational essential oils.

10. Explain how aromatherapy can be used in a massage practice.

11. Describe stone massage.

KEY TERMS

Aromatherapy

Body polishes

Body wraps

Carrier oil

Chemical, enzyme, or
   dissolving exfoliation

Clays

Dry brushing

Emollient

Essential oils

Exfoliation

Infusion

Limbic system

Manual exfoliation

Moor mud

Muds

Peat

Scrubs

Stone massage

OVERVIEW

Spa treatments are typically offered within spa establishments but can also be given by massage therapists in private practice. Spa venues range from hair salons and day spas to destination spas offering multiple-day stays and every amenity imaginable, including strategies for major lifestyle changes. Depending on the type of spa, the services can include bodywork such as massage therapy, shiatsu, and Thai massage; body treatments such as facials, body wraps, and salt glows; exercise and fitness classes; programs for nutrition, weight loss, smoking cessation, and detoxification; spiritual renewal classes such as yoga, meditation, and labyrinth walking; and cosmetic treatments for skin rejuvenation, liposuction, and plastic surgery. Many massage therapists augment their offerings with spa treatments but do not consider their practices to be spas.

Note that the terms *application, service,* and *treatment* are used interchangeably in the spa setting. Although in most health settings, the word *treatment* is reserved for approaches to healing a medical condition, the spa setting has traditionally used the term to describe spa services, for example, a seaweed body wrap treatment. This stems from their history as natural healing establishments over a century ago. See Chapter 1, *Massage Therapy Profession,* for more information on personal care settings, types of spas, and typical spa services. Also see Chapter 2, *History of Massage as a Vocation,* for a historical look at personal care and natural healing venues. There are many different spa applications and, because innovation is the hallmark of the spa industry, more are being developed all the time. Individual spas can differ greatly in what services they offer and in the equipment and supplies available. Spa staff members are expected to become familiar with and proficient at using what the spa has, and each spa provides its staff with proper training. State law or local ordinances may contain regulations related to spa treatments as a health and safety issue. These regulations should be consulted to make sure you are in compliance with the law in your particular location.

This chapter illustrates methods and techniques commonly provided by massage therapists in spa and private practice settings. The focus is on the spa applications of exfoliation, body wraps, aromatherapy, and stone massage.

EQUIPMENT AND SUPPLIES

There are certain pieces of equipment and categories of supplies practitioners are likely to encounter at any spa establishment and from which massage therapists with their own practices can choose when offering spa services.

Equipment

Equipment encompasses everything from brushes used in exfoliations to Vichy showers. The following are some examples of the equipment practitioners may use while working in a spa.

- *Hot towel cabi.* This piece of equipment stores rolled moist towels at a temperature of about 175° F. Many have a built-in UV sanitizer that keeps the towels hygienic until they can be used.

- *Wet table.* This type of table has a drain in it. Clients lie on the table for treatments involving substances that need to be rinsed off, such as muds and seaweed. Rather than have the client go to a separate shower facility, the practitioner rinses the client using a Vichy shower or other water source while the client is on the table.

- *Wet room.* This is a specially constructed room for the use of water in treatments and may contain equipment such as wet tables, Vichy showers or other handheld showers (to remove spa substance residue from clients' bodies), whirlpool tubs, or other specialty showers or hoses. The room is usually tiled on the walls and floor and also has drains in the floor. Figure 19–1■ shows a wet table and Vichy shower in a wet room.

- *Vichy shower.* This shower has multiple nozzles that hang above the client. The practitioner controls the temperature, pressure, and amount of water used to rinse off the client.

- *Small equipment.* These include bowls used for treatment substances, spatulas, eye pillows, stones for hot and cold stone treatments, music CDs, and table warmer pads.

Supplies

Everything from substances used during treatments to robes given to clients to wear in the spa are considered to be supplies. Although there are broad categories of supplies, it is important for practitioners to remember that most spas have their own lines of signature treatments and products, and it is important for spa employees to become knowledgeable about them.

FIGURE 19–1 Wet table and Vichy shower in a wet room.

Source: Goodluz/Fotolia.

- *Linens.* These include sheets used during treatments, face-rest covers, blankets, towels, washcloths, plastic sheeting using during certain treatments (like wraps), robes, or staff uniforms (these may be laundered on-site or practitioners may be expected to launder their own). Practitioners will be instructed in what the spa's protocols for handling the linen are, such as where clean ones are kept, and how to dispose of used linens.

- *Substances.* These are applied to the client's body or used as aromatherapy during the various treatments and include muds, seaweed, peat, creams, gels, exfoliation substances (salt, sugar, ground coffee, etc.), essential oils, and herbs (for herbal infusions). Practitioners will be instructed in the safe use, handling, storage, and disposal methods of each substance used within the spa.

- *Disposables.* Supplies needed during the performance of treatments, including disposable undergarments for clients, disposable spatulas to mix substances, and so forth. Disposable gloves should be available for staff use when needed for proper hygiene.

- *Toiletries.* These are offered for client cleanliness and convenience. For spas that offer showers for client use, they can include body washes, bath scrubbies and shower footwear, deodorant, shampoo, hair conditioner, hair spray, hair gel, combs, cotton swabs, and cotton balls. It may be the responsibility of practitioners to make sure these items are readily available for client use, or it may be a duty of other spa staff.

- *Cleaning supplies.* These are necessary for hygiene and sanitation, and include rubbing alcohol, bleach, and other sanitizers and disinfectants.

PURCHASING SUPPLIES

Most supplies can be purchased at local stores, beauty supply stores, natural foods stores (for herbs, some muds, and seaweed), and on the Internet. When considering what to buy, it is important for practitioners to consider that the supplies and equipment need to be able to stand up to a lot of treatments. Something may seem like a bargain but turn out not to be if it has to be replaced often. For example, towels that are inexpensive initially may end up being quite expensive in the long run if they are so thin that they wear out after just five or six uses. Thicker, plusher towels that cost more at first are more cost effective because they can last for 25 to 30 treatments. For more information on equipment and supplies, see the resources listed under Chapter 19 in Appendix E, *References and Additional Resources.*

Sanitation

As discussed in Chapter 10, *Hygiene, Equipment, Environment*, practitioners need to be aware of the risk of transferring pathogens from one client to another. Aside from the human factor, pathogens can also be found on supplies and equipment, as well as in any of the substances used in spa treatments. This is important to note because many pathogens grow in dark, warm, damp places, which makes spa treatment settings especially vulnerable to mold growth and disease transmission.

In addition to following personal health and hygiene practices, practitioners should know that it is important that everything is cleaned between clients, including linens, equipment, floors, tables, countertops, and so on. There are many good antibacterial sprays and disinfectants on the market; research them to find the ones that work best for you.

HELPING CLIENTS CHOOSE SPA TREATMENTS

Receiving spa treatments may be a totally new experience for the client, who may be feeling excited and apprehensive at the same time. It is the responsibility of practitioners to be knowledgeable about all the services they perform, to be able to answer clients' questions as completely as possible, and to give in-depth explanations of treatments, including:

- Benefits, indications, contraindications

- How the treatment is performed

- What results the client can expect

- How the client can expect to feel after the treatment

Some spa treatments involve a certain amount of nudity for the client. For example, a client may have mud from a mud wrap rinsed off with a Vichy shower and is either totally nude or covered only minimally for this process. Other treatments may involve minimal coverage of the breasts, genitals, and buttocks throughout the treatment. Although practitioners are used to this, it may be unexpected or embarrassing for a new client. Clients need to be tactfully informed about their possible levels of nudity during treatments and given the opportunity to refuse a treatment if there is anything with which they are not comfortable. Clients may also choose to receive treatments that usually involve minimal coverage but request more conservative draping. It is up to the practitioner to modify draping as necessary to make the client feel at ease. See Chapter 11, *Body Mechanics, Table Skills, General Guidelines*, for more information about draping.

Practitioner's Role

There are so many spa treatments available that it is sometimes difficult for a client to choose which one to try. Sometimes the treatment a client really wants to experience is not one he or she should receive, or perhaps there is a treatment the client does not know about that would suit his or her needs perfectly. Practitioners need to know how to elicit information from clients so they can recommend the best spa applications for them.

There are times when clients want treatments that would not be suitable. For example, a woman may have spent the morning sunbathing and arrives for an afternoon spa treatment, an exfoliation, with a sunburn. The scheduled treatment is not possible because it would be painful and damaging to the skin. It is up to the practitioner to explain this clearly and tactfully to the client. Most clients will accept the expertise of the practitioner and allow themselves to be directed to another treatment more appropriate under the circumstances or to reschedule the appointment. If clients insist on receiving treatments that are not in their best interests or could even be harmful to them, the practitioner who is employed in a spa should consult the spa supervisor for support in managing the situation. The practitioner can use conflict resolution skills if this occurs.

Health and Medical Considerations

The following questions need to be answered by the client on an intake form to get a picture of his or her health and medical history. This also will provide a good framework for designing the treatment session. Review the completed form and follow up by asking the client for clarification as needed.

- *Do you have any medical conditions?* This can include chronic and acute conditions. For example, uncontrolled hypertension and vascular disorders are contraindicated for herbal and mud wraps; pregnancy is a contraindication for certain spa applications and the use of some essential oils.

- *What prescription or over-the-counter medications do you take?* If a client is taking an analgesic (pain reliever), it could interfere with the ability to give accurate feedback about temperature and pressure; a hot stone treatment would therefore be contraindicated. Also, some essential oils inhibit the actions of certain medications.

- *Do you have any allergies?* Clients can be allergic to any and all spa treatment substances, including muds, peat, clays, ginger, essential oils, and sea products, including sea salt and sea mud. It is best if the client notes any allergies on an intake form so there is written documentation. People can develop allergies throughout their lives, so every time a client arrives for a treatment, the practitioner should check for any updates.

   A common allergy is to shellfish. Clients who are allergic to shellfish and/or iodine should *never* receive treatments with sea products such as sea salt, seaweed, and sea mud. Clients may not realize that an allergy to shellfish and/or iodine also means allergies to sea products, so it is important for the practitioner to discuss this with clients. Another common allergy is to nuts. Clients with nut allergies should not receive treatments with nut-based oils or exfoliants.

   Clients may not be aware of allergies they have, so before any treatment is performed, apply the

substance to a small area on the client's skin, usually the forearm, to see if there is an allergic reaction. Some people are allergic to latex, so ask about that before using latex gloves on the client's skin. Nonlatex alternatives are available for you to use.

Allergic reactions run a wide gamut. They can be as simple as a few localized hives and itching all the way up to a full-blown anaphylactic reaction, which interferes with the client's ability to breathe.

If a client has an allergic reaction, the most important thing the practitioner should do is to stay calm and stop the treatment immediately. The substance should be removed and the client thoroughly rinsed off. If the client's condition worsens, for example, numerous hives, impaired breathing, and/or widespread inflammation, emergency care, such as calling 911, should be initiated immediately.

- *Do you have any areas of inflammation, rashes, or other skin conditions?* Skin disorders may cause certain treatments to be contraindicated, such as exfoliations. On the other hand, there are treatments that can be soothing for some skin conditions, such as a mud wrap.

- *How often do you get sick? How fast do you recover?* If robust and not prone to illness, and provided there are no other contraindicated conditions, the client can receive just about any treatment. If, however, the client is in fragile health, then treatments using hot and cold such as stone massage would need to use less extreme temperatures or are contraindicated all together. Sedating treatments may be more beneficial; invigorating treatments could possibly deplete the client further.

- *What is your temperature tolerance?* Clients who have a low tolerance to hot temperatures may not be the best candidates for hot stone treatments, or would need the temperatures lowered. Likewise, clients who have low tolerance to cold temperatures may not be the best candidates for receiving cold stone therapy, or would need the temperatures raised.

Other Considerations

There are a few other things to consider when helping a client choose spa treatments. These are related to the client's level of spa experience, goals for the visit, and plans afterwards.

- *Have you had a spa treatment before?* If there is no prior experience, then the client may need detailed explanations of all treatments. For example, the client may ask for a wrap, but after the practitioner explains that minimal draping is involved, the client may opt for a stone massage instead.

   If the client has had spa treatments before, the practitioner should ask the client what the results were and whether the client liked it. Perhaps the client is looking to repeat a great experience or to try something new. If the client did not have good results or did not like the treatments, a different treatment should be suggested.

Practitioners should also let clients know that some spa treatment products have particular odors to them. Muds and peat have an earthy aroma; seaweed smells like the ocean. Practitioners can let clients smell the substances and, if the odor is displeasing, they can choose other treatments.

- *What are your desired goals for the treatment?* Does the client want softer, smoother skin? An exfoliation treatment followed by a seaweed wrap could be suggested. Does the client have a specific area of discomfort, such as wanting some muscle tension relief in the back? A hot stone massage on the area might be the best treatment. If the client has some sinus congestion, an inhalation treatment with eucalyptus essential oil could be performed.

- *What will you be doing after the treatment session?* Is it acceptable for the client to feel sedated afterward, or does the client need to be energized? This can determine what treatments to suggest. For example, if an important presentation is planned for later on in the day, then perhaps a relaxing body wrap that makes the client feel sleepy is not the best choice; a salt glow with peppermint essential oil may be better.

EXFOLIATION

Exfoliation is the peeling and sloughing off of dead skin cells from the surface of the body. An overabundance of dead skin cells can cause skin pores to clog with natural body oils, dirt, and debris, which can lead to dryness, flakiness, and the formation of pustules. Removal of the dead cells brightens skin color and clarity by encouraging the body to produce new skin cells. It also unclogs the follicles and pores, improves skin texture by making it smoother, and allows moisturizers, lotions, serums, and other preparations to better hydrate and nourish the skin. Exfoliation leaves the skin invigorated and increases vasodilation of skin blood vessels so that blood is brought to the surface of the body. It also energizes superficial lymphatic flow and stimulates nerve endings.

A full-body exfoliation is a powerful therapy in and of itself that can have a positive impact on the entire body. The removal of dead skin cells, the vasodilation of skin blood vessels, and the stimulation of nerve endings make it an invigorating treatment. Exfoliation can also be a prelude to another treatment, such as a mud or herbal wrap. It not only prepares the skin for the wrap, but also gives clients the benefit of receiving more than one treatment, enhancing their spa experience.

Contraindications for exfoliations include

- Skin irritations
- Rashes
- Sunburn
- Allergy to substances being used
- Contagious skin condition
- Athlete's foot—only the feet would be contraindicated; the rest of the body could be exfoliated
- Recent tattoo
- Area shaved less than 24 hours prior to treatment

Methods of Exfoliation

The term *exfoliant* encompasses both the substances and the tools used to remove dead skin cells. There are two main methods of exfoliation. The physical process of applying friction with abrasives is called **manual exfoliation**. Manual exfoliants include tools such as dry brushes, mitts, loofahs, and abrasive cloths, and natural substances such as salt, sugar, cornmeal, and ground coffee beans that are abrasive. These substances are typically mixed with water, oils, or creams before being rubbed over the surface of the skin.

The other method is **chemical, enzyme, or dissolving exfoliation**. This consists of chemicals or enzymes that work by dissolving dead skin cells, but do not overstimulate the skin the way manual abrasives can. After application, the enzymes are washed or rubbed off. Natural substances such as yogurt, milk, and papaya contain acids and enzymes that act as natural exfoliants. There are also many different commercial preparations, and the manufacturer's instructions need to be followed carefully when they are used.

Manual Exfoliation

Manual exfoliation can be done using many different tools and substances, depending on the level of abrasion needed.

DRY BRUSHING

Exfoliation using brushes or fiber tools is known as **dry brushing** or *body brushing*. Other manual exfoliation tools that can be used for dry brushing include loofahs, nylon mitts, sisal mitts (sisal is a coarse fiber), ayate cloths (a woven fiber that is less coarse than sisal), and other abrasive cloths depending on the level of abrasion desired. See Figure 19–2 ■ for examples of manual exfoliation tools. Dry brushing can be performed from mild to moderate to vigorous.

A full-body dry brushing takes about 30 minutes and can be offered as an individual treatment or in conjunction with other therapies. For example, body brushing can be done before a body wrap. When the dead skin cells are removed, the substances used in body wraps, such as mud or cream, can have a much better effect on the skin. An abbreviated version is called quick prep dry brushing. It addresses the entire body and usually only takes a total of

FIGURE 19–2 Examples of manual exfoliation tools: loofah, brushes, ayate cloth, and sisal mitt.

Source: Photoestelar/Fotolia.

10 minutes—5 minutes with the client prone and 5 minutes with the client supine.

Dry brushing and all manual exfoliation methods help to stimulate the flow of lymph. Dry brushing strokes applied to the extremities, face, neck, upper chest, abdomen, and back are done lightly to stimulate the flow of lymph in superficial lymphatic vessels. The strokes performed in dry brushing and other manual exfoliation techniques travel along the pathway of lymph flow:

- In the extremities, the strokes are performed toward the client's heart.

- Strokes on the face, neck, and upper chest are performed downward.

- Abdominal strokes are performed in a clockwise direction, then up each side to the center of the abdomen.

- Back strokes are performed downward from the neck and shoulders to the mid-back, then from the lumbar area up to the mid-back.

When using the body brush or exfoliation tool, the most efficient stroke is a brisk half-moon stroke, using a flick of the wrist. These brisk movements remove the maximum amount of dead skin cells with each stroke (see Figure 19–3 ■).

For clients who have mild edema not due to medical conditions, such as from standing for long periods of time, dry brushing may be useful. Practitioners, however, should never go beyond their scope of practice. There are specific courses of study in lymphatic drainage, including certification courses, that give practitioners the skills and tools needed to address more serious medical conditions such as lymphedema. See Chapter 23, *Lymphatic Facilitation*, for manual techniques to improve lymph flow.

SCRUBS AND BODY POLISHES

Other manual exfoliation methods are **scrubs** or *frictions* using salts, sugar, or coarser organic substances. These tend to be brisk treatments that leave the client energized. The

A

B

FIGURE 19–3 (A) A brisk half-moon stroke is an efficient technique to use with the body brush or exfoliation tool. (B) Dry brushing can help stimulate movement of lymph fluid.

Source: CandyBox Images/Fotolia.

exfoliant substance is mixed with a fluid such as water, oil, cream, milk, yogurt, vinegar, water, or a body wash. Essential oils can be added to the mixture to enhance the treatment with fragrance. These treatments remove the top layers of the skin and cause vasodilation of skin blood vessels, thus the person is left with brighter skin characterized as a "glow." Because of this, scrubs using salt and sugar are often referred to as *salt glows* and *sugar glows*.

Unlike salt, sugar has moisturizing properties; like salt, it leaves the skin soft and smooth. The salt or sugar is usually mixed with a few drops of oil and a little water, to make it the consistency of snow. The amount of water needed to make the mixture is minimal enough that it does not dissolve the salt and sugar crystals. The salt or sugar can be mixed completely with oil for the exfoliation but this makes for a messier treatment. The oil is difficult to remove from the client's body and to launder from the sheets.

Salts and sugars are particularly useful because, in addition to being abrasive, they contain glycolic acid that dissolves away dead skin cells so they can be considered chemical or enzymatic exfoliants as well. In addition, salt is an excellent substance to use in spa and hydrotherapy treatments because it can do the following:

• Act as a natural antibacterial agent

• Draw impurities out of the skin

• Ease certain skin disorders such as eczema and psoriasis

There are several major types of salts used in spa treatments. Sea salt is often used, and the salts harvested from the Dead Sea, which is located between the West Bank of Israel and Jordan, are popular. The magnesium and potassium in Dead Sea salts have cleansing, detoxification, and restorative properties, especially for the skin and muscles.

Desert mineral salts are gathered from deserts that are the remnants of prehistoric oceans. The most common desert mineral salt is borax. Borax, or sodium borate, is a complex mineral, mined near Death Valley, California, as well as in Tibet and Italy. It is naturally fine-grained so is ideal for use in body polishes. Redmond salt is another type of desert mineral salt. It gets its name from the part of the world in which it was initially discovered, Redmond, Utah. Redmond salt contains over 50 trace minerals, which gives it a slight pink color. Pink Himalayan salt is also increasing in popularity.

Epsom salt is named for the mineral-rich waters of Epsom, England. The therapeutic agent in Epsom's water is magnesium sulfate, a mineral salt. Epsom salt can be used for exfoliation; soothing, stress-reducing soaks; reducing inflammation; and calming muscle aches and pains.

Unrefined salt is always the best choice to use in spa treatments because it has no additives nor has it undergone chemical processing. Dead Sea salt, sea salt, and natural mineral salts come in different size grains. A fine- or medium-grain salt is best for a salt glow exfoliation or body polish.

Body polishes are a gentler form of exfoliation using softer granules such as those found in fine blue cornmeal or finely ground natural substances like crushed almonds or grape seed meal. A skin **emollient** such as oil, lotion, or cream can be used as part of the mixture. A skin emollient is a substance that makes the skin soft and supple. For coarser grains, the emollient should be thicker; for smaller grains, the emollient can be thinner.

Many different substances can be used for scrubs and body polishes. Just about anything that occurs in granular

form, or that can be ground into granules, can be used as long as it is natural. When using natural substances, it is best to grind them to a desired consistency and make them into a paste or slurry using water, oil, cream, milk, yogurt, vinegar, a body wash, or any other liquid of choice.

In addition, practitioners can explore the use of materials found in their geographic areas. For example, grape seeds, wine, and grape seed oil are used for scrubs at spa and bodywork practices in the Napa Valley wine country of California. The Spa at the Hotel Hershey in Hershey, Pennsylvania, offers a chocolate sugar scrub. Substances used in scrubs and body polishes include

• Coffee grounds

• Cornmeal—blue, white, yellow

• Crushed pearls

• Ground nuts—almonds, peanuts, hazel nuts, etc.

• Pulverized pumice (crushed volcanic rock)

• Salt—sea salt, Epsom salt, Dead Sea salt, desert mineral salt

• Seeds—grape, poppy, flax, sunflower, sesame

• Sugar—table sugar, raw sugar, brown sugar

• Oatmeal

• Barley

Figure 19–4 ■ shows some substances used in scrubs and body polishes.

There are several factors to consider when helping clients choose which exfoliation substances would work best for them. For delicate or sensitive skin, milder abrasives such as those used in body polishes would be appropriate. Clients with dry skin may benefit from the hydrating aspects of a sugar scrub. Salt scrubs may be useful for a client with oily skin. Pumice tends to be more abrasive than

FIGURE 19–4 Common substances for scrubs and/or body polishes.

Source: Sasimoto/Shutterstock.

PRACTICAL APPLICATION

Make and try out your own natural exfoliants for scrubs. Compare cost of supplies, ease of application, and overall effectiveness.

1. Which substances and liquids go together the best?

2. What considerations (such as allergies) do you need to keep in mind when gusing these exfoliants on clients?

3. How could you pair scrubs with other treatments to make them more effective and appealing to clients?

---

many other exfoliation substances, making it an excellent scrub for the feet.

An exfoliation can be very invigorating, so practitioners need to keep communicating with the client about pressure of application. Sometimes deeper pressure and more time are needed to exfoliate the soles of the feet, palms of the hands, elbows, and knees.

Natural exfoliation substances leave residue on the body; therefore, it may be best to use them in locations where there is access to a shower. Some spas will have wet tables or Vichy showers available for rinsing clients thoroughly. This will involve a level of client nudity and, as discussed earlier in the chapter, it is very important that practitioners explain clearly to clients how the procedure is performed and what the client can expect.

If the exfoliation is being done in a dry room with no access to a shower, the exfoliation substance can be removed using the dry room substance removal technique as described in Box 19–1 ■.

Preparing for a Scrub Treatment

Gather the supplies needed for the scrub application before the client arrives. See Figure 19–5 ■. Scrub supplies typically include

- Small, nonmetal bowl for exfoliation substance— nonmetal because the substance may react chemically with metal, changing the substance's properties.

- Natural exfoliating substance (one-quarter to one-half cup). If performing a salt glow, use 50% fine salt and 50% medium grain salt (sea salt, Epsom salt, Dead Sea salt, desert mineral salt). If performing a sugar glow, use table, brown, or raw sugar.

- Essential oil(s). If using an essential oil, a couple of drops of a carrier oil will also be needed. For more information on essential oils, see the *Aromatherapy* section in this chapter.

- Liquid to make a paste or slurry (water, milk, yogurt, oil, etc.).

- Three cloth sheets (one fitted and two flat) or two sheets (one fitted and one flat) and one large towel, approximately 30″ × 60″, can also be used. The client's drape can be a flat sheet or a large towel.

- One large towel, approximately 30″ × 60″, to be used for draping the chest area when applying the scrub to the client's abdomen.

- If there is no access to a shower, a basin of warm water and three or four towels, approximately 18″ × 30″, are needed for substance removal. A towel cabi or electric slow-cooking pot filled with moist towels can also be used. More towels may be necessary for large clients or for those with a lot of body hair.

- After the supplies are gathered, prepare the work space in this manner:

- Place three sheets, or two sheets and one large towel, lengthwise on top of the table.

- Put the exfoliation substance, liquid, and small bowl within easy reach.

- If working in a dry room and using an electric pot or cabi, turn on the warmer to heat the towels for substance removal at the end of the treatment. Moisten the towels and put them in the electric pot or cabi. If using a basin of warm water to heat and moisten the towels, place the basin in a convenient spot so it can be filled with warm water during the treatment.

| BOX 19–1 | Dry Room Substance Removal Technique |

1. Place a warm, moist towel on the exfoliated area of the body for a few seconds, patting it down firmly.
2. Remove the substance with one firm, smooth stroke, taking care not to scrub or wipe with the towel.
3. A new warm, moist towel is used for each area of the body from which the exfoliation substance needs to be removed.

FIGURE 19–5 Equipment and supplies needed for manual exfoliation using natural substances.

Source: Maxfx/Fotolia.

Performing a Scrub Treatment

To begin, the client gets on the table in supine position underneath the top sheet or large towel. He or she will be lying on top of two sheets. Throughout the application, be sure to ask the client for feedback about the amount of pressure you are using and adjust as necessary.

1. Blend the natural exfoliating substance with the fluid in the bowl until it resembles a slurry. Just enough fluid is added to make the salt or sugar the consistency of snow; if desired, an essential oil (mixed well with a couple of drops of carrier oil) can be added to the mixture.

2. Undrape one of the client's legs. Pour some water into your hands and, starting at the right foot, apply it up the client's leg.

3. Rub a small amount of the exfoliation mixture between your hands and apply to the top surface of the client's foot using small circular strokes to thoroughly exfoliate it.

4. Continue using small circular strokes up the ankle and anterior right leg, taking more exfoliation mixture as needed (Figure 19–6 ■). Redrape the leg, and repeat on the left leg.

5. Move to one side of the client's upper body and undrape the arm. Use small, circular strokes to thoroughly exfoliate the client's hand and arm, up to the shoulder. Redrape and repeat on the other arm.

6. Standing at the head of the table, accordion the large chest draping towel vertically over the client's chest area and grasp the top of the large, horizontal towel on top of the client. As you unfold the vertical towel, fold down the horizontal towel until the client's chest is draped by the vertical towel and the abdomen is undraped (Figure 19–7 ■).

FIGURE 19–6 Use small circular strokes up the ankle and leg.

Source: Pearson Education, Inc.

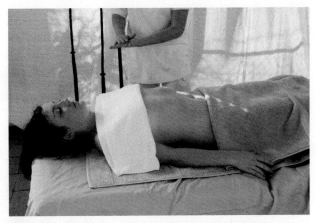

FIGURE 19–7 Cover the breasts with a towel before undraping to expose the abdomen.

Source: Pearson Education, Inc.

7. Using smaller movements and a lighter touch, stroke in a clockwise direction on the abdominal area. Finish this area by exfoliating each of the client's sides and coming back to the center of the abdomen. Pull the towel up over the client's abdomen and draping towel on the client's chest area, then gently pull the chest draping towel out from under the sheet.

8. Move to the head of the table to exfoliate the client's upper chest area. Use smaller movements and a lighter touch, working downward from the collarbone. If the client's face is to be included, a light touch is also used. With small gentle strokes, exfoliate from the chin to forehead.

9. Before the client turns over to prone position, remove the exfoliation substance (it can be left on and removed all at once at the end of the treatment, if preferred). If using a wet table or Vichy shower, rinse the client thoroughly. If working in a dry room, use the dry room substance removal technique described earlier in Box 19–1.

10. Help the client turn over. Undrape the left leg and exfoliate the bottom of the foot using small circular strokes, then continue using small circular strokes up the posterior leg, including the gluteal area, taking care to use less pressure on the back of the knee. Redrape and repeat on the right leg.

11. Move to the head of the table and undrape the client's back. Using small, circular strokes, apply the exfoliating substance to the client's neck and back (Figure 19–8 ■), moving around to the side of the table to include the lateral sides of the back. The exfoliation process is now complete.

12. If using a wet table or Vichy shower, rinse the client thoroughly. If there is a separate shower facility, help the client off the table, draping the top sheet or large towel around him or her for modesty. Guide the client to the shower and then back to the treatment table after rinsing off. While the client is in the shower,

FIGURE 19–8 Using small, circular strokes, exfoliate the client's neck and back.

Source: Pearson Education, Inc.

FIGURE 19–9 Removing the sheet from underneath the client.

Source: Pearson Education, Inc.

remove the top sheet on the massage table, uncovering the fresh, fitted sheet underneath.

13. If the exfoliation is being done in a dry room with no access to a shower, use the dry room removal technique as described in Box 19–1, then remove the sheet the client is lying on using the dry room sheet removal technique described in Box 19–2 ■ and shown in Figure 19–9 ■.

14. Whichever method is used to remove the exfoliation substance, and once the client is lying on a clean sheet, apply a moisturizing oil or lotion to the body.

Chemical Exfoliation

Another type of exfoliation uses chemical, enzyme, or dissolving exfoliants. Enzymes and alphahydroxy acids (AHA) or betahydroxy acids (BHAS) are found in commercial products. They are also found in nature as:

- Citric acid in citrus fruits
- Malic acid in apples
- Tartaric acid in grapes
- Lactic acid in dairy products like milk, cream, and yogurt
- Glycolic acid in sugar and sugar cane

> **BOX 19–2 Dry Room Sheet Removal Technique**
>
> 1. Have the client lift his or her head slightly, then reach across the client's body, grasp the sheet on both sides, and gently pull down.
> 2. With the client's head back down on the table, have him or her lift the shoulders, then lay the shoulders down, then lift the hips and lay the hips down as you continue pulling the sheet toward the foot of the table.

When these acids are applied to the skin, they loosen the keratin that holds skin cells together, allowing the cells to be easily sloughed off. Papaya (papain) and pineapple (bromelain) also contain enzymes that are effective exfoliants. Because they are nonacid enzymes, they are considered the safest for sensitive skin, unless there is an allergy to papaya or pineapple.

A chemical exfoliation can be very gentle on the skin or very aggressive, as in a medical facial peel. It is recommended that a reputable esthetician be consulted regarding the use of any over-the-counter chemical, enzyme, or dissolving exfoliation products. It is very likely that spas will carry chemical, enzyme, or dissolving exfoliation products. Spa staff members who are expected to use these on clients will receive training on how to apply them properly.

A full-body chemical, enzyme, or dissolving exfoliation treatment can be done in much the same way as a scrub application with a few modifications:

- Approximately one-half cup of the exfoliation substance with no additional liquid is needed.

- Preparation is the same with the addition of a large towel placed horizontally at the head of the table.

- The application is similar, with the exfoliation substance being applied either by hand or by painting it on the client's body with a brush. Once the exfoliation substance has been applied to both the front and back of the client, instead of being immediately removed, the practitioner wraps the two top sheets around the client securely, then wraps the towel around the client over the sheets. (Figure 19–10 ■). The client stays wrapped for about 20 minutes, after which the exfoliation substance is either rinsed off or removed using the dry room substance removal technique described in Box 19–1.

- Once the exfoliation is complete, another treatment can be performed, such as a massage or body wrap.

FIGURE 19–10 After the chemical exfoliation substance has been applied, wrap the two top sheets around the client securely.

Source: Pearson Education, Inc.

BODY WRAPS

A popular spa treatment is the **body wrap**. Its primary purpose is to detoxify the body by stimulating blood and lymph circulation. Body wraps can be used in conjunction with many different substances. Muds, peats, and seaweed are commonly used materials, as well as sheets soaked in an herbal infusion (herbal wraps). After the substance is applied, the body is wrapped in sheets, blankets, and/or a plastic covering.

New wraps are being continually developed. For example, avocado, aloe, and chocolate wraps are currently popular. Spas and individual therapists can offer regional specialties, such as a prickly pear gel wrap in the southwest. As more and more organic substances are discovered to have healing properties, innovations in body wrap materials are inevitable. Treatments also can be packaged together, such as a desert mineral salt scrub applied before a desert herbal wrap, a sea salt glow coupled with a seaweed body wrap, or a coffee scrub preceding a chocolate wrap.

It is important to begin with an exfoliation. Removing the dead skin cells enables the substance being used to work more efficiently. This can be done with any exfoliation treatment, although the quick-prep dry-brushing technique is commonly applied before a body wrap. The full-body dry brushing can be performed if clients desire a longer treatment.

There are many ways to perform wraps. Generally, each spa has its own body wrap protocols and trains their practitioners accordingly. What is presented in this chapter may or may not be consistent with how individual spas perform their wraps. However, by practicing the procedures in this chapter, practitioners, whether they work in a spa, clinic, or private practice, will acquire foundational skills, become comfortable handling supplies and equipment, and become able to discuss body wrap options with clients in a knowledgeable manner.

The body wrap treatment itself typically takes 35 to 40 minutes. The time can be extended to 60 to 90 minutes when supplemented with other bodywork treatments, such as full-body dry brushing, massage therapy, shiatsu, acupressure, or reflexology. Some body wraps use creams and gels, such as aloe vera, cocoa butter, or shea butter to smooth and hydrate the skin. An ideal way to conclude the wrap is to perform short gliding massage strokes so the body wrap substance is evenly distributed and absorbed.

Contraindications for body wraps include

- Heart conditions
- Untreated hypertension
- Allergy to iodine or shellfish (seaweed wraps)
- Inflammation
- Vascular disease, including varicose veins
- Numbness/loss of sensation in area; neuropathy
- Flare-up stages of autoimmune disorders such as lupus, rheumatoid arthritis, and multiple sclerosis (the heat from a wrap would be painful and debilitating)
- Skin conditions made worse by heat; burns
- Intolerance to heat
- Broken or irritated skin
- High body temperature (fever)
- Claustrophobia
- Pregnancy

Muds and Clays

Sometimes the terms *mud* and *clay* are used interchangeably because they can resemble each other. However, they have different constituents and different properties and need to be considered separately.

Muds are differentiated based on the soils and marine sediments from which they are derived. Inorganic muds contain mostly minerals that result from lake and river sedimentation and have very little organic material. Volcanic muds can be found near hot mineral springs. Organic muds are formed from algae, plant, and animal matter that have mixed with lime, clay, and sand in the soil. The colors of the muds depend on the amounts of various minerals in them. For instance, muds that are red contain a high amount of iron.

One of several properties of muds that can make them therapeutic is their mineral content. The minerals help with deep skin cleansing and aid in the removal of waste products by their drawing action, which also can stimulate local blood and lymphatic flow. When applied, mud forms a covering that acts as an insulator on the body, trapping heat and keeping it from radiating away and keeping water from evaporating from the body. Thus muds are excellent warming and hydrating treatments. The trapped heat also serves to increase local blood circulation.

Overall, muds are applied therapeutically to help relieve soreness in muscles and joints, and to reduce pain from tendinitis, muscle strain, joint injuries, and noninflammatory stages of arthritis and bursitis. They are also used to soothe certain skin conditions.

The therapeutic effects of both marine-based and soil-based **clays** lie in their mineral content and ability to suspend easily in an emulsion with water or other liquid. Clays draw impurities from the body, aiding deep skin cleansing and the removal of waste products. Because clays are porous and hold water molecules, they hold heat especially well, making them excellent for heat applications.

Muds and clays are categorized based on their region of origin and composition. New ones are continually being discovered, and new treatments are developed that are location specific. Table 19–1 ■ shows representative examples of muds and clays from the United States and around the world.

Peat

For the past 200 years, peat has been used therapeutically in baths and packs. **Peat** is an organic soil that contains minerals, organic material, water, and trapped air. It is formed by the decomposition of layers of plants, mainly mosses, and animal matter under bodies of water. The properties of the different peats depend on the local flora and fauna that made up the layers. Most peats used in spa therapies are a combination of moss and sedge, a marshland plant. Peats are cultivated primarily in Ireland, Austria, Germany, the Czech Republic, and other Eastern European countries.

The substances in peat that contribute to its therapeutic effectiveness are organic acids and minerals. The acids contribute to peat's ability to draw and absorb toxins from the body. Physically, peat contains micropores that allow it to take in water like a sponge. Like muds and clays, peat can form a covering that acts an insulator on the body. It keeps heat from radiating away from the body and keeps water from evaporating from the body. Thus, peats are excellent warming and hydrating treatments. The heat also increases local blood and lymph circulation.

Like mud treatments, peat applications help relieve aching muscles and joints, and pain from muscle injuries and noninflammatory arthritis. Peat applied to the skin can also have soothing effects.

Moor Mud

Moor mud is a type of peat that is also known as *black mud,* because of its appearance. It is the mineral-rich sedimentation that is deposited at the bottom of lakes and rivers fed by both hot springs and cool springs. The hot springs contribute volcanic ash to the mixture of plant material settling to the bottom of the water. The lakes from which moor mud is taken maintain a temperature around 86° F, but the combination of hot and cool water creates a great deal of circulation in the lake. This enhances the decomposition of organic material; layers and layers build up over time. The Neydharting Moor in Austria is in a glacial valley that was once a lake, and the moor has been developing there for over 20,000 to 30,000 years. Neydharting moor mud is an organic mud and is known for being pure and nutrient-rich.

Moor mud has a very low pH, usually around 3.54. The application of moor mud can assist in the regeneration of the acid mantel of the skin, which protects the body from harmful bacteria. High-grade moor muds come from Austria, Germany, Hungary, and the Czech Republic. In North

TABLE 19–1	Examples of Muds and Clays from the United States and Around the World

Mud/Clay	Location	Comments
Calistoga mud	Calistoga, CA	Volcanic mud and hot springs known for their healing properties; Native Americans first made use of the mud baths and later the Spaniards; today, many spas are located in the area
Natural red clay	Glen Ivy Hot Springs, Corona, CA	Clay known for healing and purifying; Native Americans designated the area as sacred; later the Spaniards took advantage of the healing benefits; today a spa on the site offers treatments from local mud
Dead Sea mud	Dead Sea, Israel	Mineral-rich, highly saline mud that draws impurities and retains heat; used for a wide range of skin disorders such as psoriasis and eczema; especially beneficial for muscle pain and stiffness, arthritis, and other joint pain
Rotorua thermal mud	New Zealand	Volcanic mud; silky in texture and rich in minerals and trace elements; QE Health (formerly known as the Queen Elizabeth Hospital) in Rotorua uses the mud as part of its standard care in the treatment of arthritis and other joint conditions
Muds and clays	Australia	Muds and clays found near mineral-rich, natural springs; harvested from undeveloped areas so are essentially free from chemical pollutants; sun dried after being harvested; used for over 60,000 years by Aboriginal tribes for healing, sacred and ceremonial purposes; only recently available outside Aboriginal culture
Rasul (Rhassoul)	Morocco	Lava clay mined in the Atlas Mountains of Eastern Morocco; used alone or in a combination mud and steam treatment originating in the Middle East

Sources: Data from Calistoga Spas, "The Mud Baths" (2008); Glen Ivy Hot Springs Spa, "Hot Springs Spa, History" (2008); Minton, M., "Mud: Dig It!" (2008); Williams, A., *Spa Bodywork, A Guide for Massage Therapists* (2007).

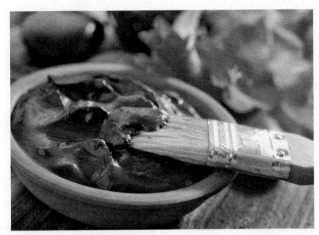

FIGURE 19–11 Hungarian Moor Mud can assist in the regeneration of the acid mantel of the skin, which protects the body from harmful bacteria.

Source: Tycoon101/Fotolia.

America, Canadian moor mud is known for its mineral-rich qualities (Figure 19–11 ■).

Seaweed and Sea Mud

Seaweed and sea mud are organic materials that have an abundance of salts, vitamins, and other trace elements essential to the body. Seaweed and sea mud have the same therapeutic benefits to the body as other muds. In addition, they are also antibacterial agents; the minerals and salts in these sea products kill certain bacteria.

The term *seaweed* has become an umbrella term for any marine plant or algae. However, seaweed is not technically a true plant. Although it does have chlorophyll, which allows it to produce oxygen like plants do, it does not have true roots, stems, or leaves. It is actually *algae*. Often, the terms *algae* and *seaweed* are used interchangeably. Algae are groups of aquatic organisms that perform photosynthesis. They are found in almost every habitat in the world. Species of algae can be anything from single-celled and microscopic, such as plankton, to multicellular and huge, such as a brown seaweed that has fronds (leaves) 200 feet long. There are many different types of seaweed. Some are harvested from beaches where they have washed up, some from the water close to shore, and some from the deep oceans.

The three major categories of seaweed are based on their colors: green, brown, and red. *Green seaweeds* are found near shores in shallow waters. One of the most common green seaweeds used in spa treatments is sea lettuce (*Ulva lactuca*), which is used to relieve inflammation and muscle soreness.

Brown seaweeds have a brown pigment that masks the green of the chlorophyll. There are two major groups of brown seaweeds used in spa treatments, the *Laminaria* species (kelp) and the *Fucus* species (wracks). Brown seaweeds are used in spa treatments and hydrotherapy treatments for detoxification, revitalization (through increased local blood and lymph circulation), slimming, and skin tightening.

The *red seaweeds* are mostly delicate and fernlike. One red seaweed, *Chondrus crispus,* actually grows in more shallow waters, especially around the British Isles. Because it is harvested extensively in Ireland, it is called Irish moss. Another name for it is carrageen (or carrageen moss). Irish moss is used in spa and hydrotherapy treatments for detoxification, revitalization (through increased local blood and lymph circulation), slimming, skin tightening, and moisturizing.

There are other algae that are not seaweed; some of these are also used in spa therapy treatments. These include spirulina, a type of blue-green or white algae, which is actually a lichen. Lichens are a combination of a fungus and another organism, usually a type of green algae, which produces food from sunlight. Spirulina and white algae treatments are used in spa treatments for detoxification, revitalization (through increased local blood and lymph circulation), slimming, skin tightening, and moisturizing.

Sea mud is collected from beaches at low tide and mixed with seawater. Like all sea products, it is used for its analgesic, warming, and sedative properties, as well as for detoxification. Sea mud can be used by itself or mixed with clays.

Preparing for a Body Wrap Treatment

Gather the supplies needed for the body wrap application before the client arrives or while he or she is undressing. Essential supplies and equipment include:

- Exfoliation tools or ingredients for a scrub.

- Mud, seaweed, or peat; or powders of any of these mixed with water; or gels or cream of any of these (one-quarter to one-half cup).

- Small, nonmetal bowl—nonmetal because mud and peat react chemically with metal, and their properties will change. Likewise, mud and peat should not be stored in metal containers.

- Three cloth sheets (one fitted and two flat).

- Insulating sheet (rubber, plastic, Mylar, etc.).

- Wool blanket.

- One extra-large towel, approximately 35″ × 65″.

- Two large towels, approximately 30″ × 60″.

- Textured washcloth or bath scrubby the client can use to remove the mud or peat if there is access to a shower.

- If there is no access to a shower, a basin of warm water and three to four towels, approximately 18″ × 30″, for substance removal are needed. A towel cabi or electric pot filled with moist towels can also be used. More towels may be necessary for large clients or for those with a lot of body hair.

- Washcloth.

- Small bowl.

- Cool water.

After the supplies are gathered, prepare the work space in this manner:

- Layer the table in the following order, as shown in Figure 19–12 ■:

  ○ Fitted sheet to protect table

  ○ One large towel placed horizontally across the head of the table

  ○ Wool blanket placed horizontally across the table, on top of the towel, leaving enough room for the head to rest on the towel

  ○ One large towel placed horizontally across the end of the table, on top of the wool blanket

  ○ Flat sheet placed horizontally on top of the wool blanket

  ○ Insulating sheet placed horizontally on top of the cloth sheet

  ○ One flat sheet placed lengthwise on top of the insulating sheet

  ○ Extra-large towel placed lengthwise on top of the flat sheet

- Place the body wrap substance (mud, peat, seaweed) in the small bowl; position the bowl within easy reach.

- If working in a dry room and using an electric pot or cabi, turn it on to warm the smaller towels for substance removal at the end of the treatment. Moisten the towels and put them in the electric pot or cabi.

If using the basin of warm water and towels, place the basin in a convenient place so it can be filled it with warm water during the treatment.

- Fill the small bowl with cool water, and place the washcloth in it. Position it within easy reach.

- Leave the room while the client gets on the table under the extra-large towel, lying prone.

- It is important to stay near the client while he or she is wrapped. Some clients may become claustrophobic or overheated and need to have the wrappings removed as soon as they start feeling uncomfortable.

Performing a Body Wrap Treatment

1. Perform a pre–body wrap exfoliation starting with the client prone and ending with the client supine.

2. Remove the sheet immediately under the client. Use the dry room sheet removal technique described earlier. Set the sheet aside. Make sure that the client's shoulders are slightly below the top of the insulating sheet.

3. Help the client sit up and quickly apply the body wrap substance to the back with long, smooth strokes, covering the area thoroughly (Figure 19–13 ■). Help the client lie back down.

4. Move to the client's left leg and ask him or her to flex the knee while draping carefully and securely. To stabilize the client's leg, gently sit on the foot. Apply the substance to the posterior leg with one smooth stroke (Figure 19–14 ■). Grasp the client's ankle and lay the leg flat.

5. Apply the substance to the client's left anterior leg with long, smooth strokes. Cover the left leg with the

FIGURE 19–12 Layers of sheets and towels on the table for a body wrap.

Source: Pearson Education, Inc.

FIGURE 19–13 Apply the body wrap substance to the back with long, smooth strokes, covering the area thoroughly.

Source: Pearson Education, Inc.

insulating sheet to prevent chilling. Move to the client's right leg and apply the substance to the posterior and anterior leg in the same manner as for the left leg. Cover the right leg with the insulating sheet to prevent chilling.

6. Move to the client's abdomen and drape one of the large towels across the client's chest area and have the client hold it firmly. Pull the bottom draping towel inferiorly until the client's abdomen is undraped. Apply the substance to the abdomen in a clockwise motion (Figure 19–15 ■).

7. Move to the client's left arm and apply the substance to the posterior and anterior arm with long, smooth strokes (Figure 19–16 ■). Cover the left arm and

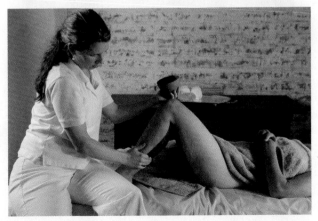

FIGURE 19–14 Apply the substance to the client's posterior leg with one smooth stroke. To stabilize the client's leg, gently sit on her foot.

Source: Pearson Education, Inc.

FIGURE 19–15 Apply the substance to the abdomen in a clockwise motion.

Source: Pearson Education, Inc.

abdomen with the insulating sheet to prevent chilling. Move to the client's right arm and apply the substance the same as for the left arm. Cover the right arm with the insulating sheet to prevent chill.

8. Move to the head of the table and apply the substance to the client's upper chest (Figure 19–17 ■).

9. Wrap the client securely with sheets. Wrap one side over the top of the body (Figure 19–18A ■) then enclose the body completely using the remaining sheet (Figure 19–18B ■).

10. Use the towel at the head of the table to wrap around the client's neck securely.

11. Make sure the client is comfortable using bolsters, pillows, or other props as needed. An extra blanket can be added for more warmth. The client should remain wrapped for 25 to 30 minutes. During this time a scalp and facial massage can be given or the client's feet can be unwrapped for a foot massage. Another option is to sit quietly at the head or foot of the table. Place a cool, moist washcloth on the client's face or forehead if needed.

FIGURE 19–16 Apply the substance to the arm with long, smooth strokes, then cover the arm and abdomen with the insulating sheet to prevent chilling.

Source: Pearson Education, Inc.

FIGURE 19–17 Apply the substance to the client's upper chest.

Source: Pearson Education, Inc.

A

B

FIGURE 19–18 Wrap the client securely with sheets.
(A) Lay one side of the sheet over the body. (B) Enclose the body with the other side of the sheet. Leave the bottom sheet flat.

Source: Pearson Education, Inc.

A

B

FIGURE 19–19 (A) Unwrap each of the layers until the client is covered by just the plastic sheet and the towels with which the client was initially draped. (B) Place a large towel lengthwise over the client, then gently pull the plastic sheet out from underneath the towel.

Source: Pearson Education, Inc.

12. When the time is up, unwrap each of the layers until the client is covered by just the plastic sheet and the towels with which he or she was initially draped (Figure 19–19A ■). Place a large towel lengthwise over the client (Figure 19–19B ■). Gently pull the plastic sheet out from underneath the towel.

13. Help the client sit up with legs hanging off the side of the table. Use a warm, moist towel to remove residue from the client's back.

14. If using a wet table or Vichy shower, rinse the client thoroughly to remove residue. If there is a separate shower facility, help the client off the table, offering

a bathrobe or draping a large towel for modesty. Give the client the textured washcloth or bath scrubby, and guide him or her to the shower and then back to the massage table after rinsing off. If working in a dry room, use the dry room substance removal technique described earlier in Box 19–1. Once the residue has been removed thoroughly from the skin, help the client off the table.

Herbal Wraps

The herbal wrap is probably the most popular and best known herbal spa treatment. It is a full-body moist heat treatment, using multiple towels or muslin sheets soaked in an herbal infusion. The herbal wrap treatment can easily be incorporated into a 60-minute treatment; the wrap itself typically takes 20 to 30 minutes. It can be an individual treatment, or it can be preceded by an exfoliation and followed by a complementary therapy.

HERBS

Herbs are invaluable additions to spa treatments in the form of infusions for wraps, inhalations, and aromatherapy applications. You may discover useful plants that are indigenous to your geographic area. For example, in the southwest, poultices can be made from prickly pear pads (after the needles are removed, of course). In the northeast, chickweed can be used for body wraps. Hayflower grows abundantly in Germany, and spas there have long incorporated it into treatments. Hayflower treatments are now becoming popular in the United States. Table 19–2 ■ lists the effects of common herbs and plants.

Organic and natural food stores are good places to find a variety of high-quality herbs; there are also many Internet sources. Herbs can be purchased either fresh or dried. If fresh plants are desired, only purchase as much as will be used for specific treatments to ensure they do not spoil before the next use. Plants can also be dried by gathering them in small bundles, tying them together with string, and hanging them upside down. Hanging them this way makes it easier to pull leaves off stems.

When the herbs are fully dried, they can be stored in glass jars with tight lids. Even dried plants do not last more than a couple of months before they lose their potency. If a continual supply of high quality, fresh plants is desired, planting an herb garden may be the solution.

TABLE 19–2	Effects of Common Herbs in Spa Treatments	
Stress Relief and Relaxation	Energizing and Balancing	Detoxification
Lavender	Chamomile	Juniper
Chamomile	Clary sage	Ginger
Clary sage	Rosemary	Grapefruit zest
Jasmine	Geranium	Eucalyptus
Marjoram	Lemongrass	Clove
Linden flowers	Orange zest	Lemon balm
Hops	Ylang ylang	Hayflower
Valerian		Oatstraw
Passionflower		Fennel
		Nettle

Sources: Data from Ody, P., *Essential Guide to Natural Home Remedies* (2002); Ody, P., *The Medicinal Herbal* (1993).

HERBAL INFUSIONS

Infusions are one of the easiest methods to prepare herbs for use in spa treatments. An **infusion** involves immersing the leaves, flowers, or berries of a fragrant plant in boiling water. The mixture is then left to stand for 15 to 30 minutes, or longer for a stronger infusion. The infusion water can then be used in simple inhalations and facial saunas (discussed in the Aromatherapy section in this chapter) and herbal wraps.

AROMATHERAPY

Aromatherapy is the therapeutic use of the preparation of fragrant essential oils extracted from plants. According to the National Association for Holistic Therapy, "Aromatherapy can be defined as the art and science of utilizing naturally extracted aromatic essences from plants to balance, harmonize and promote the health of the body, mind and spirit"[1] Aromatherapy has many effects on the body, and it is because of this that aromatherapy can be used in many different ways.

There are so many different ways scents can be used in spa and bodywork treatments, as well as in everyday life,

CRITICAL THINKING

Of the different types of substances that can be used in a body wrap treatment, such as muds, peats, seaweed, and herbal infusions, which one would you want to experience? Compare the benefits, contraindications, equipment, supplies, and procedures of each.

1. Do you have a specific condition that would benefit from this body wrap?
2. What do you think you would like about this body wrap?
3. What do you think you would not like about it?
4. How would you expect to feel after the treatment?

that aromatherapy in popular culture has come to mean anything that is scented in a pleasant way. Air fresheners, candles, and even flower-scented detergents are now called aromatherapy. Scented spray mists to freshen the face or feet, dishes of aromatic beads placed in the treatment room, and lavender-scented lubricants are all examples of what may be considered aromatherapy in the spa and bodywork realm.

One particular type of substance, however, requires more research and education. These are essential oils, and their effects can be so powerful that, to truly understand how they should be used, it is recommended that practitioners who are interested in becoming aromatherapists attend formal courses in aromatherapy. Aromatherapy is regulated in some areas, and practitioners should learn about laws that may affect them.[2] The National Association for Holistic Aromatherapy (www.naha.org) is a valuable source of information. This is an educational, nonprofit organization dedicated to enhancing public awareness of the benefits of true aromatherapy.

This section discusses basic aromatherapy concepts for practitioners who are beginners in the use of essential oils. Information on common essential oils is presented, such as characteristics, uses, and cautions, along with methods of incorporating essential oils into spa and bodywork treatments.

It is important to note that practitioners should never go beyond their scope of practice. Check with local and/or state regulations regarding the use of essential oils in the spa setting or a massage therapy practice. Some areas require that anyone who applies essential oils topically to another person be professionally licensed, such as for massage therapy, energy work, cosmetology, and other practices. Check with all pertinent regulatory bodies to be sure of compliance with laws governing the application of essential oils.

Essential Oils

Essential oils are the volatile oils that aromatic plants, trees, and grasses produce. The term *volatile* means able to vaporize easily at low temperatures. It is the volatility of essential oils that causes their scents to spread so rapidly. These oils can be obtained from any part of the plant. Usually they are distilled from the flowers, roots, rinds of fruits, stalks, sap or resin, nuts, or bark of plants. For example, sandalwood is gathered from the heart of the tree, but only after the tree is at least 40 years old. Eucalyptus is obtained from the leaves of the eucalyptus tree. Neroli, rose, jasmine, and lavender come from the plants' flowers. Various species of frankincense trees grow wild throughout western India, northeastern Africa, and southern Saudi Arabia. The oil is distilled from the gum resin that oozes from incisions made in the bark of the trees. Myrrh comes from a shrub that grows in Ethiopia, Sudan, and Somalia. The shrubs exude a resin that hardens into reddish brown tear-shaped drops—this is myrrh.

How Essential Oils Work

About 200 different essential oils have been extracted from plants for use in aromatherapy and are employed for many different purposes:

- Antiseptics against viruses, bacteria, and fungi
- Analgesics
- Act on the central nervous system to reduce anxiety and insomnia or to be stimulating and energizing
- Act on the endocrine system and metabolism
- Stimulate the immune system

Essential oil preparations that are taken internally may stimulate the immune system and function as antibiotics. Because these are pharmacological uses of essential oils, recommending internal use of essential oils is beyond the scope of practice of massage therapists and bodyworkers and is not discussed in this text.

Other essential oils that are applied to the skin activate thermal (heat) receptors and kill dermal microbes and fungi. They can also be absorbed through the skin from baths, massage treatments, and compresses. Essential oils are readily absorbed through the skin due to their lipid-solubility and the small size of the aromatic molecules. The molecules enter the bloodstream quickly and easily cross the blood–brain barrier to have an effect on the brain. The natural oiliness of the skin also enhances the uptake of essential oils.

Essential oils used for their aromas stimulate a specific part of the brain called the **limbic system**. The limbic system (Figure 19–20 ■) is located within the higher brain, or cerebrum. It is sometimes referred to as the *emotional brain* because it has a major role in a variety of emotions—pleasure, affection, passivity, fear, sorrow, sexual feelings, and anger. It is also involved in memory and *olfaction,* which is the term for the sense of smell. This is why our sense of smell evokes memories much more strongly than any of our other senses. *Olfaction bulbs,* components of the limbic system, are formed of nervous tissue, which plays a role in the brain's interpretation and differentiation of all the diverse aromas we are able to detect.

The limbic system is closely associated with the part of the brain called the hypothalamus that controls many physiological functions and plays a major role in the regulation of homeostasis. It is responsible for, among other things, controlling the autonomic nervous system and regulating emotional and behavioral patterns.

From the olfactory bulbs, the impulses travel along the olfactory tract. The olfactory tract extends into parts of the brain that identify odors, so a person can put a name to them, and to parts of the brain that distinguish different odors, so a person can sort them out. This tract extends into the part of the brain where conscious awareness of smell begins, as well as into the limbic system and hypothalamus. It is this connection to the limbic system and hypothalamus that accounts for emotional and memory-based responses to aromas.

FIGURE 19–20 The limbic system is located within the higher brain, or cerebrum.

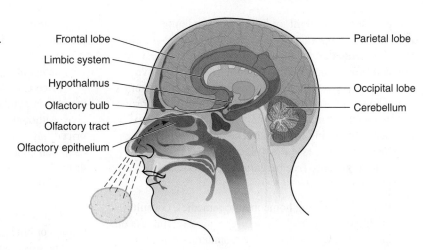

Frontal lobe
Limbic system
Hypothalmus
Olfactory bulb
Olfactory tract
Olfactory epithelium

Parietal lobe
Occipital lobe
Cerebellum

PRECAUTIONS FOR WORKING WITH ESSENTIAL OILS

Essential oils are highly concentrated and volatile, and should be handled with care. There are only two essential oils that can be applied directly to the skin—lavender and tea tree. All other essential oils must be diluted in **carrier oil**, also called *base oil,* before applying to the body. These are typically plant-based oils used to dilute essential oils for use on the skin, as in massage. They can also serve to moisturize the skin and keep essential oils on the skin longer. The carrier oil can be any high-quality vegetable oil such as:

- Sweet almond
- Apricot
- Grape seed
- Olive
- Coconut
- Sunflower
- Jojoba
- Sesame
- Canola
- Sunflower
- Safflower
- Peanut

See Table 19–3 ■ for the percentage of dilution of common essential oils expressed as a certain number of drops per ounce of carrier oil. For example, for a 1% dilution put 5–6 drops of essential oil into the carrier oil.

Additional precautions to keep in mind when working with essential oils:

- A skin test should always be done on clients and on practitioners themselves before any essential oil is used, even if the essential oil has been used before. As stated previously, people can develop allergies

throughout their lives, even to substances to which they have not previously been allergic.

- Essential oils are *never* used near the eyes.

- Pregnancy can be a contraindication, especially during the first trimester. A qualified aromatherapist can be consulted for information about essential oils that work well and those that are contraindicated. Some safe essential oils for use during pregnancy are rose, neroli, lavender, ylang-ylang, chamomile, sandalwood, spearmint, frankincense, and the citruses. A 1% dilution of essential oil to carrier oil should be used on pregnant clients, or one drop added to bath water. When in doubt, do not use essential oils.

- Use essential oils cautiously with clients who are fragile, including babies, small children, the aged, and those who have serious health problems such as asthma, epilepsy, or heart disease. No more than a 1% dilution of essential oil to carrier oil, or one drop added to bath water, should be used for these clients. When in doubt, do not use essential oils.

- Caution should be used with essential oils that can result in photosensitivity. For example, bergamot contains a natural chemical called bergaptene that causes the skin to become very sensitive to ultraviolet light. If bergamot is applied and the skin is

TABLE 19–3	Dilutions of Essential Oils in Carrier Oil	
Dilution	Drops of Essential Oil per Ounce of Carrier Oil
1%	5–6
2%	10–12
3%	15–18

exposed to sunlight, or light from sun lamps or tanning beds, the reaction can be anywhere from mild (just reddening of the skin) to severe (acute lesions and brown spots). Mild reactions usually resolve within a day or so. However, severe reactions can take weeks to resolve, with the accompanying brown spots taking months or years to completely disappear. Removing the bergaptene does not hinder the benefits of the essential oil, so it is recommended that bergaptene-free bergamot be used whenever possible.

• If a client is taking homeopathic remedies, consult a qualified aromatherapist before using essential oils on him or her. Essential oils may counteract the action of the homeopathic remedy.

PURCHASING AND CARE OF ESSENTIAL OILS

It is best to buy only pure, organic, good-quality essential oils. "Organic" means that the plant material was grown without the use of pesticides, herbicides, or fungicides made from synthetic chemicals or petrochemicals.

Avoid synthetic fragrance oils. They have no therapeutic value. Labels on bottles may say "organic," "pure," and "natural," but the oil may, in fact, be synthetic. If the label says "fragrant oil," "perfume oil," or "aromatherapy oil," it is an indication that the oils are not pure oils and have been mixed with other substances. For example, the oil may have been diluted with vegetable oils. A good way to test for this is to place a couple of drops of the essential oil on a piece of paper. If an oily stain is left behind when the essential oil evaporates, it was most likely diluted with vegetable oil.

REALITY CHECK

BARBARA

JACKIE: My client forgot to mention that she had an allergy to nuts, and she is having an allergic reaction to the KuKui nut oil I am using. What should I do?

BARBARA: Stay calm and stop the treatment. Immediately remove all of the oil and rinse the skin. If the reaction is mild and has stopped, ask your client if she would like to continue with the treatment. If so, be sure to check the ingredients on the new lubricant you use. And remember to add the information about her allergy to her health history file and document the incident in session notes.

True essential oils will have the botanical name, not just the common name, on the label. The label will also state that it is a "pure essential oil" or "100% essential oil." If the label is not clear about this information, do not buy it.

Price can also be an indication. Pure, organic oils cost more than synthetic oils or blends. Some are quite expensive. Although orange, lemon, and lime may be reasonably priced, jasmine, neroli, and rose are very costly. The bottle itself can be a guide. The best-quality oils will always be in dark glass bottles to protect them from sunlight. A product line of aromatherapy oils in clear glass bottles that are all the same price are most likely synthetic fragrance oils.

Essential oils are best stored tightly sealed in amber, brown, or blue glass bottles. Oxygen, sunlight, and heat can damage oils, causing them to lose their therapeutic properties. The average shelf life for most essential oils is 2 years, although the citrus oils have a somewhat shorter life expectancy. Unused oils that have reached the end of their shelf life should be discarded. Interestingly, the heavy, woodsy resin-type oils can last much longer (up to 6 years) and are said to actually improve with age.

Classification by Notes

Essential oils have been classified by the French perfume industry according to their *notes,* or scent characteristics, and by the rate at which they evaporate. There are top notes (T), middle notes (M), and base notes (B). Some oils are a combination of top and middle (T/M), or middle and base (M/B) notes.

Top notes have light, fresh, and uplifting qualities. They typically have antiviral properties. Because they evaporate quickly, their scents are usually not long lasting. *Middle notes* comprise the bulk of the essential oils. They have warm, soft fragrances that unfold gradually. Also known as the heart notes, they are the balancing and harmonizing scents. *Base notes* are intense, heavy, long-lasting fragrances that evaporate slowly. They are rich and relaxing and usually are the most expensive essential oils. See Table 19–4 ■ for more information on essential oils and notes.

Ten Foundational Essential Oils

With almost 200 essential oils to choose from, practitioners may not know where to start when beginning their work with aromatherapy. Some practitioners may want to learn as much as they can as fast as they can, whereas others may want to find a few they can use regularly and in many different ways.

Table 19–5 ■ lists and describes 10 essential oils that have many different uses. Purchasing these would provide a good "starter set" of essential oils without investing a large amount of money. As practitioners become more comfortable working with essential oils, they may discover that they want more oils in their collection. Or they may discover that just having these is enough for the treatments they perform.

The information in Table 19–5 provides an introduction to essential oils and does not contain in-depth descriptions.

TABLE 19–4	Essential Oils and Notes		
Note	Top Notes (T)	Middle Notes (M)	Base Notes (B)
Characteristics	Light and airy	Harmonizing	Deep
	Evaporates quickly	Soothing, soft undertones	Intense
	Penetrating or sharp scent	Scent unfolds gradually	Powerful
	Fresh smell		Long lasting
			Warm and sensuous
Examples	Peppermint (T/M)	Chamomile	Rose absolute
	Orange	Cypress	Patchouli
	Lemon	Marjoram	Vetiver
	Lime	Lavender	Jasmine
	Tangerine	Geranium	Myrrh
	Grapefruit	Dill	Frankincense
	Melissa	Celery	Sandalwood
	Lemongrass	Coriander	Benzoin
	Mandarin	Black pepper	Spikenard
	Eucalyptus (T/M)	Juniper	Cedarwood
	Basil	Thyme	
		Rose (M/B)	
		Neroli (M/B)	
		Rosemary	
		Pine	

Source: Data from Pure Essential, Inc., "Essential Oils and Perfume Notes" (2007).

TABLE 19–5	Ten Foundational Essential Oils		
Essential Oil	Characteristics	Uses	Cautions
Bergamot (T) *Citrus bergamia*	Relaxing, refreshing, uplifting, cooling; the flavor of Earl Grey tea; can be a good substitute for rose oil.	Reduces allergies, acne, psoriasis and gas; relieves anxiety; alleviates depression	Avoid exposing skin to sunlight after using this oil until after bathing or showering to remove the oil
Peppermint (T) *Mentha piperta*	Stimulating, refreshing, cooling, restorative; uplifts the mind and body; one of the most useful essential oils	Relaxes the muscles of the digestive system and stimulates bile flow; relieves gas, colic, and indigestion; refreshes tired head and feet; inhale briefly from bottle or apply one drop on a tissue and inhale to revive during travel; blend with rosemary and juniper to make a stimulating morning bath.	Can cause a burning sensation and irritate skin if too much is used or it is not diluted properly; can neutralize homeopathic medicines
Eucalyptus (T) *Eucalyptus globulus*	Energizing and stimulating; cleanses and purifies	Helps relieve respiratory congestion, colds, fevers, and pain; kills airborne bacteria	Do not use on pregnant clients, by pregnant therapists, or by people who have epilepsy; can neutralize homeopathic medicines.
Tea Tree (T) *Melaleuca alternifolia, M. linariifolia, M. uncintata*	Powerful antiseptic, antifungal, and antiviral agent	Reduces acne, cold sores, warts, and burns; cleansing agent for the skin; can be used as a vapor to kill airborne germs; helps combat foot odor and athlete's foot	May be used full strength as a first aid application; do a patch test first on extremely sensitive skin; limit usage to problem area if using undiluted

(continued)

TABLE 19–5 *(continued)*

Essential Oil	Characteristics	Uses	Cautions
Geranium (M/T) *Pelargonium graveolen*	Uplifting and calming	Soothes certain skin conditions; helps relieve PMS, cramps, menstrual and menopausal issues, tension, anxiety, and depression; is an immunostimulant, can be used as an aromatic insect repellant.	Do not use if pregnant or on pregnant clients; do not use on persons with a history of estrogen-dependent cancer
Lavender (M/T) *Lavendula augustifolia, L. officinalis, L. vera*	Most versatile and valuable essential oil; helpful in many ways for the mind and body; safe to use on children; blends easily with many other oils	Helps heal wounds, cuts, burns; relieves headaches; acts as a local anesthetic to relieve pain from sunburn, asthma, and throat infections; relieves irritability and sleeplessness; is an immunostimulant; can be used as an aromatic insect repellant.	Avoid high doses during pregnancy; can cause uterine contractions
Chamomile (Roman Chamomile) (M) *Chamaemelum nobile (formerly known as Anthemis noblis)*	Relaxing; safe to use on children	Relieves pain; increases mental clarity; decreases anxiety, nervous tension, depression, anger, and irritability; soothes sunburn, earaches, toothaches, and headaches	Can neutralize homeopathic medicines
Cypress (M) *Cupressus sempervirens*	Distilled from the twigs, needles, and cones of the cypress tree; has a spicy, smoky, pungent, pinelike scent	Antispasmodic; warming; diuretic; helps relieve edema, asthma, hot flashes; assists in balancing hormonal levels; helps relieve pain from varicose veins and hemorrhoids; decreases the appearance of thread veins; supports weight reduction	Do not use if pregnant or on pregnant clients; do not use on persons with a history of estrogen-dependent cancer
Marjoram (M) *Origanum Marjorana, Majorana hortensis*	Calming, relaxing, and sedating	Relieves pain, insomnia, headaches, constipation, and colds; increases circulation; helps regulate menstrual cycle; helps relieve anxiety; makes an excellent after-sports rub because of its pain-relieving ability	Do not use if pregnant or on pregnant clients; do not use on persons with a history of estrogen-dependent cancer
Rosemary (M) *Rosemarinus officinalis, R. coronarium*	Revives, warms, stimulates, and restores	Refreshes tired muscles and feet; increases mental concentration; perfect in pre- and postsports rubs to maintain suppleness; helps combat water retention; combats fatigue; clears a stuffy atmosphere	Do not use by or on people who are pregnant, by or on people who have epilepsy, or by people who have untreated high blood pressure; can neutralize homeopathic medicines

Sources: Data from Buckle, J., *Clinical Aromatherapy, Essential Oils in Practice* (2007); Price, S., & Price. L., *Aromatherapy for Health Professionals,* 3rd ed. (2007); Rose, J., *375 Essential Oils and Hydrosols* (1999); Shutes, J., & Weaver, C., *Aromatherapy for Bodyworkers* (2008); Tisserand, R. B., *The Art of Aromatherapy* (1985); Worwood, V. A., *The Fragrant Heavens* (1999).

The information is not intended to treat, cure, prevent, or diagnose any disease, disorder, or health condition.

BLENDING ESSENTIAL OILS

Used individually, essential oils can have powerful effects. Sometimes, though, blending different essential oils together creates a more optimal outcome. The main thing to keep in mind when considering which essential oils to blend together is the intention behind the blend. For example, if the goal is the creation of pleasant and relaxing ambiance for the treatment area, any essential oils that are soothing can be blended and placed in a diffuser. On the other hand, if a client's muscles are tense, a blend of essential oils that specifically helps muscles relax can be created.

The French perfume industry considers a well-rounded blend to contain top, middle, and base notes. Top notes can be up to 20% of the blend, middle notes are approximately

50% to 80% of the blend, whereas the deep base notes can be up to 5% of the blend. Using this as a guideline, the majority of the blend should contain middle note essential oils because they tend to harmonize with other oils the best. Because top note oils are lighter and more quickly detected by the nose, they are used in a lesser amount. Base note oils are intense and longer lasting, so they are usually used in the least amount.

For example, if a 2% well-rounded blend is desired, 10 to 12 drops of essential oil will be added to 1 ounce of carrier oil, according to Table 19–3. Of those, 2 drops might be a top note oil, 5 to 8 drops a middle note oil, and 1 to 3 drops a base note oil.

However, all three notes do not always have to be used in a blend; it all depends on the individual properties of the essential oils, what they will be used for, and the blender's preference of oils and the desired final scent.

Using Essential Oils in a Spa or Massage Therapy Practice

There are numerous ways to use essential oils for aromatherapy purposes. These include diffusers, aromastones, scented candles, scented massage oils and lotions, simple inhalation treatments, and scrubs.

- **Diffusers.** Aromatherapy diffusers come in many sizes, shapes, and styles. The basic diffuser is a ceramic pot with a small bowl to hold water and essential oils (4 to 6 drops), heated by a small candle (Figure 19–21 ■). The warmth of the candle releases the properties in the essential oils. Another type of aromatherapy diffuser uses the warmth of hot water indirectly. A plate is placed over a pot filled with hot water, and 4 to 6 drops of essential oil are placed on the plate. As the plate warms, the essential oil evaporates and diffuses into the air. There are also electric diffusers, some with fans, some made of glass. These diffusers disinfect and scent the atmosphere by releasing droplets of essential oil as a cool mist.

- **Aromastones.** Aromastones are made of porcelain or ceramic and plug into electrical outlets. Essential oil is poured directly onto the heated porcelain or ceramic surface; no water is needed.

FIGURE 19–21 Aromatherapy diffuser. The warmth of the candle releases the properties in the essential oils.

Source: Pearson Education, Inc.

- **Scented Candles.** Candles come in all different sizes and shapes and scents. They can be made of paraffin, soy wax, or beeswax. High-quality candles that burn cleanly and are scented with pure essential oils are the best to use.

- **Scented Massage Oils, Lotions, and Cream.** To prepare one application, dilute 10 to 12 drops of essential oil with 1 ounce of an unscented carrier oil, lotion, or cream. If preparing a 4 to 8 ounce bottle of oil or lotion, or a 4 to 8 ounce jar of cream, the addition of a few drops of jojoba oil, vitamin E oil, or wheat germ oil will act as a preservative.

- **Simple Inhalation Treatments.** Simple inhalation treatments using essential oils are excellent for relieving head congestion and sinus infections. Pour 1 quart of boiling water into a large bowl. Add 5 to 8 drops of the desired essential oil and stir. Cover head with a towel, and lean over water. Keep eyes closed and breathe deeply through the nose for 5 to 15 minutes, depending on your level of comfort. Rinse face with cool water, and gently blot skin dry. Essential oils can also be used in steam cabinets; just add 5 to 8 drops to the water.

- **Scrubs.** The scrubs discussed previously in this chapter can be enhanced by adding 2 to 3 drops of desired essential oil to the manual exfoliation mixture.

CRITICAL THINKING

Experiment with using aromatherapy therapy three different ways. Compare the therapeutic benefits and safety precautions of each essential oil.

1. What essential oils blend well together?

2. How would you make aromatherapy massage oils, lotions, and creams that are soothing, invigorating, or "sports blends" effective for working on tight muscles?

3. How cost effective is it to incorporate aromatherapy into a massage practice?

STONE MASSAGE

Stone massage involves the use of hot or cold stones for therapeutic purposes. Basically, a stone is a collection of minerals with a very dense structure. The main type of stone used in hot stone therapy is basalt because its chemical structure makes it ideal for retaining heat (Figure 19–22 ■). Round, smooth basalt stones are heated and then placed on or tucked around the client and used in the palms of the practitioner's hands to massage the body. Marble, jade, and sardonyx are often used for cold stone therapy because their chemical structures retain coolness. Chilled stones are applied after deep focus work or during deep tissue and trigger point therapy. The beneficial effects of stone massage and its contraindications are shown in Table 19–6 ■.

There are currently many different types of hot and cold stone therapy options. Treatments can range from simple treatments using a few stones to elaborate setups using multiple sets of stones. The stones are adaptable to a variety of modalities. There are custom sets especially for estheticians, reflexologists, practitioners of Asian bodywork, physical therapists, chiropractors, sports massage therapists, and spa practitioners.

Because of the heat involved in stone massage treatments, it is highly recommended that practitioners learn how to use them from experienced and credentialed instructors. The risk of practitioners injuring clients and themselves due to lack of proper supervised instruction is otherwise too great.

Preparing for Stone Massage

For a hot stone application, the basalt stones need to be heated in water that is 130° to 140°F for 45 to 60 minutes. They retain the heat for a relatively long time, but the body

FIGURE 19–22 Basalt is the most common type of stone used in hot stone therapy.

Source: Antonino D'Anna/Fotolia.

draws heat from the stones so newly heated stones need to be continually reapplied during a treatment.

If the stones are used at 120°F or below, they tend to lose heat rapidly and are not as beneficial. However, 110° to 120°F is a good temperature to use on people who are frail or have a low tolerance to heat. When the treatment is being learned, it is best to begin at the lower temperatures.

Cold stones are able to draw a great deal of heat away from the body. Chilling time for stones is about 15 minutes using ice or an hour using a freezer. Their temperature should be at or just above freezing (32°F) to be effective.

Both hot and cold stones can be used in the same treatment to achieve different effects. The weight of the stones also provides benefits during treatments because the weight helps heat to penetrate the body or, if cold stones are being used, to draw heat from the body more readily.

TABLE 19–6	Stone Massage: Beneficial Effects, Therapeutic Uses, and Contraindications		
Beneficial Effects of Hot Stone Massage	Beneficial Effects of Cold Stone Massage	Therapeutic Uses of Both Hot and Cold Stone Massage	Contraindications for Stone Massage
• Increases blood flow to soft tissues • Relaxes tight muscles • Makes connective tissue more pliable • Warms the joints so that they move more easily • Creates an overall sense of relaxation	• Decreases inflammation and swelling (cold acts as a vasoconstrictor) • Enhances tissue repair after deep tissue work • Slows down nerve or pain impulses • Provides analgesic effects	• Injuries both acute and chronic • Muscle spasms • Osteoarthritis, tendinitis, and bursitis (cold for acute stages; heat for noninflammatory stages) • Sprains, strains (cold for acute stages; heat for noninflammatory stages) • Headache • Stress	• Heart conditions • Hypertension • Fever • Vascular disease in area stones would be applied • Numbness or loss of sensation in area stones would be applied • Broken or irritated skin • Inflammation (contraindication for heat) • Pregnancy • Physical frailty • Intolerance to heat • Intolerance to cold

FIGURE 19–23 Hot stones placed on the sacrum, up the back, and into each of the palms.

Source: Dangubic/Fotolia.

Oil is the lubricant of choice for stone massage; lotions and creams do not provide enough glide. Because of its thickness, jojoba oil is recommended. A generous amount of oil is needed to perform stone massage because of the heat of the stones and their weight.

Performing Hot Stone Massage

1. Remove stones from hot water and dry off.

2. With the client prone and draped with an extra-large towel, approximately 35″ × 65″, place a large, flat stone under the abdomen (protected by a towel), another on the towel over the sacrum, others up the client's back, and into each of the client's palms (Figure 19–23 ▪). Let the heat penetrate into the body for a period of time.

3. Choose a pair of stones to use for massage and uncover the area to be massaged.

4. After massaging oil on the client's body, apply the stones with firm pressure and long, gliding strokes, making several passes. Keep the stones on muscle tissue, and avoid the bony areas. Strokes on the extremities should always be performed toward the shoulder.

5. When the stones start to lose their heat, return them to the heating unit, and use another pair.

6. Hot stones can be used on the client's back (Figure 19–24 ▪), posterior arms, posterior legs and gluteals (Figure 19–25 ▪), feet, and posterior neck.

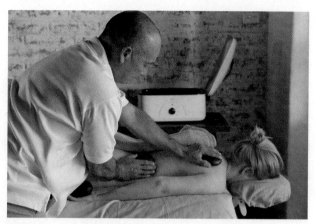

FIGURE 19–24 Hot stones used to massage the back

Source: Pearson Education, Inc.

7. Specific work can also be performed with stones (Figure 19–26 ▪).

8. When finished with the client's posterior side, help the client turn over, making sure he or she stays draped, as described in Chapter 11, *Body Mechanics, Table Skills, General Guidelines.*

9. With the client supine, place the hot hand stones in the client's hands and the toe stones between the client's toes. Cold stones can also be placed along the client's torso and on the forehead. A hot stone can be placed under the client's neck (Figure 19–27 ▪).

10. Hot stones can be used to massage the client's anterior arms, hands, anterior legs, upper chest, neck (Figure 19–28 ▪) and face (Figure 19–29 ▪).

11. Finish by removing the stones placed on the client's body and then performing some long, gliding strokes to close the treatment.

FIGURE 19–25 Hot stones used to massage the gluteals and posterior leg.

Source: Pearson Education, Inc.

FIGURE 19–26 Using hot stones for specific applications under the scapula

Source: Pearson Education, Inc.

FIGURE 19–28 Using a hot stone to massage the neck.

Source: Pearson Education, Inc.

FIGURE 19–27 A hot stone placed under the client's neck.

Source: Pearson Education, Inc.

FIGURE 19–29 Using hot stones to massage the face.

Source: Pearson Education, Inc.

When to Use Cold Stones

Chilled stones can be used in place of heated stones anywhere in a stone massage application. They can be used in combination with heated stones, tucked under the abdomen, or placed along either side of the spine when the client is supine. But they are primarily used following hot stones on a focus area. They are extremely effective when used to chill an area either before or after specific work. The cold stones draw heat from the body, so they are effective where there is inflammation or to ease the discomfort of sunburn.

As a consideration to the client, it is important to verbally announce cold stones before you apply to them to the client's body. Ask the client to take a deep breath as the stone is applied, and to let the breath out immediately after the stone is applied. Having the client focus on the breath is a way to draw attention away from the chill of the stone, and breathing deeply helps the client release muscle tension caused by the application of the cold stone. The application of chilled stones is done slowly and gradually, giving the client time to adjust to the change in temperature. Cold stones are applied with firm pressure, held in place momentarily, and then moved slowly around the area until it is thoroughly chilled.

CASE FOR STUDY

Carolina and Her First Spa Treatment

Carolina has been "burning the candle at both ends." She is working on her master's degree while struggling to keep up with increased demands in her job as a school administrator. She hasn't been eating as well as she normally does and feels depleted. She receives massage sporadically from Jaime. During their last massage, Jaime mentioned that he has learned some spa treatments and shared some of their benefits with her. Carolina has decided to take some time for herself and try one of Jaime's spa treatments.

Question:

Which spa treatments would help her feel rejuvenated?

Things to consider:

- What questions should Jaime ask Carolina to determine which treatment would be most beneficial? Be sure to ask about allergies.
- What are the benefits and indications of the various treatments?
- What are the equipment and supplies needed for the treatments?
- How are these treatments performed?

Which spa treatment do you think Jaime should recommend to Carolina?

_____

_____

_____

_____

CHAPTER HIGHLIGHTS

- Spa treatments are offered at spa establishments but can also be used by massage therapists in private practice.
- The applications that form the foundation of most spa menus are exfoliation, body wraps, aromatherapy, and stone massage.
- Spa equipment and supplies include hot towel cabi, wet table, Vichy shower, wet room, linens, substances, toiletries, cleaning supplies, and disposable gloves.
- Follow sanitation guidelines for spa application equipment and supplies because spa treatment settings are especially vulnerable to mold growth and disease transmission.
- Spa treatments need to be explained to clients in depth and include
  - Benefits, indications, and contraindications
  - How the treatment is performed
  - What results the client can expect
  - How the client can expect to feel after the treatment
  - Levels of nudity involved for certain treatments
- A health and medical history of the client is important to obtain before beginning any treatments.
- Eliciting information from clients about their likes and dislikes and previous spa treatment experiences is important, so that practitioners can recommend the best spa application for them.

- Contraindications and safety guidelines for all forms of spa applications should be observed to avoid harm to the client.
- Exfoliation is the peeling and sloughing off of dead skin cells from the surface of the body. Benefits include brightening the skin, encouraging the production of new skin cells, making the skin smoother, allowing other preparations to hydrate and nourish the skin, and stimulating superficial blood and lymph flow.
  - Manual exfoliation is the physical process of applying friction with abrasives. It includes dry body brushing, scrubs (frictions), and body polishes.
  - Chemical, enzyme, or dissolving exfoliations use chemicals or enzymes that work by dissolving dead skin cells.
- Body wraps can be used in conjunction with many different substances. Muds, peats, and seaweed are all commonly used materials, as well as sheets soaked in an herbal infusion (herbal wraps).
  - Muds help with deep skin cleansing and aid in the removal of waste products, stimulate local blood and lymphatic flow, and are excellent warming and hydrating treatments.

○ Peats draw and absorb toxins from the body, are warming and hydrating, and increase local blood and lymph circulation.

○ Seaweed and sea mud firm the skin, help eliminate toxins, stimulate blood circulation, and are moisturizing.

○ Herbs and plants used in herbal wraps can be for stress-relief and relaxation, energizing and balancing, or detoxification.

● Aromatherapy is the therapeutic use of fragrant essential oils extracted from plants.

○ Follow all precaution guidelines when working with essential oils.

○ Buy only pure, organic, good-quality essential oils.

○ Essential oils can be used in spa applications and massage practices in diffusers, lightbulb rings, aromastones, scented candles, scented oils, lotions and creams, and scrubs.

● Stone massage involves the use of hot and cold stones during a treatment.

○ Heat from warmed basalt stones applied to the body increases blood flow to soft tissues, relaxes tight muscles, and makes connective tissue more pliable.

○ Cold from chilled marble, jade, or sardonyx stones is very effective in decreasing inflammation and swelling. Cold also slows down nerve impulses, including pain impulses, which makes it an ideal analgesic.

EXAM REVIEW

Key Terms

Match the following key terms to their descriptions. For additional study, look up the key terms in the Interactive Glossary, and note other terms that compare or contrast with them.

_____ 1. Aromatherapy
_____ 2. Body polishes
_____ 3. Body wraps
_____ 4. Carrier oil
_____ 5. Chemical, enzyme, or dissolving exfoliation
_____ 6. Clays
_____ 7. Dry brushing
_____ 8. Emollient
_____ 9. Essential oils
_____ 10. Exfoliation
_____ 11. Infusion
_____ 12. Limbic system
_____ 13. Manual exfoliation
_____ 14. Muds
_____ 15. Peat
_____ 16. Scrubs
_____ 17. Stone massage

a. Substance that makes the skin soft and supple
b. Organic soil that contains minerals, organic material, water, and trapped air
c. Created by immersing the leaves, flowers, or berries of a fragrant plant in boiling water
d. Therapeutic use of fragrant essential oils extracted from plants
e. Physical process of applying friction with abrasives
f. Derived from different soils and marine sediments
g. Gentler form of exfoliation using finely ground natural substances such as crushed almonds or grape seed meal
h. Located within the cerebrum, it plays a major role in memory and the sense of smell
i. Exfoliation method using salts, sugar, or coarser organic substances
j. Exfoliation using brushes or fiber tools
k. Peeling and sloughing off of dead skin cells from the surface of the body
l. Exfoliation using substances that loosen the keratin that holds skin cells together, allowing the cells to be easily sloughed off
m. The use of hot or cold stones for therapeutic purposes
n. Treatment used for detoxification in which a substance is applied and the body is wrapped in sheets, blankets, and/or a plastic covering
o. Volatile oils that aromatic plants, trees, and grasses produce
p. Aid deep skin cleansing by drawing impurities from the body
q. Plant-based oil used to dilute essential oils for use on the skin

Memory Workout

To test your memory of the main concepts in this chapter, complete the following sentences by circling the most correct answer from the two choices provided.

1. A (Vichy) (hot cabi) shower has multiple nozzles that hang above the client.
2. It is the responsibility of practitioners in spas to be knowledgeable about all (exercises) (treatments) they provide.
3. Contraindications for certain spa applications include common allergies to foods such as (shellfish) (olives) and nuts.
4. To help clients choose spa treatments, practitioners should ask what their desired (goals) (expenses) are for the treatment.
5. The physical process of applying friction with coarse substances or textures is called (body polish) (manual exfoliation).
6. Exfoliation using brushes or fiber tools is known as (dry) (coarse) brushing or (manual) (body) brushing.
7. For a scrub, the salt or sugar is usually mixed with just enough water to make it the consistency of (oatmeal) (snow).
8. (Body polishes) (Scrubs) would be the best choice for clients who have sensitive skin.
9. Muds are categorized based on their region of origin and (density) (composition).
10. The substances in peat that contribute to its therapeutic effectiveness are organic acids and (minerals) (marine sediments).
11. After applying the body wrap substance to each extremity, it is important to cover the extremity with the insulating sheet to prevent (smearing) (chilling).
12. Seaweed and other sea products are organic materials that have abundant salts, vitamins, and other (coarse) (trace) elements essential to the body.
13. Two herbs that can be used for a detoxifying herbal wrap are (lemon balm) (sage) and (ginger) (anise).
14. Jasmine, lavender, and chamomile are all herbs that can be used for (pain) (stress) relief.
15. Harmonizing and soothing are terms used to describe essential oils that are (low) (middle) notes.
16. An essential oil that should not be used on clients with epilepsy is (eucalyptus) (lavender).
17. The main type of stone used in hot stone therapy is (marble) (basalt).
18. For clients who are frail or have a low tolerance to heat, stones should be heated to a temperature of (110°–120°F) (130°–140°F).

Test Prep

The following multiple-choice questions will help to prepare you for future school and professional exams.

1. Which of the following is one of the ways practitioners can help clients choose appropriate spa and hydrotherapy treatments?
   a. Respect client privacy by avoiding questions about medical history.
   b. Give the treatment the client asks for, even if there are contraindications.
   c. Offer the client discounts on treatments that would be ineffective for the client.
   d. Determine whether the client has any skin rashes or allergies.

2. If a client wants a body wrap but dislikes the smell of seaweed, the practitioner could:
   a. Offer the client a different treatment
   b. Explain the benefits of a seaweed treatment
   c. Refuse to do the treatment
   d. Reschedule the client for another time

3. If a client is uncomfortable with minimal draping during a treatment, the practitioner can:
   a. Reassure the client that everyone feels that way
   b. Explain that that is what the treatment requires
   c. Refuse to do the treatment
   d. Adjust coverings until the client is comfortable

4. In addition to being an exfoliant, salt is a natural:
   a. Moisturizer
   b. Detoxifier
   c. Emollient
   d. Vasodilator

5. On which of the following should dry brushing strokes be applied lightly?
   a. Abdomen
   b. Back
   c. Feet
   d. Neck

6. When making an exfoliant with natural substances, which of the following fluids can be combined with an abrasive?
   a. Milk
   b. Oil
   c. Water
   d. Any of the above

7. A therapeutic property of mud is that it is:
   a. Dehydrating to the skin
   b. Cooling to the body
   c. An effective vasoconstrictor
   d. Warming to the body

8. Which of the following describes a correct way to layer the table to prepare for a body wrap?
   a. Wool blanket, insulating sheet, cotton sheet, extra-large towel
   b. Cotton sheet, wool blanket, insulating sheet, cotton sheet
   c. Insulating sheet, cotton sheet, wool blanket, extra-large towel
   d. Cotton sheet, wool blanket, cotton sheet, insulating sheet

9. In a body wrap treatment, the typical length of time a client remains wrapped is:
   a. 10–15 minutes
   b. 25–30 minutes
   c. 30–45 minutes
   d. 45–60 minutes

10. Which of the following is used in spa treatments to relieve inflammation and muscle soreness?
    a. Spirulina
    b. Red seaweed
    c. Green seaweed
    d. White algae

11. What is the *minimum* amount of time herbs should be allowed to steep while making an infusion?
    a. 5 minutes
    b. 15 minutes
    c. 20 minutes
    d. 25 minutes

12. Essential oils are used for the purposes of:
    a. Increasing pain sensations
    b. Increasing anxiety and insomnia
    c. Stimulating the immune system
    d. Stimulating bacterial growth

13. Which of the following oils would be safe to use on a pregnant client?
    a. Cypress
    b. Bergamot
    c. Geranium
    d. Eucalyptus

14. Which of the following is a contraindication for hot stone therapy?
    a. Pregnancy
    b. Low back pain
    c. Chest congestion
    d. Headache

15. Which of the following can be used for cold stone therapy?
    a. Marble
    b. Basalt
    c. Sardonyx
    d. Both a and c

Comprehension Exercises

The following short-answer questions test your knowledge and understanding of chapter topics and provide practice in written communication skills. Explain in two to four complete sentences.

1. Explain how practitioners can communicate with clients to provide them with the best spa application possible.

2. Describe how aromatherapy can be incorporated into a massage practice.
3. Identify the beneficial effects of hot stone therapy and cold stone therapy.

For Greater Understanding

The following exercises are designed to take you from the realm of theory into the real world. They will help give you a deeper understanding of the subjects covered in this chapter. Action words are underlined to emphasize the variety of activities presented to address different learning styles and to encourage deeper thinking.

1. Visit a spa or massage practice that provides spa applications. Observe how the staff and practitioners communicate with you about such matters as choosing a treatment, contraindications, draping practices, or how best to enjoy the spa experience. What did they communicate especially well? What could they have communicated better? Report to your study partner or group about your experience, and explain how you would improve client communications.

2. Create a regional aromatherapy or body scrub treatment utilizing an herb, plant, or other substance found in your geographic area. Consider the equipment and supplies you will need, as well as the amount of time needed to perform the applications.

3. Design your own spa treatment menu based on the treatments you have developed. Think about which treatments can be successfully paired with others to offer distinctive, personalized spa experiences to clients. Discuss your spa menu with your study partner or group.

MyHealthProfessionsLab™

MyHealthProfessionsLab.com is a premium online homework management system that includes a host of features to help you study. Registered users will find:

- Powerful tools that track and analyze your results—allowing you to create a personalized learning experience
- Videos, flashcards and other learning tools to help enrich your progress
- Streaming lesson presentations and self-paced learning modules
- A space where you and your instructors can view and manage your assignments

CHAPTER

20   Seated Massage

Pearson Education, Inc.

CHAPTER OUTLINE

Learning Outcomes

Key Terms

Seated Massage Overview

History of Seated Massage

Benefits of Seated Massage

Body and Hand Mechanics

Screening for Seated Massage

Positioning for Seated Massage

Seated Massage Sessions

Preparing for Different Venues

Chapter Highlights

Exam Review

LEARNING OUTCOMES

After studying this chapter, you will have the information to:

1. Trace the history of seated massage.
2. Explain the benefits of seated massage.
3. Define on-site massage.
4. Practice good body mechanics when giving seated massage.

5. Screen for contraindications and cautions.
6. Position clients comfortably on massage chairs.
7. Perform a skillful seated massage Practice Sequence.
8. Plan for seated massage given at events and on-site.

KEY TERMS

Massage chair

Massage chair adjustments

On-site massage

Repetitive strain injuries (RSIs)

Screening interview

Seated massage

Vertical position

Workplace wellness programs

SEATED MASSAGE OVERVIEW

Massage is sometimes given with the recipient sitting on a special massage chair or on a regular chair adapted for the purpose. This is referred to as **seated massage** or *chair massage*. Being skilled in seated massage offers massage therapists more options for positioning clients and for giving massage in public venues such as community health fairs and workplaces. The massage techniques are the same for seated massage and table massage; however, there are some special considerations for client positioning and body mechanics. Seated massage is not new in the history of massage, but has regained popularity recently with the development of the portable massage chair in the 1980s.

History of Seated Massage

Throughout the centuries, massage has been given wherever it was convenient to do so, including with recipients seated on the ground, on stools, chairs, and tables. Some examples are a servant giving a foot massage to a lady sitting on a stool after a bath, a village healer treating a headache by rubbing the head of a man sitting on a tree stump, an athletic masseur rubbing the legs of an athlete sitting on a training table, and a physiotherapist in an army hospital massaging a soldier's arm while he is sitting on a chair. The body part to be massaged was easily accessed with the recipient sitting on some surface.

It was not until the early 1900s that full-body massage with the recipient lying on a padded table gained popularity. Swedish massage in particular became so popular during the twentieth century that for most people, the word *massage* conjured up a picture of someone lying on a table underneath a sheet.

That changed in the 1980s with the invention of a chair designed specifically for positioning a client for massage. The first modern **massage chair** was developed in the 1980s by David Palmer of San Francisco. The original idea of the massage chair was to make receiving massage readily available to the general public. The chair can be transported easily, allows recipients to receive massage sitting up and with their clothes on, and can be used in public areas. Massage techniques that do not need oil for their application are generally used for seated massage. A typical modern massage chair is shown in Figure 10–13.

The first massage chairs were promoted as the foundation for **on-site massage**. On-site massage means that the massage practitioner goes to where the potential clients are, thereby making massage more accessible. One of the first large corporations to provide on-site massage for its employees was Apple Computer Corporation in 1984.[1] Massage chairs are now familiar sights in a number of public places, such as in stores and day spas, at trade shows and conventions, at shopping malls and airports, and even on the street and in parks.

The availability of the massage chair has sparked renewed interest in the potential for giving massage to seated clients. In addition to massage for relaxation and rejuvenation, clinical massage applications are being adapted for the seated position. It is also used for special populations such as athletes, the elderly, and people with disabilities. Seated massage can supplement standard massage and provide additional income or may constitute a full-time massage therapy practice. Some massage therapists specialize in giving seated massage in the workplace.

BENEFITS OF SEATED MASSAGE

The benefits of seated massage are largely the same as for table massage. It promotes general relaxation, improved circulation, muscle relaxation, and mental clarity. Having a massage chair available in a massage office can be useful as an alternative or as an adjunct to table massage. Some clients may prefer massage in a chair, but more often a massage chair is used to give better positioning for certain therapeutic applications, for example, the shoulder, arm, or back.

Outside the massage therapy office, seated massage has the added benefit of being more convenient for those with less discretionary time, and the massage therapist and chair can travel easily to where potential clients are located. Some benefits are related to the specific venues where seated massage takes place.

Public Places and Events

Seated massage at airports and train stations provides a respite from the stresses of traveling. It relieves muscle tension from sitting in uncomfortable positions and gets the circulation going after long periods of sitting. It also presents a pleasurable pastime for those waiting for the next leg of their journey. Because travelers do not have to get undressed for massage, and the time is relatively short, seated massage can be squeezed in between flights or trains.

Seated massage in malls and stores is a walk-by opportunity. Shoppers not planning or scheduling a massage ahead of time have the chance to stop for a brief session. It may motivate people new to massage to give it a try. Such a public venue may seem safe and too convenient to pass up. Seated massage gives shoppers a chance to get off their feet and be rejuvenated for the rest of the day's activities.

Seated massage at trade shows can be an attraction that brings attendees to a specific booth. It serves as a break from walking exhibition halls and sitting in meetings and lectures. Besides its physical benefits, massage can help attendees stay alert for long days of meetings and networking.

Health fairs, fund-raising runs and walks, and other community events are also prime venues for seated massage. They are places to expose potential clients to massage in general and to the massage therapists in their communities. Recipients reap the overall health benefits of massage at a convenient time and place.

In the Workplace

Massage is increasingly popular in **workplace wellness programs**. These employer-sponsored programs make services and activities available to employees to improve their overall health and well-being. Seated massage, in particular, is popular with businesses exploring ways to reduce employee stress on the job and to minimize job-related injuries.

Many tasks performed by workers in the past are now done by sophisticated machines run by computers. However, many workers still sit at workstations for long periods of time performing repetitive tasks such as using computer keyboards, sorting objects, or assembling parts. Tradespeople, craftspeople, artists, and musicians repeat certain movements over and over, stressing their bodies. These repetitive movements can lead to debilitating musculoskeletal problems.

Repetitive strain injuries (RSIs) are common in a number of occupations. RSIs may involve tendinitis (inflammation of tendons), bursitis (inflammation of fluid sacs around a joint), ganglion cysts (a mass formed over a tendon), or nerve impingement. Symptoms of RSI include aching, tenderness, swelling, tingling, numbness, weakness, loss of flexibility, and spasms in the muscles affected. RSI can result in chronic pain, loss of mobility, and eventually, disability. Massage is effective for preventing and treating various forms of RSI and can be a valuable component of a comprehensive rehabilitation plan.

Tension headaches are also common at work. They have a variety of causes, including poor posture, lack of movement, mental tension, and poor nutrition. Headaches are more common toward the end of the day with the accumulation of stresses. Massage that addresses tension and trigger points in the shoulders and neck can be very effective in treating tension headaches. See Figure 22–2 for trigger points related to tension headaches.

The stress level of employees is a major wellness factor in the workplace. Meeting deadlines, working long hours, and relationships with coworkers are just some of the stressful aspects of work life. The dizzying pace of modern times, at work and in everyday life, also adds to the stress of employees. A high level of chronic stress is known to have a negative effect on health. It compromises the immune system and reduces the ability to concentrate. In the workplace, massage can be an oasis of relaxation in an otherwise stressful environment.

Massage also has been found to increase mental clarity and alertness. Studies show that workers who received seated massage got more work done and made fewer mistakes.[2,3] Practitioners can adapt massage sessions to address the needs of workers, and the use of massage chairs makes offering this service in the workplace convenient.

One study on work-site acupressure massage found that the group receiving the specific massage protocol enjoyed significant health benefits. The massage was a 20-minute session received twice weekly for a period of 8 weeks. The recipients were fully clothed. Techniques included Swedish massage, acupressure, and reflexology. Results showed that people receiving massage had a significant decrease in anxiety, an increase in emotional control, a decrease in perceived sleep disturbances, decreased blood pressure, improved cognition, and a decrease in perception of muscle tightness.[4] Training is available for massage practitioners desiring to specialize in chair massage, and information about different workshops and certificate programs can be found on the Internet.

Popularity of Seated Massage

Seated massage is popular for a number of different reasons. It takes less time than table massage and eliminates having to undress. It has immediate positive effects; recipients usually feel better right away. It may alleviate some of the physical aches and pains developed from sitting, standing, or walking for long periods of time. In contrast to other wellness practices, massage requires no practice and little effort on the part of the recipient. It complements other health practices such as exercise and stress-reduction programs.

Seated massage in the workplace helps increase good feelings about the employer and promotes loyalty. It boosts productivity and can be taken advantage of by most workers.

BODY AND HAND MECHANICS

Body and hand mechanics for giving seated massage are based on the same principles as for table massage, but are adapted for a client in a more vertical position. To summarize:

- Keep your spine and head in good alignment, shoulders down, joints stacked, and wrists in a neutral position.

- Apply pressure forward or downward by leaning into the technique with your body weight rather than just pushing with the arms.

- Use a bow-and-arrow stance for most techniques, and lower the body by bending the knees.

- Kneel if necessary to reach the arms and hands to keep your back and neck in alignment.

For more detailed information on hand and body mechanics for seated massage, see Chapter 11, *Body Mechanics, Table Skills, General Guidelines*.

SCREENING FOR SEATED MASSAGE

Before giving seated massage, screen for contraindications and cautions. When massaging repeat clients, for example at a regular workplace appointment, you may be familiar with recipients and their health histories. However, at events and places such as airports and trade shows, you may be seeing clients on a one-time basis. A brief **screening interview**

REALITY CHECK

RANDY: I'm having a hard time adapting my massage techniques to work with someone clothed sitting upright. And my back and my thumbs hurt after I do seated massage for a while. How can I get more skilled at this?

ANTONIA: Seated massage does take some getting used to at first. You have to be really aware of maintaining good body and hand mechanics until they become more natural. Seated massage requires a lot more bending of the knees, and wider stances. Many people incorporate techniques from Eastern bodywork forms such as acupressure that do not use oil or lotion. Learn the practice sequence presented in class, and then experiment with variations of techniques such as compression, kneading, and direct pressure.

will reveal important information. At a minimum, ask the recipient:

1. Have you ever had a massage before? In a massage chair?
2. Have you had any illness or injuries recently?
3. Are you taking any medication?
4. If a woman: Are you pregnant?
5. Do you wear contact lenses?
6. Are there any areas you want me to avoid when giving the massage?
7. Do you have low blood pressure or are you prone to fainting?

The answer to the first question lets you know how much instruction to offer the recipient during the session. Questions 2 and 3 may reveal general and regional contraindications or cautions for massage. See Chapter 8, *Endangerment Sites, Contraindications, Cautions*, to review contraindications.

If a woman is pregnant (question 4), ask follow-up questions to screen further for contraindications relevant to pregnancy. Some authorities consider pregnancy to be a general contraindication for seated massage, whereas others advise appropriate cautions. Techniques applied to the back

that result in heavy pressure against the abdomen should be avoided. See Chapter 18, *Special Populations and Adaptations*, for more information on contraindications for massage during pregnancy.

If the recipient wears contact lenses (question 5), be sure that the face cradle does not press against the eyes or will not displace the contact lenses. Question 6 offers the recipient the opportunity to set personal boundaries. It may also lead to further information about regional contraindications. The last question (7) is important because massage may temporarily lower blood pressure further. When lying on a massage table, this usually does not present a problem. But when sitting up, a drop in blood pressure can result in light-headedness, dizziness, or fainting. If any of these symptoms occur during the seated massage, help the recipient off the chair and have him or her lie on the ground. Elevating the legs helps bring blood pressure back to normal.

POSITIONING FOR SEATED MASSAGE

Positioning clients for seated massage takes into consideration the type of chair available, the parts of the body to be massaged, and the types of techniques to be applied. Review Chapter 11, *Body Mechanics, Table Skills, General Guidelines*, for a description of positioning recipients in regular chairs when a massage chair is unavailable. A portable tabletop device designed to offer support for the chest and head when the recipient is seated at a desk or table is shown in Figure 11–27.

Positioning in specially designed massage chairs simulates lying prone on a massage table in many ways. Of course, a big difference is that clients are in a more **vertical position** supported on their buttocks, lower legs, and chest instead of lying facedown on a horizontal surface. Done properly, positioning in a massage chair can be very comfortable and relaxing.

There are several models of massage chairs, and each has its own features for positioning a client comfortably. Standard **massage chair adjustments** include the height of the chest pad and the angle of the face cradle. Other adjustments may include the height and/or angle of the seat, the kneeling pads, and the armrest. Examine the model available to you for its adjustment features.

Note that different massage chair models have limits on body types and weights that they can accommodate safely and comfortably. For example, the maximum weight a chair can typically hold is about 300 pounds. People less than 4 feet tall or more than 6 feet tall, or with a large girth, may have trouble fitting into a particular massage chair properly. Be familiar with your chair's limitations. See Chapter 10, *Hygiene, Equipment, Environment,* for a discussion of important considerations when buying a massage chair.

To position a client for massage, first have him or her sit down and kneel on the pads provided. Check the angle of the kneeling pads and seat and the overall fit of the client in the chair. The client should be able to sit comfortably in this basic position. If kneeling is uncomfortable or painful, have the client put his or her feet flat on the floor instead. The seat may have to be adjusted to be more horizontal in this case.

Next adjust the height of the chest pad and ask the client to lean forward. Special chest pads are available to position large-breasted women comfortably. Some chairs have an additional chest pad angle adjustment. Then raise or lower the face cradle and tilt it down, so that the client's neck is flexed slightly. If the face cradle is too low, the neck will be shortened with an exaggerated curve. If it is too high, the top of the face cradle pad will not rest on the forehead, or the chin will be tilted up out of good alignment.

Last, adjust the angle of the arm rest. Ask for feedback about the overall comfort of this position. Make further adjustments as needed. Proper positioning for seated massage is shown in Figure 10–13B.

Some chairs can be adjusted to allow clients to sit facing out with their backs against the chest pad. This allows access to the front of the body for some massage applications. With this feature, anterior leg and foot massage may be added to a seated massage session.

SEATED MASSAGE SESSIONS

Seated massage sessions commonly focus on the upper body. Areas addressed include the neck and shoulders, head and scalp, upper and lower back, forearms, wrists, and hands. Techniques that are effective without the use of oil are used. The most common are petrissage (i.e., kneading and compression), friction, direct pressure, tapotement, light stroking, and joint movements. Forms of energy balancing such as polarity therapy may be incorporated into a session. Shiatsu and other forms of Asian bodywork are particularly adaptable for seated massage because they are given without lubricant and include techniques such as thumb and finger pressure, compressions, and percussion.

Before beginning sessions, ask recipients to remove obstacles to massage, for example, eyeglasses, large pieces of jewelry, ties, jackets, and sweaters. Ask permission to work on the face if the recipient is wearing makeup. Also get the recipient's consent to massage the scalp, which typically disturbs the hair.

The Practice Sequence for seated massage is designed for general relaxation and for treating common areas of muscular tension. Techniques can be added to address the needs of each specific recipient.

PRACTICAL APPLICATION

Practice positioning different people in a massage chair. Make adjustments for different body types, shapes, and sizes.

1. What adjustments are possible on the massage chair you are using? How does the chair work mechanically?

2. In what order are the adjustments made? What do you look for to determine proper positioning in the massage chair?

3. What role does the recipient play in positioning?

4. Practice a few massage techniques to see if the recipient is positioned well to receive them.

PRACTICE SEQUENCE 20–1

Seated Massage | 20 minutes

Preliminary Instructions
• Screen for contraindications and cautions.
• Ask recipient to remove jewelry, bulky clothing, eyeglasses, etc.
• Give instructions for getting onto the massage chair.
• Adjust chest pad, face cradle, and other areas as needed.

Figure 20–1 Stand behind the recipient. Lay your hands on the shoulders to establish contact. Squeeze the shoulders (upper trapezius and deltoid muscles) several times. Gradually increase the force of the squeezes.

Figure 20–2 Press the back muscles, using the palms or loose fists to apply compression. Do not hyperextend your wrists. Press along the sides as well as along the spine, but not over the spine.

Figure 20–3 Apply thumb pressure to points along the spine bilaterally from superior or inferior. Keep your joints stacked. Shift weight to apply pressure. Space points about every 2 inches.

4

Figure 20–4 Apply direct pressure to points along the shoulders. Stand to one side and use your forearm to apply broad pressure to one shoulder. Move from medial to lateral. Repeat with your elbow, pressing points about every 2 inches. Only press into muscle. Repeat on other side.

5

Figure 20–5 Standing behind the recipient, squeeze the shoulders and down the upper arms. Squeeze muscles bilaterally across the shoulders and down the upper arms. Use for finishing and transition to arms.

6

Figure 20–6 Shift to one side. Let the recipient's arm hang down. Knead upper and lower arm muscles from armpit to wrist. Afterward position the arm back on the armrest.

7

Figure 20–7 Apply thumb pressure to forearm muscles, particularly the extensors muscles. Apply circular friction to tender spots. Finish with squeezes from elbow to wrist.

Figure 20–8 Squeeze hands and fingers. Compress and broaden the hand. Squeeze along each finger.

Figure 20–9 Move joints in hands. Apply scissoring to metacarpals and figure-8s to fingers.

Figure 20–10 Stretch arm overhead. Stand to the side facing the same direction as the recipient. Hold onto the hand, and stretch the arm upward in line with the recipient's body angle. Lean into the stretch. Replace the arm on armrest. Brush off to finish before moving to the other arm.

Repeat Steps 6–10 on the other arm.

Figure 20–11 Knead neck muscles. Use one hand to knead muscles on both sides of the neck.

Figure 20–12 Press into points along the neck with your thumb, one side at a time. Apply circular friction to tender spots. Move from the base of the neck up to and across the suboccipital region.

Figure 20–13 Apply circular friction with both hands to mobilize the scalp.

Figure 20–14 Tap the head. Apply light fingertip tapotement to the head: top, sides, and back.

Figure 20–15 Brush off the back. Apply several long brushing strokes from head to hips to finish the session.

Assist the recipient as needed to get up and out of the chair.

After you perform the Practice Sequence, evaluate how well you did by filling out Performance Evaluation Form 20–1, Seated Massage. The form can be found in Appendix D, *Performance Evaluation Forms,* and at MyHealthProfessionsLab.com.

Figures source: Pearson Education, Inc./Segal Photography.

PREPARING FOR DIFFERENT VENUES

Giving seated massage in different venues involves some preparation, especially for places away from your regular office. Equipment and supplies need to be gathered and transported to the site. Space must be set up, and a method for scheduling and screening clients determined. Products for sanitizing equipment must be available, as well as a way of washing your hands between clients.

Supplies needed for seated massage events include disposable face cradle covers, something to wipe the chair after each client, hand sanitizer, and a garbage bag for used supplies. Dispose of used face cradle covers, and put on a fresh one after each massage. Antibacterial or antimicrobial disposable wipes can be used to sanitize the face support, armrests, chest pad, and leg rests of the massage chair after each session. A hand sanitizer is essential when working on-site because washroom facilities may not be available or convenient to use.

CASE FOR STUDY

Ramón Addresses Forearm Strain

Ramón gives seated massage to workers twice a month at a small office. One of his clients, Maria, works part-time as a hair stylist in addition to working at a computer for hours at the office. She is starting to experience pain in her forearms and hands from the repeated stress in her upper body. She has asked Ramón to focus on those areas during her regular seated massage.

Question:

What can Ramón do to address Maria's complaints?

Things to consider:

- What musculoskeletal structures are likely involved?
- Can Ramón consider using massage techniques that require lotion in this case?
- How would the arm be positioned most effectively for applying techniques?
- What can Ramón do to maintain good body mechanics and reduce stress on his own body?

Outline a 20-minute seated massage sequence to address Maria's complaints. Be specific about massage techniques and timing. List home care suggestions (stretches, self-massage, cold applications).

_____

_____

_____

Additional supplies include a clipboard, pen, and intake/release forms for keeping records of clients seen. Other useful items include a small table to set things on and a little tray or dish for holding clients' jewelry or eyeglasses. Depending on the setting, you may want to bring a device to play appropriate music.

The space for seated massage can be flexible. If at the workplace, it may be at the recipient's workstation, or in an empty office or cubicle or in a conference or workroom. It may be in a booth at a trade show or the lobby of a health club. It may be under a tent at a street fair or in a space at the back of a store. The only requirement is enough space for the practitioner to move around and keep good body mechanics. An ideal space would be quiet and somewhat removed from the hectic activity of the surrounding environment.

Time is also a factor. Seated massage sessions typically last from 15 to 20 minutes. A minimum 10-minute break between sessions allows for necessary transition from one client to the next. During this time, equipment is sanitized, and the face cradle cover is changed. The incoming client can be screened and given instructions.

Be sure to take regular breaks to avoid undue stress and strain. Scheduling sessions on the half-hour provides for a short break between clients. Take at least a 30-minute break after four sessions. Do no more than 5 hours of seated massage in 1 day.

With adequate preparation, taking seated massage on-the-road can run smoothly. It can be a rewarding addition to a general massage practice or may provide a specialty for a full-time seated massage business.

CRITICAL THINKING

Think about the various places where seated massage is offered other than the workplace, for example, at street fairs, in airports, at trade shows, and in shopping malls. Analyze how seated massage might be adapted to meet the needs of people in four different venues.

1. What physical and mental stresses do people in each venue face?
2. What goals for a seated massage might be appropriate to meeting their needs?
3. How might a session be adapted for the circumstances?
4. What equipment and supplies would you need to take to each venue?

CHAPTER HIGHLIGHTS

- Giving massage to a client sitting on a special massage chair or regular chair is referred to as seated massage or chair massage.
- Throughout history, massage has been given in the seated position whenever it was convenient to do so.
- The invention of the modern massage chair in the 1980s sparked an interest in seated massage that continues today.
- The benefits of seated massage are largely the same as for table massage, with the addition of convenience and accessibility.
- Massage in the workplace is useful to minimize job-related injuries and health problems, such as repetitive strain injuries, tension headaches, and high stress levels.
  - Seated massage increases mental clarity and worker productivity.
- Basic principles of good body and hand mechanics apply to seated massage.
  - Body mechanics are adapted for applying massage with the client in a more vertical position.

- Seated massage clients are screened for contraindications and cautions.
  - Important questions include information on previous massage experience, recent injuries or illnesses, medications being taken, pregnancy, contact lenses, areas to avoid, and low blood pressure.
- Positioning a client properly on a massage chair requires adjustments in the chair seat, kneeling pads, arm pad, chest pad, and face cradle.
- Massage techniques that do not require oil are used for seated massage, for example, compression and kneading (petrissage), friction, tapotement, and other forms of bodywork such as shiatsu, and polarity therapy.
- Areas of focus for seated massage include neck and shoulders, head and scalp, upper and lower back, forearms, wrists, and hands.

- Clients remove jewelry, jackets and sweaters, ties, eyeglasses, and other potential obstacles to massage. Ask permission to massage the face or scalp.
- Giving seated massage in different venues involves preparation of equipment, supplies, and the space; scheduling and screening; sanitizing and hygiene.

- At events, scheduling clients on the half hour allows time for a short break between sessions and time to sanitize equipment.
  - Take a 30-minute break after four sessions, and do no more than 5 hours of seated massage in 1 day.

EXAM REVIEW

Key Terms

To study the key terms listed at the beginning of this chapter, match the appropriate lettered meaning to each numbered key term listed. For additional study, look up the key terms in the Interactive Glossary, and note other terms that compare or contrast with them.

_____ 1. Massage chair
_____ 2. Massage chair adjustments
_____ 3. On-site massage
_____ 4. Repetitive strain injuries (RSIs)
_____ 5. Screening interview
_____ 6. Seated massage
_____ 7. Vertical position
_____ 8. Workplace wellness programs

a. The massage practitioner goes to where the potential clients are
b. Questions to ask prospective clients for massage that can reveal important information regarding health conditions and possible contraindications for massage
c. Massage given with the recipient sitting on a special massage chair or on a regular chair adapted for the purpose
d. Can be transported easily and allows recipients to receive massage sitting up and with their clothes on
e. Massage clients are supported on their buttocks, lower legs, and chest instead of lying facedown on a horizontal surface.
f. Services and activities for employees sponsored by employers to improve people's overall health and well-being
g. Can include the height of the chest pad, the angle of the face cradle, the height and/or angle of the seat, the kneeling pads, and the armrest
h. Debilitating musculoskeletal problems resulting from repeated overwork or overload

Memory Workout

To test your memory of the main concepts in this chapter, complete the following sentences by circling the most correct answer from the two choices provided.

1. The first modern massage chair was developed in the (1950s) (1980s) by (David Palmer) (Janet Travell).

2. When the massage therapist goes to where the clients are located, for example, at their workplace, it is often referred to as (on-site) (chair) massage.

3. One of the main attractions of seated massage is that it is (convenient) (relaxing) for clients.

4. Seated massage has been found to increase mental (relaxation) (alertness) that can only enhance worker productivity.

5. For office workers, tension headaches are more common toward the (middle) (end) of the day.

6. Body and hand mechanics for seated massage take into consideration the (reclining) (vertical) position of the client on the chair.

7. People with low blood pressure may be prone to (fainting) (shaking).

8. Pressing into the back of someone in a massage chair calls for more (forward) (upward) motion, rather than downward.

9. To position a client on a massage chair, tilt the face cradle slightly (downward) (upward).

10. Ask for the client's (assistance) (permission) to massage the face or scalp.

Test Prep

The following multiple-choice questions will help to prepare you for future school and professional exams.

1. One of the first large corporations to provide on-site massage for its employees in 1984 was:
   a. Boeing Aircraft
   b. Apple Computer Corporation
   c. Hartford Insurance
   d. Coca-Cola Corporation

2. For seated massage techniques, pressure is most often applied by:
   a. Pushing with the arms
   b. Bending from the waist
   c. Lifting your shoulders
   d. Leaning with your body weight

3. Pressing into the back of a seated client is best done from a:
   a. Bow-and-arrow stance
   b. Horse riding stance
   c. Kneeling stance
   d. Sitting position

4. If a client receiving seated massage suddenly feels faint or dizzy, the best action is to:
   a. Call 911
   b. Have the person stand up immediately
   c. Have the person lie on the ground with his or her feet elevated
   d. Switch to tapotement to increase his or her alertness

5. If a person with knee pain wants to receive massage in a massage chair, a good alternative for positioning is to:
   a. Raise the chest pad to take pressure off of the knees
   b. Raise the seat to take pressure off of the knees
   c. Have him place his feet flat on the floor instead of on the knee pads
   d. Adjust the angle of the knee pads to be more horizontal

6. If a pregnant woman in her third trimester signs up for seated massage at a health fair and she is otherwise healthy, the best action is to:
   a. Adjust the massage chair to fit her current shape and size and give the usual massage
   b. Let her get into the massage chair but avoid pressing hard on her back
   c. Ask her to sit in regular chair and give her a head, neck, and shoulders massage
   d. Politely refuse to give her massage because of contraindications

7. Seated massage sessions in the workplace or at community events typically last:
   a. 5 minutes
   b. 15–20 minutes
   c. 30–40 minutes
   d. 60 minutes

8. In the bow-and-arrow stance, the body is lowered by:
   a. Widening the stance and bending the knees
   b. Narrowing the stance and straightening the knees
   c. Bending at the waist
   d. Widening the stance and bending at the waist

9. A thoroughly sanitized face cradle for each seated massage client is best achieved by:
   a. Changing the disposable face cradle cover for each client
   b. Washing the face cradle after the last client
   c. Both washing the face cradle and using a clean cover for each client
   d. Sanitizing after every third client

10. As a self-care measure, take regular breaks when providing seated massage at events. A good rule of thumb is to take at least a:
    a. 30-minute break after each session
    b. 30-minute break after every four sessions
    c. 15-minute break after 2 hours of massage
    d. 30-minute break after 4 hours of massage

Video Challenge

Watch this video, which can be found at MyHealthProfessions-Lab.com, Chapter 20, and then answer the following questions.

Seated Massage

1. What type of massage techniques were used most often in the seated massage demonstration in the video?

2. For which technique applications were shifting the body weight most obvious?
3. How did the practitioner in the video keep good body mechanics when massaging the arms and hands?

Comprehension Exercises

The following short-answer questions test your knowledge and understanding of chapter topics and provide practice in written communication skills. Explain in two to four complete sentences.

1. Describe equipment, space, and time requirements for seated massage in the workplace.

2. Give four reasons for the popularity of seated massage in workplace wellness programs.
3. What screening questions are asked prior to seated massage? How do you use the information from the client's answers?

For Greater Understanding

The following exercises are designed to take you from the realm of theory into the real world. They will help give you a deeper understanding of the subjects covered in this chapter. Action words are underlined to emphasize the variety of activities presented to address different learning styles and to encourage deeper thinking.

1. Receive a seated massage offered in a public place such as a shopping mall, airport, or street fair. Describe your experience: How did the practitioner prepare you for the session? Did he or she adjust the chair? What techniques were used? How long did it last? How did you feel afterward?

2. Interview people who receive massage at their workplaces. Ask them to describe the seated massage sessions. What benefits do they experience personally?

3. Compare the features of several different massage chairs available for purchase. How many adjustments can be made? How stable and sturdy is each chair? How easy is each to transport and store? Prepare a written cost and features comparison.

MyHealthProfessionsLab™

MyHealthProfessionsLab.com is a premium online homework management system that includes a host of features to help you study. Registered users will find:

- Powerful tools that track and analyze your results—allowing you to create a personalized learning experience
- Videos, flashcards and other learning tools to help enrich your progress
- Streaming lesson presentations and self-paced learning modules
- A space where you and your instructors can view and manage your assignments

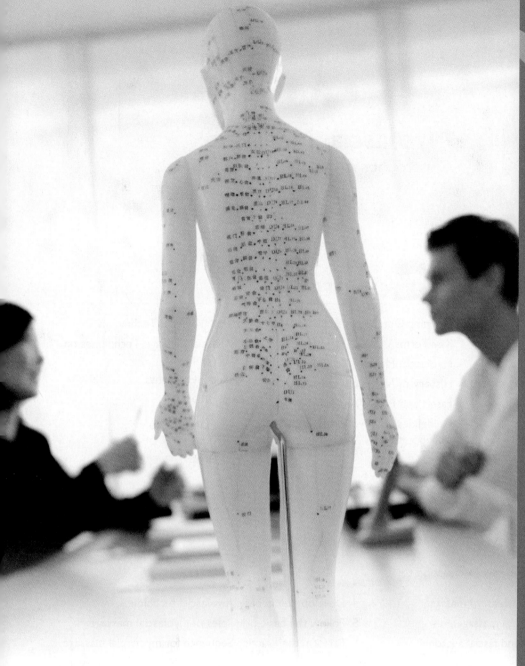

© Ralf Schultheiss/Corbis

Chapter 21
Myofascial Massage

Chapter 22
Trigger Point Therapy

Chapter 23
Lymphatic Facilitation

Chapter 24
Reflexology

Chapter 25
Asian and Energy-Based
Bodywork

P A R T

5

Tappan's Guide to Contemporary Massage and Bodywork

21 Myofascial Massage

Christopher Alvarado

Pearson Education, Inc.

CHAPTER OUTLINE

Learning Outcomes

Key Terms

Myofascial Massage Overview

History of Myofascial Massage

Fascia and Fascial Anatomy

Guidelines for Myofascial
Applications

Basic Myofascial Techniques

Myofascial Massage Techniques on
the Back

Chapter Highlights

Exam Review

LEARNING OUTCOMES

After studying this chapter, you will have information to:

1. Explain the general intent of myofascial massage.

2. Discuss the history of myofascial massage.

3. Describe the nature of fascia and fascial anatomy.

4. Develop skill in basic myofascial techniques.

5. Follow the basic principles of myofascial massage.

6. Perform the Practice Sequence for myofascial massage.

KEY TERMS

Collagen

Deep fascia

Elastin

Fascia

Fascial anatomy

Fascial restrictions

Ground substance

Melting

Myofascial massage

Subcutaneous
fascia

Thixotropy

MYOFASCIAL MASSAGE OVERVIEW

Myofascial massage addresses the body's **fascial anatomy**, that is, the fibrous connective tissue that holds the body together and gives it shape. The general intent of myofascial massage is to release restrictions in superficial fascia, in deep fascia surrounding muscles, and in fascia related to overall body alignment. Myofascial techniques stretch fascial sheets, break fascial adhesions, and leave tissues softer and more pliable. These techniques release **fascial restrictions** that limit mobility and cause postural distortion, poor cellular nutrition, pain, and a variety of other dysfunctions.

HISTORY OF MYOFASCIAL MASSAGE

The history of today's myofascial massage can be traced to earlier systems of manual therapy that focused on the fascial tissues of the body. Many of the myofascial techniques that have become part of the skill base of today's massage therapists were developed in the mid-twentieth century.

Connective tissue massage (CTM), sometimes known as *Bindegewebsmassage*, was developed by Elizabeth Dicke of Germany in the late 1920s and 1930s. CTM, as Dicke taught it, is the systematic application of light strokes without lubricants to various areas of the skin. CTM is thought to improve circulation in subcutaneous connective tissue, which results in reflex actions to other parts of the body, including the visceral organs.

Structural integration, or Rolfing, was developed by Ida Rolf (1896–1979) and taught at the Esalen Institute in California in the 1960s. Rolfing seeks to reestablish proper vertical alignment in the body by manipulating the myofascial tissue so that the fascia elongates and glides, rather than shortens and adheres. Rolf's work spawned a number of other systems of bodywork that address alignment of the structure of the body through manipulation of the deep fascia.

An osteopath named Robert Ward coined the term *myofascial release* in the 1960s to describe his system of treating the body's myofascial anatomy. In the 1980s, the term myofascial release (MFR) was adopted by a physical therapist named John Barnes as the designation for his method of freeing restrictions in the myofascial tissues. The overall intention of MFR, according to Barnes, is to relieve pain, resolve structural dysfunction, restore function and mobility, and release emotional trauma.[1]

Variations of myofascial massage approaches continue to be developed and are known variously as myofascial release, myofascial unwinding, myofascial manipulation, and myofascial massage. They all view an unrestricted myofascial system as integral to good health.

The importance of healthy myofascial tissues to overall well-being is gaining recognition in both conventional and complementary health care. The first International Fascia Research Congress (IFRC), held at the Harvard Medical School in Boston in 2007, brought together scientists and clinicians from around the world. Besides surveying the research on fascia being conducted worldwide, the conference provided a venue for scientists, educators, and therapists to share insights about fascia and their approaches to fascial tissue health. IFRC conferences continue to be held and are in the forefront of research about myofascial tissues and related manual therapy.[2]

FASCIA AND FASCIAL ANATOMY

Fascia is loose, irregular connective tissue found throughout the body. Fascia surrounds every muscle, nerve, blood vessel, and organ. It holds structures together giving them their characteristic shapes, offers support, and connects the body as a whole. It can be thought of as winding through the body in a continuous sheet.

Fascia is the soft tissue component of the connective tissue system that permeates the human body. It forms a whole-body continuous three-dimensional matrix of structural support. Fascia interpenetrates and surrounds all organs, muscles, bones and nerve fibers, creating a unique environment for body systems functioning.[3]

Fascial tissue is composed of three primary elements: ground substance, collagen, and elastin. **Ground substance** is a gel-like mucopolysaccharide, the same liquid that forms interstitial or intercellular fluid. **Collagen** fibers are long, straight proteins that are strong yet flexible. Collagen is the most common type of fiber in connective tissue. **Elastin** fibers are wavy, branched proteins that return to their original length when stretched. Fascia has been described as sparse, with a loose arrangement of collagen fibers and with greater amounts of elastin than the dense regular connective tissue found in ligaments and tendons.[4] The multidirectionality and low density of fibers in typical fascia is illustrated in Figure 21–1 ■.

Fascia has a greater amount of ground substance than other types of connective tissue. It is the immediate environment of every cell in the body and forms the interstitial spaces. It has important functions in support, protection, separation, cellular respiration, elimination, metabolism, fluid flow, and immune system function. Any restriction or dysfunction of the fascia can lead to a variety of problems, including poor exchange of cellular nutrients and wastes, pain, and loss of mobility.

Fascia displays an intriguing characteristic called **thixotropy**, that is, it can change from a more solid to a more fluid consistency as a result of movement, stretching, and increase in temperature.[5] Myofascial release techniques, and the method of their application, are based on these characteristics of fascia.

Depths of Fascia

Fascia is found at three different depths in the body (i.e., subcutaneous fascia, deep fascia, and subserous fascia). The most superficial is **subcutaneous fascia**, which forms

FIGURE 21–1 Illustration of multidirectionality and low density of fibers in typical fascia.

a continuous layer of connective tissue over the entire body between the skin and the deep fascia. **Deep fascia** is an intricate series of dense connective sheets and bands that hold the muscles and other structures in place throughout the body. *Subserous fascia* lies between the deep fascia and the serous membranes lining the body cavities. Myofascial massage focuses on the subcutaneous and deep fascia related to the musculature.

John Barnes defines another layer of fascia that he calls *deepest fascia*, which is within the dura mater of the craniosacral system (cranium, spine, and sacrum).[6] It is interesting to note that a researcher reported finding cerebrospinal fluid inside collagen fibrils, which suggests that the connective tissue framework may function as a circulatory system carrying chemical messages throughout the body.[7] There is clearly much more to learn about this important body tissue.

Fascial Structures

Fascial anatomy includes identifiable fascial structures that shape and connect the body. For example, there are the *retinaculae* or body straps at the wrist and ankle, which secure the tendons that cross there like bungee cords keeping computer cables in place. There are also seven bands that give characteristic shape to the human torso. These bands run horizontally at the level of the pubic area, the lower abdomen (iguinal), abdomen (umbilical), the chest just below

the nipples, the collar bone, the chin, and the eyes.[8] And there are fascial sheaths surrounding and linking muscles and muscle groups, for example, the large muscles of the back of the body as shown in Figure 21–2 ■. Knowledge of fascial structures helps practitioners locate and release restrictions.

The pervasiveness and interconnectedness of fascia throughout the body creates a situation in which fascial restriction in one part of the body can affect other parts as well. A metaphor often used to describe the fascia is a knitted sweater. Because all of the threads of yarn are connected, a pull in one section of the sweater may cause a pull in a spot distant from the original, or distortion of the shape of the entire sweater. Likewise, a restriction in fascia in one place in the body can cause distortion in another area.

If fascia surrounding muscle becomes rigid or adheres to other structures, it can prevent full relaxation and elongation of muscle tissue, thus restricting movement. It has been observed that "a muscle cannot regain its resting length even when contracted fibers are relaxed if the surrounding fascial membranes are binding it. . . . Techniques that address the unique characteristics of fascia must be applied to liberate contracted myofascial tissue fully."[9]

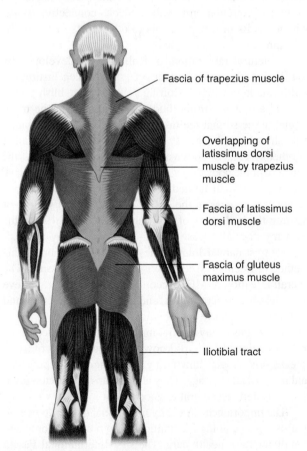

FIGURE 21–2 Fascial sheaths surrounding and linking the muscles of the back of the body.

GUIDELINES FOR MYOFASCIAL APPLICATIONS

Myofascial massage applications involve identifying and releasing myofascial restrictions. Guidelines for these applications follow from the nature of fascial tissue and fascial structures. A summary of guidelines for myofascial massage appears in Box 21–1 ■.

Myofascial restrictions are located in two primary ways, that is, by observation and palpation. Visual analysis of a client's posture can reveal areas of fascial shortening and distortion in fascial anatomy. Restrictions may also be detected through palpation of soft tissues, or feeling where tissues seem "stuck together" and resist lengthening. Knowledge of fascial structures points to likely areas for restrictions.

Choose myofascial techniques suitable for the area and for the depth of the application. Some techniques address more superficial fascia, while others penetrate to deeper fascia.

Use no lubricant, or very little, on the skin. You must be able to feel subtle restrictions in the movement of soft tissues and the letting go that occurs as fascia elongates, becomes more pliable, and fascial sheets get unstuck. These subtleties are lost if the hands are sliding over the skin. Myofascial techniques also require traction on the skin as tissues are slowly and gently pushed, pulled, and stretched.

BOX 21.1 Guidelines for Myofascial Massage

1. Use observation of posture, palpation skills, and knowledge of fascial anatomy to identify areas of fascial restriction.
2. Choose myofascial massage techniques suitable for the area and for the depth at which you are working.
3. Use no or very little lubricant so that you can feel fascial restrictions and apply techniques without sliding over the skin.
4. Make gentle contact and enter tissues slowly until a point or area of resistance is felt.
5. Shift tissues horizontally once you are at the depth you wish to affect.
   - Avoid compressing tissues into bone.
6. Hold a stretch of fascial tissues until they release, usually in 2–5 minutes.
   - Maintain a continuous stretch.
   - Release feels like "melting," softening, or "giving" in tissues.
7. Flow with the tissues. Let the direction of the stretch be determined by which way the tissues seem to want to release.
8. Exit tissues with as much care and awareness as when you entered into them.
9. Let fascial tissues rest and integrate after a stretch.

Note: This list of myofascial massage guidelines summarizes instructions from many sources cited in this chapter.

Myofascial techniques are characteristically gentle, slow, and sustained. Movements are very subtle. The stretch of tissues is typically held from 2 to 5 minutes. The elastin stretches first. The collagen barriers and bonds take longer to release, and respond later to sustained gentle pressure. When they release, a **melting**, elongation, or sinking into tissues is felt. Barnes describes it thusly:

> At first the elastic component of the fascia will release, and at some point in time the collagenous barrier will be engaged. This barrier cannot be forced (it is too strong). One waits with gentle pressure, and as the collagenous aspect releases, the therapist follows the motion of the tissue, barrier upon barrier until freedom is felt.[10]
>
> —Pearson Education

For superficial applications involving skin lifting, make gentle contact, pick up the skin, and slowly pull it away from underlying tissues (see Figure 21–3A). Feel for areas of resistance to the lifting action. Hold the tension until a subtle stretch or giving way is felt.

For deep myofascial applications, make gentle contact and enter the soft tissues slowly until a point or area of resistance is felt. Once you are at the depth you wish to effect, shift the tissues horizontally (see Figure 21–5A). Avoid compressing tissues into bone. After a time, a melting or letting go will be felt in the tissues. There will be subtle movement and lengthening.

For some applications, it makes sense to flow with the restrictions and releases, letting the tissues lead the direction. This occurs in myofascial unwinding, which addresses fascia from a more three-dimensional view. Unwinding restores structural integrity and proper alignment of tissues, and promotes improved tissue health and organ function.

Exit tissues slowly with care and awareness. Let fascial tissues rest after stretching them. Avoid overworking tissues in one area.

Myofascial applications can be integrated into a full-body massage as needed, or may be used as the primary approach in a session. For treatment of specific problems, myofascial release techniques are sometimes combined with other soft tissue approaches such as trigger point therapy, as well as exercise, nutrition, relaxation, and psychotherapy.

Contraindications

Myofascial massage is contraindicated locally if the tissues are damaged in some way, for example, if there is bruising, a wound, a burn, a fracture, local infection, or edema due to trauma. Joint diseases such as arthritis with inflammation and gout are also contraindications for manipulation of the fascia in the immediate area. General contraindications include cellulitis, fever, systemic infection, lymphedema, advanced osteoporosis, and advanced diabetes. Avoid myofascial applications if a client is taking medication that decreases sensitivity to pain, reduces the ability of blood to clot (e.g., anticoagulants), or compromises tissue integrity (e.g., steroids). See Table 8.1 Pharmacology Overview for information about classes of drugs and their actions.

BASIC MYOFASCIAL TECHNIQUES

The myofascial massage techniques presented in this chapter address subcutaneous fascia and deep fascia related to the musculature. Their intent is to make fascial tissues more pliable and to release adhesions that cause restrictions to free movement. This is accomplished by the application of stretching, pulling, and pushing movements that separate tissues mechanically. In addition, the practitioner's hand or arm impart heat, which together with the stretch, produces a softer consistency in fascial tissues (an example of thixotropy), breaks adhesions, and frees restrictions.

The quality of application of myofascial techniques is essential to their success. That includes slow and sustained stretching of fascial membranes in a direction that releases their adherence to each other. Little if any lubricant is used to prevent the hands from sliding over the skin superficially.

Myofascial technique categories include skin lifting, fascial stretching, and fascial mobilizations. There are many variations within each category. The techniques presented here are useful for learning the basics of myofascial applications and can be readily integrated into a massage session.

Skin Lifting Techniques

Skin lifting techniques free restrictions in subcutaneous fascia. They release adhering tissues and increase local superficial circulation. The skin is gently picked up with the fingers and slowly pulled away from underlying tissues. Maintain the pull until tissues are more pliable and shift direction more easily. This usually takes 2 to 3 minutes for problem areas. Do not overwork an area by staying too long at one time, or by repeated applications in one session.

Skin lifting techniques include basic lifting, lifting with directional shift, and skin rolling (Figure 21–3 ■). In basic skin lifting, the tissues are picked up vertically. While sustaining the vertical lift, you may also gently pull or push in more horizontal directions feeling for restrictions. For skin rolling, lift the skin vertically and then crawl your fingers

FIGURE 21–4 Fascial stretching techniques. (A) Cross-hand dual direction stretch. (B) Pin and stretch with the thumb and fingers.

Source: Pearson Education, Inc./Segal Photography.

along the skin pushing up from behind with the thumbs. This creates a rolling wave of tissue that moves across the surface.

Fascial Stretching Techniques

Fascial stretching techniques elongate fascial tissues in broad areas. They can be applied at different depths. For all fascial stretches, hold the tension steadily for 2 to 5 minutes until you feel the tissue give way or elongate, and avoid sliding over the skin. This category includes dual and single direction stretches and *pin-and-stretch* techniques (Figure 21–4 ■).

The cross-hand stretch is a dual direction stretch for subcutaneous fascia. Place crossed hands parallel to and adjacent to the spine, with one hand in the thoracic region and the other in the lumbar region. Engage the tissue, and slowly apply horizontal pressure to spread the tissue between the hands.

To make the cross-hand stretch a single direction stretch, anchor the skin with one hand, while the other hand pushes horizontally in the opposite direction. Hold and wait

A   B   C

FIGURE 21–3 Skin lifting techniques. (A) Basic skin lifting. (B) Lifting with directional shift. (C) Skin rolling.

Source: Pearson Education, Inc./Segal Photography.

for an elongation of tissues. For a smaller area, use a thumb to anchor the skin in place, while the fingers of the other hand pull and stretch the fascia in the opposite direction. These are also called pin-and- stretch techniques.

Fascial Mobilizations

Fascial mobilizations are used to apply a shearing force across the surface of fascial sheets to release bonding between the sheets. The general direction of this stretch is horizontal to the adhering tissues. Fascial mobilizations are entered into slowly to the depth desired followed by a horizontal stretch. The stretch is held steadily for 2 to 5 minutes until a release is felt. Fascial mobilizations can be applied with the palms, forearm, or fingertips (Figure 21–5 ■).

A reinforced palm can be used to apply pressure to a broad area such as the lower back (Figure 21–5A ■). Press into the tissue with the palm until you engage the surface

of the muscular layer, and then sift the tissues horizontally toward the pelvis. Hold until a release is felt.

Fascial mobilization over the round surface of the thigh is applied with a flat hand (Figure 21–5B ■). In this broad plane shift, the entire hand makes contact with the skin surface; however, the heel is used to engage tissues and shift the fascia around the leg toward the table. The recipient is in side-lying position for this technique.

The forearm can also be used for fascial mobilization on both flat (Figure 21–5C ■) and rounded surfaces. Note in the example of fascial mobilization around the shoulder that the proximal third of the forearm is used to engage the tissues and the upper arm is held away from the body. Avoid applying pressure with the point of the elbow (Figure 21–5D ■).

The fingertips can be used for deeper pressure in smaller areas. Pressure is applied vertically into tissues until the desired depth is attained, and then tissues are shifted more

FIGURE 21–5 Fascial mobilization techniques. (A) Fascial mobilization on the lower back using the palm. (B) Broad plane shift around the thigh using the heel of the hand. (C) Fascial mobilization on the flat upper back using the forearm. (D) Fascial mobilization around the top of the shoulder using the forearm. (E) Fascial mobilization using the fingertips.

Source: Pearson Education, Inc./Segal Photography.

horizontally (Figure 21–5E ■). Sensitive fingers can feel in which direction the fascial sheets seem to be adhering (point of resistance) or in which direction the tissues seem to want to release (point of least resistance). With experience, you will develop a kinesthetic feel for which way to go to best unwind the fascial sheets.

Be sure to let the tissues rest after myofascial massage applications (Figure 21–6 ■). This allows the tissues to integrate the changes that have occurred. Passive touch can be used as a finishing technique after redraping the area treated.

FIGURE 21–6 Allow tissues to rest after myofascial applications.

Source: Pearson Education, Inc./Segal Photography.

MYOFASCIAL MASSAGE TECHNIQUES ON THE BACK

The following Practice Sequence guides you through a session of myofascial massage of the back. Use caution and practice with light pressure at first to develop sensitivity. As you perform myofascial massage, keep in mind that areas of the back corresponding to fascial lines are usually more difficult to lift (e.g., tissues directly over the spine, the lumbar area, and the sacrum). Difficulty rolling the skin indicates an area with more adhering in subcutaneous fascia.

CRITICAL THINKING

Think about basic myofascial massage techniques and their intent (i.e., skin lifting, fascial stretching, fascial mobilization). Compare those techniques in terms of the effects they have on myofascial tissues.

1. How does each technique affect myofascial tissues?
2. Do any techniques have similar effects?
3. How would you choose one technique rather than another for a specific application?

PRACTICAL APPLICATION

Apply myofascial techniques to different areas of the body, for example, to the upper or lower extremities.

1. How does the anatomy of the area affect myofascial applications?
2. Are there positioning considerations?

3. How can basic myofascial techniques be adapted for the area?
4. Are some myofascial techniques not appropriate for certain areas?

PRACTICE SEQUENCE 21–1

Myofascial Massage of the Back | 30 minutes
Recipient prone

Preliminary Considerations
• Apply the following techniques without the use of oil or lotion.
• Do not apply pressure directly over the spinous processes.

Figure 21–7 Before removing the drape, initiate contact by placing your hands on the recipient's lumbar and upper thoracic back. Apply gentle rocking movements to the back, then undrape the back so that the skin is exposed down to the posterior superior iliac spine.

Figure 21–8 Using both hands, gently but firmly grasp the skin over a spot on the upper back, and lift the skin until tension is felt. Maintain tension for 2–3 minutes. Apply the skin lifting technique over all areas of the back, searching for areas that have more restriction than others as indicated by increased resistance to lifting.

Figure 21–9 Add movement to skin lifting by gently pulling it in a certain direction (e.g., up and forward) to feel for restrictions. Try shifting in different directions, paying attention to points of more or less resistance. If resistance is detected, hold until a fascial release is felt. *Variation:* While lifting the skin, ask the client to take a couple of slow, deep breaths. The rhythmic expansion and contraction of the thoracic cage provides subtle movement, increasing shifting of the fascia.

Figure 21–10 Apply skin rolling by lifting the skin and crawling your fingers along the skin while the thumbs gently push from behind, creating a constant "wave" of tissue that moves across the surface of the back. Perform in multiple directions over the same area.

5

Figure 21–11 Stand facing the side of the table and apply cross-handed stretches for the subcutaneous fascia. Place your hand closest to the client's head near the ilium in the lumbar area; place your other hand on the thoracic region on the same side; arms will be crossed. Engage the tissue, and gradually spread your hands farther apart until you sense tension in the tissues between your hands. Without gliding on the skin, hold that tension comfortably for 2–3 minutes until you feel your hands move further apart slightly as the tissue releases. Apply this technique in several directions on the back, and try it with one hand on the left side and the other hand on the right side of the spine.

6

Figure 21–12 Apply fascial mobilization in one direction using a palm. Stand to the side of the face cradle; place one hand over the other, and make contact with the area between the shoulder blade and the spinous processes. Press into the tissue until you engage the surface of the muscular layer beneath. Shift your engagement horizontally toward the pelvis until you feel tension in the fascial tissues. Hold that tension steadily for 2–5 minutes until you feel movement or "giving" within the tissues. *Variations* (not shown): Use both palms or a loosely held fist to apply pressure; apply in any direction and in any area of the back.

Repeat Step 6, shifting direction. If you sense the tissue wanting to shift, or resisting to shift, in one direction or another, you can choose to move either toward the direction of ease or toward the direction of most restriction. This choice is often intuitive and is related to your intent and angle of application.

7

Figure 21–13 Pin the skin and subcutaneous fascia on a spot on the back using the thumb of one hand; place the fingertips of the other hand slightly away from the first hand, engaging the fascial layer; slowly pull away from the pinning thumb. Hold tension in the tissue until a release is felt. *Variation* (not shown): Use thumbs to pin and stretch a small spot; apply in any direction.

Source: Pearson Education, Inc./Segal Photography.

8

Figure 21–14 Using the fingertips of one hand, make contact with an area on the back with high fascial restriction. To apply deep fascial mobilization, place the opposite hand on top of the first with fingers directly over each for reinforcement. Apply deep pressure through the skin and subcutaneous fascia until you reach the underlying deep fascia on top of the muscle layer. Shift your fingers away from you until tissue tension is sensed. Hold that tension 2–3 minutes or until a release is felt; apply in any direction.

9

Figure 21–15 Apply forearm to the deep fascia of the back. Stand to one side of the face cradle; use the proximal third of your ulna to engage into the long erector spinae muscles of the back; forearm is parallel to and adjacent to the spine; hold your upper arm away from and in front of your body. Be careful not to place direct pressure through the point of your elbow. Hold 2–5 minutes until you feel a release in the tissues.

10

Figure 21–16 Forearm application to engage the common fascial restrictions in the trapezius and levator scapula musculature in the top of the shoulder and back. Use a low stance when addressing the superior aspect of the shoulder, being careful not to place too much pressure on any bony structures.

11

Figure 21–17 Redrape the back, face the head of the table, and apply passive touch as finishing technique. Gently place both hands on the upper back, and hold for about 10 seconds.

After you perform the Practice Sequence, evaluate how well you did by filling out Performance Evaluation Form 21–1, Myofascial Massage of the Back. The form can be found in Appendix D: *Performance Evaluation Forms,* and at MyHealthProfessionsLab.com.

Figures source: Pearson Education, Inc./Segal Photography.

CASE FOR STUDY

Edgar and His "Solid Back"

Darren has a client named Edgar who came for massage looking for relief from tension in his back. Edgar reported in his intake interview that he recently got a job requiring lifting heavy objects. Since then he has been experiencing a lot of tension in his back. In fact, Edgar described his back as feeling like a "solid block," instead of moveable parts. Darren will focus on Edgar's back in this massage session with the goal of relieving some of the tension built up there.

Question:

How might myofascial techniques be integrated into a therapeutic massage for Edgar's back tension?

Things to consider:

- How can Darren assess the overall condition of the musculature of the back?
- How might he assess the myofascial tissues specifically?
- When is the best time to introduce myofascial techniques into the session?
- Which myofascial techniques would be most appropriate to address tension in back muscles?

Give an example of an approach to integrating myofascial techniques into a massage session to address back tension.

_____

_____

_____

CHAPTER HIGHLIGHTS

- Myofascial massage addresses the body's fascial anatomy with the intent of releasing restrictions in the superficial fascia, in deep fascia surrounding the musculature, and in fascia related to body alignment.
- Myofascial techniques release restrictions that limit mobility, cause postural distortion, poor cellular nutrition, pain, and a variety of other dysfunctions.
- The history of myofascial massage includes earlier systems of manual treatment that focus on the fascia of the body:
  - *Bindegewebsmassage* by Elizabeth Dicke in the 1920s
  - Rolfing by Ida Rolf in the 1960s
  - Myofascial release by osteopath Robert Ward in the 1960s
  - Myofascial release (MFR) by John Barnes in the 1980s
  - Other systems of myofascial massage: myofascial unwinding and myofascial manipulation
  - First International Fascia Research Congress at Harvard Medical School in 2007
- Fascia is loose, irregular connective tissue found throughout the body.
  - It surrounds muscles, nerves, blood vessels, and organs, giving them their shapes.
  - It winds through the body in a continuous sheet and supports and connects the body as a whole.

- Fascia is composed of ground substance, collagen, and elastin.
  - Sheets of fascia are formed by hydrogen bonds between collagen fibers.
- Functions of fascia include support, protection, cellular respiration, elimination, metabolism, fluid flow, and immune system function.
- Fascia has a characteristic called thixotropy, that is, it becomes more pliable with movement, stretching, and increased temperature.
- Fascia lies at three different depths in the body as subcutaneous fascia, deep fascia, and subserous fascia.
  - Barnes defines another layer called deepest fascia in the craniosacral system.
- Fascial anatomy includes structures like horizontal straps that give the body contour, and sheaths surrounding and linking muscles.
- Restrictions in the fascial web can cause distortion in other parts of the body and restrict movement.
- Myofascial massage focuses on subcutaneous and deep fascia.
- Guidelines for performing myofascial techniques:
  - Locate restrictions by visual analysis of posture and palpation.
  - Chose techniques based on the area and depth of application.

○ Use no or little lubricant to allow the feel of fascial restrictions and to get sufficient skin traction.

○ Move gently and slowly until a point of resistance is felt in the tissues.

○ Shift tissues horizontally to provide a stretch and release restrictions.

○ Hold the stretch until restrictions release (i.e., melt, soften, give), usually in 2–5 minutes.

○ Let movement flow with the tissues.

○ Exit the stretch with care and awareness.

○ Let tissues rest after the stretch.

• There are local and general contraindications for myofascial massage.

○ Local contraindications include tissues that are compromised in some way (e.g., bruising, local infection, a wound, a burn, a fracture, edema due to trauma, and inflamed joints).

○ General contraindications include cellulitis, fever, systemic infection, lymphedema, advanced osteoporosis, advanced diabetes, and medications that decrease sensitivity to pain, reduce the ability of blood to clot, or compromise tissue integrity.

• Categories of myofascial techniques include skin lifting, fascial stretching, and fascial mobilizations.

○ Myofascial techniques are applied with full palm, fingertips, thumbs, or forearm.

EXAM REVIEW

Key Terms

Match the following key terms to their descriptions. For additional study, look up the key terms in the Interactive Glossary, and note other terms that compare or contrast with them.

_____ **1.** Collagen
_____ **2.** Deep fascia
_____ **3.** Elastin
_____ **4.** Fascia
_____ **5.** Fascial anatomy
_____ **6.** Fascial restrictions
_____ **7.** Ground substance
_____ **8.** Melting
_____ **9.** Myofascial massage
_____ **10.** Subcutaneous fascia
_____ **11.** Thixotropy

a. Study of fascial structures that shape the body including retinaculae and sheaths
b. Same liquid as intercellular fluid
c. Loose irregular connective tissue found throughout the body
d. Dense connective tissue sheets and bands that hold body structures in place
e. Long, straight, strong proteins
f. Change from more solid to more liquid
g. Connective tissue between skin and deep fascia
h. Wavy, branched proteins that stretch
i. Limit mobility and cause postural distortions
j. Feeling when fascial adhesions release
k. Manual techniques that address the fascial tissues

Memory Workout

To test your memory of the main concepts in this chapter, complete the following sentences by circling the most correct answer from the two choices provided.

1. The term *myofascial release* was coined by osteopath (John Barnes) (Robert Ward) in the 1960s to describe his system of treating the body's fascial anatomy.
2. Fascia is loose, (irregular) (smooth) connective tissue found throughout the body.
3. Fascia is made up of ground substance, collagen, and (elastin) (sheaths).
4. Fascial (mobility) (restrictions) lead to a variety of problems including poor exchange of cellular nutrients, postural distortion, and pain.
5. Fascia has a characteristic called (elasticity) (thixotropy), that is, it can change from a more solid to a more gel-like consistency.
6. A metaphor often used to describe the fascia is a (knitted sweater) (unwinding flag).
7. In a technique called (myofascial mobilization) (skin lifting), the skin is gently picked up and slowly pulled away from underlying structures.
8. In myofascial mobilization techniques, tissues are shifted in a (diagonal) (horizontal) direction.
9. In the pin-and-stretch technique, one hand applies enough pressure to hold fascial tissues in place in a certain spot, and the other hand moves connected fascial tissues in the (opposite) (same) direction.
10. Dense connective sheets and bands that hold the muscles and other structures in place throughout the body are called (subserous) (deep) fascia.

Test Prep

The following multiple-choice questions will help to prepare you for future school and professional exams.

1. Typical fascial tissue is best described as:
   a. One-directional and low density
   b. One-directional and high density
   c. Multidirectional and low density
   d. Multidirectional and high density

2. The continuous layer of connective tissue over the entire body between the skin and the deep fascia is called:
   a. Subcutaneous fascia
   b. Subserous fascia
   c. Deepest fascia
   d. Craniosacral fascia

3. The primary mechanism of myofascial techniques is:
   a. Physiological
   b. Reflexive
   c. Mechanical
   d. Energetic

4. The amount of oil or lotion used for myofascial applications is best described as:
   a. Maximal
   b. Minimal
   c. Generous
   d. Thick

5. Myofascial techniques are best described as:
   a. Stretching, pulling, and pushing movements
   b. Sliding and gliding movements
   c. Vibration and pressing movements
   d. Rhythmic compression movements

6. Qualities of myofascial techniques are best characterized as:
   a. Fast and forceful
   b. Superficial and relaxing
   c. Slow and steady
   d. Rhythmic and lively

7. When myofascial restrictions release, it feels to the massage therapist like:
   a. Hardening and shortening
   b. Gathering and contracting
   c. Melting and shortening
   d. Melting and lengthening

8. Fascial tissues become more pliable with:
   a. Heat
   b. Cold
   c. Movement
   d. Both a and c

9. Which of the following is a general contraindication for myofascial massage?
   a. Myofascial pain
   b. Systemic infection
   c. Muscle tightness
   d. Fascial restrictions

10. How long would you expect to hold a myofascial technique before feeling a release of restrictions in the tissue?
    a. 10 seconds
    b. 30 seconds
    c. 2 minutes
    d. 10 minutes

Video Challenge

Watch this video, which can be found at MyHealthProfessions-Lab.com, Chapter 21, and then answer the following questions.

Myofascial Massage

1. How would you describe the elements of the myofascial massage applications demonstrated in the video (e.g., pace, depth, direction, quality of touch)?

2. What principles of good hand and body mechanics were evident in the video?
3. What depth of myofascial tissues is typically engaged by each of the myofascial techniques demonstrated in the video?

Comprehension Exercises

The following short-answer questions test your knowledge and understanding of chapter topics and provide practice in written communication skills. Explain in two to four complete sentences.

1. Explain the nature of fascia and why restrictions in fascial tissues cause health problems.

2. Describe the mechanics of myofascial mobilization techniques. Why is pressure exerted horizontally to the tissues?
3. Contrast myofascial mobilization with pin-and-stretch techniques. How do they affect myofascial tissues differently?

For Greater Understanding

The following exercises are designed to take you from the realm of theory into the real world. They will help give you a deeper understanding of the subjects covered in this chapter. Action words are underlined to emphasize the variety of activities presented to address different learning styles and to encourage deeper thinking.

1. Locate a practitioner with special training in a form of myofascial massage. Receive a myofascial session or series of sessions. Write down your experience or verbally describe it to a study partner.

2. Observe a session with a practitioner with advanced training in myofascial massage. Describe in writing the techniques and overall approach the practitioner used. Explain his or her intent in applying techniques and how tissues seemed to respond.

3. Interview someone who has received a series of myofascial massage sessions from a specially trained practitioner. Ask the person to describe the reason for receiving the sessions and how the sessions were conducted. How did the receiver think he or she benefited?

4. Visit the websites of training programs for myofascial massage. Read the information they offer on their styles of myofascial massage. Describe what you find to a study partner.

MyHealthProfessionsLab™

MyHealthProfessionsLab.com is a premium online homework management system that includes a host of features to help you study. Registered users will find:

- Powerful tools that track and analyze your results—allowing you to create a personalized learning experience
- Videos, flashcards and other learning tools to help enrich your progress
- Streaming lesson presentations and self-paced learning modules
- A space where you and your instructors can view and manage your assignments

CHAPTER

22 Trigger Point Therapy

Pearson Education, Inc.

CHAPTER OUTLINE

Learning Outcomes

Key Terms

Trigger Point Therapy Overview

History of Trigger Point Therapy

Trigger Points

Referral Patterns

Locating Trigger Points

Deactivation Techniques

Trigger Point Therapy for Tension
   Headaches

Chapter Highlights

Exam Review

LEARNING OUTCOMES

After studying this chapter, you will have information to:

1. Define trigger point therapy.

2. Discuss the history of trigger point therapy.

3. Describe trigger points and reference zones.

4. Explain the causes of trigger points.

5. Locate trigger points through palpation and client feedback.

6. Identify contraindications and cautions for trigger point therapy.

7. Apply manual trigger point deactivation techniques.

8. Perform the trigger point therapy Practice Sequence to address tension headaches.

KEY TERMS

Active TrPs

Associated TrPs

Direct pressure

Latent TrPs

Primary TrPs

Reference zone

Satellite TrP

Secondary TrPs

Trigger point therapy

Trigger points (TrPs)

TRIGGER POINT THERAPY OVERVIEW

Trigger point therapy involves the identification and deactivation of painful fibrous nodules called trigger points that occur in muscle and connective tissue. **Trigger points (TrPs)** can be felt as taut bands of tissue that elicit pain if pressed and that refer pain to other areas in predictable patterns.

Trigger points develop in muscles as a result of trauma, poor posture, repetitive strain, or overwork. TrPs cause pain, weakness, and limited flexibility in joints. They may refer pain to other areas of the body. Manual techniques such as direct pressure to TrPs are effective in deactivating the points and relieving the accompanying pain and dysfunction. Trigger point therapy can be integrated into massage sessions as needed as part of a deep tissue or sports massage.

HISTORY OF TRIGGER POINT THERAPY

Soft tissue manipulation techniques that resemble trigger point therapy can be found as far back as the nineteenth century in Europe. A Latvian named Stanley Lief is credited with developing an early form of this bodywork approach in the 1890s. Lief was a natural healer who studied physical culture with Bernarr Macfadden in the United States and was trained in chiropractic and naturopathy. He established a world-famous natural-healing resort in 1925 in Champneys in Hertfordshire, England. There he developed soft tissue manipulative methods that closely resemble what is known in the United States today as trigger point therapy.

In more recent times, physician Janet Travell of the United States is credited with popularizing the term *trigger points*. Travell published her first written work on trigger points in 1952. She used her trigger point approach to relieve the debilitating pain of President John F. Kennedy, then a senator, who had been injured in World War II. Dr. Travell was later appointed White House physician to both Presidents Kennedy and Johnson in the 1960s. These appointments brought Dr. Travell's approach to the attention of the public. With coauthor David Simons, Travell wrote the definitive books on the subject: *Myofascial Pain and Dysfunction: The Trigger Point Manual,* Volumes 1 and 2 (1992, 1999).

Trigger point therapy gained further recognition through the writing and teaching of Bonnie Prudden in the 1970s and 1980s. Prudden's two books, *Pain Erasure* (1980) and *Myotherapy* (1984), offered practical descriptions of how to locate and relieve common trigger points in different parts of the body. Prudden made trigger point therapy accessible to the general public and within the developing field of massage therapy.

Other systems of relieving trigger points have been promoted by their developers and have various names. Neuromuscular therapy (NMT) is a comprehensive approach to treating trigger points that incorporates diet, emotional help, and hydrotherapy, as well as soft tissue manipulation.

TRIGGER POINTS

Trigger points feel like nodules or taut bands of tissue in muscles and tendons. TrPs are tender to the touch and radiate pain in specific reproducible patterns when pressed. A trigger point (TrP) is defined by Travell and Simons as "a focus of hyperirritability in a tissue that, when compressed, is locally tender and, if sufficiently hypersensitive, gives rise to referred pain and tenderness, and sometimes to referred autonomic phenomena and distortion of proprioception."[1]

A trigger point is succinctly described as an "exquisitely tender spot in a taut band of the muscle." A microscopic view of the muscle would reveal tiny contraction knots along the muscle fibers. This accounts for the nodular and taut feel of TrPs.[2]

Trigger points may be categorized as latent or active, primary or secondary, satellite, or associated. **Latent TrPs** are painful only when pressed. **Active TrPs** are always tender, prevent full lengthening of the muscle, weaken the muscle, and refer pain on direct compression. **Primary TrPs** are activated by acute or chronic overload of a muscle, whereas **secondary TrPs** become active because of their reaction to a muscle containing a primary trigger point. A **satellite TrP** becomes active because it is in a muscle in a zone of reference of another TrP. **Associated TrPs** refer to secondary or satellite trigger points. Table 22–1 ■ summarizes the varieties of trigger points.

Deactivation of primary trigger points provides relief from pain and begins to restore full function to a muscle. However, associated points (i.e., secondary and satellite) must also be deactivated for fuller recovery. Trigger points can occur anywhere in the body, but some TrP locations are more common. These are at typical points of muscular stress such as the shoulders, neck, buttocks, and legs (Figure 22–1 ■).

TABLE 22–1	Varieties of Trigger Points	
Type of TrP	**Characteristic**
Latent TrP	Painful only when pressed
Active TrP	Always tender; weakens and shortens the muscle; refers pain
Primary TrP	Activated by acute or chronic muscle overload
Associated TrP	Activated by primary TrP (i.e., secondary TrP); activated by being in reference zone of primary TrP (i.e., satellite TrP)

FIGURE 22–1
Common trigger point locations, anterior and posterior.

Origin of TrPs

Trigger points may be activated by direct stimuli such as acute overload or overwork of a muscle, chilling, or gross trauma. Indirect stimuli may also activate trigger points; for example, arthritic joints, emotional distress, certain visceral diseases, and other TrPs.

People who perform repetitive, stressful tasks, such as athletes, musicians, artists, and physical laborers, are prone to trigger points. Poor posture during daily activities such as sitting at a desk or driving a car may also elicit TrPs. Forward head posture, which places the upper body in a round-shouldered, slumped forward position, is known to produce TrPs in the pectoral and posterior cervical muscles. Something as simple as repeatedly carrying a heavy purse or briefcase on the same side can cause muscle overload that leads to trigger points.

REFERRAL PATTERNS

Trigger points radiate pain in predictable patterns. The area of the body affected by a particular trigger point is called its **reference zone**, sometimes called a *referral zone*. For example,

TrPs in the neck and shoulder muscles refer pain to the head, which is experienced as a tension headache (Figure 22–2 ■). A TrP reference zone might be some distance from the TrP itself. For example, TrPs in the suboccipital muscles refer pain to an area on the side of the head above the ear.

The referred pain of myofascial trigger points is described as "dull and aching, often deep, with intensity varying from low-grade discomfort to severe and incapacitating torture. It may occur at rest or only in motion."[3] Trigger points elicit pain when pressed or may be tender and painful without pressure. Pressing an active TrP usually intensifies pain in its reference zone. The involved muscle is typically stiff and weak and may be restricted in range of motion. Stretching the muscle increases the pain felt. Muscles in the immediate area of a TrP often feel tense and ropelike. Although trigger point charts are useful for confirming common locations and referral patterns, you may find points and patterns unique to an individual client.

Other sensory, motor, and autonomic phenomena may be "triggered" by active TrPs. These include pain, tenderness, increased motor unit activity (spasm), vasoconstriction (blanching), coldness, sweating, pilomotor response (goose bumps), vasodilation (increased local circulation), and

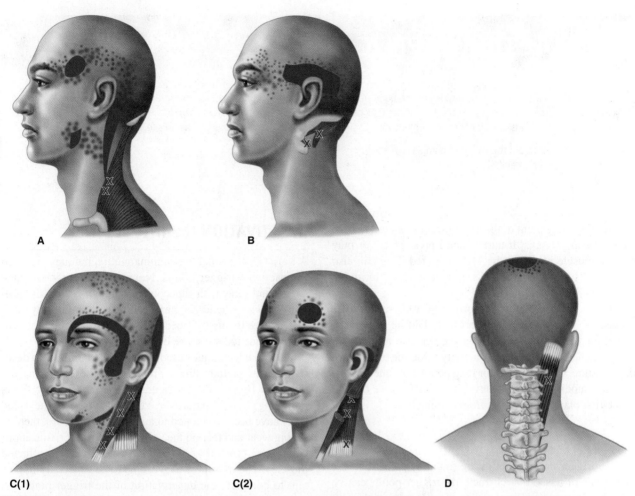

FIGURE 22–2 Locations and reference zones of trigger points that cause headaches. A. Upper trapezius. B. Suboccipitals. C. Sternocleidomastoid (SCM): (1) Superficial division, (2) Deep division. D. Splenius capitus.

hypersecretion (increased gland secretions). These effects can occur at a distance from the trigger point within the TrP's reference zone.[4]

LOCATING TRIGGER POINTS

Suspect myofascial trigger points when clients complain of muscle tension causing pain or when you find localized muscle soreness and shortening. Clients might also describe one of the common pain patterns associated with TrPs and their reference zones. The more knowledgeable you are about TrPs and their predictable referral patterns, the more easily the exact points may be located.

Massage therapists often discover latent TrPs during a massage session. Affected muscles are painful and often feel ropelike. The taut bands at exact TrP locations can be palpated. Clients can give feedback about pain referred to other areas of the body when a TrP is pressed.

CRITICAL THINKING

Think about the causes of trigger points and common locations. Create a self-care plan for the prevention and treatment of trigger points for which you are at most risk as a massage therapist.

1. Which muscles of the upper body are most susceptible to repetitive stress?
2. What self-care measures can you take to prevent TrPs from developing in those muscles?
3. What treatment can you apply to latent TrPs before they become active and cause major problems?

PRACTICAL APPLICATION

Document TrPs found in various regions of the body during a massage practice session. Use the SOAP note chart that can be found at MyHealthProfessionsLab.com to document your findings.

1. Before the session, did the recipient complain of specific muscle tension or soreness?

2. Did you find any active or latent TrPs in common trigger point locations (as shown in Figures 22–1 or 22–2)?

3. How did you identify the TrPs (e.g., by feel or client feedback)?

A client may point to the exact location of active TrPs. He or she might say, "It hurts when I press here," or may rub the muscle in which the TrP is located. You can also have clients mark painful spots on a body chart during an intake interview.

It is helpful to know the origin of a client's trigger points. Was the client in an accident? Did he fall down, or get hit with something? Does she perform a repetitive motion in her job or recreation activity? Does he or she have poor posture, or sit or stand for long periods of time? A person must modify or stop whatever it was that caused the TrP in the first place to prevent it from coming back.

Palpation of TrPs

Precise trigger point locations are found by palpation. The taut bands of tissue that characterize trigger points can be felt. Pressure on a trigger point or snapping across the taut band may elicit a *local twitch response*. This is a "visible or palpable transient contraction of fibers within the taut band."[5]

Clients can also assist in locating TrPs. They might say something like "You're almost on it, but not quite." A slight change in location or angle of pressure is often enough to find the exact point. The pain reported is frequently out of proportion to the pressure applied. Pressure directly on a TrP may elicit a *jump sign* or outcry from the recipient. Clients may report increased pain in the same area or pain referred to another area.

Feedback provided by recipients includes the exact location of TrPs, the degree of pain experienced, and the referral pattern on pressure. They can also tell when the pain diminishes, that is, when the TrP is deactivated.

CONTRAINDICATIONS AND CAUTIONS

Trigger point therapy is contraindicated for undiagnosed conditions that cause severe pain or that are related to recent accidents or trauma. It is locally contraindicated over bruises, wounds, and other instances of soft tissue damage. Caution is advised for clients taking medication that prevents blood from clotting or that compromises tissue integrity.

DEACTIVATION TECHNIQUES

A variety of manual and nonmanual techniques are used to deactivate trigger points. Nonmanual methods include stretch and spray with vapocoolant, saline injection, dry needling, and anesthetics. Nonmanual methods, especially those that require the use of needles or prescriptions for medication, are outside the scope of massage therapists.

Manual techniques used by massage therapists to deactivate TrPs include direct pressure on the TrP using the thumb or fingers, deep effleurage along the muscle fibers (stripping), and deep transverse friction at the TrP site. Hand tools have been developed to apply direct pressure, thereby saving wear and tear on the thumbs. These soft tissue applications are typically followed by a stretch of the affected muscles. The muscle stretch seems to be especially important to complete the deactivation of the trigger point and return the affected tissues to a normal state.

Direct Pressure Techniques

Direct pressure techniques involve compressing tissues directly over the taut band of the TrP. This is sometimes called *ischemic compression* because the compressed tissues become temporarily white from lack of blood, followed by increased local circulation to the spot when pressure is released.

Direct pressure into a TrP is thought to produce a mechanical barrier to the actin–myosin bonding that forms the contraction knot. In essence, direct pressure into the TrP pushes the small contractile units of the muscle cells (called sarcomeres) apart, releasing the contraction. When this happens, it is felt as a softening or releasing of the taut band.[6]

Direct pressure may be applied with the thumb or fingers, with a tool, or with a pincer technique. The amount of pressure used on the TrP is enough to engage the taut band, but not so much to cause extreme pain. Pressure is gradually increased as the sensitivity of the TrP wanes, and the tension in its taut band fades. Pressure is released when the therapist feels the TrP tension subside or when the TrP is no longer tender to pressure. This takes approximately 30–90 seconds.

FIGURE 22–3 Direct thumb pressure to a trigger point.

Source: Pearson Education, Inc./Segal Photography.

FIGURE 22–5 Use of the elbow to apply pressure to trigger points in the trapezius with the receiver in sitting position.

Source: Pearson Education, Inc./Segal Photography.

Using the right amount of pressure is essential to the successful deactivation of trigger points. The client should feel some measure of discomfort with pressure directly on the TrP. However, if you feel a protective increase of muscle tension in the area, lighten pressure a little until the discomfort does not elicit an armoring response. Causing further muscle tension is counterproductive to the goal of relieving TrPs.

The thumbs are commonly used to provide the sustained digital pressure in deactivating trigger points. Figure 22–3 ■ illustrates the use of the thumb in applying direct pressure to TrPs. Note the hand mechanics with thumb and wrist joints in alignment. Avoid pressure while the thumb is abducted.

To relieve the thumbs, other parts of the hands may be used to apply pressure, for example, the fingertips as in Figure 22–4 ■. For more heavily muscled areas, the elbow may be used. Figure 22–5 ■ shows the use of the elbow with the recipient in the seated position to deactivate TrPs in the large trapezius muscle. The elbow is also useful when working through larger muscles to affect deeper muscles in an area, for example, to reach the deeper muscles of the buttocks.

To protect the small joints of the hands from overuse, small hand tools may be used effectively for applying pressure. Find trigger points through palpation with the fingertips, and then place the tip of the tool on the point to apply pressure. If used with sensitivity, the quality of touch with the tool may be indistinguishable from using the hand directly. It is important to keep the wrists straight when using tools. Figure 22–6 ■ demonstrates the use of a wooden hand tool to apply pressure to trigger points.

In the preceding examples, the tissue containing the TrP is compressed between the practitioner's hand or hand tool and tissues underneath the point. In the pincer technique, the tissue at the TrP site is compressed between the fingers and thumb of the practitioner. For example, TrPs in the sternocleidomastoid (SCM) may be compressed using the pincer technique, as shown in Figure 22–7 ■. Take care to avoid the carotid artery located anterior to the SCM. Review endangerment sites in the anterior and posterior neck, which are illustrated in Figures 8–3 and 8–4. Sustained pressure should not be applied to blood vessels or nerves or when it induces numbness and tingling.

FIGURE 22–4 Finger pressure to a trigger point.

Source: Pearson Education, Inc./Segal Photography.

FIGURE 22–6 Use of a hand tool to apply pressure to a trigger point.

Source: Pearson Education, Inc./Segal Photography.

FIGURE 22–7 Squeezing the sternocleidomastoid (SCM) with a pincer technique.

Source: Pearson Education, Inc./Segal Photography.

Blend deep stroking or stripping, deep friction, kneading, and stretching with direct pressure to TrPs for best results. These techniques combined deactivate the TrP, separate tissues that are adhering, bring circulation back to the area, and lengthen muscles that have shortened.

TRIGGER POINT THERAPY FOR TENSION HEADACHES

Trigger point therapy has been found to be very effective in treatment of tension headaches. Practice Sequence 22–1 demonstrates a protocol used to deactivate TrPs known to refer pain to the head. It was adapted from a protocol used in a research project on treating tension headaches.[7]

 ## CASE FOR STUDY

Nikki's Neck and Shoulder Pain

Nikki has been playing the violin since childhood and now performs in a local orchestra on weekends. She practices every night for about 1 hour. During the day, she works as a receptionist in a doctor's office. Lately, she has noticed difficulty turning her head and has pains in her hands and shoulders. She is afraid she won't be able to play the violin much longer if the pain continues to worsen.

Question:

How might Nikki's massage therapist use trigger point therapy to address her complaints?

Things to consider:

- What repetitive actions or static postures are stressing Nikki's muscles?
- Where are the most likely locations for TrPs given Nikki's situation?
- What home care activities would reinforce trigger point therapy treatment?

Create a long-term plan, including trigger point therapy, to address Nikki's complaint. Include massage session plans and home care suggestions.

_____

_____

_____

PRACTICE SEQUENCE 22-1

Trigger Point Therapy for Tension Headaches | 30 minutes / Recipient supine

Preliminary Considerations
- Check for contraindications to massage in the neck and shoulders.
- Position the recipient comfortably with bolsters.
- Use oil or lotion sparingly to prevent skin friction.

1

Figure 22–8 Apply warming petrissage to cervical muscles with neck in slight traction. Traction neck with one hand holding the head; squeeze and press posterior cervical muscles with fingertips to warm tissues on both sides.

Figure 22–9 Effleurage along cervical and upper trapezius muscles from occiput to shoulder. Hold head in lateral flexion with slight rotation; slide with fist or palm from occiput to shoulder; repeat to stretch and warm tissues on both sides.

Figure 22–10 Traction neck with head in neutral position. With recipient's face directly up, hold head at occiput; pull back to create slight traction in neck.

Apply Steps 4-8 to both sides before finishing with Steps 9 and 10.

General directions for treating trigger points:
• Locate trigger points with palpation and feedback from the recipient.
• Press into TrP to engage the taut band but not cause extreme pain.
• Feel for release or softening of the band.
• Sink in deeper as the tissue allows.
• Apply for 30–90 seconds.
• Come out of pressure slowly.
• Follow up with massage and stretching of the affected muscle.

Figure 22–11 Locate and apply thumb pressure directly into suspected TrPs in upper trapezius.

5

Figure 22–12 Apply pincer pressure to TrPs in sternocleidomastoid (SCM) muscle. Turn head to side to expose SCM; locate TrPs; use pincer technique to squeeze muscle at the TrP sites.

6

Figure 22–13 Turn head for access to suboccipital muscles and locate TrPs. Use fingers or thumb to apply pressure directly into the TrPs.

7

Figure 22–14 Turn head for access to posterior cervical muscles. Locate TrPs along posterior cervical muscles, and use fingers or thumb to apply pressure.

8

Figure 22–15 Gently stretch neck muscles. Apply stretches with head in neutral position, lateral flexion, and rotation.

Repeat Steps 4-8 on other side.

9

Figure 22–16 Apply effleurage with wave motion to posterior cervical region. Use fingertips to slide along cervical muscles from base of neck to suboccipital area; push upward to create a wave in the neck as fingers pass underneath.

10

Figure 22–17 Cat paw mobilizing of shoulders toward the feet. Press downward along upper trapezius muscle from base of neck to shoulder joint, alternating rhythmic left–right pressure. Apply gentle pressure on muscles to create movement in neck and shoulders.

After you perform the Practice Sequence, evaluate how well you did by filling out Performance Evaluation Form 22–1, Trigger Point Therapy for Tension Headaches. The form can be found in Appendix D: *Performance Evaluation Forms*, and at MyHealthProfessionsLab.com.

Figures source: Pearson Education, Inc./Segal Photography.

CHAPTER HIGHLIGHTS

- Trigger point therapy involves the identification and deactivation of painful fibrous nodules in muscle and connective tissue called trigger points.
- Physician Janet Travell is credited with bringing attention to trigger point therapy in the 1950s–1970s.
  - Travell and David Simon wrote the definite work on trigger point therapy.
- Trigger points (TrPs) can be felt as taut bands of tissue that elicit pain if pressed and that refer pain to other areas in predictable patterns.
  - Latent TrPs are painful only when pressed.
  - Active TrPs are always tender, prevent full lengthening of the muscle, weaken the muscle, and refer pain on direct compression.
  - Primary TrPs are activated by acute or chronic overload of a muscle.
  - Secondary TrPs become active because of their reaction to a muscle containing a primary trigger point.

- A satellite TrP becomes active because it is in a muscle in a zone of reference of another TrP.
  - Associated TrPs refer to secondary or satellite trigger points.
- TrPs are palpated as taut bands in muscle or connective tissue.
  - TrPs feel like contracted nodules.
  - Clients can give valuable feedback about the exact location of TrPs.
- Specific TrPs refer pain to their reference zone.
- Trigger points develop in muscles as a result of trauma, poor posture, repetitive strain, or overwork.
- TrPs cause pain, weakness, and limited flexibility in joints.
  - Manual techniques such as direct pressure to TrPs are effective in deactivating the points and relieving the accompanying pain and dysfunction.

- ○ Direct pressure into the TrP produces a mechanical barrier to the actin–myosin bonding that forms the contraction knot.
- ○ Direct pressure to TrPs is sometimes called ischemic compression.
- ○ Correct pressure on TrPs engages the taut band but does not cause extreme pain.
- ○ Sustained pressure is held for 30–90 seconds.
- ○ When TrPs release, it feels like softening or sinking into tissues.

- Direct pressure is followed with broadening and stretching of the affected muscle for complete treatment.
- TrPs in the neck and shoulder regions can refer pain into the head, causing chronic tension headaches.
- Trigger point therapy can be integrated into massage sessions as needed.

EXAM REVIEW

Key Terms

Match the following key terms to their descriptions. For additional study, look up the key terms in the Interactive Glossary, and note other terms that compare or contrast with them.

_____ 1. Active TrP
_____ 2. Associated TrP
_____ 3. Direct pressure
_____ 4. Latent TrP
_____ 5. Primary TrP
_____ 6. Reference zone
_____ 7. Satellite TrP
_____ 8. Secondary TrP
_____ 9. Trigger point therapy
_____ 10. Trigger point

a. Taut tender band in muscle
b. TrP always tender and refers pain
c. TrP painful only when pressed
d. Manual therapy to address TrPs
e. Activated by acute muscle overload
f. In reference zone of primary TrP
g. Technique for compressing tissues
h. TrP from reaction to primary TrP
i. Category for secondary and satellite TrPs
j. Area of the body affected by a particular TrP

Memory Workout

To test your memory of the main concepts in this chapter, complete the following sentences by circling the most correct answer from the two choices provided.

1. The person best known for treating U.S. presidents in the 1960s, including John F. Kennedy, with trigger point therapy is (Bonnie Prudden) (Janet Travell).
2. Trigger points feel like a (taut) (loose) band of muscle or tendon tissue.
3. Trigger points refer pain to their (reference) (immediate) zone.
4. Muscles in the immediate area of a trigger point may feel tense and (wood-like) (rope-like).
5. Trigger points that are always tender, that weaken and shorten the muscle in which they are located, and that refer pain on direct compression are categorized as (satellite) (active) TrPs.
6. One of the primary causes of trigger points is (acute stress) (overstretch) of a muscle.
7. Direct pressure that causes tissues to become temporarily white from lack of blood and oxygen, is called (ischemic) (active) compression.
8. Trigger points in the shoulders and (back) (neck) are a major cause of tension headaches.
9. To save wear and tear on the thumbs, massage therapists can deactivate trigger points using (simple hand tools) (saline injections).
10. Direct pressure into a trigger point pushes the (fibers) (sarcomeres) of the muscle tissue apart, releasing the contraction.

Test Prep

The following multiple-choice questions will help to prepare you for future school and professional exams.

1. A microscopic view of a muscle with a trigger point would reveal:
   a. Tiny bacteria
   b. Dilated blood vessels
   c. Swollen lymph nodes
   d. Tiny contraction knots along the muscle fibers

2. Trigger points that are painful only when pressed are categorized as:
   a. Associated TrPs
   b. Latent TrPs
   c. Active TrPs
   d. Satellite TrPs

3. A visible or palpable transient contraction of fibers within the taut band of a trigger point when it is pressed is called:
   a. Forced contraction
   b. Spasm response
   c. Local twitch response
   d. Reflex contraction

4. A trigger point treatment technique *not* in the scope of massage therapists is:
   a. Dry needling
   b. Direct pressure
   c. Muscle stripping
   d. Stretching

5. A sign that a trigger point has released is:
   a. Softening of the taut band
   b. Sinking into the point
   c. Decreased pain felt by the client
   d. All of the above

6. For a more complete treatment, direct pressure to a trigger point is followed by:
   a. Tapotement on the affected muscle
   b. Stretching of the affected muscle
   c. Vibration in the general area
   d. Lymphatic facilitation techniques

7. When working through larger muscles to affect deeper muscles in an area, for example, to reach the deeper muscles of the buttocks, direct pressure can be applied with the:
   a. Thumb
   b. Little finger
   c. Two middle fingers
   d. Elbow

8. A trigger point that becomes active because it is in a muscle in a zone of reference of another trigger point is categorized as:
   a. Latent
   b. Active
   c. Satellite
   d. Referenced

9. The referred pain of trigger points is often described as:
   a. Dull and aching
   b. Sharp and piercing
   c. Burning
   d. Soft and light

10. Direct pressure to a trigger point is typically sustained for:
    a. 10 seconds
    b. 10–20 seconds
    c. 30–90 seconds
    d. 3 minutes

Video Challenge

Watch this video, which can be found at MyHealthProfessionsLab.com, Chapter 22, and then answer the following questions.

Trigger Point Therapy

1. In the video, what parts of the massage therapist's hand and arm are used to apply direct pressure to trigger points?

2. What principles of good hand mechanics can be seen in the trigger point therapy demonstration in the video?

3. Where is the massage therapist in the video searching for trigger points related to tension headaches?

Comprehension Exercises

The following short-answer questions test your knowledge and understanding of chapter topics and provide practice in written communication skills. Explain in two to four complete sentences.

1. Explain the causes of trigger points in muscle and connective tissue. Give two common examples.

2. Describe what trigger points feel like when palpated. What physiological basis is there for their feel?

3. Describe the use of direct pressure techniques to deactivate trigger points. How do you know when a trigger point releases?

For Greater Understanding

The following exercises are designed to take you from the realm of theory into the real world. They will help give you a deeper understanding of the subjects covered in this chapter. Action words are underlined to emphasize the variety of activities presented to address different learning styles and to encourage deeper thinking.

1. Observe a trigger point therapy session given by an experienced massage therapist. Describe the overall approach and the techniques used. How were trigger points located? How much verbal interaction was there with the client?

2. Interview someone (e.g., athlete, artist, musician, physical worker) who has received trigger point therapy from a practitioner with advanced training. Ask him or her to describe the experience. Was it painful? Effective?

3. Locate and deactivate trigger points on a practice client. Compare his or her feedback on TrP referral patterns to a commercial chart. Did the zones on the chart match your client's experience? Did you find TrPs not on the chart?

MyHealthProfessionsLab™

MyHealthProfessionsLab.com is a premium online homework management system that includes a host of features to help you study. Registered users will find:

- Powerful tools that track and analyze your results—allowing you to create a personalized learning experience
- Videos, flashcards and other learning tools to help enrich your progress
- Streaming lesson presentations and self-paced learning modules
- A space where you and your instructors can view and manage your assignments

Lymphatic Facilitation

Dale Perry

Pearson Education, Inc.

CHAPTER OUTLINE

Learning Outcomes

Key Terms

Overview of Lymphatic Facilitation

History of Lymphatic Facilitation

The Lymphatic System

Lymphatic System Vessels

Lymph Nodes

General Drainage Patterns

Indications and Contraindications

Lymphatic Facilitation Attributes
  and Strokes

Lymphatic Facilitation Applications

Integration of Lymphatic Facilitation into a Massage Session

Chapter Highlights

Exam Review

LEARNING OUTCOMES

After studying this chapter, you will have information to:

1. Define lymphatic facilitation (LF).

2. Describe the benefits of LF applications.

3. Explain lymphatic system anatomy and physiology relevant to LF applications.

4. Identify indications and contraindications for LF.

5. Distinguish between manual lymphatic drainage (MLD) and LF.

6. Apply the basic LF techniques.

7. Perform the LF Practice Sequences for the head and neck and the lower extremity.

8. State basic concepts and attributes of LF applications.

KEY TERMS

Catchments

Collector
  vessels

Cisterna chyli

Initial/terminal (I/T) lymph
  vessels

Interstitial matrix

L stroke

Long stroke

Lymph

Lymphatic facilitation (LF)

Terminus

Transport vessels

Watersheds

OVERVIEW OF LYMPHATIC FACILITATION

Lymphatic facilitation (LF) is a light and gentle massage technique used to accelerate the removal of excess fluid that collects in tissues after trauma and inflammation. Excess fluid accumulation can cause irritation to pain receptors, reduce range of motion in affected joints, reduce the delivery of nutrition to cells, and lead to restrictions in fascia. The application of LF expedites the transportation of fluids through interstitial spaces (spaces between cells and tissues in the body) and the lymph system, and away from the affected area. This action results in pain relief, increased local circulation, and increased range of motion in affected joints.

LF evolved from manual lymphatic drainage (MLD), which was designed specifically to treat a pathology known as lymphedema, an accumulation of surplus fluid in bodily tissues caused by faulty lymphatic drainage. Differences in MLD and LF are explained more fully in the following sections.

HISTORY OF LYMPHATIC MASSAGE

Enhanced circulation and lymph flow have been recognized as benefits of massage for over a century. However, due to the unique anatomy and physiology of the lymph system, manual lymphatic techniques are distinctly different from more traditional styles of massage.

Two Danish physiotherapists, Emil and Astrid Vodder, developed a unique protocol for lymphatic massage in the 1930s. It was known as the Vodder Method® of Manual Lymphatic Drainage (MLD).[1, 2] The Vodder Method took into consideration new information about how the lymphatic system works. This approach required extensive training in precise stroke application. Due to its effectiveness, it became a core element in the manual treatment of a disease called *lymphedema.*

The full treatment for lymphedema was a combination of skin care, MLD, compression bandaging, exercise, and patient self-care. This was known as *decongestive therapy.* Others further developed the approach, including Drs. Michael and Ethel Foldi of Germany, who called their system *complete decongestive therapy (CDT).* They kept Vodder's MLD in their system of CDT.[3] Drs. John and Judith Casley-Smith of Australia did further revisions to CDT and refer to their therapy as *complex decongestive therapy.* The Australian version replaced the Vodder method with one basic stroke that could be mastered in a short time by a trained massage therapist.[4] The therapeutic outcomes of these various manual lymphatic approaches turned out to be very similar. Massage techniques based on the complex structure of the lymphatic system continue to be developed for treatment of a variety of conditions that benefit from good lymph fluid circulation.

Lymphatic Facilitation Compared to Manual Lymphatic Drainage

Lymphatic facilitation was developed as an adaptation of lymphatic techniques for sports and injury rehabilitation.

An entirely different set of rules was required for reducing edema around an injury site. Athletes need to recover from injuries quickly and frequently are unable to follow the normal rest and rehabilitation patterns of nonathletes. Thus an approach different from Vodder MLD was sought. The result is an adaptation based on European and Australian approaches to lymphedema treatment, but simplified for use in treatment of injuries.

Vodder MLD involves mastering a variety of manual techniques applied in a specific order using a precise protocol. In contrast, LF is less complicated, easier to learn, more adaptable, and more easily integrated into massage sessions. LF skills are useful for massage therapists in a variety of settings. LF is not used to treat lymphedema; therefore those wishing to work in medical settings with lymphedema patients will need advanced training in MLD protocols, which are not in the scope of this textbook.

THE LYMPHATIC SYSTEM

Knowledge of the structure and function of the lymphatic system is essential for understanding lymphatic facilitation applications. The techniques themselves, and the order in which they are applied, are based on the unique character of this complex body system. It will be helpful for you to review basic lymphatic system anatomy in preparation for the following discussion, which focuses on information related to LF applications.

Lymphatic system components include a network of lymph vessels, lymph fluid, lymph nodes, the cisterna chyli, and the spleen and thymus. An overview of lymphatic system structures appears in Figure 23–1 ▪. Note that the flow of lymph fluid in the system is in an asymmetrical pattern. Lymph fluid from the legs, lower abdomen, and left side of the body flows to the thoracic duct (left lymphatic duct) and into the left subclavian vein. Lymph from the right side of the body above the diaphragm flows to the right lymphatic duct and into the right subclavian vein. Lymphatic facilitation applications direct flow toward the appropriate lymphatic duct.

Lymphatic system functions include the production and distribution of lymphocytes and the transport of fluid, hormones, waste products, and cellular debris back to the cardiovascular system from the tissues. Normally, about 10% of interstitial fluid is returned to the cardiovascular system via the lymphatic system.[5]

Another important function of the lymphatic system is immunity or resistance to disease. The lymph system houses many of the cells involved in our immune response. These include T-cells and B-cells along with monocytes that are responsible for identifying and breaking down cellular debris and pathogens.

Homeostasis

The general principle of homeostasis (i.e., maintaining a stable internal environment) is the basis of lymphatic

FIGURE 23–1
Overview of lymphatic system structures and the general direction of lymph flow from the extremities to the terminus at the thoracic ducts.

Cervical nodes

Right lymphatic duct

Thoracic duct (left lymphatic duct)

Axillary nodes

Lymphatic vessels

Secondary nodes

Cisterna chyli

Inguinal nodes

Lymphatic vessels

Secondary nodes

Secondary nodes

facilitation. LF applications reestablish a healthy balance in the internal environment of soft tissues by removing an excess accumulation of interstitial fluid.

To understand the overall goal of LF, it is useful to consider how interstitial fluid is reabsorbed into general circulation. Fluid is returned to the cardiovascular system through both blood and lymph circulation. Normally, about 90% of interstitial fluid is returned directly to the cardiovascular system via the veins, whereas 10% is the responsibility of the lymph system.

If the blood or lymph capillaries in a certain area become blocked or damaged, there will be fluid buildup in the tissues resulting in edema or swelling. This typically happens with traumatic injury and common musculoskeletal injuries such as strains and sprains. To reestablish fluid balance in the tissues and reduce edema, the lymphatic system must increase its capacity. The lymphatic system has the ability to boost its capability up to 50% for a short period of time. The skillful application of LF techniques assists fluid absorption and flow, thus reestablishing homeostatic fluid balance in tissues.

This illustrates a hypothesis formulated by physician Ernst Henry Starling in 1896. Starling's hypothesis states that to maintain a fluid balance in the body, the circulatory and lymphatic systems must be working at normal volumes. If the circulatory system becomes dysfunctional, then the lymphatic system must increase its capacity to reestablish fluid balance in the tissues.

Lymph

Lymph is the colorless fluid in the lymph vessels that contains water, protein molecules, cellular components, and fatty acids that need to be transported back into blood circulation. Before it enters the lymph system, this fluid resides in and moves through the intercellular spaces as interstitial fluid.

Molecules, proteins, and cellular wastes too large to enter blood capillaries are returned to general circulation via the lymph capillaries. Without the lymph system, this material would accumulate in the tissues, causing inflammation, irritation, and pain.

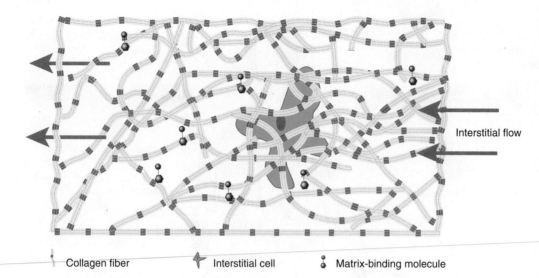

FIGURE 23-2
Interstitial matrix.

Interstitial flow

Collagen fiber   Interstitial cell   Matrix-binding molecule

Interstitial Matrix

Interstitial matrix is a more accurate description of what is often called the *interstitial space*. The word *space* implies a vacant open area between cells. However, this space is more structured than usually depicted. The interstitial matrix is created by collagen fibers that form "scaffolding" within which fluids such as water and plasma flow (Figure 23–2 ■). The interstitial matrix is referred to as a *prelymphatic channel* in many manual lymph drainage texts.[6]

The optimal delivery of nutrients and removal of waste products requires that the interstitial matrix be free of debris and restrictions. Lymphatic facilitation applications help maintain the health of this matrix by moving interstitial fluid through the system. If lymphatic vessels are damaged in a certain area, LF techniques can move fluid through the interstitial matrix into a different watershed (drainage area) to facilitate its eventual removal via the blood and lymph capillaries.

LYMPHATIC SYSTEM VESSELS

The lymphatic system is composed of hollow vessels that carry lymph from peripheral tissues back to the venous circulatory system. The smallest vessels dead-end in the interstitial spaces and are known as lymph capillaries or initial/terminal (I/T) lymph vessels. These initial vessels flow into progressively larger vessels called collector vessels and transport vessels (Figure 23–3 ■). The lymphatic vessels finally empty into two large collecting ducts in the chest.

Initial/Terminal (I/T) Lymph Vessels

The **initial/terminal (I/T) lymph vessels** are the entry point for metabolic and cellular waste, proteins, and excess fluids. They are the smallest lymph vessels, with walls that are only one cell thick. A schematic drawing of the I/T lymph vessels or initial lymphatics appears in Figure 23–4 ■.

The overlapping design of cell junctions creates one-way valves to prevent backflow of fluid into the interstitial spaces. It is at the site of the I/T lymph vessels that LF techniques have their greatest effect.

Opening of the *flaps* or *overflaps* is stimulated by several mechanisms, including variations of tissue pressure . . . and contraction of *fibrils* or *anchoring filaments* attached to the exterior cells' walls and surrounding connective tissue. . . . An increase in interstitial fluid will cause a pull on the fibrils, which will open the flaps. External mechanical stimulation to superficial connective tissue, such as gentle skin traction, may contribute to flap opening by pulling on the anchoring filaments.[7]

—Excerpt from A PRIMER ON LYMPHEDEMA CONTACT DETAILS by Deborah G. Kelly. Published by Pearson Education,© 2002.

Too much pressure (e.g., as used in standard massage) closes the flaps and slows or stops the flow of lymph into the I/T lymphatics. This is the reason that techniques designed to facilitate lymphatic flow are applied with only enough

Initial lymph vessels

Epidermis

Dermis

Collector vessels

Fascia and muscle tissue

Anastomosis

Transport vessels

FIGURE 23–3 Lymphatic system vessels and the flow of lymph.

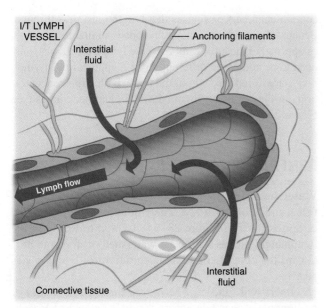

I/T LYMPH VESSEL

Interstitial fluid

Anchoring filaments

Lymph flow

Interstitial fluid

Connective tissue

FIGURE 23–4 Schematic drawing of initial/terminal (I/T) lymph vessel.

pressure to create traction and movement in the superficial skin layers.

It is estimated that 40% of all I/T lymph vessels are found in the dermis. The opening and closing of the I/T lymph vessels allows for the filling of lymph transport vessels and the removal of proteins, metabolic wastes, and cellular debris that are too large to enter venous capillaries.

Only small- and medium-size molecules, proteins, gases, amino acids, and cellular wastes are able to pass into the venous capillary system. However, these same products passing into the lymphatic system via I/T lymph vessels can be up to extra large in size. This size differential is of paramount importance in understanding the vital role the lymph system plays in removal and transport of waste products. Large complex proteins and large pathogens would likely not be removed unless the lymph system is operating optimally. Along with the interstitial matrix, I/T lymph vessel structures are the focus of lymphatic facilitation, and their importance cannot be overstressed.

Collector Vessels

As their name indicates, **collector vessels** collect lymph from the I/T lymph vessels and connect to the transport vessels or lymphangia. The collector vessel walls are generally only one or two cells thick and do not contain valves. They extend from the I/T lymph vessels found in the dermis through the subcutaneous tissue to fill the larger, more complex lymphatic transport vessels.

Transport Vessels

The **transport vessels**, or *lymphangia,* are larger than collector vessels and are constructed more like veins. Transport vessels are segmented, with each segment approximately 2 to10 cm in length. Each segment is referred to as a

lymphangion. It is bounded by a valve on each end. A continuous length of these structures is most appropriately referred to as a lymphangia.[8] It is important to note that once lymph enters this structure, manual techniques cannot change its path. They can facilitate increased transport capacity and flow but not influence direction.

Transport vessels have an outer, middle, and inner tunica (layers of tissues) similar to those found in veins. The middle layer contains smooth muscle that contracts in a peristaltic manner. MLD texts make reference to stretching these muscle layers as strokes are applied, which increases the contraction rate. It is more probable that these vessels are engaged by filling them. As LF is applied and I/T lymph vessels are filled, collector vessels deliver lymph to the transport vessels, which expand as they fill. This expansion of the vessel wall stretches the smooth muscle, and when it reaches a certain point of stretch, the muscle responds by contracting. This is referred to as a *stretch reflex.*

The contraction rate of these muscles at rest is estimated to be 4 to10 times per minute. It is possible that, through skeletal muscle contraction and increased heart rate, the contraction rate can reach 40 times per minute. The lymphangia are also stimulated by breathing and traction. With proper application of LF techniques, a substantial increase in the rate of lymphangia contraction may be achieved without increasing skeletal muscle contraction or increased heart rate. This is particularly important when working with clients who are inactive due to injury or surgery.

If a transport vessel becomes damaged or blocked, an emergency pathway is provided by a network called the *anastomosis,* shown in Figure 23–3. This system of small vessels links one lymphangion to another, providing an alternate route for lymph flow. Anastomosis structures are especially important in areas of trauma and injury.

Cisterna Chyli

Lymph collected from the below the waist watershed must first pass through the **cisterna chyli**, shown in Figure 23–1. This structure is considered the abdominal part of the thoracic duct and is located very deep in the abdomen.

Imagine that the cysterna chyli is the bulb on top of a turkey baster, and the thoracic duct is the tube of the baster. If you turn the turkey baster bulb-side down, you can approximate the relationship of the cisterna chyli to the thoracic duct in the abdomen. To clear the cisterna chyli, we simply squeeze the "bulb" and the lymph is pushed through the thoracic duct and enters the subclavian vein. This is accomplished through the action of the diaphragm in breathing and may be exaggerated through contraction of the abdominal muscles, such as when doing sit-ups. The cisterna chyli is important to consider in LF applications to the lower extremities.

Terminus

The **terminus** is located in the hollow space just lateral to the attachments of the sternocleidomastoid (SCM) muscles on the clavicle. It is at the terminus that LF techniques are applied to increase the flow of lymph into the thoracic ducts, thus clearing the area.

Stimulating the terminus also increases the uptake of fluid at I/T lymph vessel structures. This happens because the increase in fluid uptake at the terminus decreases the internal pressure of the lymphatic system as a whole, relative to the pressure in the interstitial spaces. Because of this pressure gradient differential, more fluid will enter I/T lymph vessels until the pressure is equalized.

The stimulation of the terminus is accomplished by application of L strokes, as described in the following Practice Sequences, prior to starting an LF session. Dr. Michael Foldi has suggested that this alone can increase the lymph uptake at I/T lymph vessels by up to 30% and last for several hours after the massage session.

LYMPH NODES

The primary function of lymph nodes is to house cells of immunity, filter out water, concentrate lymph, and remove nonorganic material. The significance of the nodes, when applying LF, is that they tend to slow transport. This is due to their construction. As you can see in Figure 23–5 ■, nodes

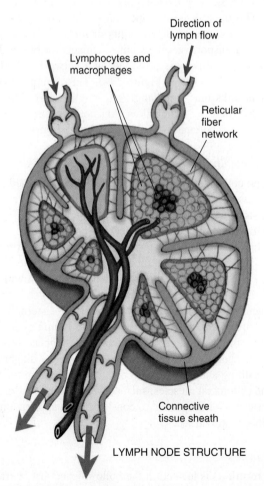

Direction of lymph flow

Lymphocytes and macrophages

Reticular fiber network

Connective tissue sheath

LYMPH NODE STRUCTURE

FIGURE 23–5 Lymph node structure.

contain chambers or sinuses that lymph must pass through. Because the structure of a lymph node is similar to a sponge, as opposed to the hollow tubes of the lymph capillaries, they need to be addressed differently in LF applications. Lymph nodes are found throughout the body, with large concentrations in the popliteal, inguinal, axilla, and neck areas (see Figure 23–1).

GENERAL DRAINAGE PATTERNS

Watersheds describe superficial drainage patterns in different areas of the body. Their boundaries are outlined as dotted lines in Figure 23–6 ■. Lymph traveling in the lymphangia moves within its watershed or drainage area toward the **catchments** or concentrations of lymph nodes nearby.

Interstitial fluid may be moved through the matrix or prelymphatic channels across watersheds using LF techniques. Long strokes or flat-hand L strokes directed perpendicular to the watershed can move fluid across these drainage areas.

INDICATIONS AND CONTRAINDICATIONS

There are many indications for the use of lymphatic facilitation. One important indication is edema or excess interstitial fluid due to trauma. This includes removing the fluid itself as well as the debris and wastes suspended in it. Pain caused by irritants in interstitial fluids may also be reduced due to improved flow of those fluids.

LF can minimize the formation of fascial adhesions during tissue repair and thereby increase range of motion in affected joints. Allergy, arthritis, sinus congestion, and psoriasis symptoms may also improve with enhanced lymph transport.

Contraindications

There are few absolute contraindications for LF. One of these is lymphedema, which is swelling caused by lymph system dysfunction that allows the accumulation of protein-rich fluid in interstitial spaces. Lymphedema often results from treatment for cancer. Complete/complex decongestive therapy is a treatment for lymphedema that encompasses manual lymphatic drainage in the protocol.

Other contraindications for LF include infection, thrombosis or blood clots, phlebitis, pitting edema, and major heart problems such as congestive heart failure. Any conditions that can be worsened by increased fluid circulation warrant caution when applying lymphatic techniques. This includes kidney disease, severe asthma, thyroid conditions, and menstruation in women. Release of waste products into circulation too rapidly during LF can cause flu-like symptoms afterward. Don't over treat in one session. Advise clients to drink several glasses of water in the hours after an LF

FIGURE 23–6
Superficial lymph drainage pathways or watersheds determine the direction of lymphatic facilitation applications.

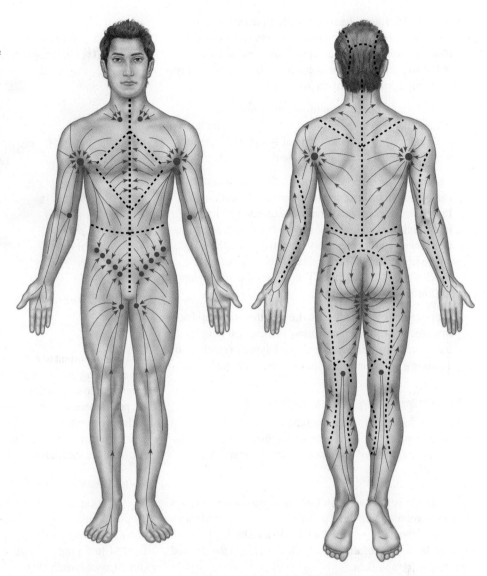

treatment to help the body with its normal job of removing waste products from the system.

It has been long speculated that massage, and specifically lymphatic massage, may cause malignant tumors to spread to other parts of the body, but at this point there is no evidence that would support that idea. Therefore, when working with a cancer patient, the therapist must discuss the merits and cautions of using LF with the individual's physician. LF may be appropriate at different stages of a cancer patient's treatment; for example, postsurgery to enhance secondary edema removal, promote decreased adhesions, and support the healing cycle. It may also be beneficial post-radiation for the same reason. If the lymph system has been compromised during treatment and lymphedema results, it is important to refer the patient to a complete decongestive therapy (CDT) specialist and not use lymphatic facilitation alone for treatment. Consultation with a cancer patient's physician is advised before providing lymphatic massage of any kind.

LYMPHATIC FACILITATION ATTRIBUTES AND STROKES

LF techniques are designed to increase the absorption of interstitial fluid at I/T lymph vessel structures, move interstitial fluid within the interstitial space or matrix, increase the rate of lymphangia contraction, and generally improve the flow of lymph fluid within lymphatic vessels. LF can also affect the direction of lymph flow in superficial tissues.

LF is effective if the strokes are applied with the correct attributes. These attributes can be summarized as light, rhythmic, slow, and applied in the direction of lymph flow. The skin stretches and releases, that is, it snaps back into place.

- **Light.** Use 4 to 5 grams of pressure so that the I/T lymph vessel structures are not closed by compression. An easy way to remember this is to put your finger on your eyelid and move the eyelid over your eye. This should approximate the pressure used for LF strokes.

- **Rhythmic.** Interstitial fluid is prompted to flow in the stroke direction by initiating a "pressure wave" inside the interstitial space that moves in the direction of the stretch. This flow is enhanced by a slow, steady rhythmic application of the strokes.

- **Slow.** The lymph system moves at a slow rate. Although 7,000 liters of blood flow through the heart in 24 hours, only about 2 liters of lymph flow through the thoracic duct during the same time period.

- **Applied in the direction of lymph flow.** Interstitial fluids and lymph are directed toward catchment areas. Practitioners may modify the stroke direction to redirect interstitial fluid around and/or away from areas of trauma. Catchment areas immediately proximal to the places where LF strokes will be applied are cleared before moving fluids toward them. This creates space for lymph to flow into.

- **Skin stretches and releases.** Letting the skin snap back into place after stretching promotes increased lymph transport by opening and closing I/T lymph vessels, and creating a "pressure wave" in the interstitial space.

L Stroke and Long Stroke

Lymphatic facilitation is a combination of Australian and European approaches. Two basic techniques that can be easily learned and applied are L strokes and long strokes.

L STROKE

The **L stroke** is applied in an L-shaped pattern. The skin is stretched when tracing the L pattern. The L stroke ends with a release of the tissue so that it returns to the starting position or snaps back. One of the stretch directions is in the desired direction of lymph flow.

FIGURE 23–7 L stroke used in lymphatic facilitation.

Source: Pearson Education, Inc./Segal Photography.

It is important to note that the skin on different clients will have varying elasticity or stretchiness. For the L stroke, the length of the stretch does not matter. It is more important that the practitioner stretches the skin within its willingness to move without increasing pressure beyond the 4 to 5 grams. Generally fingertips, finger pads, thumb pads, flat fingers, and the full hand are the tools used for the L stroke. See Figure 23–7 ■.

LONG STROKE

The LF **long stroke** resembles effleurage, but differs in its specific application. The long stroke is applied with an open hand, including the fingers and palm. Like the L stroke, it is light (4 to 5 grams pressure). The stroke direction is in the direction of lymph flow.

CASE FOR STUDY

Ravi Applies Lymphatic Facilitation for Seasonal Allergies

Ravi has a client with bad seasonal allergies that cause sinus congestion and sinus headaches. He suggests to the client that lymphatic facilitation to the head and neck might help relieve some of the allergy symptoms.

Question:

What can Ravi say to explain how lymphatic facilitation works to help alleviate allergy symptoms?

Things to consider:

- What are typical symptoms of seasonal allergies that lymphatic facilitation can address?
- How can Ravi explain the difference between standard massage and lymphatic facilitation techniques to his client?
- How might Ravi integrate lymphatic facilitation into a regular massage session?

Write a brief script that Ravi might use to explain to his client how lymphatic facilitation of the head and neck can help relieve his seasonal allergy symptoms.

_____

_____

_____

The long stroke is initiated by first engaging the skin with light (4 to 5 grams) pressure. The skin is then stretched in the direction of lymph flow with no increase of pressure. The stroke is continued in the direction of lymph flow, maintaining the initial stretch tension. The skin remains stretched as the hand slides over the skin as far as desired. It is important to not increase pressure but to maintain the stretch along the full length of the stroke.

The distance covered is generally no farther than the closest proximal joint in the extremities or the catchment area in the trunk. At the end of the long stroke, the hand is removed quickly, allowing the skin to snap back to the starting position. This can be characterized as "releasing a hot potato." See Figure 23–8 ■.

FIGURE 23–8 Long stroke used in lymphatic facilitation.

Source: Pearson Education, Inc./Segal Photography.

LYMPHATIC FACILITATION APPLICATIONS

The following Practice Sequences of lymphatic facilitation applications provide the opportunity to practice basic LF techniques. They are also models for understanding the principles of LF related to direction of application.

PRACTICE SEQUENCE 23–1

Lymphatic Facilitation for the Head and Neck

30 minutes
Recipient supine

Preliminary Instructions
• Drape appropriately for access to the neck and shoulder.
• Screen for contraindication and cautions.
• Determine cause and nature of trauma or other indications for LF.
• Sit at the head of the table to start.

Figure 23–9 Apply L stroke on both sides of the neck, from below the ear to just above the upper trapezius with the palm and flat fingers. Stretch is toward the shoulders and then down toward the back of the neck. Release; allow skin to snap back to starting position. Repeat 10 to 15 times, until you feel the tissue soften or stretch more than when you started.

1

2

Figure 23–10 Apply L stroke on terminus. Place your index and middle fingers on the left and right terminus; apply the stretch forward toward the clavicle and then follow toward the midline; stop and release the stretch as you stretch the skin over the terminus. Repeat 10 to 15 times or until you feel a change.

3

Figure 23–11 Apply L stroke under the mandible. Place your middle and ring fingers under the tip of the chin; first stretch the skin in toward the midline and then back to the lateral neck; release and return to starting position. Repeat 10 to 15 times each in three positions from the tip of the chin to the angle of the mandible.

4

Figure 23–12 Use a full hand/flat of fingers to apply L stroke to face, below the eye and to the edge of the mandible. Stroke direction is down to the shoulder and back toward the ear and then release. Repeat 10 to 15 times.

5

Figure 23–13 Using your fingertips at the edge of the eye orbit, apply L stroke down to chin and back toward the ears. Repeat 10 to 15 times.

Figure 23–14 Use flat fingers to apply L stroke in several locations to cover the entire forehead, from midline to just in front of the ears. Stroke is stretch toward the chin, back to the ears, and release. Repeat 10 to 15 times.

Figure 23–15 Apply L strokes, using flat fingers, from temples to edge of mandible. Stretch is forward toward the shoulders and down to ears and release. Repeat 10 to 15 times.

Figure 23–16 Use flat fingers to apply L strokes along lateral neck from below the ears toward the terminus and release. Repeat 10 to 15 times.

Figure 23–17 Apply long effleurage stroke to entire arm, from hand to shoulder. Brush off from shoulder to hand. Repeat on other side.

10

Figure 23–18 Stand behind recipient and use two hands to knead both sides of upper trapezius.

11

Figure 23–19 Passive touch on shoulders to end. Hold for 5 to 10 seconds.

 After you perform the Practice Sequence, evaluate how well you did by filling out Performance Evaluation Form 23–1, Lymphatic Facilitation for the Head and Neck. The form can be found in Appendix D: *Performance Evaluation Forms*, and at MyHealthProfessionsLab.com.

Figures source: Pearson Education, Inc./Segal Photography.

 CRITICAL THINKING

Think about the structure of the lymph system on the head and neck. Analyze Practice Sequence 23–1 for the head and neck presented in this chapter.

1. Why does the sequence start with L strokes on the neck and terminus?

2. Why is the order of application mandible, face, eyes, forehead, and temples?

3. What is accomplished by ending with effleurage to the entire arm and kneading the upper trapezius muscle?

PRACTICE SEQUENCE 23–2

Lymphatic Facilitation for the Lower Extremity

30 minutes
Recipient supine

Preliminary Instructions
• Drape appropriately for access to the leg.
• Screen for contraindication and cautions.
• Determine cause and nature of trauma or indications for LF.
• Stand at the side of the table facing the head.

Figure 23–20 Stand at the side facing the client. Apply L stroke to both sides of the neck with flat fingers placed just below the ears. The stretch is toward the back of the neck, and then down toward the shoulders. Release, allow skin to snap back to starting position. Repeat 10 to 15 times, until you feel the tissue soften or stretch more than when you started.

Figure 23–21 Apply L stroke on terminus. Place your index and middle fingers on the left and right terminus; apply the stretch down toward the clavicle and then follow toward the midline; stop and release the stretch as you stretch the skin over the terminus. Repeat 10 to 15 times or until you feel a change. (*Note:* Steps 1 and 2 clear the lymph vessels near the thoracic ducts, which begins the process of lymphatic drainage in the entire body.)

Figure 23–22 Clear the cisterna chyli. Instruct the recipient to take in a deep diaphragmatic breath and hold it for a moment. While holding the breath, ask the person to imagine a candle about 2 feet away. Then have him or her breathe out forcibly to "blow out the candle." Repeat 5 or 6 times. This can be done by the individual at home several times a day to continue clearing the cisterna chyli.

4

Figure 23–23 Clear the inguinal catchment area. Face the side of the table at recipient's waist. Place your upper hand parallel to the inguinal ligament with the little finger inferior. Place your other hand on top and gently press, using your top hand, straight down toward the tabletop, using a medium pressure. Maintain this pressure while stretching the skin gently toward the abdomen and then release the skin, allowing it to "snap" back to the starting position. Repeat 10 to 15 times.

5

Figure 23–24 Clear the thigh with long strokes. Start superior to the patella; place your full flat hand and fingers on the skin using light pressure; stretch the skin toward the inguinal nodes and then slide over the skin up to the inguinal node area maintaining the stretch. At the inguinal nodes quickly remove your hand(s) from the skin, allowing it to snap back to its starting position. You need only to cover the anterior thigh because the lymph from the posterior thigh passes through the anterior thigh on its way to the inguinal nodes. Repeat 10 to 15 times.

6

Figure 23–25 Clear the popliteal catchment area. Stand next to the recipient's knee, and face the head of the table. Place both hands under the person's knee with palms up and fingers interlaced. Lift up into the popliteal space until the knee begins to bend. Maintain this pressure and stretch the skin toward the trunk. When the skin is stretched as far as possible without sliding over the skin, release quickly, and allow the skin to return to the starting position. Repeat 10 to 15 times.

7

Figure 23–26 Clear the lower leg with long strokes. Start proximal to the ankle, and stroke to the knee and release. Because the area of the gastrocnemius and the soleus drain to the popliteal space, it is necessary to also cover the posterior leg from the ankle to the popliteal space. Bend the recipient's knee to allow access to the posterior leg; lower it back to the table when finished. Cover each area with 10 to 15 strokes.

Figure 23–27 Clear the tarsals, metatarsals, and toes. Stand at the end of the table, support the plantar surface of the recipient's foot with one hand, and place your other hand, thumb on the hallicus side, with palm down and encompass the dorsum. Using LF pressure, stretch the skin up toward the popliteal space and release. Repeat 10 to 15 times.

Note: Modify this protocol to meet the needs of each client. If the pathology being addressed is located at the knee, then the practitioner need only clear down to the knee and not below. This will prevent additional fluid from being pushed into an area of existing edema or inflammation and allow the most effective clearing of the area of pathology.

After you perform the Practice Sequence, evaluate how well you did by filling out Performance Evaluation Form 23–2, Lymphatic Facilitation for the Lower Extremity. The form can be found in Appendix D: *Performance Evaluation Forms,* and at MyHealthProfessionsLab.com.

Figures source: Pearson Education, Inc./Segal Photography.

INTEGRATION OF LYMPHATIC FACILITATION INTO A MASSAGE SESSION

LF can be adapted to fit into many different applications within a massage session. It is easy on the practitioner's hands and can be done in the seated position. LF can be utilized as a:

1. **"Stand-alone" treatment modality.** This would be appropriate for clients whose area of complaint is in the acute or subacute stage of healing (i.e., postsurgery, rehabilitating from muscle strains, tendinitis, bruising). It may also be appropriate to support good nutrition, spa wraps, or body cleanses.

2. **Part of a session to address specific areas.** Such areas, identified during the session, would benefit from a light mobilization of the interstitial spaces. This might include application to an area after deeper, more invasive bodywork to decrease residual soreness due to therapeutic inflammation.

3. **"Full-body" application to support wellness and the immune system.** Caution should be taken in this situation. Application for full body may cause some flu-like symptoms, depending on the level of metabolic wastes present. It is suggested that this application be done over two to three sessions to minimize this possibility.

PRACTICAL APPLICATION

Develop a lymphatic facilitation protocol for addressing swelling related to a sprained wrist. Use the Practice Sequence for the lower extremity as a model.

1. What are the first steps in this upper body protocol?

2. How might it differ from the protocol for the lower extremities?

3. In what order are different drainage areas addressed? When are L strokes and long strokes used?

CHAPTER HIGHLIGHTS

- Lymphatic facilitation (LF) is a light and gentle massage technique used to facilitate the removal of excess fluid that collects in tissues after trauma and inflammation.
  - Excess fluid accumulation can cause irritation to pain receptors, reduce range of motion in affected joints, reduce the delivery of nutrition to cells, and lead to restrictions in fascia.

- The application of LF facilitates transportation of fluids through interstitial spaces and the lymph system and away from the affected area.
  - LF applications result in pain relief, increased local circulation, and increased range of motion in affected joints.

- LF can be used for several different wellness objectives.
  - Promotes well-nourished skin by improving local lymph and interstitial circulation.
  - Keeps fascia and muscles more pliable, improves joint flexibility, and strengthens immune system function.

- LF is especially beneficial when addressing injuries and trauma.
  - Helps remove secondary edema during the acute stage of healing.
  - May increase the rate of healing by clearing out the interstitial spaces and providing for better delivery of nutrients.
  - Increases range of motion by removing edema.
  - Reduces pain by reducing the amount of nerve irritants.

- Compared to classic manual lymphatic drainage (MLD), LF techniques are simpler, easier to learn, and more easily integrated into massage sessions.
  - LF was developed by adapting lymphatic techniques for sports and injury rehabilitation.

- Features of lymphatic system anatomy and physiology important for understanding lymphatic facilitation techniques include the:
  - Nature of lymph fluid
  - General flow of lymph in the body
  - Structure of interstitial matrix
  - Lymph nodes and the process of immunity
  - Structure of lymph vessels (collector and transport)

- Cisterna chyli
- Location of the thoracic ducts and the terminus

- General lymph drainage patterns are defined by watersheds and the location of catchments or concentrations of lymph nodes in different parts of the body.

- Clients may have contraindications for LF techniques.
  - Pathologies that compromise the heart and kidneys.
  - Systemic infections.
  - Presence of thrombosis, clots, or embolism.
  - Lymphedema, for which manual lymph drainage (MLD) is indicated.

- LF techniques are designed to increase absorption of interstitial fluid and move lymph through the system.
  - Increase absorption at the I/T lymphatic vessels.
  - Move interstitial fluid through the interstitial matrix.
  - Increase the rate of lymphangia contraction.
  - Generally improve the flow of lymph within the lymph vessels and toward the thoracic ducts.

- LF strokes must be applied with the correct attributes.
  - Light, using only 4–5 grams of pressure to move superficial tissues.
  - Rhythmic application of repeated strokes.
  - Slow pace.
  - Applied in general direction of lymph flow.
  - Clear catchment areas before moving fluids toward them.
  - Clear proximal areas before distal areas.
  - Skin stretches and then releases or snaps back.

- Two basic LF strokes are the L stroke and the long stroke.
  - In the L stroke the skin is stretched in an L pattern toward the desired direction of lymph flow.
  - The long stroke resembles effleurage but is applied to stretch the skin in the desired direction of lymph flow.

- All LF sessions begin with clearing in the neck and at the terminus. This begins the facilitation of lymph flow throughout the system.

- LF is easy on the practitioner's hands and can be performed from the seated position.

EXAM REVIEW

Key Terms

Match the following key terms to their descriptions. For additional study, look up the key terms in the Interactive Glossary, and note other terms that compare or contrast with them.

_____ **1.** Catchments
_____ **2.** Collector vessels
_____ **3.** Initial/terminal vessels
_____ **4.** Interstitial matrix
_____ **5.** L stroke
_____ **6.** Long stroke
_____ **7.** Lymph
_____ **8.** Lymphatic facilitation (LF)
_____ **9.** Terminus
_____ **10.** Transport vessels
_____ **11.** Watersheds

a. Resembles effleurage but with a stretch of tissues
b. Structure of interstitial space
c. Concentration of lymph nodes
d. Superficial drainage pattern
e. Entry point for waste and excess fluid
f. LF applied here increases lymph flow into thoracic ducts
g. Colorless fluid in lymphatic vessels
h. Connect I/T vessels to lymphangia
i. Lymphangia
j. Manual therapy to enhance lymph flow
k. Applied in letter-shaped pattern

Memory Workout

To test your memory of the main concepts in this chapter, complete the following sentences by circling the most correct answer from the two choices provided.

1. Normally, about (50%) (10%) of interstitial fluid is returned to the cardiovascular system by way of the lymphatic system.
2. The lymphatic system has the ability to increase its capacity up to (50%) (90%) for a short period of time.
3. (Interstitial matrix) (catchment) is a more accurate description of the space between cells.
4. Lymphatic vessels that are segmented and that have the ability to contract are called (I/T) (transport) vessels.
5. A lymphatic structure found deep in the abdomen that pumps lymph from the lower extremities into the thoracic duct is the (cisterna chyli) (inguinal node).

6. The hollow space just lateral to the sternocleidomastoid (SCM) muscles where LF strokes are applied to clear the thoracic ducts is called the (terminus) (collector).
7. Concentrations of lymph nodes in a specific drainage area are called a (matrix) (catchment).
8. Lymphedema is a major (indication) (contraindication) for LF applications.
9. The skin (melts) (snaps) back into place when an LF stroke is released.
10. Using too much (stretch) (pressure) closes the flaps between cells of the initial/terminal lymph vessels, thus preventing fluid from being absorbed.

Test Prep

The following multiple-choice questions will help to prepare you for future school and professional exams.

1. The combination of skin care, manual lymph drainage, compression bandaging, exercise, and self-care used to treat lymphedema is called:
   a. Complex lymphatic facilitation
   b. Complete decongestive therapy
   c. Myofascial facilitation
   d. Complete lymphatic facilitation

2. Lymph is the fluid contained in the:
   a. Circulatory system
   b. Interstitial matrix
   c. Spleen
   d. Lymphatic vessels

3. Larger molecules and inorganic and organic materials are reabsorbed from interstitial spaces by way of the:
   a. Initial/terminal lymphatic vessels
   b. Blood capillary vessels
   c. Lymph nodes
   d. Watersheds

4. What percent of the lymph capillaries are found in the dermis?
   a. 60%
   b. 40%
   c. 20%
   d. 10%

5. LF applications always start at the:
   a. Temples
   b. Watershed
   c. Catchment
   d. Terminus

6. An important characteristic of LF strokes is that they:
   a. Slide over the skin
   b. Stretch the skin superficially
   c. Press into the skin
   d. Lift the skin

7. The repeated and rhythmic application of LF strokes creates a:
   a. Pressure wave inside the interstitial space
   b. Pressure wave inside the lymphangions
   c. Blockage at I/T vessels
   d. Blockage at blood capillaries

8. When applying long strokes, the skin is stretched in the direction of the:
   a. Nearest distal catchment
   b. Nearest proximal catchment
   c. Farthest distal catchment
   d. Deepest transport vessels

9. A major contraindication for LF applications is:
   a. Edema due to trauma
   b. Allergies
   c. Sinus congestion
   d. Acute infection

10. Having the client breathe out forcibly, repeated about five times, clears the:
    a. Sinuses
    b. Distal catchment areas
    c. Cisterna chyli
    d. Terminus

Video Challenge

Watch these videos, which can be found at MyHealthProfessionsLab.com, Chapter 23, and then answer the following questions.

Lymphatic Facilitation for the Head and Neck

Lymphatic Facilitation for the Lower Extremity

1. Describe the quality of touch used by the practitioners in the lymphatic facilitation demonstrations in the videos.

2. Compare the first step of the Lymphatic Facilitation for the Head and Neck Practice Sequence and the first step of the Lymphatic Facilitation for the Lower Extremity Practice Sequence as demonstrated in the videos. What is different about how the first step is applied in each massage sequence?

3. Describe the process for clearing the cisterna chyli demonstrated in the video demonstration of lymphatic facilitation in the lower extremities.

Comprehension Exercises

The following short-answer questions test your knowledge and understanding of chapter topics and provide practice in written communication skills. Explain in two to four complete sentences.

1. Contrast lymphatic facilitation and manual lymphatic drainage.

2. Describe the intent of lymphatic facilitation techniques. How do they improve lymph flow?

3. Explain why lymphatic facilitation techniques are applied using very light pressure.

For Greater Understanding

The following exercises are designed to take you from the realm of theory into the real world. They will help give you a deeper understanding of the subjects covered in this chapter. Action words are underlined to emphasize the variety of activities presented to address different learning styles and to encourage deeper thinking.

1. Receive a session of lymphatic facilitation or manual lymphatic drainage from a trained practitioner. Verbally describe your experience to a study partner. Note the techniques used and the order and direction of application.

2. Observe a session of lymphatic facilitation or manual lymphatic drainage performed by a trained practitioner. Write a report on what you saw. Note the techniques used and order of application of techniques. Did it conform to the attributes described in this chapter? (Variation: Watch a video.)

3. Interview someone who received lymphatic facilitation or manual lymphatic drainage for a particular pathology. Did this application seem appropriate for the condition? Were the results positive for the recipient? Write a report of your interview and share it with a study partner.

4. Search a research database for studies related to manual lymphatic techniques. Make a list of the studies and summarize their findings.

MyHealthProfessionsLab™

MyHealthProfessionsLab.com is a premium online homework management system that includes a host of features to help you study. Registered users will find:

- Powerful tools that track and analyze your results—allowing you to create a personalized learning experience
- Videos, flashcards and other learning tools to help enrich your progress
- Streaming lesson presentations and self-paced learning modules
- A space where you and your instructors can view and manage your assignments

24 Reflexology

Paula Stone

CHAPTER OUTLINE

Learning Outcomes

Key Terms

Overview

History of Reflexology

Zone Therapy and Guidelines

Theories about Reflexology

Sensation During and After
   Reflexology

Positioning the Receiver

Body Mechanics

Reflexology Techniques

Reflexology Session

Chapter Highlights

Exam Review

LEARNING OUTCOMES

After studying this chapter, you will have information to:

1. Trace the history of reflexology.
2. Explain theories about how reflexology works.
3. Identify areas of the feet that correspond to different parts of the body.
4. Position the client to receive a reflexology session.

5. Use good body mechanics when performing foot reflexology.
6. Apply basic foot reflexology techniques.
7. Perform a general reflexology session.

KEY TERMS

Diaphragm relaxation

Direct pressure

Fingerwalking

Foot reflexology

Guidelines

Hook-and-backup

Press-and-flex

Reflexology chart

Rolling

Stabilizing hand

Thumbwalking

Working hand

Zone therapy

OVERVIEW

Foot reflexology is based on the theory that pressure applied to specific spots on the feet produces changes in corresponding parts of the body. For example, according to reflexology theory, pressing the pads of the toes, or sinus reflex, affects the sinuses in the head. There are reflex areas on the feet that correspond to all systems and structures of the body. Compression applied to reflexes is thought to marshal the body's innate healing forces and to help normalize body functions.

Maps of the feet, like the **reflexology chart** in Figure 24–1 ■, identify the locations of reflexes on the foot. Reflex maps are also available for the entire body (body reflexology), hands (hand reflexology), ears (auricular reflexology), face (face reflexology), and eyes (iridology). This chapter focuses on foot reflexology because it is the most common form and is easily integrated into a massage session.

Foot reflexology can be incorporated into a full-body Swedish massage, or given as a specialty treatment using the theory and techniques of reflexology exclusively. Massage practitioners can train to become certified reflexologists, a specialization that fits well with a massage therapy practice.

HISTORY OF REFLEXOLOGY

The history of reflexology spans centuries and extends to the corners of the earth. Its origins can be found in ancient civilizations; however, the forerunners of modern reflexology arose in eighteenth century Europe. The theory and practice came to America where it was further developed in the twentieth century, and in due course spread worldwide in its current form.

Ancient Roots

Manipulating and pressing into the soft tissues of the feet was an ancient health practice found in many parts of the world. The oldest known records come from Asia, including India, Tibet, China, and Japan. Foot maps appeared in India about 5,000 years ago, and curious symbols can be found on the feet of some statues of the Buddha.[1] Oral tradition hints at similar practices of foot rubbing in the ancient Americas.

An early pictograph of a foot treatment was found in a physician's tomb in Saqqara, Egypt, dating from about 2500 BCE.[2] The Land of the Pharaohs was renowned throughout the ancient world for their advances in medicine and in other skilled fields. Travelers who came to ancient Egypt from faraway places included scholars, doctors, merchants, worshipers, and students seeking greater knowledge. They were from Central Africa, Greece, the Middle East (notably Arabia), and possibly as far away as Great Britain; these travelers introduced Egyptian ideas to their native communities when they returned home. Some also think that beliefs and practices from the Land of the Nile (including Egyptian foot manipulation) spread throughout Europe during the period of the Roman Empire and later became part of European folk traditions. Forms of what has become known as foot reflexology can be found today all over the world, often as part of traditional medicine or as a complementary and alternative (CAM) therapy.[3]

Reflexology in Europe

Modern reflexology had its origins in eighteenth century Europe, where it grew out of new discoveries about the nervous system and a treatment approach called *zone therapy*. Earliest known European writings related to zone therapy were published in the late 1500s by Dr. Adamus, Dr. A'tatis, and later, Dr. Ball. German physiologist Johann August Unzer advanced the concept of reflexive action and coined the term *reflex* in 1771 to explain motor reactions to applied pressure. English physiologist Marshall Hall used the term *reflex action* in 1833 to distinguish between unconscious reflexes and conscious actions.

Sir Henry Head (1861–1940) of London established that a connection exists between the skin, spinal cord, and brain. He charted the links among areas of the head and specific internal organs, mapping out what came to be known as *Head's zones*. In the early twentieth century, conventional medicine began to split into various specialty branches. Reflexive response to pressure applied to specific points, later known as reflexology, was at first associated with the nervous system and the science of neurology. Forms of pressure point treatment were practiced throughout Europe under the umbrella of neurology, particularly in Russia, Germany, Great Britain, Spain, and Italy.

PRACTICAL APPLICATION

Draw the corresponding organs and structures on a partner's feet with a washable marker. Use the reflexology charts in Figure 24–1 and the guidelines in Figure 24–3 for reference.

1. In what ways are the left and right feet different?

2. To what areas of the body do the guidelines correspond?

3. Where are the reflexes in relation to anatomical structures of the feet, for example, the metatarsal heads?

4. Where on the grid (formed by the longitudinal zones and the guidelines) are various reflexes located?

FIGURE 24–1 Reflexology chart showing location of reflexes with corresponding anatomical structures and organs affected.

Reflexology in America

The beginnings of American reflexology can be traced to the early 1900s and the system of **zone therapy** popularized by Dr. William Fitzgerald. Fitzgerald was a respected physician and prominent nose and throat surgeon at St. Francis Hospital in Hartford, Connecticut. He discovered that pressure on certain places in the body provided pain relief in other parts in predictable patterns. He mapped out his findings and summarized them in a book called *Zone Therapy* published in 1917.[4]

An eclectic natural healer, Dr. Joseph Shelby Riley is credited with refining Fitzgerald's techniques and making the first detailed diagrams of reflex points in the feet.[5] In the 1930s, a physiotherapist and masseuse named Eunice Ingham (1889–1974) worked for Dr. Riley in his St. Petersburg, Florida office. She learned about zone therapy from him and subsequently developed a system that combined compression massage of the feet with zone therapy. Working from clinical experience, Ingham created a detailed map of the feet, charting areas of the body affected at each point or reflex, and also devised special manual techniques for applying pressure to the feet. Ingham has been rightfully called the "Mother of Modern Foot Reflexology."

Ingham developed her methods in the years before World War II and afterwards traveled across the United States by car, teaching reflexology in workshops. Her primary audience in the 1950s and 1960s came from from the ranks of natural healers and massage therapists.[6, 7] Mildred Carter (1912–2005), a student of Ingham's, built on the zone therapy philosophy in fundamental ways. She identified reflex points located throughout the entire body with a focus on the reflexes in the hands and feet, used devices (rollers, dowels, massagers, and so forth), described energy flow throughout the body, and emphasized the value of nutrition and supporting therapies. Carter's earlier book, *Body Reflexology*, has been updated by her daughter, Tammy Weber, and titled *Healing Yourself with Foot Reflexology* (1997). This work integrates the principles of Asian bodywork with reflexology.[8]

Modern Professional Reflexology

By the end of the twentieth century, modern reflexology had spread to countries all over the world. Reflexology today is recognized as a bodywork specialty distinct from massage and is sometimes presented as related to energy-based Asian bodywork. Nevertheless, foot reflexology remains a popular adjunct to Swedish massage and is practiced by massage therapists, as well as reflexologists.

Reflexology is currently considered a form of complementary and alternative therapy. Classes and certification programs in reflexology are now available in both Western and Asian traditions. More detailed information about foot reflexology and practitioner organizations can be found in textbooks devoted to the subject, for instance in those resources listed in Appendix E, *References and Additional Resources*.

ZONE THERAPY AND GUIDELINES

The theory and practice of reflexology and zone therapy are interrelated. According to zone therapy, the body is divided lengthwise into 10 imaginary zones, five on each side of the body. See Figure 24–2 ■. The longitudinal zones have endpoints in the feet, hands, and top of the head.

The theory is that pressure applied anywhere in the zone affects the entire zone. Therefore, pressure applied to the feet can affect structures and organs in other parts of the body. The feet have proven an especially sensitive and easily accessed place to apply pressure for zone therapy.

Reflexology charts of the feet are derived from zone therapy and show which reflexes on the feet to press to affect specific structures and organs. Charts of the plantar surface of the feet show the 10 longitudinal zones of the body (running from toes to heel) crossed at right angles by *guidelines*.

FIGURE 24–2 Ten longitudinal zones of reflexology.

Guidelines are landmarks based on anatomical structures. The four parallel guidelines are neck/shoulder, diaphragm, waist, and pelvis. The longitudinal tendon is the one longitudinal guideline (Figure 24–3 ■). Together, the zones and guidelines form a grid of the feet, making it possible to locate any reflex on any size foot with accuracy.

Neck and Shoulder Guideline This horizontal guideline is located at the base of the toes in the webbing where the toes meet the ball of the foot. Apply pressure in this area for neck and shoulder problems. Effects on particular body areas, including isolation of muscle groups, are achieved by identifying their location within specific zones.

Diaphragm Guideline This important guideline runs along the base of the metatarsal heads of all toes from the medial to lateral foot. This guideline is also the diaphragm reflex that divides the body into the chest and abdominal cavities. Relaxing the diaphragm reflex releases tension in the thoracic region to improve breathing and digestion. Work this reflex to reduce stress and anxiety.

Waist Guideline Locate the tuberosity of the fifth metatarsal on the lateral foot, which often feels like a bulge. Then draw an imaginary horizontal line to the medial foot. This is the waist guideline.

Anatomically, the area between the diaphragm and pelvis is the abdominal cavity. The waist divides the abdominal cavity into upper and lower regions. The waist guideline serves as the landmark dividing the foot into upper and lower abdominal area reflexes. Location of the reflexes mirrors anatomical locations.

The *upper region* contains the liver, gallbladder, hepatic flexure, kidneys, adrenal glands, stomach, pancreas, duodenum, spleen, and splenic flexure. The *lower region* contains the small intestine, large intestine, ileocecal valve, appendix, kidneys, ureters, and bladder.

Pelvic Guideline This guideline is located on the heel, typically where the tougher heel changes into the softer arch. This guideline identifies the pelvic girdle, reproductive organs, and colon, and forms a bridge between the lateral and medial reflex points on the ankles.

Longitudinal Tendon The longitudinal tendon guideline is located in zone 1 between the diaphragm and pelvic guidelines. It is the only guideline that is defined by an anatomical structure in the foot. This guideline helps locate the all-important adrenal glands, kidneys, ureters, and bladder with accuracy.

THEORIES ABOUT REFLEXOLOGY

A number of theories seek to explain how reflexology works. These can be categorized as physiological or energetic. Physiological models deal with some aspect of the physical body, for example, the nervous system, circulatory system, or proprioception. Energetic theories propose that reflexology affects the flow of bioelectrical energy in and around the body. Zone therapy and systems based on Asian bodywork fall into this latter category.

Eunice Ingham believed that the techniques of reflexology dissolved crystalline deposits in the feet. These deposits were thought to interfere with nerve and blood supplies.[9] This concept has been expanded to include all types of *congestion* that might reduce or inhibit optimal functioning of body systems. The idea of congestion now takes in a number of potential *inhibiting factors*, including buildup of cellular debris, uric acid, toxins, excess fluid, and inflammation. Reflexologists do not claim to diagnose, prescribe, treat, or cure medical pathologies, and so the conceptual model of relieving congestion in the tissues has been useful for describing what is happening generally in reflexology. The compression techniques of reflexology are thought to dispel inhibiting factors, and thereby improve function of body systems. This, in turn, helps the body normalize, achieve homeostasis, and heal.

Reflexology theory related to the nervous system begins with the fact that each foot has more than 7,000 nerve endings. Compressing the soft tissues of the feet transmits nerve impulses to the spine and onward to the brain, which then communicates with the body to produce changes that support good health.

Some believe that zones are more like the energy pathways in traditional Chinese medicine (TCM), and

FIGURE 24–3 Guidelines.

Neck/Shoulder Guideline

Longitudinal Tendon Guideline

Diaphragm Guideline

Waist Guideline

Pelvic Guideline

that reflexology helps keep energy or *Qi* flowing freely. Acupoints (sites at which the Qi in energy channels is close to the surface of the body) enable reflexologists to gain access not only to the "organ energy" through reflexes, but also to the supporting "energy networks" to maintain harmony and balance in the entire body.[10] See Chapter 25, *Asian and Energy-Based Bodywork,* for more information on TCM, energy channels and acupoints.

Reflexology Research and Application

Regardless of the theory used to explain the mechanism behind reflexology, many find it to be effective for improving good health and as a complementary treatment for health challenges. Research studies indicate the effectiveness of reflexology for treatment of dozens of ailments, with pain relief leading the list. Nurses, like bodyworkers, use reflexology as a means for increasing human touch, a basic human need. Reflexology is noninvasive and can be given without clients disrobing and therefore does not compromise their privacy. The Research Analysis Document published by the International Council of Reflexologists summarizes more than 300 studies from around the world.[11] Citations can also be found in various research databases such as PubMed managed by the National Institutes of Health (www.ncbi .nlm.nih.gov/pubmed).

SENSATION DURING AND AFTER REFLEXOLOGY

Receivers report a wide variety of sensations during reflexology sessions. These include relaxation, tenderness, pain, ticklishness, electrical or energy bursts, resurfacing emotions, deep rest, and recuperation.

The completely healthy person experiences no discomfort during a reflexology session. Tenderness in the body is a sign of imbalance. Simply expressed, there is sharp pain and dull pain. Both indicate imbalance. Sharp pain is a sign of excess in energy. Dull pain is a sign of too little energy.

It is more advantageous to work the tenderness immediately on noticing it, continuing until the discomfort declines or dissipates. This assists the body to reestablish balance. There is a difference between unnecessary pain and an "Oh, it's tender, but feels like a good hurt" reaction. Countless people worldwide attest to the healing benefits of discomfort that they know instinctively is "doing something," "working," "hurts good," and similar expressions. The goal of reflexology is to encourage the body to balance, not inflict pain. Applying the correct technique helps the body achieve balance with minimal discomfort.

Reflexologists can detect conditions in the feet of which the client may or may not have conscious awareness. These include swollen areas (lymphatic or fluid), tight areas (tight foot muscles or hypertonic areas on specific reflexes), congestion (a traditional term for inorganic mineral salts and other debris trapped in the tissue), cool or warm temperatures in certain tissues, and hard knots under the skin and around joints (from tiny salt-grain size to pellet size).[12]

Possible Reasons for Tenderness and Pain

The feet reflect our lives up to the moment in time when the reflexologist touches them. Many factors in our past and present can create the sensation of tenderness and pain in the feet. Tenderness and pain signal an imbalance. Among these are

1. Imbalance (or illness) in a specific organ, gland, structure, or part of the body, or even throughout the body

2. Generalized tension and stress in the body (as from a high-stress job) or localized tension and stress in a part of the body (as in computer operators)

3. Fatigue (overuse of the feet and the body)

4. Toxicity

5. Medications and drugs (prescription and nonprescription)

6. Lymphatic or fluid congestion in the feet themselves, or in a specific organ, structure, or part of the body or throughout the body

7. Surgeries, injuries, soft tissue strain (muscles, tendons, ligaments), bruises, ill-fitting shoes

CRITICAL THINKING

Look at a reflexology chart showing the bottoms of the feet, and imagine the whole body to which they are attached. Relate the location of various body structures and organs to their reflexology points.

1. Why do reflexology charts show the right foot on the left side and the left foot on the right side?
2. Does the location of reflexes reflect the left–right asymmetry of the body? How?
3. How do reflexology charts account for the three-dimensional reality of the body?

8. Specific conditions (bunions, bone spurs, corns, thin skin)

9. Diseases such as diabetes and others (some conditions actually desensitize the feet)

10. Low pain tolerance

After the Reflexology Session

Drinking adequate amounts of pure water, rest, and foot soaks immediately following the reflexology session help the body eliminate impurities and detoxify. These restorative self-care practices assist the healing process and can avert or minimize uncomfortable aspects of cleansing. Experiences after sessions may include an increase in elimination through the skin, bowels, urination, and sometimes headaches. A past illness may flare. Deep, restful sleep may occur accompanied by feelings of calm and peace. Or conversely, unresolved emotions or situations may rise to the surface. These experiences can be viewed as part of the spiritual, mental, emotional, and physical healing process and usually resolve within 2 to 3 days. Suggest to receivers that they seek a physician's advice for any medical concerns they might have.

POSITIONING THE RECEIVER

Perform foot reflexology with the recipient lying supine as during standard Swedish massage. If the session is devoted entirely to reflexology, the receiver might be more comfortable in a semireclining position propped up with pillows on the massage table. Some massage tables have hinged tops that can be adjusted to create a back rest for a semireclining client. Recliner chairs that tilt back and lift the legs are also used for reflexology.

A bolster placed under the knees will take the pressure off knee joints. It can also raise the receiver's legs for better body mechanics for the practitioner (Figure 24–4 ■).

FIGURE 24–4 Client and therapist positioning for foot reflexology.

Source: Pearson Education, Inc./Segal Photography.

BODY MECHANICS

Regardless of the position of the receiver, the practitioner should observe proper body mechanics, including good head, neck, and back alignment. Sitting on a chair is preferred when performing reflexology. Avoid bending the back and neck to reach the recipient's feet. Adjust table height, place bolsters under the legs, and fix practitioner chair or stool height to achieve proper alignment. Review good body mechanics for sitting, as shown in Figure 11–12.

REFLEXOLOGY TECHNIQUES

Reflexology techniques described in this chapter are designed to stimulate reflex areas on different parts of the feet. They can be categorized as compression, friction, and joint mobilization techniques. Compression techniques include thumb- and fingerwalking, thumb and finger rolling, hook-and-backup, press-and-flex, and direct pressure. Friction techniques add motion to direct pressure. Dorsal fulling is a unique fascial technique. And joint mobilizations stimulate reflexes through movement at joints.

For many reflexology techniques, one hand stabilizes the foot, while the other hand applies the technique. The hand applying the technique is called the **working hand**. The hand providing a brace or backstop is called the **stabilizing hand**.

REALITY CHECK

ESTEBAN

NADIA: My hands hurt after practicing reflexology and trigger point therapy—especially my thumbs. Is this normal, and I just have to get used to it? Is there anything I can do about it?

ESTEBAN: There could be a few things going on to cause your hands to hurt. Maybe you're pressing too hard or using poor hand mechanics. Be sure that your wrist and thumb joints are in good alignment when you apply pressure. Then see how little pressure you can use and still get good results. You need to apply adequate pressure, but people often press harder than they need to be effective. Harder doesn't mean better. And when your hands hurt after practicing massage, soak them in ice water for about ten minutes to reduce swelling and inflammation. You can also try doing more to condition your hands. Getting the strength for doing massage develops over time. Get a hand strengthening device, and use it daily to build up the strength you need.

Walk and Roll

Specialized finger techniques, called thumbwalking and fingerwalking, apply direct pressure quickly and systematically to the reflexes on the plantar foot and ankles.

To practice **thumbwalking**, stabilize the foot with one hand (stabilizing hand) while the working hand performs the technique. Starting at the heel of the foot on the medial side, "walk" your thumb up the foot to the toes. To do this, bend the thumb at the first joint, press into the tissues, then straighten the thumb and move to the next spot. This action is repeated as the thumb "walks" in line along the foot. Pressure is applied with the edge of the thumb just to the side of the nail or the center of the thumb (see Figure 24–5 ■).

Thumbwalking is rhythmical and steady, much like the action of a sewing machine needle as it travels over a piece of cloth. The application of pressure is controlled by using the four fingers of the working hand in opposition to the thumb as leverage. The stabilizing hand assists by pressing the foot into the thumb as the thumb is "walking."

Thumbwalking is especially beneficial on the *spinal reflex,* located on the medial edge of the foot. Divide the foot into segments. Thumbwalk each segment in parallel lines from heel to toes for thorough coverage.

The walking technique can also be applied with the fingers. **Fingerwalking** is useful for applying pressure to larger areas (such as the flat ankle bones of the pelvic reflex, as shown in Figure 24–6 ■), small areas of the foot (all sides of the toes), and for the smaller feet of children. Thumb- and fingerwalking are quick and effective ways to work the reflexes on the entire plantar surface of the foot.

Rolling is an alternative to walking. Hold the thumb or fingertip on a reflex. Then rotate your entire hand to roll your thumb or finger into the reflex. This can be performed

FIGURE 24–6 Fingerwalking the pelvic reflex.

Source: Pearson Education, Inc./Segal Photography.

on a single reflex, such as the *shoulder reflex,* or over a larger area, such as the *spinal reflex* or *neck/shoulder reflex,* or the *brain reflex* on the tips of toes.

Hook-and-Backup

The **hook-and-backup** technique is used to apply deep pressure to a specific area or reflex. Locate the area you wish to press, place your thumb directly on the spot, and bend the first joint to apply pressure. Then pull the thumb to the side across the spot to deepen the pressure, as shown in Figure 24–7 ■. Sustain pressure for a few seconds, and then repeat one to three times. This technique is useful on small reflexes, such as the spleen, gallbladder, sigmoid colon, and ileocecal valve/appendix.

Press-and-Flex

Reflexes can also be worked by the **press-and-flex** technique. Deep pressure is applied by moving the foot into the finger or thumb. Position the thumb or finger on a reflex. Flex the foot toward the thumb or finger, and hold the position for a few seconds (Figure 24–8 ■). Repeat one to three times. Press-and-flex is a highly effective method for working the spinal reflex, chest reflex, visceral organ reflexes, and flexures of the colon reflexes.

Direct Pressure and Friction

Direct pressure is a compression technique in which the finger or thumb applies sustained pressure on a specific reflex point. It is effective for small reflexes such as the

FIGURE 24–5 Thumbwalking the spinal reflex on the medial edge of the foot.

Source: Pearson Education, Inc./Segal Photography.

FIGURE 24–7 Hook-and-backup technique for the gallbladder reflex.

Source: Pearson Education, Inc./Segal Photography.

head, brain, sinus, and reproductive organs. Hold for a few seconds and repeat one to three times on each point. Direct pressure applied to the sinus reflex by squeezing firmly is shown in Figure 24–9 ■.

Direct pressure applied to a reflex can be enhanced with *circular friction*. This is a deep friction technique made by adding small circular movements to pressure at a specific point. This additional movement is thought to improve circulation to the reflex.

Dorsal Fulling

Dorsal fulling can be thought of as a type of fascial technique applied to the lymphatic reflex on the top of the foot. For this application, the skin is stretched without applying a lot of pressure into the tissues. To begin, position all eight fingers on the dorsum of the foot near the base of the toes.

FIGURE 24–9 Direct pressure applied to a sinus reflex on the tip of a toe.

Source: Pearson Education, Inc./Segal Photography.

Stretch the skin toward the toes using light pressure, release it, and then move the fingers toward the ankle to a new row (Figure 24–10 ■). Repeat the skin stretch moving rhythmically row-by-row from the base of the toes (chest/back reflex) to the ankle (groin reflex). Dorsal fulling affects the entire back, as well as the muscular, nervous, lymphatic, and respiratory systems.

Joint Movements

Several reflexology techniques employ free joint movements. Reflexes in the area of joint movements are stimulated by the action. Examples of reflexology joint movement techniques are the spinal twist (Figure 24–13) and toe rotations (Figure 24–21).

The **diaphragm relaxation** technique is an example of a joint movement used to deepen thumb pressure. Position the thumb under the metatarsal head of the big toe. Extend the toe toward the dorsum. Lift the toe and flex over the thumb toward the plantar surface (Figure 24–11 ■). Release and repeat one to three times. Reposition the thumb moving laterally, and repeat. Cover the entire diaphragm reflex, which is located under all the metatarsal heads from the medial to the lateral foot.

FIGURE 24–8 Press-and-flex technique for the pelvic organ reflexes near the medial ankle.

Source: Pearson Education, Inc./Segal Photography.

FIGURE 24–10 Dorsal fulling for the back, ribs, and lymphatic reflexes.

Source: Pearson Education, Inc./Segal Photography.

FIGURE 24–11 Diaphragm relaxation technique. (A) Place the thumb on the metatarsal head of the big toe. (B) Bend the toe into hyperextension. (C) Lift and flex the toe over the thumb.

Source: Pearson Education, Inc./Segal Photography.

Adjuncts to Reflexology

Basic reflexology techniques can be combined with massage, shiatsu, and joint movements to work reflexes and zones. Reflexology sessions—either for relaxation or therapeutic outcomes—are readily combined with various types of foot soaks (before and after the session) to soften the feet and assist with detoxification. Therapeutic-grade essential oils and special lotions for reflexology further support the healing process.

REFLEXOLOGY SESSION

The basic reflexology routine described in this section works the entire body. It relaxes tight muscles to ease tension-related pain. It prepares the body for protocols for specific health challenges.

The following Practice Sequence can be used to practice reflexology techniques or for a general reflexology session. Keep a reflexology chart and client notes handy for reference.

PRACTICE SEQUENCE 24–1

| General Reflexology Session | 30 minutes
Recipient semireclining or lying on massage table |

Preliminary Instructions

- Before beginning, conduct a verbal screening for general contraindications for massage (e.g., fever or extreme nausea).
- Ask about any structural problems with the feet and any contagious foot conditions such as athlete's foot. Do not perform reflexology on a foot if it might cause structural damage or spread contagious skin conditions.
- Place a bolster under recipient's knees and raise the legs so that you can keep your spine in good alignment while applying techniques.
- Sit at the feet of the recipient.
- You may wear latex (or nonlatex substitute) gloves for protection in certain cases.
- If a foot soak is used prior to the reflexology session, towel dry the feet thoroughly and sprinkle with cornstarch or nontalcum foot powder. Reflexology techniques require that pressure be applied without gliding or slipping over the skin.

1

A   B   C

Figure 24–12 Warm-up (5 minutes). Warm up the soft tissues of the feet with a variety of kneading, sliding, and joint movement techniques. Check for structural abnormalities or problem skin conditions. (A) Compress and knead the foot. (B) Metatarsal loosener. (C) Ankle jostling.

2

Figure 24–13 Spinal Twist. Apply three quick rhythmical twists at each of the pelvic, waist, and diaphragm guidelines. Repeat 3–4 times. The rhythmical movement stretches soft tissues surrounding the spinal reflex, releases spinal tension, and creates space.

Reflex: Lumbar and Thoracic Vertebral Segments

Figure 24–14 Spinal Reflex. Thumbwalk the spinal reflex from the sacrum to C-1 (i.e., heel of the foot to the top of the big toe), and back down again. Adjust stabilizing and working hand positions as needed while moving up and down the spinal reflex. Use multidirectional thumbwalking for maximum coverage at each segment and thumb rolling for deeper pressure as desired. Bend knee to lay foot on lateral edge. This key reflex affects the central nervous system.

Reflex: Entire Spine

Figure 24–15 Neck and Occipital Ridge. Apply thumb compression across the area at the base of the big toe. One hand stabilizes the toes, while the thumb of the opposite hand applies pressure. Bend the toe into the thumb for added pressure. Eases tension and improves blood and nerve supply in the neck and head. (May be repeated beneath each toe between the neck and diaphragm guidelines for greater coverage.)

Reflex: Neck, Occipital Ridge, Head

Figure 24–16 Lymphatic Drainage on Dorsum with Ankle Rotation. With the fingers of both hands, gently stretch the skin on the top of the foot toward the toes. Begin at base of the toes and apply the stretch row by row ending at the ankle joint (groin reflex). Then rotate the ankle using the fingers. Works the entire back affecting many body systems—muscular, nervous, lymphatic, and respiratory.

Reflex: Back, Ribs, Lymph (axillary, inguinal), Groin, Reproductive

Figure 24–17 Bidirectional Thumb Pressure on Plantar Surface. Apply bidirectional thumb pressure over the entire bottom of the foot. Start with your elbows out to the sides and then push them down to aid in applying pressure at the thumbs. Cover the chest and abdominal reflexes.

Reflex: Anterior Chest, Abdominal and Pelvic Cavities

7

Figure 24–18 Medial Pelvis/Hip. Press-and-flex medial ankle by positioning fingers as in fingerwalking the ankle. Roll the ankle into the movement.

Reflex: Medial Pelvis (uterus, prostate, hip muscles)

8

Figure 24–19 Lateral Pelvis/Hip. Press-and-flex lateral ankle by positioning fingers as in fingerwalking the ankle. Roll the ankle laterally into the fingers.

Reflex: Lateral Pelvis (ovaries, testicles, hip muscles)

9

Figure 24–20 Diaphragm. Place the thumb on a spot along the diaphragm guideline, then flex the toe above that spot to apply pressure into the thumb. Work the diaphragm guideline from medial to lateral. This eases breathing, improves the flow of blood, nerve supply, and bioelectrical energy.

Reflex: Diaphragm

10

Figure 24–21 Toe Rotations. Rotate each toe from the big toe to the little toe. Toe rotations ease neck muscle tension; tips of toes are brain reflexes.

Reflex: Head, Neck

Figure 24–22 Gentle foot compression to end a session.

11

Repeat Steps 1–11 on the other foot. Return to tender areas for additional work. Finish with foot massage (see Practice Sequence 16–3, Foot Massage).

After you perform this massage sequence, evaluate how well you did by filling out Performance Self-Evaluation Form 24–1, General Reflexology Session. The form can be found in Appendix D: *Performance Evaluation Forms*, and at MyHealthProfessionsLab.com.

Figures source: Pearson Education, Inc./Segal Photography.

CASE FOR STUDY

Larry Uses Reflexology for Client's Aches and Pains

Before his regular massage appointment, Larry's client complained of added stress, constipation, and shoulder and neck tension. Larry knew that the client enjoyed work on his feet and seemed to respond positively to pressure applied there. Larry suggested to the client that about 30 minutes of the 1-hour massage this week be spent on foot reflexology. The client agreed to try foot reflexology for its therapeutic effects.

Question:
How does Larry integrate foot reflexology into the massage session?

Things to consider:
- When would the 30 minutes of reflexology occur? At the beginning, middle, or end of the session?
- How would the client be positioned for the foot reflexology application?
- How would Larry use the reflexology charts to locate likely spots for addressing the client's complaints?

Write a brief description of the 1-hour massage organization and the best approach to integrate reflexology into this session.

_____

_____

_____

CHAPTER HIGHLIGHTS

- Foot reflexology is based on the theory that pressure applied to specific spots on the feet stimulates corresponding areas in other parts of the body.
  - The pressure is thought to marshal the body's innate healing forces and to help normalize body function.

- Reflexology is a distinct form of bodywork with its own theory and techniques. Professional reflexologists seek certification.
- The history of reflexology is ancient and reaches to the corners of the earth.
  - Evidence of foot treatments similar to reflexology have been found in ancient cultures.
  - Eunice Ingham combined compression massage of the feet with zone therapy to develop modern reflexology. Ingham taught reflexology throughout the United States in the 1950s–1960s.
  - Since that time, reflexology has spread to many different countries throughout the world.

- Zones and guidelines form a grid of the feet, making it possible to locate any reflex on any size foot with accuracy.
  - According to zone therapy theory, the body is divided into 10 longitudinal zones, and pressure anywhere in a zone stimulates the entire length of the zone.
    - Direct pressure within a zone on the feet affects corresponding structures and organs within that zone throughout the body.
  - Guidelines are horizontal markers on the feet that help locate specific reflex areas.
    - The four parallel guidelines are neck/ shoulder, diaphragm, waist, and pelvis.
    - The longitudinal tendon is the one longitudinal guideline.

- Foot, hand, and ear reflexology charts identify reflexes and corresponding parts of the body.
- Explanations of how reflexology works are generally outside the realm of biomedicine at this time. There are several alternative theories of reflexology.
  - Eunice Ingham believed that reflexology dissolved crystals in the feet and improved blood and nerve supply.
  - Mildred Carter incorporated principles of traditional Asian medicine into her system of reflexology.
  - Theories related to the nervous system suggest that pressure to reflexes transmits nerve impulses to the brain that then effect changes in the body.
  - Zone therapy states that pressure applied within zones on the feet affects everything in the entire zone.
  - Some believe that reflexologists access acupoints to gain entry to "organ energy" and supporting energy networks.

- The recipient of reflexology may be lying in a supine position, or semireclining on a massage table, or sitting in a recliner chair.
- Practitioners sit on chairs or stools and practice good sitting body mechanics while performing reflexology.
- For the practitioner to maintain good body mechanics, adjustments are made to the table height, bolster placement, and the practitioner's chair height.
- Reflexology techniques include thumb- and finger-walking and rolling, hook-and-backup, press-and-flex, direct pressure, friction, and joint mobilization. Dorsal fulling is a fascial technique.
- Reflexology techniques can be combined with foot massage and joint movements for greater therapeutic benefit.

EXAM REVIEW

Key Terms

Match the following key terms to their descriptions. For additional study, look up the key terms in the Interactive Glossary, and note other terms that compare or contrast with them.

_____ 1. Diaphragm relaxation
_____ 2. Direct pressure
_____ 3. Fingerwalking
_____ 4. Foot reflexology
_____ 5. Guidelines
_____ 6. Hook-and-backup
_____ 7. Press-and-flex
_____ 8. Reflexology chart
_____ 9. Rolling
_____ 10. Stabilizing hand
_____ 11. Thumbwalking
_____ 12. Working hand
_____ 13. Zone therapy

a. Hand applying the technique
b. Apply deep pressure with press and pull
c. Map of feet with reflex areas
d. Apply pressure rhythmically and quickly with thumb
e. Flex big toe over thumb pressure
f. Zone therapy on the feet
g. Hand providing backstop
h. Apply pressure rhythmically and quickly with fingers
i. Moving your hand deeper into the reflex point
j. Compression into specific point
k. Popularized by Fitzgerald in 1900
l. Landmarks to locate anatomical structures
m. Moving body into deep pressure

Memory Workout

To test your memory of the main concepts in this chapter, complete the following sentences by circling the most correct answer from the two choices provided.

1. Foot reflexology is based on the theory that pressure applied to specific (spots) (joints) on the feet produces a change in a corresponding part of the body.
2. Physician William Fitzgerald popularized a treatment called (meridian) (zone) therapy, which is the theoretical base for modern reflexology.
3. Eunice Ingham developed a system of manual therapy that combined zone therapy with (compression massage) (shiatsu).
4. According to zone therapy, the body is divided into 10 (latitudinal) (longitudinal) zones.

5. These zones have endpoints in the hands, feet, and (chest) (top of the head).
6. Ingham believed that reflexology dissolved (toxic) (crystalline) deposits in the feet.
7. Today, the term (congestion) (hypertonic) refers to any number of factors that inhibit optimal body functioning.
8. The best technique to apply pressure quickly and systematically to points along the bottoms of the feet is (thumbwalking) (hook-and-backup).
9. Athlete's foot is (an indication) (a contraindication) for foot reflexology.
10. A type of fascial technique applied to the top of the foot is called (dorsal fulling) (diaphragm relaxation).

Test Prep

The following multiple-choice questions will help to prepare you for future school and professional exams.

1. In the 1930s–1940s modern foot reflexology was developed in the United States by:
   a. Joseph Riley
   b. William Fitzgerald
   c. Eunice Ingham
   d. Ida Rolf

2. The primary technique in foot reflexology is:
   a. Vibration of the sole of the feet
   b. Stroking the tops and bottoms of the feet
   c. Joint movement of the toes
   d. Direct pressure to areas on the feet

3. According to zone therapy theory, pressure applied anywhere in the zone affects the:
   a. Entire zone
   b. Adjacent zone
   c. Entire body
   d. Corresponding area of the brain

4. The diaphragm guideline that divides the body into the chest and abdominal cavities is located:
   a. At the base of the toes in the webbing where the toes meet the ball of the foot
   b. On the heel, typically where the tougher heel changes into the softer arch
   c. Along the base of the metatarsal heads of all toes from the medial to lateral foot
   d. Along the longitudinal tendon in the foot

5. In positioning the receiver of reflexology, a bolster is usually placed:
   a. Under the ankles
   b. Under the knees
   c. Behind the neck
   d. Behind the lower back

6. According to reflexology theory, where would you apply pressure to work the sinuses?
   a. At the heels of both feet
   b. At the heel of the left foot
   c. On the toe pads of both feet
   d. On the arches of both feet

7. On which foot is the corresponding reflex area for the heart?
   a. Left foot
   b. Right foot
   c. Left ankle
   d. Both feet

8. On which foot is the corresponding reflex area for the kidneys?
   a. Left foot only
   b. Right foot only
   c. Outside ankles
   d. Bottoms of both feet

9. Which of the following best describes the use of lubricant when applying reflexology techniques like thumbwalking?
   a. Plentiful
   b. Sparingly
   c. Enough for sliding
   d. None

10. Which of the following techniques is best for applying deep pressure to a specific reflex on the bottom of a foot?
    a. Thumbwalking
    b. Fingerwalking
    c. Hook-and-backup
    d. Tapotement

Video Challenge

Watch this video, which can be found at MyHealthProfessionsLab.com, Chapter 24, and then answer the following questions.

Reflexology

1. How is the receiver positioned in the video?
2. What warm-up techniques are shown in the video? Is lotion used?

3. Describe where the stabilizing hand is placed when the practitioner is applying thumbwalking to the spinal reflexes as demonstrated in the video. What does this accomplish?

Comprehension Exercises

The following short-answer questions test your knowledge and understanding of chapter topics and provide practice in written communication skills. Explain in two to four complete sentences.

1. Briefly explain the general theory and technique of foot reflexology.

2. Describe client positioning for foot reflexology. How does this help the practitioner maintain good body and hand mechanics?

3. Describe the thumbwalking technique in detail.

For Greater Understanding

The following exercises are designed to take you from the realm of theory into practical applications. They will help give you a deeper understanding of the information covered in this chapter. Action words are underlined to emphasize the variety of activities presented to address different learning styles and to encourage deeper thinking.

1. Receive a reflexology session from a certified practitioner. Notice how he or she conducts the session. What did reflexology feel like? Did you notice any reaction to the techniques in the rest of your body? Write up or discuss your findings with a study partner.

2. Observe a certified practitioner perform reflexology. Notice the person's body mechanics and the techniques used. Describe what you saw to a study partner. (Alternative: View an instructional video.)

3. Review a clinical study about reflexology. What was the study trying to find out? How was it conducted? What were the findings? Conclusions? Write a summary of the research.

4. Develop a note-taking chart specifically for reflexology sessions using a basic SOAP model. Include blank foot charts. Use your note format to document at least three general reflexology sessions. Share your notes with a study partner.

MyHealthProfessionsLab™

MyHealthProfessionsLab.com is a premium online homework management system that includes a host of features to help you study. Registered users will find:

- Powerful tools that track and analyze your results—allowing you to create a personalized learning experience
- Videos, flashcards and other learning tools to help enrich your progress
- Streaming lesson presentations and self-paced learning modules
- A space where you and your instructors can view and manage your assignments

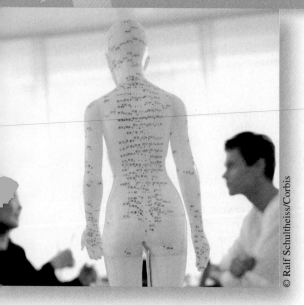

CHAPTER

25 Asian and Energy-Based Bodywork

Will Parks – Acupressure Massage Integration
Beverly Shoenberger – Polarity Therapy

© Ralf Schultheiss/Corbis

CHAPTER OUTLINE

Learning Outcomes

Key Terms

Energy-Based Bodywork

Eastern Bodywork Forms

Traditional Chinese Medicine
  Overview

Acupressure Massage Integration

Qi Gong

Ayurveda

Ayurvedic Massage

Hatha Yoga

Thai Massage

Polarity Therapy

Basic Polarity Movements

Some Final Thoughts on Polarity
  Therapy

Chapter Highlights

Exam Review

LEARNING OUTCOMES

After studying this chapter, you will have information to:

1. Define energy-based bodywork.
2. Describe forms of bodywork from China, India, and Thailand.
3. Explain key concepts of traditional Chinese medicine.
4. Integrate acupressure and massage to promote both physical and energetic well-being.
5. Describe qi gong exercises.

6. Explain key concepts of Ayurvedic philosophy.
7. Describe Ayurvedic massage.
8. Describe yoga postures.
9. Explain the theory underlying Thai massage.
10. Describe a Thai massage session.
11. Explain the theory and principles of polarity therapy.
12. Give a basic polarity therapy session.

KEY TERMS

Acupoints

Acupressure massage
  integration (AMI)

Ayurveda

Chinese body clock

Eastern bodywork

Energy-based bodywork

Energy channels

Energy flow

Five Elements

Hatha yoga

Polarity therapy

Qi

Qi gong

Removing obstructions

Thai massage

Traditional Chinese
  medicine (TCM)

Yin and Yang

ENERGY-BASED BODYWORK

Energy-based bodywork refers to forms of manual therapy in which the chief intention is to enhance the free flow of energy or life force in and around the physical body. Although some of the techniques of energy-based bodywork appear similar to Swedish massage (for example, direct pressure and sliding techniques), the theory behind the practice is significantly different. Also different is the method of technique application. The energy-based bodywork systems explored in this chapter include traditional Eastern or Asian bodywork and an offshoot called polarity therapy that was developed by an American in the early twentieth century. Energy-based bodywork can be integrated with Swedish massage for sessions that address both structure and energy.

EASTERN BODYWORK FORMS

Eastern bodywork refers to traditional forms of manual therapy from the continent of Asia. The term distinguishes these forms from Western massage as developed in Europe and America in the past few centuries. Three forms of Eastern bodywork that are particularly popular in Western countries are Asian bodywork therapies from China and Japan, Ayurvedic massage from India, and Thai bodywork from Thailand. This chapter provides a survey of these popular Eastern bodywork forms to familiarize massage therapists with some of their basic concepts and techniques.

Eastern bodywork forms developed within cultures with roots that go back thousands of years in time. They predate modern science and are embedded in whole systems of medicine. These systems are based on certain beliefs about the nature of the universe, of human beings, and of health and healing. There are differences as well as some striking similarities in these beliefs.

One overarching similarity is the holistic view of human beings as body, mind, and spirit. Unlike the relatively recent interest of Western medicine in the concept, a holistic perspective is nothing new to these ancient systems of medicine. Another similarity of the Eastern forms is their consideration of human beings as essentially part of nature and as influenced by their relationships to the natural world. They also incorporate some notion of energy or life force that flows in, around, and through the physical body.

Ancient systems of medicine used herbs, temperature therapy, physical exercise, and manual therapy as mainstays of treatment. In these systems manual therapies and related exercises are used to balance life energy and remove obstructions to its free flow.

As we explore Eastern forms of massage and bodywork that are so different from Western approaches, keep an open mind and heart. Understand that they come from worldviews different from Western thinking and have endured for centuries. You do not have to accept the ideas presented in this chapter as "true" in the sense of scientifically proven facts. They are ways of thinking about health and disease that grew out of a particular culture long ago and that continue to evolve. These theories have spawned practices and treatments that are accepted today as valuable and effective approaches to health and healing.

Truly understanding these systems takes years of study and practice. This introduction provides a broad overview. In studying these forms, we enlarge our understanding of the world.

TRADITIONAL CHINESE MEDICINE OVERVIEW

Traditional Chinese medicine (TCM) is thought to have originated in the barren lands north of the Yellow River in China. Long ago, the inhabitants of this area used herbs, acupuncture, *anmo* (body manipulation), and other methods to heal various ailments. Over the centuries, these folk healing practices became formalized into a system of medicine unique to China. Eventually these practices spread to Korea and Japan.

The earliest known text on Chinese medicine is the *Huang Di Nei Jing,* or the *Yellow Emperor's Classic of Internal Medicine.* It is traditionally ascribed to the legendary Yellow Emperor, Huang Di, who is thought to have lived around 2500 BCE. The concepts of Yin and Yang, Qi or energy, Five Elements, energy channels, and acupoints were developed over time to form the foundation of traditional Chinese medicine. An ancient drawing of energy channels is shown in Figure 25–1 ■. The aim of TCM is to restore and maintain natural balance and harmony in the body, mind, and spirit.

Yin and Yang

The concepts of **Yin and Yang** are used to illustrate the relatedness and interconnectedness of all. The Ying/Yang symbol has been described as two comets chasing each other (Figure 25–2 ■). It reminds one of the movement and constant change of the universe, which is a fundamental idea in TCM. Yin and Yang are always considered in relationship to each other.

Yin is represented by the dark side of the Yin/Yang symbol. The Chinese character for Yin depicts the shady side of a hill. Yin is the dark, deep, dense aspect of the universe. It is characterized as feminine, interior, still, substantial, cool, and contracting in contrast to Yang.

Yang is represented by the light side of the Yin/Yang symbol. The Chinese character for Yang depicts the sunny side of a hill. Yang is the light, energetic, and spacious or heavenly aspect of the universe. Yang is characterized as masculine, exterior, moving, insubstantial, warm, and expanding in contrast to Yin.

Notice that there is a dot of Yang in the Yin side of the symbol, and a dot of Yin in the Yang side. This symbolizes that nothing is pure Yin or Yang, but that these aspects are

FIGURE 25–1 Ancient drawing of energy channels and acupoints.

continually morphing and changing in relationship to each other.

FIVE PRINCIPLES OF YIN/YANG

Five principles explain the relationship of Yin and Yang. The principle of *interdependence* reminds us that these are relative concepts that cannot exist in isolation. The principle of *mutual/supporting relationship* points out that Yin and Yang must be in constant dynamic balance. The principle of *opposition* means that Yin and Yang control and restrict each other. *Intertransformation* explains that Yin and Yang are not static, but are constantly transforming into each other. Last, Yin and Yang are *infinitely divisible* and can exist in small or large amounts in everything.

FIGURE 25–2 Yin/Yang in traditional Asian medicine.

THE BODY IN TERMS OF YIN/YANG

In TCM, the human body is considered in terms of Yin and Yang. Yang corresponds to the back, head, exterior, and lateral/posterior aspects of the limbs. Yang organs, which are hollow, transform, digest, and excrete impure products of food and fluids. Yin corresponds to the front, interior, medial/interior aspects of the limbs. Yin organs, which are solid, store the pure essences extracted from food by the Yang organs. Each of the energy channels described later in this chapter is also designated as Yin or Yang.

Qi

Qi (pronounced *chee*) refers to the energy of the universe. In a larger sense, everything in the universe is Qi, sometimes referred to as Big Qi. When Big Qi condenses, it becomes material, and when it disperses, it becomes nonmaterial.

The Chinese character for Qi depicts rice cooking in a pot with steam escaping. Qi is the rice and the steam, the material and the energy. Qi condensed becomes material, forming rocks, trees, raindrops, birds, and human beings. Qi dispersed becomes energy, sunshine, starlight, and the movement of the wind. This is similar to the idea of quantum physics, in which matter and energy are seen as interchangeable, merely vibrating at different frequencies.

In a more narrow sense, Qi is the *life force* or *life energy* that flows through the body and makes people alive. This energy is extracted from the food we eat and the air we breathe. This useable Qi circulates through the body in a network of energy channels bringing life and health.

Qi's functions in the body are summarized as transforming, transporting, holding, protecting, and warming. Disease is the result of disharmony or disruption of these functions.

BALANCING QI

TCM focuses on harmonizing and balancing Qi and enhancing its flow throughout the body. If Qi is deficient, you tonify or strengthen it. If it is in excess in some place, you disperse it. If it is stagnant, you move it. If it is sinking, you uplift it. If it is rebellious, you rectify or calm it. Bodywork based in TCM uses manual techniques to tonify, disperse, move, uplift, and rectify Qi as needed to create harmony and balance.

Another goal of TCM is to harmonize the ease and flow of Qi along with the other fundamental substances: Shen or *Spirit,* Jing or *Essense,* Xue or *Blood,* and Jin/Ye or *Fluids.* Qi, Spirit, and Essence are known as the "Three Treasures" in Chinese medicine, and harmony among them is considered essential for good health.

The Five Elements

In TCM, the **Five Elements**, or *Five Elemental Energies*, are Wood, Fire, Earth, Metal, and Water. The Five Elements are a way of thinking about nature, human beings, and relationships among all natural phenomena. They are used in a metaphorical sense and do not refer to the chemical elements found in Western science.

The Five Elements are used in TCM to explore the causes of imbalances that lead to poor health and disease. They have relationships to Yin and Yang, energy channels, and other TCM concepts. Table 25–1 ■ lays out some of these important relationships.

Wood Wood is a Yang element. Wood energy is expanding. The Wood element is evident in spring when seeds germinate and young plants push out of the ground. It is seen at sunrise, heard in shouting, and felt in anger. Wood is associated with green, wind, sour taste, and sight. Balanced Wood energy results in benevolence, discernment, and patience. Unbalanced Wood energy can lead to being argumentative, timid, rigid, or unable to make decisions.

Fire Fire is the most Yang element. Fire energy is fusing. The Fire element provides heat and light and is evident in summer. It affects our ability to feel warm both physically and emotionally. The Fire element is associated with laughter, joy, sweat, and bitter taste. Fire affects a person's capacity for love, passion, self-realization, and confidence. Unbalanced Fire energy may appear as being guarded, vulnerable, controlling, or apathetic.

Earth Earth is a Yin element felt in late summer when the weather is humid and damp. Earth energy is moderating. It is felt in the change of seasons and has a transformative quality. Earth energy allows for being rooted, secure, and centered to flow with changes. Earth is heard in singing, tasted in sweet, and smelled in fragrant. Balanced Earth energy is displayed in integrity, altruism, and adaptability.

Individuals with unbalanced Earth energy tend to be selfish, martyrs, self-sufficient or needy, stubborn, or wishy-washy.

Metal Metal is a Yin element felt most in autumn and associated with letting go. Metal energy is condensing. It is felt at dusk, in grief, and heard in crying. Metal has a pungent taste and rank smell. It is related to a sense of smell, dryness, and mucus. Individuals with balanced Metal energy appear inspired, receptive, and discriminating. Unbalanced Metal energy can appear as vanity, anguish, zealotry, or despondency.

Water Water is the most Yin element and the most yielding. Water energy is conserving. The Water element is felt in the cold, dark, quiet winter, and at night. It is related to body fluids such as blood, sweat, tears, saliva, and urine. Water is associated with hearing, fear, the sound of groaning, rotten smell, and salty taste. Body parts influenced by Water energy are the bones, ears, kidneys, and bladder. Balanced Water energy manifests as wisdom, concentration, and contemplation. Imbalance in Water energy may appear as extreme recklessness, scattered attention, profound conservativeness, or physical or emotional isolation.

SHENG AND KO CYCLES

Relationships among the Five Elements are described in the Sheng and Ko cycles. In these cycles, the Five Elements are seen as supporting one another and also as being controlled by each other in predictable patterns. These relationships are summarized in Figure 25–3 ■.

TABLE 25–1 Attributes of Major Energy Channels According to Traditional Chinese Medicine

Energy Channel	Symbol	Yin/ Yang	Element	Acupoints*	Flow	Body Clock	Connects With
Lung	Lu	Yin	Metal	11 × 2	Chest to hand	3 A.M.–5 A.M.	LI
Large Intestine	LI	Yang	Metal	20 × 2	Hand to head	5 A.M.–7 A.M.	Lu
Stomach	St	Yang	Earth	45 × 2	Head to foot	7 A.M.–9 A.M.	Sp
Spleen	Sp	Yin	Earth	21 × 2	Foot to chest	9 A.M.–11 A.M.	St
Heart	Ht	Yin	Fire	9 × 2	Chest to hand	11 A.M.–1 P.M.	SI
Small Intestine	SI	Yang	Fire	19 × 2	Hand to head	1 P.M.–3 P.M.	Ht
Bladder	Bl	Yang	Water	67 × 2	Head to foot	3 P.M.–5 P.M.	Ki
Kidney	Ki	Yin	Water	27 × 2	Foot to chest	5 P.M.–7 P.M.	Bl
Pericardium	Pc	Yin	Fire	9 × 2	Chest to hand	7 P.M.–9 P.M.	TW
Triple Warmer	TW	Yang	Fire	23 × 2	Hand to head	9 P.M.–11 P.M.	Pc
Gallbladder	GB	Yang	Wood	44 × 2	Head to foot	11 P.M.–1 A.M.	Lv
Liver	Lv	Yin	Wood	14 × 2	Foot to chest	1 A.M.–3 A.M.	GB
Conception Vessel	CV	Yin		24 midline front		Anytime	6 Yin Primary Channels
Governing Vessel	GV	Yang		28 midline back		Anytime	6 Yang Primary Channels

*(x 2 = bilateral).

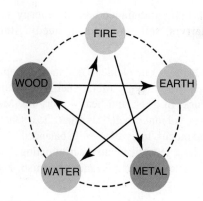

FIGURE 25–3 Sheng and Ko cycles.

Sheng Cycle The Sheng cycle is also called the creation, generating, or promoting cycle. In the Sheng cycle, each Element supports the next. For example, Wood feeds Fire, which creates ash residue, which becomes Earth. Metal originates deep within the Earth and is then found in trace amounts in the Water that springs from the ground. Water nourishes the trees or Wood, and the cycle continues.

Ko Cycle The Ko cycle is also called the controlling or acting cycle. Each Element controls another and is also controlled by another Element. Metal, such as an ax, will control Wood. Wood controls Earth, such as the trees covering the ground or the roots of trees holding the soil to prevent erosion. Earth can dam or channel Water. Water will control or extinguish Fire. Fire will melt the metal blade of the ax. Overall, the Ko cycle balances the Sheng cycle to avoid unrestrained growth.

Certain Elements, if especially strong, can either nourish or control another Element. If especially weak, it will fail to nourish or can be easily overcome. The balanced cyclic relationship of the Elements maintaining one another is considered to foster the healthiest life. The therapies of TCM, including bodywork and exercises like qi gong, aim to restore natural balance and equilibrium among the Five Elements.

Energy Channels

Qi travels through the body in a network of **energy channels** or meridians. Every part of the body is enlivened, nourished, and warmed by Qi flowing through this network. There are 12 primary energy channels, 8 extraordinary vessels, and various other channels. Two extraordinary vessels are especially important, the Conception Vessel (CV) and the Governing Vessel (GV). The paths of the 12 primary channels and the CV and GV vessels are traced in Figure 25–4 ■.

Each energy channel is named for a body organ it affects and is considered either Yin or Yang. Each is associated with one of the Five Elements. There are a number of acupoints or spots on the channel where Qi is more easily accessed. Each channel flows in a certain direction and connects and communicates with other channels. Important attributes of the 12 primary channels and 2 extraordinary vessels are summarized in Table 25–1

CHINESE BODY CLOCK

The channels flow through the body according to a natural, rhythmic cycle called the **Chinese body clock**. The day is divided roughly into 2-hour periods, and during that 2 hours, a certain primary channel is most active. During the next 2-hour period a different channel is most active—and so on throughout the day. For example, the Stomach channel is most active from 7 A.M.–9 A.M., followed by the Spleen channel from 9 A.M.–11 A.M. and the Heart channel from 11 A.M.–1 P.M. The channels cycle through their peak periods in a consistent pattern every day (see Table 25–1).

TCM practitioners use the knowledge of the location of channels, and the flow of Qi within them, to diagnose energy imbalances and to plan treatment. Also taken into consideration are the correspondences to Yin/Yang, the Five Elements, and the location of acupoints.

Acupoints

Acupoints are places in the body where Qi collects and where it can be accessed and influenced. There are 365 classic acupoints located along the primary energy channels. In the ancient practice of acupuncture, acupoints are stimulated by inserting needles. Acupoints can also be stimulated by applying pressure, as in the manual therapies of acupressure and shiatsu.

Acupoints are designated by the name of the energy channel on which they are found and by a number, indicating their place in the sequence of points on that channel. For example, GB-20 is located on the Gallbladder energy channel and is the 20th acupoint from the beginning of that channel. Each acupoint can also be located in reference to anatomical structures in the area. GB-20 is located in the suboccipital area in a recess between the sternocleidomastoid and trapezius muscles. Each acupoint also has a Chinese name. GB-20 is also known as *Fengchi* or Wind Pond. Refer to Figure 25–4 for the location of acupoints along the primary channels.

Acupoints are useful in the diagnosis and treatment of energy imbalances. Certain acupoints have been associated with treating specific ailments. Pressing GB-20 has been found to be effective for treating tension headaches, stiff neck or shoulders, dizziness, vertigo, and insomnia. Table 25–2 ■ lists some useful acupoints for common ailments.

However, it is important to remember that in TCM acupoints are not used as "pills" that treat disease. So pressing a point will not automatically cure an ailment or remove symptoms. Acupoints are treated as part of a broad approach that aims for harmony and balance in Yin/Yang, the Five Elements, and Qi. Acupoints are selected specifically to support a person's movement into greater balance.

TABLE 25–2	Useful Acupoints		
Acupoint	Name	General Location	Indications
Lu-1	Central Treasury	Lateral chest, between ribs 1-2	Lung congestion, asthma
Lu-7	Broken Sequence	Lateral interior forearm, proximal to thumb	Common cold, asthma, stiff neck, dry throat and eyes, worry and sadness
LI-4	Tiger's Mouth	Dorsal side of thumb web	Frontal headache, toothache, hay fever symptoms, excessive sweating (contraindicated during pregnancy)
LI-11	Crooked Pond	Distal humerus on lateral side just above elbow crease	Sore throat, skin eruptions, hypertension, elbow pain
LI-15	Shoulder Bone	Depression in center of deltoid muscle when arm is raised	Shoulder pain and dysfunction
LI-20	Welcome Fragrance	Groove at lateral edge of nostril	Nasal congestion, nosebleed, sneezing, facial paralysis, facial tics
St-36	3 Mile Point	Just below lateral knee	Stomach pain, indigestion, vomiting, diarrhea, knee/wrist pan, postpartum dizziness, energy deficiency
St-40	Bountiful Bulge	Lower leg midway between knee and ankle and lateral to tibial crest	Upper respiratory congestion, asthma, heavy feeling, mental disturbance
Sp-6	Yin Intersection	Just above medial ankle bone on posterior edge of tibia	Abdominal pain, menstrual disorders, medial knee pain, diarrhea, sexual dysfunction, urination problems (contraindicated during pregnancy)
SI-3	Back Stream	Ulnar side of hand, just proximal to the fifth metacarpal head (little finger side)	Stiff neck, shoulders or back, occipital headache, weak spine, convulsions, lacking courage
Bl-10	Celestial Pillar	Suboccipital region lateral to cervical spine at hair line	Tension headache
Bl-40	Entrusting Middle	Back of knee in center at crease	Lower back pain, hip problems, abdominal pain, vomiting, diarrhea, burning urination
Bl-60	Kunlun Mountain	Depression between lateral ankle and Achilles tendon	Occipital headache, chronic stiff neck, shoulders or back, heel pain (contraindicated during pregnancy)
Pc-6	Inner Gate	Inner forearm above wrist crease	Nausea, vomiting, hiccups, chest pain, insomnia, agitation, nervousness
TW-5	Outer Gate	Back of forearm just above wrist	Fever and chills, headache, ear problems, red/swollen eyes, pain in ribs
GB-20	Wind Pond	Suboccipital region	Tension headache, stiff neck or shoulders, dizziness, vertigo, and insomnia
GB-21	Shoulder Well	Highest point on the shoulder	Tension headache, stiff shoulder (contraindicated during pregnancy)
GB-30	Jumping Round	Hip	Sciatica, lumbar pain, frustration
GB-34	Sunny Side of Mountain	Depression anterior and inferior to head of fibula	Numbness, weakness or pain in lower extremities, bitter taste in mouth, frequent sighing or irritability

 PRACTICAL APPLICATION

Use a washable marker to trace the primary energy channels of Traditional Chinese Medicine on a practice partner. Locate the useful acupoints described in Table 25–2.

1. Where does each channel begin and end?
2. What path does each channel take as it flows through the body?
3. What anatomical landmarks help you locate specific acupoints?

A. Lung

B. Large intestine

C. Stomach

D. Spleen

E. Heart

F. Small intestine

G. Bladder

H. Kidney [2 images]

FIGURE 25–4

Twelve primary energy channels and the Conception and Governing Vessels of Traditional Chinese Medicine. Acupoints are denoted by numbers along the energy channels.

I. Pericardium

J. Triple warmer

K. Gallbladder

L. Liver

M. Conception Vessel (CV)

N. Governing Vessel (GV)

FIGURE 25–4 *(continued)*

KYO AND JITSU

Shiatsu, an Asian bodywork form from Japan, uses the concepts of Kyo and Jitsu to indicate acupoints (called *tsubos* in Japanese) and surrounding tissues with an imbalance of Ki (same as Qi). Kyo is energy deficiency and is felt in the tissues as a soft, hollow spot with no tone. Jitsu is energy excess and is felt in the tissues as hardness, resistance, or sensitivity. Figure 25–5 ■ summarizes characteristics of kyo and jitsu.

Areas of kyo and jitsu are treated differently with manual techniques. When a kyo or deficient point is found, the practitioner presses into the spot and holds it for 7 to 10 seconds. The intention is to tonify or strengthen the area. When an area of jitsu or excess is found, the spot is pressed for 3 to 5 seconds and then released. This is repeated about 10 times or until a change is felt. The intention is to disperse the excess energy and sedate the area.

Assessment and Treatment in Traditional Chinese Medicine

A TCM practitioner uses various methods of assessment to locate energy imbalances and disharmony in Yin/Yang

	Kyo	Jitsu
Definition	Energy deficiency	Energy excess
Palpation	Soft, hollow, toneless spot	Hard, sensitive, resistant spot
Technique	Press into point and hold for 7–10 seconds	Press into point for 3–5 seconds, then release. Repeat 10 times.
Intention	To draw energy; to strengthen and tonify the area	To disperse excess energy; sedate the area

FIGURE 25–5
Kyo and jitsu—concept of energy deficiency and excess from shiatsu.

and the Five Elements. This is very different from diagnosis in Western medicine, which looks at organic disease processes.

The traditional pillars of assessment are looking, touching, smelling, listening, and asking. For example, the TCM clinician observes a person's physical appearance, general demeanor, and movement. He or she looks at the condition of the hair and skin, and listens to the quality of the voice. The tongue is fully assessed, including its shape, color, and coating. Energy pulses on each hand are felt. This is different from the cardiovascular pulse. Clients are asked about their physical and emotional state. An assessment of energy imbalances is made from this information.

In some forms of shiatsu, a *hara* diagnosis is conducted by feeling the abdominal area (roughly the area below the ribs and the sternum to just above the pubic bone). Diagnostic areas for each of the 12 primary meridians are found in this region. The practitioner palpates the abdomen to detect meridians that are out of balance or show signs of kyo or jitsu. He or she then applies pressure to acupoints along those energy meridians to correct imbalances found.

TREATMENT OF ENERGY IMBALANCES

Treatment of energy imbalances in TCM can take several forms. Acupuncture with thin needles inserted at acupoints is perhaps the most recognizable treatment. Different Asian bodywork therapies (ABT) are also familiar in the West. These include tuina and acupressure from China, and amma and shiatsu from Japan. Tuina and amma are more massage-like, whereas acupressure and shiatsu rely on direct pressure to acupoints.

Other common TCM treatments are Chinese herbs, *moxibustion* (burning mugwort), *guasha* (scraping the skin), and cupping (glass vacuum jar). Moxibustion warms the

vessels when there are symptoms of cold, guasha moves Qi and Blood when there is stagnation, and cupping also unblocks stagnation. Qi gong, a form of active exercise, is also used to stimulate and balance Qi. Qi gong is performed for prevention, as well as treatment of energy imbalances, and is discussed further in a later section of this chapter.

Acupuncture is a licensed profession in many states. Asian bodywork practitioners may also need state licenses. This differs from state to state. TCM practitioners are certified through the National Certification Commission for Acupuncture and Oriental Medicine (NCCAOM).

ACUPRESSURE MASSAGE INTEGRATION

Massage therapists can integrate principles and techniques of acupressure with standard Swedish massage to address both the physical and energetic wellness of their clients. **Acupressure massage integration (AMI)** utilizes the massage therapist's knowledge of Western anatomy, energy pathways, and location of key acupoints. In an AMI session, both Swedish massage techniques and ABT finger pressure techniques are applied systematically for their wellness effects.

The intent of AMI is to balance the body's vital energy (Qi) overall, release tension, and improve circulation. Acupressure techniques can tonify areas of Qi deficiency and disperse excess Qi that is pooling in one place. Stimulating specific acupoints restores Qi, strengthens weaknesses, relieves common ailments, and prevents health problems.

Acupressure massage integration combines some of the theory and techniques of Chinese massage with Swedish massage techniques. It uses Swedish massage style manipulations to balance the free flow of Qi in the body.

Basic AMI Approach

The basic approach in acupressure massage integration is to apply massage techniques region by region along major energy pathways, feeling for signs of deficiency (kyo) or excess (jitsu), and pressing important acupoints. When areas needing attention are found, appropriate techniques are performed to restore energy balance and flow.

When integrating acupressure and massage, practitioners are aware of both the physical condition of the musculature and signs of energy balance or imbalance. Manual techniques are applied to the body's soft tissues along classic energy pathways and to key acupoints.

Practitioners aim for certain effects when applying techniques. Keeping your intention in mind during AMI guides the energy as needed. Your intention may be to increase **energy flow** generally in energy channels, to stimulate key acupoints, or to address specific areas of energy deficiency or excess. It is an important principle that energy follows intention.

AMI uses a combination of Swedish massage and Asian bodywork techniques. Effleurage or sliding techniques are used to spread oil or lotion. When applying effleurage, especially over energy pathways, palpate for areas of deficiency (kyo) or excess (jitsu). Petrissage or lifting and pressing techniques influence energy flow in broad areas. Cross-tissue and circular fiber applied with the fingertips or knuckles addresses smaller areas with more specificity.

The thumb or elbow is used to apply pressure to key acupoints. When areas of energy deficiency or excess are found, pressure is applied to the points to reestablish the free and harmonious flow of energy. The discussion of kyo and jitsu earlier in this chapter describes the difference in treating an area of deficiency and an area of excess.

Any number of massage technique variations may be effective for AMI. Rather than following a precise protocol, it is more important to keep in mind the intent of the techniques and choose those that will accomplish your goals. It is also essential in AMI to apply techniques specifically to energy pathways and acupoints.

Principles for Applying Pressure to Acupoints

There are four general principles for applying direct pressure to acupoints. These are (1) weight transfer, (2) stacking the joints, (3) perpendicularity, and (4) good back and neck alignment.

Weight Transfer In acupressure applications, weight transfer refers to applying pressure by shifting the body weight into the point of contact rather than pushing from the shoulders and arms. Pressure through weight transfer has a more comfortable feel to the receiver than that created by tensing the arm and hand muscles. Weight transfer performed using the whole body ensures that the connection between the giver and the receiver involves the entire person.

Stacking the Joints Applying pressure through the joints from bone to bone is called stacking the joints. For example,

FIGURE 25–6 Correct alignment for stacking the joints to apply thumb pressure to acupoints.

Source: Pearson Education, Inc./Segal Photography.

in applying thumb pressure, the thumb's joints are stacked in line with the wrist, elbow, and shoulder joints. This way the bones absorb much of the force of pressure rather than the joints themselves. When pressure is applied across a joint at an angle, or if the joint is bent, the joint structures and surrounding muscles are stressed. This can cause damage if repeated over time. Correct alignment for stacking the joints to apply thumb pressure is illustrated in Figure 25–6 ■.

Perpendicularity Applying pressure straight into an acupoint at a 90-degree angle, called perpendicularity, achieves maximum effect. If the line of application is less than or more than 90 degrees, the skin usually slips in one direction or another, lessening the pressure applied to the point itself. This has been likened to trying to pour water into a vase with a narrow neck. Unless you pour the water from directly overhead, some of the water will spill out.

Good Back and Neck Alignment Along with the other three principles, good body alignment ensures that back and neck muscles are not stressed when applying techniques. It is particularly important not to bend from the waist or let the head drop forward.

AMI Practice Sequences for the Back, Arm, and Neck–Head–Face

The principles of acupressure massage integration can be practiced on different parts of the body. Practice sequences for the back, the arm, and the neck–head–face complex are included in this chapter. Before practicing a sequence, take time to review the flow of the channels and the location of specific acupoints involved. Figure 25–7 ■ shows the location of key energy channels and acupoints used in the practice sequences for the back, shoulder, arm, and the neck–head–face complex.

It is common for forms of Asian bodywork to be given on a mat on the floor. This is how it would have been done in Asian countries. Acupressure massage integration can

A   B

FIGURE 25–7 Locations of key energy meridians and acupoints for the back, shoulder, arm, neck, head, and face.

Source: Pearson Education, Inc.

be easily adapted for a recipient lying on a massage table. The table is set lower than for Western massage to make it easier to maintain good body mechanics when applying direct pressure into acupoints.

The sequences presented here offer some ideas for addressing major meridians and acupoints on a few different parts of the body. Swedish massage techniques can be added for warming, smooth transitions, and finishing as desired. The important point is to be conscious of meridian and acupoint locations and to work with the intention to balance energy, as well as to address areas of kyo and jitsu.

PRACTICE SEQUENCE 25–1

AMI for the Back | 20 minutes
Recipient prone

Preliminary Considerations:
• Adjust table height for good body mechanics.
• Screen the recipient for contraindications.
• Position the recipient comfortably in the prone position, and undrape the back.

Primary Energy Meridians Affected:
• Bladder—Inner and Outer (BI)
• Gallbladder (GB)

Key Acupoints:
BI-10, GB-20, GB-21, GB-30

Figure 25–8 Effleurage to the entire back to apply oil. Stand at the side of the table near the recipient's hips to apply oil to the back; feel for areas of kyo and jitsu.

Perform Steps 2–19 on one side, and then repeat on the other side.

Figure 25–9 Effleurage hand over hand along spinal muscles. Stand at the side directly facing the table and reach over to massage the opposite side; (A) one hand slides up the back and (B) the other hand slides down alternately. Repeat several times; deepen pressure as muscles are warmed.

A

B

3

A

B

Figure 25–10 Pull-ups to side of torso from iliac crest to shoulder. Slide palms up the side of the torso, alternating hands while lifting the soft tissues; (A) cover the oblique abdominal muscles, slide fingers between the ribs, (B) pull up over the scapula and tops of the shoulders.

4

Figure 25–11 Fingertip kneading from shoulder to hip along the paraspinal muscles. Use fingertips to press and lift soft tissues along the side of the spine over the Inner and Outer Bladder meridians.

5

Figure 25–12 Thumb petrissage to the paraspinal muscles up the back from hip to shoulders. Use the thumbs to press into the soft tissues while sliding away from the spine; pressure on Inner then Outer Bladder meridians; focus on upper back between spine and medial border of scapula.

Figure 25–13 Thumb petrissage back down the same side of the spine from shoulder to sacrum.

Figure 25–14 Thumb press the sacral notches; four notches and four presses; may be done over the drape.

Figure 25–15 Thumb petrissage and direct fingertip pressure along iliac crest to muscle attachments.

Figure 25–16 Press with (A) fingertips into GB-30; or (B) with thumb into GB-30; press 2–3 times.

A

B

10

Figure 25–17 Fingertips knead along paraspinal muscles from the sacrum to the top of the shoulder; one hand on the inner bladder meridian and the other hand on the outer bladder meridian. Take note of tightness.

11

A

B

Figure 25–18 (A) Thumb press across top of shoulder. (B) Repeated pressing to GB-21 to disperse energy; massage the top of the shoulder.

12

Figure 25–19 Thumb press Inner and Outer Bladder meridians in upper back between shoulder blades; press into areas of kyo or excess found there.

13

Figure 25–20 Stripping effleurage over the shoulder area. Use the thumbs sliding away from each other to apply a form of stripping effleurage to the shoulder area.

Figure 25–21 Rhythmic sliding compression down the spine and effleurage with palms back to the head. Place palms on either side of the spine and then slide to hips, compressing tissues rhythmically along the way; return to head with simple effleurage with palms.

Figure 25–22 Press with fingertips into Bl-10 and GB-20 at the base of the skull; press individually and then with fingertips to all points along the occipital ridge at the same time.

Figure 25–23 Pull-ups from shoulder to buttocks.
(A) Move across the shoulder, fingertips between the ribs.
(B) Move along the oblique abdominal muscles to the iliac crest.

A

B

17

A

B

Figure 25–24 (A) Alternating thumb petrissage to paraspinal muscles from sacrum to shoulder. Search for areas of muscle tightness or energy imbalance, especially in the mid back. (B) Use thumb presses or deep friction to tense spots.

18

A

B

Figure 25–25 (A) Thumb presses between shoulder blades on inner and outer bladder meridian acupoints. (B) Apply friction to areas of muscle tightness.

19

Figure 25–26 Stripping effleurage to shoulder as smoothing and transition technique. Apply with thumbs sliding away from each other.

Repeat Steps 2–19 on the opposite side.

Finish the sequence with Steps 20–25 applied bilaterally to the back.

Figure 25–27 Rhythmic sliding compression down both sides of the spine, with palmar friction back up to shoulders.

Figure 25–28 Open palmar friction moving back and forth over the lumbar and thoracic regions.

Figure 25–29 Fingertip kneading along the paraspinal muscles from shoulders to buttocks. Check to make sure all areas of tension have been relieved and that tissues are supple and pliable.

Figure 25–30 Circular palmar petrissage back up the spine from buttocks to shoulders. Tissues lift as hands trace circles in soft tissues.

Figure 25–31 Hourglass effleurage around the tops of shoulders and base of the neck.

Figure 25–32 Superficial friction with palms along back. Hands are perpendicular to the spine; apply friction with palms, shifting hands back and forth as they move first down the spine to the hips and back up to the shoulders.

After you perform the Practice Sequence, evaluate how well you did by filling out Performance Evaluation Form 25–1, AMI for the Back. The form can be found in Appendix D, *Performance Evaluation Forms,* and at MyHealthProfessions.com.

Figures source: Pearson Education, Inc./Segal Photography.

PRACTICE SEQUENCE 25–2

AMI for the Anterior Arm

10 minutes
Recipient supine

Preliminary Instructions
• Adjust table height for good body mechanics.
• Screen the recipient for contraindications.
• Position the recipient comfortably in the supine position, and undrape the arm and chest.
• Stand on same side you are working.

Primary Energy Meridians Affected
• Heart (Ht)
• Large Intestine (LI)
• Lung (Lu)
• Pericardium (P)
• Triple Burner (TB)

Key Acupoints:
GB-21, Ki-27, LI-4, LI-11, LI-15, Lu-1, Lu-2, Lu-5, TB-5, SI-3

A   **B**   **C**

1

Figure 25–33 (A) Effleurage to entire arm to apply oil or lotion. (B) Apply with flat palms and fingers from recipient's hand to top of shoulder and neck, and upper chest. (C) Press GB-21 when in the upper shoulder.

A   **B**   **C**

2

Figure 25–34 Finger press acupoints under the clavicle: (A) Ki-27, (B) Lu-2, (C) Lu-1.

Figure 25–35 Fingertip rake over sternum and pectoralis muscles from midline to lateral chest. Adjust for women. Apply over the skin or drape.

3

4

Figure 25–36 Reverse pull-ups (palms up) from hip to armpit. Reach under the back and pull up with the fingertips around the sides of the ribs.

5

Figure 25–37 Alternate thumb petrissage to pectoralis major. Apply along edge and muscle belly.

6

Figure 25–38 Fingertip rake over pectoralis major from sternum to shoulder. Pull arm out from the body to access the muscle.

7

Figure 25–39 Thumb, knuckle slides, and kneading (as appropriate) to energy meridians in the upper arm in 5 lines. Apply along (A) Heart, (C) Pericardium, (E) Lung, (G) Triple Burner, and (H) Large Intestine meridians. Thumb press to (B) Lu-5, (D) LI-11, and (F) LI-15.

Figure 25–40 Apply kneading and deep stroking to lower arm muscles. (A) Knead muscle bellies. (B) Thumb press TB-5. Stroke along the (C) Lung, (D) Small Intestine, and (E) Triple Burner meridians. (F) Thumb press LI-11.

Figure 25–41 General hand massage. Include (A) metacarpal mobilizations and (B) gentle finger pulls. (C) Press LI-4, SI-3.

10

Figure 25–42 Shake the arm and then brush entire arm with fingertips to finish.

Repeat Steps 1–10 on the other arm.

After you perform the Practice Sequence, evaluate how well you did by filling out Performance Evaluation Form 25–2, AMI for the Anterior Arm. The form can be found in Appendix D: *Performance Evaluation Forms,* and at MyHealthProfessionsLab.com.

Figures source: Pearson Education, Inc./Segal Photography.

 PRACTICAL APPLICATION

On a practice partner, use a washable marker to trace the energy meridians and mark the acupoints used in AMI Practice Sequence 25–2. Practice the sequence, being precise about where techniques are applied.

1. What major energy pathways are located in the anterior arm?

2. Where are important acupoints located?
3. What manual techniques are described in the Practice Sequence to affect these meridians and acupoints?
4. Can you suggest other technique approaches to affect those meridians and acupoints?

PRACTICE SEQUENCE 25–3

AMI for the Neck–Head–Face

15 minutes
Recipient supine

Preliminary Instructions
• Adjust table height for good body mechanics.
• Screen the recipient for contraindications.
• Position the recipient comfortably in the supine position; support the neck as needed.
• Sit at the head of the table for the entire sequence.

Primary Energy Meridians Affected:
• Bladder—Inner and Outer (Bl)
• Gallbladder (GB)
• Small Intestine (SI)
• Stomach (St)
• Triple Burner (TB)

Key Acupoints:
B-1, Bl-10, GB-1, GB-20, GB-21, GV-26, LI-20, SI-18, SI-19, St-2, St-3, St-6, St-7, TB-23

1

Figure 25–43 Rhythmic compression to shoulders. Stand at the head and place one hand on each shoulder. Gently mobilize the shoulders, pushing one side and then the other in "cat paw" movement.

2

Figure 25–44 Effleurage with fingertips to tops of both shoulders and neck. Feel for which side is most tense and work on that side first.

Perform Steps 3–9 on both sides of the neck before proceeding to Step 10.

3

Figure 25–45 Pinch the sternocleidomastoid (SCM) muscle at points along its length. Turn head to side to expose the side of the neck. Starting at the superior attachment, pinch along the SCM muscle between the thumb and the curled index finger. *Note:* Be careful to lift the muscle only and not blood vessels in the area.

4

Figure 25–46 Press into the top side of the clavicle near the manubrium along the Stomach meridian.

Figure 25–47 (A) Thumb slide along the top of the clavicle to the shoulder, and then with fingertips go up the neck to the base of the skull. (B) Press GB-20.

A

B

Figure 25–48 (A) Slide with fingertips along the path of the Gallbladder meridian (scalene muscles) to GB-21. (B) Press into GB-21 with fingertips. Address points of kyo or jitsu found in the area.

A

B

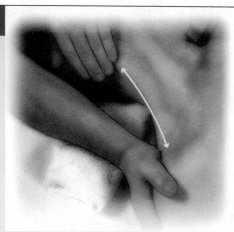

Figure 25–49 Stretch neck in lateral flexion. Place one hand on the head and the other hand on the shoulder and apply the stretch.

A

B

Figure 25–50 (A) Slide the hand up the shoulder and neck to GB-20 and Bl-10. (B) Fingertip press or circular friction to those acupoints.

Figure 25–51 Press with fingertips around the ear over the pathways of Gallbladder and Triple Burner meridians. Using three or four fingers in a row, press in several places around the ear in a fan shape.

Reminder: Repeat Steps 3–9 on both sides of neck.

Figure 25–52 (A) Thumb slides to forehead in 2–3 rows, and along the eyebrow to the outer edge. (B) Press into TB-23. Recipient is facing directly upward.

Figure 25–53 Press Bladder meridian points along upper orbital ridge with fingertips, from B-1 on the inside corner of the eye to GB-1 on the outside corner of the eye.

Figure 25–54 (A) Thumb slide down nose to (B) St-2. Press points along the cheekbone: (C) LI-20, (D) St-3, (E) SI-18, (F) St-7, to (G) SI-19 in the jaw joint.

Figure 25–55 (A) Thumb slides above upper lip; to begin, fingers are placed near the ears, and thumbs begin at midline above the upper lip at GV-26. (B) Thumb slides below lower lip and up the sides of the face to the temples.

Figure 25–56 (A) Pinch along jaw line from midline to lateral aspect. (B) Press St-6 at masseter attachment.

A

B

Figure 25–57 (A) Massage the ears between thumb and fingers. (B) Gently pull on ears.

A

B

16

A   B   C

Figure 25–58 Apply neck stretches. Lift the head with two hands to apply (A) rotations, (B) lateral flexion, and (C) forward flexion.

17

Figure 25–59 Finish gently holding the head. Place palms of hands lightly over the ears for a few seconds. Slowly remove hands.

After you perform the Practice Sequence, evaluate how well you did by filling out Performance Evaluation Form 25–3, AMI for the Neck–Head–Face. The form can be found in Appendix D: *Performance Evaluation Forms*, and at MyHealthProfessionsLab.com.

Figures source: Pearson Education, Inc./Segal Photography.

CASE FOR STUDY

Kareem Applies Acupressure Massage Integration to the Legs

Kareem has a client named Don who is experiencing tension in his legs and feet. The standard massage Kareem is using has had some relaxing effects, but he feels he can get better results by incorporating some acupressure into the sessions. Don is open to the idea and gives Kareem permission to use AMI for a few sessions.

Question:

How might Kareem apply AMI to Don's legs?

Things to consider:

- What energy meridians run through the legs and feet?
- What important acupoints are located there?
- What massage and acupressure techniques can be adapted to the AMI session?
- Of what importance is intention to the application?

Plan an AMI session for addressing Don's legs. Map out important energy meridians and acupoints, and describe techniques that might be used.

_____

_____

_____

QI GONG

Qi gong means *energy exercise* in Chinese. The overall objective of these ancient exercises is to stimulate the healthy and balanced flow of Qi in the body. Practiced regularly, qi gong aims to prevent illness, improve health, and promote longevity.

Qi gong is also a body–mind practice that develops coordination, body awareness, and concentration. It focuses the mind and coordinates posture, breathing, and movement. Performed regularly, qi gong improves overall well-being and can be a valuable self-care practice for massage practitioners. It is a useful supplement to Asian Bodywork Therapy because it has the same goal, that is, to improve the flow of Qi in the body's energy channels.

Two examples of simple qi gong forms from the Dao Yin Shen Gong style illustrate basic qi gong principles. They are Gliding Phoenix and Spring for the Crane and Deer. See Figures 25–60 ■ and 25–61 ■.

Qi Gong Forms

Qi gong exercises consist of a variety of choreographed movements that involve bending, stretching, reaching, stepping, and other movements designed to harmonize the flow of Qi. Each movement, sometimes referred to as a form, has its own benefits. Different forms are strung together for a continuous flow of movement. Qi gong is often performed to music to pace the movements and inspire a gentle, flowing quality. The slow and fluid movements of qi gong bring the mind into a meditative state for rejuvenation and relaxation.

Individual qi gong forms are designed to stimulate specific energy channels and acupoints. Some exercises also aim at specific therapeutic effects, for example, to improve range of motion in a certain area, or to improve function of a certain organ. Some have a more general effect on overall health.

BREATHING

Qi gong movements are coordinated with deep, even abdominal breathing. Breathing is through the nose and is gentle and quiet. Most upward and inward movements of the arms and head are done on the inhalation, whereas most downward and outward movements occur on the exhalation. The breath sets the pace for the rhythmic movement of qi gong, alternating in and out, up and down.

AYURVEDA

Ayurveda refers to the traditional health and healing practices of India. The term Ayurveda combines two Sanskrit words, *ayu,* or life, and *veda,* or knowledge. Thus Ayurveda is knowledge of life, or more to the point, knowledge of the principles of living a long and healthy life. It is one of the oldest systems of health and healing in the world.

Ayurveda is said to have been passed down to mortals from Brahma the creator to the seers on earth, who started an oral tradition passed on from generation to generation. This knowledge has been written down through the ages, first in the ancient text of the *Rig Veda* (c.1700 BCE), and later in two treatises from about 1000 BCE called the *Charaka Samhita* (medicine) and *Sushrut Samhita* (surgery). Through the centuries, Ayurdeva has evolved and been transformed by various influences, including Muslim invasions of the eleventh century, healing traditions within different areas of India, and most recently by modern science and technology.

FIGURE 25–60

Gliding Phoenix.

Beginning position: Legs straight and together, arms at sides of body.

1. Rise up onto the balls of the feet, keeping the legs naturally straight, and rotate your head to the left fully; raise arms to the sides at a 45-degree angle and rotate the arms externally to full extension, bringing scapulae toward the spine (inhale).

2. Lower your heels to the ground, and lower arms to the side of the body naturally; return head to center (exhale).

Perform movements 1 and 2 to the right side. (Left and right = 1 cycle). Perform two breathing cycles.

FIGURE 25–61

Spring for the Crane and Deer.

Beginning position: Legs straight and together, arms at sides of body.

1. Gradually raise arms to sides at shoulder height and flex wrists to press Tia Yuan, Da Ling, and Shen Men points; hands should be hooked with thumb over index finger; rotate head left (inhale).

2. Step the right foot back crossed behind the left foot and bend the knees; elbows sink down and wrists flex; hands face forward; keep looking left. Lower the body and the hands; end in a squat looking left (exhale).

3. Gradually raise your body, straighten right leg behind left leg, keeping left leg bent softly; raise wrists and arms from front of body to sides of ears with hooked hands, thumb over index finger; extend arms to full extension (inhale).

4. Release tension and relax, softly lower arms and palms from front to sides of body; right foot returns to center. End with hands at sides and legs together (exhale).

Alternate left and right sides (one cycle). Perform two cycles.

Ayurvedic Health Practices

Many Ayurvedic practices focus on enhancing overall health and on prevention of illness and disease. Some practices aim toward increasing longevity. Another aspect is the treatment of physical and mental disorders. An underlying goal is the achievement of our full potential as human beings. Thus Ayurveda spans the entire scope of the wellness perspective and is holistic in nature.

Ayurvedic health practices include a vegetarian diet, cleansing and detoxifying the body, movements and postures (hatha yoga), breathing exercises, meditation, and massage. Sources of further information about Ayurveda can be located in Appendix E, *References and Additional Resources*.

Ayurveda is a complex philosophy of health and healing unique to India. A complete description of this philosophy is not within the scope of this text. However, a few basic concepts relevant to Ayurvedic massage are explored here. Table 25–3 ■ is a glossary of some basic terms used in Ayurveda.

TABLE 25–3	Glossary of Basic Ayurvedic Terms
Term	**Meaning**
Ayurveda	Knowledge of long and healthy life
Chakras	Seven energy centers: Root, Sacral, Solar Plexus, Heart, Throat, Third Eye, Crown
Dhatus	Types of tissues or fluids in the body: lymph, blood, muscle, bone, fat, marrow, and sexual fluids
Doshas	Three governing principles: Vata, Pitta, Kapha
Elements	Components of all matter: earth, air, fire, water, and ether
Koshas	Five body sheaths: Physical body, subtle energy, mind, intellect, bliss
Malas	Waste products of digestion: urine, feces, sweat
Marma point	Subtle junctions between consciousness and matter
Nadis	Energy channels for Prana flow
Prakriti	Constitution: Vata, Pitta, Kapha, Vata-Pitta, Pitta-Kapha, Vata-Kapha, Sama
Prana	Subtle energy
Shakti	Creative spiritual life force or love
Srotas	Sixteen circulatory channels in the body 1–3 control flow of water, food, and breath 4–10 support major tissues of the body 11–13 control waste removal 14 carries thought from heart to mind 15–16 carry menstrual fluid and lactate
Vayu	Subtle energy

The Physical Body—Koshas, Doshas, and Chakras

In Ayurveda, human beings are seen as having a material body, as well as subtle energy bodies that surround and move through the physical aspect. A person has five layers or sheaths called *koshas*. These sheaths range from the physical body on the outside to pure consciousness at the center (Figure 25–62 ■). Ayurvedic massage touches the physical body and the outer layer of subtle energy directly, while affecting the deeper layers indirectly.

PHYSICAL BODY—KOSHA 1

The outermost kosha is the *annamaya* or physical body. The physical body is composed of the three *doshas* or principles, seven *dhatus* or tissues, and three *malas* or waste products. These evolved from the five basic elements of the universe: earth, air, fire, water, and ether.

Within the physical body are 16 *srotas* or channels that allow for the circulation or movement of substances such as air, food, lymph, blood, urine, feces, sweat, and cellular-level nutrients. Also circulating through the srotas are the three doshas called *Vata, Pitta,* and *Kapha.*

Vata Vata, also called Vayu, is the wind principle, composed of the elements of air and ether or space. It is associated with bodily movement and the nervous system. Vata is located primarily in the pelvic and leg regions, and its seat is the colon.

Pitta Pitta is the bile principle, composed of the elements of fire and water. It is associated with digestion, thirst, courage, and thinking. Pitta is located primarily in the abdominal region and in blood and skin, and its seat is the stomach.

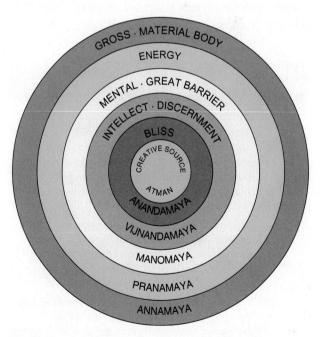

FIGURE 25–62 Five layers or sheaths called koshas in Ayurvedic philosophy.

Kapha Kapha is the mucus principle, composed of the elements of earth and water. It is responsible for lubrication and controls patience. Kapha is located primarily in the upper body, and its seat is the lungs.

Constitutional Types The proportion of the three doshas differs from person to person. A person's innate natural healthy dosha mix is his or her *prakriti* or body constitution. There are seven constitution types:

1. Vata
2. Pitta
3. Kapha
4. Vata-Pitta
5. Pitta-Kapha
6. Vata-Kapha
7. Sama

In the rare Sama constitutional type, the three doshas are found in equal proportion. The doshas are in dynamic relationship to each other. When they are in proper balance, the result is health. When they are imbalanced, there is dysfunction and disease. The main goal of Ayurvedic medicine and health practices is to maintain and restore balance according to an individual's unique constitutional makeup. Major characteristics of the three major constitutional types or prakriti are listed in Table 25–4 ■.

SUBTLE ENERGY—KOSHA 2

The next kosha is the *pranamaya,* which regulates the flow of subtle energy in the body. It is in the pranamaya kosha that the *prana* or subtle energy (also known as the *ten vayus*) flows through nonphysical channels called *nadis.* Nadis lead to important energy centers called *chakras.*

TABLE 25–4	The Three Major Doshas— Basic Constitutional Types
Dosha	**Characteristics**
Vata	Thin frame, very tall or short, odd proportions, narrow hips and shoulders, dry skin and hair, cold hands and feet, high metabolism, quick, endurance poor, aversion to cold weather, tendency for irregular bowels, painful joints, acute allergies, and worry.
Pitta	Medium frame, medium height, proportionate, medium hips and shoulders, oily skin and hair, competitive, hot, fiery, endurance medium, aversion to hot weather, tendency for heartburn, skin rashes, inflammatory diseases, irritability.
Kapha	Large frame, solid build, broad hips and shoulders, easy going, low metabolism, endurance strong, hold weight and water, methodical, tendency for allergies and congestion, and resists change.

There are seven chakras or concentrations of nadis at different levels of the spine and in the head. Chakra means wheel and refers to the whirling centers of energy at each level. These centers receive, process, and distribute energy to balance the body, mind, and spirit. The chakras are arranged from gross (bottom, lower functions, physical) to subtle (top, higher functions, mind and awareness). See Figure 25–63 ■.

The First Chakra Called the Root Chakra or *Muladhara,* it is located at the base of the spine in the perineum. It is governed by the earth element, and its qualities are groundedness, patience, stability, and security. Essential oils associated with it are cinnamon, garlic, and sandalwood, and its herb is mugwort.

The Second Chakra Called the Sacral Chakra or *Svadhisthana,* it is located just below the naval and toward the center of the body. It is governed by the water element, and its qualities are well-being, sexuality, sensuality, pleasure, and abundance. It is the seat of the emotions. Associated essential oils are jasmine and orange blossom, and its herb is cedar.

The Third Chakra Called the Solar Plexus Chakra or *Manipura,* it is directly below the sternum at the solar plexus. It is governed by the fire element, and its qualities are self-worth, self-esteem, and confidence. Associated essential oils are lemon, grapefruit, and juniper, and its herb is rosemary.

7 the Crown Chakra

6 the Third Eye Chakra

5 the Throat Chakra

4 the Heart Chakra

3 the Solar Plexus Chakra

2 the Sacral Plexus Chakra

1 the Root Chakra

FIGURE 25–63 The seven chakras or energy centers in Ayurvedic philosophy.

Source: Courtesy of Rev. Larissa Dahroug, Reiki/MT, Clear & Balanced Energy Work.

The Fourth Chakra Called the Heart Chakra or *Anahata,* it is located in mid-chest. It is governed by the air element, and its qualities are love, peace, unity, purity, and innocence. Associated essential oils are rose, carnation, and lily of the valley, and its herb is lavender.

The Fifth Chakra Called the Throat Chakra or *Vishuddha,* it is located at the throat. It is governed by the ether element, and its qualities are communications, creativity, truthfulness, and integrity. Associated essential oils are chamomile and gardenia, and its herb is wintergreen.

The Sixth Chakra Called the Third Eye or *Ajna,* it is located mid-forehead. It is governed by awareness, and its qualities are intuition, discernment, wisdom, imagination, and knowledge. Associated essential oils are camphor and sweet pea, and its herb is sage.

The Seventh Chakra Called the Crown Chakra or *Sahasrar,* it is located on the top of the head. Its qualities are enlightenment, grace, beauty, serenity, and being one with the universe. Associated essential oils are violet, lavender, and lotus, and its herbs are frankincense and myrrh.

A major goal of the various Ayurvedic health practices is to move the creative spiritual life force or shakti from the Root Chakra to the Crown Chakra or twelve petal lotus. This completes the harmony of body, mind, and spirit.

INNERMOST KOSHAS 3–5

Beyond the physical body and the first subtle energy sheath are the mental (*manomaya*), intellect and discernment (*nanamaya*), and the causal (*anandamaya*) sheaths. At the center of the five sheaths is pure consciousness.

Marma Points

Marma points are Ayurvedic pressure points. They are considered part of the subtle body, and occur at the junction of the five organic principles of vessels, muscles, ligaments, bones, and joints. The 107 marma points are considered to be junctions between consciousness and matter. They are the locus of *prana* or the vital life force. See Figure 25–64 ■ for major marma point locations.

Marma points are addressed in different ways in different approaches to Ayurvedic massage. During a massage session, stimulation of marma points can be used to release tension in a congested area. For example, gentle circular stroking of a marma point with the index or middle finger is employed to release toxins from the area.

Systematic treatment of marma points is called *marma chikitsa.* Marma point therapy is considered a specialization requiring advanced training.

AYURVEDIC MASSAGE

The goal of Ayurvedic massage is to balance the physical and energetic processes that lead to a healthy vibrant life. It begins with attention to physical well-being, which in turn affects subtle energy and ultimately spiritual consciousness.

REALITY CHECK

GABRIEL: I have a hard time relating to theories of energy flow in Eastern bodywork. I don't feel energy when I touch people during massage sessions. How do I know anything worthwhile is happening when I practice Eastern bodywork?

KELLY: Those of us from Western cultures aren't as sensitive to the presence of energy as practitioners from Asian cultures. We don't have a concept of Qi, Prana, or life force that compares. Western thinking focuses more on the material aspects. When considering Eastern bodywork, I try to keep an open mind to what others have found over centuries of studying these practices. As far as feeling energy, I have tried to be more aware of energy in my hands as I work. I'm slowly developing a consciousness of its existence. But even if I don't feel energy flowing, I can see physical changes happening like clients relaxing, and muscles letting go of tension. So I can see the effects of these techniques on that level, and if I get the health benefits I'm going for, I don't feel a need to believe all of the theory to value the approach. On the other hand, it is interesting to hear about another culture's perspective. We all experience life so differently.

The effects of massage in the physical body are familiar to Western massage therapists. These effects include good blood and lymph circulation, muscle relaxation, connective tissue pliability, overall tissue health, and general relaxation. When there is balance in the physical body, effects can occur at deeper levels.

Once balance in the physical body is restored, channels of circulation called *srotas* help to balance the three *doshas*—Vata, Pitta, and Kapha. At this point Ayurvedic massage begins to move the ten *vayus* or *pranas* that carry life force to both the physical and energetic bodies. Once the vayu function is optimal, the *nadi* system is activated. There are 72,000 nadis in the body that carry subtle energy. Specifically they carry consciousness to the *chakra* system and into the brain centers, where body, mind, and spirit are purified. The goal of this process is full human potential, whereby consciousness is lively in each and every cell.

FIGURE 25–64
Major marma point locations.

The subtle-body system and the physical body begin to function as one, resulting in perfect physical, mental, and spiritual health.[1]

Varieties of Ayurvedic Massage

Just as there are variations and specializations within massage in Western cultures, several varieties of Ayurvedic massage applications can be identified. These include *Garshana* or dry lymphatic skin brushing, *Abhyanga* or classic herbal oil massage, and *Vishesh* or deep muscular massage. *Udvartana* is an herbal paste and exfoliating lymphatic massage, whereas the Ayruvedic facial focuses on nourishing the skin and overall energetic balance. Ayurvedic massage is given as part of *panchakarma* or detoxification therapy supervised by an Ayurvedic physician. Two popular adjunct modalities are *Swedana* or herbal steam bath and *Shirodhara* or pouring herbal oil over the forehead.

Several modern spa offerings incorporate knowledge of Ayurvedic practices. These include aromatherapy, stone massage, medicated steam therapy, and various types of herbal showers and baths. Classic Ayurvedic massage is given with oils individualized to a client's prakriti or constitutional type.

CRITICAL THINKING

Think about the theoretical foundations for different forms of Eastern bodywork, especially concepts related to energy, energy channels, and special points. Analyze how these theories are applied in traditional bodywork of different parts of Asia: China, India, and Thailand.

1. How do each of these theories explain the intent of bodywork sessions?
2. What manual techniques were developed to address health goals?
3. How would you describe what is common in these systems? What is unique in each system?

Massage Oils

The composition of massage oils in classic Ayurvedic massage is very important. Massage oils are carefully chosen and mixed according to the recipient's constitutional type, the season of the year, and any therapeutic goals. Base oils typically used for Ayruvedic massage are sesame, coconut, almond, olive, mustard, or corn. Some modern blends use a jojoba base.

Essential oils are mixed into the base oil to achieve specific therapeutic goals, for example, relaxation, warming, moisturizing the skin, or relieving congestion. Essential oils are highly concentrated liquids distilled from plant materials such as grasses, leaves, flowers, needles, fruit peels, and roots. They contain volatile aromatic compounds, that is, the distinct scent and essence of the plant. Essential oils are potent. They are used sparingly and are measured by numbers of drops. They should never be applied to the skin in undiluted form. Be aware of the properties of each essential oil to be put into a mixture.

Some common Ayurvedic oil blends can be purchased premade. For example, a blend especially for relaxation might consist of a base oil enhanced with lavender, rosewood, champa, and tangerine essential oils. A blend for energizing massage might consist of a base oil augmented with mint, lavender, orange, bergamot, and lime essential oils. Ideally massage oil mixtures are heated and applied warm. This ensures deeper penetration and feels soothing.

Essential oils are the focus of the science and art of aromatherapy. Consult aromatherapy or Ayurvedic references for further information about specific essential oils and their uses. Study essential oils to determine their safe use in different circumstances, and be especially careful during pregnancy. See Chapter 19, *Spa Treatments*, for more information about essential oils.

Massage Applications

Ayurvedic techniques for oil massage include sliding or rubbing, kneading, squeezing, and tapping. Rubbing with oil is performed with a flat palm molding to the contour of the body. Fingertips can be used to apply circles in small areas and around joints. Kneading relaxes muscles and resembles kneading bread dough. Squeezing or wringing is performed

FIGURE 25–66 Ayurvedic massage. Sliding circles at the seat of Vata, recipient in side-lying position.

Source: Pearson Education, Inc./Segal Photography.

on the limbs moving proximal to distal. Tapping is applied with cupped hands and is used to activate the nervous system. Fingers and thumbs can be used to stimulate specific points and in small areas.

Ayurvedic massage techniques themselves are familiar to Western massage therapists, but the intent of the application would be quite different. See Figures 25–65 ■, 25–66 ■, and 25–67 ■.

The pressure applied during massage varies according to a recipient's constitutional type. Vata types tend to prefer lighter pressure, Pitta types medium pressure, and Kapha types heavier pressure.

Different traditions of Ayurvedic massage apply techniques in different parts of the body in their own unique way. One approach to full-body Ayurvedic massage moves from region to region in a systematic sequence. Starting on the back of the body, the lower limbs are massaged from

FIGURE 25–65 Ayurvedic massage. Long sweeping stroke from foot around shoulder and down the arm, recipient prone.

Source: Pearson Education, Inc./Segal Photography.

FIGURE 25–67 Ayurvedic massage. Pressing the ansa marma on the front and back of the shoulders with recipient supine.

Source: Pearson Education, Inc./Segal Photography.

CASE FOR STUDY

Paul Applies Eastern Bodywork to Enhance a Massage Session

Paul has a client named Jeff who is experiencing tension in his legs and feet. The Swedish massage Paul is using has some relaxing effects, but he feels he can get better results by integrating some Eastern bodywork techniques in the sessions. As a martial artist, Jeff is open to the idea and gives Paul permission to use Eastern bodywork techniques for a few sessions to see the results.

Question:

How might Paul approach integrating Eastern bodywork for the desired effects?

Things to consider:

- What energy channels run through the hips, legs, and feet?
- Where are special points located there?
- What Eastern bodywork techniques can be adapted for an integrated bodywork session?
- Of what importance is intention to the application?

Plan a massage therapy session incorporating Eastern bodywork theory and techniques for addressing Jeff's therapeutic goals. Describe a possible approach, being specific about concepts and techniques.

_____

_____

_____

pelvis to toes, then the spine from sacrum to neck, and then the upper limbs from shoulder to fingers. On the front of the body, massage is applied from pelvis to toes, navel to chest, and then collarbone to fingertips.

Some Ayurvedic massage sessions routinely include massage in the side-lying position. The client might start prone, turn to one side, turn to the other side, and end supine. Ayurvedic head and face massage has its own special application.

In another approach called *marma point massage,* strokes are applied in sequence, with special attention to important marma points. If congestion is felt at a marma point, additional techniques are applied to move energy at that point.

Seasonal massage sessions focus on special needs during each of the four seasons. An example is a Vata balancing massage given in winter. Essential oils would be chosen to balance the dry sluggishness of winter months. For a Pitta constitutional type, these might include bergamot, cypress, geranium, lemongrass, and mogra or Indian jasmine. For other constitutional types the mix might be different.

Ayurvedic massage sessions are typically preceded by a brief interview to determine constitutional type, contraindications including skin allergies, and a recipient's specific goals for the massage. Client preferences are also taken into consideration.

HATHA YOGA

Yoga literally means "joining," and refers to various practices that aim to reunite an individual to pure consciousness. Yoga in its totality is essentially a spiritual practice; however, one aspect called **hatha yoga** has gained popularity in the West as a health and fitness exercise. Hatha yoga is an

excellent complement to Ayurvedic massage and a beneficial self-care practice for massage therapists.

Five important aspects of hatha yoga are relaxation, physical exercises or postures called *asanas,* proper breathing, proper diet, and positive thinking and meditation. The postures are exercises in mind–body coordination and also build strength and flexibility while calming the mind.

A basic relaxation posture is *Savasana* or the corpse pose. Lie on your back on a mat with your feet apart and arms comfortably away from the body, palms upward. Close your eyes and take several deep abdominal breaths (Figure 25–68 ■). Let your mind grow calm and clear.

The Sun Salutation or *Surya Namaskar* is a good beginning series of postures that can be used later as a warm-up to more difficult postures. It is traditionally performed at dawn, but can be used at any time for limbering and waking up. It begins in a standing position, followed by continuous movement from one posture to the next (Figure 25–69 ■).

Hatha yoga postures are performed on floor mats from standing, sitting, and lying positions. Traditional postures have varying degrees of difficulty and can be modified for all abilities and ages.

THAI MASSAGE

Traditional bodywork from Thailand is called *nuad boran,* known in the West as **Thai massage**. It has been practiced in Thailand for centuries, passed down through different lineages. It is thought to have come to Thailand originally from India along with Buddhism. Thai massage has become a popular form of bodywork in the West in recent years. The intent is to stimulate the body's self-healing processes and to correct energy imbalances.

FIGURE 25–68

Hatha yoga corpse pose—savasana.

Source: Pearson Education, Inc./Segal Photography.

Thai massage is based on Ayurvedic medicine. It incorporates knowledge of energy meridians or *sen* lines, pressure points, and hatha yoga postures. It is performed on the floor on a mat. Both giver and receiver are clothed, and no oil is applied. It can be thought of as a combination of pressure techniques, joint mobilizations, and assisted yoga-like stretching.

Sen lines are similar to nadis in the Ayurvedic tradition. They also have similar names, for example, *Sen Pingala* is the same as the *Pingala Nadi*. Sen lines are pathways that carry subtle energy. Many pressure points along sen lines are identical with marma points. The exact location of sen lines varies among different lineages of Thai massage. See Figure 25–70 ■ for an example of a sen line diagram. These diagrams are found on many Buddhist temple walls, such as the famous Wat Po Temple in Bangkok, where the tradition of Thai massage is preserved.

Thai massage sessions typically begin at the feet and move toward the head. The practitioner uses the palms, fingers, thumbs, forearm, and elbow to apply pressure along sen lines and to pressure points. Joint mobilizations and assisted yoga-like stretches are interspersed. The session is systematic and flowing from one region to the next. Figures 25–71 ■ to 25–73 ■ are examples of Thai massage techniques.

POLARITY THERAPY

Polarity therapy is a holistic health practice that includes gentle energy-based bodywork. Polarity techniques involve simple touching and gentle movements designed to release obstructions to the free flow of energy in the body. In polarity therapy sessions, the practitioner might rest his or her hands in various places, gently rock the body, or press into points rhythmically to free energy flow.

Polarity therapy was developed in the early 1900s by Randolph Stone (1890–1981), an eclectic natural healer trained in the fields of chiropractic, naturopathy, and osteopathy when they were relatively new. Stone also studied Chinese acupuncture and herbal remedies and Ayurvedic medicine of India. He spent many years in India learning Ayurvedic healing practices, and his writings include concepts from Ayurveda such as the energy centers called chakras, five elements, and balancing these forces with exercise. From his studies, Stone came to believe that there is a subtle form of life energy that permeates the body and gives it health, and that disease is a result of obstruction to that energy flow. He developed a system for improving energy flow that includes exercise, nutrition, self-awareness, love, and gentle bodywork. After Stone's retirement in 1973, Pierre Pannetier carried on his work. Several different schools of polarity therapy have sprung up over the years. The American Polarity Therapy Association (APTA) was founded in 1985 to set professional standards for polarity therapy practitioners (www.polaritytherapy.org).

Polarity Therapy Theory

The effects of polarity therapy can be explained both in esoteric terms related to Ayurveda and energy, and in physiological terms of Western science. Both ways of looking at polarity therapy are valid within their own theoretical frameworks. It is useful to consider these very different approaches in establishing a basis for polarity techniques presented later in the chapter.

Energy is a central concept in polarity therapy; therefore it is explored first. Health is often equated with being full of energy, whereas illness is associated with its absence. When practitioners apply polarity techniques, they often report feeling a tingling in their hands that they equate with the movement of energy. The degree and pattern of this tingling vary with the state of health of the area being touched and with changes taking place. The giver and receiver often note simultaneous changes in their sense of energy. The receiver may report feeling freer, lighter, or more relaxed. The practitioner notes a balancing or strengthening of the tingling, and a sense of shift or increase in energy felt. Polarity therapists view these changes as a response to unblocking the life energy.

FIGURE 25–69
Hatha yoga Sun Salutation.

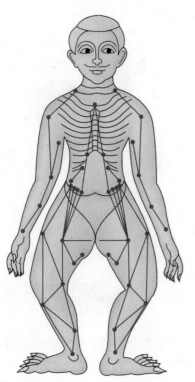

FIGURE 25–70 Sen lines in traditional Thai massage.

FIGURE 25–72 Wide angle pose (upavistha konasana in hatha yoga), assisted by practitioner on the left during Thai massage session.

Source: Pearson Education, Inc./Segal Photography.

FIGURE 25–71 Press along sen lines and marma points on inner forearm.

Source: Pearson Education, Inc./Segal Photography.

FIGURE 25–73 Reclining hand to foot pose variation (sputa padangushtasana in hatha yoga), and elbow press to marma points on the foot bottom during Thai massage session.

Source: Pearson Education, Inc./Segal Photography.

Western science would note objective changes taking place in the recipient. These include signs of deep relaxation: flushed cheeks, drop in blood pressure, increased salivation, slower heart rate, teary eyes, and rumbling stomach. These are objective signs of the relaxation response of the parasympathetic nervous system.

Some of these physiological changes can be explained with a closer examination of polarity therapy techniques. For example, in one technique a very light oscillating pressure is applied over the pressure-sensitive baroreceptors in the carotid arteries on the sides of the neck. It is probable that this is sufficient to activate the neurological reflex that slows heart rate and lowers blood pressure.

Polarity techniques that involve rocking motions of the limbs and torso stimulate mechanoreceptors in joints. It appears that when these receptors are stimulated, a reflex response is activated that lowers muscle tone, increases circulation, and results in endorphin release.

The rhythmic quality of other polarity techniques can induce a light hypnotic state. This brings calming and peace of mind. Sometimes this state of quiet awareness allows people to see their problems from a broader perspective or allows hidden feelings to surface. Polarity therapy can be a valuable adjunct to psychotherapy.

Many polarity techniques are as easily set within the framework of modern science as they are within Ayurvedic and energy theories. It is as if the basic principle that Stone sought transcends all ideas, ancient or modern, and is instead embodied in the actual experience of the hands-on work, rather than in the particular theories used to explain it. Energy is simply an abstract metaphor, one way of looking at the results obtained through polarity therapy. Neurological reflex is another abstract metaphor, a way of explaining a mechanism we cannot see, except in its effects.

Principles of Polarity Therapy

Polarity therapy is based on concepts of energy, love, removing obstructions, and understanding. These concepts guide the application of the gentle polarity techniques.

Energy Polarity therapy practitioners develop an awareness of feeling energy in their hands. These sensations can be picked up and amplified with practice. For example, rub your hands together to wake up the nerve endings, and bring your awareness to your palms. Then hold your palms about six inches apart, and focus your awareness on how they feel. Experiment with moving your palms closer and farther apart. Note changes in the feeling and a sense of the palms plugging into each other energetically.

Love Another important polarity therapy concept is *love*. Love in this sense is not a sentimental attachment or affection. It can be thought of as caring for someone else with no agenda or objective in mind, not even that of healing or helping. It is an attitude of surrender or openness. It is getting out of the way and letting the body's tendency to wholeness and healing take place.

FIGURE 25–74 Feeling the palms "plugging into each other."

Source: Pearson Education, Inc./Segal Photography.

One way to explore this quality of love is a simple front-to-back polarity technique. Have the recipient sit up straight but relaxed. Stand on the person's left side, and place your left hand over his or her heart and the right hand on the upper back between the shoulder blades (Figure 25–74 ■). Move your hands around slowly until you feel a sense of the palms "plugging in" to each other, as if they are connected by a flow of energy. Simply hold your hands in place and feel the connection. Note any reaction in the recipient. After a few minutes, slowly withdraw your hands.

Removing Obstructions Another principle of polarity is **removing obstructions** to the free flow of energy. An energy obstruction can be seen in the body where there is holding, tension, or misalignment. An alert polarity practitioner begins assessing clients visually as soon as they arrive. Obstructions can be further detected through palpation.

To develop skill in locating energy obstructions, practice the *tummy rock* technique. Have the recipient lie supine with the hands at his or her sides. Stand at the right side and place your right hand lightly on his or her abdomen below the navel (Figure 25–75 ■). Become aware of his or her breathing pattern, skin temperature, and muscular tension. Make certain that your own hand and arm muscles are completely relaxed, and that your breathing is calm. Increase the pressure slightly, and introduce a wavelike movement by pressing first with the heel and then the fingers of your hand, repeating the motion gently. Place your hand on the person's forehead, and feel for a sensation of plugging in. Gently rock the abdomen while keeping the hand on the forehead still. Note any tingling in your own hands, and watch for subtle changes in the recipient such as deeper breathing or muscle relaxation. These are signs of removing obstructions.

FIGURE 25–75 Tummy rock to release energy blocks in the torso and head.

Source: Pearson Education, Inc./Segal Photography.

Understanding The fourth principle is understanding, a concept that invites the practitioner to be open to the recipient's experience and to the effects of polarity therapy. Each recipient will react to polarity therapy differently, and understanding calls for knowledge of the broader picture of what might be happening physiologically and psychologically in a session.

Polarity is a gentle art. Nothing is ever forced. The recipient is experiencing the effects of past actions and present decisions. The giver is not there to rescue the receiver, but to plant seeds of letting go and trusting, and to be an accepting observer. This attitude protects the practitioner from taking on the recipient's ailments in a misguided attempt to heal. A commonsense approach emphasizes a caring attitude, acceptance, and trust that whatever happens is from a clearing of obstructions and is for the best.

BASIC POLARITY MOVEMENTS

Polarity students are typically taught a general session of a series of movements that serve to stimulate and balance the entire body. The gentle holding, rocking, and probing techniques form a generally relaxing session and also aid the practitioner in locating areas that appear to be obstructed and in need of further attention.

Some of these techniques are derived from osteopathy, craniopathy, and chiropractic of the 1930s and 1940s. Some were derived by Stone from observations made by psychics, from his study of acupuncture, and from Egyptian medicine. Some were derived from theories of harmonic resonance, that is, that certain parts of the body vibrate harmonically when other areas are worked. All in all, the techniques form a fascinating and rich array of moves that must be experienced in order to be appreciated. Practice Sequence 25–4 ■ illustrates and explains some basic polarity therapy techniques.

PRACTICE SEQUENCE 25–4

General Session of Polarity Therapy

30 minutes (abbreviated version)
Recipient supine

Preliminary Instructions
• To begin, sit on a chair at the head of the table.

Figure 25–76 Hand position for the cradle. Overlap the last three fingers of your left hand on the last three fingers of your right hand, palms up, to form a cradle.

1

2

Figure 25–77 The cradle. Rest your hands on the table, supporting the recipient's head in your palms. Your index fingers extend along the grooves beside the sternocleidomastoid muscle. Rest your thumbs on your index fingers rather than over the receiver's ears. Hold 1–2 minutes, or until a current is strongly felt.

3

Figure 25–78 Neck stretch. Rest the receiver's head on the palm of your right hand, taking a firm hold on the base of the skull. Your left hand rests lightly on the forehead. With firm, steady pressure from the right hand only, apply gentle traction toward you. As the recipient exhales, release slightly; as he or she inhales, increase the traction slightly. *Note:* This move is contraindicated if there is any neck pain during the movement.

4

Figure 25–79 Tummy rock. Standing on the recipient's right side, rest your left hand on the forehead and your right hand on the abdomen halfway between the navel and the pubic bone. Rock the abdomen gently, trying to tune in to the person's natural "rocking rhythm."

5

Figure 25–80 Leg pull. Grasp both feet behind the heels, and gently pull legs straight toward you several inches above the table. Rest the legs back on the table gently, and place your hands over the feet for a few moments before proceeding.

Steps 6–7 are performed first on right foot then on left foot before proceeding to Step 8.

6

Figure 25–81 Inside ankle press. Place the heel of your left hand on the ball of the recipient's right foot, with your fingers lightly grasping the toes. With the heel resting in your right hand, gently press spots around the inner ankle bone (medial malleolus) with your thumb. Keeping your left hand in place, press on the ball of the foot to flex the ankle forward (dorsiflexion). Alternate between pressing an ankle point and flexing the ankle in rhythmic motion. Continue pressing around the ankle bone until the points are pain free.

7

Figure 25–82 Outside ankle press. Now, support the heel of the recipient's right foot with your left hand. With your left thumb, find any tender areas along the area under the outside ankle bone (lateral malleolus). With your right hand, press the top of the foot downward (plantarflexion), giving a good stretch. Rhythmically alternate pressing and stretching the foot.

Reminder: Repeat Steps 6 and 7 on both sides before moving on.

Steps 8–12 are performed in sequence on the right side and are then repeated on the left side before proceeding to Step 13.

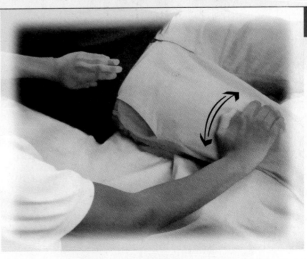

8

Figure 25–83 Pelvis and knee rock. Hold the feet again for a moment, and move to the person's right side. Place your left hand on the lower right abdomen, just above the thigh crease, with the fingers pointing down toward the feet. Place your right hand just above the knee. Very gently apply pressure with the right hand in a rhythmic fashion, rocking the leg for 10–30 seconds. Allow the leg to slow and then to be still. Continue holding for 30 seconds or so, again being aware of any sensations you feel. Slowly remove your hands.

9

Figure 25–84 Arm–shoulder rotations. Holding the receiver's right wrist and controlling movement from the wrist, gently rotate the shoulder in a small circle. The shoulder blade elevates and depresses slightly with the movement. Repeat 10 times.

10

Figure 25–85 Thumb web–forearm stimulation. Using the thumb and finger of your left hand, squeeze the webbing between the recipient's thumb and finger, concentrating on any tender areas. Press the pad of your right thumb into a point 1 inch below the elbow crease and a half-inch from the inside of the arm. Stimulate the two points alternately in a rhythmic movement about 10 times.

11

Figure 25–86 Elbow milk–abdomen rock. Place your left hand under the recipient's right elbow and lay your thumb across the elbow crease. Milk upward with your thumb. Place your right hand lightly along the bottom edge of the rib cage and gently rock the abdomen. Alternate milking and rocking, about 10–12 times each for about a minute.

12

Figure 25–87 Pelvic rock. Place your right hand over the recipient's left hip bone. Place your left hand over the right shoulder. Stabilizing the shoulder girdle with your left hand, gently rock the trunk with the right. Gradually increase the rocking movement for 20 seconds and then gradually decrease. Hold for a moment before moving on.

Reminder: Perform Steps 8–12 on both sides before moving on.

13

Figure 25–88 Occipital press. Sitting at the recipient's head, turn the head slightly to the left. Using the second finger of your right hand, perform circular friction to the suboccipital muscles to the right of the midline. Your left hand should be supporting the person's head by resting lightly on the left side of the forehead. Your index finger should rest gently on the spot known in India as the "third eye," the area between and just above the eyes. The hand on the back of the head should feel as though it were plugged into the palm of the hand on the forehead. Hold and feel for a sensation of tingling. When a steady, gentle pulsation is felt in the hands, or a minute or so has passed, turn the head to the other side and repeat, switching hands.

14

Figure 25–89 Cranial polarization. Lightly place both thumbs on the anterior fontanel, with both index fingers touching on the "third eye" and the remaining fingers across the forehead. It is important that you relax your hands, arms, and shoulders as much as possible, and that your breathing is relaxed and your posture comfortable. Hold for about 1 minute, or until a steady gentle pulsation is felt.

15

Figure 25–90 Navel–third eye. Move to the recipient's right side. Lightly place your left thumb pad between the eyebrows and your right thumb in the navel, with the thumbs pointing toward each other. Hold 1 minute, and then lift the hands very slowly, initiating movement from the thumbs, rather than the shoulders.

16

A   **B**

Figure 25–91 Brushing off to finish—back. In a quiet voice ask the person to sit up with legs off the side of the table. (A) Standing behind the recipient, place your hands on the shoulders. (B) With a sweeping motion, brush your hands across the spine, then down to the sacrum, and out to the crest of the hips. Repeat several times.

17

Figure 25–92 Brushing off to finish—front. Move to the front and place the person's hands on his or her knees. (A) Place your hands on the shoulders. (B) With a sweeping motion, brush down the arms to the knees and down the legs. Repeat several times.

After you perform the Practice Sequence, evaluate how well you did by filling out Performance Evaluation Form 25–4, General Session of Polarity Therapy. The form can be found in Appendix D: *Performance Evaluation Forms,* and at MyHealthProfessionsLab.com.

Figures source: Pearson Education, Inc./Segal Photography.

CASE FOR STUDY

Carmina Explains Polarity Therapy to a Client

Carmina integrates some polarity techniques into her regular massage sessions. A new client, who is not familiar with energy bodywork, asks Carmina to explain what she is doing. Carmina had performed the cradle, tummy rock, and elbow milk/abdominal rock during the massage session. These techniques seemed strange to the client, and she seems a little concerned about why the techniques were included in a massage.

Question:

How can Carmina explain these polarity techniques so that the client understands and appreciates their benefits?

Things to consider:

● What was different about these techniques from what the client had experienced in massage?
● How would you explain energy flow and relate that concept to the techniques?
● What might be the result of trying to say too much? How much does the client really need to know to benefit from the techniques?

Write your response to the client:

_____

_____

_____

Notes on the Practice Sequence

If you decide to explore these techniques, remember the primary principle of openness. If you get confused, let yourself laugh. If you find the rhythm difficult, remember to let your breathing relax and let your shoulders down. If you are relaxed and accept yourself, the receiver will benefit, regardless of your skill level. Do the best you can in a simple way, and be kind to yourself. Although you are not "the healer," you may find yourself being healed while giving polarity. You may find that in the circle of love and self-acceptance, your own obstructions begin to disappear, and you are no longer sure who is "giving" polarity to whom.

You may integrate any of these movements into a Swedish full-body massage. You may find some techniques useful for beginning or ending a session, or before the receiver turns over from prone to supine. During a full-body session, you may sense energy blockages and use one or more of these basic techniques to try to allow energy to flow freely

again. Once you are familiar with the techniques, you can insert them where it seems like the right thing to do.

SOME FINAL THOUGHTS ON POLARITY THERAPY

The unique gift of polarity therapy is its simplicity. Behind the techniques and esoterica is an opening and surrendering to life and to being at home with our natural energies. The ideal supplement to this brief introduction would be to receive a session from a professional polarity therapist, as it is very difficult to convey the experience of polarity in writing. Polarity therapy is truly an art form, requiring much study and dedicated practice to master the rhythm and quality of touch that are so important to the effects. In addition, the hands-on work is only a small part of the therapy, which usually includes basic nutritional guidance, exercise, and support for emotional balancing.

PRACTICAL APPLICATION

Integrate at least four polarity therapy techniques into a Swedish massage session. Experiment with how they might be used for different effects.

1. Which techniques might be effective opening or closing moves for a massage?

2. Which techniques might be especially useful in a relaxation massage?

3. How can polarity techniques be integrated smoothly into the sequence of the session?

CRITICAL THINKING

Think about the concept of *flow* and its relationship to good health. Identify the different ways that the general idea of *flow* appears in discussing the effects of massage and bodywork. Analyze how each technique in the abbreviated polarity therapy form enhances *flow* in some way.

1. What types of substances and nonmaterial forces *flow* in the living human body?

2. What mechanisms of massage techniques discussed in Chapter 3, *Effects and Benefits of Massage*, are at work in polarity therapy?

3. What is it about each polarity technique that facilitates removal of obstructions to *flow*? Is it hand position, hand placement, the quality of touch, the practitioner's intention, or some combination?

CHAPTER HIGHLIGHTS

- Energy-based bodywork refers to forms of manual therapy in which the chief intention is to enhance the free flow of energy in and around the physical body.

Eastern Bodywork

- Eastern bodywork refers to traditional forms of manual therapy from the continent of Asia.
- Three popular forms of Eastern bodywork are Asian bodywork therapies from China and Japan, Ayurvedic massage from India, and Thai bodywork from Thailand.
  - Their applications and theory are very different from Swedish massage.
  - They predate modern science and are embedded in whole systems of medicine.
- Similarities in Eastern bodywork forms: holistic view, human beings as part of nature, notion of energy or life force.
- These Eastern manual therapies are used to balance energy and remove obstructions to its free flow.

Traditional Chinese Medicine

- Traditional Chinese medicine (TCM) originated in China as folk medicine and later evolved into a formalized system of medicine.
  - Earliest known text on TCM is the *Yellow Emperor's Classic of Internal Medicine* written about 500 BCE.
- The Yin/Yang symbol has been described as two comets chasing each other.
  - Yin is a dark, deep, dense aspect of the universe; feminine, interior, still, substantial, cool, and contracting in contrast to Yang; the front, interior, medial/interior aspects of the limbs; solid organs that store pure essences extracted from food by the Yang organs.
  - Yang is a light, energetic, and spacious or heavenly aspect of the universe; masculine, exterior, moving, insubstantial, warm and expanding in contrast to Yin; the back, head, exterior, and lateral/posterior aspects of the limbs; hollow organs that transform, digest, and excrete impure products of food and fluids.
  - Five principles of Yin/Yang: interdependence, supporting, opposition, intertransformation, infinitely divisible.
- Qi refers to the life energy of the universe.
  - Chinese character for Qi depicts rice cooking in a pot with steam escaping.
  - TCM harmonizes and balances Qi and enhances its flow throughout the body.
  - TCM tonifies, disperses, moves, uplifts, and rectifies Qi.
- The Five Elements or *Five Elemental Energies* are Wood, Fire, Earth, Metal, and Water.
  - Wood is Yang, expanding, spring, sunrise, green, wind, and sour taste.
  - Fire is most Yang, fusing, heat, light, summer, laughter, sweat, bitter taste.
  - Earth is Yin, late summer, transformative, rooted, sweet, fragrant.
  - Metal is Yin, autumn, letting go, grief, pungent, dry.
  - Water is most Yin, winter, yielding, conserving, fear, wisdom, salty.
- Sheng and Ko cycles describe relationships among the Five Elements.
  - Sheng is the creation, generating, or promoting cycle.
  - Ko cycle is the controlling or acting cycle.
- Qi travels through the body in a network of energy channels or meridians.
  - There are 12 primary energy channels.

- ○ Each channel flows in a certain direction and connects and communicates with other channels.
- ○ The channels flow through the body according to a natural, daily rhythmic cycle called the Chinese body clock.

- Acupoints are places on energy channels where Qi collects and where it can be accessed and influenced.
  - ○ There are 365 classic acupoints.
  - ○ Acupoints are useful in the diagnosis and treatment of energy imbalances.

- In Japanese shiatsu, the concepts of Kyo and Jitsu indicate acupoints with imbalance of Ki (same as Qi).
  - ○ Kyo means energy deficiency; kyo acupoints feel hollow and soft; kyo acupoints are pressed for 7–10 seconds to tonify them.
  - ○ Jitsu means energy excess; jitsu acupoints feel hard and sensitive; jitsu acupoints are pressed for 3–5 seconds, released, and that press-release repeated about 10 times.

- The traditional pillars assessment in TCM are looking, touching, smelling, listening, and asking.
- Massage can be integrated with the theory and techniques of acupressure to address both the physical and energetic wellness of their clients.
- Acupressure massage integration applies massage techniques region by region along major energy pathways, feeling for signs of deficiency (kyo) or excess (jitsu), and pressing important acupoints; energy balance is restored in areas of kyo and jitsu.
- Qi gong consists of choreographed movements that involve bending, stretching, reaching, stepping, and other movements designed to harmonize the flow of Qi.

Ayurveda

- Ayurveda means knowledge of life and is the traditional health and healing practices of India.
- In Ayurvedic theory, human beings are seen as having a material body, as well as subtle energy bodies that surround and move through the physical aspect.
- The physical body has 16 channels or *srotas* for the circulation of substances such as air, food, lymph, blood, urine, feces, sweat, and cellular level nutrients, and the three principles or *doshas* called Vata, Pitta, and Kapha.
- A person's innate natural healthy dosha mix is his or her body constitution or *prakriti.*
  - ○ Seven constitution types: Vata, Pitta, Kapha, Vata-Pitta, Pitta-Kapha, Vata-Kapha, and Sama.
- Energy centers called *chakras* receive, process, and distribute energy to balance body, mind, and spirit.

- ○ Chakras from bottom to top (gross to subtle) are Root, Sacral, Solar Plexus, Heart, Throat, Third Eye, and Crown Chakras.

- A major goal of the various Ayurvedic health practices is to move the creative spiritual life force or *shakti* from the Root Chakra to the Crown Chakra or twelve petal lotus.
- Marma points are Ayurvedic pressure points; the junctions between consciousness and matter.
- In classic Ayurvedic massage, oils are carefully chosen and mixed according to the recipient's constitutional type, the season of the year, and any therapeutic goals.
  - ○ Ayurvedic techniques for oil massage include sliding or rubbing, kneading, squeezing, and tapping.
- Hatha yoga is an Ayurvedic health practice consisting of relaxation, physical exercises or postures called *asanas,* proper breathing, proper diet, and positive thinking and meditation.

Thai Massage
- Thai massage is a combination of pressure techniques, joint mobilizations, and assisted yoga-like stretching; both giver and receiver are clothed.

Polarity Therapy
- Polarity therapy is a holistic bodywork approach that involves simple touching and gentle movements such as rocking and pressing.
- Polarity techniques are designed to release obstructions in the free flow of energy through the body, thus supporting health and healing.
- Objective changes in the body observed during polarity sessions indicate deep relaxation and include flushed cheeks, drop in blood pressure, increased salivation, muscle relaxation, slower heart rate, and grumbling in the digestive system associated with the activity of peristalsis.
- Western science may find physiological reasons for some of these effects, such as stimulation of nerve centers and mechanoreceptors in joints.
- The basic principles of polarity therapy are related to the concepts of energy, love, working with obstructions, understanding.
- Polarity techniques include gentle holding, rocking, and probing movements that are combined into relaxing sessions.
- Some techniques aid the practitioner in locating areas that appear to be obstructed and in need of further attention.
- Polarity techniques may be used alone or integrated into traditional Swedish massage.

EXAM REVIEW

Key Terms

Match the following key terms to their descriptions. For additional study, look up the key terms in the Interactive Glossary and note other terms that compare or contrast with them.

_____ 1. Acupoints
_____ 2. Acupressure massage integration (AMI)
_____ 3. Ayurveda
_____ 4. Chinese body clock
_____ 5. Eastern bodywork
_____ 6. Energy-based bodywork
_____ 7. Energy channels
_____ 8. Energy flow
_____ 9. Five Elements
_____ 10. Hatha yoga
_____ 11. Polarity therapy
_____ 12. Qi
_____ 13. Qi gong
_____ 14. Removing obstructions
_____ 15. Thai massage
_____ 16. Traditional Chinese medicine (TCM)
_____ 17. Yin and Yang

a. Manual therapies from Asia
b. Life force or energy
c. Way of thinking about relationships among natural phenomena
d. Energy approach by Randolph Stone
e. Ayurvedic health practice consisting of relaxation, postures called *asanas,* and meditation
f. Pressure, joint movements, and assisted yoga
g. Points where Qi is easily accessed
h. Manual therapy that aims to balance energy
i. Healing practices from ancient China
j. Natural, daily, rhythmic cycle of Qi flow
k. Free unobstructed movement of energy
l. Restoring free flow of energy
m. Traditional healing from India
n. Illustrates the relatedness and interconnectedness of all
o. Pressure applied to acupoints to balance energy
p. Pathways for Qi flow
q. Ancient Chinese energy exercises

Memory Workout

To test your memory of the main concepts in this chapter, complete the following sentences by circling the most correct answer from the two choices provided.

1. An overarching similarity in forms of Eastern bodywork is a (holistic) (mechanistic) perspective, and some notion of (fluid) (energy) that flows throughout the physical body.
2. (Yin) (Yang) is the light, energetic, and spacious or heavenly aspect of the universe.
3. In TCM, if Qi is stagnant, you (move) (uplift) it.
4. In Shiatsu, (kyo) (jitsu) is a point of energy deficiency.
5. Pressure is most effectively applied to an acupoint at a (45-) (90-) degree angle.
6. In qi gong, most downward and outward movements occur on the (inhalation) (exhalation).
7. In Ayurvedic theory, medium frame and height, aversion to hot weather, and tendency to inflammatory diseases describes the (Pitta) (Kapha) constitutional type.

8. The goal of Ayurvedic health practices is to move the creative spiritual life force or shakti from the (Root) (Sacral) Chakra to the (Crown) (Third Eye) Chakra.
9. In Ayurveda, the (vata) (marma) points are considered to be the locus of the vital life force or prana.
10. Traditional Thai massage is based in principles of (Chinese medicine) (Ayurveda).
11. Noticeable changes during polarity therapy include (deep relaxation) (shallow breathing).
12. The style of touch in polarity therapy may induce a light (traumatic) (hypnotic) state.
13. A typical polarity therapy session ends with (the cradle) (brushing off).
14. Polarity can be described as a (gentle) (martial) art.

Test Prep

The following multiple-choice questions will help to prepare you for future school and professional exams.

1. Which principle of Yin/Yang reminds us that these are relative concepts that cannot exist in isolation?
   a. Infinite divisibility
   b. Mutual supporting
   c. Interdependence
   d. Intertransformation

2. Qi dispersed becomes:
   a. Energy, sunshine, the movement of the wind
   b. Material, rocks, trees, rain drops, human beings
   c. Wood, fire, earth, metal, water
   d. Kyo and jitsu

3. The Yin element felt in late summer and in the change of seasons, and that has a transformative quality, is:
   a. Water
   b. Earth
   c. Wood
   d. Metal

4. Wood feeds Fire, which creates ash residue, which becomes Earth, is an example of the:
   a. Qi cycle
   b. Body clock cycle
   c. Sheng cycle
   d. Ko cycle

5. Tiger's mouth, or LI-4 acupoint, is found on the:
   a. Inside ankle
   b. Dorsal thumb web
   c. Side of the nose
   d. Top of the shoulder

6. The energy channel that runs down the posterior body in double rows on the back is the:
   a. Lung channel
   b. Bladder channel
   c. Large Intestine channel
   d. Gallbladder channel

7. In Ayurveda, the term *chakra* meaning *wheel* refers to the:
   a. Concentration of acupoints on an energy pathway
   b. Kapha body constitutional type
   c. System of nadis that carries vital energy
   d. Whirling centers of energy at seven levels in the body

8. In Ayurvedic massage, what is mixed into base oils to achieve specific therapeutic goals?
   a. Essential oils
   b. Minerals
   c. Herbs
   d. Vital energy

9. Postures or *asanas* are a major component of:
   a. Qi gong
   b. Acupressure massage integration
   c. Hatha Yoga
   d. Chinese medicine

10. In Thai massage, the pathways that carry energy are called:
    a. Meridians
    b. Sen lines
    c. Nadis
    d. Marma

11. The original theory of polarity therapy was heavily influenced by:
    a. European folk remedies
    b. Ayurvedic medicine from India
    c. Western medicine from Europe
    d. Mayan healing practices from Central America

12. The principle of *love* in polarity therapy refers to:
    a. Sympathy for the client
    b. Attitude of surrender and openness
    c. Sentimental caring
    d. Affectionate touch

13. If the recipient feels pain during the *neck stretch* technique, it means that:
    a. Energy is flowing freely
    b. The technique may be contraindicated
    c. You should pull harder
    d. You should pull on the exhale instead of the inhale

14. The rocking movements in polarity therapy are performed:
    a. Forcefully and rhythmically
    b. Gently and rhythmically
    c. Gently with uneven rhythm
    d. With moderate force and with uneven rhythm

Video Challenge

Watch these videos, which can be found at MyHealthProfessionsLab.com, Chapter 25, and then answer the following questions.

AMI for the Back

1. What principles of good alignment are demonstrated in the AMI segment of the video?
2. What manual techniques are applied over energy meridians?

3. How does the massage therapist in the video apply pressure to acupoints?

Qi Gong for Self-Care

4. What do you notice in the video about the quality of movement in the qi gong form? How would you describe it?

5. Where is the practitioner looking during the qi gong form demonstrated in the video? How does that affect spinal alignment?

6. What do you notice about the stances in the various qi gong moves demonstrated in the video? How might practicing these stances benefit massage therapists' body mechanics while giving massage?

General Session of Polarity Therapy

7. What do you notice about positioning, draping, and the use of bolsters in the polarity therapy session in the video?

8. In the video, what position is the practitioner in for techniques applied to the head? What principles of good body mechanics do you see?

9. What did the practitioner do in the video to help the recipient sit up for the finishing techniques of brushing off?

Comprehension Exercises

The following short-answer questions test your knowledge and understanding of chapter topics and provide practice in written communication skills. Explain in two to four complete sentences.

1. Compare and contrast the theories of TCM energy channels, Ayurvedic nadis, and Thai sen lines. What are the similarities and differences? What is their role in their respective forms of Eastern bodywork?

2. Compare qi gong and yoga as body–mind practices. What are the goals of each? How do they differ in practice?

3. How do the applications of the manual techniques in different forms of Eastern bodywork differ?

4. Describe the visible physiological changes that might be observed in a polarity therapy session as energy blockages are released.

5. Describe three different general types of polarity therapy techniques. Give specific examples of each type from the abbreviated session.

For Greater Understanding

The following exercises are designed to take you from the realm of theory into the real world. They will help give you a deeper understanding of the subjects covered in this chapter. Action words are underlined to emphasize the variety of activities presented to address different learning styles and to encourage deeper thinking.

1. Receive a bodywork session from a practitioner who specializes in an Eastern bodywork form. Compare and contrast your experience with Swedish massage.

2. Integrate knowledge of TCM energy channels and acupoints into a Swedish massage. Apply sliding techniques along energy channel lines, and press important acupoints as you address different regions. Focus on your intent to balance energy as you apply techniques.

3. Practice qi gong exercises or hatha yoga postures. Relate these practices to associated forms of Eastern bodywork.

4. Receive a polarity therapy session from a certified practitioner. Be aware of any feelings of energy flow as the practitioner performs various techniques. Discuss your experience with the practitioner and later with a study partner.

5. Practice the polarity routine described in this chapter. Be aware of how your hands feel and any movement of energy that you sense. Were you aware of energy flow or obstruction in any part of the body or during a specific technique? Discuss your and the recipient's experiences afterward.

MyHealthProfessionsLab™

MyHealthProfessionsLab.com is a premium online homework management system that includes a host of features to help you study. Registered users will find:

- Powerful tools that track and analyze your results—allowing you to create a personalized learning experience
- Videos, flashcards and other learning tools to help enrich your progress
- Streaming lesson presentations and self-paced learning modules
- A space where you and your instructors can view and manage your assignments

Pearson Education/PH College/Haskell Photography

Chapter 26
Career Plans and Employment

Chapter 27
Private Practice and Finances

Chapter 28
Business Ethics

PART

6

Foundations of Career and Practice Development

26 Career Plans and Employment

Tyler Olson/Fotolia.

CHAPTER OUTLINE

Learning Outcomes

Key Terms

Follow Your Dream

Vision

Identity

Getting Employment

Chapter Highlights

Exam Review

LEARNING OUTCOMES

After studying this chapter, you will have information to:

1. Develop a career plan for the first year after graduation.

2. Create a vision and identity for a massage practice.

3. Identify the benefits and drawbacks of employment and self-employment.

4. Design a résumé, business card, and brochure.

5. Locate and secure employment as a massage therapist.

KEY TERMS

Employee

Income goal

Independent contractor

Mission statement

Practice identity

Private practice

Résumé

Self-employed

Sole proprietor

Vision

FOLLOW YOUR DREAM

Career plans begin with a dream—imagining the possibilities for your future as a massage therapist. Making that dream come true takes planning, effort, and perseverance. Career plans provide direction to achieving success step-by-step.

As described in Chapter 1, there are many career possibilities for massage therapists. Some work full-time and some part-time. Some look for certain settings such as spas, health clubs, integrative health care clinics, or private practice. Some prefer to focus on specific populations such as athletes, the elderly, people with certain diseases, or those in rehabilitation from musculoskeletal injuries. Others focus on a specific type of massage and bodywork, such as Swedish massage, energy-based bodywork, reflexology, or seated massage. Most massage therapists choose eclectic practices with a variety of clients and types of massage. There are many options.

A good place to begin career plans is to formulate your practice vision and identity. Focus for now on the first year after graduation. You can always revise the plan later as you become more experienced and your vision evolves, but it is important to make a decision and choose a place to start.

VISION

All aspects of your practice flow from your vision. Your **vision** is how you see your practice in its broad scope. It includes whether you work full-time or part-time, your practice format, the setting you are working in, your clients, what kind of massage you offer, and your income goals. The clearer the vision, the more likely you will be to achieve your career dreams one year after graduation and for each year of your practice into the future. A worksheet for outlining your practice vision is provided in Figure 26–1 ■.

Part-Time or Full-Time Work

Massage therapists can have successful careers working full-time or part-time. Full-time work can be thought of as earning most or all of your income doing massage therapy. However, it is not as simple as a 40-hour workweek. For a private practice, figure full-time work in terms of client load at about 15 to 20 clients per week, spending 90 minutes on setup, massage, and cleanup for an hour appointment. That comes to 22 to 30 hours per week. Add in another 1 to 2 hours per day for related activities, such as client notes, bookkeeping, and marketing your practice. Full-time employment may be 4 to 5 days per week, seeing several clients each day at a place such as a spa, health club, or other facility.

It is important to keep in mind that because massage therapy is physically and emotionally demanding, taking more than 20 clients per week for 1-hour massage can put you at risk for injury, stress, and burnout. Although some massage therapists may be able to handle more clients per week safely, massage therapists starting out are wise to build

their stamina gradually and learn their limits. Take control of your own well-being, and set a schedule that is full yet reasonable. Figure on at least 1 day of rest per week and a minimum of 2 to 3 weeks of vacation per year. When you plan your budget for the year, figure in your scheduled holidays and vacation time.

Part-time work as a massage therapist can be a fulfilling way to supplement other income. Some massage therapists choose part-time work because they have another job that they do not want to give up, family responsibilities, or other time commitments. Part-time work ranges anywhere from 1 to 10 clients per week and accounts for part of your income or part of a total household income. You might work 2 nights at a spa or take a few private clients per week. There are a variety of options for the part-time massage therapist.

Some massage therapists start out working part-time while keeping a steady job doing something else, and then gradually develop a full-time practice. Some work part-time in two different careers or jobs, or part-time while pursuing advanced education. Formulating a career plan takes into consideration whether working full-time or part-time as a massage therapist is the goal and how best to go about making that happen. Flexible scheduling is a major benefit of a career in massage therapy.

Employment or Private Practice

Work formats include regular employment and self-employment in private practice. Many massage therapists combine part-time employment with a private practice for a full-time career. Each work format has its upsides and downsides.

Regular employment can be found in spas, resorts, massage chain stores, integrative health care clinics, and other settings that offer massage. The Internal Revenue Service (IRS) glossary says that an **employee** "works for an employer. Employers can control when, where, and how the employee performs the work."[1] Employers set prices, assign work schedules, book clients, provide equipment and supplies, advertise services, and generally take care of the business side of the practice. Employers may also dictate the type of massage offered to clients, set a dress code, or impose other restrictions. Massage therapist employees perform massage as scheduled and, in some cases, may be required to do other work such as paperwork, cleaning, or staffing a reception desk.

The upsides of regular employment are a stable hourly wage; low or no expenses for space, equipment, and supplies; potential for health insurance and vacation benefits; and having much of the business of massage taken care of by the employer. In addition, employers pay a portion of Social Security taxes (FICA). Downsides include no control over massage fees, less time flexibility, and less control over the schedule and work environment. Employees do not take home all of the fees that clients pay, but also do not have the extra expenses, responsibilities, and risks that self-employed massage therapists do.

FIGURE 26–1
Vision worksheet.

Vision of Massage Therapy Practice for

_____
Name of massage therapist / Practice

Dates _____ to _____
        Month/Day/Year   Month/Day/Year

Size

☐ Full-time—hours/clients per week _____

☐ Part-time—hours/clients per week _____

Format

☐ Employee (preferred setting: _____)
☐ Self-employed (private practice—sole proprietor/independent contractor)
☐ Combination
        _____ % employed (# days/clients per week _____)

        _____ % self-employed (#days/clients per week _____)

Mission Statement (Purpose/Focus and Competitve Edge)

_____

_____

_____

_____

    Annual Income Goal

☐ <$5,000   amount $ _____

☐ $ 5,000–10,000   amount $ _____

☐ $10,000–20,000   amount $ _____

☐ $20,000–30,000   amount $ _____

☐ $30,000–40,000   amount $ _____

☐ $40,000–50,000   amount $ _____

☐ >$50,000   amount $ _____

You are considered **self-employed** if you carry on your practice as a sole proprietor or an independent contractor. Self-employment is sometimes referred to as being in **private practice**. Legal structures for private practices are discussed further in Chapter 27, *Private Practice and Finances*.

As a **sole proprietor**, you are the legally recognized business owner—the employer and employee rolled into one. This form of practice offers maximum flexibility for creating your own workspace, choosing clientele, controlling the type of massage offered, setting the schedule, and determining fees. You also have sole responsibility for building an adequate client base, complying with government regulations, completing paperwork and bookkeeping, and paying required taxes. Being a sole proprietor means being a self-starter and self-motivator and taking responsibility for getting things done.

An **independent contractor** performs services for another person or business, but is not an employee. Independent contractors are self-employed. They are contracted to accomplish a certain result, but are not under the direct control of an employer. An example of an independent contract situation for a massage therapist would be if a business hired a massage therapist to come to its office or workplace to give chair massage to employees on Employee Appreciation Day.

Some businesses use the independent contractor format rather than taking on the added expense of hiring massage therapists as employees. This applies to massage therapists who hire other massage therapists to expand their practices. The United States has labor laws that define when this is legal and when it is not, that is, when persons can be considered independent contractors and when they must be treated as employees.

CASE FOR STUDY

Roberta and Her Dream Practice

Roberta has participated in sports all her life, from junior soccer to high school volleyball. She loves to work out and enjoys being around athletes. Her dream practice as a massage therapist is to work with athletes either in a health club, professional sports setting, or private practice.

Question:

What can Roberta do to increase her chances of achieving her dream practice after graduation?

Things to consider:

- What expertise will potential employers and clients look for on her résumé?
- Could her grades in any particular subjects be important to a potential employer?

- How important might it be for her to keep up her own fitness level?
- What part-time jobs might she get for general experience in sports settings?
- What kind of volunteer work might she do to demonstrate experience with sports massage to a potential employer?
- What type of specialty training might she seek out?
- How can she create a professional identity to match her dream?
- What might her mission statement look like?

Ideas for realizing Roberta's dream practice:

_____

_____

_____

Just declaring someone an independent contractor does not make him or her one in the eyes of the law. The courts have developed a strategy called the "dominant impression test" to distinguish between employees and independent contractors. No single factor determines status, but several factors taken together are considered for their overall effect. The following are some factors that help define employment:

- Instructions given about when, where, and how to perform the work

- Training provided

- Integration into the business operation

- Services rendered personally by the worker

- Set work hours and schedule

- Oral or written reports required

- Significant tools, material, and equipment furnished

- Right to discharge the worker at will

- Work performed on the business premises

- Ongoing relationship

- Working for or supplying services to only one business

Why is it important for massage therapists to understand the difference between employees and independent contractors? One reason is to know if you are being treated fairly and legally by a potential employer. Massage therapists can be taken advantage of by employers who are just trying to avoid the responsibility and expense of having additional employees. Another reason is that if you want to expand your business by hiring other massage therapists, you will want to know the applicable labor laws. The U.S. government imposes monetary penalties on businesses that misrepresent employee status. Consult a lawyer for advice on whether a dominant impressions test for a certain situation points to employment or an independent contractor arrangement. Internal Revenue Service (IRS) Form SS-8 lists a series of questions to help determine if a person is an employee or independent contractor for federal employment tax and income tax withholding purposes.[2]

How do you determine which format is best for you starting out in your career? Only you can decide, but these are some factors to consider. Look for employment if you want to focus on clients rather than business tasks, or if you are looking for steady work with some benefits. Employment gives you immediate income with minimal or no startup costs. Also, if you have little work or business experience, you can learn the basics by working for someone else first.

Consider self-employment if you are self-motivated and like your independence. It helps to have prior business experience, good contacts or a natural ability to network, and the necessary skills to build a business from the ground up. Startup money is important to get a practice off and running. Private practices are not built in a day, but hard work and perseverance can lead to satisfying results.

Some massage therapists have short-term and longer-term plans, which might entail starting out with part-time employment while building knowledge and skills with an eye toward building a private practice in the future. Table 26–1 ■ compares different work formats.

TABLE 26–1 Comparison of Employment and Self-Employment Requirements, Upsides, and Downsides

Work Format	Requirements	Upsides	Downsides
Employment	• Successful interview • Meet employer expectations and obey policies • Cooperate with coworkers • Be reliable in attendance • Satisfy customers and employer	• Stable hourly wage • Low overhead • Employer pays portion of FICA • Employer advertises and schedules clients • Employer handles government regulations such as business or massage establishment license • Potential health insurance & vacation benefits • Shared client-base building with employer	• No control over fees, schedule, environment • Less time flexibility • Imposed dress code
Self-Employment Sole proprietor Independent contractor	• Business skills • Self-motivation • Discipline • Perseverance • Patience • Ability to satisfy clients	• Control over fees, policies and procedures, and type of massage offered • Create own environment • Personal choice about clientele • Set own schedule	• Income less predictable • Expenses for space, equipment, and supplies • Keep own records • Build own client base • Provide own health insurance • Pay self-employment tax

Mission Statement

A useful approach to clarifying your vision is to write a **mission statement**. A mission statement consists of one to three sentences defining the purpose of your practice and your main strategy for achieving competitive advantage. It answers the questions, "What is the focus of this practice?" and "Why would clients come to me (or why would an employer hire me) instead of someone else?"

A good mission statement narrows your focus and keeps you on a straight path toward your goal. A personal mission statement can lead you to employment in a particular setting or working with a certain type of client. A mission statement for a private practice serves as a reference point for the many decisions that must be made, and it defines who you are as a massage therapist. In a combined practice, your mission statement may have two different parts, or you may maintain a coherent mission throughout your practice. Box 26–1 ■ contains some examples of mission statements.

Your mission statement directs your path; therefore, it is worth taking time to create one that truly reflects your current interests and talents. Write several drafts of your statement until it seems right for you at this time in your career.

Income Goal

An **income goal** specifies how much money you need or want from the practice in a certain time period, such as a year. This figure will guide you in many important choices, such as whether to work full-time or part-time, whether to accept a certain job, or how many clients need to be scheduled per week. Income goals go hand in hand with mission

statements in filling out the vision of a viable massage therapy practice.

Because massage therapists work both part-time and full-time, the range for potential income is wide. Income goals should be as realistic as possible. For example, a

REALITY CHECK

KELLY

MAURICE: I'm trying to write a vision for my future practice, but can't quite get a clear picture. I just want to get a job as a massage therapist when I graduate. Isn't that enough?

KELLY: I would encourage you to look further than just getting a job someplace where you may or may not be happy in the longer term. Let yourself dream a little about your ideal situation after you graduate. What type of settings are you attracted to? What settings would you not like to work in? Look around at massage therapists who have built practices that you admire. Find a role model about whom you can say, "Yes, that's what I want to be doing in the future." Your vision will become clearer to you as you get a sense of the possibilities.

BOX 26–1 **Examples of Mission Statements**

Employed

- My mission as a massage therapist is to apply my training to help clients achieve optimal wellness within the spa environment. Continuing education and active membership in professional associations keep my knowledge and skills about massage and bodywork in spas up-to-date and responsive to consumer trends.
- My mission as a massage therapist is to apply my skills as part of an integrative team of health professionals in a medical practice environment. Advanced training in manual methods of pain management and musculoskeletal conditions provide me with knowledge and skills necessary to treat patients in rehabilitation.

Self-Employed

- My mission as a massage therapist is to apply my knowledge and skills to help clients achieve optimal wellness. Affordable massage therapy is offered in a clean, pleasant, and relaxing environment. This is a community-centered and family-based private practice welcoming people of all ages.

- My mission is to help clients heal from illness and injury through massage therapy. Advanced approaches to healing through manual therapies are applied in a caring and competent manner. Collaboration with other health professionals ensures safe and effective treatment.
- The mission of Office Oasis Massage is to relieve the stress of office workers by providing high-quality chair massage at a convenient time and place. In addition to relaxation, therapeutic applications focus on muscular aches and pains resulting from sitting at a desk for a major part of the workday. We create an oasis for rejuvenation in the midst of the workplace.
- The mission of Gold Medal Sports Massage is to improve athletes' performance and to prevent and treat sports-related injuries through massage therapy. Athletes receive personal attention from highly skilled sports massage professionals who understand their needs and competitive drive. We earn the athletes' confidence by producing observable results.

---

person in private practice has to build a client base, so the income for the first year or two will probably be less than it will be once the practice matures.

Projecting your personal expenses for the first year helps you determine how much money you need to bring in. That involves calculating, month by month, such expenses as rent, food, transportation, health care, personal services, recreation, loan payments, and other essentials. Be as realistic and detailed as possible. These projections will vary for different people because the cost of living differs in different parts of the country and for cities and smaller towns.

For the first year, figure in startup costs for the practice. Startup costs are discussed in detail in Chapter 27, *Private Practice and Finances*. Take into consideration the income from another job or business and whether you share personal expenses with someone else. When all things are considered, determine how much you need to make from the massage therapy practice to pay the bills and have some discretionary money.

IDENTITY

Practice identity flows from your vision and is the image you project to the world. It includes such things as business name and logo, credentials, résumé, business cards and stationery, and a website. It includes your dress and office decoration. Even the color and quality of your sheets and the music you play reflect your practice identity.

Business Name and Logo

Your business name should take into consideration your vision and your potential market. It could be as simple as your name, for example, Robin P. Jones or Alex Lipinsky. A practice name could include your location, for example, Granite City Massage Therapy. Or it might contain some natural characteristic you want associated with your practice, for example, sky, water, clouds, rain, or earth. It might suggest the type of massage and bodywork you offer, such as quiet space, workplace oasis, or relief center. If you are choosing a business name that is not your own name, check with state or local authorities, and the U.S. Patent and Trademark Office to make sure the name is not already taken (www.uspto.gov).

A *logo* is a symbol that identifies you and your practice at a glance. Your logo could be original artwork that you commissioned, paid for, and trademarked, or it could be chosen from clip art in the public domain. Printers usually have books of clip art from which people can choose a design or graphic for their business cards and stationery. Some people use stylized versions of their initials for their logos. Your business name and logo are used on business cards, stationery, brochures, and your website.

Credentials

Information about credentials and the ethics related to their use are found in Chapter 1, *The Massage Therapy Profession*, and in Chapter 28, *Business Ethics*. Remember that credentials are titles awarded for achievements and meeting professional standards. Use them correctly to advertise yourself to potential clients, other health professionals, and the general public. Credentials can be sought and earned to build an identity in concert with your mission.

Résumé

A **résumé** is a written summary of education, experience, achievements, professional memberships, and other information relevant to application for a job, volunteer position, or other occasion where someone wants a snapshot of your identity. A résumé contains selected pieces of information and not your entire personal history. It is formatted so that the reader can easily scan it at a glance for pertinent information.

It is important to have an up-to-date résumé on hand. In addition to accompanying job applications, résumés can be displayed on websites for massage therapy practices, among other uses. Figure 26–2 ▪ shows typical categories and content for massage therapists' résumés.

The basic elements of a résumé include general information such as name, address, phone number, email and/or website address. Current practice is *not* to include your age, year of birth, marital status or family information, or Social Security number.

Name
Mailing Address
City, State, Zip Code
Telephone Number
E-mail Address/Website

RÉSUMÉ

[Optional: Mission Statement or Employment Goal]

EDUCATION (reverse chronological order)

Certificate/Date   School Name
                                     Massage Program Name
                                     City/State

Degree/Date   College Name
                                     City/State
                                     Major/Minor

Diploma/Date   High School Name
                                     City/State

EMPLOYMENT (reverse chronological order)

Dates   Employer or Self-Employed
                                     City/State
                                     Job title/Responsibilities

Dates   Employer or Self-Employed
                                     City/State
                                     Job title/Responsibilities

PROFESSIONAL AFFILIATIONS, LICENSE, CERTIFICATIONS, HONORS

Date   Massage License, State, Number
Date   Certification Name, Organization, City/State
Date   Professional Organization Membership, Level
Date   Award, Organization

VOLUNTEER EXPERIENCE

Date   Organization
                                     City/State
                                     Responsibilities

Date   Organization
                                     City/State
                                     Responsibilities

LEISURE ACTIVITIES

Activities

References available upon request.

FIGURE 26–2
Sample of résumé content.

A detailed résumé contains dates, places, degrees, job titles, and credentials. It shows the depth of your knowledge and skills, past responsibilities and accomplishments, areas of expertise, and other elements for your identity as a massage therapist.

Education and training are listed in reverse chronological order. This section lists dates of attendance or graduation, school name and place, name of the course of study or program, and the degree or certificate earned. Program accreditation can be indicated. Sometimes formal education like college attendance is separated from massage therapy training.

Work experience is also listed in reverse chronological order. This section lists dates, employers' names, job titles and responsibilities, and special achievements. It is often useful to list your military service and record. Massage therapy experience and other types of work may be separated into two different sections.

Credentials, including occupational licenses and specialty certifications, professional memberships, and special awards and achievements, are listed to build your identity further. Potential employers will be looking for required licenses and training in desired specialties. Professional memberships show a level of commitment to the profession, and awards indicate outside recognition of your achievements.

Volunteer experience is important for those with limited work experience and also shows an altruistic commitment to the community. Volunteer work relevant to massage therapy includes activities such as outreach programs and officer or committee work in professional associations. Community volunteer experience might include work with the American Red Cross, a local food pantry, or an animal shelter.

Optional information includes hobbies, leisure activities, and other interests. These further define you as a person and may help your résumé stand out in a pile of otherwise similar résumés.

RÉSUMÉ DESIGN

Good résumés are simple in design and concise—one or two pages. They use a consistent format for margins and headings and leave plenty of white space to avoid looking crowded. The font chosen for the text is easily readable. Word processing features such as bold, italics, underlining, and capital letters are used conservatively to prevent too much visual distraction.

Remember that résumés are designed to be read at a glance. The main divisions within a well-organized résumé stand out and are easily located. Reverse chronological order is used for items such as education and work experience, so that the most recent items are on top, and work history is traced backward by skimming down the list.

Unfamiliar abbreviations, symbols, or initials after a name are avoided, and entries are spelled out fully for the reader. For example, the initials *LMP,* used in some states, should be spelled out as *Licensed Massage Practitioner.* The same applies to organization names; for example,

AMTA should be spelled out as *American Massage Therapy Association,* and *ABMP* as *Associated Bodywork and Massage Professionals.*

Grammatical style is consistent, especially elements such as verb tense and punctuation. Grammar, spelling, and typographical errors are avoided by looking over the résumé carefully. Remember that your résumé is part of your identity and should reflect your best efforts.

BUILDING AN IMPRESSIVE RÉSUMÉ

The résumé can serve as a vehicle for planning professional growth. A look at your current résumé can bring to mind ideas for what education, work or volunteer experience, certification, or other additions would make it more attractive to a potential employer or client. Seek opportunities that demonstrate professional development and add them as they are completed. Use your mission statement as a guide. Keep the résumé in electronic form so that it can be updated easily and as often as needed.

Be sure that everything that appears on your résumé is true, and there is nothing misleading. Honesty and accuracy are expected in an ethical massage therapist.

Business Cards and Stationery

Business cards may be the single most important marketing device for building a client base. Business cards give clients and prospective clients essential information about you and how to contact you for appointments. They reflect who you are as a massage therapist.

A business card packs a lot of information into 2.5 × 3 inches of space. A typical card has your name and/or business name, address if you have an office, phone number to call for appointments, and other contact information such as email address and website. It may list the type of massage and bodywork you offer and important certification and license information. The design may include a logo or graphic element. A sample business card design is shown in Figure 26–3 ■.

As with résumés, readable and simple business cards are best. Use fonts large enough for everyone to read. Do not let design elements and color detract from the essential information. However, a unique and attractive design may make a favorable impression.

FIGURE 26–3 Sample of a business card design.

Remember that most clients want to think that their massage therapist is professional, trustworthy, and competent. A well-designed business card communicates that impression.

A spa, health club, massage chain, clinic, or other business that employs massage therapists may provide standard business cards with its name and logo. Because you still have to build a client base at a place of employment, business cards are important to have available there, too.

Although stationery may not be important for massage therapists who are employed full-time, anyone in private practice should have stationery on hand for official correspondence. The design, color, and general impression should match business cards, brochures, and website elements to present a coherent identity. Although an increasing percentage of communication is done through email, business stationary is still needed from time to time for certain types of correspondence related to a massage practice.

Brochures and Websites

Brochures and websites give potential clients more detailed information about massage therapists and their private practices. With word processing programs and digital photography, a massage therapist can create attractive brochures that reflect a practice identity. A simple trifold brochure can be printed on standard 8.5 × 11 heavyweight paper and copied in color.

A typical brochure for a massage therapy practice might have a cover page with the name and/or business name, address, phone number to call for appointments, and other contact information such as email address and website. Photos of the massage therapist, the reception area and massage room, and other relevant images can be included. Other ideas include descriptions of the type of massage and bodywork offered, more detail on credentials, possible goals for massage sessions, policies, appointment times, and fees. Plan on updating a brochure about once per year.

Websites serve the same general purpose as brochures and may be more accessible to potential clients. Someone thinking about making an appointment with you may want to check your website for a better sense of you and your practice. Potential employers may also check out your website. Websites can hold more information than brochures, such as complete résumés, testimonials, fuller explanations of services, and more photos. They can have special features such as links to other sites that have information about the type of massage therapy you offer.

Developing technology is making website creation more user-friendly and economical. Check out websites for other massage therapists as you plan your website design to see what the options are. Make sure that your website reflects your practice identity and that your image and information is consistent throughout your marketing materials. Website designers can be hired to help you set up your website. Some professional associations offer website hosting as a service to members. More information about marketing a private practice can be found in Chapter 27, *Private Practice and Finances.*

GETTING EMPLOYMENT

Getting employment as a massage therapist is a step-by-step process that begins with finding the job opening and then interviewing successfully. It entails locating openings, filling out job applications, submitting résumés, writing cover letters, presenting references, getting interviews, and interviewing well.

Your school's placement department may have a listing of local employers and openings for massage therapists. Job postings for massage therapists can also be found in places such as local newspapers, professional journals and magazines, and some websites listing employment opportunities. Networking with other massage therapists can lead to hearing about job opportunities.

As you survey the job market, think about the vision for your practice and whether it leads you toward certain types of jobs or settings. If possible, narrow your search to the types of jobs that best fit your career plan. You can also be proactive in identifying where you would like to work, such as a specific spa or massage chain location, and then inquiring about how to go about getting a job there.

Once a potential job situation is identified, your focus is on getting a job interview. Steps to the interview typically involve filling out a job application and/or submitting a résumé and references. These steps may be completed online for larger employers.

CRITICAL THINKING

Analyze the identity or image of several different massage practices in your area. Look at résumés, business cards, brochures, and websites.

1. What do they say to potential clients about the massage therapist and his or her practice?

2. Is the image presented consistent with the reality of the practice?
3. Can you think of ways to create a more attractive identity for this practice?
4. What ideas would you consider using to create the identity of your own future practice?

A job application is a preprinted form used by companies to get essential information for screening job applicants. It gives employers a standard format to more easily compare applicants and narrow down the pool before looking at résumés. Even though much of the information asked for may be on your résumé, do not write in "see résumé." The purpose of the form is for employers to easily see relevant information to determine if they want to look at your résumé. If the application is incomplete, they may not look any further. Fill in all information neatly and accurately. An employer may also want to see if you can read and follow directions, and how good are your written communication skills, such as grammar and spelling.

If the application asks why you want the job, take time to think about your answer. Let the employer know that you understand the job requirements, that you are familiar with the company and want to work there, and that you are a good match for the job. Be honest about your schooling and credentials. Misrepresentation is not only unethical but may also have legal consequences. Many states require massage therapists to disclose prior criminal offenses to obtain licenses. Do not lie about past convictions on your job application. That is fraud and would later be grounds for immediate dismissal.

A potential employer may also ask for your résumé. If possible, submit it with a cover letter written in business letter format on good stationery. In the letter, introduce yourself, detail your qualifications, and state your interest in the job. Try to find out who is actually doing the hiring, and address the letter to that person. Show your knowledge about the company and the nature of the job. An employer will be impressed that you did your homework. Be sure to include your contact information and good times to call you. As mentioned previously, this step is sometimes completed online for larger employers.

References are good to have. These are people who know you personally, can recommend your work, and give a prospective employer information about you. References can be former employers, coworkers, people from volunteer and community work, teachers, or anyone who can give relevant information about your work, character, and factors relevant to the job. Never use family members as references. Later in your career, satisfied clients may also be willing to write letters of recommendation.

Keep two to three letters of reference on hand to include with a résumé or take to an interview. Prospective employers may want to contact your references personally for verification and for further information. It is a good idea to call your references to ask their permission to use their names and to let them know what job you've applied for and when they might expect to be contacted by the employer.

Your answering machine or voice mail message should be one that you would want a prospective employer to hear. Remember that employers may call to arrange an interview or to ask questions.

Once prospective employers know that you are a job candidate, they notice how you dress and act. The impression

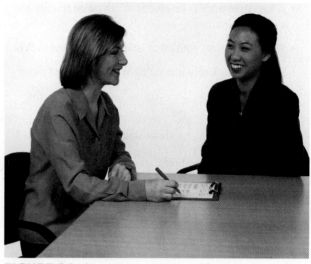

FIGURE 26–4 Appear professional and organized for a job interview.
Source: Dorling Kindersley Limited.

you make stays with you. Even before a job interview, appear neat and well groomed to a potential employer, for example, when dropping off a résumé or inquiring about a place like a spa or clinic (Figure 26–4 ■).

Realize that employers often use the Internet to check job applicants. Internet search engines can find your name in newspaper articles, official notices, and other website postings. Social networking sites may also be able to be accessed by others. Be aware of your Internet profile, and do not post anything that might be embarrassing if seen by a potential employer.

A direct call to a manager or person hiring for a job may be useful. You can inquire if your information was received and if you need to send anything else. This gives the person a chance to hear your voice and talk to you personally.

Successful Job Interviews

Job interviews are a two-way street. The massage therapist is evaluating whether the job offers what he or she is looking for, and the employer is determining whether the massage therapist has the knowledge and skills for the position and will fit well into the work environment.

Before going for an interview, write down questions you would like answered about the job, benefits, pay, and other important factors. The following are things you might want to consider.

- What types of clients/patients come to the spa/clinic/office? What are they looking for from massage therapy? Does that fit your knowledge and skills, mission and identity?

- What exactly will your duties be? Will anything else in addition to doing massage therapy be required?

- How many massages will you be expected to do in a day? How much time will you have between massages?

- What paperwork is involved? Will you be required to write SOAP notes?

- Will you interact with other health professionals? Who?

- What is your likely schedule? What days and times?

- What is the dress code? Are uniforms required and provided?

- What are the policies about sick days and vacations?

- Who will your supervisor be?

- What are the terms of your wages? Is this true employment, or would you be hired as an independent contractor? How often are you paid? What is the policy about tips?

- Are there any benefits (e.g., health insurance, 401k or other retirement plan, vacation pay)?

- Do they have an employee policy manual?

- Are there any additional perks (e.g., use of spa or health club, free parking)?

To further prepare for the interview, plan what you will wear. Choose clothes that fit well into the environment in which you would be working. Find out in advance if you will be expected to give the interviewer a massage. If so, arrive dressed appropriately or be ready to change into proper clothes for giving massage.

Review the materials you sent to the employer. Bring copies to the interview so that you can refer to them if you forget something. Bring letters of recommendation if you did not send them before. Also bring your massage therapy license if one is required in the employer's geographic area. Arrange any papers you bring to the interview neatly in a folder so that you appear organized. To boost confidence and practice your verbal responses, role-play the interview with another massage therapist or friend.

On the day of the interview, arrive a little early to settle in and relax. Greet the interviewer by name if you know it. Be prepared to answer the following common interview questions:

- "Tell me a little about yourself and your background in massage."

- "How did you hear about this job?"

- "What types of massage therapy are you trained in?"

- "What makes you qualified for this job?"

- "Why do you want this job?"

- "How do you think you'll fit in here?"

- "When are you available to work?"

- "What are your salary requirements?"

A massage therapist is often asked to give a massage to the interviewer or someone else connected to the employer. This is reasonable because the employer is hiring the massage therapist for his or her skills. Before the massage session, ask if the employer or hiring person would like you to do a health history interview, or if the person receiving the massage has a file you can review. Even if the employer or interviewer says to go ahead with the massage without a health history, do a brief verbal screening for contraindications and ask the person to clarify what he or she wants from the massage. It is important to know the employer or interviewer's expectations so you can plan the session accordingly. He or she may be looking for specific things in your massage.

Be very careful in responding to questions and requests. A potential employer may be testing to see how well you keep professional boundaries, or how you handle inappropriate behavior. Be confident and act professionally at all times.

ILLEGAL INTERVIEW QUESTIONS

It is wise to be informed about interview questions that courts have determined to be discriminatory in nature and illegal to ask. Federal and state laws attempt to ensure that job candidates are hired based solely on their qualifications for the job. Discrimination in hiring typically is prohibited based on certain factors such as marital status, family responsibilities, plans for pregnancy, child care arrangements, age, gender, sexual orientation, nationality, ethnic background, and disability. Comments about one's weight, height, and grooming are also not appropriate. See the National Labor Relations Board (www.nlrb.gov) and the U.S. Equal Employment Opportunity Commission (www.eeoc.gov) websites and similar agencies in your state for further information on illegal hiring practices.

Appropriate questions are directly related to job qualifications and are usually general in nature. The following are acceptable questions:

- "Do you have any responsibilities that will limit what days or times you can work?"

- "Are you prepared to perform four or five massages in a day?"

- "If you are hired, could you provide verification of your right to work in the United States?"

- "Do you have training in working with the elderly?"

If you think the interviewer has asked an illegal question, you have various options for responding. It may have been an innocent mistake by an untrained interviewer or a truly discriminatory inquiry.

Depending on the situation, you can steer your answer more toward what you think the interviewer is trying to get at or what you want the person to know about you. For example, a good response to "How old are you?" might be "After I finished high school I completed my massage training and am well prepared for the responsibilities of this job." Or you could respond "Is there an age requirement for the job?" This question steers the interviewer back to job qualifications.

PRACTICAL APPLICATION

Role-play job interviews with a study partner or friend. Use specific job postings to add some reality to the exercise. Write out expected questions and even some illegal questions for your interviewer to ask. Practice your responses aloud. Rehearse your responses until you have confidence in your ability to answer them well.

Keep in mind that the purpose of a job interview is not only to answer questions posed by the interviewer, but also to ask questions that will allow you to determine if the job you are applying for is right for you. What questions will you ask your interviewer to find out more about the job expectations, the working environment, clients, benefits, and so on?

Now switch roles with your study partner.

1. Critique each other's answers to the interview questions. Constructively brainstorm together about how your answers could be improved.
2. Take careful note of which types of questions were the most difficult to answer, and plan to practice these until you are satisfied that you can answer them well.

If you feel there is potential for illegal discrimination for some reason, it is wise to practice your responses to illegal questions. Planning ahead and good communication skills will help you complete job interviews with confidence.

AFTER THE INTERVIEW

If the job is offered to you after the interview, your possible responses are yes, no, or I have to think about it. Before you accept a job offer, be sure that the job meets your requirements in terms of your vision and income goals. If you have done your homework and are sure the job is everything you have been looking for, do not be afraid to say yes right away.

If you have any doubts, take time to talk it over with friends or family and think about your decision.

If the job is not offered to you right away, feel free to call back in a day or two to see how things stand. They may have hired someone else or may have more interviews to do. Calling to inquire shows continued interest and keeps your name visible.

If you do not get the job, call and ask if the employer or hiring person would share with you why you were not hired or what would have made you a more desirable candidate. The company may have found someone more qualified or who was available for more days or hours. Take it as a learning experience to increase your chances of success in the future.

CHAPTER HIGHLIGHTS

- A massage therapist's career plans begin with formulating the vision and identity of a future practice.
  - The practice may be full-time or part-time and may consist of regular employment, self-employment, or a combination of the two.
  - The mission statement defines the purpose of the practice and the main strategy for achieving a competitive advantage.
  - Income goals specify how much money is needed or wanted from the practice in a certain period of time, such as a year.

- Practice identity flows from the vision and is the image projected to the world.
  - Business cards present a lot of information in a small space and are important for building a client base.
  - Brochures and websites are useful for displaying more detailed information.

- Getting employment as a massage therapist entails locating openings, filling out job applications,

submitting résumés, writing cover letters, presenting references, getting interviews, and interviewing well.
  - A résumé summarizes relevant education, experience, and professional achievements and is essential when looking for employment.
  - A cover letter for a résumé should explain why you are qualified for the job and reflect your suitability for the place of employment.
  - References provide outside verification of your past performance and give you credibility.

- Job interviews are for massage therapists to evaluate whether the jobs offer what they are looking for and for employers to determine if the massage therapists have the qualifications for the positions.
- Preparation for an interview involves writing your questions about the job and practicing answers to probable questions from the interviewer.
  - Giving a massage is often part of a job interview for massage therapists.

○ Project confidence and be professional at all times. Be aware of illegal questions from interviewers and respond tactfully.

- Accept a job offer right away if you are sure you want it, but do not be afraid to say no or ask for time to think about it if you are not sure.

○ Call the employer if you do not hear back from the company within a few days.

○ If you do not get the job, try to find out why, and consider it a learning experience for future success.

EXAM REVIEW

Key Terms

To study the key terms listed at the beginning of this chapter, match the appropriate lettered meaning to each numbered key term listed below. For additional study, look up the key terms in the Interactive Glossary, and note other terms that compare or contrast with them.

_____ **1.** Employee
_____ **2.** Income goal
_____ **3.** Independent contractor
_____ **4.** Mission statement
_____ **5.** Practice identity
_____ **6.** Private practice
_____ **7.** Résumé
_____ **8.** Self-employed
_____ **9.** Sole proprietor
_____ **10.** Vision

a. Defines the purpose of your practice and describes your main strategy for achieving competitive advantage
b. The image you project about your practice
c. You carry on your practice as a sole proprietor or an independent contractor; also called private practice
d. How much money you need or want from your practice in a certain time period
e. The legally recognized owner of a one-person business
f. Someone who works for an employer
g. How you see your practice in its broad scope
h. Written summary of education, experience, achievements, professional memberships, and other information relevant to application for a job
i. You carry on your practice as a sole proprietor or an independent contractor; also called self-employed
j. Performs services for another person or business, but is not an employee

Memory Workout

To test your memory of the main concepts in this chapter, complete the following sentences by circling the most correct answer from the two choices provided.

1. Employees have less (control) (security) than self-employed massage therapists have.
2. You are considered self-employed if you carry on your practice as a sole (proprietor) (employer) or an independent (contractor) (employee).
3. A mission statement consists of one to three sentences defining the (layout) (purpose) of your practice and your main strategy for achieving (competitive) (therapeutic) advantage.
4. As with résumés, (elaborate and trendy) (readable and simple) business cards are best.

5. Massage therapists in private practice should have (stationery) (notepads) on hand for official written correspondence.
6. Websites serve the same general purpose as (business cards) (brochures).
7. A job application is a preprinted form used by companies to get essential information for (screening) (interviewing) job applicants.
8. Misrepresentation on a job application is not only unethical, but may have (legal) (emotional) consequences.
9. References are people who know you personally and who can (recommend) (describe) your work.

10. It is (illegal) (reasonable) for a potential employer to ask for a massage as part of a job interview.

11. Federal and state laws attempt to ensure that job candidates are hired based solely on their (qualifications) (aspirations) for the job.

12. If a job is not offered to you right away after an interview, feel free to call back in a (day) (month) or two to see how things stand.

Test Prep

The following multiple-choice questions will help to prepare you for future school and professional exams.

1. Which of the following offers immediate income with minimum startup costs?
   a. Sole proprietor
   b. Employee
   c. Independent contractor
   d. Private practice

2. Which of the following is *not* part of a mission statement for a massage therapy practice?
   a. Focus of the practice
   b. Purpose of the practice
   c. Income goal
   d. Competitive advantage

3. A logo is:
   a. Part of your practice identity
   b. A symbol that identifies your practice at a glance
   c. Original or clip art
   d. All of the above

4. On a résumé, education and work experience are typically listed in:
   a. Chronological order
   b. Reverse chronological order
   c. Alphabetical order
   d. Order of importance

5. The single most important marketing device for building a client base will most likely be your:
   a. Diploma
   b. Résumé
   c. Business card
   d. Brochure

6. Which of the following would *not* be appropriate to list as your references as part of a job application?
   a. Family members
   b. Teachers
   c. Former employers
   d. Satisfied clients

7. Which of the following is *not* appropriate for a prospective employer to do during a job interview?
   a. Ask about your qualifications for the job
   b. Ask for a sample massage session
   c. Ask about your marital status and children
   d. Ask about your ability to work a certain schedule

8. If you have limited job experience, which of the following would likely impress a prospective employer the most as evidence of your character and sense of responsibility?
   a. Music or other collection
   b. Professional image you project
   c. Good grades in school
   d. Volunteer work in the community

Video Challenge

Watch this video, which can be found at MyHealthProfessionsLab.com, Chapter 26, and then answer the following questions.

Career Plans and Employment

1. What were the initial visions of the massage therapists interviewed in the video of their future practices? How did they change with time?

2. What does the massage therapist in the video say about having small goals? How did that lead her in the direction she wanted to go?

3. According to the video, how should you prepare for a job interview?

Comprehension Exercises

The following short-answer questions test your knowledge and understanding of chapter topics and provide practice in written communication skills. Explain in two to four complete sentences.

1. What is the purpose of developing a vision of your future massage therapy practice? What are the essential elements of that vision?

2. Compare employees and independent contractors. What does the government look for in determining which category best fits a particular job? What is the dominant impression test?

3. What are some questions you might have for a potential employer during a job interview? Why would you be asking questions at this time?

For Greater Understanding

The following exercises are designed to take you from the realm of theory into the real world. They will help give you a deeper understanding of the subjects covered in this chapter. Action words are underlined to emphasize the variety of activities presented to address different learning styles and to encourage deeper thinking.

1. Write a mission statement for your future massage therapy practice. Take into account your current interests, talents, and employment goals. Write your mission statement in positive language so that it may inspire you and keep you on track to meet your overall career goals.

2. Develop a personal budget for a year listing projected expenses and total income, including income from various jobs and contributions from spouse or family. Given your circumstances, determine how much money you need to make from your massage therapy practice to cover bills and have some discretionary income. This is your income goal for your massage therapy practice.

3. Develop a list of job opportunities for massage therapists in your area. How many job postings could you find? How many fit your vision for your practice?

MyHealthProfessionsLab™

MyHealthProfessionsLab.com is a premium online homework management system that includes a host of features to help you study. Registered users will find:

- Powerful tools that track and analyze your results—allowing you to create a personalized learning experience
- Videos, flashcards and other learning tools to help enrich your progress
- Streaming lesson presentations and self-paced learning modules
- A space where you and your instructors can view and manage your assignments

Private Practice and Finances

CHAPTER OUTLINE

Learning Outcomes
Key Terms
Private Practice
Business Plan Overview
Description of the Business
Marketing

Management
Finances
Health Insurance Billing and
 Reimbursement
Chapter Highlights
Exam Review

Pearson Education, Inc.

LEARNING OUTCOMES

After studying this chapter, you will have information to:

1. Develop a business plan for a private practice in massage therapy.
2. Create a marketing strategy to build a client base.
3. Organize a massage practice office.
4. Enter into contracts with knowledge and forethought.
5. Establish policies for practice management.

6. Create a filing system for keeping client records.
7. Project startup costs for a massage therapy practice.
8. Project first-year income and expenses.
9. Design a bookkeeping system for tax purposes.
10. Manage practice finances on a daily basis.

KEY TERMS

Advertising
Business plan
Cash reserve
Contract

Estimated tax
Fixed costs
Marketing
Private practice

Promotions
Salary draw
Self-employment
 (SE) tax

Startup costs
Variable costs

PRIVATE PRACTICE

A self-employed massage therapist is said to have a **private practice**. A private practice can be small and part-time, with a few clients per week, or it can be large and full-time and serve many clients each week. A private practice in massage therapy has much in common with other small businesses that sell products and services to the public. For example, a massage therapy practice is regulated as a business and has responsibilities for keeping financial records for tax purposes. It also markets services to the public to build a client base. This chapter provides an overview of the business side of having a private practice in massage therapy.

BUSINESS PLAN OVERVIEW

A **business plan** spells out the details of putting the practice vision into operation. A business plan has four major parts: description of the business, marketing, management, and finances. The major elements of a business plan for a massage therapy practice are summarized in Box 27–1 ■. Further information about developing a business plan is available from the U.S. Small Business Administration (www.sba.gov). The remainder of this chapter discusses these elements in more detail.

DESCRIPTION OF THE BUSINESS

The vision developed in your career plan (see Chapter 26, *Career Plans and Employment*) lays the foundation for the description of your private practice, that is, your business. The mission statement is a good opening for the description. Express the size of the business in terms of whether it is full-time or part-time, how many clients are planned on average per week, and the total number of clients per year. State your income and profit goals. Looking at the income and profit goals in relation to the number of clients is essential. Remember that income from clients minus business expenses and taxes is the real profit from the practice. It is the profit that you put into your pocket. Do the math to see if your expectations about how much money you will make from your practice are realistic. Finances are discussed in more detail later in the chapter.

Legal Structure

The concept of sole proprietor was introduced in Chapter 26, *Career Plans and Employment*, to distinguish employment from self-employment. Sole proprietor is the most common legal structure chosen for massage therapy practices, especially when starting out. Other choices are partnership and corporation. Major differences in the three structures have to do with who owns the business, who takes profits and losses, who is responsible for legal matters, and what taxes apply. Box 27–2 ■ summarizes the characteristics of the three possible legal structures.

BOX 27–1 **Private Practice Massage Therapy Business Plan**

Section 1: Description of the Business
- Vision
  - Mission
  - Size (full-time or part-time; number of clients per week or month)
  - Income and profit goals
  - Legal structure (sole proprietor, partnership, corporation)
- Location
  - Home, space rental, or traveling practice
  - Applicable ordinances and zoning laws

Section 2: Marketing
- Market research
- Client sources
- Advertising and promotions
  - Business card
  - Brochure
  - Website
  - Other

Section 3: Management
- License, insurance, contracts
- Policies
- Office space
- Appointments
- Client records

Section 4: Finances
- Startup budget
- First-year budget
- Bookkeeping
- Taxes
- Banking

It is outside the scope of this text to delve deeply into the pros and cons of partnerships and corporations for massage therapy practices. If you want to know more, someone experienced in business, such as a lawyer or accountant, can help sort out the issues. Information is also available from the U.S. Small Business Administration.

For the purposes of this text, a sole proprietor legal structure will be assumed. A sole proprietor makes all decisions, takes all profits and losses, is personally liable for lawsuits, and pays income taxes on business profits as personal income.

Location

Location can make or break a business. Marketing research can tell you where your potential clients are and how much competition will be in a certain area. Municipal ordinances regulating massage therapy and local zoning laws may limit where a massage therapy business can be located.

Options for massage therapy practice locations include a home office, space in a commercial building or within

BOX 27-2   Options for Legal Structures*

Sole Proprietor

- Owned by one person who makes all decisions and who takes all profits and losses.
- Owner is personally liable for any lawsuits that arise from the business.
- Registered in the state as a sole proprietor.
- Owner pays income taxes on the business profits as personal income.

Partnership

- Two or more owners who make decisions and share profits.
- All partners are liable for lawsuits that arise from the business.
- Legal contract called a "partnership agreement" defines the responsibilities of each partner.
- Partners pay income taxes on their share of the profits as personal income.

Corporation

- A corporation is a legal entity or "person" under the law and is composed of stockholders operating under one company name. Stockholders own the corporation and elect a board of directors to manage the company.
- The corporation is liable for lawsuits that arise from the business. Stockholders have limited liability and cannot have their personal assets taken to pay a judgment from a lawsuit.
- Corporations are registered by states in the United States and must abide by that state's laws related to corporations. Laws differ in different states.
- Main disadvantage in some types of corporations is that corporate profits are taxed twice—once as a corporation and again as dividends to individual stockholders on their personal income tax.
- Types of corporations
  - *C Corporation* sells ownership as shares of stock; limited liability for stockholders; income taxed twice.
  - *Subchapter S Corporation* limits the number of stockholders to 75; has limited liability; income taxed only once as personal income of the owners.
  - *Professional Corporation* for professionals in practice together; special rules apply.
  - *Nonprofit Corporation* or 501c (3) set up with mission to improve society; tax exempt; no profits shared by stockholders.
  - *Limited Liability Company* (LLC) combines best features of partnerships and corporations; limited personal liability; income taxed once.

*See U.S. Small Business Administration (www.sba.gov) and U.S. Internal Revenue Service (www.irs.gov) for more information about legal structures for businesses.

another business space, or a storefront. These options may be limited by law in some locations, for example, in some places home businesses are prohibited. Each of these potential places has advantages and disadvantages to consider.

Many massage therapists have satisfying practices in their homes. The main advantages here are low overhead and a short commute. Home-based practices require a separate space dedicated to massage and, ideally, separate entrances and bathrooms. Mixing of personal and business space should be avoided as much as possible. Having strangers in their homes may not appeal to some massage therapists. In addition, zoning laws may prohibit home businesses, or a variance may be required. Check your homeowner's or renter's insurance for any clauses regarding a business run out of a home, and be sure you are covered for all "slip and fall" types of occurrences on your property. Despite all the potential difficulties, home-based practices can be quite successful with careful planning.

Renting space is another option. A room in an office building or within another business may be all you need. Rooms within spas, salons, health clubs, and medical offices can offer a nice reception area and give valuable exposure to potential clients. Sometimes massage therapists rent rooms to other massage therapists. If an acceptable schedule can be worked out, sharing space with another massage therapist is a good startup alternative. Note that this is not a legal partnership, but simply a space-sharing arrangement.

Storefront rental is a larger financial commitment. The advantage is that foot traffic in the area may result in more clients as people walk by and see your business signs. You can design the space as you like it and even rent space to other massage therapists or other compatible businesses. It is also a more complex situation, complete with a landlord, more possible legal restrictions, more initial financial outlay for altering the space to fit your needs, more upkeep expenses, and usually a greater monthly financial liability. A storefront may be a good option for a suburban or small-town practice.

An alternative to having a fixed location is to have an on-the-road practice in which you go to your clients' locations. You can see private clients in their own homes, or in places such as hotels and resorts, nursing homes, or the workplace. An individual client may contract with you for massage, or you may have an arrangement as an independent contractor to provide massage to patrons or employees of another business in its space. A traveling practice eliminates overhead for space, but requires a means of transportation and possibly special equipment for easy transport.

MARKETING

A market is defined as a group of people with the potential interest of buying a given product or service. **Marketing** is the process of identifying these potential customers and meeting their needs and wants. In marketing yourself, you identify potential clients who want what you have to offer.

In a sense, everyone is a potential client, so you must decide to whom to market your services. Options are to try to appeal to a broad, diverse market or to narrow your focus to a group with specific needs. A practical strategy when starting out is to market to a broader audience and narrow your focus later, if you want to, once your client base has grown. You might also create a profile of your ideal client to help you streamline your marketing efforts and attract clients in line with your skills and interests. Once you identify your ideal client, marketing involves finding out where they look for services and building a presence where they will find you.

Marketing also takes into consideration your competitive advantage, which is the reason people would come to you for massage instead of someone else. Factors that may give you an advantage are quality, expertise, price, location, variety of services, special skills, convenience, or environment. From the business point of view, it is useful to think of clients as customers or consumers.

Market Research

Market research is the process of collecting relevant information for identifying and reaching potential customers. The following are basic market research questions for massage therapists.

- Who are my potential clients? Who is interested in receiving the massage therapy that I offer?

- What do they hope to gain by receiving massage?

- Who in my area can afford massage?

- How do potential clients find out about massage therapists in the area?

- Who else is providing massage in the area? Who do they seem to be targeting or attracting?

- Is there an untapped or underserved market in the area?

- What are my strengths and/or preferences in massage therapy, and how do they match with potential markets?

- How can I develop my own niche or loyal client base?

- Who is the target audience for my massage practice?

Answers to these questions are found in a variety of sources. To begin with, the Wellness Massage Pyramid discussed in Chapter 1, *Massage Therapy Profession*, offers insight into the broad range of reasons that people might need or want massage therapy. Consumer research conducted by associations and organizations provides insight about massage consumers. An example is the annual *Massage Therapy Consumer Survey Fact Sheet* from the American Massage Therapy Association.

Magazine and journal articles can show what the general public is looking for from massage therapy and the latest trends. Organizations or support groups for people with certain illnesses or disabilities may promote massage to their members. The local library, phone book, or Internet search can uncover information about who in a geographic area is already providing massage and whom they are targeting, as well as potential competing practices at spas, salons, health clubs, YMCAs, integrative health care facilities, chiropractic offices, and other places.

Once potential clients are identified, you can make decisions about how best to reach them and position your practice as the best choice for their needs.

Building a Client Base

A primary source of clients in a personal service like massage is word of mouth, that is, recommendations from other clients, friends, and family. Referrals from health professionals such as personal trainers, chiropractors, physical therapists, and doctors can also be important. A strong referral network steers potential clients in your direction and vouches for the quality of your work.

Professional associations and independent groups offer special massage therapist locator services to the general public. Potential clients often check the Internet to locate massage therapists in their areas, and so subscribing to one of these services may be beneficial.

Networking in the community helps potential clients get to know you. Many massage therapists join their local chamber of commerce, or service clubs such as Rotary International and Lions Clubs International. Besides being supporting members, massage therapists can give presentations about massage to these community organizations. Special-interest groups such as sports clubs, senior centers, and support groups are also open to having speakers come to talk to them. Good presentation skills, as discussed in Chapter 3, *Professional and Personal Development*, are useful in marketing private practices.

Getting your name and face out to the public is the key. People need to know that you are in the area and how to contact you for an appointment.

Advertising and Promotions

Advertising is a paid public announcement providing information about a product or service to potential customers. Ads may be in print or electronic media and range in size from what can fit on the side of a pen to an outdoor billboard.

The purpose of advertising is to attract potential clients to a specific business or person and convince them that their needs or wants can be fulfilled by the service advertised. Ads remind potential clients of needs or wants and may even create a desire for the service that did not exist before. Ads convince potential clients that a certain business or person is the right one to fulfill their desires.

The most cost-effective advertising investments for a startup massage practice are business cards, brochures, websites, and online directories. In smaller towns, ads in the local newspaper or in the yellow pages phone directory may be worthwhile. Small circulation newspapers or magazines for specific target audiences such as an ethnic or other narrowly defined group can be effective. Visible signs with basic information also let potential customers know that you are in the area. Perhaps the most expensive and least effective advertising for most small practices are big-city newspapers, and television and radio ads, unless there are local channels or stations that serve the immediate area in which your practice is located. Advertising opportunities can be found in a variety of public places. For example, a public sports facility may have advertising space around a lobby bulletin board, or a local movie theater may show ads for community businesses on the screen before the feature starts. Some fund-raising groups sell space in ad books or souvenir programs and encourage their supporters to do business with sponsors who bought ads. These types of advertising build awareness of your existence and can make your name familiar in the community over a period of time. Buy such ads in places where you think your potential clients will see them. When someone thinks of massage therapy, your name will come up in association.

An increasing number of people look for massage therapists through online search engines. You can build an attractive profile in online directories such as Yahoo and White Pages. Some directories such as YELP and Citysearch include reviews and ratings from customers. It is good to check your reviews frequently to be aware of your current online image and to identity aspects of your practice that clients appreciate, as well as areas for improvement. Good ratings and positive comments attract clients, whereas poor ratings and negative experiences of others keep them away. Directory listings typically have links to your website so potential clients can get further information.

Social media can also help clients find you online. Build a Facebook, or similar social networking site, profile that presents your massage therapy practice favorably. Create a professional image as you would in print media, and keep it up to date. Paid Facebook advertising can be targeted to a specific audience using demographics such as age, gender, income level, education, etc., so you can tailor your efforts to the clients you want to attract. Twitter is another avenue for creating a public profile and keeping in touch with clients. Tweets can be used to educate, inform, and otherwise keep clients interested in massage therapy and you as their massage therapist. Topics might be recent research on benefits of massage, health tips related to massage, something you learned at a conference, a volunteer experience you had, or other engaging information. As a general rule, social media content should be about 80% educational, useful, or fun and only 20% promotional.

Keep your personal and business profiles completely separate, and track your Internet presence periodically. Social networking is becoming a powerful tool for marketing, but must be managed wisely to avoid pitfalls that may negatively impact your practice. Also be aware of changes in the popularity of different networking sites, and choose a site most likely to be used by your ideal clients.

Promotions are ways to encourage people to pick up the telephone and make those appointments. Promotions include giving discounts to new clients for their first massage, or a discounted package for a series of sessions, for example, five sessions for the cost of four. Some massage therapists offer seasonal discounts around the holidays or for special groups such as teachers, police, and firefighters. Gift certificates can also bring in new clients.

Commercial promotion websites like Groupon help you reach large numbers of clients with discount offers. These promotions have benefits and drawbacks. The benefits are reaching a large audience easily and possibly gaining new clients. However, be prepared for a spike in appointments and reduced income for the number of massages given. Massage therapists can be overwhelmed with a rapid increase in business and become at risk for burnout. Clients who take advantage of these discounts may not become regular clients at the full price for a massage. It would be wise to be clear about your contract with the promotions company, including legal obligations, and make sure that the program fits with your overall business plan.

Advertising and promotion ideas abound in a free market environment. A lot can be learned from becoming more aware of how other businesses market their services. Some methods may work for a massage therapy practice, and some may not. Box 27–3 ■ lists some ideas for building a client base.

In any case, care must be taken in marketing and advertising to avoid unethical practices. Many of the ethical pitfalls in this area of business are discussed in Chapter 28, *Business Ethics*. To summarize ethical advertising:

• Tell the truth and avoid deception

• Be professional

• Do not make guarantees

• Use testimonials sparsely

• List prices honestly

• Honor copyright and trademark rights

MANAGEMENT

Management involves activities necessary to keep the business running smoothly, such as obtaining licenses and insurance, defining policies, and negotiating contracts. Massage office design and upkeep, making appointments, and maintenance of client files are also important management functions. All the behind-the-scenes operations that make it possible for the massage therapist to provide a therapeutic experience for clients fall into the category of management. This section discusses some of the basic management details of a massage therapy practice.

BOX 27–3   Building a Client Base

Sources of Clients

- Word of mouth from other clients, friends, and family
- Referrals from other health professionals
- Referrals from massage therapist locator services
- Networking in the community (chambers of commerce, service groups, special-interest groups)
- Online directory
- Social media

Advertising

- Business cards
- Signs on a place of business
- Yellow Pages phone book
- Website
- Brochure
- T-shirts, caps, pens, bags, or other objects with name and contact information for a business
- Refrigerator magnets with business name and information
- Signage on cars and vans
- Printed signs for placement on bulletin boards or in windows
- Advertisements in newspapers, magazines, or newsletters
- Direct-mail coupons
- Announcements on local radio or television stations
- Digital ads on social media websites

Promotions

- Discount for new clients
- Packages of sessions at special price
- Seasonal promotions
- Discount for special groups
- Gift certificates

Licenses and Insurance

Certain licenses may be required to start a private massage practice. First, an occupational license to practice massage therapy must be obtained from the state or local government where applicable. This applies to employment, as well as to having a private practice.

Second, a business license may be required by a city or county. Some places have special massage establishment licenses and space requirements. Zoning may limit where a massage business can be located. Before you sign a rental contract, make sure that massage is legally allowed in that location, and get the required permits.

Insurance protects you financially. *Professional liability insurance* covers you for liability for incidents arising from the massage therapy itself. Criminal acts or actions outside the scope of massage therapy as legally defined are usually excluded. Injuries occurring when practicing without a required license may also not be covered. Read your professional liability insurance policy to clearly understand what it includes.

Massage therapy association membership typically includes professional liability insurance at professional member levels.

Premise liability insurance, also called "slip and fall" insurance, is for accidents to clients and visitors on the business premises not related to massage. *Renter's insurance* covers the cost of equipment, supplies, and other objects lost or damaged due to fire, theft, or flood.

Contracts

Setting up a private practice usually entails some legal agreements or contracts. Examples are rental agreements, phone and Internet service, credit cards, linen service, cleaning service, and bills of sale. Independent contractor agreements are used when a massage therapist provides massage services to another business. It is important to understand the basic elements of contracts to ensure that agreements entered into support your business plans and expectations.

A **contract** is a legal written agreement between two or more people. The terms of a contract may be upheld in court if one party is considered to have breached or violated the agreement. Lawsuits arise when agreements are either not clear or have not been kept.

A contract must have a clear statement of the terms of the agreement, that is, person A agrees to this, and person B agrees to that. The length of the agreement should be specified from beginning date to ending date. What happens if one party breaches the agreement may be clarified, such as arbitration or mediation. Grounds for termination and method of termination should be spelled out. Acknowledgment of understanding of the agreement, the date of the agreement, and parties to the agreement and their signatures appear on the contract. Guidelines for legal agreements include the following:

- Always put contracts in writing, and have them signed and dated by all legally responsible parties.

- Never sign a significant contract, for example, partnership, rental, or lease, without a lawyer looking it over first.

- Always read contracts before you sign them, so that you know what you are agreeing to. You will be held responsible whether you have read it or not.

- If you write the contract, use the simplest language possible so all parties understand what they are agreeing to; avoid legalese when possible.

- Have legal counsel review the contract if it involves a significant amount of money.

- Don't be afraid to suggest changes to a contract presented to you. If all parties agree to a change, simply strike out the words you do not want, write in alternate terms if appropriate, and have each party initial the change.

- For a contract involving a lot of money, add a witness, who is a neutral party, to the signing of the agreement.

Massage therapists who work as independent contractors usually have a stock contract that they fill in for different situations. This contract is an agreement by a massage therapist to provide massage services for a separate legal entity. It states the fee per massage session or time worked, date(s) of service, place, and how and when payment is made. It may stipulate conditions such as how clients are solicited and scheduled, reporting mechanisms, and type of massage provided. There may be a cancellation provision. Both parties sign the contract and keep copies for future reference.

Verbal agreements may be legally binding but are hard to enforce. People may have different understandings of the agreement or may remember details differently. Always get agreements related to your business in writing and signed. Laws related to contracts vary by state.

Practice Policies

Practice policies clarify expectations and specific points of the agreement between the massage therapist and the client. Policies set the ground rules for what happens given a particular situation. They should be given to clients and signed as part of the general client contract.

There are many types of policies. Pricing policies list fees for different services, and posting them may be required by law. Payment policies specify when payment is due, for example, before or after a session. Method of acceptable payment is clarified, for example, cash, check, debit card, or credit card. Other financial policies include insufficient funds/returned check policy and a health insurance reimbursement policy. Some massage therapists have a satisfaction or money-back guarantee.

Late arrival policies clarify what happens when a client comes late for an appointment. One approach is that clients pay for the time periods they have scheduled. If clients are late, their massages end at the originally designated times, and the clients owe the originally agreed-upon fees. Another approach may be that a client who is over 30 minutes late for an appointment does not receive a massage and is charged as if he or she were a no-show.

A cancellation policy may be that 24-hour notice is required or $25 will be charged for the missed appointment. It may also be that no penalty is incurred if the time slot is subsequently filled. A missed appointment policy may be that clients pay in full for missed appointments or, alternatively, that clients pay 50 percent of the original fee for missed appointments.

Conduct policies clarify to clients that the massage provided is nonsexual massage and that any attempt to sexualize a session will be grounds for termination of the massage without a refund of fees. Hygiene policies might specify that clients are expected to come for massage clean and free of strong scents from products like perfumes and cologne or that clients are expected to shower immediately prior to a massage.

A health history disclosure and update policy might be that clients agree to disclose medical conditions and medications as requested to screen for contraindications. They might also be expected to keep the massage therapist updated on any changes in medical conditions and medications.

A termination policy might state that the massage therapist reserves the right to terminate a session if he or she believes that the safety or health of the client or massage therapist would be threatened if the session were continued. A confidentiality and privacy policy reiterates that the massage therapist will not talk to anyone, including health care providers and insurance companies, without the client's permission. It also states that client health and session records will be kept secure and only seen by those needing to see them.

A scope of practice statement defines what type of massage therapy is offered and for what purposes. It is good to make clear that the massage therapist applies massage only within his or her scope of practice and will refer clients as needed to an appropriate massage therapist or health care professional. Explanation of scope of practice is often followed by a consent form.

Waiver of liability can be attached to a policies document. In waivers, clients agree to hold the massage therapist harmless for unpredictable negative reactions or results. This may benefit the massage therapist in the event of a lawsuit, but waivers do not usually hold in cases of proven negligence.

Clearly stating policies in writing promotes greater understanding of expectations and defines important aspects of the therapeutic relationship. Signed copies should be kept in clients' files and additional copies be given to them to take home. A summary of types of policies important to a massage therapy practice appears in Box 27–4 ■.

BOX 27–4 Types of Policies Important for a Massage Therapy Practice

Financial Policies

- Pricing/fees
- Payment due
- Methods of payment
- Insurance reimbursement
- Insufficient funds or returned checks
- Satisfaction or money back guarantee

Client Behavior Policies

- Late arrival
- No-show or missed appointment
- Cancellation
- Conduct or unacceptable behavior
- Hygiene
- Health history disclosure and update

General Practice Policies

- Schedule of days and times for appointments
- Services and types of massage therapy offered
- Scope of practice
- Referral
- Termination
- Confidentiality
- Consent for massage applications
- Waiver of liability

Massage Practice Office Space

Massage practice spaces have some common requirements whether in the home or in a commercial building. There should be space set aside for a reception area, massage therapy room, business office, and bathrooms.

The reception area is where clients are greeted and can wait if they are early for an appointment. A reception area typically has one or two chairs, a small table, lamp, and decorations. Framed certificates may hang on the wall. The area should be inviting, comfortable, and partitioned off from the massage therapy room.

The massage therapy room must be large enough for all the equipment and supplies needed for massage sessions. At a minimum, it should hold a massage table and sitting stool on wheels, with adequate space for movement around the table. Storage cabinets hold linens, lotions, and other supplies, and a covered container keeps dirty linens separate. An accessible tabletop is necessary for lubricants, small hand tools, hot packs, and other objects used during massage. A step stool may be useful for short or less mobile clients to get onto the table.

The room should also have a chair and clothes rack for clients' belongings. A small wall mirror is useful for clients to check their hair or makeup after massage. Anatomy charts, certificates, or artwork may be hung on the walls. The floor covering should be easily washable.

Office space is set aside for working on and keeping financial records, client files, and other aspects of the business side of the practice. Office furniture includes a desk and chair and a locking file cabinet. Basic office equipment includes a telephone with voice mail capabilities or an answering machine, with optional computer, printer, and copier. Many massage therapists use their mobile phones with voice mail instead of a landline phone. Storage space is needed for office and cleaning supplies. Figure 27–1 ■ shows a basic layout for a massage therapy office.

A bathroom should be accessible for client use. Some massage ordinances also require showers. Check local massage ordinances for requirements related to massage establishments.

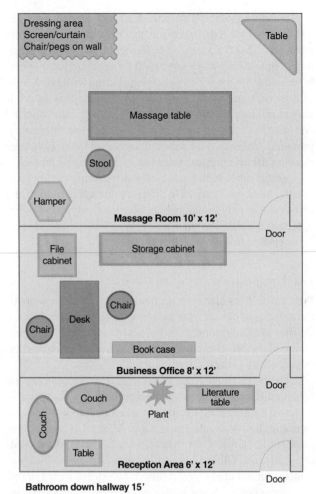

FIGURE 27–1 Basic massage practice office area.

Appointments

Making and keeping appointments is an important time-management function. A massage therapist should have a separate appointment book for his or her private practice. This can also serve as a supporting document for tax purposes.

PRACTICAL APPLICATION

Visit several massage therapy practices and carefully observe the offices. Sketch their office spaces using approximate dimensions. Answering the following questions will help you focus on the elements that constitute a well-designed massage therapy office space.

1. What colors, smells, lighting, or other factors do you remember from your visits to massage therapy offices? Which ones made a favorable or unfavorable impression on you?

2. What was it about the offices' atmosphere, comfort, and safety practices that impressed you?

3. Which elements did the offices have in common?

4. What were the elements that left you with a positive impression?

Now design your own massage office space. Include reception area, massage room, business office, and location of bathrooms. Incorporate elements that will positively influence clients coming to you for massage.

An appointment book can be the pencil-and-paper variety or can be in electronic form. A drawback of electronic record keeping is the potential for a glitch that wipes out appointment information. On the other hand, a traditional appointment book can be lost. Keeping a backup of all electronic information is vital for responsible record keeping.

Some website services offer the capability for clients to schedule their appointments online, and the services then send out email or text message appointment reminders to the clients. Check the reliability of specific service providers before signing a contract; for example, contact other businesses with that particular provider to see how the service is working for them. These websites can be difficult or confusing if not designed to be user-friendly. Although online appointment scheduling may be convenient for certain groups of clients, others may prefer personal contact by telephone for making appointments. Choose the best option or blend of options for the clients you wish to attract and keep.

Generally, the days of the week and times appointments are scheduled should be consistent and a matter of policy. Resist the temptation when starting out to take appointments whenever clients want them. If clients are informed of your days and times of operation, they generally find a time that works for them. Switching appointment times to fit clients' schedules should be kept to a minimum.

Leave at least 30 minutes between appointments if you have one massage room in a location. If traveling to an appointment, plan enough time for travel plus setup and takedown.

Client Records

Create a folder with essential information for each regular client. File folders with fasteners at the top keep papers in order. On one side of the folder, attach a cover sheet with contact information such as name, address, telephone number, and e-mail address. A signed policy agreement and waiver, and HIPAA confidentiality statement, if applicable, are underneath. On the other side, fasten the initial health history form and SOAP notes for massage sessions. Billing and payment records are usually kept in separate files from session records (Figure 27–2 ■).

Client records must be kept secure and locked to ensure client confidentiality and in some cases may entail compliance with HIPAA regulations. HIPAA rules apply only to health care providers that electronically store, process, or transmit medical records, medical claims, remittances, or certifications. See Chapter 5, *Ethics and the Therapeutic Relationship*, for general information on confidentiality and HIPAA.

HIPAA requires covered entities to inform patients/clients about their privacy rights and how their information will be used. Providers must get permission in writing to contact insurance companies and other third parties interested in the health records. Providers must implement procedures to ensure the confidentiality of records, and train employees to comply. In an office or clinic with more than

FIGURE 27–2 Client files are kept in alphabetical order in locked file cabinets.

Source: Pearson Education, Inc.

one employee, a person must be designated as responsible for seeing that privacy policies are followed.

Patients/clients have the right to see their records and obtain copies upon request. They may ask for corrections to records if they find mistakes.

Patient/client records must be secured, and only those who need to see them should have access. For example, hard copies of records should be kept in locked files, preferably in isolated records rooms, and electronic files should be protected by passwords on office computers. Patients/clients must give written consent for the use and disclosure of information for treatment, billing, and other health care operations.

Electronic systems are available for client records. Computer programs for keeping client files have been developed and can be found on the Internet and in advertisements in professional journals. Back up electronic files daily for preservation in case of file corruption, and use passwords for client record security.

Keep accurate, honest, adequate client records. Keep client records secure and confidential. Abide by laws related to record keeping, for example, those set forth by HIPAA if your practice is a covered entity. Schedule record keeping into your practice time. Doing paperwork is an important part of a massage therapy practice.

FINANCES

The financial viability of a massage therapy practice is fundamental to its success. That means setting income goals and profit projections, budgeting for income and expenses, tracking money coming in and going out, and paying taxes. Once you understand the basics of business finances and put them into practice, it can be rewarding to watch your massage therapy business grow and prosper.

Income and profit goals are part of the vision for your private practice. *Gross* income means how much money is collected from clients, whereas *net* income is what is left over after expenses and taxes. After subtracting expenses from income, a negative number means the business had a *loss* for the year, and a positive number shows your *profit*. The concept is simple, but keeping expenses low enough in relation to income to generate a profit is the challenge of having a private practice. More about planning for profit is discussed later in the chapter in the section on figuring the first-year budget.

Startup Costs

Startup costs are the initial expenses involved in setting up a massage therapy practice. Many of these costs are incurred before the first client walks in the door. Startup costs include buying basic equipment such as a massage table and related equipment, linens, and lotions; getting a license to practice; securing professional liability insurance; printing business cards; purchasing basic office supplies; establishing telephone service and an answering machine; and paying a security deposit and the first month's rent. Other costs fall into the "nice to have" category rather than the essential things. Nonessential expenses can be put off until money is available.

Startup costs are related to the type of private practice being developed. Some types of practices have lower startup costs than others. Typical categories of startup costs for a massage practice are listed in Box 27–5 ■.

Startup cash may come from a variety of sources. Some massage therapists use their personal savings or borrow from family members. Some work at other jobs with steady income, and start out as part-time massage therapists, gradually building their practices. A smaller number of massage therapists take out loans from banks or credit unions. Some startup costs can be covered by credit cards, but these often incur high interest payments that eat into profits. Starting out with the least amount of debt at the lowest interest rate is a good financial goal.

First-Year Budget

The first-year budget forecasts income and expenses for the initial 12 months of operation. Month-by-month budgeting is usually the most useful. Develop a month-by-month chart or spreadsheet that shows monthly expenses and projected income from the practice.

Projecting income for the first year can be tricky. Income will be a factor of the number of clients seen per week multiplied by the fees collected per session. Research the going rate for massage in your area, and price your sessions competitively for the market you are in. When starting out, you might want to consider staying on the lower end of the cost range to attract clients, especially if there is a lot of massage available in your area. On the other hand, if you

---

BOX 27–5 **Typical Startup Cost Categories**

Licensing Costs
- Occupational license (application, exam, fingerprinting, other)
- Massage establishment license
- Business permit or license

Professional Association Membership

Insurance
- Professional liability
- Premise liability ("slip and fall")
- Health insurance
- Auto insurance
- Other insurance

Business Checking Account

Communication Services
- Phone installation or connection
- Computer connection to Internet

Massage Equipment
- Massage table and accessories
- Massage chair and accessories
- Heater for hot packs
- Freezer for cold packs
- Other equipment

Office Furniture and Equipment
- Light fixtures
- Computer and printer
- Sound system for music
- Answering machine

Supplies
- Linens (sheets and towels)
- Oils
- Hot and cold packs
- Appointment book/system
- Forms and folders for client records
- Miscellaneous office supplies
- Decorations for office

Marketing and Advertising
- Business cards
- Brochures
- Website
- Stationary

Legal and Professional Fees
- Attorney
- Bookkeeper
- Accountant
- Other

Office Setup
- Security deposit
- First month's rent
- Communications installation
- Utilities deposit

CRITICAL THINKING

Write a business plan for your future massage therapy practice. Refer back to your notes about your practice identity and mission statement in writing your business plan. Present your plan to the class, and solicit feedback and suggestions. Review and revise your plan as you think of better approaches.

Now list the startup costs for a private practice you currently have in mind. Ask yourself these questions:

1. How do you plan to get the money needed for the startup?
2. Are there any ways to reduce startup costs to increase your profits in the beginning?

---

are one of a few massage therapists, or if you have a unique service, you may want to charge the average rate or more.

Expect a gradual growth in clients and massage sessions over the initial 12-month period. Figure no more than six clients per week in the first 6 months, gradually working up to 10 to 15 per week by the end of the year. Be conservative. Allow for cancellations. It is better to have more income than predicted. Remember to plan for vacation time, holidays, and sick days during the first year. Projecting 4 weeks of downtime is recommended. The following is an example of projecting income from client fees for the first year using an average number of clients per week and building over a period of 12 months (52 weeks).

2 clients × 4 weeks = 8 clients

4 clients × 8 weeks = 32 clients

6 clients × 16 weeks = 96 clients

10 clients × 20 weeks = 200 clients

0 clients × 4 weeks = 0 clients

Using this example, and assuming that each client visit was for an hour's massage, there were a total of 336 clients × $60 per hour, equaling $20,160 in gross income from client fees. Adjust your projected income as the year progresses and your client load numbers become more accurate. Lower numbers may spur you to rethink your marketing plan; higher numbers will be a cause for celebration.

Projecting monthly expenses allows you to determine how much income you need to break even, or make a profit, in any given month. **Fixed costs**, sometimes called *overhead,* are expenses you have whether you see clients or not, for example, rent and utilities. Fluctuating operating expenses, or **variable costs**, such as laundry, oil and lotions, disposable covers, and other massage supplies, depend on the number of clients seen.

Some experts recommend putting enough money in the bank to cover at least 3 months' fixed costs before you start your practice. This is called a **cash reserve** and should be figured in startup costs. Ideally, a cash reserve should be built up and maintained throughout a practice to cover unforeseen events such as illnesses or family emergencies. Deficits in 1 month can be made up in subsequent months, or profits in 1 month can help offset expected expenses in coming months. By the end of the year, income hopefully will outpace expenses to yield a profit.

A **salary draw** is the money taken out of the practice monthly for your personal use. Some experts recommend not expecting a salary draw for the first six months of a new practice. This allows for income to be put back into the business to cover operating expenses and build the cash reserve. To make this possible, some massage therapists build up savings, borrow money, depend on a spouse or family for support, or keep part-time jobs to cover personal expenses until their practices starts turning a good profit.

Keeping expenses low is paramount. Income minus expenses predicts your cash flow, or how much cash you have on hand at any one time. If your expenses outpace your income, and you have no savings to back you up, your practice will eventually fail. Careful monitoring of income and expenses can help you make adjustments as your practice evolves. Consider the first-year budget as a working plan for developing the business side of your practice. A sample spreadsheet for developing a first-year budget is shown in Figure 27–3 ■.

Income Taxes

Massage therapists pay income tax on the profits from their private practices, in addition to taxes related to employment. This means that they must keep accurate records of income from their private clients, as well as receipts from business expenses.

The following information is an overview of the subject of income taxes; however, a professional tax preparer is recommended for specific questions about any individual situation. The Internal Revenue Service (IRS) has information booklets on matters related to taxes that are updated every year (www.irs.gov). Some IRS publications and forms that massage therapists may find useful are listed in Box 27–6 ■.

The *tax year* for sole proprietor businesses like massage therapy practices is the calendar year beginning January 1 and ending December 31. *Taxable income* is the total income from a massage therapy practice minus qualified business expenses. All fees collected, as well as tips, are considered taxable income. Tips are taxable income for employed massage therapists as well.

PROJECTED INCOME

Source	Jan	Feb	Mar	April	May	June	July	Aug	Sept	Oct	Nov	Dec
Massage fees												
Tips												
Miscellaneous												
Monthly Totals												

PROJECTED EXPENSES

Expense	Jan	Feb	Mar	April	May	June	July	Aug	Sept	Oct	Nov	Dec
Loan payment												
Rent												
Phone												
Utilities												
Bank fees												
Equipment												
Massage supplies												
Office supplies												
Linen service/Laundry												
Cleaning												
Bookkeeper												
Legal/Professional												
Insurance												
Memberships												
Continuing Education												
Business travel												
Estimated taxes												
Salary draw												
Miscellaneous												
Monthly Totals												

FIGURE 27–3 Sample budget spreadsheet form for first year of business.

BOX 27.6	Useful IRS Publications and Forms*

IRS Publications

- Your Federal Income Tax—For Individuals (Publication 17 & 17SP [Spanish version])
- Starting a Business and Keeping Records (Publication 583)
- Tax Guide for Small Businesses (Publication 334)
- Instructions for Schedule C Profit or Loss from Business
- Business Expenses (Publication 535)
- Tax Withholding and Estimated Tax (Publication 505)
- Reporting Tip Income (Publication 531)
- Employee's Daily Record of Tips & Report to Employers (Publication 1244)
- Travel, Entertainment, Gift & Car Expenses (Publication 463)
- Business Use of Your Home (Publication 587)

Forms for Filing Income Taxes

- Form 1040 Individual Income Tax Return
- Schedule C Profit or Loss from Business (sole proprietorship)
- Schedule SE (Form 1040) Self-Employment Tax
- Form 1065 (partnership)
- Form 2553 Election by a Small Business Corporation
- Form 1120S U.S. Income Tax Return for an S Corporation

*IRS forms and publications can be obtained online from www.irs.gov, or by calling the IRS toll free number, or from the U.S. Post Office during tax season. Tax laws are changed yearly, so obtain the latest publication available.

Massage therapists who do not sell products usually use the *cash method* of accounting. Under the cash method, income is reported in the tax year it is received, and expenses are deducted in the tax year they are paid for. A different system called the *accrual method* is sometimes used by businesses. In the accrual method, income is reported in the tax year it is earned, even though payment may be received in a later year, and expenses are deducted in the tax year they are incurred, whether or not they are paid in that year. (See IRS Publication 583, *Starting a Business and Keeping Records*.)

Qualified business expenses reduce the amount of taxable income. Most expenses related to maintaining a practice/business are deductible, for example, equipment and supplies, office rent, continuing education, and license fees. Mileage to and from clients' homes or other travel may be deductible; however, travel to and from a place of employment is not deductible. Keeping good records and receipts related to business expenses is essential for an accurate calculation of deductions, and it is extremely important if you are audited by the IRS. Check with a tax preparer for further information on allowed deductions. (See IRS Publication 535, *Business Expenses*.)

Form 1040 is used to file U.S. income taxes for individuals and covers both employment and self-employment. Form 1040 is a summary form to which other forms and schedules are attached, for example, W-2 forms to report

CASE FOR STUDY

Shay and his Startup Plans

Shay wants to build a private massage practice after graduation, but realizes that will take money he does not have right now. He is willing to get part-time employment as a massage therapist as he builds his own business. His mission is "to apply my knowledge and skills to help clients achieve optimal wellness. Affordable massage therapy is offered in a clean, pleasant, and relaxing environment. This is a community-centered and family-based private practice welcoming people of all ages."

Question:

What strategies can Shay use to minimize startup costs and build his own private practice over time?

Things to consider:

- How can Shay decide how many days to devote to employment and how many to building his private practice during the first year?

- Employment in what type of setting(s) would contribute most to his long-range plans for his private practice?
- What are the options for his initial private practice location to minimize overhead?
- How can he build a solid client base for his private practice successfully and ethically?
- In what ways can he best and most inexpensively get his name out into the community?
- What could his contingency plans be if (a) his private practice grows more rapidly than expected or (b) his private practice grows more slowly than expected?

Ideas for Shay to accomplish his first-year goals:

_____

_____

_____

MARIA

REALITY CHECK

BARRY: I have some great ideas for a private practice but the financial aspects and record keeping seem too complicated. Do you have any suggestions for how to approach this side of having a private practice?

MARIA: Going into private practice is essentially starting a small business. Keep things simple, and get some help with record keeping and taxes. Set aside time every week to put income and expenses in a bookkeeping ledger, and keep all expense receipts. Consider it part of your practice, like seeing a client. Look ahead to tax time, and track all deductible expenses and taxable income. Consider using a computer program for record keeping. In learning how to use the program, you will get a better picture of the financial side of having a private practice. Finally, hire an accountant to fill out your income tax forms, especially in the first year. It will be well worth the cost, and it is a deductible business expense.

wages and tips from employment. Schedule C reports small business income and expenses. Form 1099 is similar to a W-2 form from an employer but is used to report income as an independent contractor.

Various other forms are attached to the 1040 as needed to complete the filing. A tax preparer can help you figure out which forms are required for a specific case. (See IRS Publication 17, *Your Federal Income Tax for Individuals.*)

Self-employment (SE) tax is a Social Security and Medicare tax for individuals who work for themselves. Also called FICA, this tax applies to Social Security coverage for retirement, disability, survivor, and Medicare benefits. SE tax applies if your net earnings from self-employment are $400 or more. SE tax is in addition to your regular income tax and was 15.3% percent in 2014 up to $117,000 in net income. Some SE tax may be claimed as a business expense, but rules change yearly. (See Schedule SE [Form 1040], *Self-Employment Tax.*)

Estimated tax payments may be due to the IRS four times a year in April, June, September, and January. This is another financial matter to discuss with your tax preparer, preferably at the beginning of the tax year and every quarter thereafter. Estimated tax payments, similar to withholding for employment income, estimate the tax that will be owed at the end of the year. Because you are your own employer, you have the responsibility for paying estimated tax. Estimated tax payments should appear on the budget as an expense. (See IRS Publication 505, *Tax Withholding and Estimated Tax.*)

Using a tax preparation professional is recommended unless you have all income from regular employment or an otherwise simple tax situation. Costs for tax preparation are qualified business expenses.

Tax preparation is made easier with a good bookkeeping system. The tax preparer takes the numbers provided by you and fills in tax forms. An accountant who is a tax preparer can also give you advice on deductions and other ways to reduce income tax owed at the end of the year. Setting up a bookkeeping system is addressed later in this chapter.

Income taxes are an integral part of the financial planning of a private practice in massage therapy—not an afterthought. Good planning can reduce any confusion and stress surrounding bookkeeping and taxes. It is all part of the business side of having a massage therapy practice.

Bookkeeping

Bookkeeping involves keeping accurate records of income and expenditures for tax purposes and tracking payments made by clients, as well as calculating how the business side of the practice is doing financially. The bookkeeping system chosen for a specific practice depends on how large the practice is and how skilled the massage therapist is with numbers.

Bookkeeping Systems One choice for bookkeeping is a simple handwritten ledger. The advantage of pencil-on-paper systems is that they are inexpensive and easy to learn. The process of making entries by hand can lead to a better understanding of how ledgers work. It is estimated that "half of all new businesses use hand-posted ledgers the first year, and some never see a need for anything else."[1] For most sole proprietor massage therapists, a handwritten bookkeeping system is adequate.

Published bookkeeping ledgers typically have a page for listing details of daily expenditures and daily receipts or income. There is sometimes a section for expenditures broken out by category of deduction such as rent, postage, and telephone. Keeping running totals for expenditures and income provides a check of profits at a glance and is handy at tax time (Figure 27–4 ■).

Often these record books include additional useful information such as a tax calendar, allowable deductions, instructions for making entries, calculation of net worth, and tax information sheets. The *Dome Simplified Weekly/ Monthly Bookkeeping Record* is an example of a handwritten system available from office supply stores.[2]

Computer programs for bookkeeping are also available. Some programs are designed specifically for massage therapists' needs. Computer programs do essentially the same things as hand-posted ledgers. Their advantages are that they are faster, provide clean-looking reports, and do the math for you. Some software programs integrate banking and bookkeeping and can generate totals and reports easily. Mastering the software may take some time, but for larger practices, bookkeeping by computer may make sense.

Accountants and bookkeepers can also be hired to help track finances. *Accountants* are trained in the principles of setting up and auditing financial accounts and are responsible for reporting financial results in accordance with government and regulatory authority rules. Accountants can set up bookkeeping systems and prepare taxes. *Bookkeepers* record day-to-day transactions in systems chosen by the business owner. They take care of the paperwork involved in recording expenditures and receipts and may also balance the checkbook. Bookkeepers still have to be provided with necessary checks, bills, receipts, and other records from the business.

Tracking Client Payments Massage fees collected plus tips received equal income from a private practice. A simple way to track client payments is to keep a handwritten receipt book. A typical receipt lists the amount of money received, method of payment (cash, check, or charge), date, service rendered, client's name, and the person who took the payment and filled out the receipt. The client gets one copy, and a carbon copy stays in the receipt book. The receipt book can serve as a supporting document for bookkeeping and tax reporting purposes.

As a backup record, a daily accounting of income can be made right in an appointment book. For each appointment kept, write the amount the client paid plus tip. Also note when appointments are canceled or missed. This provides a valuable cross-check and record of the daily activity of the practice.

One-write systems are useful for offices with more than one massage therapist or for tracking payment histories of individual clients. These systems include a running daily income ledger for the office, individual client ledger cards that can be filed alphabetically, and individual receipts for each transaction. These are sometimes called pegboard systems.

There are also computer systems for tracking client payments. Whatever system is used, receipts should be entered into the bookkeeping system daily.

Banking

It is important to keep a separate business checking account for a private practice. This keeps personal and business finances clearly separate and makes bookkeeping simpler. There is also less chance of confusion if audited for income taxes.

Compare fees and features for business accounts before choosing a bank. Choose a bank convenient for making frequent deposits. Establishing a banking relationship may be useful if seeking a business loan or for credit card processing in the future.

A few important rules apply to banking. First, pay all business bills by check (including electronic checks), from a petty cash account, or a credit card designated for the business. Second, deposit all income, checks, and cash into the business account. Third, when taking money out of the business account for personal use, write a check payable to

FIGURE 27–4
Sample of a weekly
bookkeeping ledger.

Week of _____ 2___ ___ ___
Month/Day to Month/Day

Total Receipts for the Week*

Day	Notes — Fees & Tips	$ Amount	
Sun			
Mon			
Tues			
Wed			
Thurs			
Fri			
Sat			
	Total This Week		
	Previous Total		
	Total for Year to Date		

*A receipt book or notations in an appointment book serve as supporting documents for the daily receipt totals in the ledger.

Expenditures for the Week*

Date	Paid To	Check#/Credit	$ Amount	

*Receipts for goods and services purchased, reflected in cancelled checks and credit card bills, are support documents for expenditures listed.

Expenditures by Deduction Category*

#	Category	Total This Week	Previous Total	Total for Year to Date	
1	Rent				
2	Phone				
3	Utilities				
4	Linen service/laundry				
5	Equipment				
6	Massage supplies				
7	Office supplies				
8	Advertising				
9	Travel				
10	Professional dues				
11	Continuing education				
12	Miscellaneous				

*Expense categories are set up by an accountant or bookkeeper and reflect the usual expenses of the business.

yourself and write "personal draw" on the memo line. This way personal draws or withdrawals can be tracked more easily.

Set aside time every month to balance the business bank account and review financial records. It is recommended that bank statements and canceled checks be kept for at least 7 years.

HEALTH INSURANCE BILLING AND REIMBURSEMENT

Few insurance companies cover massage therapy in their policies. As a result of public demand and changes in health care regulations, some of the more progressive managed care plans (Health Maintenance Organizations [HMOs],

Preferred-Provider Organizations [PPOs]) cover massage therapy if the client has a referral and a prescription from a medical doctor or if the treatment is part of a prescribed physical therapy regimen. In a small number of states in the United States (Maryland, New Hampshire, Utah, Washington) coverage of massage therapy is mandated in health care plans offered by employers. Many automobile insurance policies include Personal Injury Protection (PIP) clauses, which cover massage therapy services. Workers' Compensation claims frequently will be covered if prescribed by a medical doctor. Medicare and Medicaid generally do not cover massage therapy.

A massage therapist who is an employee of a health care business, such as a physical therapy or chiropractic practice, a spa, or a licensed massage therapy business, most likely will not have to assume the task of dealing with insurance companies. That will be handled by an administrative staff member or possibly the owner of the business. To maintain the records required for insurance company reimbursement to the business, however, the massage therapist needs to be capable of certain tasks, such as conducting and recording client assessments, keeping charts current, writing treatment plans, and in general, keeping accurate and up-to-date records.

For the massage therapist in his or her own practice, the decision to accept clients with insurance coverage requires careful thought. The additional paperwork, record keeping, billing, and waiting for reimbursement (which may never arrive or be severely discounted when it does) can become a financial quagmire for a small business. The massage therapist must gain entry to the list of approved providers of the HMO or PPO to have services covered, which often are paid at a reduced rate. It is important to have the client sign a medical release form so that there can be communication between the insurance company, the massage practitioner, and the client's other health care providers. Equally vital is keeping the physician's prescription for the client in a secure file.

Massage therapists who accept clients using insurance to pay their bills should be educated about relevant insurance company policies and procedures. It is dishonest and illegal to misrepresent the nature of treatment or the number of sessions given to a client. Adequate records should be kept to substantiate charges billed. It is unethical, and may be illegal in some places, to charge insurance companies more than clients who are paying out of pocket.

Massage therapists are not considered primary health care providers (PHCPs); therefore, a diagnosis from a PHCP is usually necessary for insurance billing. These referrals are for a specific pathology, and massage billed to an insurance company should be related to treatment for the stated condition. "According to standard insurance definitions, treatment is warranted until the condition is corrected or maximum improvement is made" and also includes instruction for self-care and prevention of future occurrences of the same problem.[3] Massage sessions for maintenance and prevention are not usually included in insurance plans and should not be billed as treatment.

Standardized Forms and Billing Codes

A standardized form, the CMS-1500, is used for billing all insurance companies, as well as Medicare and Medicaid. Using one form instead of many different types is efficient and a time-saver for health care professionals. To ensure legibility (and readability by the optical character recognition software that scans each form), the form should be filled out in black ink using a typewriter or computer. It is important to be sure that each client's intake form and other documentation contain all the information required on the CMS-1500 form.

Filling out a CMS-1500 form requires knowledge of the U.S. ICD-10-CM (International Classification of Disease, 10th Revision, Clinical Modification) codes, CPT (current procedural terminology) codes, and place of service codes. Because they change frequently, actual code numbers are not listed or discussed in this text. You can ask the referring physician's office to email or fax the prescription and applicable code to you to ensure that it is correct.

- *ICD-10-CM Codes* Every health condition (diseases, symptoms, complaints, etc.) can be assigned a category and given a code using this system first instituted by the World Health Organization (WHO) and published in the United States by the National Center for Health Statistics, a component of the Centers for Disease Control and Prevention (CDC). A diagnosis, and thus an ICD-10-CM code, can be provided only by a physician. Be sure when accepting a client's prescription that the ICD-10-CM code is included. You will need to enter it on the CMS-1500 form.

- *CPT Codes* All services health care practitioners provide to patients, such as medical, surgical, and diagnostic procedures, are assigned a five-digit alphanumeric code. Developed, maintained, and copyrighted by the American Medical Association (AMA), these codes provide a uniform way of communicating information to insurance companies, who then determine the amount of reimbursement to be paid to practitioners based on the coding. CPT codes change frequently, and there are a specific few that apply to massage therapy. When submitting bills to insurance companies, it is important to use only those codes that are within your scope of practice. Code books can be purchased from the AMA (www.ama-assn.org), but it may be more cost-effective and efficient simply to verify the proper codes to use with each insurance company you are billing.

- *Place of Service Codes* These are generally two-digit codes that indicate where the provided services took place, such as office, hospital, rehabilitation facility, and so on.

Billing insurance companies (and getting paid) can be difficult and stressful. The following are a few keys to success.

- Verify that the client's insurance company reimburses for massage therapy.
- Provide accurate documentation.
- Use correct code numbers.

- Follow the doctor's prescription.
- Stay within your scope of practice.
- Fill out the CMS-1500 form correctly and fully.

In addition, inform your clients in writing that they will be responsible for any charges not paid by their insurance companies.

CHAPTER HIGHLIGHTS

- A self-employed massage therapist is said to have a private practice with a business side, much like other businesses.
- A business plan spells out the details of a practice and includes sections on business description, marketing, management, and finances.
- A business description explains the practice vision and identity, as well as legal structure and plans for location.
  - Most massage therapists start out as sole proprietors, with office locations in the home, in a commercial space, or traveling to the clients' homes or workplaces to give massage.

- Marketing is the process of identifying potential clients and their needs or wants using market research.
- In building a client base, it is important to find ways to make yourself visible to the public and provide contact information.
  - Business cards are a key tool for obtaining new clients.
  - Online directory listings and social media sites create a presence on the Internet.
  - Paid advertising may help, as well as promotions to encourage people to make appointments.

- Management includes activities necessary to run the business.
  - Acquiring necessary licenses, insurance, and contracts lays the foundation.
  - Written policies clarify expectations related to fees, hours of operation, payment, conduct, scope of practice, client health information and confidentiality, and other aspects of the client relationship.

- Massage practice spaces typically have a reception area, massage therapy room, office, and bathrooms.
  - Spaces should be attractive, comfortable, and safe and comply with local ordinances.

- Appointments may be listed by hand in an appointment book or in electronic form.

- Client records with basic information, health histories, and session notes should be kept well organized and secure.
  - HIPAA rules apply to covered entities and can be found at the Health and Human Services website (www.hhs.gov/ocr/hipaa).

- A good financial goal is to start out in practice with the least amount of debt as possible at the lowest interest rate.
- Planning a first-year budget helps forecast income and expenses and is essential for making good financial decisions.
  - Tracking monthly income and expenses closely is essential for financial viability.
  - Keeping fixed and variable costs to a minimum maximizes profits in the end.
  - A salary draw is the money taken out of the business for your personal use.

- Income taxes must be paid annually on profits from the business.
  - Taxable income for a sole proprietor is the total income (fees and tips) from the practice minus qualified business expenses.
  - Self employment (SE) tax is an additional social security and Medicare tax for self-employed individuals.
  - Estimated taxes are paid to the IRS four times per year.
  - The IRS publishes many useful instruction booklets.
  - Hiring a professional tax preparer is recommended for massage therapists with private practices.

- Bookkeeping systems record financial transactions related to the practice.
- Financial records should be kept up-to-date and accurate.
  - Set aside time every month to balance the business bank account and review financial records.

- Some insurance plans cover massage therapy, including automobile insurance policies with PIP clauses and Workers' Compensation. Medicare and Medicaid generally do not cover massage therapy at this time.

- A physician's prescription for massage therapy is necessary for insurance claims to be paid.
- When billing insurance companies for massage services, company policies and procedures should be followed and treatment reported honestly.
  - ○ It is unethical, and may be illegal in some places, to charge insurance companies more than clients who are paying out of pocket.
  - ○ Accurate and up-to-date records need to be kept to support insurance claims and substantiate charges billed.

- ○ The CMS-1500 form is a standardized form used to bill all insurance companies. Massage providers need to be familiar with ICD-9-CM codes, CPT codes, and place of service codes in order to fill out forms correctly.

- Clients should be informed in writing that they will be responsible for charges not paid by their insurance companies.

EXAM REVIEW

Key Terms

Match the following key terms to their descriptions. For additional study, look up the key terms in the Interactive Glossary, and note other terms that compare or contrast with them.

_____ 1. Advertising
_____ 2. Business plan
_____ 3. Cash reserve
_____ 4. Contract
_____ 5. Estimated tax
_____ 6. Fixed costs
_____ 7. Marketing
_____ 8. Private practice
_____ 9. Promotions
_____ 10. Salary draw
_____ 11. Self-employment tax
_____ 12. Startup costs
_____ 13. Variable costs

a. Self-employed massage therapist
b. Expenses such as rent and utilities
c. Process of identifying potential customers and meeting their needs and wants
d. Money taken out of the practice on a regular basis for your personal use
e. Spells out the details of putting your practice vision into operation
f. Fluctuating operating expenses
g. A Social Security and Medicare tax for individuals who work for themselves
h. Paid announcement about a service
i. The initial expenses involved in setting up a massage therapy practice
j. An official written agreement between two or more people
k. Include giving discounts to new clients for their first massage
l. Putting enough money in the bank to cover at least 3 months' fixed costs
m. Payments sent to the IRS four times a year

Memory Workout

To test your memory of the main concepts in this chapter, complete the following sentences by circling the most correct answer from the two choices provided.

1. Income from clients minus (personal) (business) expenses equals the real profit from the practice.
2. The main advantages of a (home) (storefront) practice are low rent and a short commute.
3. (Promoting) (Marketing) is the process of identifying potential clients and meeting their needs and desires.
4. Advertising is a (free) (paid) public announcement providing information about goods and services to potential clients.
5. (Gift certificates) (Fee schedules) are an example of a promotion to attract clients.
6. To help avoid lawsuits, contracts should be (written down) (made verbally in good faith).

7. Practice (policies) (brochures) clarify expectations and points of agreement between the massage therapist and the client.
8. Reception areas should be (open to) (partitioned from) the massage therapy room.
9. Starting out with the least amount of (income) (debt) at the lowest interest rate is a good financial goal.
10. Money put away to cover fixed costs when starting out, or later in case of emergency, is called (a cash reserve) (petty cash).
11. Money taken out of the practice for personal use is called a (salary draw) (business expense).
12. (Taxable) (Spendable) income includes all fees collected plus tips received.
13. Charging more for a massage when an insurance company is paying the bill is considered (unethical) (good business).

Test Prep

The following multiple-choice questions will help to prepare you for future school and professional exams.

1. The most common legal structure for massage practices starting out is:
   a. Sole proprietor
   b. Partnership
   c. Limited Partnership
   d. Corporation

2. A primary source of clients in a personal service like massage is:
   a. Newspaper advertising
   b. Radio advertising
   c. Word of mouth from satisfied clients
   d. Direct mailing advertising

3. Insurance that covers you for liability for incidents arising from massage therapy itself is called.
   a. Premise liability insurance
   b. Catastrophic insurance
   c. "Slip and fall" insurance
   d. Professional liability insurance

4. How often should electronic files and records be backed-up?
   a. At least once a week
   b. At least monthly
   c. Daily
   d. Biweekly

5. Money left over after expenses are paid is called.
   a. Gross income
   b. Net income
   c. Profit
   d. Both b and c

6. Expenses incurred whether you see clients or not are called.
   a. Fixed costs
   b. Variable costs
   c. Startup costs
   d. Reserve

7. When you are self-employed, estimated tax payments are typically sent to the IRS.
   a. Two times a year
   b. Four times a year
   c. When taxes are filed
   d. When requested in writing

8. In addition to regular income tax, massage therapists in private practice pay an additional tax to cover Social Security and Medicare. This tax is referred to as:
   a. Reserve tax
   b. Variable tax
   c. Net income tax
   d. Self-employment tax

Video Challenge

Watch this video, which can be found at MyHealthProfessionsLab.com, Chapter 27, and then answer the following questions.

Private Practice and Finances

1. What do the massage therapists interviewed in the video say about who helped them get started in their practices? What kind of help did they get?

2. What ideas for marketing and advertising a massage therapy practice are presented in the video?
3. What does the video say about the importance of figuring startup costs and developing a first-year budget?

Comprehension Exercises

The following short-answer questions test your knowledge and understanding of chapter topics and provide practice in written communication skills. Explain in two to four complete sentences.

1. List the four sections of a business plan, and explain what information goes into each section. Why is a business plan important for starting and maintaining a successful massage therapy practice?

2. Define *market research*. List at least five useful market research questions.
3. Explain why a good bookkeeping system is essential for a massage therapy practice. What are the elements of a good bookkeeping system?

For Greater Understanding

The following exercises are designed to take you from the realm of theory into the real world. They will help give you a deeper understanding of the subjects covered in this chapter. Action words are underlined to emphasize the variety of activities presented to address different learning styles and to encourage deeper thinking.

1. Conduct market research for the area in which you plan to open a private practice. Who is already practicing in the area? What kind of massage therapy are they offering? How do they advertise their services? What type of competitive advantage might you develop?

2. List the startup costs for a private practice you currently have in mind. How do you plan to get the money needed for the startup? Are there any ways to reduce startup costs to increase your profits in the beginning?

3. Develop a first-year budget for a private practice you currently have in mind. Use a month-by-month format. List all fixed and variable expenses you can think of. Determine your cash flow for each month.

MyHealthProfessionsLab™

MyHealthProfessionsLab.com is a premium online homework management system that includes a host of features to help you study. Registered users will find:
- Powerful tools that track and analyze your results—allowing you to create a personalized learning experience
- Videos, flashcards and other learning tools to help enrich your progress
- Streaming lesson presentations and self-paced learning modules
- A space where you and your instructors can view and manage your assignments

Business Ethics

28

iStockphoto/© Pashalgmatov

CHAPTER OUTLINE

Learning Outcomes

Key Terms

Business Ethics

Local and State Regulations

Advertising

Claims for Massage Therapy

Copyrights, Trademarks, and
    Patents

Fees and Pricing

Tips and Gifts

Selling Products

Referrals

Client Base

Defamation

Safety and Welfare
    of Clients

Reporting Unethical Behavior

Beyond Graduation—An Invitation

Chapter Highlights

Exam Review

LEARNING OUTCOMES

After studying this chapter, you will have information to:

1. Follow consumer protection laws.

2. Present your credentials honestly.

3. Make truthful claims for massage therapy.

4. Abide by copyright and trademark laws.

5. Set fair policies related to money.

6. Sell products with integrity.

7. Make and take referrals properly.

8. Increase client base ethically.

9. Report unethical behavior appropriately.

KEY TERMS

Business ethics

Copyright

Deceptive advertising

Defamation

Endorsements

Guarantee

Massage establishment
    ordinances

Occupational license

Qualifying statements

Trademarks

BUSINESS ETHICS

Business ethics are moral and legal considerations related to commercial transactions (i.e., buying and selling of goods and services) and fair treatment of consumers. Because public safety and financial interests are involved, state and local governments enact business practices and consumer protection laws that give many ethical principles legal force.

Massage therapists, and the spas and clinics that employ them, are selling massage as a health service to customers. So in addition to treating people ethically as *clients* in the therapeutic relationship, they should also be treated fairly as *consumers* who pay money for advertised services.

Because massage therapy consumers are also clients, business ethics related to massage practices are stricter in some ways than in other commercial venues. The ethics of the therapeutic relationship give the massage therapist a fiduciary responsibility not necessarily present in other business transactions. For example, salespeople in clothing stores, or servers in restaurants, do not have the same responsibilities to their customers as massage therapists do to their clients. It is a responsibility of all massage therapists to put their clients' well-being above their own personal gain. This is a departure from usual business thinking.

Health professionals usually speak of having a *practice* rather than a *business*. The concept of a practice blends the professional aspects related to relationships with clients and the business aspects of the operation. The professional and business sides together make up a massage therapy practice.

A massage therapist's practice is the totality of his or her work. A practice may range from 5 to 20 regular private clients a week. It may include work in several locations, for example, a few clients at a home office, a few days as an employee of a spa, and a shift at a chiropractor's office. Or a person may be a practicing massage therapist for 20 hours per week and a spa manager for 20 hours. A small, part-time practice may include 2 days' work at a spa. Depending on where they work and the hats they are wearing, massage therapists can have more or less involvement in the business side of massage.

LOCAL AND STATE REGULATIONS

It is a basic ethical principle that massage therapists comply with local and state laws. Therefore, knowledge of applicable laws is fundamental to developing ethical massage practices. There are four general types of laws to be aware of: those related to occupational licenses, zoning ordinances, business licenses, and special massage establishment licenses.

An **occupational license** is a credential issued by a government that gives a person permission to practice a profession in its jurisdiction. In the United States, state governments issue occupational licenses, although in the absence of a state license, some cities and counties issue their own occupational licenses. Forty-six states plus the District of Columbia currently regulate massage therapy. Usually states have specific educational requirements and possibly others, such as passing a written examination and not having a criminal record. Licensing laws also specify scope of practice and advertising policies. Having a license for one location does not automatically mean that you can practice in a different place. Having a current occupational license, if it is required in the location where you are working, is a basic ethical principle. More on occupational licensing can be found in Chapter 1, *Massage Therapy Profession*.

A zoning ordinance is a law that specifies what type of housing or what kind of business can be in a particular location. For example, some areas are zoned for residential housing (e.g., single- or multifamily) and some for certain types of businesses such as retail or manufacturing. Massage businesses are sometimes zoned in light industrial or adult entertainment areas, especially if a locality has had problems with massage parlors. Zoning for massage should be checked before signing a lease or other contract for practice space. Some places prohibit small businesses, such as massage therapy practices, from operating out of private homes. Zoning variances that allow exceptions to the law may be available if applied for and approved. Zoning ordinances are passed by local governments like towns, cities, or counties.

A business license may be required by a town or city government to operate a commercial enterprise in that jurisdiction. This way, government agencies know who is doing business in their area and can ensure that the businesses are complying with all related laws.

Some local governments have enacted special **massage establishment ordinances**, primarily to try to stop massage parlors being used as a cover for prostitution. In localities where a massage establishment license is required, even health clubs and spas must have a license to offer massage therapy. Because an establishment is a place with an address, massage therapists who work for someone else or who have home visit practices are usually exempt from getting massage establishment licenses.

Establishment ordinances cover a variety of topics such as where the business can be located, hours of operation, shower and toilet facilities, sanitation, posted prices, and other factors related to the business operation. Some have requirements for STI (sexually transmitted infection) tests for persons performing massage, for clothes that may not be worn (e.g., see-through garments), unlocked massage room doors, unannounced inspection, prohibitions on serving liquor, and other regulations obviously aimed toward curbing prostitution, and not for legitimate massage therapists.

As offensive as some of these laws are, massage therapists must work for their revision rather than avoid getting licenses to operate their practices. It has become easier to change restrictive establishment and zoning laws as more states adopt occupational licensing that limits the practice of massage to trained and ethical practitioners.

ADVERTISING

Advertising involves disseminating information about your massage therapy practice to potential clients. Advertising takes many forms and includes handing out business cards, putting flyers on community bulletin boards, displaying brochures, putting ads in newspapers and magazines, having a telephone directory Yellow Pages listing, or posting a website on the Internet. Possibilities for advertising are discussed in more detail in Chapter 27, *Private Practice and Finances*.

The ethical principles of advertising are based on values of honesty and integrity. **Deceptive advertising** involves misleading the public about credentials, the nature of the service, its benefits, or how much it costs. The Federal Trade Commission (FTC) defines deceptive advertising as a "representation, omission or practice that is likely to mislead the [reasonable] consumer."[1] Consumer protection laws are designed to protect the public from unsafe products and services, and from deceptive advertising. Local regulations and licensing laws may also affect how massage therapy may be advertised.

Professional Image

The words and images used in advertising should convey a sense of professionalism, such as the ad shown in Figure 28–1 ■. Some of the ethical principles of therapeutic relationships also apply to advertising, for example, those related to professional boundaries and confidentiality.

Using sexual suggestion in advertising text or images is highly unethical and may also be illegal. Unfortunately, many allusions to relaxation and pleasurable touch, which are perfectly ethical benefits of massage, also have sexual overtones. In the United States, the word *masseuse* has become associated with prostitution, so *massage therapist* is the preferred term for a professional massage practitioner.

Ads in big city phone books are instructive of what to avoid in advertising. For example, "taste of paradise, female masseuse, 24 hours, outcalls available" with a photo of a seductive-looking woman in a flirtatious pose does not say "professional massage" to the reader. Another example of the type of advertising to avoid is "Angela's magic hands, full-body sensual massage, beautiful female masseuses, 'it doesn't get any better than this,' " with a photo of a woman's hands with long nails. "Jeannie Pampers, 'get pampered at your own place' " is less obvious but still suggestive.

Photos should show professional massage with good draping. If using photos of actual clients, get written permission to use their photos or names. Professional associations and photo dealers may have stock photos that can be used in ads.

Giving the wrong impression in advertising can result in unwanted calls from people looking for prostitution. Have colleagues, family, or friends review your ads to evaluate their professional image. What seems cute or clever to you may give the wrong impression about your massage therapy practice. This holds true for websites as well as print ads.

CREDENTIALS

Credentials are professional designations or titles given to massage therapists by organizations such as schools, certification commissions, licensing agencies, and other legitimate institutions. Credentials should be represented honestly in advertising. The general public, clients, employers, and other health professionals rely on credentials to assess a person's training and qualifications.

Obviously, it is unethical to lie about your credentials. It is more likely that a massage therapist would mislead the public by being vague about qualifications or by wording his or her qualifications incorrectly in an advertisement. The ethical question to ask is, "Will the public be misled about my qualifications if I use this wording?" Massage therapists are recognized health professionals; thus, they should display their credentials using the same conventions as other similar professions.

The credential received on graduation from an entry-level massage program is usually a *certificate of completion* or a *diploma*. The correct way to word that credential in advertising would be "Graduate of ABC Massage School" or "Diploma from ABC Professional Massage Program."

Certification and *certified* are perhaps the most ambiguous terms used as credentials by massage therapists. Being "certified" is currently used to mean anything from completing a weekend workshop in some massage technique, to finishing a 500-hour program, to completing extensive training in a specialty, passing an examination, and keeping up with continuing education. Such inconsistency can be confusing to the general public.

In addition, other health professions generally reserve the term *certification* for lengthy programs aimed at competence in a specialty. Consequently, when practitioners refer to themselves as "certified" in a particular massage approach, most people expect them to have considerable training and expertise in the method. If their "certification"

Green Space Massage Therapy

For Relaxation, Rejuvenation & Therapeutic Benefits

Licensed massage therapists

- Swedish massage
- Sports massage
- Shiatsu
- Reflexology

432 Grove Ave.   Green Space, MI 23456

Call for an appointment: 321-654-7895

FIGURE 28–1 Massage therapy advertising should convey a professional image.

PRACTICAL APPLICATION

Knowing the correct ways to maintain a professional image and advertise your massage therapy practice is often a matter of knowing what *not* to do. In your community, observe what other massage therapists do to promote their massage practices. Keep your eyes and ears open for examples of good and bad advertising, professional and unprofessional images, appropriate and inappropriate use of credentials, and the use of guarantees, endorsements, and claims made in advertising.

Ask yourself whether the examples you find in your community reflect well or ill upon the massage practitioner. Take note of good examples that you might emulate, without violating another practitioner's copyright, trademark, or patent.

1. Find examples of deceptive advertising in a newspaper or magazine. What makes the advertisements misleading?
2. Find examples of professional and unprofessional advertising for massage in newspapers, magazines, and the telephone book. What makes some examples unprofessional?
3. Find examples of credentials displayed both correctly and questionably in advertising by massage therapists. What makes the use of credentials questionable?
4. Find examples of guarantees, endorsements, and claims made in advertising. Analyze their legitimacy. Should the massage therapist have such elements in his or her advertising? Would you?

is based on a weekend workshop, then calling themselves certified would be misleading.

Board certification and *national certification* are understood as being conferred after one completes a program of study, passes a written and/or performance examination, and meets other criteria. Adherence to a code of ethics, continuing education, and a certain amount of experience are often required. This level of certification is given by an independent, nonprofit organization or commission whose mission is to provide these credentials for the benefit of the public. Passing a profession's "boards" is often a prerequisite for getting an occupational license.

So when is it ethical for a massage therapist to say that he or she is *certified*? Certification boards usually designate titles for those certified by their organization, for example, "Board Certified Massage Therapist" (NCBTMB) or "Certified Rolfer" (Rolf Institute). Some use the word *registered* to mean much the same thing, as in "Registered Polarity Practitioner" (American Polarity Therapy Association). In any case, the title designates the practitioner as having acquired competence and continuing education in the subject, and using the title exactly as it is given is correct.

On the other hand, it is misleading to say that you are certified after a one-day workshop in a certain technique, whether or not the presenter or organization giving the workshop says that you are certified. It is more accurate to say that you have completed so many hours of training in a particular subject. The certificate you receive at the end of the workshop is just that, a certificate of completion for the course of study.

The use of initials after a name is also a matter of judgment. Initials after a name are generally understood to signify an earned academic degree, board certification, or licensing. Academic degrees are AA, BS, MS, PhD, or some variation. BCMT means Board Certified Massage Therapist (formerly *Nationally Certified in Therapeutic Massage and Bodywork [NCTMB]*). In some states, LMT is used to

designate Licensed Massage Therapist. In Canadian provinces, RMT is used to mean Registered Massage Therapist. There are other variations for initials used by massage therapists, and it is wise to check on which designations are correct in your situation.

Initials should not be used to signify an occupation. The initials "MsT" (used to mean "massage therapist") and "CMT" (used to mean having a diploma from a massage program) are misleading. Information should be spelled out if using only initials or abbreviations would be confusing, for example, use the terms *massage therapist*, or *graduate massage therapist*. It may be more informative to spell out *licensed massage therapist* followed by the license number in states or local areas where licensing is required. Some states require a person's license number to appear on all advertising.

Guarantees and Endorsements

Honesty in advertising means describing the service or product truthfully and avoiding unfounded guarantees and claims. A **guarantee** is a promise that something will work as stated, usually with the implication that the money will be refunded if it does not.

The problem with making guarantees is that no one can predict the outcome of a particular massage session or series of sessions. There are too many variables involved. Statements like "guaranteed to reduce stress" or "guaranteed relief after one session" border on fraudulent. Using a ploy such as "guaranteed to work or your money back" is not appropriate for a professional health service. Some have suggested that massage therapists might use "satisfaction guaranteed or your money back" to show confidence in their service. The therapeutic result is not guaranteed, but the client's satisfaction, which is easier to substantiate, is ensured.

Endorsements or testimonials are anecdotes from someone besides the massage therapist, usually clients, about how well the massage worked for them. The Federal

Trade Commission defines an endorsement as "any advertising message . . . which consumers are likely to believe reflects the opinions, beliefs, findings, or experience of a party other than the sponsoring advertiser."[2]

Some examples of massage therapy endorsements are: "My tension headaches went away after one massage." "I shaved 10 minutes off my marathon time with sports massage." "My insomnia dissolved, and I sleep like a baby after receiving massage from ABC Massage." Endorsements may be made by individuals, organizations, or experts. Keep a release statement signed by the person or organization quoted for any endorsement used in advertising. The statement should say that you have permission to use the name and the quote of the individual or organization for the purpose of promoting your massage practice.

Although these statements by particular clients may be true, they may also be misleading. FTC policy states that endorsements "may not contain any representations which would be deceptive, or could not be substantiated if made directly by the advertiser." Making claims for massage therapy is discussed in a following section.

Endorsements are best used sparingly, if at all. They are not a substitute for the results of research on the effects of massage. Acceptable strategies for advertising are discussed in Chapter 27, *Private Practice and Finances*.

Prices and Bait Advertising

If a price is stated in an advertisement, the massage therapist must honor it in most cases. Exceptions would be if it is an obvious typographical mistake by the printer of a one-time ad (e.g., $6 instead of $65 for an hour-long massage) and would present an undue financial hardship. A mistake on a brochure should be fixed by hand and/or by having the brochure reprinted. It is wise to add in print that prices are subject to change to allow for raising prices in the future, especially in a brochure that someone may keep for a period of time.

If offering a special price or discount, the conditions should be clearly stated. For example, include the time period for the offer (e.g., November 20 through December 24, 2015), the specific service covered, and special conditions such as "daytime appointments only."

Bait advertising is unethical and illegal. Bait advertising is "an alluring but insincere offer to sell a product or service which the advertiser in truth does not intend or want to sell."[3] The purpose of bait advertising is to generate leads to potential customers, or to sell something else at a higher price, which is called bait and switch. For example, it would be unethical to advertise $10 for a 30-minute massage, and then pressure the client to switch to a $60 hour massage instead. Other ethical considerations related to pricing are discussed later in the chapter.

CLAIMS FOR MASSAGE THERAPY

Claims that massage therapists make for their work must be honest and truthful. This includes claims made in advertising or directly spoken to a client, and those stated explicitly or implied. Exaggerated claims, like promising a client that massage can cure pain in five sessions, are almost always unfounded and dishonest.

CASE FOR STUDY

Rafi the Natural Salesman

Rafi is a natural salesman and promoter, and he is putting those skills to use in building his massage practice. In his advertising, he claims that his massage can cure a variety of modern-day ills and always includes six endorsements from satisfied clients. He figures that getting potential clients to make appointments is most important and that all his customers can only benefit from getting massage.

Question:

Is Rafi's style of advertising ethical?

Things to consider:

- Are there any legal implications with Rafi's style of advertising related to claims for massage and the use of endorsements?
- Would this style of advertising be permitted under massage therapy licensing laws?

- If Rafi's ads are successful in attracting clients, aren't they acceptable from a business point of view?
- How does his style of advertising live up to values of honesty, integrity, and professionalism?
- Is this situation covered in a code of ethics or standards of practice for massage therapists?
- Who might be affected by this style of advertising, either positively or negatively?
- What is Rafi's major motivation with this style of advertising?
- What are the most important considerations in this situation?
- What decision would maintain the highest standards?

Your reasoning and conclusions:

_____

_____

_____

Furthermore, the FTC requires that claims made in advertising are substantiated claims, that is, "that advertisers and ad agencies have a reasonable basis for advertising claims before they are disseminated."[4] Businesses are required to possess information substantiating claims such as "research shows" or "doctors recommend."

Scientific research is perhaps the most reliable evidence for claims about the various benefits of massage. Legitimate claims may also be backed by knowledge in textbooks and articles, logical deduction from facts, and personal experience. However, claims are legitimately made for massage therapy itself and not for how it will affect any particular client.

Massage therapists are admonished to "accurately inform clients, other health practitioners, and the public of the scope and limitations of their discipline," and to "acknowledge the limitations of and contraindications for massage and bodywork and refer clients to appropriate health professionals."[5] For example, a client who comes for massage to lose weight or "melt fat" would be better referred to a nutritionist or personal trainer.

It is the responsibility of massage therapists to become knowledgeable about the potential effects and benefits of massage and to stay up-to-date on the latest research and knowledge in the field. This can be accomplished through reading and studying journals, pursuing continuing education, and looking up research on various topics of interest. Massage therapists who practice critical thinking examine evidence for the benefits of massage and do not accept everything they read or hear without question.

Qualify claims about massage therapy by citing sources of information. **Qualifying statements** that can be made when speaking to clients include "in a pathology and massage text it says . . . ," "a recent research study found that . . . ," "from my experience I've noticed that . . . ," "according to the manufacturer, this product . . . ," and "other clients have reported that. . . ." Having to qualify statements forces massage therapists to become more aware of how they know what they know. It is wise to check out claims made by vendors selling something or claims for new or unique techniques. Do not make claims you cannot reasonably substantiate or that you know or suspect are false.

COPYRIGHTS, TRADEMARKS, AND PATENTS

Copyright, trademarks, and patents offer legal protection for intellectual property rights. It is a matter of ethics that these protections be respected by individuals and businesses.

Copyright laws protect written, musical, and artistic works from unauthorized use and are designated by the symbol ©. Copyrights are administered in the United States by the U.S. Copyright Office at the Library of Congress in Washington, DC (www.copyright.gov).

According to copyright laws, a person cannot copy brochures, flyers, pamphlets, business logos, artwork, books or significant parts of books, and other materials written or prepared by someone else without the author's or copyright holder's express permission. A work receives copyright protection immediately from the time it exists in fixed form. Protected use includes reproduction, derivative works, and distribution of copies. Authors and artists may sign over copyright for their work to someone else, such as a publisher.[6]

When developing advertising materials and other documents, copyrighted works may be used for ideas and for reference, but should not be copied exactly and used as one's own. For example, it would be unethical to take someone else's unique brochure and just replace that person's name with yours without permission.

Some brochures are available for purchase and have a space for printing a business name and contact information. It is all right to buy these brochures for distribution, but unethical to copy them rather than ordering more from the publisher.

Fair use of a copyrighted work is allowed. "Fair use" allows limited use of copyrighted materials for education and research purposes. This does not apply to whole works or significant parts of works such as whole chapters in a book. Any use that takes away from the copyright holder's potential market for selling the work is not fair use. For example, if an author creates drawings of self-massage techniques to give to clients for home care and makes them available for purchase in notepad format, it would be unethical and illegal for you to photocopy them for your clients. If however, they are published in a book, and the author clearly states that they may be copied for clients, then this use does not violate copyright law.

Trademarks offer exclusive use of a name or symbol to identify unique goods and services and use the symbol™ or ® for registered trademarks. Trademarks distinguish a particular brand or company from others. Trademarks are handled by the U.S. Patent and Trademark Office in Washington, DC. States in the United States (www.uspto.gov) and Canadian provinces may also have laws that protect trademarks such as names and logos for businesses that operate within their jurisdictions.

Trademarks include unique business names like "Wellspring Massage Therapy" or "Morristown Spa and Massage," along with the logo or identifying design used on documents and in advertising. Trademarks for services are also called *service marks* (sm). The business that uses the name or logo first and consistently on materials associated with the business has the right to the trademark. Most states have offices where the names of businesses can be researched to see if they are already in use. It is wise to register the name of your practice or business to protect it from use by someone else.

Artwork for logos and text for advertising may be in the "public domain" meaning that they are commonly available or have been created for pubic distribution. Books of stock logos are available at printing companies, and professional associations may have text and designs for advertising available for general use. Using words and artwork in the public domain is an ethically safe and economical alternative to developing your own unique materials.

Massage and bodywork systems such as Rolfing®, Jin Shin Do®, and Feldenkrais Method® are registered trademarks. Massage therapists may not use trademarked names in their advertising or descriptions of their work unless they hold credentials from the trademark organizations that allow them to use the designation.

Patents are protections for inventions and include utility and design patents. The inventor of a massage tool, machine, or other product related to massage may apply for a patent from the U.S. Patent and Trademark Office. Patented inventions may not be copied by others for sale.

FEES AND PRICING

The exchange of money is an integral part of massage therapy practices and must be done with honesty and integrity. Key principles are fair compensation, clarity, and consistency.

Fair compensation is determined partially by the usual rate for massage in a particular location. What are others charging? Generally speaking, massage costs more in big cities than in rural areas or areas with lower costs of living. A house call usually costs more than in-office massage. A massage therapist with more training and/or experience may command a rate at the higher end of the scale than one just out of school. In many ways "fair" is determined by what the market will bear, that is, what people are willing to pay.

Once established, a pricing policy should be clearly stated in promotional materials and posted prominently in the place of business. Simplicity is best, but different rates for different session lengths (usually 30, 60, or 90 minutes), or sessions for which special training is required (e.g., lymphatic drainage massage or sports massage), are appropriate.

Be sure that policies regarding when payment is expected and what form it can take (cash, check, credit/debit card) are clear. Tell clients before a session begins what rate will be charged. If a session goes longer than expected, it is the massage therapist's responsibility, and the client would not ordinarily be charged extra.

Consistent pricing is a matter of fairness. Charging one person less than another can be complicated, even when offering discounts for friends and family. Treating discounted sessions with less professionalism is unethical.

Special pricing such as sliding scales and prepaid plans require careful thought. Sliding scales are problematic and are avoided by most practitioners. If a sliding scale is adopted, establish objective guidelines, for example, based on a person's or family's income. Prepaid plans can be good for marketing, but be sure to state the terms clearly. An example of a prepaid plan is a package of six prepaid sessions for the price of five sessions. Make time limits clear, like "must be used within 1 year" or by a certain expiration date.

Charging more for a massage when an insurance company is paying is considered unethical and may also be illegal. Although it is true that practices using third-party payments have more paperwork to complete, those costs are typically absorbed in general operation costs.

TIPS AND GIFTS

Tips are gratuities (i.e., given in gratitude) over and above the cost of a massage session given directly to the massage therapist. Whether a tip is given and the amount is

---

CASE FOR STUDY

Chloe's Pricing System

Chloe is just beginning to build her massage therapy practice. She worries about being competitive with other massage therapists in the area and has difficulty asking for money from clients. The going rate for massage seems so high to her. She never publishes her rates and changes her rates according to what she thinks the client can afford or will be willing to pay.

Question:

Is Chloe's pricing system ethical?

Things to consider:

- Are there any legal implications for Chloe's pricing system? Do local licensing laws require posting rates?
- Does Chloe have the right to charge what she wants for her massage?

- How does her system of pricing live up to values of fairness and integrity?
- Is this situation covered in a code of ethics or standards of practice for massage therapists?
- Who might be affected by her system of pricing?
- What is Chloe's major motivation for this pricing system?
- What are alternative pricing strategies?
- What are the most important considerations in this situation?
- What decision would maintain the highest standards?

Your reasoning and conclusions:

_____

_____

_____

_____

determined at the discretion of the client. Accepting tips in an ethical way calls for some careful thought.

Soliciting or accepting tips for massage therapy poses ethical questions not relevant to other service occupations. Complicating factors are that massage therapy is given in a variety of settings with different customs related to tipping (e.g., spas, salons, medical settings, and private offices), that massage therapists may have independent practices or may be employees, and that massage involves a therapeutic relationship with clients, which presents special responsibilities.

Accepting tips can be ethical if they do not negatively influence the therapeutic relationship, if they are truly optional, and if tippers and nontippers receive the same level of care. Tips are most appropriate in settings where it is customary to give gratuities for services, such as at salons, spas, hotels, and resorts.

In places where tipping is customary, owners of the businesses are usually not tipped. Employees or independent contractors who receive less than the cost of the massage are commonly tipped. In private massage practices, where the practitioner sets the price of the massage, tips should not be expected.

Tips for massage are problematic in settings such as medical clinics, chiropractic offices, and private practices. Tipping health professionals is not customary. Tipping may be confusing and awkward for clients in settings considered to be health care related, rather than personal service related.

It is appropriate to let clients know if tipping is customary in a certain setting. A sign that states "Tips appreciated" lets clients know that it is a place where tips are accepted. However, clients must never feel that they need to give a tip to receive high-quality service. Tips should never be solicited personally by massage therapists.

Turn down tips that have expectations attached and tips that are too large. Tips that seem too large (e.g., $30 for a $60 massage) may involve transference on the part of the client or may be an attempt to gain favor. Such tips cross professional boundaries and should not be accepted. On the other hand, a client who offers a larger than usual tip in appreciation for pain relief or doing well in a big race after receiving sports massage may simply be expressing his or her gratitude, and accepting the tip causes no harm. These are judgment calls for the massage therapist to make. It is acceptable to adopt a "no tipping" policy in a private practice.

Gifts are a similar situation. Nonmonetary gifts that are tokens given in appreciation or at special times like the holidays may be appropriate to accept. Gifts given to gain favor compromise the therapeutic relationship and cross boundaries and should be politely refused. Never accept a gift from a client whom you suspect has a romantic interest in you. Gifts with high monetary value are also inappropriate to accept. Trust your intuition to tell you that something does not seem right, or ask advice about it from a colleague or friend who understands the professional implications involved.

REALITY CHECK

ROB

SASHA: I really look forward to getting tips from my clients at the health club. I count on that added income. I have some stingy clients who never tip, and I don't feel like giving them my best. Should I drop some hints to them about leaving a tip? Maybe they don't know I expect one.

ROB: Given your expectations, I can understand why you feel the way you do. But let's look at this from an ethical point of view. First, your clients probably view you as a health professional and may not think of tipping you anymore than they would a physical therapist. Calling them "stingy" sounds really judgmental. Does the health club have a tipping policy displayed at the appointment desk? Soliciting tips directly, even by hinting, is unacceptable. Tipping is always at the discretion of the client. It is unethical to tie the level of service you provide to the tip you may or may not receive afterward. This is all about expectations and attitude. I suggest figuring your projected income without any tips. At the health club, I'd prefer to get paid at a good rate, like the other professionals working there, and not worry about tips.

According to the IRS, tips are taxable income and should be reported when filing income tax returns. Monetary gifts would be considered tips. Keep a record of all tips received.

SELLING PRODUCTS

Some massage therapists sell products in conjunction with their massage practices. Massage-related products include massage oils and lotions, tools for self-massage such as foot rollers, support pillows, hot and cold packs, and books and videos. Having products for sale can be a valuable service to clients and is not unethical as long as clients do not feel pressured to buy them from you. Your role as a massage therapist would be to inform clients about the benefits of the products with the opportunity to buy them, if desired. There are clearer boundaries if products for sale are not displayed in the massage room, but are in a reception or sales area (Figure 28–2 ■).

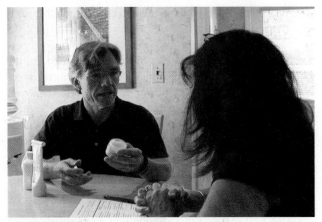

FIGURE 28–2 Educate clients about products related to massage therapy and the clients' health goals without pressuring them to buy.

Source: Pearson Education, Inc.

Selling products is often part of a spa or salon business, and employees may be expected to "push" the products for sale. This is problematic for massage therapists who are cautioned not to use the power differential in the therapeutic relationship for their personal gain. As stated earlier, educating clients and making products available is acceptable; however, talking clients into products they may not want or need is not.

Be particularly aware of your conflict of interest if you are part of a multilevel marketing program. It is not ethical to use your massage clients to meet sales goals. Clients who feel pressured into buying products outside their interest in receiving massage may also feel taken advantage of and seek massage elsewhere.

Be especially mindful if you are selling nutritional supplements, herbal preparations, or vitamins. Do not confuse being trained in selling a product by its manufacturer or distributor with having professional education in nutrition. To keep clear boundaries between your massage practice and nutritional sales, make separate appointments to talk to clients about these other products, preferably in a space different from the massage office.

Know that your massage clients may see you as a health expert and may therefore give unwarranted trust in your judgment about nutrition. Make it clear that you are not an expert in nutrition unless you have additional academic training and credentials in that field. If clients feel that you are prescribing supplements for a specific medical condition, you may be perceived as practicing medicine without a license. You may also be liable if the client has a negative reaction to a product you sold to him or her.

REFERRALS

It is expected that massage therapists make referrals to other health professionals when clients have needs outside the therapists' scope of practice, or when massage may not be the best treatment for a specific condition. A client's needs may also be beyond a particular massage therapist's training or expertise, and referral to a massage therapist with advanced or specialized training might be best for the client.

Keeping a list of other health professionals (including doctors, chiropractors, naturopathic physicians, acupuncturists, physical therapists, athletic trainers, and massage therapists) that you believe are competent and ethical is a good practice. When making referrals give the client two or three names from which to choose. Become familiar with websites that list certified practitioners of specific massage and bodywork systems or that list massage therapists and their specialties. Refer clients to those sites if appropriate.

It is unethical for health practitioners to reward each other for referrals in a quid pro quo manner with either money or gifts. For example, it would be unethical for a massage therapist to accept $10 for every referral she makes to a local chiropractor. This violates the principle of avoiding conflict of interest. Massage therapists are advised to "refuse any gifts or benefits which are intended to influence a referral, decision or treatment that are purely for personal gain and not for the good of the client."[7] The same principles apply when accepting referrals. Do not accept clients on referral that have conditions outside your scope, and do not reward referrals made to you. Clients should be able to trust that referrals are made in their best interests and not for monetary gain. A thank-you note for referrals is an appropriate acknowledgment. However, because of confidentiality issues, you might consider omitting the name of the client and just give a simple "thank you for a recent referral."

CLIENT BASE

Building a base of regular clients is the foundation of success for massage therapists, whether they are in private practice or employed somewhere like a spa. Clients will come back to massage therapists whom they respect and trust, and who give them good service.

There are a few ethical pitfalls in attracting and keeping clients. Previous sections have discussed making false claims and exceeding scope of practice. Another pitfall is trying to build yourself up by speaking poorly of another massage therapist. A wise person once said, "You don't make yourself taller by cutting down your neighbor." It is better to concentrate on the quality of what you offer than criticize a colleague to a client.

If you are employed somewhere like a spa or clinic, the clients you see there are shared by you and the larger business. It is considered unethical, and may be a violation of an employment agreement, to solicit clients seen at an employer's place for your private practice. For example, it would be unethical to say to a client, "Why don't you come for massage at my home office instead of here?" The temptation is there because you might make more money by seeing a client in your own space.

The issue of "stealing" clients can be a murky one; after all, clients have free choice regarding from whom they receive massage. They also can get attached to their massage therapists, much the same as they do to the people who cut their hair. What if a regular client requests to see you at your place for the sake of convenience? If your employment agreement explicitly prohibits seeing the company's clients at another place, then this would be unethical.

What if you are leaving an employer and your clients want to keep seeing you for massage? It would be unethical to actually make an appointment for your private practice while on your employer's premises. However, providing information about your practice, if directly asked by a client, would in most circumstances be all right. Then the client can take the initiative to call you if he or she prefers to continue as your client. The key principles here are "no solicitation," the "client's initiative," and any prior employment agreement. In complex cases like these, it is best to apply the ethical decision-making model described in Chapter 5, *Ethics and the Therapeutic Relationship*, to determine the most ethical path.

DEFAMATION

Defamation is a legal term for injury to a person or an organization's reputation. Defamation is known as *libel* if written and as *slander* if spoken. It is highly unethical to defame the character or reputation of a client or another massage therapist or health professional.

Defamation can also result in a civil lawsuit if the person defamed experiences a loss of some kind. A court may award a plaintiff monetary damages if the statements were untrue and/or made with malice or intent to harm. To avoid such issues, do not repeat malicious gossip.

Defamation laws differ slightly in different jurisdictions but usually include accusations of criminal conduct and allegations that negatively affect a person's business or profession. Stating that a person has a disease or has engaged in certain sexual activity, thus damaging his or her reputation, may also be defamation.

Descriptive statements and opinions about situations are two different things. For example, it would be better to say to a coworker that a client came for massage smelling like beer and talking with a slur than to call him a "drunk" or "lush." If the descriptive statement was made in confidence as a matter of information to protect other massage therapists, or to describe to a supervisor why you refused to work with a client at a specific appointment, it might not qualify as defamation with damages. A court of law would make its own judgment.

Remember that a client may ask to see his or her records, so what is written in them should be thought out carefully to avoid accusations of libel. It is an especially sensitive situation to report perceived misbehavior by a client, or to record something not related to the massage

CASE FOR STUDY

Rochelle and Client Choice

Rochelle started out giving massage at a local beauty salon as an independent contractor. There was a verbal agreement that she could use a spare room for appointments and split the receipts 60/40 with the salon owners. After a while, Rochelle decided that she would leave the salon and take a job at a local spa that offered better working conditions and employee benefits. She would receive a bit less income from each massage, but she figured that it was to her advantage overall. Another massage therapist is taking Rochelle's place at the salon. Massage rates are a little higher at the spa than at the salon.

Question:

Is it ethical for Rochelle to solicit her salon clients to come to the spa for massage instead of to the salon?

Things to consider:

- Are there any legal implications in this situation?
- Was there an explicit or implicit agreement with the salon about whose customers the massage clients were?

- What values are involved in a decision to solicit those clients?
- Is this situation covered in a code of ethics or standards of practice for massage therapists?
- Who might be affected by Rochelle's solicitation, either positively or negatively?
- What is Rochelle's major motivation for soliciting these clients?
- What are alternative courses of action?
- What are the most important considerations in this situation?
- What decision would maintain the highest standards?

Your reasoning and conclusions:

_____

_____

_____

_____

itself that was told in confidence in a session. It is wise to stick with accurate objective descriptions and tell a coworker or colleague immediately after something unusual happens.

It is also defamation to criticize or malign another massage therapist or health professional. If you do not trust the competence of a colleague, and for some reason wish to reveal your view to someone else, state the facts and then your opinion separately. For example, "Two of my clients have complained about massage therapist 'G' using too much pressure and bruising them. I believe that she is being insensitive."

SAFETY AND WELFARE OF CLIENTS

Massage therapists are responsible for the safety and well-being of their clients during massage sessions and while clients are on the premises. It is unethical to put clients in danger through carelessness.

Provide regular maintenance for massage tables, chairs, and other equipment. Make sure surfaces are sanitary and massage procedures hygienic. Massage offices should be well lighted and free from obstacles that could cause accidents.

Massage therapists are guilty of negligence if an accident or injury is caused by their carelessness. If the cause is something a trained practitioner is expected to know, the massage therapist may be guilty of malpractice.

To protect themselves and their clients financially, massage therapists should carry accident (slip and fall) insurance, as well as professional liability insurance. Carrying certain types of insurance may be a condition for maintaining a license to practice.

REPORTING UNETHICAL BEHAVIOR

What should massage therapists do when they suspect another massage therapist of unethical behavior? What kinds of actions are important to report? How much evidence is enough to accuse someone of wrongdoing? To whom do they report their suspicions? These are some important questions to ask before accusing someone of something that may affect that person's future as a massage therapist.

Before reporting suspected unethical behavior, a person should be clear about the facts of the case and reasonably sure that something unethical happened. If the unethical behavior is relatively minor, and the person unaware that he or she is behaving unethically, talking to the offender about the situation may be the best response. For example, if someone starts talking inappropriately about a client, make a statement such as, "This seems like gossip to me; I'd rather not continue this conversation."

Reminding a coworker or colleague of an ethical principle may be enough to stop the unethical behavior. For example, if coworkers are leaving client files open on a desk, remind them that files are confidential and should be kept secure. Friendly reminders are usually accepted well.

If, however, the situation involves physical or emotional harm to a client, or to another health professional, then more formal action may be required. Professional associations, certification commissions, and licensing agencies have procedures for reporting misconduct by professionals. Unethical conduct can result in disciplinary action against the offender, which ranges from letters of reprimand, to probation, to losing a membership or license. These actions would follow due process, investigation, and a hearing.

Passing along secondhand information is less desirable than convincing the person harmed, or a firsthand witness, to file a complaint. However, if the allegations are serious enough, and there is strong evidence for them, then they could be reported with or without firsthand information. The organization or agency receiving the report can determine if it wants to follow through with a hearing.

Where does someone report suspected unethical behavior? Serious crimes such as physical and sexual assault should be reported to the local police. The appropriate state agency should be contacted in the case of a licensed massage therapist. If misconduct involves a business practice such as deceptive advertising or a payment dispute, then a complaint can also be filed with the Better Business Bureau. The Federal Trade Commission has a complaint procedure in place for consumer protection (www.ftc.gov). Local and state governments may also have procedures for consumer complaints. Upholding the integrity of the profession by acting ethically and expecting proper behavior of colleagues is an important aspect of being a massage therapist.

CRITICAL THINKING

If your state has occupational licensing, explain in writing the process for reporting misconduct by a massage therapist. Then answer the following questions:

1. In your state, what constitutes professional misconduct?

2. What disciplinary actions might happen to a massage therapist who is proven to have engaged in misconduct?

3. How do the standards of practice and code of ethics for massage practitioners protect both the practitioner and the consumer?

BEYOND GRADUATION—AN INVITATION

The journey to becoming a successful massage therapist in some ways never ends. Beyond graduation loom the challenges of getting employment or setting up a private practice. But the reward of having meaningful and satisfying work that sustains you through the years is worth the effort.

The following "invitation" is based on similar oaths from other health professions. It summarizes important ideas to keep in mind as you start out in your new chosen profession.

Invitation to Massage Therapists

Welcome into the ranks of therapeutic massage and bodywork professionals.

May you remember your days at school with fondness and appreciation.

May you honor your teachers and all who helped you through your training.

May you serve others with compassion and humility.

May you always hold the best interests of your clients above your own personal gain.

May you behave honestly and honorably in your practice.

May you continue to seek knowledge and skill in your profession—there is always more to learn.

May you join your colleagues in protecting the practice of massage therapy.

May you value always the healing benefits of touch.

And overall, may you find fulfillment and meaning in the work of your hands.

PJB

CHAPTER HIGHLIGHTS

- Business ethics are moral and legal considerations related to commercial transactions.
- Business practices and consumer protection laws give ethical principles legal force.
- A massage therapy practice blends professional aspects related to client relationships with business aspects of the operation; in this sense, a client is also a customer.
- Massage therapists must comply with local and state laws, including occupational licensing laws, zoning ordinances, and business license and establishment license requirements.
- Design advertising to be professional and avoid deception.
  - Display credentials honestly and correctly.
  - Limit guarantees or promises about massage therapy, and use endorsements and testimonials sparingly.
  - Advertised prices must be honored, discounts defined clearly, and bait advertising avoided.
- Claims for massage therapy must be honest and truthful and backed up by research if possible.
  - Qualify claims by citing sources of information such as textbooks or experience.
- Copyright, trademark, and patent laws protect intellectual property rights. Never claim another person's work as your own, and do follow principles of fair use.
  - Massage therapists may not use trademarked names for massage and bodywork unless they hold proper authorization.
- Charging more for a massage when an insurance company is paying is considered unethical and may also be illegal.
- Accepting tips or gifts is acceptable under certain circumstances.
  - Tips are taxable income to be reported when filing income tax returns.

○ Refuse tips and gifts if there are unethical expectations attached, and never accept gifts from clients who may have romantic intentions.

- Selling products as part of a massage practice may be ethical if done properly.
  ○ Educating clients about useful products is acceptable, but pressuring them to buy is not.
  ○ Massage clients should not be used to meet sales quotas.
  ○ Special care about scope of practice is warranted when selling nutritional products.

- Refer clients to other qualified health professionals for treatment beyond the scope of a massage therapist's own knowledge and skills.
  ○ Receiving money or gifts from another health professional for referrals is considered a conflict of interest and is unethical.

- When building a client base, emphasize the quality of your service, rather than criticizing other massage therapists.
- Do not solicit clients of an employer's business for your own private practice.

- Defamation—injury to another's reputation—is called libel if written and slander if spoken. Defamation can result in a civil lawsuit if the person defamed experiences a loss.
  ○ It is safer to keep to descriptive statements of something that happened rather than give interpretations or opinions.
  ○ Clients are entitled to see their records, so massage therapists should be especially careful about what is written in them.

- It is unethical to put clients in danger through carelessness or negligence.
  ○ Keep premises and equipment clean and well maintained.

- Massage therapists should talk to each other about minor or unintentional unethical behaviors.
- Report suspected serious unethical behavior by other massage therapists to proper authorities, such as a state licensing agency or the local police.
- Acting ethically and expecting proper behavior of colleagues is an important aspect of being a professional massage therapist.

EXAM REVIEW

Key Terms

Match the following key terms to their descriptions. For additional study, look up the key terms in the Interactive Glossary, and note other terms that compare or contrast with them.

_____ **1.** Business ethics
_____ **2.** Copyright
_____ **3.** Deceptive advertising
_____ **4.** Defamation
_____ **5.** Endorsements
_____ **6.** Guarantee
_____ **7.** Massage establishment ordinance
_____ **8.** Occupational license
_____ **9.** Qualifying statements
_____ **10.** Trademarks

a. Anecdotes from someone besides the massage therapist about how well the massage worked for them
b. Credential issued by a government that gives a person permission to practice a profession in its jurisdiction
c. Local government regulations that cover hours of operation, sanitation, and other aspects of a massage therapy business
d. A promise that something will work as stated, usually with the implication that the money will be refunded if it does not
e. Moral and legal considerations related to commercial transactions and fair treatment of consumers
f. Citing sources of information to substantiate claims about the benefits of massage therapy
g. Offer exclusive use of a name or symbol to identify unique goods and services
h. Protects written, musical, and artistic works from unauthorized use
i. Misleading the public about credentials, the nature of the service, its benefits, or how much it costs
j. Legal term for injury to a person or an organization's reputation

Memory Workout

To test your memory of the main concepts in this chapter, complete the following sentences by circling the most correct answer from the two choices provided.

1. Business ethics are moral and legal considerations related to (commercial) (banking) transactions.
2. Massage therapists can mislead the public by being (truthful) (vague) about their qualifications or by wording their qualifications (incorrectly) (in Latin).
3. Information should be (left) (spelled) out completely if using initials after a name would be misleading.
4. The FTC states that endorsements "may not contain any representation which would be deceptive, or could not be (broadcast) (substantiated)."
5. Advertising something for a certain price, and then pressuring the client/customer to buy something more expensive is called (bait) (smart) advertising.

6. Claims about massage should be qualified by citing (sound bites) (sources) of information.
7. Massage therapists may not use (trademarked) (copyrighted) names for forms of bodywork, unless they have earned the appropriate credentials.
8. Tips that should be turned down are ones with (gratitude) (expectations) attached, or that are too (large) (small).
9. Do not confuse being trained in selling a nutritional product by its manufacturer or distributor with having (sales experience) (professional education) in nutrition.
10. It is unethical for health professionals to (reward) (thank) each other for referrals.
11. It is unethical to (solicit) (talk to) clients seen first at an employer's business.

Test Prep

The following multiple-choice questions will help to prepare you for future school and professional exams.

1. Consumer protection laws are designed to:
   a. Ensure a minimum level of training for professionals
   b. Regulate where certain types of businesses can be located
   c. Protect the public from unsafe products and deceptive advertising
   d. Protect employees from unfair employment situations

2. When a seller makes a promise that something will work as stated, with the implication that the money will be refunded if it does not, it is called:
   a. Endorsement
   b. Guarantee
   c. Testimonial
   d. Bait advertising

3. Which of the following is the most ethical method of advertising to clients that you have graduated from a massage therapy program?
   a. Spelling out "Graduate of ABC Massage Therapy School"
   b. Using the initials "GMT" after your name to designate "graduate massage therapist"
   c. Using the initials "CMT" after your name to designate "certified massage therapist"
   d. Any of the above

4. Which of the following offers legal protection for the exclusive use of a name or symbol to identify unique goods and services?
   a. Copyright
   b. Trademark
   c. Patent
   d. Licensing

5. When is it ethical to pressure massage clients to buy goods you have for sale?
   a. When you must meet a sales goal
   b. When you are sure that they will benefit from the product
   c. When you need to reduce inventory
   d. Never

6. Slander is:
   a. Gossiping about someone
   b. Publicly criticizing someone's behavior
   c. Causing injury to someone's reputation by something written
   d. Causing injury to someone's reputation by something spoken

7. If an accident or injury results from carelessness, it is called:
   a. Libel
   b. Negligence
   c. Unfortunate
   d. An act of God

8. When is it ethical to give reduced service to a client who never leaves a tip?
   a. At spas where tipping is customary
   b. When a "tips accepted" sign is clearly visible
   c. When saving energy for clients who do tip
   d. Never

Video Challenge

Watch this video, which can be found at MyHealthProfessionsLab.com, Chapter 28, and then answer the following questions.

Business Ethics

1. What are the ethical principles related to advertising discussed in the video?

2. What do the massage therapists in the video say regarding when accepting tips is ethical and when to turn them down?
3. What types of products might massage therapists sell to clients? What are some ethical principles related to selling products mentioned in the video?

Comprehension Exercises

The following short-answer questions test your knowledge and understanding of chapter topics and provide practice in written communication skills. Explain in two to four complete sentences.

1. What types of laws must massage therapists be aware of for building ethical practices? What is the over-reaching ethical principle related to laws?

2. What does the law say about making claims for a product or service? How do you qualify claims made for massage? Give an example.
3. When is it *not* ethical to accept tips from clients? What is the ethical principle related to soliciting tips?

For Greater Understanding

The following exercises are designed to take you from the realm of theory into the real world. They will help you give a deeper understanding of the subjects covered in this chapter. Action words are underlined to emphasize the variety of activities presented to address different learning styles and to encourage deeper thinking.

1. Tell the class or a study partner about a time you were treated unfairly or dishonestly in a business transaction. Analyze what happened in ethical and legal terms. Were consumer protection laws or any other laws broken?

2. Speak to the class or a study partner about a time you were given a gift that didn't feel right to you (i.e., with expectations attached or too costly given your relationship with the person). Analyze the person's motivation and your response. Was the outcome positive or negative? Would you act differently today?

3. Tell the class or study partner about a time you felt pressured to buy something. Analyze the motivation of the seller and how you felt being pressured.

4. Obtain a copy of an employment agreement for a massage therapist at a spa or clinic. Analyze provisions for soliciting clients, and discuss it in terms of fairness or unfairness.

MyHealthProfessionsLab™

MyHealthProfessionsLab.com is a premium online homework management system that includes a host of features to help you study. Registered users will find:

- Powerful tools that track and analyze your results—allowing you to create a personalized learning experience
- Videos, flashcards and other learning tools to help enrich your progress
- Streaming lesson presentations and self-paced learning modules
- A space where you and your instructors can view and manage your assignments

Organizations and Publications

ORGANIZATIONS

Alliance for Massage Therapy Education (AFMTE)
1232 Bonefish Court
Fort Pierce, FL 34949
(855) 236–8331
www.afmte.org

American Massage Therapy Association (AMTA)
500 Davis Street, Suite 900
Evanston, IL 60201
(877) 905–0577
www.amtamassage.org

American Organization for Bodywork Therapies of Asia
   (AOBTA)
P.O. Box 343
West Berlin, NJ 08091
(856) 809–2953
www.aobta.org

American Polarity Therapy Association (APTA)
122 North Elm Street, Suite 504
Greensboro, NC 27401
(336) 574–1121
www.polaritytherapy.org

Associated Bodywork & Massage Professionals (ABMP)
25188 Genesee Trail Road
Golden, CO 80401
(800) 458–2267
www.abmp.com

Canadian Massage Therapists Alliance (CMTA)
16-1724 Quebec Avenue
Saskatoon SK S7K 1V9
(306) 384–7077
www.crmta.ca

Canadian Touch Research Center
760 Saint-Zotique Street East
Montreal, Quebec, Canada H2S 1M5
(514) 272–2254
www.ccrt-ctrc.ca

Center for Compassionate Touch
610 East University Street
Springfield, MO 65807
(417) 844–8514
www.compassionate-touch.org

Commission on Massage Therapy Accreditation (COMTA)
5335 Wisconsin Avenue, NW, Suite 440
Washington, D.C. 20015
(202) 888–6790
www.comta.org

Federation of State Massage Therapy Boards (FSMTB)
10801 Mastin Boulevard, Suite 420
Overland Park, KS 66223
(913) 681–0380
www.fsmtb.org

International Institute of Reflexology, Inc.
5650 First Avenue North
P.O. Box 12642
St. Petersburg, FL 33733-2642
(727) 343–4811
www.reflexology-usa.net

International Loving Touch Foundation (infant massage)
   Certified Infant Massage Instructor (CIMI®) Training
2122 S.E. Division Street
Portland, OR 97202
(800) 929–7492 or (503) 253–8482
www.lovingtouch.com

International Spa Association (ISPA)
2365 Harrodsburg Road, Suite A325
Lexington, KY 40504
(888) 651–4772
www.experienceispa.com

Massage Therapy Foundation (MTF)
500 Davis Street, Suite 950
Evanston, IL 60201
(847) 869–5019
www.massagetherapyfoundation.org

National Center of Complementary and Alternative
Medicine (NCCAM)
National Institutes of Health
9000 Rockville Pike
Bethesda, Maryland 20892
(888) 644–6226
www.nccam.nih.gov

National Certification Board for Therapeutic Massage and
Bodywork (NCBTMB)
1333 Burr Ridge Parkway
Burr Ridge, IL 60527
(800) 296–0664
www.ncbtmb.com

National Certification Commission for Acupuncture and
Oriental Medicine (NCCAOM)
76 South Laura Street, Suite 1290
Jacksonville, FL 32202
(904) 598–1005
www.nccaom.org

National Association of Nurse Massage Therapists
(NANMT)
P.O. Box 406
Long Beach, MS 39560
(855) 366–2668
www.nanmt.org

Therapeutic Touch® International Association
TTIA Box 130
Delmar, NY 12054
(518) 325–1185
www.therapeutic-touch.org

Rolf Institute® of Structural Integration
5055 Chaparral Court, Suite 103
Boulder, CO 80301
(800) 530–8875 or (303) 449–5903
www.rolf.org

The Stone Institute LLC—Reflexology
2025 Zumbehl Road #20
St. Charles, MO 63303
(636) 724–8686
www.thestoneinstitute.org

TouchPro International (Chair Massage)
153 Buena Vista Avenue E
San Francisco, CA 94117
(800) 999–5026
www.TouchPro.com

Touch Research Institutes (TRI)
University of Miami Miller School of Medicine
Mailman Center for Child Development
Miami, FL
(305) 243–6781
www.miami.edu/touch-research

PERIODICAL PUBLICATIONS

Peer-Reviewed Journals

International Journal of Therapeutic Massage & Bodywork: Research, Education & Practice (Open access publication of the Massage Therapy Foundation)
    www.massagetherapyfoundation.org
Journal of Bodywork and Movement Therapies
    www.elsevier.com

Trade Publications

Massage Therapy Journal
    www.amtamassage.org/journal/home.html
Massage & Bodywork
    www.massageandbodywork.com
Massage Magazine
    www.massagemag.com
Massage Today
    www.massagetoday.com

Code of Ethics and Standards of Practice for Massage Therapists

CODE OF ETHICS—NATIONAL CERTIFICATION BOARD FOR THERAPEUTIC MASSAGE & BODYWORK

Revised October 2008
©2007 National Certification Board
for Therapeutic Massage & Bodywork

NCBTMB certificants and applicants for certification shall act in a manner that justifies public trust and confidence, enhances the reputation of the profession, and safeguards the interest of individual clients. Certificants and applicants for certification will:

I. Have a sincere commitment to provide the highest quality of care to those who seek their professional services.

II. Represent their qualifications honestly, including education and professional affiliations, and provide only those services that they are qualified to perform.

III. Accurately inform clients, other health care practitioners, and the public of the scope and limitations of their discipline.

IV. Acknowledge the limitations of and contraindications for massage and bodywork and refer clients to appropriate health professionals.

V. Provide treatment only where there is reasonable expectation that it will be advantageous to the client.

VI. Consistently maintain and improve professional knowledge and competence, striving for professional excellence through regular assessment of personal and professional strengths and weaknesses and through continued education training.

VII. Conduct their business and professional activities with honesty and integrity, and respect the inherent worth of all persons.

VIII. Refuse to unjustly discriminate against clients and/or health professionals.

IX. Safeguard the confidentiality of all client information, unless disclosure is requested by the client in writing, is medically necessary, is required by law, or necessary for the protection of the public.

X. Respect the client's right to treatment with informed and voluntary consent. The certified practitioner will obtain and record the informed consent of the client, or client's advocate, before providing treatment. This consent may be written or verbal.

XI. Respect the client's right to refuse, modify, or terminate treatment regardless of prior consent given.

XII. Provide draping and treatment in a way that ensures the safety, comfort, and privacy of the client.

XIII. Exercise the right to refuse to treat any person or part of the body for just and reasonable cause.

XIV. Refrain, under all circumstances, from initiating or engaging in any sexual conduct, sexual activities, or sexualizing behavior involving a client, even if the client attempts to sexualize the relationship unless a preexisting relationship exists between an applicant or a practitioner and the client prior to the applicant or practitioner applying to be certified by NCBTMB.

XV. Avoid any interest, activity, or influence which might be in conflict with the practitioner's obligation to act in the best interests of the client or the profession.

XVI. Respect the client's boundaries with regard to privacy, disclosure, exposure, emotional expression, beliefs, and the client's reasonable expectations of professional behavior. Practitioners will respect the client's autonomy.

XVII. Refuse any gifts or benefits that are intended to influence a referral, decision, or treatment, or that are purely for personal gain and not for the good of the client.

XVIII. Follow the NCBTMB Standards of Practice, this Code of Ethics, and all policies, procedures, guidelines, regulations, codes, and requirements promulgated by the National Certification Board for Therapeutic Massage and Bodywork.

STANDARDS OF PRACTICE—NATIONAL CERTIFICATION BOARD FOR THERAPEUTIC MASSAGE & BODYWORK

Revised October 2009
©2007 National Certification Board
for Therapeutic Massage & Bodywork

Background

The purpose of the National Certification Board for Therapeutic Massage and Bodywork (NCBTMB) is to foster high standards of ethical and professional practice in the delivery of services through a recognized credible certification program that assures the competency of practitioners of therapeutic massage and bodywork.

These Standards of Practice ensure that certificants and applicants for certification are aware of, and committed to, upholding high standards of practice for the profession. Also, the Standards of Practice are meant to assist members of the general public, including consumers, other health care professionals, and State and Municipal Regulatory Agencies or Boards with understanding the duties and responsibilities of NCBTMB certificants and applicants for certification.

The NCBTMB developed and adopted the Standards of Practice to provide certificants and applicants for certification with a clear statement of the expectations of professional conduct and level of practice afforded the public in, among other things, the following areas: Professionalism, Legal and Ethical Requirements, Confidentiality, Business Practices, Roles and Boundaries, and Prevention of Sexual Misconduct. These Standards of Practice were approved and ratified by the NCBTMB Board of Directors, representatives of the certificant population, and key stakeholders of the NCBTMB.

Preamble

These Standards of Practice for the profession of therapeutic massage and bodywork are the guiding principles by which certificants and applicants for certification conduct their day-to-day responsibilities within their scope of practice. These principles help to assure that all professional behaviors are conducted in the most ethical, compassionate, and responsible manner. Through these Standards of Practice, NCBTMB seeks to establish and uphold the highest standards, traditions, and principles of the practices that constitute the profession of therapeutic massage and bodywork. The Standards are enforceable guidelines for professional conduct, and therefore, are stated in observable and measurable terms intended as minimum levels of practice to which certificants and applicants for certification are held accountable. Upon submission of the application for the National Certification Examinations, each applicant for certification must agree to uphold and abide by the NCBTMB Code of Ethics, Standards of Practice, and applicable policies. Certificants

or applicants for certification's failure to comply with the Code of Ethics and the Standards of Practice as provided herein constitutes professional misconduct and may result in sanctions, or other appropriate disciplinary actions, including the suspension or revocation of certification.

NCBTMB certificants and applicants for certification are obligated to report unethical behavior and violations of the Code of Ethics and/or the Standards of Practice they reasonably and in good faith believe have been performed by other NCBTMB certificants and applicants for certification to NCBTMB.

These Standards of Practice reflect NCBTMB's clear commitment that certificants and applicants for certification provide an optimal level of service and strive for excellence in their practice. This includes remaining in good standing with NCBTMB, committing to continued personal and professional growth through continuing education, and understanding and accepting that personal and professional actions reflect on the integrity of the therapeutic massage and bodywork profession and NCBTMB. Certificants and applicants for certification are responsible for showing and maintaining professional compliance with the Standards of Practice.

NCBTMB requires certificants and applicants for certification to conduct themselves in a highly professional and dignified manner. NCBTMB will not consider and/or adjudicate complaints against certificants and applicants for certification that are based solely on consumer related issues or are based on competitive marketplace issues.

As the therapeutic massage and bodywork profession evolves, so, too, will the Standards of Practice. The Standards of Practice are, therefore, a live and dynamic document and subject to revision in keeping with the changing demands and expectations of the therapeutic massage and bodywork profession.

Standards of Practice

STANDARD I: PROFESSIONALISM

The certificant or applicant for certification must provide optimal levels of professional therapeutic massage and bodywork services and demonstrate excellence in practice by promoting healing and well-being through responsible, compassionate, and respectful touch. In his/her professional role the certificant or applicant for certification shall:

a. Adhere to the NCBTMB Code of Ethics, Standards of Practice, policies, and procedures

b. Comply with the peer review process conducted by the NCBTMB Ethics and Standards Committee regarding any alleged violations of the NCBTMB Code of Ethics and Standards of Practice

c. Treat each client with respect, dignity, and worth

d. Use professional verbal, nonverbal, and written communications

e. Provide an environment that is safe and comfortable for the client and which, at a minimum, meets all legal requirements for health and safety

f. Use standard precautions to ensure professional hygienic practices and maintain a level of personal hygiene appropriate for practitioners in the therapeutic setting

g. Wear clothing that is clean, modest, and professional

h. Obtain voluntary and informed consent from the client prior to initiating the session

i. If applicable, conduct an accurate needs assessment, develop a plan of care with the client, and update the plan as needed

j. Use appropriate draping to protect the client's physical and emotional privacy

k. Be knowledgeable of his/her scope of practice and practice only within these limitations

l. Refer to other professionals when in the best interest of the client and practitioner

m. Seek other professional advice when needed

n. Respect the traditions and practices of other professionals and foster collegial relationships

o. Not falsely impugn the reputation of any colleague

p. Use the initials NCTMB only to designate his/her professional ability and competency to practice therapeutic massage and bodywork, or the initials NCTM only to designate his/her professional ability and competency to practice therapeutic massage

q. Remain in good standing with NCBTMB

r. Understand that the NCBTMB certificate may be displayed prominently in the certificant's principal place of practice

s. Use the NCBTMB logo and certification number on business cards, brochures, advertisements, and stationery only in a manner that is within established NCBTMB guidelines

t. Not duplicate the NCBTMB certificate for purposes other than verification of the practitioner's credentials

u. Immediately return the certificate to NCBTMB if certification is revoked

v. Inform NCBTMB of any changes or additions to information included in his/her application for NCBTMB certification or recertification.

STANDARD II: LEGAL AND ETHICAL REQUIREMENTS

The certificant or applicant must comply with all the legal requirements in applicable jurisdictions regulating the profession of therapeutic massage and bodywork. In his/her professional role the certificant or applicant shall:

a. Obey all applicable local, state, and federal laws

b. Refrain from any behavior that results in illegal, discriminatory, or unethical actions

c. Accept responsibility for his/her own actions

d. Report to the proper authorities any alleged violations of the law by other certificants or applicants for certification

e. Maintain accurate and truthful records

f. Report to NCBTMB any criminal conviction of, or plea of guilty, nolo contendere, or no contest to, a crime in any jurisdiction (other than a minor traffic offense) by him/herself and by other certificants or applicants for certification

g. Report to NCBTMB any pending litigation and resulting resolution related to the certificant or applicant for certification's professional practice and the professional practice of other certificants or applicants for certification

h. Report to NCBTMB any pending complaints in any state or local government or quasi-government board or agency against his/her professional conduct or competence, or that of another certificant, and the resulting resolution of such complaint

i. Respect existing publishing rights and copyright laws, including, but not limited to, those that apply to NCBTMB's copyright-protected examinations.

STANDARD III: CONFIDENTIALITY

The certificant or applicant for certification shall respect the confidentiality of client information and safeguard all records. In his/her professional role the certificant or applicant for certification shall:

a. Protect the confidentiality of the client's identity in conversations, all advertisements, and any and all other matters unless disclosure of identifiable information is requested by the client in writing, is medically necessary, is required by law or for purposes of public protection

b. Protect the interests of clients who are minors or who are unable to give voluntary and informed consent by securing permission from an appropriate third party or guardian

c. Solicit only information that is relevant to the professional client/therapist relationship

d. Share pertinent information about the client with third parties when required by law or for purposes of public protection

e. Maintain the client files for a minimum period of four years

f. Store and dispose of client files in a secure manner.

STANDARD IV: BUSINESS PRACTICES

The certificant or applicant shall practice with honesty, integrity, and lawfulness in the business of therapeutic massage and bodywork. In his/her professional role the certificant or applicant shall:

a. Provide a physical setting that is safe and meets all applicable legal requirements for health and safety

b. Maintain adequate and customary liability insurance

c. Maintain adequate progress notes for each client session, if applicable

d. Accurately and truthfully inform the public of services provided

e. Honestly represent all professional qualifications and affiliations

f. Promote his/her business with integrity and avoid potential and actual conflicts of interest

g. Advertise in a manner that is honest, dignified, accurate and representative of services that can be delivered and remains consistent with the NCBTMB Code of Ethics and Standards of Practice

h. Advertise in a manner that is not misleading to the public and shall not use sensational, sexual, or provocative language and/or pictures to promote business

i. Comply with all laws regarding sexual harassment

j. Not exploit the trust and dependency of others, including clients and employees/coworkers

k. Display/discuss a schedule of fees in advance of the session that is clearly understood by the client or potential client

l. Make financial arrangements in advance that are clearly understood by and safeguard the best interests of the client or consumer

m. Follow acceptable accounting practices

n. File all applicable municipal, state, and federal taxes

o. Maintain accurate financial records, contracts and legal obligations, appointment records, tax reports, and receipts for at least four years.

STANDARD V: ROLES AND BOUNDARIES

The certificant or applicant for certification shall adhere to ethical boundaries and perform the professional roles designed to protect both the client and the practitioner, and safeguard the therapeutic value of the relationship. In his/her professional role the certificant or applicant for certification shall:

a. Recognize his/her personal limitations and practice only within these limitations

b. Recognize his/her influential position with the client and not exploit the relationship for personal or other gain

c. Recognize and limit the impact of transference and countertransference between the client and the certificant

d. Avoid dual or multidimensional relationships that could impair professional judgment or result in exploitation of the client or employees and/or coworkers

e. Not engage in any sexual activity with a client

f. Acknowledge and respect the client's freedom of choice in the therapeutic session

g. Respect the client's right to refuse the therapeutic session or any part of the therapeutic session

h. Refrain from practicing under the influence of alcohol, drugs, or any illegal substances (with the exception of a prescribed dosage of prescription medication which does not significantly impair the certificant)

i. Have the right to refuse and/or terminate the service to a client who is abusive or under the influence of alcohol, drugs, or any illegal substance.

STANDARD VI: PREVENTION OF SEXUAL MISCONDUCT

The certificant or applicant for certification shall refrain from any behavior that sexualizes, or appears to sexualize, the client/therapist relationship. The certificant or applicant

for certification recognizes the intimacy of the therapeutic relationship may activate practitioner and/or client needs and/or desires that weaken objectivity and may lead to sexualizing the therapeutic relationship. In his/her professional role the certificant or applicant shall:

a. Refrain from participating in a sexual relationship or sexual conduct with the client, whether consensual or otherwise, from the beginning of the client/therapist relationship and for a minimum of six months after the termination of the client/therapist relationship unless a preexisting relationship exists between a certificant or applicant for certification and client prior to the certificant or applicant for certification applying to be certified by NCBTMB

b. In the event that the client initiates sexual behavior, clarify the purpose of the therapeutic session, and, if such conduct does not cease, terminate or refuse the session

c. Recognize that sexual activity with clients, students, employees, supervisors, or trainees is prohibited even if consensual

d. Do not touch the genitalia

e. Only perform therapeutic treatments beyond the normal narrowing of the ear canal and normal narrowing of the nasal passages as indicated in the plan of care and only after receiving informed voluntary written consent

f. Only perform therapeutic treatments in the oropharynx as indicated in the plan of care and only after receiving informed voluntary consent

g. Only perform therapeutic treatments into the anal canal as indicated in the plan of care and only after receiving informed voluntary written consent

h. Only provide therapeutic breast massage as indicated in the plan of care and only after receiving informed voluntary consent from the client.

Glossary of Terms Used in This Document

Acceptable Accounting Procedures: Rules, conventions, standards, and procedures that are widely accepted among financial accountants.

Boundary: A boundary is a limit that separates one person from another. Its function is to protect the integrity of each person.

Competency: Study and development of a particular professional knowledge base and skills associated with and applied in practice within that knowledge base.

Countertransference: A practitioner's unresolved feelings and issues which are unconsciously transferred to the client.

Dignity: The quality or state of being worthy, honored or esteemed.

Dual Relationships: An alliance in addition to the client/therapist relationship, such as social, familial, business, or any other relationship that is outside the therapeutic relationship.

Genitalia, Female: Labia majora, labia minora, clitoris, and vaginal orifice.

Genitalia, Male: Testes, penis, and scrotum.

Impugn: To assail by words or arguments, oppose or attack as false.

Integrity: Honesty. Firm adherence to a code of values.

Multidimensional Relationships: Overlapping relationships in which therapist and client share an alliance, in addition to the therapeutic relationship.

Progress Notes: Notes written, by a practitioner certified by NCBTMB, and kept in a separate client file that indicates the date of the session, areas of complaint as stated by client, and observations made and actions taken by the practitioner.

Scope of Practice: The minimum standards necessary for safe and effective practice and the parameters of practice determined by the certificant's professional training and education, and, when applicable, regulatory bodies.

Sexual Activity: Any verbal and/or nonverbal behavior for the purpose of soliciting, receiving, or giving sexual gratification.

Sexual Harassment: Sexual harassment consists of unwelcome sexual advances, requests for sexual favors, and other verbal or physical conduct of a sexual nature when: 1. Submission to such conduct is made either explicitly or implicitly a term or condition of an individual's employment; 2. Submission to, or rejection of, such conduct by an individual is used as the basis for employment decisions affecting such individuals; or 3. Such conduct has the purpose or effect of unreasonably interfering with an individual's work performance or creating an intimidating, hostile, or offensive working environment.

Therapeutic Breast Massage: Manipulation of the nonmuscular soft tissue structure of the breast up to and including the areola and nipple.

Transference: The displacement or transfer of feelings, thoughts, and behaviors originally related to a significant person, such as a parent, onto someone else, such as a massage therapist (or doctor, psychotherapist, teacher, spiritual advisor).

Goal-Oriented Planning

LONG-TERM PLANNING—INITIAL SESSION AND ONGOING EVALUATION

1. Gather information from the client.
   - Review intake form.
   - Review health history form.
   - Conduct interview.

2. Collect information through observation and measurement.
   - Observe client (e.g., general posture, motion, expression, stress level).
   - Conduct tests and measurements related to stated goals or complaint.

3. Assess the overall situation and establish long-term goals.
   - Identify wellness goals that can be addressed with massage.
   - Identify problems for which massage is indicated.
   - Identify contraindications and cautions.
   - Prioritize goals together with the client.

4. Develop an action plan to achieve long-term goals.
   - Suggest frequency and length of massage sessions.
   - Determine general massage approaches to use.
   - Set a date for evaluating progress on specific goals.
   - Suggest home care to help achieve goals (e.g., self-massage, hot and cold applications, stretching, exercises, relaxation techniques).

5. Implement the long-term plan.
   - Make appointments.
   - Provide client with information or tools for home care.

6. Evaluate progress toward long-term goals.
   - Write SOAP notes to document the long-term plan.
   - Adjust the long-term plan as needed to achieve original client goals and/or set new or modified goals.
   - Set date for evaluating progress toward long-term goals.

INDIVIDUAL SESSION PLANNING

1. Gather information from the client, and review previous documentation.
   - Review intake and health history forms.
   - Review notes from previous sessions.
   - Conduct presession interview.
     - Ask about changes in health status or medications.
     - Ask about progress or regression since previous session.

2. Collect information through observation and measurement.
   - Observe the client (e.g., general posture, motion, expression).
   - Palpation and simple measurements during the session.

3. Assess the situation and set session goals.
   - Identify current client state and next step to reach long-term goals.
   - Prioritize goals for the session.
   - Determine cautions and contraindications for this session.

4. Develop a general plan for the session.
   - Plan session organization, including body areas to be addressed, and in what order to apply massage.
   - Choose general approach to use in the session (e.g., relaxation massage, trigger points, myofascial massage, lymph drainage massage, polarity therapy).
   - Determine use of adjunct methods (e.g., hot or cold applications, aromatherapy, electronic vibration device).

5. Implement the session plan.
   - Apply massage and related techniques.

6. Evaluate progress toward the session goals.
   - Ongoing evaluation during session.
   - Postsession evaluation (e.g., postsession observations, postsession client interview).
   - Ongoing adjustments during the massage session.
   - Write SOAP notes to document the session.

TREATMENT PLANNING—FOR TREATMENT AND RECOVERY FROM ILLNESS OR INJURY

1. Gather information from client related to the illness, injury, or complaint.
   - Review intake form.
   - Review medical history.
   - Review medical diagnosis if available.
   - Conduct initial interview.
     - Onset of condition
     - Symptoms
     - Degree of pain
     - Functional limitations
     - Activities of daily living (ADL) affected
     - First aid or home remedies applied
     - What seems to make it better or worse

2. Collect information related to the illness or injury through observation and measurement.
   - Observe general state of client (e.g., facial expression, voice quality, energy level).
   - Take measurements relative to the complaint or diagnosed condition (e.g., standing posture, sitting posture, walking gait, body mechanics, range of motion at specific joints).
   - Visual observation of skin (e.g., color, bruises, swelling, pitting, scars, moles, wounds, rashes).
   - Palpation of soft tissues in specific areas (e.g., texture [degree of oiliness or dryness], temperature, pliability, firmness, adhesion, fibrosis, puffiness, springiness).
   - Palpation of muscle and tendon structures (e.g., firmness, shape, tension, atrophy or wasting, taut bands in muscle tissue, trigger points, taut tendons).
   - Palpation of movement (e.g., ease of movement, crepitations).
   - Orthopedic tests for specific pathologies.

3. Assess the situation and set treatment goals.
   - Determine the condition of tissues.
   - Determine function or loss of function.
   - Identify contraindications and cautions for massage therapy.
   - Determine how massage can alleviate symptoms or facilitate healing.
   - Set anatomical, physiological, and/or functional treatment goals.

4. Develop a treatment action plan.
   - Suggest the frequency and length of massage sessions.
   - Choose a general approach to reach goals (e.g., Swedish massage, myofascial massage, neuromuscular therapy, lymphatic massage, foot reflexology, polarity therapy).
   - Set a date for evaluating progress on specific goals.
   - Suggest home care (e.g., self-massage, hot and cold applications, stretching, exercises, relaxation techniques).

5. Implement the treatment plan.
   - Make appointments.
   - Provide client with information or tools for home care.

6. Evaluate progress toward healing and recovery.
   - Adjust the treatment plan as needed to achieve goals for healing and recovery.
   - Write SOAP notes to document the treatment plan.

Performance Evaluation Forms

INSTRUCTIONS

Use these Performance Evaluation Forms to track your progress in learning massage techniques and to prepare for upcoming practical exams. Rate yourself, or have a practice partner rate you, on how well you performed the techniques and Practice Sequences presented throughout this text. The instructor can also use these forms to measure your accomplishments.

There is a Performance Evaluation Form in this appendix for individual Swedish massage techniques, joint movements, and every Practice Sequence in this text. If you prefer, the Performance Evaluation Forms can be downloaded from MyHealthProfessionsLab.com.

HOW TO EVALUATE YOUR PERFORMANCE

Before the performance evaluation, look over the form to see what elements are listed. This helps identify what the evaluator will be looking for. Review the chapters for descriptions of techniques listed and other important information related to their application. Make notes about points you want to remember. Review the video for the Practice Sequence or techniques you are going to evaluate. Look closely for items mentioned on the evaluation form.

When practicing for a practical exam, add items emphasized by your instructor in class if you do not see them listed on the form. Note that some elements are common to almost all forms, for example, client communication, positioning, draping, and body mechanics. Others are unique to a particular form of massage and bodywork.

Evaluation is done by using a rating scale from 0 to 5. Although this is somewhat subjective, it provides a measurement for seeing progress over time. Be honest about how you are doing. Work on skills that need improvement. Aim for achieving ratings of good (4) or excellent (5) for all items listed.

PERFORMANCE EVALUATION FORM 10–1

Hygienic Hand Washing

Student: _____ Date: _____

Scoring Key: 0 = incorrect; 1 = very poor; 2 = poor; 3 = adequate; 4 = good; 5 = excellent

1. Wet hands and forearms up to elbows. Water flows from elbows to hands and off of fingertips.

   0   1   2   3   4   5

2. Scrub nails to loosen dirt. Clean the surface and under the nails.

   0   1   2   3   4   5

3. Apply soap and create soapy lather up to the elbows. Include finger and thumb webs.

   0   1   2   3   4   5

4. Rub hands and arms for at least 15 seconds.

   0   1   2   3   4   5

5. Rinse off soap from fingertips to elbows. Water flows off of elbows.

   0   1   2   3   4   5

6. Dry hands thoroughly with paper towels.

   0   1   2   3   4   5

7. Use the same paper towel to turn off the faucet, and if applicable, open the door handle to the massage room.

   0   1   2   3   4   5

8. Discard the paper towel in a proper receptacle.

   0   1   2   3   4   5

Total points _____ / 8 = _____ Average Rating

Evaluated by: _____

PERFORMANCE EVALUATION FORM 12–1
Individual Swedish Massage Techniques

Student: _____ Date: _____

Scoring Key: 0 = incorrect; 1 = very poor; 2 = poor; 3 = adequate; 4 = good; 5 = excellent

Effleurage

1. Basic sliding effleurage.

    0   1   2   3   4   5

2. Stripping.

    0   1   2   3   4   5

3. Shingles effleurage.

    0   1   2   3   4   5

4. Bilateral tree stroking.

    0   1   2   3   4   5

5. Three-count stroking of the trapezius.

    0   1   2   3   4   5

6. Horizontal stroking.

    0   1   2   3   4   5

7. Mennell's superficial stroking.

    0   1   2   3   4   5

8. Nerve strokes.

    0   1   2   3   4   5

9. Knuckling.

    0   1   2   3   4   5

Petrissage

10. Basic two-handed kneading.

    0   1   2   3   4   5

11. One-handed kneading.

    0   1   2   3   4   5

12. Circular two-handed petrissage.

    0   1   2   3   4   5

13. Fingers-to-thumb petrissage.

    0   1   2   3   4   5

14. Skin lifting.

    0   1   2   3   4   5

15. Compression.

    0   1   2   3   4   5

16. Rolling.

    0   1   2   3   4   5

Friction

17. Superficial warming friction with the palms.

    0   1   2   3   4   5

18. Superficial warming friction—sawing (ulnar friction).

    0   1   2   3   4   5

19. Superficial warming friction with the knuckles.

    0   1   2   3   4   5

20. Cross-fiber deep friction.

    0   1   2   3   4   5

21. Circular deep friction.

    0   1   2   3   4   5

22. Deep transverse (Cyriax) friction.

    0   1   2   3   4   5

Tapotement

23. Hacking.

    0   1   2   3   4   5

24. Rapping.

    0   1   2   3   4   5

25. Cupping.

    0   1   2   3   4   5

26. Clapping.

    0   1   2   3   4   5

27. Slapping.

    0   1   2   3   4   5

28. Tapping.

    0   1   2   3   4   5

29. Quacking.

    0   1   2   3   4   5

30. Squishes.

    0   1   2   3   4   5

Vibration

31. Fine vibration with electric device.

    0   1   2   3   4   5

32. Deep vibration with the fingertips.

    0   1   2   3   4   5

33. Light effleurage with vibration.

    0   1   2   3   4   5

34. Shaking—coarse vibration.

    0   1   2   3   4   5

35. Jostling—coarse vibration.

    0   1   2   3   4   5

Touch without movement

36. Passive touch.

    0   1   2   3   4   5

37. Direct static pressure with thumb or fingers.

    0   1   2   3   4   5

38. Ischemic compression.

    0   1   2   3   4   5

Total points _____ / 38 = _____ Average Rating

Evaluated by: _____

PERFORMANCE EVALUATION FORM 13–1
Joint Movements

Student: _____ Date: _____

Scoring Key: 0 = incorrect; 1 = very poor; 2 = poor; 3 = adequate; 4 = good; 5 = excellent

Neck

1. Simple mobilizing movements of the neck.

   0   1   2   3   4   5

2. Finger push-ups.

   0   1   2   3   4   5

3. Suboccipital release.

   0   1   2   3   4   5

4. Wave movement.

   0   1   2   3   4   5

5. Stretch in lateral flexion.

   0   1   2   3   4   5

6. Stretch in rotation.

   0   1   2   3   4   5

7. Stretch in forward flexion.

   0   1   2   3   4   5

8. Cross-arm stretch.

   0   1   2   3   4   5

Shoulder girdle

9. Wagging the arm.

   0   1   2   3   4   5

10. Shaking the arm.

   0   1   2   3   4   5

11. Passive shoulder roll.

   0   1   2   3   4   5

12. Scapula mobilizing.

   0   1   2   3   4   5

13. Horizontal flexion.

   0   1   2   3   4   5

14. Overhead stretch.

   0   1   2   3   4   5

Elbow

15. Wagging the arm.

    0   1   2   3   4   5

16. Pronate and supinate the hand.

    0   1   2   3   4   5

17. Circling the forearm.

    0   1   2   3   4   5

18. Overhead stretch.

    0   1   2   3   4   5

Wrist

19. Passive movement through range of motion.

    0   1   2   3   4   5

20. Wagging.

    0   1   2   3   4   5

21. Flexion.

    0   1   2   3   4   5

22. Extension.

    0   1   2   3   4   5

Hand

23. Mobilizing knuckles with figure-8s.

    0   1   2   3   4   5

24. Scissoring metacarpals.

    0   1   2   3   4   5

25. Hyperextend the fingers.

    0   1   2   3   4   5

Chest

26. Gentle rocking of rib cage.

    0   1   2   3   4   5

27. Overhead stretch.

    0   1   2   3   4   5

Hip

28. Rocking the leg.

    0   1   2   3   4   5

29. Passive movement through range of motion.

    0   1   2   3   4   5

30. Knee to chest flexion.

    0   1   2   3   4   5

31. Straight leg flexion.

    0   1   2   3   4   5

32. Diagonal adduction.

    0   1   2   3   4   5

33. Hyperextension.

    0   1   2   3   4   5

Knee

34. Wag the leg.

    0   1   2   3   4   5

35. Leg toss.

    0   1   2   3   4   5

36. Circling the lower leg.

    0   1   2   3   4 5

37. Heel to buttocks stretch.

    0   1   2   3   4   5

Ankle

38. Dorsiflexion of foot.

    0   1   2   3   4   5

39. Passive movement of ankle through its full range of motion.

    0   1   2   3   4   5

40. Side-to-side mobilizing.

    0   1   2   3   4   5

41. Stretch in dorsiflexion.

    0   1   2   3   4   5

42. Stretch in plantarflexion.

    0   1   2   3   4   5

Foot

43. Figure-8s with toes.

    0   1   2   3   4   5

44. Scissoring metatarsals.

    0   1   2   3   4   5

45. Uncurling toes with effleurage.

    0   1   2   3   4   5

46. Stretch toes in hyperextension.

    0   1   2   3   4   5

47. Widening stretch at metatarsals.

    0   1   2   3   4   5

48. Fingers between toes.

    0   1   2   3   4   5

Methods of Stretching

49. Simple static stretch.

    0   1   2   3   4   5

50. Contract–relax–stretch (CRS).

    0   1   2   3   4   5

51. CRS using reciprocal inhibition.

    0   1   2   3   4   5

52. Active assisted stretch.

    0   1   2   3   4   5

Total points _____ / 52 = _____ Average Rating

Evaluated by: _____

PERFORMANCE EVALUATION FORM 14–1

Full-Body Swedish Massage

Student: _____   Date: _____

Scoring Key: 0 = incorrect; 1 = very poor; 2 = poor; 3 = adequate; 4 = good; 5 = excellent

1. Professional demeanor.

    0   1   2   3   4   5

2. Client communication: health history interview, explanations, feedback.

    0   1   2   3   4   5

3. Positioning and draping.

    0   1   2   3   4   5

Recipient Prone

4. Back—apply oil, application of massage techniques.

    0   1   2   3   4   5

5. Lower limbs and buttocks—apply oil, application of massage techniques.

    0   1   2   3   4   5

6. Finish and transition—rock and light effleurage over drape; turn over.

    0   1   2   3   4   5

Recipient Supine

7. Lower limbs—apply oil, application of massage techniques.

    0   1   2   3   4   5

8. Upper limbs and chest—apply oil, application of massage techniques.

    0   1   2   3   4   5

9. Abdomen—apply oil, application of massage techniques.

    0   1   2   3   4   5

10. Neck and shoulders—apply oil, application of massage techniques.

    0   1   2   3   4   5

11. Face and head—application of massage techniques.

    0   1   2   3   4   5

12. Finish—brush off front, hold feet, announce end of session.

    0   1   2   3   4   5

13. Safety, use of pressure, avoidance of endangerment sites.

    0   1   2   3   4   5

14. Body/hand mechanics and ease of movement around the table.

    0   1   2   3   4   5

15. Overall application (timing, pacing, rhythm, flow, quality of touch).

    0   1   2   3   4   5

Total points _____ / 15 = _____ Average Rating

Evaluated by: _____

PERFORMANCE EVALUATION FORM 15–1
Head and Face Massage

Student: _____ Date: _____

Scoring Key: 0 = incorrect; 1 = very poor; 2 = poor; 3 = adequate; 4 = good; 5 = excellent

1. Positioning and draping.

    0   1   2   3   4   5

2. Client communication: health history interview, explanations, feedback.

    0   1   2   3   4   5

3. Initial contact—stroking face with palms.

    0   1   2   3   4   5

4. Forehead area—effleurage to forehead, circular friction to temples, squeeze along eyebrows.

    0   1   2   3   4   5

5. Eyes and nose area—stroke over eyelids, slide along nose, pressure under zygomatic arch.

    0   1   2   3   4   5

6. Mouth area—slide around mouth, knead chin, circular friction over masseter muscle.

    0   1   2   3   4   5

7. Ears—rub outer ears, pull ears, circular friction around base of ears.

    0   1   2   3   4   5

8. Head—move scalp with friction, circular friction over head muscles, head press.

    0   1   2   3   4   5

9. Finish with passive touch over face.

    0   1   2   3   4   5

10. Body/hand mechanics and ease of movement around the table.

    0   1   2   3   4   5

11. Safety, use of pressure, avoidance of endangerment sites.

    0   1   2   3   4   5

12. Overall application (timing, pacing, rhythm, flow, quality of touch).

    0   1   2   3   4   5

Total points _____ / 12 = _____ Average rating

Evaluated by: _____

PERFORMANCE EVALUATION FORM 15–2

Massage of the Neck Region

Student: _____   Date: _____

Scoring Key: 0 = incorrect; 1 = very poor; 2 = poor; 3 = adequate; 4 = good; 5 = excellent

1. Positioning and draping.

    0   1   2   3   4   5

2. Client communication: health history interview, explanations, feedback.

    0   1   2   3   4   5

3. Apply oil to neck and shoulders and warming effleurage with soft fist.

    0   1   2   3   4   5

4. Upper trapezius muscle—effleurage with soft fist, and direct pressure to tender points.

    0   1   2   3   4   5

5. Scalene and SCM muscles—effleurage with fingertips.

    0   1   2   3   4   5

6. Stretch neck and shoulder in lateral flexion—slow and sustained.

    0   1   2   3   4   5

7. Wave-like neck mobilizing technique.

    0   1   2   3   4   5

8. Suboccipital muscles—circular friction and direct pressure to tender points.

    0   1   2   3   4   5

9. Stretch neck in forward flexion with cross-armed stretch.

    0   1   2   3   4   5

10. Traction neck in neutral position.

    0   1   2   3   4   5

11. Finishing technique—head cradle.

    0   1   2   3   4   5

12. Body mechanics and ease of movement around the table.

    0   1   2   3   4   5

13. Safety, use of pressure, avoidance of endangerment sites.

    0   1   2   3   4   5

14. Overall application (timing, pacing, rhythm, flow, quality of touch).

    0   1   2   3   4   5

Total points _____ / 14 = _____ Average rating

Evaluated by: _____

PERFORMANCE EVALUATION FORM 15–3
Upper Back and Shoulder Massage

Student: _____   Date: _____

Scoring Key: 0 = incorrect; 1 = very poor; 2 = poor; 3 = adequate; 4 = good; 5 = excellent

1. Positioning and draping.

   0   1   2   3   4   5

2. Client communication: health history interview, explanations, feedback.

   0   1   2   3   4   5

3. Initial contact—apply oil to entire back and shoulders with bilateral tree stroking.

   0   1   2   3   4   5

4. Warming one side of upper back—shingles effleurage and deep circular effleurage.

   0   1   2   3   4   5

5. Paraspinal muscles in upper back—circular friction with fingertips.

   0   1   2   3   4   5

6. Shoulder blade area—knuckle friction between and over scapula.

   0   1   2   3   4   5

7. Scapula mobilizing technique—press along medial border.

   0   1   2   3   4   5

8. Upper trapezius muscle—kneading, effleurage, direct pressure.

   0   1   2   3   4   5

9. Finishing technique for one side—shingles effleurage.

   0   1   2   3   4   5

10. Finishing techniques for whole upper back—two-hand circular petrissage and bilateral tree stroking.

   0   1   2   3   4   5

11. Body mechanics and ease of movement around the table.

   0   1   2   3   4   5

12. Overall application (safety, timing, pacing, rhythm, flow, quality of touch).

   0   1   2   3   4   5

Total points _____ / 12 = _____ Average rating

Evaluated by: _____

PERFORMANCE EVALUATION FORM 15–4

Low Back Massage

Student: _____ Date: _____

Scoring Key: 0 = incorrect; 1 = very poor; 2 = poor; 3 = adequate; 4 = good; 5 = excellent

1. Positioning and draping.

     0   1   2   3   4   5

2. Client communication: health history interview, explanations, feedback.

     0   1   2   3   4   5

3. Initial contact and warming—apply oil to entire back and shoulders with bilateral tree stroking.

     0   1   2   3   4   5

4. Paraspinal muscles on one side of low back—deep circular friction.

     0   1   2   3   4   5

5. Quadratus lumborum and paraspinal muscles—thumb stripping in both directions.

     0   1   2   3   4   5

6. Quadratus lumborum and paraspinal muscles—direct pressure to points and repeat thumb stripping.

     0   1   2   3   4   5

7. Finish one side of low back with lifting effleurage from opposite side.

     0   1   2   3   4   5

8. After both sides of low back—finish with bilateral tree stroking to entire back.

     0   1   2   3   4   5

9. Body/hand mechanics and ease of movement around the table.

     0   1   2   3   4   5

10. Overall application (safety, timing, pacing, rhythm, flow, quality of touch).

     0   1   2   3   4   5

Total points _____ / 10 = _____ Average rating

Evaluated by: _____

PERFORMANCE EVALUATION FORM 15–5

Massage of the Upper Extremities

Student: _____ Date: _____

Scoring Key: 0 = incorrect; 1 = very poor; 2 = poor; 3 = adequate; 4 = good; 5 = excellent

1. Positioning and draping.

    0   1   2   3   4   5

2. Client communication: health history interview, explanations, feedback.

    0   1   2   3   4   5

3. Initial contact and warming—apply oil to entire arm.

    0   1   2   3   4   5

4. Wagging the arm.

    0   1   2   3   4   5

5. Stretch upper extremity with the arm in lateral flexion.

    0   1   2   3   4   5

6. Tendons at shoulder—squeeze along upper arm, apply friction and stripping to tendons.

    0   1   2   3   4   5

7. Triceps muscle—elbow positioned upward, deep effleurage.

    0   1   2   3   4   5

8. Forearm—squeezing, stripping, friction to tendons at elbow, repeat stripping, draining.

    0   1   2   3   4   5

9. Wrist and metacarpals—friction over wrist bones, broadening hand, thumb slides between metacarpals, broadening across palm.

    0   1   2   3   4   5

10. Fingers—mobilizing figure-8s at knuckles, squeeze along fingers.

    0   1   2   3   4   5

11. Stretch wrist—flexion and extension at wrist.

    0   1   2   3   4   5

12. Finish and reconnect arm—effleurage to entire arm.

    0   1   2   3   4   5

13. Body/hand mechanics and ease of movement around the table.

    0   1   2   3   4   5

14. Safety, use of pressure, avoidance of endangerment sites.

    0   1   2   3   4   5

15. Overall application (timing, pacing, rhythm, flow, quality of touch).

    0   1   2   3   4   5

Total points _____ / 15 = _____ Average rating

Evaluated by: _____

PERFORMANCE EVALUATION FORM 15–6
Chest and Abdominal Massage

Student: _____   Date: _____

Scoring Key: 0 = incorrect; 1 = very poor; 2 = poor; 3 = adequate; 4 = good; 5 = excellent

1. Positioning and draping.

    0   1   2   3   4   5

2. Client communication: health history interview, explanations, feedback.

    0   1   2   3   4   5

3. Initial contact and warming—apply oil to chest and effleurage to pectoral muscles.

    0   1   2   3   4   5

4. Pectoral muscles—friction along inferior clavicle, effleurage and direct pressure to attachments.

    0   1   2   3   4   5

5. Mobilizing techniques for the chest—pressing down on shoulders, cat paw, rib cage.

    0   1   2   3   4   5

6. Rib cage and diaphragm—rake ribs, thumbs slide along diaphragm attachment.

    0   1   2   3   4   5

7. Abdomen—clockwise effleurage with reinforced hand, vibration, repeat effleurage in circles.

    0   1   2   3   4   5

8. Abdomen finish—petrissage center, light effleurage in circle, passive touch.

    0   1   2   3   4   5

9. Body/hand mechanics and ease of movement around the table.

    0   1   2   3   4   5

10. Overall application (safety, timing, pacing, rhythm, flow, quality of touch).

    0   1   2   3   4   5

Total points _____ / 10 = _____ Average rating

Evaluated by: _____

PERFORMANCE EVALUATION FORM 16–1

Hip and Buttocks Massage

Student: _____   Date: _____

Scoring Key: 0 = incorrect; 1 = very poor; 2 = poor; 3 = adequate; 4 = good; 5 = excellent

1. Positioning and draping.

     0   1   2   3   4   5

2. Client communication: health history interview, explanations, feedback.

     0   1   2   3   4   5

3. Initial contact and warming—apply oil to entire leg and hip.

     0   1   2   3   4   5

Recipient Prone—Massage

4. Gluteal muscles—deep effleurage, rhythmic compression with fist, circular friction to attachments.

     0   1   2   3   4   5

5. Deep rotator muscles—direct pressure with elbow, slide with knuckles along muscles.

     0   1   2   3   4   5

6. Hip attachments and finish—deep friction with knuckles around hip attachments, circular effleurage with palm, reconnect to leg with effleurage.

     0   1   2   3   4   5

Recipient Supine—Joint Movements

7. Rocking rotation for passive movement at the hip.

     0   1   2   3   4   5

8. Passive movement at hip with leg bent at knee—full range of motion.

     0   1   2   3   4   5

9. Stretch at hip—flexion and lateral flexion with knee bent.

     0   1   2   3   4   5

10. Finish with effleurage and rocking.

     0   1   2   3   4   5

11. Body/hand mechanics and ease of movement around table.

     0   1   2   3   4   5

12. Overall application (safety, timing, pacing, rhythm, flow, quality of touch).

     0   1   2   3   4   5

Total points _____ / 12 = _____ Average rating

Evaluated by: _____

PERFORMANCE EVALUATION FORM 16–2 (RECIPIENT SUPINE)
Thigh and Lower Leg Massage

Student: _____ Date: _____

Scoring Key: 0 = incorrect; 1 = very poor; 2 = poor; 3 = adequate; 4 = good; 5 = excellent

1. Positioning and draping.

   0   1   2   3   4   5

2. Client communication: health history interview, explanations, feedback.

   0   1   2   3   4   5

3. Initial contact and warming—apply oil and warming effleurage to entire leg.

   0   1   2   3   4   5

4. Thigh region—deep effleurage with reinforced palms entire thigh, kneading quadriceps muscles.

   0   1   2   3   4   5

5. Medial thigh—adductors kneading, reposition leg, adductors effleurage, return position.

   0   1   2   3   4   5

6. Anterior and lateral thigh—forearm effleurage to quadriceps, palmar effleurage to illiotibial band, horizontal stroking of thigh, circular friction over lateral/medial attachments at the knee.

   0   1   2   3   4   5

7. Lower leg region—broadening effleurage, squeeze posterior muscles, knuckling friction to tibialis anterior.

   0   1   2   3   4   5

8. Finish with effleurage of entire leg, and redrape leg.

   0   1   2   3   4   5

9. Body/hand mechanics and ease of movement around table.

   0   1   2   3   4   5

10. Overall application (safety, timing, pacing, rhythm, flow, quality of touch).

    0   1   2   3   4   5

Total points _____ / 10 = _____ Average rating

Evaluated by: _____

PERFORMANCE EVALUATION FORM 16–2 (RECIPIENT PRONE)
Thigh and Lower Leg Massage

Student: _____ Date: _____

Scoring Key: 0 = incorrect; 1 = very poor; 2 = poor; 3 = adequate; 4 = good; 5 = excellent

1. Positioning and draping.

   0   1   2   3   4   5

2. Client communication: health history interview, explanations, feedback.

   0   1   2   3   4   5

3. Initial contact and warming—apply oil and warming effleurage to entire leg.

   0   1   2   3   4   5

4. Thigh region—longitudinal and horizontal effleurage.

   0   1   2   3   4   5

5. Medial and posterior thigh—petrissage to adductors, forearm effleurage to hamstrings.

   0   1   2   3   4   5

6. Stretch quadriceps—heel to buttocks.

   0   1   2   3   4   5

7. Lower leg region—effleurage/petrissage posterior muscles, thumb slide to Achilles tendon.

   0   1   2   3   4   5

8. Foot region—mobilizing ankle with dorsiflexion and sliding with fist over foot bottom, finishing with effleurage over entire leg.

   0   1   2   3   4   5

9. Body/hand mechanics and ease of movement around table.

   0   1   2   3   4   5

10. Overall application (safety, timing, pacing, rhythm, flow, quality of touch).

   0   1   2   3   4   5

Total points _____ / 10 = _____ Average rating

Evaluated by: _____

PERFORMANCE EVALUATION FORM 16–3
Foot Massage

Student: _____   Date: _____

Scoring Key: 0 = incorrect; 1 = very poor; 2 = poor; 3 = adequate; 4 = good; 5 = excellent

1. Positioning and draping.

   0   1   2   3   4   5

2. Client communication: health history interview, explanations, feedback.

   0   1   2   3   4   5

3. Initial contact and warming—apply oil to entire foot and ankle, mobilizing ankle.

   0   1   2   3   4   5

4. Metatarsals—thumb slides between metatarsals.

   0   1   2   3   4   5

5. Joint movements—scissoring action between metatarsals, figure-8s at toe knuckles.

   0   1   2   3   4   5

6. Toes—squeeze along length of each toe, straighten toes with sliding posterior surface.

   0   1   2   3   4   5

7. Plantar foot—effleurage with fist to foot bottom, circular friction with knuckles, transverse friction to plantar aponeurosis with thumb.

   0   1   2   3   4   5

8. Finish with joint movement and tapotement—pull from sides to broaden foot, slap foot bottom.

   0   1   2   3   4   5

9. Body/hand mechanics.

   0   1   2   3   4   5

10. Overall application (safety, timing, pacing, rhythm, flow, quality of touch).

   0   1   2   3   4   5

Total points _____ / 10 = _____ Average rating

Evaluated by: _____

PERFORMANCE EVALUATION FORM 17–1
Hot Application on Upper Back

Student: _____ Date: _____

Scoring Key: 0 = incorrect; 1 = very poor; 2 = poor; 3 = adequate; 4 = good; 5 = excellent

1. Positioning and draping.

    0   1   2   3   4   5

2. Client communication: health history interview, explanations, feedback.

    0   1   2   3   4   5

3. Check heat source for temperature.

    0   1   2   3   4   5

4. Place heat barrier on upper back—sheet or towel of appropriate thickness.

    0   1   2   3   4   5

5. Instructions about effects of heat and how to give feedback if the application becomes too hot.

    0   1   2   3   4   5

6. Apply heat source, cover, and ask for feedback—apply more heat barriers if necessary.

    0   1   2   3   4   5

7. Get feedback every 3–4 minutes about heat intensity—add or take away barriers to maintain therapeutic heat level.

    0   1   2   3   4   5

8. Remove heat and check skin for redness.

    0   1   2   3   4   5

9. Body/hand mechanics and ease of movement around the table.

    0   1   2   3   4   5

10. Overall application (safety, timing, pacing, rhythm, flow, quality of touch).

    0   1   2   3   4   5

Total points _____ / 10 = _____ Average Rating

Evaluated by: _____

PERFORMANCE EVALUATION FORM 17–2

Cold Application for Knee

Student: _____ Date: _____

Scoring Key: 0 = incorrect; 1 = very poor; 2 = poor; 3 = adequate; 4 = good; 5 = excellent

1. Positioning and draping.

    0   1   2   3   4   5

2. Client communication: health history interview, explanations, feedback.

    0   1   2   3   4   5

3. Place cold barrier on knee—sheet or towel of appropriate thickness.

    0   1   2   3   4   5

4. Instructions about effects of cold, and how to give feedback if the cold becomes too intense.

    0   1   2   3   4   5

5. Apply cold source, cover, and ask for feedback—apply more cold barriers if necessary.

    0   1   2   3   4   5

6. Get feedback every 3–4 minutes about cold intensity—add or take away barriers to maintain therapeutic cold level.

    0   1   2   3   4   5

7. Remove cold source, and check for redness and swelling.

    0   1   2   3   4   5

8. Body/hand mechanics and ease of movement around the table.

    0   1   2   3   4   5

9. Safety, use of pressure, avoidance of endangerment sites.

    0   1   2   3   4   5

10. Overall application (safety, timing, pacing, rhythm, flow, quality of touch).

    0   1   2   3   4   5

Total points _____ / 10 = _____ Average Rating

Evaluated by: _____

PERFORMANCE EVALUATION FORM 17–3
Ice Massage for Elbow

Student: _____   Date: _____

Scoring Key: 0 = incorrect; 1 = very poor; 2 = poor; 3 = adequate; 4 = good; 5 = excellent

1. Positioning and draping.

   0   1   2   3   4   5

2. Client communication: health history interview, explanations, feedback.

   0   1   2   3   4   5

3. Massage forearm muscles—kneading, muscle stripping, transverse friction over tendons, direct pressure to tender points.

   0   1   2   3   4   5

4. Instructions about effects of ice, stages of feeling cold, and how to give feedback if the cold becomes too intense.

   0   1   2   3   4   5

5. Ice massage to tendons around elbow—continuous circular movement of ice, medium pressure, 10 minutes.

   0   1   2   3   4   5

6. Get feedback periodically about cold intensity and stages of feeling.

   0   1   2   3   4   5

7. Remove cold source, and apply superficial friction with towel.

   0   1   2   3   4   5

8. Body/hand mechanics and ease of movement around the table.

   0   1   2   3   4   5

9. Safety, use of pressure, avoidance of endangerment sites.

   0   1   2   3   4   5

10. Overall application (safety, timing, pacing, rhythm, flow, quality of touch).

   0   1   2   3   4   5

Total points _____ / 10 = _____ Average Rating

Evaluated by: _____

PERFORMANCE EVALUATION FORM 18–1
Postevent Sports Massage for Run/Walk Event

Student: _____   Date: _____

Scoring Key: 0 = incorrect; 1 = very poor; 2 = poor; 3 = adequate; 4 = good; 5 = excellent

1. Positioning the recipient.

   0   1   2   3   4   5

2. Client communication—health history interview, explanations, feedback.

   0   1   2   3   4   5

Athlete Supine

3. Initial contact and leg mobilizing.

   0   1   2   3   4   5

4. Thigh muscles—broaden/lift, knead, shake, jostle.

   0   1   2   3   4   5

5. Stretch hamstrings—knee to chest.

   0   1   2   3   4   5

6. Knee—circular friction to tendons.

   0   1   2   3   4   5

7. Lower leg muscles—position leg, squeeze.

   0   1   2   3   4   5

8. Ankle and foot mobilizing—joint movements at ankle, foot, and toes.

   0   1   2   3   4   5

9. Foot muscles—squeeze/press.

   0   1   2   3   4   5

10. Finish—light strokes from hip to foot.

   0   1   2   3   4   5

Athlete Prone

11. Stretch quadriceps—heel to buttocks.

    0   1   2   3   4   5

12. Buttocks muscles—compressions with fist.

    0   1   2   3   4   5

13. Thigh muscles—compressions, lift and wring, shaking, jostling.

    0   1   2   3   4   5

14. Lower leg muscles—shake, squeeze.

    0   1   2   3   4   5

15. Ankle—dorsiflex and press into foot bottom.

    0   1   2   3   4   5

16. Finish leg—light strokes from ankle to hip.

    0   1   2   3   4   5

17. Upper body—compressions over back and shoulders.

    0   1   2   3   4   5

18. Finish session—brush off from shoulders to feet.

    0   1   2   3   4   5

19. Body/hand mechanics and ease of movement around the table.

    0   1   2   3   4   5

20. Overall application (safety, timing, pacing, rhythm, flow, quality of touch).

    0   1   2   3   4   5

Total points _____ / 20 = _____ Average Rating

Evaluated by: _____

PERFORMANCE EVALUATION FORM 18–2

Pregnancy Massage in Side-Lying Position

Student: _____ Date: _____

Scoring Key: 0 = incorrect; 1 = very poor; 2 = poor; 3 = adequate; 4 = good; 5 = excellent

1. Positioning and draping.

    0   1   2   3   4   5

2. Client communication: health history interview, explanations, feedback.

    0   1   2   3   4   5

3. Apply oil and effleurage to top leg.

    0   1   2   3   4   5

4. Hip and leg muscles—effleurage, petrissage.

    0   1   2   3   4   5

5. Feet—squeeze, press, joint movement.

    0   1   2   3   4   5

6. Back and shoulders—warming effleurage.

    0   1   2   3   4   5

7. Paraspinal muscles—circular friction.

    0   1   2   3   4   5

8. Shoulder and neck muscles—effleurage, petrissage.

    0   1   2   3   4   5

9. Finish back—superficial friction.

    0   1   2   3   4   5

10. Arm—effleurage, petrissage.

    0   1   2   3   4   5

11. Finish side—passive touch.

    0   1   2   3   4   5

12. Assist recipient in turning over or in getting off the table.

    0   1   2   3   4   5

13. Body/hand mechanics and ease of movement around the table.

    0   1   2   3   4   5

14. Safety, use of pressure, avoidance of endangerment sites.

    0   1   2   3   4   5

15. Overall effectiveness (timing, pacing, rhythm, flow, quality of touch).

    0   1   2   3   4   5

Total points _____ / 15 = _____ Average Rating

Evaluated by: _____

PERFORMANCE EVALUATION FORM 18–3
Infant Massage

Student: _____ Date: _____

Scoring Key: 0 = incorrect; 1 = very poor; 2 = poor; 3 = adequate; 4 = good; 5 = excellent

1. Positioning the infant supine and prone.

    0   1   2   3   4   5

2. Communication—eye contact, talking, smiling.

    0   1   2   3   4   5

3. Quality of touch—gentle, firm.

    0   1   2   3   4   5

Infant Supine

4. Fingertip circle over head.

    0   1   2   3   4   5

5. Thumb slides over forehead and along nose.

    0   1   2   3   4   5

6. Apply oil with butterfly strokes across the chest.

    0   1   2   3   4   5

7. Squeeze and milk the arms.

    0   1   2   3   4   5

8. Thumb strokes to palm and fingers.

    0   1   2   3   4   5

9. Squeeze and milk the legs.

    0   1   2   3   4   5

10. Thumb strokes to foot bottoms.

    0   1   2   3   4   5

11. Stroking to abdomen clockwise.

    0   1   2   3   4   5

12. Shoulder movement—cross arms and open out.

    0   1   2   3   4   5

13. Hip and leg movement—bend and straighten legs.

    0   1   2   3   4   5

Infant Prone

14. Circular fingertip friction along paraspinal muscles.

    0   1   2   3   4   5

15. Scoop from shoulders to heels.

    0   1   2   3   4   5

16. Turn baby over and finish supine with passive touch to head—eye contact and smile.

    0   1   2   3   4   5

17. Body/hand mechanics and ease of movement.

    0   1   2   3   4   5

18. Overall application (safety, timing, pacing, flow, quality of touch).

    0   1   2   3   4   5

Total points _____ / 18 = _____ Average Rating

Evaluated by: _____

PERFORMANCE EVALUATION FORM 18–4
Massage for the Elderly in Semireclining Position

Student: _____ Date: _____

Scoring Key: 0 = incorrect; 1 = very poor; 2 = poor; 3 = adequate; 4 = good; 5 = excellent

1. Positioning and draping.

    0   1   2   3   4   5

2. Client communication: health history interview, explanations, feedback.

    0   1   2   3   4   5

3. Establish contact and mobilize the feet.

    0   1   2   3   4   5

4. Apply lotion to foot and leg.

    0   1   2   3   4   5

5. Thigh muscles—compressions, effleurage, petrissage.

    0   1   2   3   4   5

6. Lower leg muscles—knead, press.

    0   1   2   3   4   5

7. Passive movements to leg—rocking, knee flexion.

    0   1   2   3   4   5

8. Apply lotion to arm.

    0   1   2   3   4   5

9. Arm muscles—squeezes.

    0   1   2   3   4   5

10. Hands—thumb strokes to back of hand and palm.

    0   1   2   3   4   5

11. Mobilizing hand and wrist joints.

    0   1   2   3   4   5

12. Finish arm—long effleurage and brush off.

    0   1   2   3   4   5

13. Shoulders—knead.

    0   1   2   3   4   5

14. Neck muscles—knead.

    0   1   2   3   4   5

15. Upper and lower back—superficial friction.

    0   1   2   3   4   5

16. Scalp mobilizing and circular friction over temples.

    0   1   2   3   4   5

17. Connecting with light tapotement over head, arms, legs.

    0   1   2   3   4   5

18. Finish session with brush off from head to feet.

    0   1   2   3   4   5

19. Body/hand mechanics and ease of movement around the table/chair.

    0   1   2   3   4   5

20. Overall application (safety, timing, pacing, flow, quality of touch).

    0   1   2   3   4   5

Total points _____ / 20 = _____ Average Rating

Evaluated by: _____

PERFORMANCE EVALUATION FORM 18–5

Gentle Hand and Arm Massage

Student: _____ Date: _____

Scoring Key: 0 = incorrect; 1 = very poor; 2 = poor; 3 = adequate; 4 = good; 5 = excellent

1. Positioning the recipient.

   0   1   2   3   4   5

2. Client communication: health history interview, explanations, feedback.

   0   1   2   3   4   5

3. Quality of touch—gentle, firm, adapted to recipient's condition.

   0   1   2   3   4   5

4. Apply lotion to entire arm.

   0   1   2   3   4   5

5. Upper arm—stroke and knead.

   0   1   2   3   4   5

6. Lower arm—stroke and knead.

   0   1   2   3   4   5

7. Joint mobilizing with pressing and rolling.

   0   1   2   3   4   5

8. Hand and fingers—thumb circles over wrist, squeeze hand and fingers, thumb slides.

   0   1   2   3   4   5

9. Joint mobilizing wrist, hand, and fingers.

   0   1   2   3   4   5

10. Connecting arm with gentle squeezes from shoulder to hand.

   0   1   2   3   4   5

11. Finish session holding hands.

   0   1   2   3   4   5

12. Overall application (safety, timing, pacing, flow, quality of touch).

   0   1   2   3   4   5

Total points _____ / 12 = _____ Average Rating

Evaluated by: _____

PERFORMANCE EVALUATION FORM 20–1
Seated Massage

Student: _____ Date: _____

Scoring Key: 0 = incorrect; 1 = very poor; 2 = poor; 3 = adequate; 4 = good; 5 = excellent

1. Positioning the recipient on the massage chair.

   0   1   2   3   4   5

2. Client communication—health history interview; explanations, feedback.

   0   1   2   3   4   5

3. Establish contact and squeeze shoulders.

   0   1   2   3   4   5

4. Upper back—compressions and thumb pressure to paraspinal muscles.

   0   1   2   3   4   5

5. Shoulders—broad forearm compression and elbow pressure to points.

   0   1   2   3   4   5

6. Finish shoulders and transition to arms—squeeze along shoulders and down arms bilaterally.

   0   1   2   3   4   5

7. Arm—position arm hanging down, knead, reposition.

   0   1   2   3   4   5

8. Forearm—thumb pressure, circular friction, squeezes.

   0   1   2   3   4   5

9. Wrist, hand, fingers—circular friction, squeezes.

   0   1   2   3   4   5

10. Joint mobilizing wrist, hand, and fingers.

    0   1   2   3   4   5

11. Stretch arm overhead.

    0   1   2   3   4   5

12. Neck muscles—kneading, thumb pressure, and circular friction to points.

    0   1   2   3   4   5

13. Scalp mobilization and light tapotement to head.

    0   1   2   3   4   5

14. Finish session with brush off from head to hips.

    0   1   2   3   4   5

15. Body/hand mechanics and ease of movement around the massage chair.

    0   1   2   3   4   5

16. Overall application (safety, timing, pacing, rhythm, flow, quality of touch).

    0   1   2   3   4   5

Total points _____ / 16 = _____ Average Rating

Evaluated by: _____

PERFORMANCE EVALUATION FORM 21–1
Myofascial Massage of the Back

Student: _____   Date: _____

Scoring Key: 0 = incorrect; 1 = very poor; 2 = poor; 3 = adequate; 4 = good; 5 = excellent

1. Positioning and draping.

    0   1   2   3   4   5

2. Client communication: health history interview, explanations, feedback.

    0   1   2   3   4   5

3. Initial contact—place hands over sheet on upper and lower back, and rock gently.

    0   1   2   3   4   5

4. Skin lifting—simple lift and lift adding movement, slow steady lift 1 to 2 minutes per spot.

    0   1   2   3   4   5

5. Skin rolling—skin lift and roll, slow steady movement in multiple directions over same spot.

    0   1   2   3   4   5

6. Cross-handed stretch for subcutaneous fascia—hold for 2 to 3 minutes or until tissues release.

    0   1   2   3   4   5

7. Fascial mobilization in 1 direction using palm—engage tissues, shift horizontally, hold tension steadily for 2 to 5 minutes until a shift is felt, move from spot to spot.

    0   1   2   3   4   5

8. Facial mobilization shifting direction—engage tissues, shift horizontally in direction of resistance or least resistance, shift direction as tissues dictate.

    0   1   2   3   4   5

9. Pin and stretch—pin tissues with one hand while the other pulls away, slow steady tension, hold for 2 to 3 minutes or until tissues release.

    0   1   2   3   4   5

10. Deep fascial mobilization—use reinforced fingertips or forearm; engage deep fascia, shift tissues horizontally, hold steady for 2 to 5 minutes or until tissues release.

    0   1   2   3   4   5

11. Finish with redraping and passive touch—letting tissues rest.

    0   1   2   3   4   5

12. Body/hand mechanics and ease of movement around table.

    0   1   2   3   4   5

13. Safety, use of pressure, avoidance of endangerment sites.

    0   1   2   3   4   5

14. Overall application (timing, pacing, rhythm, flow, quality of touch).

    0   1   2   3   4   5

Total points _____ / 14 = _____ Average Rating

Evaluated by: _____

PERFORMANCE EVALUATION FORM 22–1

Trigger Point Therapy for Tension Headaches

Student: _____   Date: _____

Scoring Key: 0 = incorrect; 1 = very poor; 2 = poor; 3 = adequate; 4 = good; 5 = excellent

1. Positioning and draping.

   0   1   2   3   4   5

2. Client communication: health history interview, explanations, feedback.

   0   1   2   3   4   5

3. Initial contact and warming neck—gently squeeze posterior cervical muscles, effleurage along cervical and shoulder muscles, traction with head in neutral position.

   0   1   2   3   4   5

4. Locating TrPs—checking common trigger point locations in cervical and shoulder muscles, using feedback from recipient.

   0   1   2   3   4   5

5. General treatment of TrPs—pressing, monitoring pain, slow application, hold for 30 to 90 seconds and repeat, follow up with massage and stretching.

   0   1   2   3   4   5

6. Direct pressure to TrPs in upper trapezius—locating, applying direct pressure.

   0   1   2   3   4   5

7. Pincer technique to SCM muscle—turn head, avoid endangerment site.

   0   1   2   3   4   5

8. Direct pressure to TrPs in posterior and suboccipital muscles—using fingertips or thumbs, position head for access.

   0   1   2   3   4   5

9. Stretches for neck muscles—forward flexion, lateral flexion, rotation, traction.

   0   1   2   3   4   5

10. Finishing—wave-like movement in posterior cervical muscles, cat paw.

    0   1   2   3   4   5

11. Body/hand mechanics.

    0   1   2   3   4   5

12. Overall application (safety, timing, pacing, rhythm, flow, quality of touch).

    0   1   2   3   4   5

Total points _____ / 12 = _____ Average Rating

Evaluated by: _____

PERFORMANCE EVALUATION FORM 23–1

Lymphatic Facilitation for the Head and Neck

Student: _____ Date: _____

Scoring Key: 0 = incorrect; 1 = very poor; 2 = poor; 3 = adequate; 4 = good; 5 = excellent

1. Positioning and draping.

   0   1   2   3   4   5

2. Client communication: health history interview, explanations, feedback.

   0   1   2   3   4   5

3. L stroke on both sides of neck—finger placement, L direction, snap back, repetitions.

   0   1   2   3   4   5

4. L stroke on terminus—finger placement, L direction, snap back, repetitions.

   0   1   2   3   4   5

5. L stroke under mandible—finger placement, L direction, snap back, repetitions.

   0   1   2   3   4   5

6. L stroke on face—hand placement, L direction, snap back, repetitions.

   0   1   2   3   4   5

7. L stroke near eyes—finger placement, L direction, snap back, repetitions.

   0   1   2   3   4   5

8. L stroke on forehead—finger placement, L direction, snap back, repetitions.

   0   1   2   3   4   5

9. L stroke on temples and side of head—finger placement, L direction, snap back, repetitions.

   0   1   2   3   4   5

10. L stroke on lateral neck toward terminus—finger placement, L direction, snap back, repetitions.

   0   1   2   3   4   5

11. Finishing—effleurage to arms, kneading shoulders, passive touch.

   0   1   2   3   4   5

12. Principles of lymphatic facilitation—light touch; slow, gentle repetitions; appropriate direction; skin snaps back.

   0   1   2   3   4   5

13. Body/hand mechanics.

   0   1   2   3   4   5

14. Overall application (safety, timing, pacing, rhythm, flow, quality of touch).

   0   1   2   3   4   5

Total points _____ / 14 = _____ Average Rating

Evaluated by: _____

PERFORMANCE EVALUATION FORM 23–2

Lymphatic Facilitation for the Lower Extremity

Student: _____ Date: _____

Scoring Key: 0 = incorrect; 1 = very poor; 2 = poor; 3 = adequate; 4 = good; 5 = excellent

1. Positioning and draping.

   0   1   2   3   4   5

2. Client communication: health history interview, explanations, feedback.

   0   1   2   3   4   5

3. L stroke on both sides of neck—finger placement, L direction, snap back, repetitions.

   0   1   2   3   4   5

4. L stroke on terminus—finger placement, L direction, snap back, repetitions.

   0   1   2   3   4   5

5. Clearing the cisterna chyle—instruction for forceful breaths, 5–6 breaths.

   0   1   2   3   4   5

6. Clearing the inguinal catchment area—hand placement, direction of movement, repetition.

   0   1   2   3   4   5

7. Clearing the thigh with long strokes—full hand placement, skin stretch, slide, snap back, repetitions.

   0   1   2   3   4   5

8. Clearing the popliteal catchment area—hand placement under knee, lift and stretch, release and return to start, repetitions.

   0   1   2   3   4   5

9. Clearing the lower leg with long strokes—full hand placement, skin stretch, slide, snap back, repetitions.

   0   1   2   3   4   5

10. Clearing the tarsals, metatarsals, and toes—hand placement, skin stretch, snap back, repetitions.

    0   1   2   3   4   5

11. Principles of lymphatic facilitation—light touch, slow gentle repetitions, appropriate direction, skin snaps back.

    0   1   2   3   4   5

12. Body/hand mechanics and ease of movement around the table.

    0   1   2   3   4   5

13. Safety, use of pressure, avoidance of endangerment sites.

    0   1   2   3   4   5

14. Overall application (safety, timing, pacing, rhythm, flow, quality of touch).

    0   1   2   3   4   5

Total points _____ / 14 = _____ Average Rating

Evaluated by: _____

PERFORMANCE EVALUATION FORM 24–1

General Reflexology Session

Student: _____ Date: _____

Scoring Key: 0 = incorrect; 1 = very poor; 2 = poor; 3 = adequate; 4 = good; 5 = excellent

1. Positioning the recipient.

   0   1   2   3   4   5

2. Client communication—health history interview, foot examination for structural and skin problems, explanations, feedback.

   0   1   2   3   4   5

3. Warm-up—variety of massage and joint movement techniques.

   0   1   2   3   4   5

4. Spinal twist—three quick twists at pelvis, waist, and diaphragmatic guidelines.

   0   1   2   3   4   5

5. Spinal reflex—thumb rolling sacrum to C-1, foot position on lateral edge.

   0   1   2   3   4   5

6. Bidirectional thumb pressure on plantar surface—elbows flap, apply in horizontal lines from base of toes to heel.

   0   1   2   3   4   5

7. Pressure along diaphragm guidelines—apply medial to lateral.

   0   1   2   3   4   5

8. Lymphatic drainage on dorsum ending with ankle rotation—stretch dorsum skin row by row, end at ankle joint, use fingers to rotate ankle.

   0   1   2   3   4   5

9. Press-and-flex medial and lateral ankle—finger position, roll ankle into pressure points.

   0   1   2   3   4   5

10. Press-and-flex on shoulder reflex—roll foot into pressure points.

    0   1   2   3   4   5

11. Hook and backup on the hypothalamus/pituitary gland reflex—thumb position, pressure application.

    0   1   2   3   4   5

12. Toe rotations—rotate each toe, compress tip with snap, work from medial to lateral.

    0   1   2   3   4   5

13. Finish with general foot massage.

    0   1   2   3   4   5

14. Knowledge of reflex and guideline locations.

    0   1   2   3   4   5

15. Overall application (safety, timing, pacing, rhythm, flow, quality of touch).

    0   1   2   3   4   5

Total points _____ / 15 = _____ Average Rating

Evaluated by: _____

PERFORMANCE EVALUATION FORM 25–1

A M I for the Back

Student: _____   Date: _____

Scoring Key: 0 = incorrect; 1 = very poor; 2 = poor; 3 = adequate; 4 = good; 5 = excellent

1. Positioning and draping.

    0   1   2   3   4   5

2. Client communication—health history interview, explanations, feedback.

    0   1   2   3   4   5

3. Oil application and warm-up—effleurage to entire back.

    0   1   2   3   4   5

4. Hand-over-hand effleurage to entire back—reach to opposite side, stroke up and down the back alternately, parallel to spine.

    0   1   2   3   4   5

5. Pull-ups around side of torso from iliac crest to the shoulder—flat palms.

    0   1   2   3   4   5

6. Circular fingertip kneading along paraspinal muscles—hip to shoulders.

    0   1   2   3   4   5

7. Alternate thumb petrissage along paraspinal muscles—shoulder to sacrum.

    0   1   2   3   4   5

8. Thumb press sacral notches.

    0   1   2   3   4   5

9. Press GB-30—with fingertips, 2–3 times.

    0   1   2   3   4   5

10. Fingertip kneading along paraspinals on Inner and Outer Bladder meridians—sacrum to top of shoulder.

    0   1   2   3   4   5

11. Thumb press across top of shoulder—press GB-21 repeatedly, finish with kneading.

    0   1   2   3   4   5

12. Thumb press between shoulder blades Inner and Outer Bladder meridians—press into areas of kyo or excess.

    0   1   2   3   4   5

13. Effleurage over upper shoulder area.

    0   1   2   3   4   5

14. Rhythmic sliding compression down the paraspinal muscles, sliding back to start—palms on either side of spine, compression movement from shoulders to sacrum.

    0   1   2   3   4   5

15. Press points at base of skull—Bl-10, BG-20 and all points with spread fingertips.

    0   1   2   3   4   5

16. Pull-ups from shoulder to buttocks—reach across, pull up around torso, fingertips between ribs.

    0   1   2   3   4   5

17. Thumb petrissage to paraspinal muscles from sacrum to shoulder—search for tightness in mid-back area, thumb presses or deep friction to tight spots.

    0   1   2   3   4   5

18. Thumb presses between shoulder blades to acupoints on Inner and Outer Bladder meridians.

    0   1   2   3   4   5

19. Rhythmic sliding compression from shoulders to hips, palmar friction back to start—palms on either side of spine, compression movement from shoulders to sacrum.

    0   1   2   3   4   5

20. Effleurage to entire back.

    0   1   2   3   4   5

21. Fingertip kneading along paraspinal muscles from shoulders to buttocks.

    0   1   2   3   4   5

22. Circular palmar petrissage over entire back—tissues lift.

    0   1   2   3   4   5

23. Hourglass effleurage around tops of shoulders.

    0   1   2   3   4   5

24. Superficial friction with palms over paraspinal muscles.

    0   1   2   3   4   5

25. Overall application (safety, timing, pacing, rhythm, flow, quality of touch).

    0   1   2   3   4   5

Total points _____ / 25 = _____ Average Rating

Evaluated by: _____

PERFORMANCE EVALUATION FORM 25–2

AMI for the Anterior Arm

Student: _____ Date: _____

Scoring Key: 0 = incorrect; 1 = very poor; 2 = poor; 3 = adequate; 4 = good; 5 = excellent

1. Positioning and draping.

    0   1   2   3   4   5

2. Client communication: health history interview, explanations, feedback.

    0   1   2   3   4   5

3. Oil application and warm-up—effleurage to entire arm, shoulder, neck, press GB-21.

    0   1   2   3   4   5

4. Finger press acupoints under clavicle—Ki-27, Lu-2, Lu-1.

    0   1   2   3   4   5

5. Fingertip rake over sternum and pectoral muscles—midline to lateral chest, adjust for women, over skin or drape.

    0   1   2   3   4   5

6. Reverse pull-ups from hips to armpit—palms up, around sides of torso.

    0   1   2   3   4   5

7. Pectoralis major—alternate thumb petrissage to pectoralis major along edge and muscle belly; rake over muscle from sternum to shoulder.

    0   1   2   3   4   5

8. Sliding and kneading over energy meridians in upper arm—Heart, Pericardium, Lung, Large Intestine, Triple Burner; thumb press to Lu-5, LI-11, and LI-15.

    0   1   2   3   4   5

9. Knead forearm along energy meridians—Lung, Small Intestine, Triple Burner; thumb press LI-11 and TB-5.

    0   1   2   3   4   5

10. General hand massage—include metacarpal mobilizing and gentle finger pulls; thumb press LI-4 and SI-3.

    0   1   2   3   4   5

11. Finish—shake arm and then brush from shoulder to hand.

    0   1   2   3   4   5

12. Overall application (safety, timing, pacing, rhythm, flow, quality of touch).

    0   1   2   3   4   5

Total points _____ / 12 = _____ Average rating

Evaluated by: _____

PERFORMANCE EVALUATION FORM 25–3

AMI for the Neck–Head–Face

Student: _____ Date: _____

Scoring Key: 0 = incorrect; 1 = very poor; 2 = poor; 3 = adequate; 4 = good; 5 = excellent

1. Positioning and draping.

   0   1   2   3   4   5

2. Client communication: health history interview, explanations, feedback.

   0   1   2   3   4   5

3. Warm-up with rhythmic compression to shoulders—cat paw.

   0   1   2   3   4   5

4. Bilateral effleurage to tops of shoulders and neck with fingertips.

   0   1   2   3   4   5

5. Clavicle area—press near manubrium to stomach meridian; thumb slide along top of clavicle and up the neck; press GB-20.

   0   1   2   3   4   5

6. Slide fingertips along Gall Bladder meridian (scalenes)—press GB-21.

   0   1   2   3   4   5

7. Stretch neck in lateral flexion—one hand on head and the other hand on the shoulder.

   0   1   2   3   4   5

8. Fingertip pressure to GB-20 and Bl-10—fingertips slide along neck into position.

   0   1   2   3   4   5

9. Press around ear into pathways of Gall Bladder and Triple Burner meridians—spread fingers, press in several places.

   0   1   2   3   4   5

10. Thumb slides to forehead in 2–3 rows—press TB-23.

    0   1   2   3   4   5

11. Press Bladder meridian points along upper orbital ridge with fingertips, from Bl-1 to GB-1.

    0   1   2   3   4   5

12. Press points along nose and cheekbones—slide down nose to St-2 then LI-20, St-3, SI-18, St-7, to SI-19 on jaw joint.

    0   1   2   3   4   5

13. Slide over upper lip, lower lip, and up sides of face to temples—begin at GV-26.

    0   1   2   3   4   5

14. Pinch along jaw line from chin to masseter attachment—press St-6.

    0   1   2   3   4   5

15. Massage and gently pull the ears.

    0   1   2   3   4   5

16. Stretch neck in rotation, lateral and forward flexion.

    0   1   2   3   4   5

17. Finish—place palms lightly over the ears.

    0   1   2   3   4   5

18. Overall application (safety, timing, pacing, rhythm, flow, quality of touch).

    0   1   2   3   4   5

Total points _____ / 18 = _____ Average rating

Evaluated by: _____

PERFORMANCE EVALUATION FORM 25–4

General Session of Polarity Therapy

Student: _____ Date: _____

Scoring Key: 0 = incorrect; 1 = very poor; 2 = poor; 3 = adequate; 4 = good; 5 = excellent

Polarity Therapy Techniques

1. The cradle.

   0   1   2   3   4   5

2. Neck stretch.

   0   1   2   3   4   5

3. Tummy rock.

   0   1   2   3   4   5

4. Leg pull.

   0   1   2   3   4   5

5. Inside ankle press (right foot).

   0   1   2   3   4   5

6. Outside ankle press (right foot).

   0   1   2   3   4   5

7. Inside ankle press (left foot).

   0   1   2   3   4   5

8. Outside ankle press (left foot).

   0   1   2   3   4   5

9. Pelvis and knee rock (right side).

   0   1   2   3   4   5

10. Arm shoulder rotation (right side).

   0   1   2   3   4   5

11. Thumb web—forearm stimulation (right side).

   0   1   2   3   4   5

12. Elbow milk—abdominal rock (right side).

   0   1   2   3   4   5

13. Pelvic rock (right side).

   0   1   2   3   4   5

14. Pelvis and knee rock (left side).

   0   1   2   3   4   5

15. Arm shoulder rotation (left side).

   0   1   2   3   4   5

16. Thumb web—forearm stimulation (left side).

    0   1   2   3   4   5

17. Elbow milk—abdominal rock (left side).

    0   1   2   3   4   5

18. Pelvic rock (left side).

    0   1   2   3   4   5

19. Occipital press.

    0   1   2   3   4   5

20. Cranial polarization.

    0   1   2   3   4   5

21. Navel-third eye.

    0   1   2   3   4   5

22. Brushing off to finish—back and front.

    0   1   2   3   4   5

Polarity Therapy Session

23. Client positioning and instructions.

    0   1   2   3   4   5

24. Client communication: health history interview, explanations, feedback.

    0   1   2   3   4   5

25. Practitioner body mechanics.

    0   1   2   3   4   5

26. Transitions from technique to technique.

    0   1   2   3   4   5

27. Quality of touch and energy sensitivity.

    0   1   2   3   4   5

28. Overall effect.

    0   1   2   3   4   5

Total points _____ / 28 = _____ Average Rating

Evaluated by: _____

References and Additional Resources

References are the sources of quotes and specific content in the chapters.

Additional Resources are valuable sources for further information.

CHAPTER 1

References

[1]U.S. Department of Health and Human Services. (2002). White House Commission on Complementary and Alternative Medicine Policy. Retrieved from http://www.whccamp.hhs.gov

[2]Harstad Strategic Research. (2013). National consumer survey of 610 adults 21 years and older, conducted January 6–9, as cited in *Massage Therapy Fast Facts* (March 2013) from Associated Bodywork & Massage Professionals.

[3]ORC International 2014 annual survey of 1003 adults 18 years and older living in the continental United States, as cited in *AMTA Consumer Survey Fact Sheet* (October 2014) from American Massage Therapy Association.

[4]Nahin, R. L., Barnes, P. M., Stussman, B. J., & Bloom, B. (2009). Costs of complementary and alternative medicine (CAM) and frequency of visits to CAM practitioners: United States, 2007. *National Health Statistics Report*, U.S. Department of Health and Human Services, Number 18, July 30, p. 1.

[5]National Center for Complementary and Alternative Medicine. (2004). *NCCAM Newsletter*, 11 (3).

[6]Samueli Institute. (2011). *Complementary and Alternative Medicine Survey of Hospitals 2010: Summary of Results*, also sponsored by Health Forum, an American Hospital Association Company.

[7]U.S. Department of Labor, Bureau of Labor Statistics, Occupational Outlook Handbook. Retrieved from http://bis.gov/ooh/healthcare/massage-therapists.html

[8]International Spa Association (ISPA). (2014). Retrieved from http://www.experienceispa.com

[9]American Organization of Bodywork Therapies of Asia (AOBTA). Retrieved from http://www.aobta.org

[10]ORC International 2014 annual survey of 1003 adults 18 years and older living in the continental United States, as cited in *AMTA Consumer Survey Fact Sheet* (October 2014) from American Massage Therapy Association.

[11]ORC International 2014 annual survey of 1003 adults 18 years and older living in the continental United States, as cited in *AMTA Consumer Survey Fact Sheet* (October 2014) from American Massage Therapy Association.

Additional Resources

American Massage Therapy Association (AMTA) (http://www.amtamassage.org)

Associated Bodywork and Massage Professionals (ABMP) (http://www.abmp.com)

American Organization of Bodywork Therapies of Asia (AOBTA) (http://www.aobta.org)

American Polarity Therapy Association (APTA) (http://www.polaritytherapy.org)

Bonnie Prudden Myotherapy® (http://www.bonnieprudden.com)

Commission on Massage Therapy Accreditation (COMTA) (http://www.comta.org)

Federation of State Massage Therapy Boards (http://www.fsmtb.org)

Healthcare Policy Consortium (IHPC) of the Collaboration for Healthcare Renewal Foundation (http://www.ihpc.org)

International Association of Infant Massage (IAIM) (http://www.iaim.net)

International Spa Association (ISPA) (http://experienceispa.com)

Jin Shin Do® (http://www.jinshindo.org)

Massage Therapy Foundation (MTF) (http://www.massagetherapyfoundation.org)

National Association of Nurse Massage Therapists (NANMT) (http://www.nanmt.org)

National Center of Complementary and Alternative Medicine at the National Institutes of Health, Washington, DC (http://www.nccam.nih.gov)

National Certification Board for Therapeutic Massage and Bodywork (NCBTMB) (http://www.ncbtmb.org)

National Certification Commission for Acupuncture and Oriental Medicine (NCCAOM) (http://www.nccaom .org)

Rolf Institute® of Structural Integration (http://www.rolf.org)

Touch Research Institute at the University of Miami (TRI) (http://www.miami.edu/touch-research)

U.S. Department of Education (http://www.ed.gov)

White House Commission on CAM Policy Report (http:// www.whccamp.hhs.gov)

CHAPTER 2

References

[1] Johnson, W. (1866). *The anatriptic art* (pp. 4–5). London, England: Simpkin, Marshall & Co.

[2] Taylor, G. (1900). *Health by exercise . . . showing what exercises to take . . . including the process of massage* (p. 40). New York, NY: The Improved Movement Cure Institute. (Original work published 1860)

[3] M'Lean, T. (1914.) *Picturesque representations of the dress and manners of the Chinese.* London, England: Howlett & Brimmer.

[4] Joya, M. (1958). *Mock Joya's things Japanese.* Tokyo, Japan: Tokyo News Service.

[5] Johnson, 1866.

[6] Zhang, Y. (Director). (2000). *Shower* [Film]. Sony Pictures Entertainment, Inc.

[7] Livingston, H., & Maroni, A. (1945). *Everyday beauty culture.* Bloomington, IL: McKnight & McKnight.

[8] College of Swedish Massage. *Catalogue,* c.1939

[9] Benjamin, P. J. (2001). Genuine Swedish massage applied to slim down. *Massage Therapy Journal, 40*(2), 152–154; Benjamin, P. J. (2002). Breast massage: Old becomes new again. *Massage Therapy Journal, 41*(1), 154–158.

[10] Graham, D. (1902). *A treatise on massage: Its history, mode of application and effects* (3rd ed., p. 19). Philadelphia, PA: Lippincott.

[11] Graham, 1902, p. 28.

[12] Johnson, 1866.

[13] Murphy, M. C. (1914). *Athletic training* (p. 161). New York, NY: Scribner's.

[14] Murphy, 1914, p. 21.

[15] McKenzie, R. T. (1915). *Exercise in education and medicine* (2nd ed., p. 170). Philadelphia, PA: Saunders.

[16] Frierwood, H. T. (1953, September–October). The place of health service in the total YMCA program. *Journal of Physical Education,* p. 21.

[17] Williams, R. J. (1943). Second annual national YMCA health service clinic. *Journal of Physical Education, 30.* 3030

[18] Thomas, N. (2003). *Cook: The extraordinary voyages of Captain James Cook* (p. 342). New York, NY: Walker & Company.

[19] Perrone, B., Stockel, H. H., & Krueger, V. (1989). *Medicine women, curanderas, and women doctors.* Norman, OK: University of Oklahoma Press.

[20] Graham, 1902, p. 21.

[21] Johnson, 1866, pp. 12–19.

[22] Johnson, 1866, p. 8.

[23] Graham, 1902, p. 52.

[24] Graham, 1902, pp. 51–52.

[25] Mitchell, S. W. (1877). *Fat and blood and how to make them.* Philadelphia, PA: J. B. Lippincott & Co.

[26] Ellison, M. A. (1909). *Manual for students of massage* (3rd ed., p. 138). London, England: Bailliere, Tindall, and Cox.

[27] Ellison, 1909, pp. 143–144.

[28] Ellison, 1909, p. 138.

[29] Roth, M. (1851). *The prevention and cure of many chronic diseases by movements.* London, England: John Churchill.

[30] Nissen, H. (1899). *A manual of instruction for giving Swedish movement and massage treatment* (p. 3). Philadelphia, PA: F. A. Davis.

[31] Erz, A. A. (c. 1924). Ad for book *The medical question: The truth about official medicine and why we must have medical freedom.* Butler, NJ: Nature Cure Publishing.

[32] American Association of Naturopathic Physicians. Retrieved from http://www.naturopathic.org/content .asp?pl=16&sl=57&contentid=57

[33] Puderbach, P. (1925). *The massage operator* (p. 7). Butler, NJ: Dr. Benedict Lust.

[34] Puderbach, 1925, p. 7.

[35] Kellogg, J. H. (1895). *The art of massage: Its physiological effects and therapeutic applications* (pp. v–vi). Battle Creek, MI: Modern Medicine Publishing.

[36] Armstrong, D., & Armstrong, E. M. (1991). *The great American medicine show: Being an illustrated history of hucksters, healers, health evangelists, and heroes from Plymouth Rock to the present.* New York, NY: Prentice Hall.

[37] Benjamin, P. J. (1986, Fall). National historian's report: Annual convention programs. *Massage Therapy Journal,* pp. 8–9.

[38]AMTA National Historian's Report. (1987, Fall). AMTA membership 1943–1987. *Massage Therapy Journal,* pp. 12–15.

Additional Resources

Barclay, J. (1994). *In good hands: The history of the chartered society of physiotherapy 1894–1994* (p. 3). London, England: Butterworth-Heinemann.

Benjamin, P. J. (2015). *The emergence of the massage therapy profession in North America: A history in archetypes.* Toronto, ON: Curties-Overzet.

Calvert, R. N. (2002). *The history of massage: An illustrated survey from around the world.* Rochester, VT: Healing Arts Press.

Esalen Institute (http://www.esalen.org).

Ling, P. H. (1840). Notations to the general principles. In *The collected works of P. H. Ling.* (1866). Stockholm, Sweden. Translated by Lars Agren and Patricia J. Benjamin and published in *Massage Therapy Journal,* Winter 1987.

Murphy, W. (Ed.). (1995). *Healing the generations: A history of physical therapy and the American Physical Therapy Association.* Lyme, CT: Greenwich Publishing Group.

CHAPTER 3

References

[1]Makely, S. (2005). *Professionalism in health care: A primer for career success* (2nd ed., pp. xiv–xv). Upper Saddle River, NJ: Prentice Hall.

[2]Makely, 2005, p. 5.

[3]McIntosh, N. (1999). *The educated heart: Professional guidelines for massage therapists, bodyworkers and movement teachers* (p. 25). Memphis, TN: Decatur Bainbridge Press.

[4]Benjamin, B. E., & Sohnen-Moe, C. (2003). *The ethics of touch.* Tucson, AZ: SMA.

[5]Bloom, B. S., (Ed.). (1984). *Taxonomy of educational objectives: Book 1 cognitive domain* (2nd ed.). Boston, MA: Addison-Wesley Publishing.

[6]Levine, M. (2002). *A mind at a time* (p. 203). New York, NY: Simon & Schuster.

[7]McCormick, A. R., & McCormick, M. D. (1997). *Horse sense and the human heart: What horses can teach us about trust, bonding, creativity and spirituality* (p. 84). Deerfield Beach, FL: Health Communications.

[8]Goleman, D. (1995). *Emotional intelligence: Why it can matter more than IQ* (pp. 28–29). New York, NY: Bantam Books.

[9]Goleman, 1995.

[10]McCormick & McCormick, 1997, p. 99.

[11]*American heritage dictionary of the English language* (4th ed.). (2000). New York, NY: Houghton Mifflin.

[12]Bixler, S., & Dugan L. S. (2001). *5 steps to professional presence: How to project confidence, competence, and credibility at work* (p. 7). Avon, MA: Adams Media Corporation.

[13]Cole, K. (2002). *The complete idiot's guide to clear communication.* Indianapolis, IN: Alpha.

[14]Cole, 2002.

[15]Cole, 2002.

[16]Cole, 2002.

[17]Cole, 2002.

[18]Booher, D. (1994). *Communicate with confidence: How to say it right the first time and every time* (p. 151). New York, NY: McGraw-Hill.

[19]Cole, 1994, pp. 158–159.

[20]Booher, 1994.

[21]Hahn, P. R. (2003). *The everything writing well book: Master the written word and communicate clearly.* Avon, MA: Adams Media Corporation.

CHAPTER 4

References

[1]Heckler, R. S. (1997). *Holding the center: Sanctuary in a time of confusion* (p. 96). Berkeley, CA: Frog.

[2]National Heart, Lung, and Blood Institute, retrieved May 2014 from http://www.nhlbi.nih.gov/guidelines/obesity/BMI/bmicalc.htm

[3]Schlosberg, S. (2005). *The ultimate workout log* (p. 14). Boston, MA: Houghton Mifflin Company.

[4]Chuen, L. K. (1991). *The way of energy: Mastering the Chinese art of internal strength with chi kung exercise.* New York, NY: Simon & Schuster.

[5]Mipham, S. (2003). *Turning the mind into an ally* (p. 24). New York, NY: Penguin Putnam.

[6]Simpkins, C. A., & Simpkins, A. (2000). *Simple Confucianism: A guide to living virtuously.* Boston, MA: Tuttle.

[7]Marieb, E. N. (2009). *Essentials of human anatomy and physiology* (9th ed.). Upper Saddle River, NJ: Pearson Prentice Hall.

Additional Resources

Bloom, B. (Ed.). (1956). *Taxonomy of educational objectives: Handbook I. Cognitive domain.* New York, NY: Longman.

Choose My Plate, U.S. Department of Agriculture (http://www.choosemyplate.gov).

Csikszentmihalyi, M. (1997). *Finding flow: The psychology of engagement with everyday life.* New York, NY: Basic Books.

Greene, E., & Goodrich-Dunn, B. (2004). *The psychology of the body.* Philadelphia, PA: Lippincott Williams & Wilkins.

Kagan, J., Snidman, N., Arcus, D., & Reznick, J. S. (1998). *Galen's prophecy: Temperament in human nature.* Boulder, CO: Westview Press.

Seiger, L., Kanipe, D., Vanderpool, K., & Barnes, D. (1998). *Fitness and wellness strategies* (2nd ed.). New York, NY: McGraw-Hill.

Travis, J. W., & Ryan, R. S. (2004). *Wellness workbook* (3rd ed.). Berkeley, CA: Celestial Arts.

CHAPTER 5

References

[1]Taylor, K. (1995). *The ethics of caring* (p. 5). Santa Cruz, CA: Hanford Mead.

[2]Taylor, 1995, p. 233.

[3]*National Certification Board for Therapeutic Massage and Bodywork (NCBTMB) Code of Ethics.* (2008).

[4]*NCBTMB Code of Ethics*, 2008.

[5]*NCBTMB Code of Ethics*, 2008.

[6]Purtilo, R. (1993). *Ethical dimensions in the health professions* (2nd ed.). Philadelphia, PA: W. B. Saunders.

[7]Benjamin, B. E., & Sohnen-Moe, C. (2003). *The ethics of touch* (p. 9). Tucson, AZ: SMA.

[8]Benjamin & Sohnen-Moe, 2003, p. 243.

[9]Greene, E., & Goodrich-Dunn, B. (2004). *The psychology of the body* (p. 17). Philadelphia, PA: Lippincott Williams & Wilkins.

[10]Benjamin & Sohnen-Moe, 2003, p. 112.

[11]Greene & Goodrich-Dunn, 2004, p. 13.

[12]McIntosh, N. (2005). *The educated heart: Professional guidelines for massage therapists, bodyworkers, and movement teachers* (2nd ed., p. 17). Philadelphia, PA: Lippincott, Williams & Wilkins.

[13]Greene & Goodrich-Dunn, 2004, p. 55.

[14]Benjamin & Sohnen-Moe, 2003, p. 39.

[15]McIntosh, 2005.

[16]Report of the Sexual Abuse Task Force of the AMTA Council of Schools, January, 1991.

[17]*NCBTMB Code of Ethics*, 2008.

[18]Illinois Massage Licensing Act [225 ILCS 57/], 2003.

[19]Kisch, R. M. (1998). *Beyond technique: The hidden dimensions of bodywork.* Dayton, OH: BLHY Growth Publications.

[20]Juhan in Kisch, 1998.

Additional Resources

American Massage Therapy Association (http://www.amtamassage.org)

Associated Bodywork and Massage Professionals (http://www.abmp.com)

HIPAA Guidelines (http://www.hhs.gov/ocr/hipaa)

National Certification Board for Therapeutic Massage and Bodywork (http://www.ncbtmb.org)

National Certification Commission for Acupuncture and Oriental Medicine (http://www.nccaom.org)

CHAPTER 6

References

[1]Juhan, D. (1987). *Job's body: A handbook for bodywork* (p. 35). Barrytown, NY: Station Hill Press.

[2]Walton, T. (2006, Summer). Cancer & massage therapy: Essential contraindications. *Massage Therapy Journal, 45*(2), 119–133.

[3]Benjamin, P. J. (2012). Historical overview. In T. Dryden & C. Moyer (Eds.), *Massage therapy: Integrating research and practice.* Champaign, IL: Human Kinetics.

[4]Moraska, A., & Chandler, C. (2008). Changes in clinical parameters in patients with tension-type headache following massage therapy: A pilot study. *Journal of Manual & Manipulative Therapy, 16*(2), 106–112.

[5]Menard, M. B. (2009). *Making sense of research: A guide to research literacy for complementary practitioners* (2nd ed.). Toronto, ON: Curties-Overzet Publications.

[6]Yates, J. (2004). *A physician's guide to therapeutic massage* (3rd ed., p. 30). Toronto, ON: Curties-Overzet Publications.

[7]Cyriax, J. H., & Cyriax, P. J. (1993). *Illustrated manual of orthopedic medicine* (2nd ed.). Boston, MA: Butterworth & Heinemann.

[8]Kania, A. (2012). Scars in massage therapy. In T. Dryden & C. Moyer (Eds.), *Massage therapy: Integrating research and practice* (pp. 173–183). Champaign, IL: Human Kinetics.

[9]Greene, E. (1996). Study links stress reduction with faster healing. *Massage Therapy Journal, 35*(1), 16.

[10]Juhan, 1987, pp. 69–70.

[11]Yates, 2004, pp. 72–74.

[12]Schleip, R., Klingler, W., & Lehmann-Horn, F. (2005). Active fascial contractility: Fascia may be able to contract in a smooth muscle-like manner and thereby influence musculoskeletal dynamics. *Medical Hypotheses, 65,* 273–277.

[13]Ernst, E. (1998). Does post exercise massage reduce delayed onset muscle soreness? A systematic review. *British Journal of Sports Medicine, 32,* 212–214.

[14]Howatson, G., & van Somerson, K. A. (2008). The prevention and treatment of exercise-induced muscle damage. *Sports Medicine, 38,* 483–503.

[15]Yates, 2004, p. 51.

[16]Crosman, L. J., Chateauvert, S. R., &Weisburg, J. (1985). The effects of massage to the hamstring muscle group on range of motion. *Massage Journal, 59–62*.

[17]Field, T. (2000). *Touch therapy.* London, England: Churchill Livingstone.

[18]Ottenbacher, K. J., Muller, L., Brandt, D., Heintzelman, A., Hojem, P., & Sharpe, P. (1987). The effectiveness of tactile stimulation as a form of early intervention: A quantitative evaluation. *Developmental and Behavioral Pediatrics, 8,* 68–76.

[19]Field, 2000, pp. 123–169.

[20]Rich, G. J. (2002). *Massage therapy: The evidence for practice.* New York, NY: Mosby.

[21]Rapaport, M. H., Schettler, P., & Bresee, C. (2010). A preliminary study of the effects of a single session of Swedish massage on hypothalamic-pituitary-adrenal and immune function in normal individuals. *Journal of Alternative and Complementary Medicine, 16*(10), 1079–1088.

[22]Yates, 2004, p. 30.

[23]Wood, E. C., & Becker, P. D. (1981). *Beard's massage* (3rd ed.). Philadelphia, PA: W. B. Saunders.

[24]Sefton, J. M., Yarar, C., Berry, J. W., & Pascoe, D. D. (2010). Therapeutic massage of the neck and shoulders produces changes in peripheral blood flow when assessed with dynamic infrared thermography. *Journal of Alternative and Complementary Medicine, 16*(7), 723–732.

[25]Shoemaker, J. K., Tiidus, P. M., & Mader, R. (1997). Failure of manual massage to alter limb blood flow: Measures by Doppler ultrasound. *Medicine and Science in Sports and Exercise, 29,* 610–614.

[26]Hinds, T., McEwan, I., Perkes, J., Dawson, E., Ball, D., & George, K. (2004). Effects of massage on limb and skin blood flow after quadriceps exercise. *Medicine and Science in Sports and Exercise, 36,* 1308–1313.

[27]Barr, J. S., & N. Taslitz. (1970). Influence of back massage on autonomic functions. *Physical Therapy, 50.*

[28]Cady, S. H., & Jones, G. E. (1997). Massage therapy as a workplace intervention for reduction of stress. *Perceptual and Motor Skills, 84*(1), 157–158.

[29]Mitchell, J. K. (1894). The effect of massage on the number and haemoglobin value of the red blood cells. *American Journal of Medical Science, 107,* 502–515.

[30]Pemberton, R. (1939). Physiology of massage. In *American Medical Association Handbook of Physical Therapy* (3rd ed.). Chicago, IL: Council of Physical Therapy.

[31]Drinker, C. K., & Yoffey, J. M. (1941). Lymphatics, lymph and lymphoid tissue: Their physiological and clinical significance. Cambridge, MA: Harvard University Press.

[32]Elkins, E. C., Herrick, J. F., Grindlay, J. H., Mann, F. C., & DeForest, R. E. (1953). Effects of various procedures on the flow of lymph. *Archives of Physical Medicine, 34,* 31.

[33]Mortimer, P. S., Simmonds, R., Rezvani, M., Robbins, M., Hopewell, J. W., & Ryan, T. J. (1990). The measurement of skin lymph flow by isotope clearance: Reliability, reproducibility, injection dynamics, and the effects of massage. *Journal of Investigative Dermatology, 95,* 666–682.

[34]Kelly, D. G. (2002). *A primer on lymphedema.* Upper Saddle River, NJ: Prentice Hall.

[35]Martini, F. H., & Bartholomew, M. S. (1999). *Structure & function of the human body.* Upper Saddle River, NJ: Prentice-Hall.

[36]Ironson, G., Field, T., Scafidi, F., Hashimoto, M., Kumar, M.,Kumar, A., . . . Fletcher, M. A. (1996). Massage therapy is associated with enhancement of the immune system's cytotoxic capacity. *International Journal of Neuroscience, 84,* 205–217.

[37]Zeitlin, D. et al. (2000). Immunological effects of massage therapy during academic stress. *Psychosomatic Medicine, 62,* 83–87.

[38]Stringer, J., Swindell, R., & Dennis, M. (2008). Massage in patients undergoing intensive chemotherapy reduces serum cortisol and prolactin. *Journal of Psychosocial Oncology, 17,* 1024–1031.

[39]DeDomenico, G., & Wood, E. C. (1997). *Beard's massage* (4th ed.). Philadelphia, PA: W. B. Saunders.

[40]Curties, D. (1999). *Breast massage.* Toronto, ON: Curties-Overzet Publications.

[41]Brown, C. C. (Ed.). (1984). *The many facets of touch.* Johnson & Johnson Baby Products Company.

[42]Diego, M. A., Field, T., Hernandez-Reif, M., Shaw, J. A., Rothe, E. M., Castellanos, D., & Mesner, L. (2002). Aggressive adolescents benefit from massage therapy. *Adolescence, 37,* 597–607.

[43]Juhan, 1987, pp. 53–55.

[44]Montageu, A. (1978). *Touching: The human significance of the skin* (2nd ed.). New York, NY: Harper & Row.

[45]Juhan, 1987, p. 40

[46]Juhan, 1987, p. 34

[47]American Massage Therapy Association. (2013). AMTA Consumer Survey Fact Sheet.

[48]Hasson, D., Arnetz, B., Jelvis, L., & Edelstam, B. (2004). A randomized clinical trial of the treatment effects of massage compared to relaxation tape recordings on diffuse long-term pain. *Psychotherapy and Psychosomatics, 73,* 17–24.

[49]Walach, H., Guthlin, C., & Konig, M. (2003). Efficacy of massage therapy in chronic pain: A pragmatic randomized

[50] trial. *Journal of Alternative and Complementary Medicine, 9,* 837–46.

[50] Rattray, F. S. (1994). *Massage therapy: An approach to treatments.* Toronto, ON: Massage Therapy Texts and MA Verick Consultants.

[51] Yates, 2004.

[52] Yates, 2004, pp. 82–83.

[53] Travell, J. G., & Simons, D. G. (1983). *Myofascial pain and dysfunction: The trigger point manual.* Baltimore, MD: Williams & Wilkins.

[54] Yates, 2004, pp. 78–81.

[55] Bauer, W. C., & Dracup, K. A. (1987). Physiological effects of back massage in patients with acute myocardial infarction. *Focus on Critical Care, 14*(6), 42–46.

[56] Fakouri, C., & Jones, P. (1987). Relaxation: Slow stroke back rub. *Journal of Gerontological Nursing, 13*(2), 32–35.

[57] Fraser, J., & Kerr, J. R. (1993). Psychophysiological effects of back massage on elderly institutionalized patients. *Journal of Advanced Nursing, 18,* 238–245.

[58] Robbins, G., Powers, D., & Burgess, S. (1994). *A wellness way of life* (2nd ed.). Madison, WI: Brown & Benchmark.

[59] Field, 2000, pp. 106–122.

[60] Field, T. M., Fox, N., Pickens, J., Ironsong, G., & Scafidi, F. (1993). Job stress survey. Unpublished manuscript. Touch Research Institute, University of Miami School of Medicine. Reported in *Touchpoints: Touch Research Abstracts, 1*(1).

[61] Field, 2000, pp. 123–169.

[62] Kaard, B., & Tostinbo, O. (1989). Increase of plasma beta endorphins in a connective tissue massage. *General Pharmacology, 20*(4), 487–489.

[63] Moyer, C. A., Rounds, J., & Hannum, J. W. (2004). A meta-analysis of massage therapy research. *Psychological Bulletin, 130,* 3–18.

[64] Rich, G. J. (Ed.). (2002). *Massage therapy: The evidence for practice* (pp. 50–52, 57–83). New York, NY: Mosby.

[65] Greene, E., & Goodrich-Dunn, B. (2004). *The psychology of the body* (p. 111). Philadelphia, PA: Lippincott, Williams & Wilkins.

[66] Martini & Bartholomew, 1999, p. 173.

[67] Knaster, M. (1996). *Discovering the body's wisdom* (pp. 123–124). New York, NY: Bantam.

[68] Price, C. J. (2012). Massage for adults with a history of sexual trauma. In T. Dryden & C. Moyer (Eds.), *Massage therapy: Integrating research and practice* (pp. 165–172). Champaign, IL: Human Kinetics.

[69] Yates, 2004, p. 39.

Additional Resources

Basics of Research Literacy, online continuing education course offered through Massage Therapy Foundation (http://www.massagetherapyfoundation.org/research-literacy-courses/)

Cochrane Collaboration (http://www.cochrane.org)

Dychtwald, K. (1977). *Body-mind.* New York, NY: Jove Publications.

International Journal of Therapeutic Massage & Bodywork: Research, Education, & Practice (http://www.ijtmb.org)

Journal of Bodywork and Movement Therapies (http://www.journals.elsevier.com/jouranl-of-bodywork-and-movement-therapies/)

Massage Therapy Foundation (http://www.massagetherapyfoundation.org)

Mulvihill, M. L., Zelman, M., Holdaway, P., Tompary, E., & Raymond, J. (2006). *Human diseases, a systemic approach* (6th ed.). Upper Saddle River, NJ: Pearson Prentice Hall.

National Center for Complementary and Alternative Medicine (http://www.nccam.nih.gov)

National Library of Medicine (http://ncbi.nlm.nih.gov/PubMed)

Nurse-Healers–Professional Associates International (http://www.therapeutic-touch.org)

Touch Research Institute (TRI) at the University of Miami, School of Medicine (http://www.miami.edu/touch-research).

Werner, R. (2012). *Massage therapist's guide to pathology* (5th ed.). Philadelphia, PA: Lippincott Williams & Wilkins.

CHAPTER 7

References

[1] Sackett, D. L., Straus, S. E., Richardson, W. S., Rosenberg, W., & R. B. Haynes. (2000). *Evidence-based medicine: How to practice and teach EBM.* Edinburgh, Scotland: Churchill Livingston.

[2] Kahn, J. (2012). Integrating research in clinical practice. In T. Dryden & C. Moyer (Eds.), *Massage therapy: Integrating research and practice* (pp. 223–231). Champaign, IL: Human Kinetics.

[3] Field, T. (2000). *Touch therapy* (p. vii.). London, England: Churchill Livingston.

[4] Finch, P. M. (2007). The evidence funnel: Highlighting the importance of research literacy in the delivery of evidence informed complementary health care. *Journal of Bodywork and Movement Therapies, 11*(1), 78–81.

[5.]Yates, J. (1999). *A physician's guide to therapeutic massage* (2nd ed.). Vancouver, BC: Massage Therapists Association of British Columbia.

[6.]Yates, 1999, pp. 3–4.

[7.]Bucci, C. (2012). *Condition specific massage therapy.* Philadelphia, PA: Lippincott, Williams & Wilkins.

[8.]Hammer, W. I. (1993). The use of transverse friction massage in the management of chronic bursitis of the hip and shoulder. *Journal of Manipulation and Physical Therapy, 16*(2), 107–111.

[9.]De Bruijin, R. (1984). Deep transverse friction: Its analgesic effect. *International Journal of Sports Medicine, 5*(suppl.), 35–36.

[10]Quinn, C., Chandler, C., & Moraska, A. (2002). Massage therapy and frequency of chronic tension headaches. *American Journal of Public Health, 92*(10), 1657–1660.

[11]Preyde, M. (2000). Effectiveness of massage therapy for subacute low back pain: A randomized control trial. *Canadian Medical Association Journal, 162*(13), 1815–1820.

[12]Cherkin, D. C., Eisenberg, D., Sherman, K. J., Barlow, W., Kaptchuk, T. J., Street, J., & Deyo, R. J. (2001). Randomized trial comparing traditional Chinese medical acupuncture, therapeutic massage, and self-care education for chronic low back pain. *Archives of Internal Medicine, 161*(8), 1081–1088.

[13]Nelson, D. (2012). Fibromyalgia. In T. Dryden & C. Moyer (Eds.), *Massage therapy: Integrating research and practice* (pp. 185–193). Champaign, IL: Human Kinetics.

[14]Sunshine, W., Field, T. M., Quintino, O., Fierro, K., Burman, I., & Schanberg, S. (1996). Fibromyalgia benefits from massage therapy and transcutaneous electrical stimulation. *Journal of Clinical Rheumatology, 2*(1), 18–22.

[15]Field, T. (2000). *Touch therapy* (p. 68–73). London, England: Churchill Livingston.

[16]Field, T., Diego, M., Cullen, C., Hernandez-Reif, M., Sunshine, W., & Douglas, S. (2002). Fibromyalgia pain and substance P decrease and sleep improves after massage therapy. *Journal of Clinical Rheumatology, 8*, 72–76.

[17]Brattberg, G. (1999). Connective tissue massage in the treatment of fibromyalgia. *European Journal of Pain 3*(3), 235–244.

[18]Lemstra, M., & Olszynski, W. P. (2005). The effectiveness of multidisciplinary rehabilitation in the treatment of fibromyalgia: A randomized control trial. *Clinical Journal of Pain 21*(2), 166–174.

[19]Ekici, G., Bakar, Y., Akbayrak, T., & Yuksei, I. (2009). Comparison of manual lymph drainage and connective tissue massage in women with fibromyalgia: A randomized controlled trial. *Journal of Manipulative Physiological Therapeutics, 32*(2), 127–133.

[20]Longworth, J. D. (1982). Psychophysiological effects of slow stroke back massage in normotensive females. *Advances in Nursing Science, 4*, 44–61.

[21]Curtis, M. (1994). The use of massage in restoring cardiac rhythm. *Nursing Times, 90*(38), 36–37.

[22]Hernandez-Reif, M., Field, T., Krasnegor, J., Hossain, Z., Theakston, H., & Burman, I. (2000). High blood pressure and associated symptoms were reduced by massage therapy. *Journal of Bodywork Movement Therapy, 4*, 31–38.

[23]Moyer, C. A., Rounds, J., & Hannun, J. W. (2004). A meta-analysis of massage therapy research. *Psychological Bulletin, 130*, 3–18.

[24]Bauer, W. C., & Dracup, K. A. (1987). Physiological effects of back massage in patients with acute myocardial infarction. *Focus on Critical Care, 14*(6), 42–46.

[25]Heidt, P. (1981). Effects of Therapeutic Touch on anxiety level of hospitalized patients. *Nursing Research, 30*(1), 32–37.

[26]Werner, R. (2012). *A massage therapist's guide to pathology* (5th ed.). Philadelphia, PA: Lippincott Williams & Wilkins.

[27]Archer, P. (2007). *Therapeutic massage in athletics* (p. 300). Philadelphia, PA: Lippincott Williams & Wilkins.

[28]Kelly, D. G. (2002). *A primer on lymphedema.* Upper Saddle River, NJ: Prentice Hall.

[29]Zanolla, R., Monzeglio, C., Balzarini, A., & Martino, G. (1984). Evaluation of the results of three different methods of postmastectomy lymphedema treatment. *Journal of Surgical Oncology, 26*, 201–213.

[30]Bunce, I. H., Mirolo, B. R., Hennessy, J. M., Ward, L. C., & Jones, L. C. (1994). Post-mastectomy lymphedema treatment and measurement. *Medical Journal Australia, 161*, 125–128.

[31]Hamner, J. B., & Fleming, M. D. (2007). Lymphedema therapy reduces the volume of edema and pain in patients with breast cancer. *Annals of Surgical Oncology 14*(6), 1904–1908.

[32]Vignes, S., Porcher, R., Arrault, M., & Dupuy, A. (2007). Long-term management of breast cancer-related lymphedema after intensive decongestive physiotherapy. *Breast Cancer Research and Treatment, 101*(3), 285–290.

[33]Field, 2000, pp. 201–205.

[34]Hernandez-Reif, M., Field, T., Ironson, G., Beutler, J., Vera, Y., Hurley, J., . . . Fraser, M. (2005). Natural killer cells and lymphocytes increase in women with breast cancer following massage therapy. *International Journal of Neuroscience, 115*(4), 495–510.

[35]Corwin, E. J. (1996). *Handbook of pathophysiology.* Philadelphia, PA: Lippincott.

[36]Field, T., Hentleff, T., Hernandez-Reif, M., Martinez, E., Mavunda, K., Kuhn, C., & Schanberg, S. (1998). Children with asthma have improved pulmonary functions after massage therapy. *Journal of Pediatrics, 132*(5), 854–858.

[37]Witt, P. L., & MacKinnon, J. (1986). Trager psychophysical integration: A method to improve chest mobility of patients with chronic lung disease. *Physical Therapy, 66*(2), 214–217.

[38]Beeken, J. E., Parks, D., Cory, J., & Montopoli, G. (1998). Effectiveness of neuromuscular release massage therapy on chronic obstructive lung disease. *Clinical Nursing Research, 7*(3), 309–325.

[39]Culpepper-Richards, K. (1998). Effect of a back massage and relaxation intervention on sleep in critically ill patients. *American Journal of Critical Care, 7*(4), 288–299.

[40]Mitchinson, A. R., Kim, H. M., Rosenburg, J. M., Geisser, M., Kirsh, M., Ciktir, D., & Hinshaw, D. B. (2007). Acute postoperative pain management using massage as an adjuvant therapy. *Archives of Surgery, 142*(12), 1158–1167.

[41]Frazer, J., & Kerr, J. R. (1993). Psychophysiological effects of back massage on elderly institutionalized patients. *Journal of Advanced Nursing, 18,* 238–245.

[42]Fakouri, C., & Jones, P. (1987). Relaxation: Slow stroke back rub. *Journal of Gerontological Nursing, 13*(2), 32–35.

[43]Walton, T. (2006). Cancer and massage therapy: Essential contraindications. *Massage Therapy Journal, 45*(2), 119–133.

[44]Rhiner, M., Ferrell, B. R. R., Ferrell, B. A., & Grant, M. M. (1993). A structured non-drug intervention program for cancer pain. *Cancer Practice, 1,* 137–143.

[45]Sims, S. (1986). Slow stroke back massage for cancer patients. *Nursing Times, 82,* 47–50.

[46]Weinrich, S. P., & Weinrich, M. C. (1990). The effect of massage on pain in cancer patients. *Applied Nursing Research, 3,* 140–145.

[47]Hernandez-Reif et al., 2005.

[48]Ferrell-Torry, A. T., & Glick, O. J. (1993). The use of therapeutic massage as a nursing intervention to modify anxiety and the perception of cancer pain. *Cancer Nursing, 16*(2), 93–101.

[49]MacDonald, G. (1995, Summer). Massage for cancer patients: A review of nursing research. *Massage Therapy Journal,* 53–56.

[50]Chamness, A. (1996). Breast cancer and massage therapy. *Massage Therapy Journal, 35*(1), 44–46.

[51]Hernandez-Reif, M., Ironson, G., Field, T., Hurley, J., Katz, G., Diego, M., . . . Burman, I. (2004) Breast cancer patients have improved immune and neuroendocrine functions following massage therapy. *Journal of Psychosomatic Research, 57*(1), 45–52.

[52]Bunce, 1994.

[53]Curties, D. (1999). *Breast massage.* Toronto, ON: Curties-Overzet Publications.

[54]Curties, D. (1999). *Massage therapy and cancer.* Toronto, ON: Curties-Overzet Publications.

[55]Vignes, S., Porcher, R., Arrault, M., & Dupuy, A. (2007). Long-term management of breast cancer-related lymphedema after intensive decongestive physiotherapy. *Breast Cancer Research and Treatment, 101*(3), 285–290.

[56]Walton, 2006.

[57]Post-White, J. E. (2012). Cancer. In T. Dryden & C. Moyer (Eds.), *Massage therapy: Integrating research and practice* (pp. 201–202). Champaign, IL: Human Kinetics.

[58]Deng, G. E. M., Frenkel, L., Cohen, B. R., Cassileth, D. I., Abrams, J. L., Capodice, K. S. Courneya, T., . . . Sagar, S. (2009). Evidence-based clinical practice guidelines for integrative oncology: Complementary therapies and botanicals. *Journal of the Society for Integrative Oncology 7*(3), 85–120.

[59]Field, T., & Hernandez-Reif, M. (2001). Sleep problems in infants decrease following massage therapy. *Early Child Development Care, 168,* 95–104.

[60]Field, T., Schanberg, S. M., Scafidi, F., Bauer, C. R., Vega-Lahr, N., Garcia, R., . . . Kuhn, C. (1986). Tactile/kinesthetic stimulation effects on preterm neonates. *Pediatrics, 77*(5), 654–658.

[61]Wheeden, A., Scafidi, F., Field, T., Ironson, G., Valdeon, C., & Bandstra, E. (1993). Massage effects on cocaine-exposed preterm neonates. *Developmental and Behavioral Pediatrics, 14*(5), 318–322.

[62]Gonzalez, A. P., Vasquez-Mendoza, G., Garcia-Vela, A., Guzman-Ramirez, A., Salazar-Torres, M., & Romero-Gutierrez, G. (2009). Weight gain in preterm infants following parent-administered Vimala massage: A randomized controlled trial. *American Journal of Perinatology, 26*(4), 247–252.

[63]Massaro, A. N., Hammad, T. A., Jazzo, B., & Aly, H. (2009). Massage with kinesthetic stimulation improves weight gain in preterm infants. *Journal of Perinatology, 29*(5), 352–357.

[64]Kelmanson, I. A., & Adulas, E. I. (2006). Massage therapy and sleep behavior in infants born with low birth weights. *Complementary Therapies in Clinical Practice, 12*(3), 200–205.

[65]Procianoy, R. S., Mendes, E. W., & Silveira, R. C. (2010). Massage therapy improves neuro-development outcome at two years corrected age for very low birth weight infants. *Early Human Development, 86*(1), 7–11.

[66]Shipwright, S. (2012). Pediatrics. In T. Dryden & C. Moyer (Eds.), *Massage therapy: Integrating research and practice* (pp. 73–83). Champaign, IL: Human Kinetics.

[67]Joachim, G. (1983). The effects of two stress management techniques on feelings of well-being in patients with inflammatory bowel disease. *Nursing Papers, 15*(5), 18.

[68]Field, T., Morrow, C., Valdeon, C., Larson, S., Kuhn, C., & Schanberg, S. (1992). Massage reduces anxiety in child and adolescent psychiatric patients. *Journal of the American Academy of Child and Adolescent Psychiatry, 31*(1), 125–131.

[69]Price, C. (2012). Massage for adults with a history of sexual trauma. In T. Dryden & C. Moyer (Eds.), *Massage therapy: Integrating research and practice* (pp. 165–172). Champaign, IL: Human Kinetics.

[70]Benjamin, B. E. (1995). Massage and body work with survivors of abuse: Part I. *Massage Therapy Journal, 34*(3), 23–32.

[71]Moyer et al., 2004.

[72]Karpen, M. (1995, April/May). Dolores Kreiger, PhD, RN: Tireless teacher of Therapeutic Touch. *Alternative & Complementary Therapies,* 142–146.

[73]Karpen, 1995.

[74]Keller, E., & Bzdek, V. M. (1986). Effects of Therapeutic Touch on tension headache pain. *Nursing Research, 35*(2), 101–106.

[75]Denison, B. (2004). Touch the pain away: New research on therapeutic touch and persons with fibromyalgia syndrome. *Holistic Nursing Practice, 18*(3), 142–151.

[76]Newshan, G., & Schuller-Civitella, D. (2003). Large clinical study shows value of therapeutic touch program. *Holistic Nursing Practice, 17*(4), 189–192.

[77]Cherkin et al., 2001.

[78]Preyde, 2000.

[79]Munk, N. (2013). Case reports: A meaningful way for massage practice to inform research and education. *International Journal of Therapeutic Massage and Bodywork, 6*(3), 3–5.

Additional Resources

Born, B. A. (2005) *The essential massage companion: Everything you need to know to navigate safely through today's drugs and diseases.* Berkley, MI: Concepts Born.

Canadian Massage Therapy Research Network (http://www.cmtrn.ca)

Canadian Touch Research Center (http://www.ccrt-ctrc.ca)

Cochrane Collaboration (http://www.cochrane.org)

Massage Therapy Foundation (http://www.massagetherapyfoundation.org)

Massage Therapy Practice Magazine (http://www.massagetherapypractice.com)

Massage Therapy Research Consortium (http://www.massagetherapyresearchconsortium.com)

Menard, M. B. (2003). *Making sense of research: A guide to research literacy for complementary practitioners.* Toronto, ON: Curties-Overzet Publications.

National Center for Complementary and Alternative Medicine (http://www.nccam.nih.gov)

National Library of Medicine (http://www.ncbi.nlm.nih.gov/PubMed)

Nurse-Healers–Professional Associates International (http://www.therapeutic-touch.org)

Persad, R. (2001). *Massage therapy & medications.* Toronto, ON: Curties-Overzet Publications.

Rattray, F., & Ludwig, L. (2000). *Clinical massage therapy: Understanding, assessing and treating over 700 conditions.* Toronto, ON: Talus Incorporated.

Touch Research Institute (http://www.miami.edu/touch-research)

Werner, R. (2012). *Massage therapist's guide to pathology* (5th ed.). Philadelphia, PA: Lippincott Williams & Wilkins.

CHAPTER 8

Additional Resources

Benjamin, P. J. (2007). Hidden hardware: What's under your client's skin? *Massage Therapy Journal, 46*(1), pp. 106–115.

Mulvihill, M. L., Zelman, M., Holdaway, P., Tompary, E., & Raymond, J. (2006). *Human diseases, a systemic approach* (6th ed.). Upper Saddle River, NJ: Pearson Prentice Hall.

Persad, R. (2001). *Massage therapy & medications.* Toronto, ON: Curties-Overzet Publications.

Rattray, F., & Ludwig, L. (2000). *Clinical massage therapy: Understanding, assessing and treating over 70 conditions.* Toronto, ON: Talus Incorporated.

Werner, R. (2012). *Massage therapist's guide to pathology* (5th ed.). Philadelphia, PA: Lippincott Williams & Wilkins.

Wible, J. (2004). *Pharmacology for massage therapy.* Philadelphia, PA: Lippincott Williams & Wilkins.

Yates, J. (2004). *A physician's guide to therapeutic massage* (3rd ed.). Toronto, ON: Curties-Overzet Publications.

CHAPTER 9

References

[1]Yates, J. (2004). *A physician's guide to therapeutic massage* (p. 13).Toronto, ON: Curties-Overzet.

[2]Biel, A. (2001). *Trail guide to the body: How to locate muscles, bones, and more* (2nd ed., p. 14). Boulder, CO: Books of Discovery.

[3]Chaitow, L. (1997). *Palpation skills: Assessment and diagnosis through touch* (p. 9). New York, NY: Churchill Livingston.

[4]Biel, 2001. p. 18.

[5]Hoppenfeld, S. (1976). *Physical examination of the spine and extremities* (p. 21). Upper Saddle River, NJ: Prentice Hall.

[6]Foster, M. A. (2013). *Therapeutic kinesiology: Musculoskeletal systems, palpation, and body mechanics.* Upper Saddle River, NJ: Pearson.

[7]Thompson, D. L. (2005). *Hands heal: Communication, documentation, and insurance billing for manual therapists* (3rd ed., p. 139). Philadelphia, PA: Lippincott Williams & Wilkins.

Additional Resources

Fremgen, B. F., & Frucht, S. S. (2009). *Medical terminology: A living language* (4th ed.). Upper Saddle River, NJ: Pearson Prentice Hall.

Lowe, W. (2006). *Orthopedic assessment in massage therapy.* Sisters, OR: Daviau-Scott.

Rice, J. (2008). *Medical terminology: A word-building approach* (6th ed.). Upper Saddle River, NJ: Pearson Prentice Hall.

Holey, E., & Cook, E. (2003). *Evidence-based therapeutic massage: A practical guide for therapists.* London, England: Churchill Livingston.

Norkin, C. C., & White, D. J. (2009). *Measurement of joint motion: A guide to goniometry* (4th ed.). Philadelphia, PA: F.A. Davis.

U.S. Department of Health and Human Services, HIPAA Privacy Rules (http://WWW.hhs.gov/ocr/hipaa)

Werner, R. (2012). *Massage therapist's guide to pathology* (5th ed.). Philadelphia, PA: Lippincott Williams & Wilkins.

CHAPTER 10

Additional Resources

Dixon, M. W. (2001). *Body mechanics and self-care manual.* Upper Saddle River, NJ: Prentice Hall.

Frye, B. (2000). *Body mechanics for manual therapists: A functional approach to self-care and injury prevention.* Stanwood, WA: Freytag Publishing.

McIntosh, N. (1999). *The educated heart: Professional guidelines for massage therapists, bodyworkers and movement teachers.* Memphis, TN: Decatur Bainbridge Press.

Standards of Practice. (2008). National Certification Board for Therapeutic Massage and Bodywork (http://www.ncbtmb.org).

U.S. Department of Health and Human Services, Centers for Disease Control and Prevention (http://www.cdc.gov.).

CHAPTER 11

Additional Resources

Dixon, M. W. (2001). *Body mechanics and self-care manual.* Upper Saddle River, NJ: Prentice Hall.

Frye, B. (2000). *Body mechanics for manual therapists: A functional approach to self-care and injury prevention.* Stanwood, WA: Freytag Publishing.

Standards of Practice. (2008). National Certification Board for Therapeutic Massage and Bodywork (http://www.ncbtmb.org).

CHAPTER 12

References

[1]Kellogg, J. H. (1895). *The art of massage: Its physiological effects and therapeutic applications.* Battle Creek, MI: Modern Medicine Publishing.

[2]Hoffa, A. J. (1900). *Technik der massage* (3rd ed., p. 2). Verlagsbuchhandlung, Stuttgart: Ferdinand Enke. Translation by F. M. Tappan and Ruth Friedlander.

[3]Rattray, F., & Ludwig, L. (2000). *Clinical massage therapy* (p. 41). Toronto, ON: Talis Incorporated.

[4]Cyriax, J. H., & Cyriax, P. J. (1993). *Illustrated manual of orthopedic medicine* (2nd ed.). Boston, MA: Butterworth & Heinemann.

[5]Kellogg, 1895, p. 52.

[6]Kellogg, 1895, p. 53.

Additional Resources

Werner, R. (2005). *A massage therapist's guide to pathology* (3rd ed.). Philadelphia, PA: Lippincott, Williams & Wilkins.

CHAPTER 13

References

[1]Roth, M. (1851). *The prevention and cure of many chronic diseases by movement.* London, England: Churchill.

[2]Foster, M. A. (2013). *Therapeutic kinesiology: Musculoskeletal systems, palpation, and body mechanics* (p. 64). Upper Saddle River, NJ: Pearson.

[3]Werner, R. (2008). *A massage therapist's guide to pathology* (4th ed.). Philadelphia, PA: Lippincott Williams & Wilkins.

Additional Resources

Norkin, C. C., & White, D. J. (2009). *Measurement of joint motion: A guide to goniometry* (4th ed.). Philadelphia, PA: F.A. Davis.

CHAPTER 14

Additional Resources

Born, B. A. (2005). *The essential massage companion.* Berkley, MI: Concepts Born.

Werner, R. (2005). *A massage therapist's guide to pathology.* Philadelphia, PA: Lippincott Williams & Wilkins.

CHAPTER 15

References

[1]Curties, D. (1999). *Breast massage.* Toronto, ON: Curties-Overzet Publications.

Additional Resources

Born, B. A. (2005). *The essential massage companion.* Berkley, MI: Concepts Born.

Japanese hand massage (Video). (2001). With Shogo Mochizuki. Boulder, CO: Kotobuki Publications.

Lowe, W. (2006). *Orthopedic assessment in massage therapy.* Sisters, OR: Daviau-Scott.

Werner, R. (2012). *A massage therapist's guide to pathology* (5th ed.). Philadelphia, PA: Lippincott Williams & Wilkins.

CHAPTER 16

Additional Resources

Born, B. A. (2005). *The essential massage companion.* Berkley, MI: Concepts Born.

Lowe, W. (2006). Orthopedic *assessment in massage therapy.* Sisters, OR: Daviau-Scott.

Werner, R. (2012). *A massage therapist's guide to pathology* (5th ed.). Philadelphia, PA: Lippincott Williams & Wilkins.

CHAPTER 17

References

[1]Barclay, J. (1994). *In good hands: The history of the chartered society of physiotherapy 1894–1994* (p. 3). London, England: Butterworth-Heinemann.

[2]Belanger, A. Y. (2002). *Evidence-based guide to therapeutic physical agents.* Philadelphia, PA: Lippincott Williams & Wilkins.

[3]Fowlie, L. (2006). *An introduction to heat and cold as therapy* (pp. 38–39). Toronto, ON: Curties-Ovezet Publications.

Additional Resources

Benjamin, P. J. (2004, Spring). Massage and sweatbaths among the ancient Maya. *Massage Therapy Journal, 148–154.*

Croutier, A. L. (1992). *Taking the waters: Spirit, art, sensuality.* New York, NY: Abbeville Press.

Fowlie, L. (2006) *An introduction to heat and cold as therapy.* Toronto: Curties-Overzet Publications.

Hayes, K. W., & Hall, K. D. (2011). *Manual for physical agents.* Upper Saddle River, NJ: Prentice Hall.

Hecox, B., Mehreteab, T. A., & Weisberg, J. (1994). *Physical agents: A comprehensive text for physical therapists.* Upper Saddle River, NJ: Prentice Hall.

Knight, K. L. (1995). *Cryotherapy in sport injury management.* Champaign, IL: Human Kinetics.

Persad, R. S. (2001). *Massage therapy & medications: General treatment principles.* Toronto: Curties-Overzet.

CHAPTER 18

References

[1]Baskwill, A. (2012). Pregnancy and labor. In T. Dryden & C. Moyer (Eds.), *Massage therapy: Integrating research and practice* (pp. 85–102). Champaign, IL: Human Kinetics.

[2]Field, T., Hernandez-Reif, M., Taylor, S., Quintino, O., & Burman, I. (1997). Labor pain is reduced by massage therapy. *Journal of Psychosomatic Obstetrics and Gynecology, 18,* 286–291.

[3]Gach, M. R. (1990). *Acupressure's potent points: A guide to self-care for common ailments.* New York, NY: Bantam Books.

[4]Ibid.

[5]Shipwright, S. (2012). Pediatrics. In T. Dryden & C. Moyer (Eds.), *Massage therapy: Integrating research and practice* (pp. 73–83). Champaign, IL: Human Kinetics.

[6]Thompson, D. L. (2012). Massage and older adults. In T. Dryden & C. Moyer (Eds.), *Massage therapy: Integrating research and practice* (pp. 103–113). Champaign, IL: Human Kinetics.

[7]Holliday-Welsh, D. M., Gessart, C. E., & Renier, C. M. (2009). Massage in the management of agitation in nursing home residents with cognitive impairment. *Geriatric Nursing 30,* 108–117.

[8]Nelson, D. (1994). *Compassionate touch: Hands-on care-giving for the elderly, the ill and the dying.* New York, NY: Station Hill Press.

[9]Ibid., p. 43.

Additional Resources

American Society on Aging (http://www.asaging.org)

Archer, P. (2007). *Therapeutic massage in athletics.* Philadelphia, PA: Lippincott Williams & Wilkins.

Benjamin, P. J., & Lamp, S. P. (2005). *Understanding sports massage* (2nd ed.). Champaign, IL: Human Kinetics.

Born, B. A. (2005). *The essential massage companion.* Berkley, MI: Concepts Born.

Center for Compassionate Touch (http://www .compassionate-touch.org)

Center to Advance Palliative Care (http://www.capc.org)

Curties, D. (1999). *Breast massage.* Moncton, NB, Canada: Curties-Overzet Publications.

Day-Break Geriatric Massage Institute (http://www .daybreak-massage.com)

Ellis, V., Hill, J., & Campbell, H. (1995). Strengthening the family unity through the healing power of massage. *Journal of Hospice & Palliative Care, 12,* pp. 19–20.

Fanslow, C. (1984). Touch and the elderly. In C. C. Brown (ed.), *The many facets of touch.* Skillman, NJ: Johnson & Johnson Baby Products Company.

Field, T. (2000). Enhancing growth. In *Touch therapy.* New York, NY: Churchill Livingston.

Field, T. (2001). *Touch.* Cambridge, MA: MIT Press.

Howdyshell, C. (1998). Complementary therapy: Aromatherapy with massage for geriatric and hospice care for a holistic approach. *Hospice Journal, 13,* 69–75.

Infant massage lessons for dads: The power of a father's touch (Video). (2003) with John G. Louis. Acuforce International, Inc.

International Loving Touch Foundation (http://www .lovingtouch.com)

International Association of Infant Massage Instructors (http://www.iaimi.com)

Massage for sports health care: For enhanced athletic performance and recovery (Video). (1998). Champaign, IL: Human Kinetics. (http://www.humankinetics.com)

Mulvihill, M. L., Zelman, M., Holdaway, P., Tompary, E., & Raymond, J. (2006). *Human diseases, a systemic approach* (6th ed.). Upper Saddle River, NJ: Pearson Prentice Hall.

National Council on Aging (NCOA) (http://www .ncoa.org)

National Hospice and Palliative Care Organization (http:// www.nhpco.org)

National Hospice Foundation (http://www.hospiceinfo.org)

National Institute on Aging at the National Institutes of Health (http://www.nia.nih.gov)

Nelson, D. (2001). *From the heart through the hands: The power of touch in caregiving.* Forres, Scotland: Findhorn Press.

Remington, R. (2002). Hand massage in the agitated elderly. In G. J. Rich (ed.), *Massage therapy: The evidence for practice.* New York, NY: Mosby.

Schneider, V. (1982). *Infant massage: A handbook for loving parents.* New York, NY: Bantam Books.

Stillerman, E. (1992). *Mother-massage: A handbook for relieving the discomforts of pregnancy.* New York, NY: Delta/Delcorte.

U.S. Administration on Aging (AoA) (http://www .aoa.gov)

Werner, R. (2012). *A massage therapist's guide to pathology* (5th ed.). Philadelphia, PA: Lippincott Williams & Wilkins.

Wible, J. (2004). *Pharmacology for massage therapy.* Philadelphia, PA: Lippincott Williams & Wilkins.

CHAPTER 19

References

[1]National Association for Holistic Aromatherapy (NAHA). (2005). *About aromatherapy.* Retrieved from http://www .naha.org/explore-aromatherapy/about-aromatherapy

[2]NAHA. (2005). *Aromatherapy regulation.* Retrieved from http://www.naha.org/explore-aromatherapy/regulations

Additional Resources

Ahava—Dead Sea mud (http://www.ahava.com)

Buckle, J. (2007). *Clinical aromatherapy, essential oils in practice.* New York, NY: Churchill Livingstone.

Calistoga Spas. (2008). *The Mud Baths.* Retrieved from http://www.calistogaspas/mud-baths

Glen Ivy Hot Springs Spa. (2008). *Hot Springs Spa, History.* Retrieved from http://www.glenivy.com/index .php/resort/C8

Innovative Spa (http://www.innovativespa.com)

Massage Warehouse and Spa Essentials (http://www .massagewarehouse.com)

Minton, M. (2008b). *Mud: Dig it!* Retrieved from http:// www.massagemag.com/spa/treatment/mud/php

Ody, P. (1993). *The medicinal herbal.* New York, NY: Dorling Kindersley.

Ody, P. (2002). *Essential guide to natural home remedies.* London, England: Kyle Cathie Limited.

Price, S., & Price, L. (2007). *Aromatherapy for health professionals* (3rd ed.). Philadelphia, PA: Churchill Livingstone Elsevier

Pure Essential, Inc. (2007). *Essential oils and perfume notes.* Retrieved from http://www.essential-oil.org/essential_ oils_notes.asp

QE Health (formerly the Queen Elizabeth Hospital) in Rotorua (http://www.rotoruanz.com/attractions/ spa_wellness.php) (http://www.qehealth.co.nz)

Rose, J. (1999). *375 essential oils and hydrosols.* Berkeley, CA: Frog Ltd.

Shutes, J., & Weaver, C. (2008). *Aromatherapy for bodyworkers.* Upper Saddle River, NJ: Pearson Prentice Hall

Spa Elegance (http://www.spaelegance.com)

SpaEquip (http://www.spaequip.com)

Tisserand, R. B. (1985). *The art of aromatherapy*. Essex, England: Saffron Walden: C. W. Daniel Company Ltd.

Torf Spa—organic moor mud from Europe (http://www.torfspa.com)

Universal Companies (http://www.universalcompanies.com)

Water Werks (http://www.vichyshower.com)

Williams, A. (2007). *Spa bodywork, a guide for massage therapists*. Philadelphia, PA: Lippincott, Williams & Wilkins.

Worwood, V. A. (1999). *The fragrant heavens*. Novato, CA: New World Library.

CHAPTER 20

References

[1]Palmer, D. (1995). The death of on-site massage? *Massage Therapy Journal, 34*(3), 119–120.

[2]Field, T. M., Fox, N., Pickens, J., Armstrong, G., & Scafidi, F. (1993). Job stress survey. Unpublished manuscript, Touch Research Institute, University of Miami School of Medicine. Reported in *Touchpoints: Touch Research Abstracts, 1*(1).

[3]No author. (1996, July/August). Massage helps lower stress of working, taking final exams. *Massage, 62* 148.

[4]Hodge, M., Robinson, C., Boehmer, J., & Klein, S. (2002). Employee outcomes following work-site acupressure and massage. *Massage therapy: The evidence for practice*. New York, NY: Mosby.

Additional Resources

Japanese chair massage (Video). (2002). By Shogo Mochizuki. Boulder, CO: Kotobuki Publications.

TouchPro Institute (http://www.touchpro.org)

CHAPTER 21

References

[1]Knaster, M. (1996). *Discovering the body's wisdom*. New York, NY: Bantam Books.

[2]International Fascia Research Congress. Retrieved from http://www.fasciacongress.org

[3]International Fascia Research Congress. Retrieved from http://www.fasciacongress.org/about.htm

[4]Cantu, R. I., & Grodin, A. J. (1992). *Myofascial manipulation: Theory and clinical application*. Gaithersburg, MD: Aspen.

[5]Juhan, D. (1987). *Job's body: A handbook for bodywork* (p. 68). Barrytown, NY: Station Hill Press.

[6]Barnes, J. F. (1987, September). Myofascial massage, *Physical Therapy Forum*.

[7]Erlingheuser, R. F. (1959). Circulation of cerebrospinal fluid through connective tissue system, *Academy of Applied Osteopathy Yearbook*, as mentioned in Juhan (1987), pp. 72–73.

[8]Schultz, R. L., & Feitis, R. (1996). *The endless web: fascial anatomy and physical reality*. Berkeley, CA: North Atlantic Books.

[9]Scheumann, D. W. (2002). *The balanced body: A guide to deep tissue and neuromuscular therapy* (2nd ed., p. 45). Philadelphia, PA: Lippincott, Williams & Wilkins.

[10]Barnes, J. F. (1987, September). Myofascial massage, *Physical Therapy Forum*.

Additional Resources

Chaitow, L. (1996). *Modern neuromuscular techniques*. London, England: Churchill Livingston.

Findley, T. W., & Schleip, R. (2007). *Fascial research: Basic science and implications for conventional and complementary health care*. New York, NY: Elsevier.

International Journal of Therapeutic Massage & Bodywork: Research, Education, & Practice (http://www.ijtmb.org)

Journal of Bodywork and Movement Therapies (http://www.journals.elsevier.com/jouranl-of-bodywork-and-movement-therapies/)

Manheim, C. (2001). *The myofascial release manual* (3rd ed.). Thorofare, NJ: Slack Inc.

Schleip, R., Klingler, W., & Lehmann-Horn, F. (2005). Active fascial contractility: Fascia may be able to contract in a smooth muscle-like manner and thereby influence musculoskeletal dynamics. *Medical Hypotheses, 65*, 273–277.

CHAPTER 22

References

[1]Travell, J. G., & Simons, D. G. (1999). *Myofascial pain and dysfunction: The trigger point manual, Vol. 1. Upper half of the body* (2nd ed., p. 4). Baltimore, MD: Williams & Wilkins.

[2]Mense, S., & Simons, D. G. (2001). Myofascial pain caused by trigger points. In *Muscle pain: Understanding its nature, diagnosis, and treatment* (pp. 250–251). Philadelphia, PA: Lippincott Williams & Wilkins.

[3]Travell & Simons, 1999, p. 13.

[4]Travell, J. G., & Simons, D. G. (1992). *Myofascial pain and dysfunction: The trigger point manual, Vol. 2. The lower extremities*. Baltimore, MD: Williams & Wilkins.

[5]Archer, P. (2007). *Therapeutic massage in athletics* (p. 136). Philadelphia, PA: Lippincott Williams & Wilkins.

[6]Archer, 2007, p. 138.

[7]Quinn, C., Chandler, C., & Moraska, A. (2002). Massage therapy and frequency of chronic tension headaches. *American Journal of Public Health, 92*(10), 1657–1661.

Additional Resources

Benjamin, P. J. (2006, Summer). Loosen the grip: How massage can soothe chronic tension headaches. *Massage Therapy Journal, 45*(2), 50–59.

Chaitow, L. (1996). *Modern neuromuscular techniques.* London, England: Churchill Livingston.

International Journal of Therapeutic Massage & Bodywork: Research, Education, & Practice. (http://www.ijtmb.org)

Journal of Bodywork and Movement Therapies (http://www.journals.elsevier.com/jouranl-of-bodywork-and-movement-therapies/)

Prudden, B. (1984). *Myotherapy: Bonnie Prudden's complete guide to pain-free living.* New York, NY: Ballantine Books.

Travell, J. G., & Rinzler, S. H. (1952). The myofascial genesis of pain. *Postgraduate Medicine, 11,* 425–434.

CHAPTER 23

References

[1]Kurz, I. (1986a). *Textbook of Dr. Vodder's manual lymphatic drainage: Vol. II. Therapy* (3rd ed.). Heidelberg, Germany: Karl F. Haug.

[2]Kurz, I. (1986b). *Textbook of Dr. Vodder's manual lymphatic drainage: Vol. III. Treatment* (3rd ed.). Heidelberg, Germany: Karl F. Haug.

[3]Foldi, E., & Foldi, M. (1999). *Textbook of Foldi School.* Austria: Self-published, English translation by Heida Brenneke.

[4]Casley-Smith, J. R., & Casley-Smith, J. R. (1994). *Modern treatment of lymphedema.* Adelaide, Australia: Henry Thomas Laboratory, Lymphoedema Association of Australia.

[5]Martini, F. H., & Bartholomew, E. F. (2000). *Essentials of anatomy and physiology* (2nd ed.). Upper Saddle River, NJ: Prentice Hall.

[6]Swartz, M. A., & Fleury, M. E. (2007). Interstitial flow and its effects in soft tissues. *Annual Review of Biomedical Engineering, 9,* 229–256.

[7]Kelly, D. G. (2002). *A primer on lymphedema* (p. 5). Upper Saddle River, NJ, Prentice Hall.

[8]Archer, P. (2007). *Therapeutic massage in athletics* (pp. 57–58). Philadelphia, PA: Lippincott Williams & Wilkins.

Additional Resources

Pishinger, E. A. (1991). *Matrix and matrix regulation: Basis for a holistic theory in medicine.* Portland, OR: Medicina Biologica.

International Journal of Therapeutic Massage & Bodywork: Research, Education, & Practice. (http://www.ijtmb.org)

Journal of Bodywork and Movement Therapies (http://www.journals.elsevier.com/jouranl-of-bodywork-and-movement-therapies/)

CHAPTER 24

References

[1]Issel, C. (1993). *Reflexology: Art, science, and history.* Sacramento, CA: New Frontier Publishing.

[2]Byers, D. C. (2001). *Better health with foot reflexology* (revised ed.). St. Petersburg, FL: Ingham Publishing.

[3]Stone, P. (2004). *History of reflexology.* St. Charles, MO: Author.

[4]Fitzgerald, W. H., & Bowers, E. F. (1917). *Zone therapy.* Columbus, OH: I. W. Long.

[5]Issel, 1993.

[6]Benjamin, P. J. (1989a, Spring). Eunice Ingham and the development of foot reflexology in the United States. Part one: The early years–to 1946. *Massage Therapy Journal,* 38–44.

[7]Benjamin, P. J. (1989b, Winter). Eunice Ingham and the development of foot reflexology in the United States. Part two: On the road 1946–1974. *Massage Therapy Journal,* 49–55.

[8]Carter, M., & Weber, T. (1997). *Healing yourself with foot reflexology.* New York, NY: Penguin Putnam.

[9]Ingham, E. D. (1938). *Stories the feet can tell: Stepping to better health.* Rochester, NY: Author.

[10]Tibshraeney-Morten, L. (2008). *Moving the energy: Reflexology and meridian theory* (p. 266). Seminole, FL: JLM Publishing.

[11]International Council of Reflexologists. Retrieved from http://www.icr-reflexology.org

[12]Stone, P. (2010). *Reflexology.* Upper Saddle River, NJ: Prentice Hall.

Additional Resources

American Commission for Accreditation of Reflexology Education and Training (http://www.acaret.org)

American Reflexology Certification Board (http://www.arcb.net)

International Council of Reflexologists (http://www.icr-reflexology.org)

Kunz, K., & Kunz, B. (2007). *Complete reflexology for life.* New York, NY: Dorling Kindersley Limited.

Stone, P. (2004). A snapshot of the history of reflexology. *Massage Therapy Journal* online edition. Retrieved from http://www.amtamassage.org

Stone, P. (2006, Summer). Keeping step: Your guide to adding reflexology to your business. *Massage Therapy Journal* online edition. Retrieved from http://www.amtamassage.org

CHAPTER 25

References

[1]Douillard, J. (2004). *The encyclopedia of Ayurvedic massage* (p. 1). Berkeley, CA: North Atlantic Books.

Additional Resources

American Organization for Bodywork Therapies of Asia (http://www.aobta.org)

American Polarity Therapy Association (http://www.polaritytherapy.org)

Beresford-Cooke, C. (1999). *Shiatsu theory and practice.* Edinburgh, Scotland: Churchill Livingstone.

Capra, F. (1999). *The tao of physics: An exploration of the parallels between modern physics and eastern mysteries.* Boston, MA: Shambhala Publications.

Gordon, R. (1979). *Your healing hands: The polarity experience.* Santa Cruz, CA: Unity Press.

Jarmey, C., & Mojay, G. (1991). *Shiatsu: The complete guide.* London, England: Thorsons.

Jarrett, L. (2000). *Nourishing destiny: The inner tradition of Chinese medicine.* Stockbridge, MA: Spirit Path Press.

Johari, H. (1996). *Ayurvedic massage: Traditional Indian techniques for balancing body and mind.* Rochester, VT: Healing Arts Press.

Jwing-Ming, Y. (2005). *Qigong massage: Fundamental techniques for health and relaxation.* Boston, MA: YMAA Publication Center.

Kuhn, A. (2004). *Natural healing with qigong: Therapeutic qigong.* Boston, MA: YMAA Publication Center.

Maciocia, G. (1998). *The foundations of Chinese medicine: A comprehensive text for acupuncturists and herbalists.* Edinburgh, Scotland: Churchill Livingstone.

Masunaga, S., & Ohashi, W. (1977). *Zen Shiatsu: How to harmonize yin and yang for better health.* Tokyo, Japan: Japan Publications.

Moyers, B. *The mystery of chi, Volume 1: Healing and the mind* (Video). Video series. Ambrose Video.

Namikoshi, T. (1981). *The complete book of shiatsu therapy.* Tokyo, Japan: Japan Publications.

National Certification Commission for Acupuncture and Oriental Medicine (http://www.nccaom.org)

Ni, M. (1995). *The yellow emperor's classic of medicine: A new translation of the Nei Jing Suwen with commentary.* Boston, MA: Shambhala.

Parks, W. (2007). *Integrating acupressure with Will Parks* (Video).

Siedman, M. (1982). *Like a hollow flute: A guide to polarity therapy.* Santa Cruz, CA: Elan Press.

Sills, F. (2002). *The polarity process: Energy as a healing art.* Berkeley, CA: North Atlantic Books.

Stone, R. (1987). *Dr. Randolph Stone's Polarity Therapy: The complete collected works.* Harlan Tarbell, Illustrator. Sebastopol, CA: CRCS Publications.

Tedeschi, M. (2000). *Essential anatomy for healing and the martial arts.* Tokyo, Japan: Weatherwill.

Wang, J. (1994). *The history of massage in mainland China* (Video). American Organization for Bodywork Therapies of Asia (AOBTA), Video 13, Boston, MA: Convention.

Wang, J. (1999). To treat before sick. From *Pulse,* Voorhees, NJ: AOBTA.

Yang, J. M. (2005). *Qigong massage: Fundamental techniques for health and relaxation.* Boston, MA: YMAA Publication Center.

Yuen, J. (2001). *Light on the essence of Chinese medicine: The Nei Jing Su Wen.* Boston, MA: New England School of Acupuncture.

CHAPTER 26

References

[1]Internal Revenue Service. *Glossary of common terms.* Retrieved from http://www.irs.gov/Individuals/HCTC:-Glossary-of-Common-Terms

[2]Internal Revenue Service. Form SS-8, *Determination of Worker Status for Purposes of Federal Employment Taxes and Income Tax Withholding.* Retrieved from http://www.irs.gov/pub/irs-pdf/fss8.pdf

Additional Resources

Internal Revenue Service (http://www.irs.gov)

Makely, S. (2005). *Professionalism in health care: A primer for career success* (2nd ed.). Upper Saddle River, NJ: Prentice Hall.

Mariotti, S. (2007). *Entrepreneurship: Starting and operating a small business.* Upper Saddle River, NJ: Prentice Hall.

National Employers Association (http://neasa-sa.com)

National Labor Relations Board (http://www.nlrb.gov)

U.S. Equal Employment Opportunity Commission (http://www.eeoc.gov)

CHAPTER 27

References

[1]Kamoroff, B. B. (2003). *Small time operator: How to start your own business, keep your books, pay your taxes, and stay out of trouble* (p. 42). Laytonville, CA: Bell Springs Publishing.

[2]Piccoine, N. (1990). *Dome simplified weekly bookkeeping record: A simple, complete, and practical business record as required by federal and state laws.* Warwick, RI: Dome Publishing.

[3]Benjamin, B. E., & Sohnen-Moe, C. (2003). *The ethics of touch* (p. 207). Tucson, AZ: SMA.

Additional Resources

American Massage Therapy Association. (2005). *Massage therapy consumer survey fact sheet.* Evanston, IL: Author.

Internal Revenue Service. (2005). *Business expenses,* IRS Publication 535.

Internal Revenue Service. (2006). *Self-employment tax,* Schedule SE (Form 1040).

Internal Revenue Service. (2006). *Starting a business and keeping records,* IRS Publication 583.

Internal Revenue Service. (2006). *Tax withholding and estimated tax,* IRS Publication 505.

Internal Revenue Service. (2005). *Your federal income tax— For individuals,* IRS Publication 17.

Kamoroff, B. B. (2003). *Small time operator: How to start your own business, keep your books, pay your taxes, and stay out of trouble.* Laytonville, CA: Bell Springs Publishing.

Internal Revenue Service (http://www.irs.gov)

Madison-Mahoney, V. (updated 2008) *Manipulate your future: Comprehensive guide to massage therapy insurance billing.* (http://www.thebodyworker.com/massage-insurance-billing.htm)

Mariotti, S. (2007). *Entrepreneurship: Starting and operating a small business.* Upper Saddle River, NJ: Prentice Hall.

U.S. Small Business Administration (http://www.sba.gov)

CHAPTER 28

References

[1]Federal Trade Commission. (1983). *FTC statement on deception.* Retrieved from http://www.ftc.gov/bcp/policystmt/ad-decept.htm

[2]Federal Trade Commission. (1980). *FTC guides concerning use of endorsements and testimonials in advertising.* Retrieved from http://www.ftc.gov/sites/default/files/attachments/press-releases/ftc-publishes-final-guides-governing-endorsements-testimonials/091005revisedendorsementguides.pdf

[3]Federal Trade Commission. (2002). *Guides against bait advertising.* Retrieved from http://www.ftc.gov/bcp/guides/baitads-gd.htm

[4]Federal Trade Commission. (1984). *FTC policy statement regarding advertising substantiation.* Retrieved from http://www.ftc.gov/guides/ad3subst.htm

[5]National Certification Board for Therapeutic Massage and Bodywork. (2008). *Code of ethics.* Retrieved from http://www.ncbtmb.org/download/ncbtmb-code-ethics-2-page

[6]U.S. Copyright Office. (2000). *Circular 1: Copyright basics.* Retrieved from http://www.copyright.gov/circs/circ01.pdf

[7]National Certification Board for Therapeutic Massage and Bodywork. (2008). *Code of ethics.* Retrieved from http://www.ncbtmb.org/download/ncbtmb-code-ethics-2-page

Additional Resources

Benjamin, B. E., & Sohnen-Moe, C. (2003). *The ethics of touch.* Tucson, AZ: SMA.

Better Business Bureau (http://www.bbb.org)

Federal Trade Commission (http://www.ftc.gov)

Internal Revenue Service (http://www.irs.gov)

National Certification Board for Therapeutic Massage and Bodywork (http://www.ncbtmb.com)

U.S. Copyright Office (http://www.copyright.gov)

U.S. Patent and Trademark Office (http://www.uspto.gov)

Interactive Glossary

This interactive glossary defines terms used in the text and also suggests relationships between them. Look for the directions *See*, ***Compare to***, and ***Contrast with***; these point to specific connections with other terms. ***See*** refers to some link with another term, ***Compare to*** refers to a similarity, and ***Contrast with*** refers to a major distinction. Students can sharpen their understanding and critical thinking skills by studying these word associations.

Abdominal breathing is a method of breathing focusing on movements of the diaphragm; also called diaphragmatic breathing. During inhalation the diaphragm pushes downward, allowing the lungs to fill with air; the abdominal wall expands, while the chest and shoulders remain relatively still. During exhalation the diaphragm relaxes, and the abdominal wall contracts slightly, pushing the air out. Used for relaxation and in body–mind practices such as qi gong. See *Qi gong*.

Accountability is a trait in which individuals accept responsibility for their actions, do not make excuses for repeated mistakes, and apologize sincerely for and correct mistakes that they have made. See *Work ethic*.

Accreditation is recognition awarded to institutions or education programs by a nongovernmental organization that sets standards of excellence; accredited schools have undergone a peer evaluation to confirm that the accreditation standards are met. Contrast with *Certification*.

Active assisted stretch is a method of stretching in which a practitioner provides additional force in the direction of an active stretch being performed by a recipient. See *Stretching*. Contrast with *Simple static stretch* and *Contract–relax–stretch*.

Active listening is a communication skill that involves reflecting back to the speaker what the listener thinks was said; accomplished by paraphrasing or restating the words to clarify their meaning. Contrast with *Affirmative listening*.

Active movements are initiated and powered voluntarily by a person with no or some assistance from a practitioner. Types of active movements are free, assistive, and resistive. Contrast with *Passive movements*.

Active range of motion (AROM) refers to the evaluation of motion at a joint while a person actively moves that joint through its range; observations include degree of motion possible, restrictions or shortening, and

any discomfort experienced; used to collect objective information for *Goal-oriented planning*.

Active trigger points are always tender, prevent full lengthening, weaken the muscle, and refer pain on direct compression. See *Trigger point therapy* and *Trigger points*.

Activities of daily living (ADLs) are common physical activities performed in everyday life that contribute to living independently; examples are getting up out of a chair, dressing and undressing, climbing stairs, eating, and getting into and out of a bathtub. See *Special population*.

Acupoints are part of the theory of Asian bodywork therapy that refers to places along energy channels where Qi can collect and be accessed and influenced by applying pressure; also called acupuncture points and acupressure points. There are 365 classic acupoints located along the major energy channels. See *Acupressure*, *Energy channels*, *Qi*.

Acupressure is a Western term for a form of Asian bodywork therapy based on Chinese medicine in which energy channels and acupuncture points (acupoints) are stimulated to balance the flow of energy or Qi. See *Asian bodywork therapies*.

Acupressure massage integration (AMI) is a bodywork adaptation in which principles and techniques of acupressure are integrated with standard Swedish massage to address both the physical and energetic wellness of clients. See *Acupressure* and *Swedish massage*.

Adaptations are adjustments or changes to the way things are normally done in a massage therapy session to meet the unique needs of an individual client. See *Special population*.

Affirmative listening is a communication skill that involves letting the speaker know that you are paying attention; accomplished by occasional verbal cues and body language. Contrast with *Active listening*.

Age-appropriate elders are people over age 70 who show some of the typical signs of aging. Contrast with *Robust elders* and *Frail elders*.

Aleiptes is a historical term used in ancient Greece to describe the people in the gymnasium who rubbed athletes with oil.

Alternative therapy refers to methods or systems of healing outside mainstream medicine. Contrast with *Complementary therapy* and *Integrative health care*.

American Organization for Bodywork Therapies of Asia (AOBTA®) is a professional membership association that certifies ABT practitioners and instructors and promotes excellence in ABT education. See *Asian bodywork therapies*.

Ammashi is a historical term for a practitioner of traditional Japanese massage; occupation for the blind in nineteenth- and twentieth-century Japan. See *Asian bodywork therapies*.

Anatomical position is the body posture used when describing the positions and relationships of structures in the human body; in the anatomical position, a person is standing erect with arms at the sides, legs together, toes pointing forward, palms of the hands facing forward, and the head is centered with eyes looking straight ahead. Contrast with *Posture analysis*.

Anecdote is a general descriptive story about the treatment of a condition and the outcomes for one patient or client. Contrast with *Case study* and *Scientific method*.

Anmo is a term from Chinese medicine meaning to press or rub, and it refers to Chinese massage; three categories of anmo are Pu Tong Anmo or general massage, Tuina Anmo or push grab massage, and Dian Xue Anmo or cavity press massage. Compare to *Acupressure* and *Acupressure massage integration*.

Aromatherapy is the therapeutic use of the preparation of fragrant essential oils extracted from plants. See *Ayurvedic massage*.

Asian bodywork therapies (ABTs) are forms of massage and bodywork whose theoretical basis is traditional Asian (Chinese) medicine. See *Acupoints* and *Energy channels*.

Assertive behavior is a confident authoritative manner that demands obedience or attention. See *Intervention model*.

Assessment refers to the practitioner's conclusions from the subjective and objective information gathered during goal-oriented planning; for primary health care providers it includes a diagnosis of the problem; from a wellness perspective it may identify long- and short-term goals for the client; written in the A section of *SOAP notes*.

Assisted movement is a type of active movement in which a person initiates the movement, while another person helps him or her complete it. See *Active movements*.

Associated trigger point is a term referring to secondary or satellite trigger points. See *Trigger point therapy*, *Trigger points*, *Secondary trigger points*, and *Satellite trigger points*.

Attendance is an aspect of work ethic reflected in showing up when expected or when scheduled for work. See *Reliability* and *Work ethic*.

Ayurvedic massage is a system of soft tissue manipulation based in traditional theories of health and disease from India (i.e., Ayurvedic medicine). See *Massage and bodywork traditions*.

Bait advertising is an attractive but insincere offer to sell a product or service that the advertiser does not intend or want to actually sell; purpose is to generate leads to potential customers, or to sell something else at a higher price, an illegal practice called bait and switch. See *Business ethics*.

Bath attendant is a historical term describing persons who assisted patrons of public baths and natural healing resorts; included giving a superficial rubdown after a bath; late nineteenth- and early twentieth-century Europe and North America. Contrast with *Masseuse*.

Benefits are positive outcomes. The benefits of massage are experienced by recipients when the effects of massage support their general health and well-being. Contrast with *Effects of massage*.

Biomechanical analysis is the examination of the body in motion; takes into account principles of motion and the structure and function of the human body, especially the muscle and skeletal systems; a branch of kinesiology and an important aspect of sports medicine; used to collect objective information for goal-oriented planning. See *Gait analysis*.

Biomechanics is the study of movement in living organisms. See *Biomechanical analysis*.

Bipedal locomotion is the act of moving from one place to another on two feet. See *Gait analysis*.

Blinded is an element of research design in which subjects do not know who is receiving the treatment being studied. See *Scientific method* and *Randomized control trial*.

Board certification refers to a credential given by a nongovernmental, nonprofit organization that attests to a person's competency in a given profession; usually involves qualifying by education and/or experience, passing a written examination and/or performance evaluation, and abiding by a code of ethics; is renewed periodically and usually requires a certain amount of continuing education and/or work hours; sometimes referred to as *national certification*. Compare to *Certification*.

Body awareness is the ability to sense where your body is in space while at rest and in motion and to coordinate movement with mind; entails an integration of body and mind so that a person exists as an embodied being. See *Proprioceptors*.

Body-centered therapy refers to methods of healing that work primarily through the physical body, but that affect the whole person—body, mind, emotions, and spirit. See *Holistic*.

Body charts are diagrams of the human figure that are marked by clients to locate problem areas and to indicate the nature of a complaint; offer a visual and kinesthetic way to give subjective information. See *Interview skills*.

Body mechanics refers to the posture and biomechanics of the practitioner when performing massage. Good body mechanics protect the practitioner from injury and maximize the efficiency of technique applications. Compare to *Self-care*.

Body–mind effects of massage result from the interplay of body, mind, and emotions in health and disease. Compare to *Effects of massage* and *Holistic*.

Body language is communication through physical presence; includes posture, hand gestures, eye contact, and facial expression. See *Communication skills*.

Body–mind practices are physical exercises useful for improving various aspects of physical fitness with the added benefit of developing coordination, body awareness, concentration, and relaxation; examples are yoga, tai chi, qi gong, and pilates. See *Self-care*.

Body polish is a gentle form of exfoliation using soft granules such as those found in crushed almonds or grape seed meal. See *Exfoliants* and *Exfoliation*.

Body systems are a level of body organization characterized by several organs and tissues working together to perform specific body functions; for example, the cardiovascular system. Contrast with *Cells*. See *Effects of massage*.

Bodywork is a general term for practices involving touch and movement in which the practitioner uses manual techniques to promote health and healing of the recipient. The healing massage techniques described in this text are considered forms of bodywork. Compare to *Manual therapy* and *Massage*.

Body wraps are spa services that involve applying a substance to the body, after which the person is wrapped in sheets, blankets, and/or a plastic covering; the primary purpose is to detoxify the body by stimulating blood and lymph circulation. Contrast with *Exfoliation*.

Bolsters are long narrow pillows or cushions used to support or prop clients into position for massage. See *Positioning* and *Bracing*.

Boundaries refer to practices that clearly delineate and maintain practitioner and client roles within the therapeutic relationship. See *Therapeutic relationship*.

Boundary crossing is a transgression of personal or professional boundaries that may or may not be experienced as harmful. See *Personal boundaries* and *Professional boundaries*.

Boundary violation is a transgression of personal or professional boundaries that causes harm; leaves a sense of being violated, which is stronger than feeling annoyed or uncomfortable; personal or professional integrity is compromised in some way. See *Personal boundaries* and *Professional boundaries*.

Bow and arrow stance is a leg position used when facing the head or foot of the table; both feet face the direction of movement, the front leg is bent more than the rear leg, and the torso is upright; power is generated by shifting the weight from the back leg to the front leg while keeping the back in alignment. See *Body mechanics*. Contrast with *Horse riding stance*.

Bracing refers to offering a counterresistance to prevent movement in the opposite direction when applying force to the body; for example, having a seated client lean into pillows to brace against pressure during massage of the back. See *Positioning* and *Stabilizing hand*.

Business ethics is the study of moral behavior relative to commerce and consumers. Contrast with *Professional ethics*.

Business license is a document that grants permission to operate a commercial enterprise in a certain legal jurisdiction; allows government agencies to know who is doing business in their area, and can ensure that they are complying with all related laws. Compare to *Massage establishment license*.

Business plan is a document that spells out the details of putting a business or practice vision into operation; four major parts: a description of the business, marketing, management, and finances. See *Private practice*.

CAM is an acronym for complementary and alternative medicine. See *Alternative therapy* and *Complementary therapy*.

Carrier oils are base oils in which essential oils must be diluted before applying to the body. See *Aromatherapy* and *Ayurvedic massage*.

Case series consists of multiple case reports about a specific treatment for a particular condition. See *Case study* and *Case report*.

Case study is a type of research that involves the detailed observation and analysis of the treatment of a condition and the outcomes for one patient or client; includes pre- and posttreatment measurement. See *Case report*; contrast with *Anecdote*.

Case report is a written summary of a case study; includes background information (introduction and literature review), client description (subject), measurement of variables pre- and posttreatment, and discussion of results. See *Case study*.

Cash reserve is money set aside to cover emergencies and deficits in income at certain time periods; recommended to have at least three months' fixed costs in reserve when starting a massage practice; should be figured in startup costs. See *Startup costs* and *First year budget*.

Catchments are concentrations of lymph nodes; major catchment areas include the inguinal and axillary lymph nodes. Lymphatic facilitation techniques direct lymph fluids toward catchment areas. See *Lymphatic facilitation* and *Watersheds*.

Cautions are areas of potential danger that require thoughtful consideration and possible modifications of technique application. Compare to *Contraindications* and *Endangerment sites*.

Cells are the basic unit of all living organisms and make up all tissues and organs in the body. Contrast with *Body systems*.

Centered refers to finding your focal point or point of organization from which being and movement occur and to staying there; has a physical and psychological dimension; opposite is being scattered, off balance, and moving from the periphery. Compare to being *Grounded*.

Certificate program is a course of study in a particular subject for which a certificate of completion is awarded. Contrast with *Certification*.

Certification is a type of credential given after extensive education in a specific subject and may also include examinations, continuing education, and renewal. Contrast with *Certificate program*.

Chinese body clock is a concept in Chinese medicine that refers to the natural, rhythmic cycle of the flow of Qi in the body's energy channels; at a specific time of day, each channel has a peak flow when its Qi is at its maximum and a valley when its Qi is at its minimum. See *Energy channels* and *Qi*.

Chronological age refers to the number of years a person has been alive. Contrast with *Physiological age*.

Client-centered massage focuses on the recipient's unique situation, needs, and goals as the basis for treatment planning, as opposed to recipe-based or formula massage. Compare to *Evidence-based practice* and *Principle-based therapy*.

Clinical massage therapy describes applications of massage for the treatment of pathologies; also called *Medical massage*.

Clinical reasoning is the cognitive process used to plan treatment for a health problem or medical condition; involves problem definition, information collection, data analysis, therapeutic application planning and implementation, and outcomes evaluation. See *Goal-oriented planning*.

Clinical supervision is formal consultation with a specially trained supervisor about problems and ethical issues that come up in the therapeutic relationship; an opportunity for massage therapists to process what is happening in their practices and their experiences with clients. See *Professional ethics* and *Therapeutic relationship*.

Codes of ethics list the acceptable and encouraged moral behavior of members of a profession. Compare to *Standards of practice*.

Cold packs are temperature therapy devices for applying cold to the body; can be ice or some other material that maintains a cold temperature. See *Cryotherapy* and *Temperature therapy*. Contrast with *Hot packs*.

Collagen is a fibrous structural protein found in bones, cartilage, and connective tissue; binds structures together and gives them strength; the most abundant protein in the body. See *Fascia* and *Fascial anatomy*. Contrast with *Elastin*.

Collector vessels collect lymph from the I/T vessels and connect to the transport vessels or lymphangia; are generally only one or two cells thick and do not contain valves. See *Lymphatic facilitation*. Contrast with *Initial/terminal lymph vessels* and *Transport vessels*.

Colostomy bag is a medical device attached to the outside of the body to collect feces directly from the colon after a person has undergone a colostomy. See *Special population*.

Comforting touch is a term used in reference to massage for the terminally ill and dying; refers to touching another person with the intention of providing physical and emotional comfort. Compare to *Nurturing touch* and *Palliative care*.

Communication skills are the means of information exchange among people and include verbal (i.e., speech and writing) and nonverbal (i.e., body language, facial expression, touch) methods. See *Listening* and *Interview skills*.

Communication through touch is achieved by the contact and different qualities of touch applied during massage, or before or after the session when greeting or saying good-bye to a client. See *Contact, Touch,* and *Qualities of touch*.

Compassion is the awareness of the suffering of others coupled with the wish to relieve it; combines empathy with a dedication to service to others. See *Empathy* and *Emotional intelligence*.

Complementary therapy refers to healing methods that are used as secondary treatments to enhance the effectiveness of primary treatments and that contribute to a patient's recovery. See *CAM*. Compare to *Alternative therapy* and *Integrative health care*.

Competencies is an educational term referring to applications of knowledge and skills essential to the practice of a profession; define education in terms of what a practitioner can actually do, rather than just having completed a number of hours in certain subjects. See *Accreditation*.

Competitive advantage is a marketing concept that identifies the reasons customers would come to someone for a service or product instead of going elsewhere; competitive advantage factors for massage therapists include quality, expertise, price, location, selection or variety, level of service, convenience, and environment. See *Marketing* and *Mission statement*.

Concentration is the ability to sustain attention on something for a period of time; length of time for concentration before being distracted is called attention span; can be improved with practice. See *Meditation*.

Confidentiality is an ethical principle that upholds a client's right to privacy and prohibits giving information about a client to others without the client's permission. See *HIPAA privacy rules* and *Therapeutic relationship*.

Conflict resolution is a social skill used in solving problems or differences between two people or groups; options for resolution include collaboration, accommodation, compromise, avoidance, and force. See *Social skills*.

Conscious self-care refers to taking personal responsibility for seeking physical and emotional aid when needed from colleagues, a supervisor, or friends and family; supports health and well-being related to the practice of a profession such as massage therapy. See *Self-care*.

Contact refers to the sense presence of the massage therapist's hands on the client's body. When contact is good, the client feels a full, confident, deliberate, and warm connection to the massage therapist. Compare to *Touch*; See *Qualities of touch*.

Contemporary massage and bodywork is a general category for systems of manual therapy that were developed in the twentieth century (e.g., myofascial massage, trigger point therapy, polarity therapy). See *Bodywork* and *Massage therapy*.

Continuing education is education beyond entry-level training in an occupation or profession; often needed for license or certification renewal. See *Professionalism*.

Continuing session notes are a form of documentation that record the session-by-session history of a client's visits. See *SOAP notes*.

Continuity offers a sense of continuous touch throughout a massage session; avoids abrupt removal of touch. See *Organization*. Compare to *Flow*.

Contract is a legal agreement between two or more people; may be verbal or written; the terms of a contract may be upheld in court if one party breaches or violates the agreement; lawsuits arise when agreements are either not clear or have not been kept. See *Business ethics*.

Contract–relax–stretch (CRS) is a facilitated stretching technique in which the practitioner gets into position to apply the stretch, but first asks the client to contract the muscle to be stretched against a resistance. Immediately following the targeted muscle's relaxation, the stretch is applied. See *Resisted movements* and *Stretching*.

Contraindications are conditions or situations that make receiving massage inadvisable because of the harm that it might do. See *Do no harm*. Compare to *Cautions*.

Control group is an element of experimental research design; subjects who do not receive the treatment being studied, or who receive a placebo, or a different treatment than the experimental group. Contrast with *Experimental group*.

Copyright laws protect written, musical, and artistic works from unauthorized use; designated by the symbol ©; copyrights are administered in the United States by the U.S. Copyright Office at the Library of Congress in Washington, D.C. Compare to *Patents* and *Trademarks*.

CPT codes are medical codes used to process insurance claims; acronym for Current Procedural Terminology. Contrast with *SOAP notes*.

Countertransference is a psychological phenomenon that occurs when a practitioner responds to a client as if the practitioner were relating to someone important in his or her past (e.g., mother) and transferring those positive or negative feelings onto the therapeutic relationship. Contrast with *Transference*.

Courtesy is polite behavior that is expected in social situations; shows respect for others and exhibits thoughtfulness about their feelings, comfort, and safety; good manners. See *Social skills*.

Credentials refers to titles, certificates, or other forms of recognition that testify to the accomplishments of the person holding them; allow others to evaluate a person's background in a given field; are awarded by schools, organizations, or government agencies to individuals meeting their criteria for the credential. See *Professional associations* and *Professionalism*.

Critical thinking is a higher-level thinking process that aims to discover the truth about something; weighs reasons to believe against reasons to doubt; looks for objective evidence, confirmation of claims, errors, distortions, false information, and exaggerations; looks beneath the surface for authenticity and honesty; takes into consideration the thinker's own prejudices and beliefs. See *Intellectual skills*.

Cryotherapy refers to temperature therapy modalities below body temperature (e.g., cold packs and ice). See *Temperature therapy*. Contrast with *Thermotherapy*.

Cyriax friction is a form of deep transverse friction popularized by James Cyriax and used in rehabilitation of injuries. See *Deep friction* and *Deep transverse friction*.

Dan Tian is a concept in Chinese medicine that refers to a place just below the navel and about one-third of the way from front to back; the physical and energetic center of the body that provides a point of organization and balance. See *Qi gong*.

Deceptive advertising is advertising that misleads the public about the nature of goods or services offered for sale, their benefits, prices, or credentials; violates values of honesty and integrity; violates consumer protection laws. See *Business ethics*.

Deep fascia is an intricate series of dense connective sheets and bands that hold the muscles and other structures in place throughout the body. See *Fascia* and *Fascial anatomy*. Contrast with *Subcutaneous fascia*.

Deep friction is a type of friction in which the practitioner's fingers do not move over the skin, but instead move the skin over the tissues underneath. Cross-fiber and circular friction are types of deep friction. Contrast with *Superficial friction*. Compare to *Deep transverse friction*.

Deep transverse friction is a specific type of deep friction used in rehabilitation to break adhesions, facilitate healthy scar formation, and treat muscle and tendon lesions. It is performed across the tissues, causing broadening and separation of fibers. Deep transverse friction was popularized by James Cyriax. See *Cyriax friction*.

Defamation is a legal term for injury to a person or an organization's reputation; known as libel if written and as slander if spoken. See *Business ethics*.

Defense mechanisms are behaviors or thoughts that help people cope with unwanted feelings such as fear, anxiety, guilt, and anger; common types are projection, denial, repression, displacement, and resistance; often unconscious. See *Professional ethics* and *Social skills*.

Demonstrations are a method of presentation that show an audience how something is done or how something works by actually performing the action while giving a verbal description or explanation. Contrast with *Explanation* and *Persuasion*.

Diaphragm relaxation is a reflexology technique in which thumb pressure on the diaphragm reflex is deepened by flexing the recipient's toe over the point of pressure. See *Foot reflexology*. Compare to *Press-and-flex*.

Diploma is a document that states that a specific person has successfully completed a course of study; typically designates the school name, location, course of study, number of hours completed, and date of graduation, and is signed by school officials. Contrast with *Certification*.

Direct pressure or direct static pressure, is the application of force to compress tissues in a specific spot; it is applied with a thumb, finger, elbow, or knuckle. It can be considered a form of compression without movement and has also been called static friction. See *Touch without movement* and *Swedish massage.*

Direct therapeutic effects of clinical massage focus on the healing of a diagnosed medical condition or easing of its symptoms. Contrast with *Indirect therapeutic effects.*

Disability is a physical or mental condition that severely limits a person's ability to perform daily life activities. See *Special population.*

Discharge notes are a form of documentation containing a final summary of a client's progress, and any comments about the course of treatment. See *Documentation.*

Do no harm is one of the most basic ethical principles of giving therapeutic massage; it means avoiding actions that may harm clients and protecting their health and safety. See *Cautions, Contraindications,* and *Endangerment sites.*

Documentation is the process of writing session records for future reference; also called note-taking or charting; may refer to the documents themselves; kept on paper or in electronic form. See *SOAP notes.*

Draping refers to the use of sheets, towels, or other materials to cover recipients of massage to preserve their privacy and modesty, to maintain professional boundaries, and for warmth. Compare to *Boundaries.*

Dry brushing is an exfoliation technique using brushes or fiber tools. See *Exfoliation.* Contrast with *body polish.*

Dual relationship is any relationship other than the primary one of practitioner and client. See *Professional ethics.* Compare to *Boundaries* and *Therapeutic relationship.*

Duties are obligations to act in a particular way; responsibilities that arise out of being in a certain position in relationship to others, or as the result of some action. See *Professional ethics.*

Eastern bodywork refers to traditional forms of manual therapy from the continent of Asia. See *Bodywork* and *Massage Therapy.*

Eclectic practitioners combine two or more systems of massage and bodywork into their own unique approach to manual therapy. See *Bodywork* and *Massage therapy.*

Effectiveness of a massage performance refers to the degree to which intended goals are achieved and to which the recipient is satisfied. Compare to *Effects of massage.*

Effects of massage refer to changes that occur in the body, mind, and emotions of the recipient as a result of soft tissue manipulation. See *Long-term effects, Multiple-dose effects, Short-term effects,* and *Single-dose effects.*

Effleurage is a Western massage technique category that includes movements that slide or glide over the body with a smooth, continuous motion. See *Swedish massage* and *Western massage.*

Elastin is a protein found in elastic fibers that make up flexible body tissues such as the skin and fascia; more elastin fibers in a tissue results in greater ability for that tissue to stretch and then return to its original length when the stretch is released. See *Fascia.* Contrast with *Collagen.*

Elders are adults age 70 years and older. See *Chronological age.* Contrast with *Physiological age.*

Emollient is a substance that makes the skin soft and supple. See *Body polish.*

Emotional distress refers to feelings or emotions typically considered to be negative (e.g., isolation and loneliness, grief, depression, fear, and anger). See *Emotional intelligence.*

Emotional intelligence is defined by a set of skills related to five domains: knowing one's emotions, managing emotions, motivating oneself, recognizing emotions in others, and handling relationships; works with intellectual and physical skills for full maturity and success as a professional. Compare to *Social skills.*

Empathy is recognizing emotions in others; is the basis for creating rapport, and is the root of caring. See *Emotional intelligence.* Compare to *Compassion.*

Empirical means based on observation and/or measurement. See *Research.*

Employee is a person who works for an employer who controls when, where, and how the employee performs the work; defined by IRS and U.S. Labor Laws. Contrast with *Self-employed* and *Independent contractor.*

Endangerment sites are areas of the body where delicate body structures are less protected and, therefore, may be more easily damaged when receiving massage. See *Do no harm.* Contrast with *Contraindications.*

Endorsements are anecdotes from someone besides the advertiser about how well a product or service worked for them; reflects the opinions, beliefs, findings, or experience of a party other than the sponsoring advertiser; also called *Testimonials.* See *Business ethics.*

Energetic effects of massage refer to balancing and improving the flow of energy in the body through soft tissue manipulation. Compare to *Acupressure* and *Polarity therapy.* Contrast with *Mechanical effects.*

Energy-based bodywork refers to forms of manual therapy in which the chief intention is to enhance the free flow of energy or life force in and around the body. See *Acupressure, Ayurvedic massage,* and *Polarity therapy.*

Energy channels are part of the theory of Asian bodywork therapy that refers to the pathways for the flow of Qi in the body; there are 12 major energy channels; called meridians in some forms of Asian bodywork therapy. See *Chinese body clock* and *Qi.*

Energy flow is part of the theory of polarity therapy that states that all natural healing techniques are effective because they support the individual's innate capacity for health by stimulating the free and balanced flow of life energy; polarity therapy techniques are designed to have a positive effect on the subtle life energy of the body. See *Polarity therapy.* Compare to *Removing obstructions.*

Environment for massage includes the room, air quality, lighting, sound, dressing arrangements, equipment, and overall cleanliness and neatness of the space in which a session is given. See *Business plan.*

Equipment refers to items used in a massage practice that are relatively costly and that last for several years, such as massage tables and massage chairs. See *Business plan* and *Startup costs.*

Ergonomics is the applied science of equipment and furniture design intended to maximize productivity by reducing fatigue, discomfort, and overwork injuries. See *Repetitive strain injuries, Worker productivity,* and *Workplace wellness programs.*

Esalen massage is a genre of bodywork based on a simplified form of Swedish massage, whose main purpose is to enhance nonverbal connection with the inner self and with others. It emphasizes the sensual aspects of massage. It was developed at the Esalen Institute in Big Sur, California, in the 1970s as part of the human potential movement. See *Human potential movement.*

Essential oils are volatile plant oils extracted from certain aromatic plants that have both physiological and psychological effects on the human body and mind. See *Aromatherapy.*

Estimated tax payments are paid to the IRS quarterly (four times a year) based on the amount of income tax expected to be owed at the end of the year; similar to withholding for employment income; estimated tax payments should appear on the annual budget as an expense. See *First year budget* and *Income tax.*

Ethical decision-making model is a step-by-step process of thinking through an ethical question or ethical dilemma; involves critical thinking and problem solving; takes into consideration both external and internal standards in making an ethical choice of action. Compare to *Critical thinking.*

Ethical dilemmas are a type of ethical question in which two or more principles are in conflict and where something of value will be compromised regardless of the choice of action; involves selecting the lesser harm or greater good. Contrast with *Ethical questions.*

Ethical judgment is consistency in making good ethical decisions; strengthened by awareness, learning, and experience; improves with critical thinking and evaluating results. Compare to *Ethical decision-making model.*

Ethical questions are problems related to the morality of certain actions; require judgment to determine the most ethical choice. See *Ethical decision-making model.*

Ethical standards are statements designating the generally accepted and encouraged moral behavior of members of a profession; appear as codes of ethics and standards of practice documents developed by professional associations. See *Codes of ethics.*

Ethics is the study of the nature of moral behavior, of right and wrong; examines choices for behavior, and uses a decision-making process to determine the degree of morality of certain actions. See *Business ethics* and *Professional ethics.*

Event is a term used in sports massage to describe massage applications that help the athlete prepare for and recover from a specific competitive event. See *Interevent, Preevent, Postevent,* and *Sports massage.*

Evidence-based practice is founded on verifiable objective evidence for the effectiveness of certain therapies; considers scientific research, the practitioner's experience and judgment, and the recipient's values and preferences. Compare to *Client-centered massage* and *Principle-based therapy.*

Exfoliants are substances or processes that remove dead skin cells. See *Body polish.*

Exfoliation is the process of peeling and sloughing off dead skin cells from the surface of the body. See *Spa* and *Scrubs.*

Experimental group is an element of research design; subjects who receive the treatment being studied. See *Scientific method.* Contrast with *Control group.*

Explicit agreements are understandings between people that are spoken or written; agreements that are in the open and can be verified. Compare to *Contract.* Contrast with *Implicit agreements.*

Fascia is loose, irregular connective tissue found throughout the body; composed of three primary elements: ground substance, collagen, and elastin. Fascia holds structures together giving them their characteristic shapes, offers support, and connects the body as a whole. See *Collagen, Elastin,* and *Fascial anatomy.*

Fascial anatomy includes fascial structures that shape the body such as the body straps or retinaculae that give the body contour, and fascial sheaths that surround muscles and link muscle groups. See *Fascia* and *Myofascial massage.*

Fascial restrictions are places where fascial tissues are less pliable, shortened, or adhering. Fascial restrictions limit mobility and cause postural distortion, poor cellular nutrition, pain, and a variety of other dysfunctions. See *Myofascial massage.*

Fiduciary is a legal term used to describe a relationship in which person A has placed a special trust in person B, who is then obligated to watch out for person A's best interests. See *Business ethics, Duty,* and *Therapeutic relationship.*

Fingerwalking is a variation of the reflexology technique of *thumbwalking* in which the fingertips are used to apply pressure while they "walk" along an area of the body. See *Foot reflexology.* Compare to *Thumbwalking.*

Finishing techniques are used at the end of a massage session to reconnect parts of the body that have been worked on more specifically, or to further sedate or stimulate the recipient; effleurage, tapotement, and passive touch are common finishing techniques. See *Organization.* Contrast with *Opening techniques.*

First impressions are the thoughts, beliefs, and feelings about others formed immediately on meeting them for the first time. See *Professional demeanor* and *Professional image.*

First-year budget   is a document that forecasts income and expenses for the initial twelve months of operation of a business or practice. See *Business plan* and *Startup costs*.

Five Elements   within the context of traditional Chinese medicine are Wood, Fire, Earth, Metal, and Water; Five Element Theory describes relationships among the elements as a way of using natural phenomena to explore and treat our psyche, spiritual state, anatomy, physiology, and the dynamics of the disease process as a whole; the Five Elements are used to describe flow of Qi and the cycle of life. See *Ko Cycle* and *Sheng Cycle*.

Fixed costs   are expenses incurred whether a massage therapist sees clients or not, for example, rent and utilities; sometimes called overhead. See *First-year budget*. Contrast with *Variable costs*.

Flow   is the continuous, gentle sense of movement or quality of a massage session achieved through an orderly sequence and smooth transitions from one part of the body to the next. See *Transition techniques*. Contrast with *Pacing* and *Rhythm*.

Folk and native massage traditions   are found all over the world among families, tribes, and villages. They are based on tradition and experience and often involve herbal remedies, rituals, and religious beliefs. See *Massage and bodywork traditions*.

Foot reflexology   is based on the theory that pressure applied to specific areas on the feet, called reflexes, produces a change in a corresponding part of the body. See *Reflexology*.

Form 1040   is an IRS form used to file U.S. income taxes for individuals; covers both employment and self-employment; a summary form to which other forms and schedules are attached; must be filed annually by April 15. See *Income tax*.

Frail elders   are people over age 70 who look and feel fragile to the touch. Contrast with *Robust elders* and *Age-appropriate* elders.

Free active movements   or free exercises are performed entirely by a person with no assistance from a practitioner. See *Active movements*.

Friction   is a massage technique category that includes movements that rub one surface over another repeatedly and includes superficial and deep friction. See *Deep friction*, *Superficial friction*, and *Swedish massage*.

Full-body Swedish massage   refers to a massage session lasting from 30 to 90 minutes, in which traditional Swedish massage techniques are combined into a routine to address the whole body. These sessions are generally wellness oriented and aim to improve circulation, relax the muscles, improve joint mobility, induce general relaxation, promote healthy skin, and create a general sense of well-being. Contrast with *Acupressure* and *Acupressure massage integration*.

Full-time   work is earning most or all of your income in one job or occupation; for massage therapists full-time is 15–20 clients per week or working 4–5 days in employment, or some comparable combination. Contrast with *Part-time*.

Gait analysis   is the examination of biomechanics while walking or running; looks at normal gait and deviations from normal; used to collect information for goal-oriented planning. See *Biomechanics* and *Bipedal locomotion*.

General contraindications   are conditions or situations that make receiving *any* massage inadvisable because of the harm that it might do. See *Contraindications*. Contrast with *Local contraindications*.

General membership organization   is an organization that welcomes practitioners of different forms of massage and bodywork; can be further categorized into *professional associations* and *member services organizations*. Contrast with *Specialty associations*.

Gentle art   describes the quality of polarity therapy in which nothing is ever forced; the giver invites the receiver to enter a deeply relaxed state and invites the muscles to relax. See *Polarity therapy*. Compare to *Love* and *Understanding*.

Goal-oriented planning   is a type of session planning that focuses on meeting specific client needs, rather than giving a standardized massage routine; client goals provide the focal point for organizing massage sessions and choosing appropriate techniques. See *Session planning*.

Gong   is a Chinese word that can be translated to mean exercise. See *Qi gong*.

Greek gymnasia   were centers in ancient Athens and Sparta run by the state for free men and youths that contained facilities for exercises, frictions, and baths. Compare to *Roman baths* and *Turkish baths*.

Ground substance   is a gel-like mucopolysaccharide, the same liquid that forms interstitial or intercellular fluid. See *Fascia*.

Guarantee   is a promise that something will work as stated, usually with the implication that the money charged will be refunded if it does not. See *Business ethics*. Contrast with *Endorsement*.

Guidelines   are landmarks used in foot reflexology to help in locating specific reflexes on the feet; five important guidelines are neck/shoulder, diaphragm, waist, pelvic, and the longitudinal tendon. See *Foot reflexology*. Compare to *Reflexology chart*.

Hand mechanics   are body mechanics that minimize strain on the fingers, thumb, and wrist. See *Self-care*. Compare to *Body mechanics*.

Hatha yoga   is an Ayurvedic practice that includes relaxation, physical exercises or postures called *asanas*, proper breathing, proper diet, and positive thinking and meditation. See *Body–mind practices*. Compare to *Thai massage*.

Healing   means enhancing health and well-being. It is the process of regaining health or optimal functioning after an injury, disease, or other debilitating condition. "To heal" means to make healthy, whole, or sound; restore to health; or free from ailment. See *Wellness Massage Pyramid*.

Health care   settings are places where patients are treated for illnesses and injuries. Compare to *Wellness center*.

Health history is an interview of a client taken during the initial visit that provides information about medical conditions and health issues to be aware of before giving massage; may be verbal or written on a form. See *Contraindications* and *Do no harm.*

Health-service operator is a historical term used in the YMCA for practitioners trained in physical therapeutics or physiotherapy; included massage, hydrotherapy, electro-therapy, light, relaxation techniques, and exercise; goals focused on health, fitness, and general well-being; early to mid-twentieth-century North America. Compare to *Bath attendant* and *Masseur.*

High-risk pregnancies include those in which the mother or fetus is at higher than normal risk for complications or negative developments. See *Pregnancy* and *Trimesters.*

HIPAA privacy rules specify how medical records must be secured, who may have access to medical records, and under what conditions records may be shared with others; an acronym for the Health Insurance Portability and Accountability Act of 1996. See *Confidentiality.*

Holistic refers to those approaches to health and healing that take into account the wholeness of human beings, including body, mind, emotions, and spirit. See *Holistic massage.*

Holistic massage refers to forms of massage that take into account the wholeness of human beings (i.e., body, mind, emotions, and spirit). See *Holistic.*

Holistic self-care plan includes those activities that support development as a massage therapist and minimize factors that lead to illness and injury, for example, having a plan for physical, mental, and emotional health and fitness, and avoiding undue stress and burnout. See *Conscious self-care.*

Home-visit practice refers to a massage therapy business in which the massage therapist travels to clients' homes to provide massage; convenient for clients. See *Business plan* and *Private practice.*

Hook-and-backup is a reflexology technique used to apply deep pressure to a specific area or reflex; the thumb is placed directly on the targeted spot, bending at the first joint to apply pressure, and then pulled to the side across the spot to deepen the pressure. See *Foot reflexology.* Compare to *Direct pressure.* Contrast with *Thumbwalking.*

Horse riding stance is a leg position used when facing the table directly; both feet face the table with head and back in alignment; knees are bent equally to lower the body into position; weight is shifted from side to side as techniques are applied. See *Body mechanics.* Contrast with *Bow and arrow stance.*

Hospice programs provide compassionate care at the end of life; typically involve a team-oriented approach to medical care, pain management, and emotional and spiritual support tailored to the needs of the dying; are provided in freestanding facilities, hospitals, nursing homes, and other long-term care facilities. Compare to *Palliative care.*

Hospital-based massage is a specialty in which massage is integrated into the regular hospital setting such as in the pediatric ward, cancer unit, or cardiac care. See *Treatment.* Contrast with *Hospice.*

Hot packs are temperature therapy devices for applying heat to the body; may be wet or dry applications. See *Temperature therapy* and *Thermotherapy.* Contrast with *Cold packs.*

Human meaning of different body regions refers to the special significance individuals give to certain parts of the body. This may be related to what each region allows him or her to do and to be in this world, or there may be significant social and emotional associations. See *Holistic.*

Human potential movement was a historical social movement in the 1960s–1970s in the United States that advocated exploring the limits of human potential and spawned many forms of massage and bodywork. See *Esalen massage.*

Hydrotherapy is the use of water in different forms for its therapeutic effects. See other hydrotherapy facilities, *Sauna, Steam room,* and *Whirlpool bath.* See also *Temperature therapy.*

Hygienic hand washing is a thorough hand-washing procedure that can prevent the transfer of pathogens during massage. Compare to *Sanitation.*

Hypothalamus is the part of the brain that controls many physiological functions; plays a major role in the regulation of homeostasis. See *Aromatherapy.*

Hypothesis is an unproven theory about how something works or what will happen in a certain situation; element of research design: statement about the relationship between two or more variables; forms the basis of a scientific study. See *Research literacy* and *Scientific method.*

Ice massage involves rubbing ice directly on the skin using an ice cube or ice cup; applied in a circular motion until the area is numb. See *Cryotherapy.* Contrast with *Cold pack.*

Implicit agreements are understandings between people that may be unspoken and unwritten; agreements assumed or taken for granted. Contrast with *Explicit agreements.*

Income goal is part of a business plan that specifies the desired net income for a projected annual budget. See *Business plan* and *First-year budget.*

Income tax is a tax paid to a government based on income from employment and/or profits from a business; taxable income from a private practice equals gross income minus qualified business expenses; tips are considered taxable income; U.S. income tax is filed annually with the Internal Revenue Service on Form 1040. See *Estimated tax* and *Self-employment tax.*

Independent contractor is a form of self-employment in which a person performs services for another person or business, but is not an employee; is contracted to accomplish a certain result, but is not under the direct control of an employer. See *Self-employed.* Contrast with *Employee.*

Indication is a term used in the treatment model to mean that when a specific medical condition is present, a particular modality is indicated or advised to alleviate the condition. Massage is indicated as a treatment for a number of medical conditions. Contrast with *Contraindications*.

Indirect therapeutic effects of clinical massage focus on enhancing the effectiveness of a primary treatment, or creating a more favorable environment for healing. Contrast with *Direct therapeutic effects*.

Infant massage involves soft tissue manipulation and joint movements designed to enhance the growth and development of newborns and children. See *Tactile stimulation*.

Informed voluntary consent is a procedure used to ask for explicit permission from a client to touch a certain body area or perform a specific technique. See *Boundaries* and *Professional ethics*.

Infusions are liquids produced by steeping herbs or botanicals in boiling water; oil may be used for an infusion in place of water. See *Body wraps*.

Initial note is a type of documentation that includes the client's stated reason for massage or their complaint, related subjective and objective information, agreed-upon long-term goals, and a general plan. See *Long-term planning* and *Documentation*.

Initial/terminal (I/T) lymph vessels are the smallest lymph vessels with walls that are only one cell thick; the entry point for metabolic and cellular waste, proteins, and excess fluids. See *Lymphatic facilitation*. Contrast with *Collector vessels* and *Transport vessels*.

Intake is the process of gathering relevant information from a new client. See *Goal-oriented planning* and *Interview skills*.

Intake notes are comprehensive records that include the client's stated reason for massage or specific complaint, related subjective and objective information, agreed-upon long-term goals, and a general plan is the process of gathering relevant information from a new client. See *Communication skills* and *Interview skills*.

Integrative health care is an approach to healing in which mainstream medicine and alternative healing methods are offered as equal options for treating patients. Contrast with *CAM*.

Integrative medicine center is a health care facility that offers a team approach to the treatment of illness and injury; includes a variety of Western medical health care providers, traditional and indigenous healers, and CAM practitioners in a collaborative effort. Contrast with *Wellness center*.

Intellectual skills are thinking or cognitive abilities; six levels identified by educators include knowledge, comprehension, application, analysis, synthesis, and evaluation. Contrast with *Emotional intelligence*.

Intention is the aim that guides the action, that is, what the practitioner hopes to accomplish; refers to effects the practitioner is aiming for when applying techniques. See *Goal-oriented planning*.

Interconnections refer to the anatomical and physiological wholeness and integrity of the human body; important to keep in mind during regional and full-body massage. See *Holistic*.

Interevent is a sports massage application given between events at competitions; gives attention to psychological recovery and also readiness for the upcoming performance; combines preevent, postevent, and recovery sports massage to meet an athlete's needs. See *Sports massage*. Compare to *Postevent, Preevent, Recovery*.

Interstitial space refers to the area between cells that is structured by collagen fibers and that contains fluid and various molecules to be returned to circulation; sometimes called the matrix. See *Lymphatic facilitation* and *Matrix*.

Intervention model is a procedure used to clarify a possible misunderstanding of intention by a client (e.g., sexual intent), and to make a decision whether to stop or continue with a massage session. See *Boundaries, Professional ethics,* and *Sexual misconduct*.

Interview skills are communication skills used to elicit useful information from clients; used in initial client interviews and taking health histories. See *Intake*.

Introduction is a social process in which one person presents another person to a third person giving some basic information such as name and other relevant facts; also self-introduction to another person. See *Social skills*.

Intuition is a direct perception of the truth, independent of any rational process; lets us respond to our environment without calling rational problem solving into play; related to instinct. Contrast with *Intellectual skills*.

Jitsu is a concept from Asian bodywork therapy that describes an area of energy excess; felt in the tissues as hardness, resistance; manual techniques are applied to disperse the excess energy and sedate areas of jitsu. See *Acupressure massage integration*. Contrast with *Kyo*.

Joint manipulations sometimes called adjustments or chiropractic adjustments, refer to techniques that take a joint beyond its normal range of motion and that are specific attempts to realign a misaligned joint, usually using a thrusting movement. Joint manipulations are not part of Western massage and are not within the scope of this text. Contrast with *Joint movements*.

Joint movements are techniques that involve motion in the joints of the body and include mobilizing techniques and stretching. See *Mobilizing techniques* and *Stretching*.

Kinesiology is the study of human movement; it looks at the combined action of the muscular, skeletal, and nervous systems that result in movement. Compare to *Biomechanics*.

Ko Cycle is a concept within the Five Element Theory that looks at relationships among the Five Elements; also called the controlling or acting cycle; each Element controls another and is also controlled by another Element. The Ko Cycle balances the Sheng Cycle to avoid unrestrained growth. See *Five Elements*. Contrast with *Sheng Cycle*.

Kyo is a concept from Asian bodywork therapy that describes an area of energy deficiency; felt in the tissues as a soft, hollow spot with no tone; manual techniques are applied to strengthen or tonify kyo areas. See *Acupressure massage integration*. Contrast with *Jitsu*.

Latent trigger points are painful only when pressed. See *Trigger point*. Contrast with *Active trigger points*.

Limbic system is located within the cerebrum and plays a major role in a variety of emotions, such as pleasure, fear, sorrow, sexual attraction, and anger; also involved in memory and olfaction. See *Aromatherapy* and *Hypothalamus*.

Listening means making a conscious effort to hear what someone is trying to communicate; allows you to gather information, understand others better, and take in new ideas; helps build good relationships. See *Active listening* and *Affirmative listening*.

Local contraindications are conditions or situations that make receiving massage on a particular part of the body inadvisable because of the harm that it might do. See *Contraindications*. Contrast with *General contraindications*.

Logo is a symbol or graphic that identifies a person or business at a glance; can be original artwork or clip art in the public domain; if original, can be registered as a trademark for protection of use. See *Trademarks*.

Long stroke is a lymphatic facilitation technique similar to effleurage but applied with light pressure and stretching of the skin in the desired direction of lymph flow; applied with repetition and "snap back"; generally used on the extremities. See *Lymphatic facilitation*. Contrast with *L-stroke*.

Long-term effects of massage refer to changes that start during a massage session and that last for a longer period of time, such as a few days or weeks. Or they may be more lasting changes that occur from massage received regularly over a period of time. See *Effects of massage*. Contrast with *Short-term effects*.

Long-term planning is a form of goal-oriented planning in which the goal is to accomplish a client's specific health objectives over a series of massage sessions; long-term refers to more than one massage session, or the interval between an initial session and a progress session to check the extent to which goals have been reached. See *Goal-oriented planning*. Contrast with *Session planning*.

Love is a basic principle in polarity therapy that recognizes a caring so powerful that it carries with it no agenda, no end result that must be obtained. The practitioner does his or her work simply, always responding to the felt need, and yet without attachment to healing. See *Polarity therapy*. Compare to *Understanding*.

Lower body regions for the purposes of massage, are commonly identified as hips and buttocks, upper and lower legs, and feet. See *Regional massage*. Contrast with *Upper body regions*.

L-stroke is a lymphatic facilitation technique in which the skin is stretched tracing the L pattern; applied with repetition and "snap back"; moves lymph toward desired direction and catchment area. See *Lymphatic facilitation*. Contrast with *Long stroke*.

Lubricants are topical substances used in some massage sessions to enhance the effects of techniques and to minimize skin friction. Common lubricants include vegetable and mineral oils, jojoba, lotions, and combinations of these substances. See *Flow*.

Lymph is a clear fluid that contains water, protein molecules, cellular components, and fatty acids that need to be transported back into blood circulation; the fluid in lymphatic vessels. See *Lymphatic facilitation*.

Lymphatic facilitation (LF) is a light and gentle massage technique used to facilitate the removal of excess fluid that collects in tissues after trauma and inflammation; assists the function of the lymphatic system by the application of slow, light, and repetitive strokes that help move lymph fluid through the system of vessels and nodes. See *Long stroke* and *L-stroke*.

Maintenance is a sports massage application with the goals of enhancing recovery from strenuous exertion, treating debilitating conditions, and helping the athlete maintain optimal health. See *Sports massage*. Compare to *Recovery*, *Rehabilitation*, and *Remedial massage*.

Manual therapy refers to healing methods applied with the practitioner's hands touching or moving the recipient's body. See *Bodywork* and *Massage*.

Marketing is the process of identifying potential customers or clients and meeting their needs and wants. See *Business ethics* and *Business plan*.

Massage is the intentional and systematic manipulation of the soft tissues of the body to enhance health and healing; joint movements and stretching are commonly performed as part of massage; primary characteristics of massage are touch and movement. See *Swedish massage* and *Western massage*.

Massage and bodywork traditions are systems of manual therapy that have been passed down from generation to generation within groups of people; these traditions are typically defined as originating from a specific ethnic group, geographic location, or civilization. Compare to *Asian bodywork therapies*, *Ayurvedic massage*, *Swedish massage*, and *Western massage*.

Massage chair is a specially designed piece of equipment that provides comfortable support for receiving massage in a seated upright position; includes support for the legs, arms, and face. See *On-site massage* and *Seated massage*.

Massage chair adjustments include the height of the chest pad; the angle of the face cradle; and the height and/or angle of the seat, the kneeling pads, and the armrest. See *Positioning*.

Massage establishment license is a business license to operate a commercial space where customers come for massage; typically requires revealing the owner(s), detailing hygiene and safety standards, posting services and prices, and affirming that all practitioners in the establishment have the required occupational licenses. See *Business license*. Compare to *Zoning ordinance*.

Massage operator is a historical term for massage practitioner in early twentieth-century United States. Contrast with *Masseuse and Masseur*.

Massage therapist refers to a person who has graduated from a massage therapy program and has met accepted standards for competency in the field; has obtained occupational licensing where required and/or national certification; and upholds the ethical standards of the profession. Contrast with *Practitioner*.

Massage therapy is a general term for health and healing practices involving touch and movement, which are based in massage and related manual techniques. It is sometimes used synonymously with the term *bodywork*. The term *massage therapy* has been adopted by some massage practitioners to define their profession, which is a licensed profession in many states. See *Manual therapy*.

Masseur is the historical French term for a male massage therapist; twentieth-century Europe and North America. Contrast with *Masseuse*.

Masseuse is the historical French term for a woman massage therapist; twentieth-century Europe and North America; corrupted in mid-twentieth-century United States by association with prostitution. Contrast with *Masseur*.

Matrix is a descriptive term for *interstitial space*; referred to as a prelymphatic channel in many manual lymph drainage texts; structured by collagen fibers that form "scaffolding" within which fluids carrying nutrients, gases, wastes, and inorganic and organic material flow. See *Interstitial space* and *Lymphatic facilitation*.

Mechanical effects of massage refer to changes that occur on the gross level of the physical structure and that result from the physical forces of massage, such as compression, stretching, shearing, broadening, and vibration of body tissues. Contrast with *Energetic effects, Mind–body effects, Physiological effects*, and *Reflex effects*.

Mechanotherapy is a historical term for a tradition of bodywork also known as medical gymnastics and physical therapeutics; cure of diseases through movement including active and passive exercises; sometimes used machines to perform movements; early twentieth-century Europe and North America. Compare to *Bodywork* and *Massage therapy*.

Medical gymnast is a historical term for a practitioner trained in medical gymnastics or Swedish movement cure; used active and passive movements to treat disease; late nineteenth- and early twentieth-century Europe and North America. See *Swedish movement cure*.

Medical massage See *Clinical massage therapy*.

Medical rubbing is a term from the eighteenth and nineteenth centuries for frictions and rubbing used in conventional medical treatments. Compare to *Massage*.

Medical spa is a type of spa that integrates spa services with conventional and complementary therapies for healing mind and body. See *Spa*.

Meditation is a practice designed to improve the ability to concentrate or pay focused attention; basic meditation technique involves choosing something like a word or object to place attention on, and when the mind wanders, bringing it back to the object of attention. See *Concentration*.

Melting refers to the feeling of softening or "giving" in myofascial tissues as adhesions are broken, and tissues become softer and more pliable with the application of myofascial techniques. See *Fascial restrictions* and *Myofascial massage*.

Member services organization is a general membership organization whose major mission is to provide benefits such as professional liability insurance, group health insurance, publications, and information of interest to their members, may also promote the interests of members related to licensing and legislation. Contrast with *Professional associations*.

Mind–body effects of massage refer to the interplay of mind, body, and emotions during massage applications, for example, in the relaxation response. Contrast with *Energetic effects, Mechanical effects, Physiological effects*, and *Reflex effects*.

Mineral spring spa is a type of spa located at a natural mineral or hot springs site, which uses the spring water in treatments offered. See *Spa*.

Mission statement is a part of the vision outlined in a business plan that defines the purpose of the business and the main strategy for achieving competitive advantage; states the focus of the business. See *Vision* and *Competitive advantage*.

Mobility refers to the ability to go from place to place independently. See *Disability* and *Special population*.

Mobility restrictions are limits to the ability to go from place to place by walking, running, or other forms of locomotion; may be due to overuse and shortening of muscles, lack of use, aging, recuperation from an extended illness or injury, or a sedentary lifestyle. See *Bipedal locomotion* and *Disability* and *Special population*.

Mobilizing techniques are free and loose nonspecific joint movements within the normal range of joint motion. Compare to *Stretching*. Contrast with *Joint manipulations*.

Modality is a method of treating a medical condition; massage is considered a modality in the tradition of physiotherapy, along with other modalities such as ice packs, hot packs, ultrasound, or whirlpool baths. See *Hydrotherapy* and *Temperature therapy*.

MRSA stands for methicillin-resistant *Staphylococcus aureus*, which is a drug-resistant bacterial infection typically found on the skin but that can occur elsewhere in the body. See *Sanitation*.

Muds are derived from soils and marine sediments and applied to the body for deep skin cleansing and the removal of waste products; their drawing action also can stimulate local blood and lymphatic flow. See *Body wraps*. Contrast with *Peat*.

Multiple-choice questions are inquiries that give clients a choice of descriptors in answer to a question; gives clients choices that they might not have thought of themselves and have meaning for the interviewer. See *Interview skills*. Contrast with *Open-ended questions* and *Rating scale*.

Multiple-dose effects   of massage refer to changes that occur over time from repeated massage applications. See *Effects of massage*. Contrast with *Single-dose effects*.

Myofascial massage   is a general term for manual techniques aimed at releasing restrictions in superficial fascia, in deep fascia surrounding muscles, and in fascia related to overall body alignment; restores mobility in the body's fascia and softens connective tissue that has become rigid; also called myofascial release and myofascial unwinding. See *Fascia* and *Fascial restrictions*.

Natural healing   refers to a philosophy that shows preference for methods of healing derived from nature, the belief in an innate healing force, and a holistic view of human life. See *Natural healing arts* and *Massage and bodywork traditions*.

Natural healing arts   are methods of healing derived from nature, for example, nutritious food, herbs, water therapy, exercise, relaxation, fresh air, sunshine, and massage. See *Natural healing*.

Naturopathic physician's office   is a health care facility offering naturopathic medicine. See *CAM*.

Net income   refers to all of the money earned in a private practice, including fees and tips, minus business expenses and taxes; results in a *profit* if income is more than expenses. See *First-year budget* and *Income tax*. Contrast with *Salary draw*.

Neuromuscular therapy (NMT)   is a form of contemporary massage focused on deactivating myofascial trigger points. See *Trigger point therapy*.

Neutral position   refers to a hand position in which the wrist is neither flexed nor extended. See *Hand mechanics* and *Self-care*.

Nonverbal communication   is connecting with another person without using words; touch is a form of nonverbal communication that can convey comfort, nurturing, and caring. See *Comforting touch*, *Nurturing touch*, and *Palliative care*.

Nurturing touch   is a term used in reference to massage for the terminally ill or dying; refers to touching another person with the intention of satisfying the innate human need for touch by another person. Compare to *Comforting touch*, *Palliative care*, and *Touch deprivation*.

Nutrition   refers to the intake of food and drink to nourish the body and mind. See *Self-care*.

Obesity   is defined as having a body mass index (BMI) of 30 or above. Compare to *Physical fitness*.

Objective information   refers to what the practitioner observes about the client during goal-oriented planning; includes observations, qualitative and quantitative measurements, and results of orthopedic tests; written in the O section of *SOAP notes*. See *Goal-oriented planning*.

Observation   is the act of noticing a client's condition using the eyes, ears, nose, and hands; used to collect

information for goal-oriented planning. See *Objective information*.

Occupational licensing   is permission granted to qualified practitioners to accept compensation for massage in a specific governmental jurisdiction; is awarded by the government agency that regulates professions in the jurisdiction; is required to practice. Compare to *Certification*.

On-site massage   refers to a massage practice format in which the practitioner goes to where the potential clients are (e.g., at work, in stores, at airports, on the street), making massage more accessible; typically given with the client on a specially designed massage chair. See *Massage chair* and *Seated massage*.

Open-ended questions   are inquiries that steer clients to specific topics, but leave space for them to answer in their own words; rather than dictating the form of response, the interviewer listens to what the client has to say in answer to a simple question. See *Interview skills*. Contrast with *Multiple-choice questions* and *Rating scales*.

Opening techniques   refer to the initial touching of the recipient during a massage session; used to establish contact and sometimes also to apply oil and warm tissues. See *Organization* and *Warming techniques*.

Optimism   is an aspect of emotional intelligence that means expecting that things will turn out all right in the end, despite setbacks and difficulties; an optimistic attitude helps a person persevere when the going gets rough; contrast with being pessimistic, or expecting failure. See *Emotional intelligence*.

Organization   of a session refers to the overall structure of a massage session into beginning, middle, and end; the progression from one section of the body to another and the ordering of techniques into sequences; organization includes the use of opening techniques, transitions, and finishing techniques. See *Session* and *Session Planning*.

Organs   are anatomical structures composed of different types of tissue that work as a unit to perform specific functions in the body, for example, the heart. Compare to *Body systems*.

Orthopedic tests   are methods of assessing pathology in musculoskeletal structures, movement and locomotor disorders, and sources of soft-tissue pain and dysfunction; used to gather objective information in treatment planning. See *Objective information* and *Goal-oriented planning*.

Pacing   refers to the speed of performing techniques, which may vary from very slow to very fast for different effects. Contrast with *Continuity*, *Flow*, and *Rhythm*.

Palliative care   refers to methods of reducing symptoms and discomfort associated with certain diseases or their treatment; also care given to the terminally ill or dying for physical comfort and emotional support. Compare to *Hospice*. Contrast with *Treatment*.

Palpation   is the act of sensing information about the client through touch; is about the "feel" of tissues and of movement at joints; used to collect objective information for goal-oriented planning. See *Objective information* and *Palpatory sensitivity*.

Palpatory sensitivity is the ability to use the sense of touch to locate anatomical structures, feel the condition of the tissues, and feel changes in tissues. See *Objective information.*

Part-time work is earning a portion of your income from a particular job or occupation; for a massage therapist, part-time ranges anywhere from one to ten clients per week, or one or two days or nights at a place of employment, or some comparable combination. Contrast with *Full-time.*

Passive movements are body movements initiated and controlled by the practitioner, while the recipient remains relaxed and receptive. Contrast with *Active movements.*

Passive range of motion (PROM) refers to the evaluation of motion at a joint while it is passively moved through its range by a therapist; observations include degree of motion possible, restrictions or shortening, and any discomfort experienced; used to collect objective information for *Goal-oriented planning.*

Passive touch is simply laying the fingers or one or both hands on the body. Passive touch may impart heat to an area, have a calming influence, or help balance energy. See *Finishing techniques* and *Touch without Movement.*

Patents are legal protections for inventions and include utility and design patents; administered by the U.S. Patent and Trademark Office; patented inventions may not be copied by others for sale. Compare to *Copyright* and *Trademarks.*

Peat is organic soil that contains minerals, organic matter, water, and trapped air; has therapeutic properties when applied to the skin. Contrast with *Muds.*

Peer-reviewed journals are journals that only publish research reports that meet certain standards and that have been evaluated by experts in the field; different from trade magazines. See *Research literacy.*

Perpendicularity is one of the general principles for applying pressure to acupoints; means applying pressure directly into an acupoint at a 90-degree angle. Compare to *Stacking the joints* and *Weight transfer.*

Personal boundary is a limit established by a person to maintain his or her own integrity, comfort, or well-being. See *Boundaries* and *Boundary crossing.*

Personal care settings are places where personal grooming, relaxation, and rejuvenation services to patrons are provided. Compare to *Spa.*

Personal hygiene involves looking neat and smelling clean to inspire the confidence and trust of clients. See *Professional demeanor* and *Professional image.*

Personal temptation is an attraction to unethical actions. Contrast with *Ethical dilemmas.*

Person-centered massage refers to maintaining awareness of the whole person during a session, as opposed to focusing strictly on the pathology (i.e., pathology centered). Compare to *Client-centered massage.*

Petrissage is a massage technique category that includes movements that lift, wring, or squeeze soft tissues in a kneading motion; or press or roll the soft tissues under or between the hands. See *Swedish massage* and *Western massage.*

Phasic muscles are movers that cause movement against gravity; tend to weaken when postural muscles are shortened. Contrast with *Postural muscles.*

Physical effects of aging are the changes that occur in the mind–body as people get older; examples include decreased strength, slower nerve conduction, less efficient circulation, loss of tissue elasticity, thinner and dryer skin, loss of bone mass, diminished senses, and less efficient immune system. See *Chronological age* and *Physiological age.*

Physical fitness refers to optimal function of the physical body; elements include cardiovascular fitness, muscular strength and endurance, flexibility, and body composition. See *Conscious self-care* and *Self-care.*

Physical impairments commonly encountered in massage practices include visual, hearing, speech, size, and mobility challenges. Contrast with *Disability.*

Physiological age describes the age of an individual according to his or her overall state of health and disease compared to typical age characteristics; influenced by genetic makeup, lifelong health habits, and unique life events such as car accidents and diseases; example is a 60-year-old person having the body of a typical 50-year-old. Contrast with *Chronological age.*

Physiological effects of massage refer to biochemical processes at the cellular, tissue, organ, and organ system levels that result from massage applications. Contrast with *Energetic effects, Mechanical effects, Mind–body effects,* and *Reflex effects.*

Pilot study is a preliminary research project conducted to test a research design or to determine if a larger study is worth conducting; usually small sample of subjects. See *Randomized control trial.*

Plan refers to the activities and applications chosen to achieve results for meeting client goals; a final step in goal-oriented planning; written in the P section of *SOAP notes.* See *Goal-oriented planning.*

Polarity therapy is a form of bodywork that uses simple touch and gentle rocking movements with the intention to balance life energy, to remove obstructions to the free flow of energy, and to encourage relaxation. It was developed by Randolph Stone in the mid-twentieth century. See *Removing obstructions.*

Policies are rules set down to guide the operation of a business or practice; practice policies for massage therapists include pricing, late arrivals, missed appointments, conduct, and confidentiality. See *Private practice* and *Therapeutic relationship.*

Portable massage table is one that can be carried from place to place or set up and taken down easily. See *Equipment.*

Positioning the receiver refers to placing the recipient of massage in a position (e.g., supine, prone, side-lying, seated) to maximize his or her comfort and safety. Bolsters and other props may be used to support specific body areas. See *Bolsters.*

Postevent is a sports massage application given after an athlete competes; the primary goal is physical and psychological recovery of the athlete and may include first aid for minor injuries. See *Sports massage*. Contrast with *Interevent* and *Preevent*.

Posttest is an element of research design; measurement taken after the application of treatment. Contrast with *Pretest*.

Postural muscles are muscles that stabilize and support the body against gravity; tend to shorten and tighten under strain and are overworked if upright posture is unbalanced. Contrast with *Phasic muscles*.

Posture analysis is the evaluation of body alignment; evaluation of standing, sitting, and sleeping postures; used to collect information for goal-oriented planning. See *Objective information*. Contrast with *Gait analysis*.

Power differential refers to the difference in authority between a massage therapist and a client in the therapeutic relationship; massage therapists have more power in the relationship by virtue of training, experience, and perception of greater authority. See *Professional ethics* and *Therapeutic relationship*.

Practice clients are family and friends of students who agree to allow students of massage to practice techniques on them; a type of dual relationship; special type of client for whom professional boundaries and ethical considerations apply. See *Professional ethics*.

Practice identity is that part of a business plan that creates the image you project to the world; includes business name and logo, credentials, résumé, business cards and stationery, website, dress, and office decoration. See *Business plan*.

Practitioner refers to someone trained in massage techniques and who uses massage in the practice of his or her profession. See *Massage therapist*.

Preevent is a sports massage application given before an athlete competes; the purpose of preevent massage is to help the athlete prepare physically and mentally for the upcoming event; may be part of the athlete's warmup routine. See *Sports massage*. Contrast with *Interevent* and *Postevent*.

Pregnancy refers to the time a woman carries a fetus before birth, which is normally for 9 months after fertilization. See *Pregnancy massage*, *Pregnancy posture*, and *Trimesters*.

Pregnancy massage refers to massage and bodywork adapted to meet the needs of pregnant women and relieve some of the discomforts related to the pregnant state. See *Adaptations* and *Special population*.

Pregnancy posture refers to the typical posture of a pregnant woman; may be described as head forward, chest back, belly out, hips tilted forward, locked knees, and feet turned out; causes stress on the body. See *Pregnancy*, *Pregnancy massage*, and *Trimesters*.

Press-and-flex is a reflexology technique in which direct pressure is applied to reflexes by moving the foot into the finger or thumb. See *Foot reflexology*. Compare to *Direct pressure*.

Pressure is related to the force used in applying techniques and to the degree of compaction of tissues as techniques are applied. The amount of pressure used in massage will depend on the intended effect and the tolerance or desires of the recipient. See *Cautions*.

Pretest is an element of research design; measurement taken before the application of treatment. Contrast with *Posttest*

Primary trigger points are trigger points activated by acute or chronic overload of a muscle. See *Trigger points* and *Trigger point therapy*. Contrast with *Secondary trigger points*.

Principle-based therapy refers to treatment plans that take into consideration the pathology being treated, the condition of the individual, and the therapeutic potential of different treatment methods; allows for variation; different from protocol or formula approaches. Compare to *Client-centered massage* and *Evidence-based practice*.

Private practice refers to self-employment as a heath care practitioner; combines both the business and professional sides of being a practitioner. Contrast with *Employee*.

Private-practice settings are places where massage is given; settings include one-room massage office, massage clinic with two or more rooms, in an office building or a storefront; a dedicated massage room can be set aside in a residence for a home-based practice where not prohibited by zoning laws. See *Private practice*.

Problem solving is a systematic approach to finding a solution to a problem using critical thinking skills; starting point is some issue, question, or dilemma for which there are choices for responding; time and effort are taken to gather information needed to make an informed choice or formulate a solution; information gathered is analyzed and evaluated, and finally a solution is determined. See *Intellectual skills*.

Professional associations are nonprofit organizations run by elected leadership, whose mission is to promote their profession, to represent their members and the profession in the larger world, to offer services to members, and to set standards; typically have an IRS designation as 501(c)(6) corporations (United States), that is, nonprofit professional association. Contrast with *Member services organization*.

Professional boundaries are limits that clarify the nature of the therapeutic relationship and the roles of massage therapist and client; five types of professional boundaries are physical, emotional, intellectual, sexual, and energetic. See *Boundaries*.

Professional demeanor refers to the appearance, language, and behavior of practitioners, all of which meet professional standards and inspire trust and respect. Compare to *Professional image*.

Professional ethics is the study of moral behavior related to a certain occupation. See *Therapeutic relationship*, *Confidentiality*, and *Dual relationship*.

Professional image means projecting a professional presence in dress, grooming, posture, and language; identifies a person as someone clients can have confidence in and trust; should be clean, neat, modest, and appropriate for the work setting. See *Personal hygiene*.

Professionalism is a state of mind, a way of being, knowing, and doing that reflects a sense of being individuals who value their work and hold themselves to the highest standards of their occupations; projecting a professional image. Compare to *Professional demeanor* and *Professional image*.

Professional library includes the resources practitioners have accessible within their own offices, including some basic sources of information about conditions, pathologies, and special populations commonly encountered in their massage practices. See *Professionalism*.

Progress notes are for special sessions that reevaluate a client's progress related to his or her long-term goals; contain more assessment information than regular session notes and may identify new goals and plans. See *Documentation*.

Promotions are methods to encourage people to act to buy goods or services; includes discounts, specials, and gift certificates. Contrast with *Advertising*.

Prone refers to the positioning of a client lying facedown on a massage table. Contrast with *Semireclining* and *Supine*.

Proprioceptors are sensory organs embedded in tendons and muscles that detect the amount of stretch or tension that is occurring. See *Body awareness* and *Kinesiology*.

PSOAP is a variation of a SOAP note that separates the problem, complaint, or referral diagnosis into the first P section; recommended if one routinely accepts referrals from health care providers. See *SOAP notes*.

Psychotherapy is a health profession that treats problems and disorders related to the mind and emotions; sometimes referred to as "talk therapy"; outside the scope of practice of massage therapists. See *Defense mechanisms* and *Transference*.

Punctuality is an aspect of work ethic that means showing up for work on time or early. See *Work ethic*. Compare to *Attendance*.

Qi is a term from traditional Chinese medicine that means life force or energy; everything in the universe is produced and sustained by the movements and the changes of Qi; Qi is a continuous form of energy that takes material form when it condenses and nonmaterial form when it disperses; also spelled "chi" and referred to as "ki" in Japanese. See *Acupressure*, *Energy channels*, and *Qi gong*.

Qi gong is a Chinese term that means energy exercise, or exercise based on the theory of the natural energy of Qi; exercises consist of a variety of choreographed movements that involve bending, stretching, reaching, stepping, and other movements designed to harmonize the flow of Qi in the body. See *Energy channels*, *Gong*, and *Qi*.

Qualifying statements are explanations that accompany claims for a product or service and identify the source of information for the claim; sources may include reading, logic, experience, hearsay, or scientific research. See *Advertising* and *Business ethics*.

Qualitative refers to measurement of variables in a research study using word-based assessments. Contrast with *Quantitative*.

Qualities of touch are related to contact and vary from soft and gentle to hard and rough. See *Contact* and *Touch*.

Quantitative refers to measurement of variables in a research study using numerical data. Contrast with *Qualitative*

Randolph Stone (1890–1981) was the man who originally developed polarity therapy in the mid-1900s; he was trained in the natural healing methods of chiropractic, naturopathy, and osteopathy and studied healing methods from India. See *Polarity therapy*.

Range of motion refers to the direction and distance a joint can move to its full potential. See *Joint movements* and *Kinesiology*.

Randomized control trial (RCT) is a type of research study that uses randomly divided experimental and control groups to examine possible cause-and-effect relationships among variables. Contrast with *Case study*; compare to *Pilot study*.

Rating scales are rough measurements of things from the client's subjective view; use numbers to measure the degree or level of the client's experience of some factor related to their goals; example: a scale from 1 to 10. See *Interview skills*. Contrast with *Multiple-choice questions* and *Open-ended questions*.

Recipe-based massage is a formulaic massage in which every client receives exactly the same treatment (i.e., the same techniques applied in the same way) for a particular medical condition. Contrast with *Principle-based massage*.

Reciprocal inhibition is a facilitated stretching technique in which the practitioner gets into position to apply the stretch, but first asks the client to contract the target muscle's antagonist against a resistance; target muscle relaxes as its antagonist contracts; immediately following the antagonist's relaxation, the stretch is applied. See *Stretching*. Compare to *Resisted movements*.

Reconstruction aide is a historical term for a practitioner trained to help rehabilitate wounded soldiers using corrective exercise and massage; antecedent of physical therapists; active in early twentieth century during and after World War I. Contrast with *Bath Attendant* and *Masseuse*.

Recovery is a sports massage application that focuses on enhancing the physical and mental recovery from strenuous physical activity. See *Sports massage*. Contrast with *Maintenance* and *Rehabilitation*.

Reference zone is a trigger point therapy concept meaning the area of the body that feels pain or has another reaction when its related trigger point is activated. See *Active trigger points*, *Satellite trigger points*, and *Trigger points*.

Reflex effects of massage refer to functional changes in the mind and body mediated by the nervous system, and also the largely unexplained phenomenon in which pressing or massaging one part of the body is believed to have a normalizing effect on an entirely different part of the body. See *Reflexology*. Contrast with *Energetic effects, Mechanical effects, Mind–body effects,* and *Physiological effects*.

Reflexology is a form of bodywork based on the theory of zone therapy, in which specific spots on the feet or hands are pressed to stimulate corresponding areas in other parts of the body. See *Foot reflexology*.

Reflexology chart is a diagrammed map of the feet showing the location of reflexes on the feet according to the theory of reflexology; identifies which part of the body is affected by pressing a specific spot on a foot. See *Foot reflexology* and *Reflexology*.

Regional massage is focused on a particular area of the body, which provides an opportunity for greater specificity. See *Specificity*. Contrast with *Full-body Swedish massage*.

Rehabilitation refers to massage applications to treat injuries; a sports massage application to facilitate healing after a disabling injury. Contrast with *Event, Maintenance, Recovery,* and *Remedial massage*.

Relaxin is a hormone excreted in the first trimester of pregnancy that softens ligaments in the body, causing joints to become more mobile; helps prepare the woman's body for delivery later on; results in unstable joints for the duration of the pregnancy. See *Pregnancy massage* and *Trimesters*.

Reliability is an aspect of a work ethic that means people can depend on you to do what you say you are going to do, when you are supposed to do it; if you are reliable, people will have trust and confidence in you. See *Work ethic*. Compare to *Accountability*.

Remedial massage is a sports massage application that focuses on improving debilitating conditions and minor injuries. See *Sports massage*. Contrast with *Event, Maintenance,* and *Rehabilitation*.

Removing obstructions is a basic principle in polarity therapy referring to eliminating barriers to the free flow of energy; an obstruction is an area of the body where there seems to be a stagnation or a holding pattern that interferes with a free flow of energy. See *Energy flow* and *Polarity therapy*.

Repetitive strain injuries (RSIs) are musculoskeletal injuries caused by repeated stress on specific muscles and joints; result in aching, tenderness, swelling, tingling, numbness, weakness, loss of flexibility, and spasms in the muscles affected; can result in chronic pain, loss of mobility, and eventually, disability. See *Ergonomics, Seated massage,* and *Workplace wellness programs*.

Research is the systematic examination of a phenomenon based on careful observations using measurements; methodical, objective, and focused study of a particular subject or question. See *Research literacy*.

Research literacy refers to knowledge and skills needed to understand and use scientific research; includes an understanding of the scientific method, locating research articles, and reading, analyzing, and evaluating research studies. Compare to *Evidence-based practice* and *Principle-based therapy*.

Resisted movements are a type of active movement in which a person initiates the movement, while a second person offers resistance, thereby challenging the muscles used; sometimes used in rehabilitation to restore strength to a muscle. Contrast with *Assisted movements*.

Résumé is a document that provides a summary of training, experience, and credentials in an occupation or profession; used to present qualifications for a job, volunteer position, or whenever a summary of past accomplishments is required; also known as CV (curriculum vitae). Contrast with *Transcript*.

Rhythm refers to a recurring pattern of movement with a specific cadence, beat, or accent and may be described as smooth, flowing, or uneven. Contrast with *Flow* and *Pacing*.

Rights are claims to certain treatment or to protection from certain treatment; expected to be honored by others, and enforced by standards or laws if necessary. See *Professional ethics*. Compare to *Duties*.

Robust elders are people age 70 and older who show few outward signs of impaired health, look younger than their chronological ages, are mentally sharp, and are physically active. Contrast with *Age-appropriate* and *Frail elders*.

Rocking motions are basic polarity therapy techniques involving small, gentle oscillations of a small area of the body, or large, vigorous oscillations that move the entire body; rocking motions induce relaxation, lower muscle tone, reduce pain, and encourage an increase in the active range of motion afterward. See *Polarity therapy*. Compare to *Energy flow*.

Rolling is a reflexology technique in which a thumb or finger is rolled into a reflex point to apply pressure. See *Foot reflexology*. Contrast with *Fingerwalking* and *Thumbwalking*.

Roman baths were public institutions in the ancient Roman Empire that consisted of a space for undressing, an exercise court, a warm room, a type of steam room, and a cold pool; might also have a swimming pool. Compare to *Greek gymnasia* and *Turkish baths*.

Rubber is a historical term for an unschooled massage practitioner who gave rubdowns to athletes; learned their skills on the job, or from other rubbers; early twentieth-century Europe and North America. Compare to *Masseuse* and *Masseur*.

Rubdown is a term used in athletic venues for superficial skin friction with the hand, a brush, a coarse towel, or a horsehair glove; popular in the nineteenth and early twentieth centuries. Contrast with *Swedish massage*.

Salary draw is the money taken out of a business or practice monthly for the owner's personal use. Contrast with *Net income*.

Sanitation refers to taking precautions that prevent the spread of disease and to following good hygiene practices. See *Do no harm*.

Satellite trigger points are trigger points that become active because they are in a muscle in a zone of reference of another trigger point. See *Associated trigger point* and *Reference zone*.

Sauna   is a thermohydrotherapy facility; typically a wood-lined room heated without steam, and with very dry air; patrons sit on wooden benches. See *Thermotherapy*. Contrast with *Steam room*.

Schedule C   is an IRS income tax form that reports small business income and expenses; attaches to *Form 1040*. See *Income tax*.

Scientific method   is a systematic way of testing theories through gathering and analyzing relevant information to see if it supports the theory in question. It is based on observations rather than on authority or anecdotes. See *Hypothesis* and *Research literacy*.

Scope of practice   describes the legally allowed, or professionally defined, methods used by a certain profession, as well as its intention in performing them. Different professions have different scopes of practice as defined by law or by the profession. Massage techniques fall within the scope of practice of several professions. See *Professional ethics*.

Screening interview   is conducted to check for contraindications and cautions before giving massage to a new client. See *Intake notes*.

Scrubs   are manual exfoliation methods using salts or coarser organic substances. See *Exfoliants*. Contrast with *Body polish*.

Seated massage   refers to massage given with the recipient seated in an ordinary or a special massage chair; called on-site massage when the chair is taken to a public place such as an office or commercial establishment; also called chair massage. See *Massage chair* and *On-site massage*.

Secondary trigger points   are trigger points that become active because of their reaction to a muscle containing a primary trigger point. See *Trigger point therapy* and *Trigger points*. Contrast with *Primary trigger points*.

Self-awareness   is an aspect of emotional intelligence that involves recognizing a feeling as it happens and its accompanying emotion or impulse to act. See *Emotional intelligence*.

Self-care   refers to actions massage practitioners take for their own well-being and to promote their longevity in the profession; includes physical self-care such as physical fitness and good body mechanics and emotional self-care such as in dealing with grief, anger, and confusion. See *Conscious self-care* and *Holistic self-care plan*.

Self-disclosure   is revealing personal information about the self; self-disclosure by a therapist can be a boundary crossing in the therapeutic relationship. See *Professional boundaries*.

Self-employed   describes operating a business as a sole proprietor or independent contractor; a person is his or her own employer; called being in private practice for a massage therapist. See *Private practice* and *Independent contractor*. Contrast with *Employee*.

Self-employment tax   (SE tax) is a Social Security and Medicare tax for self-employed individuals; applies to Social Security coverage for retirement, disability, survivor, and Medicare benefits; SE tax must be paid if net earnings from self-employment are $400 or more; SE tax is in addition to the regular income tax. See *Income tax*.

Self-reflection   is an aspect of critical thinking that takes into consideration the thinker's own prejudices and beliefs in determining the truth about something. See *Critical thinking*.

Semireclining   refers to the positioning of a client who is supine on a massage table into a half-sitting position by placing pillows under the upper body; the upper body is at about a 45-degree angle to the lower body. Contrast with *Side-lying*, *Prone*, and *Supine*.

Service   is a value in which we hold our clients' well-being above our own desire for money, power, and worldly recognition; means that the primary motivation for being a massage therapist is to help people achieve their personal wellness goals. See *Professional ethics* and *Values*.

Session   refers to a period of time in which massage is given to a recipient by a practitioner. Sessions have logical organization, have a wellness or a treatment purpose, and generally vary from 10 minutes to 2 hours. See *Goal-oriented planning* and *Session planning*.

Session planning   is the logical process of thinking through a specific massage session; includes collecting relevant information, assessing the situation and setting goals, choosing massage applications, performing the massage, and evaluating results. See *Goal-oriented planning*.

Sexual misconduct   refers to any sexualizing of the relationship between a massage therapist and a current client; can occur before, after, or during a massage session, and can be perpetrated by the massage therapist or by the client; forms of sexual misconduct range from those involving speech and body language to inappropriate touch to sexual contact to sexual assault. See *Intervention model*.

Sheng   is a Chinese term meaning "life." See *Dao Yin Yang Shen Gong*. Compare to *Sheng Cycle*.

Sheng Cycle   is a concept within the Five Element Theory that looks at relationships among the elements; also called the creation, generating, or promoting cycle; in the Sheng Cycle, each Element supports the next, for example, the Ko Cycle balances the Sheng Cycle to avoid unrestrained growth. See *Five Elements*. Contrast with *Ko Cycle*.

Shiatsu   is a general term for Japanese bodywork based on Chinese meridian theory and Western science, in which *tsubo* (i.e., acupoints) are pressed to balance the flow of energy or *ki*. Compare to *Acupressure*.

Short-term effects   of massage are physiological and psychological changes that occur during a massage session. See *Effects of massage*. Contrast with *Long-term effects*.

Side-lying   refers to the positioning of a client on his or her left or right side for massage; pillows under the upper arm and leg support the body for client comfort. Contrast with *Prone*, *Semireclining*, and *Supine*.

Simple static stretch   is a passive stretch characterized by slow, sustained, and even application. See *Passive movements* and *Stretching*.

Simplified notes are forms of documentation that contain minimum information; used at venues such as health fairs, trade shows, sports events, and outreach events where people receive a short standard massage routine and will not be seen again by the practitioner. Contrast with *SOAP notes*.

Single-dose effects of massage refer to changes that occur from one massage application. See *Effects of massage*. Contrast with *Multiple-dose effects*.

Skilled touch refers to abilities related to physical contact; four dimensions important to massage therapists include contact, qualities, communication, and palpation. See *Contact* and *Palpation*.

SOAP notes are a standard form for documenting therapeutic sessions; SOAP is an acronym for Subjective, Objective, Assessment, and Plan. See *Documentation*. Contrast with *Simplified notes*.

Sobardoras are traditional Hispanic healers trained by apprenticeship to use massage in treating ailments; also use ritual, herbal remedies, and bone-setting manipulation techniques; part of the healing tradition of curanderas. Contrast with *Masseuse* and *Masseur*.

Social skills are methods of interacting with other people that promote harmony, understanding, and connection, while peacefully solving problems such as disagreements, misunderstandings, and reconciliation after harm done; primary goal is building good relationships. See *Conflict resolution* and *Emotional intelligence*.

Sole proprietor is a form of self-employment in which a person is the legally recognized business owner, the employer and employee combined. See *Self-employment*.

SOTAP is a form of documentation for therapeutic sessions; variation of SOAP notes; acronym for Subjective, Objective, Treatment, Assessment, and Plan; provides a separate T section for recording the massage and related techniques used in the session. See *Documentation*. Contrast with *SOAP notes*.

Spa refers to a business that offers personal care services in an environment that focuses on overall well-being and renewal of mind, body, and spirit; emphasis on natural therapies and spa treatments using natural substances. See *Personal care*.

Special population is a group of people with some distinctive life circumstance that sets them apart from a normal adult population; includes athletes, pregnant women, infants, the elderly, and people with various physical impairments and diseases. See *Adaptations* and *Disability*.

Specialty associations are organizations composed of practitioners of a particular style of massage or bodywork or those who work in a particular setting. Contrast with *General membership organization*.

Specialty certification refers to certification in a specific massage and bodywork system; involves some combination of education, skill development, internship, written and performance tests, ethical code, continuing education, and/or periodic renewal. See *Certification*.

Specificity refers to targeting a specific muscle or small area and applying massage techniques to structures there; different from broad or general massage applications. See *Palpatory sensitivity*.

Sports, fitness, and recreation centers are facilities whose main purpose is to provide opportunities for physical exercise and sports, but which also provide support services like massage. Contrast with *Integrative medicine* and *Wellness center*.

Sports massage is the science and art of applying massage and related techniques to ensure the health and well-being of the athlete and to enhance athletic performance; major applications of sports massage are recovery, remedial, rehabilitation, maintenance, and event (i.e., pre-, inter-, and postevent). See *Special population*.

Sports medicine center refers to a rehabilitation facility specializing in athletic injuries and improvement of sports performance. Contrast with *Integrative medicine* and *Wellness center*.

Stabilizing hand refers to the hand providing a brace or backstop during the application of reflexology techniques. See *Foot reflexology* and *Bracing*. Contrast with *Working hand*.

Stacking the joints is one of the general principles for applying pressure to acupoints; means lining the joints up so that pressure travels from bone to bone and not across joints. Compare to *Perpendicularity* and *Weight transfer*.

Standards of practice are documents developed by professional associations that outline acceptable ethical professional conduct. Contrast with *Codes of ethics*.

Startup costs are the initial expenses involved in setting up a business like a massage therapy practice. See *First-year budget*.

Steam room is a hydrotherapy facility; typically a room tiled from floor to ceiling and with benches for sitting; steam comes out from jets in the walls and fills the space with wet heat. See *Hydrotherapy* and *Thermotherapy*. Contrast with *Sauna*.

Stone massage involves the use of hot or cold stones applied to the body for therapeutic purposes. See *Spa*.

Stress-control strategies include good time management, adequate rest and relaxation, and anxiety reduction techniques, including massage. See *Holistic self-care plan*.

Stretching is a type of joint movement performed to the limit of a joint's normal range in a specific direction. Stretching elongates the muscles and connective tissues that cross the joint and helps relax the muscles involved. See *Joint movements*. Contrast with *Mobilizing techniques*.

Subcutaneous fascia is a continuous layer of connective tissue over the entire body between the skin and the deep fascia. See *Fascia* and *Myofascial massage*. Contrast with *Deep fascia*.

Subjective information refers to what clients report to the therapist during goal-oriented planning; includes complaints and comments about their conditions and how they feel; written in the S section of *SOAP notes*. Contrast with *Objective information*.

Substantiated claims   for a product or service have a credible basis or evidence in their support; unsubstantiated claims for products or services are illegal according to consumer protection laws. See *Advertising* and *Business ethics*.

Superficial friction   is a type of friction in which the hand rubs briskly back and forth over the skin to improve circulation in superficial tissues and to create heat. Contrast with *Deep friction*.

Supine   refers to the positioning of a client lying faceup on a massage table. Contrast with *Prone* and *Semireclining*.

Swedish massage   is a genre of bodywork that includes traditional European massage, Swedish movements, hydrotherapy, heat lamps, and other modalities; techniques include effleurage, petrissage, friction, tapotement, vibration, and touch without movement; a popular form of massage in health clubs, spas, and resorts. Contrast with *Swedish movement cure*. Compare to *Western massage*.

Swedish Movement Cure   refers to Pehr Ling's system of medical gymnastics that was developed in the early 1800s and that, along with Mezger's massage, was the forerunner of today's Swedish massage. See *Swedish massage*.

Systematic review   involves the analysis of a number of experimental research studies to determine the strength of evidence for use of a particular treatment for a certain condition; also called *meta-analysis*.

Table skills   include a variety of actions required to position and drape a client properly on a massage table. See *Draping* and *Positioning*.

Tactile stimulation   refers to the stimulation of the tactile nerves in the skin through touch and movement; essential for the healthy growth and development of infants; provided by infant massage. See *Infant massage*.

Tapotement   is a massage technique category consisting of brisk percussive movements that are performed in rapid, rhythmic fashion; forms include hacking, rapping, cupping, clapping, slapping, tapping, and pincement. See *Swedish massage* and *Western massage*.

Technique   refers to the technical aspects of the application of massage or how the body moves while performing massage; a broader concept of the term *technique* also includes the intent. See *Intention*.

Telltack   is a historical term for a practitioner of a vigorous type of bodywork given at the Turkish baths or hammam; nineteenth- and twentieth-century Middle East, Near East, Europe, and North America. See *Turkish baths*.

Temperature therapy   involves the application of hot and cold modalities for their therapeutic effects (e.g., hot packs, ice). See *Hydrotherapy*.

Tenting   is a technique that prevents clients from getting rolled up in the drape. See *Table skills*.

Terminus   refers to the hollow space just lateral to the left and right attachments of the sternocleidomastoid (SCM) muscles on the clavicle; at the terminus lymphatic facilitation techniques are applied to increase the flow of lymph into the thoracic ducts, thus clearing the area. See *Lymphatic facilitation*.

Tissues   of the body form when like cells group together to perform one activity, for example, muscle cells combine to form muscle tissue; come together to form body organs. See *Organs* and *Body systems*.

Thai massage   is traditional bodywork from Thailand; its intent is to stimulate the body's self-healing processes and to correct energy imbalances. Compare to *Ayurvedic massage*. Contrast with *Swedish massage*.

Therapeutic relationship   is a model for understanding the separate and unique roles of the practitioner and the client in the therapeutic setting. See *Boundaries* and *Standards of Practice*.

Therapeutic Touch   is a form of manual therapy in which the energy field of the recipient is rebalanced, thus promoting health and healing. See *Energetic effects*.

Thermotherapy   refers to temperature therapy modalities above normal body temperature (e.g., hot packs). See *Temperature therapy*. Contrast with *Cryotherapy*.

Thixotropy   is a characteristic of fascia in which fascial tissues can change from a more solid to a more liquid gel consistency. Fascia becomes more pliable with movement, stretching, and increase in temperature. See *Fascia* and *Myofascial massage*.

Thumbwalking   is a reflexology technique performed by bending the thumb at the first joint, pressing into the tissues, and then straightening the thumb, moving from spot to spot on the foot; action is repeated as the thumb "walks" in line along the foot. See *Foot reflexology*. Compare to *Fingerwalking*. Contrast with *Hook-and-backup*.

Time management   is a personal skill of scheduling daily and weekly activities to reflect personal priorities; involves identifying goals and priorities for a certain period of time and plotting a schedule accordingly; includes keeping to the schedule developed. See *Holistic self-care plan*.

Tips   are gratuities (i.e., given in gratitude) over and above the cost of a service; given directly to the person providing the service; given at the discretion of the person receiving the service; are taxable income reported to the IRS on income tax forms. See *Income tax*.

Topical substance   is a liniment, oil, lotion, cream, or combination of these used in massage. See *Lubricants*.

Touch   means "to come into contact with"; massage practitioners touch their clients or patients in many ways, but primarily with their hands; touch may happen on a physical or an energetic level. See *Palpation*, *Tactile stimulation*, and *Touch deprivation*.

Touch deprivation   is a physical and psychological condition resulting from a lack of healthy, pleasurable touch; can lead to emotional distress; can be relieved by the caring touch of massage. See *Nurturing touch* and *Palliative care*.

Touch without movement   is a massage technique in which the practitioner comes in contact with the recipient either physically or energetically, but no perceptible movement occurs that fits into the five traditional classic massage categories. Two common types of touch without movement are passive touch and direct static pressure. See *Swedish massage* and *Western massage*.

Trademarks   offer exclusive use of a name or symbol to identify unique goods and services; use the symbol ™ or ® for registered trademarks; distinguish a particular brand or company from others; handled by the U.S. Patent and Trademark Office in Washington, DC; may also be regulated on the state (United States) or provincial (Canada) level. Compare to *Copyright*.

Traditional Chinese medicine (TCM)   is a system of healing based on ancient Chinese medicine and includes concepts such as yin/yang, the Five Elements, energy (Qi), and energy channels. Compare to *Acupressure* and *Qi gong*.

Trained masseuses   is a historical term for massage practitioners who took courses of study in private schools and hospital programs in the early 1900s, differentiating themselves from the many untrained massage practitioners of the time. Compare to *Masseuses* and *Masseurs*.

Transcript   is a detailed record of a student's performance while in school, including specific subjects studied, grades, attendance, date of graduation, honors, school information, and other facts; an original transcript carrying the school seal is usually required for official purposes such as obtaining a license to practice. Contrast with *Diploma*.

Transference   is a psychological phenomenon that occurs when a client responds to a practitioner as if the client were relating to someone important in his or her past (e.g., father), and transferring those positive or negative feelings onto the therapeutic relationship. Contrast with *Countertransference*.

Transition techniques   serve to provide continuity and flow from one section of the body to another during a massage session. See *Organization*. Contrast with *Finishing techniques*.

Transport vessels,   or lymphangia, are lymph system vessels that carry lymph fluid from the collector vessels to the thoracic ducts; are segmented with each segment referred to as a lymphangion, which is bounded by a valve on each end and which contracts to move fluid through the vessel. See *Lymphatic facilitation*. Contrast with *Collector vessels* and *Initial/terminal lymph vessels*.

Treatment   refers to interventions aimed at alleviating a specific medical condition. Contrast with *Palliative care*.

Treatment model   is a concept that explains the intention of using specific interventions or modalities to alleviate medical conditions. Contrast with *Wellness model*.

Treatment planning   is a form of goal-oriented planning in which the goal is alleviation of symptoms, or facilitation of healing of a pathological condition; used for medical, clinical, and orthopedic massage applications; sometimes called a *Plan of care*. See *Goal-oriented planning*.

Trigger point therapy   involves the identification and deactivation of painful fibrous nodules in muscle and connective tissue called trigger points; manual TrP techniques include ischemic compression, deep friction, deep stripping, and stretching. See *Trigger points*.

Trigger points   are small, hyperirritable spots in muscle or related connective tissue that are felt as taut bands of tissue that elicit pain if pressed and that refer pain to other areas in predictable patterns. See *Reference zone* and *Trigger point therapy*.

Trimesters   refers to the three stages of pregnancy, each trimester lasting about 3 months; the first, second, and third trimesters each have specific implications for the mother and the fetus related to massage applications. See *Pregnancy* and *Pregnancy massage*.

Triptai   is a historical term used in ancient Greece for someone who specialized in rubbing; massage has been called the *anatriptic art*; *anatriptic* means to "rub up" or toward the body's center. See *Greek gymnasia*. Compare to *Rubber*.

Turkish baths   are public institutions modeled after Roman baths, which were brought to the West from the Middle East during the Renaissance Period; became popular in large cities in Europe and America. Compare to *Roman baths*.

Understanding   is a basic principle of polarity therapy referring to the practitioner being open to the recipient's experience and to the effects of polarity therapy; it calls for knowledge of the broader picture in terms of the physiological and psychological reactions happening in a session. See *Polarity therapy*. Compare to *Love*.

Universal precautions   are procedures that aim to prevent the transmission of serious communicable disease; also called standard or sanitary precautions. See *Sanitation*.

Upper body regions,   for the purposes of massage, are commonly identified as face, head, neck, upper and lower back, shoulders, arms and hands, and chest and abdomen. See *Regional massage*. Contrast with *Lower body regions*.

Values   are principles, traits, or qualities considered worthwhile or desirable; protected by ethical standards and codes of ethics. See *Ethics* and *Ethical standards*.

Variable costs   are fluctuating operating expenses and depend on the number of clients seen; examples: laundry and massage supplies. Contrast with *Fixed costs*.

Verbal skills   describe the ability to communicate by means of the spoken word; includes good articulation and voice quality; delivery of spoken word more important than content in some cases. See *Communication skills* and *Voice quality*.

Vertical position   is the common position during seated massage; clients are supported on their buttocks, lower legs, and chest instead of lying facedown on a horizontal surface. See *Massage chair* and *Seated massage*.

Vibration   is a Western massage technique category that includes oscillating, quivering, or trembling movements; or movement of soft tissues back and forth, or up and down, performed quickly and repeatedly. Vibration may be described as fine or coarse (e.g., shaking, jostling). See *Swedish massage* and *Western massage*.

Vision is an element of a business plan that describes the broad scope of the proposed business; for a massage practice, it would include mission, size, format, location, and income goals. See *Business plan.*

Voice quality is an aspect of verbal communication that includes the pitch, tone, volume, clarity, and richness of the sound of someone's speech; can affect a person's image or how they are perceived by others. See *Communication skills* and *Professional image.*

Warming techniques are used to raise the temperature of tissues, increase superficial circulation, and prepare an area for more specific massage applications. See *Opening techniques* and *Organization.* Contrast with *Finishing techniques.*

Watersheds describe superficial lymphatic drainage patterns in different areas of the body. Lymph traveling in the lymphangia moves within its watershed or drainage area toward the catchments or concentrations of lymph nodes nearby. See *Catchments* and *Lymphatic facilitation.*

Weight transfer is one of the general principles for applying pressure to acupoints; means applying pressure by shifting the body weight into the point of contact rather than pushing from the shoulders and arms. Compare to *Perpendicularity* and *Stacking the joints.*

Wellness refers to a condition of optimal physical, emotional, intellectual, spiritual, social, and vocational well-being. See *Wellness profession.*

Wellness center refers to a facility that offers fitness activities, rehabilitation programs, massage therapy, and classroom instruction in preventing disease and developing a healthy lifestyle; often connected to a hospital. Contrast with *Integrative medicine center.*

Wellness massage is massage performed with the intention of promoting the receiver's general well-being; it goes beyond the treatment of specific conditions to help the receiver achieve high-level wellness. See *Wellness Massage Pyramid.*

Wellness Massage Pyramid is a model for understanding the possible contributions of massage therapy to high-level wellness. Pyramid levels from the base to the top are treatment, recovery, prevention, neutral zone, health maintenance, personal growth, and life enjoyment. See *Wellness massage.*

Wellness model is a concept that explains good health and well-being as aimed at living a healthy, vibrant, and meaningful life; it goes beyond the idea of health as the absence of disease and emphasizes personal responsibility; also called the wellness perspective. See *Wellness.* Contrast with *Treatment model.*

Wellness movement is a twentieth-century phenomenon within health care and fitness that emphasizes taking responsibility for health and well-being and that addresses holistic health of body, mind, emotions, and spirit. See *Holistic* and *Wellness Massage Pyramid.*

Wellness profession is a profession or occupation with a scope of practice that spans the breadth of the wellness model from treatment and recovery to personal growth and life enjoyment; focus is on attaining high-level wellness. See *Wellness.*

Western massage refers to forms of soft tissue manipulation developed in Europe and North America over the past 200 years. Compare to *Swedish massage.* Contrast with *Asian bodywork therapies* and *Ayurvedic massage.*

Whirlpool bath is a hydrotherapy device consisting of a water-filled tub that has air or water jets causing movement or churning of the water; typically contains hot water; may be private or communal; may be large enough to sit or lie down in or small enough for a part of the body. See *Hydrotherapy* and *Thermotherapy.*

Worker productivity refers to the amount and quality of work employees can accomplish in a certain period of time; is affected negatively by work time lost due to illness or injury. See *On-site massage* and *Workplace wellness programs.*

Work ethic is an attitude that positions one's job as a high priority in life and that promotes applying oneself to high-quality performance; taking pride in one's work. See *Accountability, Attendance, Punctuality,* and *Reliability.*

Working hand refers to the hand applying a reflexology technique. See *Foot reflexology.* Contrast with *Stabilizing hand.*

Workplace wellness programs are employer-sponsored programs that make services and activities available to employees to improve their overall health and well-being. See *On-site massage* and *Worker productivity.*

Written correspondence is a form of communication that utilizes basic writing skills such as correct spelling, punctuation, grammar, sentence construction, and organization of thought; forms include memos, e-mails, and business letters. See *Communication skills.*

Yang is the masculine principle in Chinese medicine; the light, energetic, and ethereal aspect of the universe; characterized as exterior, moving, nonsubstantial, warm, expanding, and opposing but also supporting Yin; the Chinese character for Yang is a hillside in full sun. Contrast with *Yin.* .

Yin is the feminine principle in Chinese medicine; the dark, deep, dense aspect of the universe; characterized as interior, still, substantial, cool, and contracting in contrast to Yang; the Chinese character for Yin depicts the shady side of a hill or mountain. Contrast with *Yang.*

Zone therapy is a foundation theory of reflexology stating that pressure on certain places in the body provides therapeutic reactions in other parts of the body in predictable patterns; there are 10 longitudinal zones running from the head to the hands and feet. See *Foot reflexology, Reflexology,* and *Reflexology chart.*

Zoning ordinance is a local law that specifies what type of housing or what kind of business can be in a certain location. Compare to *Massage establishment license.*

Index

Note: Page numbers with *f* indicate figures; those with *t* indicate tables.

A

AAMM. *See* American Association of Masseurs and Masseuses (AAMM)
Abdomen. *See* Chest and abdomen
Abdominal breathing, 141, 607
ABHES. *See* Accrediting Bureau of Health Education Schools (ABHES)
Abhyanga (herbal oil massage), 612
ABMP. *See* Associated Bodywork & Massage Professionals (ABMP)
ABT. *See* Asian bodywork therapies (ABT)
Accommodation, in conflict resolution, 58
Accreditation, 11, 13, 13*t*
Accrediting Bureau of Health Education Schools (ABHES), 11
Accrediting Commission for Career Schools and Colleges of Technology (ACCSCT), 11
Accrual method, 658
ACCSCT. *See* Accrediting Commission for Career Schools and Colleges of Technology (ACCSCT)
Acne vulgaris, 174, 175*f*
Active assisted stretch, 292, 293*t*
Active listening, 62–63
Active meditation, 82
Active movements, 291
Active range of motion (AROM), 208, 209*f*
Active TrPs, 527, 527*t*
Acupoints, 580–583, 581*t*, 582–583*f*
  ancient drawing of, 578*f*
  applying pressure to, principles of, 585
  Kyo and Jitsu, 583, 584*f*
  overview of, 580
  useful acupoints for common ailments, 581*t*
Acupressure massage integration (AMI), 584–606
  applying pressure to acupoints, 585
  basic approach to, 585
  neck and back alignment in, 585
  overview of, 584
  perpendicularity in, 585
  practice sequence for arm, 585–586, 586*f*, 594–599
  practice sequence for back, 585–586, 586*f*, 587–594
  practice sequence for neck-head-face, 585–586, 586*f*, 599–606
  stacking the joints in, 585, 585*f*
  weight transfer in, 585

Acupuncture
  abbreviation for (ACU), 196*t*
  acupoints in, 580–583, 581*t*, 582–583*f*
  board certification for, 12
  as CAM therapy, 4, 5*f*
  for energy imbalances, 584
  in health care settings, 7, 8
  as licensed profession, 584
  in polarity therapy, 615, 619
  in 1970s revival of massage therapy, 38
  in traditional Chinese medicine, 577
Acute inflammation, 173
ADA. *See* Americans with Disabilities Act (ADA)
Adaptations, 421. *See also* Special populations
Adjunct modalities, 3
Advertising, 651–652
  credentials, 669–670
  deceptive, 669
  ethics in, 669–671
  guarantees and endorsements, 670–671
  prices and bait advertising, 671
  professional image in, 669–670
Aerobics, 38
Affirmative listening, 62
AFMTE. *See* Alliance for Massage Therapy Education (AFMTE)
Age-appropriate elders, 442
AHA. *See* Alphahydroxy acids (AHA)
Ajna (Third Eye Chakra), 610*f*, 611
Aleiptes, 29
Alexander the Great, 26
Allergic reactions, 236–237
Allergies, 176
Allergies, spa applications and, 468
Alliance for Massage Therapy Education (AFMTE), 11
Alphahydroxy acids (AHA), 474
Alternating one-handed kneading, 275, 275*f*
AMA. *See* American Medical Association (AMA)
America. *See* United States
American Association of Masseurs and Masseuses (AAMM), 35, 37
American Hospital Association, 5
American Journal of Nursing, Nursing Research, 161
American Massage Therapy Association (AMTA), 10*t*, 11, 14, 15, 17, 35, 39, 641
American Massage & Therapy Association (AM&TA), 35, 38
American Medical Association (AMA), 662

American Naturopathic Association (ANA), 36
American Organization for Bodywork Therapies of Asia (AOBTA), 10*t*, 16
American Physical Therapy Association, 35
American Polarity Therapy Association (APTA), 16, 615
Americans with Disabilities Act (ADA), 456
American Women's Physical Therapeutic Association, 35
Amma, 8, 38, 584
Ammashi, 26
Amputees and prosthesis, 459–460
AMTA. *See* American Massage Therapy Association (AMTA)
AM&TA. *See* American Massage & Therapy Association (AM&TA)
ANA. *See* American Naturopathic Association (ANA)
Anahata (Heart Chakra), 610*f*, 611
Analgesia, 140–141
Analysis, in intellectual skills, 51, 51*t*
Anandamaya, 609*f*, 611
Anastomosis, 543
Anatomy. *See also* Organ systems
  charts, in presentations, 63
  contraindications and, 173
  do no harm principle and, 167
  education in, 10, 28, 30, 33, 34
  empirical knowledge and, 124
  massage based on understanding of, 3
  palpation and, 206
  person-centered massage and, 182–183
  reliable information for, 183
  as shared knowledge, 10
  Swedish massage and, 269
  in treatment planning, 201
Anatriptic art, 32
Ancient civilizations, massage in, 26–28, 40. *See also* Public baths
  China, 26
  Greece, 26
  India, 26
  Japan, 26
Ancient roots of reflexology, 559
Andrews, Harry, 30, 30*f*
Ankle, joint movements to, 303–304, 303*f*
Annamaya, 609–610, 609*f*
Anterior neck, endangerment sites, 167, 169*f*
Anxiety, 142
AOBTA. *See* American Organization for Bodywork Therapies of Asia (AOBTA)
Apotherapeia, 29

Appendicitis, 173
Apple Computer Corporation, 497
Application, in intellectual skills, 51, 51*t*
Appointments, 654–655
Appropriate touch, 105
APTA. *See* American Polarity Therapy Association (APTA)
Arm, AMI for, 585–586, 586*f*, 594–599
Arm-shoulder rotations, 622
Aromastones, 487
Aromatherapy, 481–487
  essential oils in, 482–487
  overview of, 481–482
Artificial joint replacements, 174
Art of Massage: Its Physiological Effects and Therapeutic Applications, The (Kellogg), 37
Asanas, 614
Asian bodywork therapies (ABT), 3, 584. *See also* Eastern bodywork
Assessment, 201
Assisted movements, 291
Associated Bodywork & Massage Professionals (ABMP), 10*t*, 11, 14, 15, 17, 39, 639
Associated TrPs, 527, 527*t*
Asthmatic children, 159
Atherosclerosis, 176, 177*f*
Athletes, 421–429. *See also* Sports massage
Athlete's foot, 174
Athletic masseurs, 29–30
Attention span, 52
Autistic children, 159
Autonomic nervous system, 135–136
Autonomy, 93
Avoidance, in conflict resolution, 58
Axilla, endangerment sites, 169, 170*f*
Ayurveda, 607–611
  chakras, 609*t*, 610–611, 610*f*, 615
  doshas, 609, 609*t*, 610, 610*t*, 611
  glossary of terms, 609*t*
  health practices, 608
  koshas, 609–611, 609*t*
  marma points, 611, 612*f*
  overview of, 607
Ayurvedic massage, 3, 611–614
  applications, 613–614, 613*f*
  goal of, 611
  massage oils in, 613
  varieties of, 612

B

Back, 353–359
  alignment, 585
  AMI for, 585–586, 586*f*, 587–594
  anatomy of, 353–354, 353*f*
  hot packs on, practice sequence for, 406–408

Back (*continued*)
massage applications for, 354
massage for hospitalized patients, 157
myofascial massage techniques on, 518–521
practice sequence for, 354–359
relaxation of, 354
sedating effleurage of, 354
Back Stream acupoint, 581*t*
Bait advertising, 671
Balfour, William, 32
Banking, 660–661
Barbershops, massage offered in, 6, 6*t*
Barnes, John, 514
Basalt, 488, 488*f*
Base oils, 483
Basic research. *See also* Research literacy
defined, 124
design elements, 127*f*
Basic sliding effleurage, 270–271, 270–271*f*
Basic two-handed kneading, 274–275, 275*f*
Bath attendant, 28, 28*f*, 30
Battle Creek Sanitarium, 37, 401
Beauty culture, 28
Beauty salons, massage offered in, 6, 6*t*
Beneficence, 94
Benefits of massage, 124
Bergamot, 485*t*
"Best-case" exercises, 102–103
Betahydroxy acids (BHAS), 474
Beyond Technique: The Hidden Dimensions of Bodywork (Kisch), 110
BHAS. *See* Betahydroxy acids (BHAS)
Bidirectional thumb pressure on plantar surface, in reflexology sessions, 569
Bilateral tree stroking, 272, 272*f*
Biltz Sanitarium, 401, 402*f*
Biofeedback, 4, 5*f*, 141
Biomechanical analysis, 210–211
Bipedal locomotion, 383
Black mud, 476
Bladder acupoint, 582*f*
Blankets, 235
Bleeding and bruising, 176–177
Blood circulation, 136–137, 137*f*
Blood poisoning (lymphangitis), 176
Blood pressure (BP), 76, 137–138, 176
BMI. *See* Body mass index (BMI)
Board certification, 12, 13, 13*t*
Body alignment, 585
Body and hand mechanics, in seated massage, 498
Body awareness, 74–75
Body brushing, 469
Body-centered therapy, massage as, 123
Body charts, 204
Body composition, 80
Body language, 60–62, 61*f*
crossed arms and legs, 61
defined, 60
distance between people who are talking, 60–61
eye contact, 61
hand gestures, 61
listening, 62–63
posture, 60
smile, 61
Body mass index (BMI), 80, 85, 458
Body mechanics, defined, 246. *See also* Hand and body mechanics

Body–mind effects, 144, 145
Body–mind practices, 80–82
meditation, 81–82, 81*f*
Pilates, 81, 81*f*
qi gong, 81
tai chi, 81
yoga, 80
Body polishes, 471–472, 471*f*
Body Reflexology (Carter), 561
Bodywork, 3, 39. *See also* Eastern bodywork; Massage
Bodyworkers. *See* Massage therapists and bodyworkers
Body wrap treatments, 475–481
contraindications for, 475
equipment and supplies for, 477
herbal, 481, 481*t*
muds and clays, 475–477
overview of, 475
performing, 478–481, 479–480*f*
preparing for, 477–478
table for, 478, 478*f*
Boils, 174
Bolsters, 233, 235, 235*f*
Bookkeeping, 660
systems, 660
tracking client payments, 660
Boundaries, in therapeutic relationship, 101
boundary crossing, 101
personal boundaries, 101
staying in bounds, 109–110
Boundary crossing, 101
Boundary violation, 101
Bountiful Bulge acupoint, 581*t*
Bow and arrow stance, 248
BP. *See* Blood pressure (BP)
Bracing, 256, 256*f*
Brazelton Neonatal Behavioral Assessment Scale, 158
Breast massage for breast cancer, 158
Breasts, large, 458
Breathing, in Qi gong, 609
Brochures, 640
Broken Sequence acupoint, 581*t*
Brooklyn School for Massage and Physiotherapy, 36
Bruising, 177
Brushing off to finish-back/front, 624
Burke's Gymnasium, 30–31
Burns, 174
Business cards, 639–640, 639*f*
Business ethics, 92, 667–681. *See also* Advertising
beyond graduation, 680
claims for massage therapy, 671–672
client base, 675–676
copyrights, trademarks, and patents, 672–673
defamation, 676–677
defined, 668
fees and pricing, 673
local and state regulations, 668
referrals, 675
reporting unethical behavior, 677
safety and welfare of clients, 677
selling products, 674–675
tips and gifts, 673–674
Business letter, 64, 66*f*
Business name, 637
Business plan, 648
Buttocks. *See* Hips and buttocks

C

Calories, 84, 85
CAM. *See* Complementary and alternative medicine (CAM)
Cancer, 157–158, 177–178
Candles, scented, 487

Cardiac arrhythmias, 176
Cardiovascular (CV) system, 136–138
blood circulation, 136–137, 137*f*
blood pressure, 137–138
clinical massage and, 156
disorders, 176
effects of massage on, 136–138
red blood cells, 138
venous return, 137
Cardiovascular endurance, 76–77
Cardiovascular fitness, 76–77, 77*f*, 78*f*
Career plans, 633. *See also* Employment
income goal, 636, 637
mission statement, 636, 637
practice identity, 637–640
pursuing, 633
vision, 633–637
Carotid bruit, 176
Carrier oil, 483, 484*t*
Carter, Mildred, 561
Case reports, 161
Case series, 126
Case study, 126
Cash method of accounting, 658
Cash reserve, 657
Casley-Smith, John and Judith, 540
Catchments, 544
Cautions, 173. *See also* Contraindications and cautions, principles for
CDC. *See* Disease Control and Prevention (CDC)
CDT. *See* Complete decongestive therapy (CDT)
CE. *See* Continuing education (CE)
Celestial Pillar acupoint, 581*t*
Cellular level activity, 133
Cellulitis, 174
Celsus, 32
Centered, 74
Central Treasury acupoint, 581*t*
Certified Infant Massage Instructors (CIMI®), 16
Certified Rolfer (Rolf Institute), 670
Chair massage. *See* Seated/chair massage
Chakras, 609*t*, 610–611, 610*f*, 615
Chamomile, 486*t*
Character armor, 142
Chartered Society of Trained Masseuses, 402
Chemical exfoliation, 474–475
Chest and abdomen, 367–372
abdominal massage, 139
anatomy of, 367, 367*f*
joint movements to, 300–301, 300*f*, 301*f*
massage applications for, 367–372
Chinese baths, 27
Chinese body clock, 580
Chinese herbology, 12. *See also* Herbal therapies
Chinese medicine, 3
Chinese medicine clinics, 6*t*, 8
Chiropractic adjustments, 161, 291
Chiropractic treatment, 6*t*, 7–8
Chronic obstructive pulmonary disease (COPD), 156
CIMI®. *See* Certified Infant Massage Instructors (CIMI®)
Circling the forearm, 298
Circling the lower leg, 303
Circular friction, 278, 278*f*
Circular two-handed petrissage, 275–276, 276*f*
Cisterna chyli, 541*f*, 543
Clapping, 280–281, 280*f*
Classmates, relationship with, 50
Class work, ethics in, 50

Clays. *See* Muds and clays
Cleaning supplies, for spa treatments, 467
Client, sexual misconduct by, 106
Client base, 650, 652, 675–676
Client-centered massage, 153
Client payments, tracking, 660
Client records, 655
Client safety and welfare, 677
Clinical massage therapy, 151–165
back massage for hospitalized patients, 157
for cancer patients, 157–158
cardiovascular applications, 156
case reports, 161
chiropractic adjustment, 161
client-centered massage, 153
concepts in, 153
defined, 152
evidence-based practice, 152, 152*f*
lymphatic applications, 156
musculoskeletal applications, 154–155
overview of, 152
pediatric applications, 158–159
psychological, 160
respiratory applications, 156–157
therapeutic outcomes, 153–154
Therapeutic Touch, 160–161
Clinical reasoning, 198
Club spas, 6
CMS-1500, 662–663
Cochrane Collaboration, The, 127
Cochrane Database of Systematic Reviews, The, 127
Code of Ethics (NCBTMB), 92, 93, 101, 103, 111
Codes of ethics, 94–95
Cold applications, 409–413. *See also* Cold packs
cold packs, 409
contraindications for, 409
guidelines for safe use of, 409
ice massage for elbow, 412–413
for knee, 410–412
overview of, 409
Cold packs, 3, 409
Cold showers, 403, 404
Cold stone massage, 490
Collaboration, in conflict resolution, 58
Collagen, 513
Collector vessels, 542*f*, 543
Color, 238
Colostomy bag, 460, 461*f*
Commercial health clubs, massage offered in, 6*t*, 7
Commission on Massage Therapy Accreditation (COMTA) (USDE recognized), 10–11, 10*t*, 40
Common sense, 53
Communication skills, 59–66
body language, 60–62, 61*f*
presentations, 63–64
verbal skills, 59–60
written communication, 64–66
Communication through touch, 76
Compassion, 55, 92
Complementary and alternative medicine (CAM), 4, 5, 5*f*, 37
Complete decongestive therapy (CDT), 540
Comprehension, in intellectual skills, 51, 51*t*
Compression techniques, 276–277, 277*f*
Compromise, in conflict resolution, 58
Compromised immunity, 177
COMTA. *See* Commission on Massage Therapy Accreditation (COMTA) (USDE recognized)

Concentration, 52–53
Conception Vessel (CV), 579t, 580, 582f, 583f
Confidentiality, 93, 111
Conflict resolution, 57–59
    approaches to, 58
    defined, 57–58
    major conflicts, 58
    minor conflicts, 58
    tips for successful, 58–59
Connective tissue, 130–131, 131f
Constitution types, 610
Contact, 75–76, 75f
Contact lenses, 178
Contemporary massage and bodywork. *See also individual headings*
    lymphatic facilitation (LF), 539–557
    myofascial massage, 512–525
    polarity therapy, 615, 618–625
    reflexology, 558–575
    trigger point therapy, 526–538
Continuing education (CE), 11–12, 13, 13t
Continuing session notes, 213
Continuity, 312
Contract-relax-stretch (CRS), 292, 293t
Contracts, 652–653
Contraindication
    defined, 173
    when to use, 121
Contraindications and cautions, principles for, 173–178
    acute inflammation, 173
    bleeding and bruising, 176–177
    cancer, 177–178
    cardiovascular disorders, 176
    compromised immunity, 177
    decreased sensation, 176
    edema, 177
    increased sensitivity to touch, 176
    loss of structural integrity, 173–174
    osteoporosis, 177, 178f
    personal appliances, 178
    severe distress, 173
    skin conditions, 174–176, 175f, 176f
    spreading disease by circulation, 176
Conventional medical settings, massage offered in, 6t, 7
Conventional wisdom, 124
Cook, James, 31–32
Copyrights, 672–673
Corpse pose (savasana), 614
Cottrell, Clark, 37
Countertransference, 100
Country resorts, 37
Courtesy and good manners, 56
CPT codes, 662
CPT® Committee of the American Medical Association, 18
Cradepathy, 37
Cradle, 619–620
Cranial polarization, 623
Cream, scented, 487
Credentials, 12–14, 13t, 637–638, 669–670
    board certification, 12, 13
    occupational licensing, 13–14
    school diploma, 12, 13
    specialty certifications, 12–13
Critical thinking, 51–52, 52t
Crooked Pond acupoint, 581t
Cross-arm stretch, 296
Crossed arms and legs, 61
Cross-fiber friction, 278, 278f
Crown Chakra (Sahasrar), 610f, 611

CRS. *See* Contract-relax-stretch (CRS)
Cruise ship spas, 6
Cryotherapy, 402, 402t. *See also* Hydrotherapy
    contraindications for, 409
Cupping, 280–281, 280f, 584
Curanderas, 32
Current procedural terminology (CPT) codes, 662
Currie, James, 401–402
Cypress, 486t
Cyriax, James, 279
Cyriax friction, 279

D
Dao Yin Shen Gong style, 607
Day spas, 6
De Arte Gymnastica (Mercurialis), 33
Deactivation techniques, 530–532
Deceptive advertising, 669
Decongestive therapy, 540
Decreased sensation, 176
Deep fascia, 514
Deep friction, 278, 278f
Deep transverse friction, 279
Deep vibration, 282, 282f
Defamation, 676–677
Defense mechanisms, 100–101
    defined, 100
    denial, 100
    displacement, 101
    projection, 100
    repression, 101
    resistance, 101
Defibrillators, 460
Deficiency needs related to illness and injury, in WMP, 3, 4f
Delayed gratification, 55
Delayed-onset muscle soreness (DOMS), 133
Demonstrations, 63
Denial, 100
Depressed adolescent mothers, 159
Depression, 142
Dermatitis, 174
Description of business, 648–649
    legal structure, 648, 649
    location, 648–649
Destination spas, 6
DHHS. *See* U.S. Department of Health & Human Services (DHHS)
Diabetic children, 159
Diagonal abduction, 302
Diaphragm guideline, in zone therapy, 562, 562f
Diaphragm relaxation technique, 566, 567f, 569
Diastolic pressure, 76
Diffusers, 487, 487f
Digestive system, 139, 139f
Dilutions of essential oils, in carrier oils, 483, 484t
Diplomate in Asian Bodywork Therapy (Dipl. A.B.T.–NCCAOM), 12
Direction guidelines, 261
Direct pressure
    defined, 284
    in reflexology, 565–566, 566f
    in trigger point therapy, 530–532, 531f, 532f
Direct therapeutic outcomes, 153
Disabilities. *See* Impairments and disabilities
Discharge notes, 213
Disease, spreading by circulation, 176
Disease Control and Prevention (CDC), 662

Displacement, 101
Disposables, for spa treatments, 467
Dissolving exfoliants, 474. *See also* Chemical exfoliation
Distance between people who are talking, 60–61
Documentation. *See also* SOAP notes
    importance of, 212
    legal and ethical issues in, 219
    simplified, 216, 217, 218f, 219f
    system of, designing, 217, 218, 219
DOMS. *See* Delayed-onset muscle soreness (DOMS)
Do no harm principles, 167–187
    contraindications and cautions, 173–178
    endangerment sites, 167–173, 168f
    medications, 178–182
    person-centered massage, 182–183
    resources for practitioner, 183
Dorsal fulling, 566, 566f
Dorsiflexion, 303, 304
Doshas, 609, 609t, 610, 610t, 611
Drag, 294
Drainage patterns (watersheds), 544, 545f
Draping, 256–258
    for arm massage, 258f
    defined, 256
    in full-body Swedish massage, 312
    for leg massage, 259f
    for woman's chest, 260f
Dress, 47
Drugless doctors, 36–37
Dry brushing, 469–470, 470f
Dry room sheet removal technique, 474, 474f
Dry room substance removal technique, 472
Dual relationship, 102–103
    defined, 102
    evaluating, 102–103
    "worst-case" and "best-case" exercises in, 102–103
Duran, Diego, 401
Duties, 93–94

E
Earth element, 579
Eastern bodywork. *See also individual headings*
    acupressure massage integration, 584–606
    Ayurveda, 607–611
    Ayurvedic massage, 611–614
    hatha yoga, 614
    overview of, 577
    Qi gong, 607–609
    Thai massage, 614–615
    Traditional Chinese medicine (TCM), 577–584
Edema, 155, 177
Education, scope of practice and, 110–111
Effects of massage, 121–125
    benefits, 124
    defined, 121
    holistic view of, 121, 123–124
    knowledge of, 124–125
    massage techniques and, 121
    mechanisms explaining, 144–145, 144t
    physiological, 129–140
    psychological, 141–144
    research literacy on, 125–129
    summary of, 122–123t
    time, dose and, 121
Effleurage, 3, 270–274
    basic sliding, 270–271, 270–271f
    bilateral tree stroking, 272, 272f

horizontal stroking, 273, 273f
knuckling, 273, 273f
light, with vibration, 282
Mennell's superficial stroking, 270, 270f
nerve strokes, 273
overview of, 270
sedating, of back, 354
shingles, 271, 271f
stripping, 271, 271f
three-count stroking of the trapezius, 272–273, 272f
of toes, 304
wringing, 273
Elastin, 513
Elbow
    endangerment sites, 169, 170f
    ice massage for, 412–413
    joint movements to, 298, 299f
Elbow milk-abdomen rock, 622
Elderly, 441–451
    age-appropriate elders, 442
    cautions and adaptations, 444
    frail elders, 442
    guidelines for, 443
    overview of, 441–422
    physiological age, 442
    positioning, 442–443
    practice sequence, 445–451
    robust elders, 442
    semireclining position, 444–445
Electronic vibration devices, 282
Ellison, Mary Anna, 33
Email, 64
Emollient, 471
Emotional boundaries, 49
Emotional intelligence, 53–55
    defined, 54
    handling relationships, 55
    human emotions, range of, 54f
    managing emotions, 54–55
    motivating yourself, 55
    recognizing emotions in others, 55
    self-awareness, 54
Emotional release, 141, 142–143
Emotions
    managing, 54–55
    range of, 54f
    recognizing in others, 55
Empathy, 55, 62
Empirical knowledge, 124
Employee/employer, defined by IRS, 633
Employment. *See also* Career plans
    defining, factors in, 635
    getting, 640–643
    job interviews, successful, 641–643
    part-time *vs.* full-time work, 633
    vs. self-employment, 633, 634–635, 636t
Endangerment sites, 167–173, 168f
    anterior neck, 167, 169f
    elbow and wrist, 169, 170f
    head and face, 167, 168f
    inguinal or groin area, 171, 172f
    major veins in extremities, 171, 172f
    popliteal area, 171, 172f
    safety principles around, 173
    shoulder and axilla, 169, 170f
    thoracic cage, 169
    torso, 169, 171, 171f
    vertebral column, 167, 169, 170f
End feel, 294, 294f
Endocrine system, 136
Endorsements, 670–671
Energetic boundaries, 49
Energetic effects, 145
Energetic theories, 562
Energy, in polarity therapy, 618

Energy-based bodywork, 577
Energy channels, 580, 582–583f
    ancient drawing of, 578f
    attributes of, 579t
    Chinese body clock in, 580
    defined, 580
Energy flow, 585
Energy imbalances in TMC, 584
Enjoyment of life, in WMP, 3–4, 4f
Enthusiasm, 46
Entrusting Middle acupoint, 581t
Enzymes, 474. See also Chemical exfoliation
Epsom salt, 471
Equality, 92
Equipment, 230–233
    alternatives to tables and chairs, 233
    defined, 230
    massage chairs, 231–233, 232f
    massage tables, 230–231, 230f
    portable tabletop, 230, 256, 257f
    set up and care, 233
    for spa treatments, 466
Erection during massage, 106
Esalen Institute, 38
Esalen massage, 38, 403
Essential oils, 482–487
    base oils, 483
    blending, 486–487
    care of, 484
    carrier oils, 483, 484t
    classifications of, by notes, 484, 485t
    dilutions of, in carrier oils, 483, 484t
    foundational, 484–486, 485–486t
    limbic system and, 482, 483f
    overview of, 482
    precautions for working with, 483–484
    purchasing, 484
    purposes of, 482
    using, in spa or massage therapy practice, 487
Establishment license, 14
Estimated tax payments, 659
Ethical decision making, 96–98
Ethical decision-making model, 96–98
Ethical dilemmas, 96
Ethical judgment, 98–99
Ethical questions and dilemmas, 96
Ethical standards, 17
Ethics, 91–99. See also Business ethics; Therapeutic relationship
    arousal during massage, handling, 106, 140
    boundaries, 50
    business, 92
    class work, 50
    codes and standards, 94–95
    in decision making, 96–98
    defined, 49
    in documentation, 219
    duties in, 93–94
    in judgment, development of, 98–99
    law and, 95–96
    for massage student, 49–50
    nature of, 92
    overview of, 92
    professional, 49, 92
    professionalism, 49–50
    relationship with classmates, 50
    relationship with school, 50
    rights in, 93
    unethical behavior, vulnerability to, 94
    values in, 92–93
    work, 46
Eucalyptus, 485t
Europe, reflexology in, 559

European massage, 3
Evaluation, in intellectual skills, 51, 51t
Events sports massage, 421, 422–428
    defined, 421
    interevent massage, 422
    postevent massage, 422–423
    practice sequence, 423–428
    preevent massage, 422
Evidence, levels of, 125, 126–127
Evidence-based practice (EBP), 152, 152f
Evidence funnel, 152
Exercises, 291
Exfoliation, 469–475
    chemical, 474–475
    contraindications for, 469
    dry room sheet removal technique, 474, 474f
    dry room substance removal technique, 472
    manual, 469–472
    overview of, 469
    scrub treatment, 472–474
Experimental study, 127
Explicit agreements, 99–100
Extended care facilities, 6t, 7
External validity, 128
Extremities, endangerment sites, 171, 172f
Eye contact, 61

F
Face. See Head and face
Face cradle adjustment, 254–255, 255f
Fairness, 92
Fascia, 130–131, 131f, 513–514, 514f
Fascial mobilizations, 517–518, 517f
Fascial restrictions, 513, 515
Fascial stretching, 516–517, 516f
Fascial structures, 514, 514f
Federal Trade Commission (FTC), 669, 671
Federation of State Massage Therapy Boards (FSMTB), 10t, 13, 14
Fees and pricing, 673
Feldenkrais Method®, 38
Fetal position, 430, 430f
Fibromyalgia syndrome (FMS), 154, 155f
Fibrosis, 130
FICA (Social Security and Medicare tax), 633, 659
Fidelity, 94
Fiduciary responsibility, 99
Field, Tiffany, 17, 158
Fight-or-flight response, 136
Figure-8s, 300, 300f, 304, 304f
Finances, 655–661. See also Income taxes
    banking, 660–661
    bookkeeping, 660
    first-year budget, 658–659
    startup costs, 658
Finger push-ups, 295
Fingers-to-thumb petrissage, 276, 276f
Fingerwalking, 565, 565f
Finishing techniques, 312
Fire element, 579
First impressions, 56
First trimester considerations, 432
First-year budget, 658–659
Fitness
    history of (See Sports and fitness, history of)
    settings for massage, 6–7, 6t, 7f
Fitzgerald, William, 561
501(c)(6) designation, 14

Five Elements, 578–580
    Earth, 579
    Fire, 579
    Ko cycle, 579, 580, 580f
    Metal, 579
    overview of, 578–579
    Sheng cycle, 579–580, 580f
    Water, 579
    Wood, 579
Fixed costs, 657
Flexibility
    defined, 134
    effects of massage on of joints, 134
    physical fitness and, 77–79, 78–79f
Flexion
    dorsiflexion, 303, 304
    forward, 296, 296f
    horizontal, 298
    knee to chest, 302, 302f
    lateral, 296
    plantar, 303, 304
    straight leg, 302, 302f
    of wrist, 299, 299f
Floors, 237
Flow, 55, 312
Floyer, John, 401
FMS. See Fibromyalgia syndrome (FMS)
FNIC. See Food and Nutrition Information Center (FNIC)
Foldi, Ethel, 540
Folk practices, 3
Food and Nutrition Information Center (FNIC), 84, 85
Food groups, 84, 85t
Foot
    anatomy of, 384, 385f
    joint movements to, 304–305, 304f
    reflexology, 559
Force, in conflict resolution, 58
Form 1040, 658–659
Form 1099, 659
Form SS-8, 635
Forward flexion, 296, 296f
Foundational essential oils, 484–486, 485–486t
Fractures, 174, 174f
Frail elders, 442
Franklin, Benjamin, 125
Free active movements, 291
Free passive joint movements, 291
Fresh air, 238
Friction, 3, 277–279
    circular, 278, 278f
    cross-fiber, 278, 278f
    Cyriax, 279
    deep, 278, 278f
    overview of, 277
    parallel, 278
    in rehabilitation, 279
    sawing or ulnar, 277, 278f
    superficial warming, 277, 277f
FSMTB. See Federation of State Massage Therapy Boards (FSMTB)
FTC. See Federal Trade Commission (FTC)
Full-body Swedish massage, 310–338
    continuity and flow, 312
    draping, 312
    elements of, summary of, 311t
    guidelines for, 311
    order of techniques, 312
    overview of, 311
    practice sequence, 313–335
    rhythm, pacing, specificity, and pressure, 313

sequence of body regions, 312
Fuller, Thomas, 33
Full-time work, part-time vs., 633

G
Gait analysis, 211, 211f
Galen, 32
Gallbladder acupoint, 583f
General contraindications, 173
Geranium, 486t
Gifts, 657, 673–674
Gliding Phoenix, 607f
Goal-oriented planning, 197–199
    clinical reasoning in, 198
    defined, 197–198
    steps in, 198–199
Goals of massage therapy, in WMP, 3–4, 4f
Golgi tendons, 134, 135f
Good attendance, 46
Governing Vessel (GV), 579t, 580, 582f, 583f
Graham, Douglas, 32, 33
Granger, John, 37
Gratitude, 94
Greeting first-time client, 56–57, 57f
Grooming, 48. See also Personal grooming and rejuvenation
Grounded, 74
Ground substance, 513
Growth and development, 140
Growth levels, in WMP, 3, 4f
Guarantees, 670–671
Guasha, 584
Guided imagery, 5f, 141
Gymnastique medicinale et chirurgicalein, 32
Gymnastique Medicinale (Tissot), 33

H
Hacking, 280, 280f
Half-moon stroke, 470, 470f
Half-sitting position, 431
Hammam, 27
Hand
    care, 246–247
    gestures, 61
    joint movements to, 299–300, 300f
Hand and body mechanics, 246–252
    for different techniques, 247, 248f
    hand and wrist care, 246–247
    preventing injury and overuse, 246–247
    principles of, 246
    for seated/chair massage, 251–252
    for table massage, 248–251
Hand kneading
    alternating one-handed kneading, 275, 275f
    basic two-handed kneading, 274–275, 275f
    one-handed kneading, 275, 275f
Handshake, 56–57, 57f
Hand tools, 3
Hand washing, 227–230
Hatha yoga, 614
    aspects of, 614
    in Ayurvedic health practices, 608
    reclining hand to foot pose (sputa padangushtasana), 617f
    savasana (corpse pose), 614
    in stress reduction, 141
    Sun Salutation (Surya Namaskar), 614, 616f
    wide angle pose (upavistha konasana), 617f
Head and face, 340–347
    anatomy of, 341, 342f
    bridge of nose, 343

cheekbones, 343
ears, 343
endangerment sites, 167, 168f
eyebrow area, 342
eyelids, 342
massage applications for, 341, 342–347
mouth and jaw, 343
movements and muscles, 341t
practice sequence for, 343–347
scalp, 343
Healing Yourself with Foot Reflexology (Weber), 561
Health care, history of, 31–36
in native cultures, 31–32
sobardoras, 32
timeline, 36
Western medicine, 32–35
Health care settings, 6t, 7–8, 8f
Health history, 173
Health Information Portability and Accountability Act (HIPAA). *See* HIPAA privacy rules
Health insurance billing and reimbursement, 661–663
standardized forms and billing codes, 662–663
Health maintenance, in WMP, 3, 4f
Health/medical history, 202–203
Health service operators, 31, 31f
Health Service Operators Society, 31
Hearing aids, 178
Hearing challenges, 59
Hearing impairment, 457
Heart acupoint, 582f
Heart Chakra (Anahata), 610f, 611
Heart rate (HR), 76–77
Heel to buttocks stretch, 303, 303f
Height issues, 457–458
Herbal therapies. *See also* Herbs
Abhyanga (herbal oil massage), 612
in Ayurvedic massage, 612
board certification for, 12
in CAM therapy, 4
contraindications for, 468
drugless doctors' use of, 36
infusions, 467, 475, 481
Shirodhara (pouring herbal oil over forehead), 612
showers and baths, 612
sobardoras' use of, 32
Swedana (herbal steam bath), 612
Udvartana (herbal paste and exfoliating lymphatic massage), 612
wraps, 6, 469, 475, 481
Herbs. *See also* Herbal therapies
in ancient systems of medicine, 577
in Asian bodywork therapies, 8, 577, 584
in Crown Chakra, 611
in Heart Chakra, 611
in hydrotherapy, 401
in liniments, 236
in polarity therapy, 615
in Root Chakra, 610
in Sacral Chakra, 610
in scrubs, 471
in Solar Plexus Chakra, 610
in spa treatments, 467, 481, 481t
in Third Eye Chakra, 611
in Throat Chakra, 611
Herpes simplex, 174, 175f
High blood pressure, 176
Higher-level thinking, 51–52, 52t
critical thinking, 51–52, 52t
problem solving, 52, 52t
Hip. *See* Hips and buttocks

HIPAA privacy rules, 93, 95, 111, 212, 215, 220
Hippie counterculture movement, 38
Hippocrates, 32, 401
Hips and buttocks
anatomy of, 377, 378f
joint mobilizing and stretching, 378
joint movements to, 301–302, 301f, 302f
massage applications for, 378–383
practice sequence for, 379–383
use of elbow and forearm, 378
use of fist, 378
Hispanic healers (sobardoras), 32
History of Cold Bathing to the Ancient and Modern, The (Floyer), 401
Hives, 174–175, 175f
Holistic Nursing Practice, 161
Holistic self-care plan, 86, 86f
Holistic view of effects, 121, 123–124
Home-based practices, massage offered in, 6t, 8
Home care, scope of practice and, 110–111
Home Handbook of Domestic Hygiene and Rational Medicine (Kellogg), 401
Homeostasis, 540–541
Home visit practice, 8
Home visit practices, massage offered in, 6t, 8
Honesty, 92
Hook-and-backup, 565, 566f
Horizontal flexion, 298
Horizontal stroking, 273, 273f
Horse riding stance, 248
Horse sense, 53
Hospital-based massage, 6t, 7
back massage, 157
Hot and cold packs, 3
Hot applications, 405
Hot packs, 405–408
guidelines for safe use of, 406
overview of, 405
on upper back, practice sequence for, 406–408
Hot stone massage, 489, 489f, 490f
Hot towel cabi, 466
Hot tub, 403–404
HR. *See* Heart rate (HR)
Huang Di, 577
Huang Di Nei Jing, 577
Hugs, 57
Human emotions, range of, 54f
Human meaning, 340
Human Potential Movement, 38
Humidity, 238
Hunting reaction, 409
Hydropathy, hydrotherapy *vs.,* 401–402
Hydrotherapy, 3, 401–417
cold applications, 409–413
defined, 401
facilities, 403–405
general effects of, 403, 403t
healing properties of water, 402–403
history of, 401–402
hot applications, 405 (*See also* Hot packs)
vs. hydropathy, 401–402
temperature ranges in, 403, 403t
temperature sensations in, 402, 402t
water cure, 401
Hygiene, 227
Hygienic hand washing, 227–230

Hyperextension, 299, 300, 302, 304
Hypothesis, 125

I
IAIM®. *See* International Association of Infant Massage (IAIM®)
ICD-10-CM codes, 662
Ice massage, 412–413
Ideal weight, 85–86
IJTMB. See International Journal of Therapeutic Massage & Bodywork (IJTMB)
Illness in WMP, deficiency needs related to, 3, 4f
Image detractors, 48
Immune function, 156
Immunity, 138–139
Impairments and disabilities, 456–461. *See also* Special populations
amputees and prosthesis, 459–460
colostomy bag, 460, 461f
hearing impairment, 457
height issues, 457–458
large breasts, 458
mobility challenges, 458–459
obesity, 458
pacemakers and defibrillators, 460
speech impairment, 457
visual impairment, 456–457
Impetigo, 174
Implicit agreements, 99–100
IMSTAC. *See* Integrative Massage and Somatic Therapies Accreditation Council (IMSTAC)
Inappropriate touch, 105
Income, taxable, 657, 674
Income goal, 636–637
Income taxes, 657–660. *See also* Internal Revenue Service (IRS)
accrual method, 658
cash method of accounting, 658
estimated tax payments, 659
qualified business expenses, 658
self-employment (SE) tax, 659
taxable income, 657, 673–674
tax preparation professionals, 662
tax year, 657
Increased sensitivity to touch, 176
Independent contractor, 634
Indication, 121
Indirect therapeutic outcomes, 153
Individual session planning, 200–201
Infant massage, 436–441
applications, 436
infants of depressed adolescent mothers, 159
overview of, 436
practice sequence, 437–441
for preterm infants, 158–159
Infection control, 239–240
MRSA, 240
universal precautions, 239–240
Inflammation, 129, 173
Information, collecting, 202–211
objective, 205–212
subjective, 202–205
Informed voluntary consent, 105–106
Infusions, herbal, 481
Ingham, Eunice, 37, 561
Inguinal or groin area, endangerment sites, 171, 172f
Inhalation treatments, 487
Initial/terminal (I/T) lymph vessels, 542–543, 542f, 543f
Injury in WMP, deficiency needs related to, 3, 4f
Inner Gate acupoint, 581t
Inside ankle press, 621
Instinct, 53

Insurance, 652. *See also* Health insurance billing and reimbursement
Intake interview, 203–205
body charts used in, 204
guidelines for, 204–205
multiple-choice questions used in, 204
open-ended questions used in, 203
rating scales used in, 204
skills needed for, 203
Intake notes, 213
Integrative Massage and Somatic Therapies Accreditation Council (IMSTAC), 11
Integrative medicine center, massage offered in, 6t, 7
Integrity, 92
Integumentary system, 131–132, 132f
Intellectual boundaries, 49
Intellectual skills, 50–53
concentration, 52–53
defined, 50
higher-level thinking, 51–52, 52t
levels of, 50–51, 51t
Intelligent hands, 53
Interconnections, 340
Interevent massage, 422
Internal Revenue Service (IRS). *See also* Income taxes
employee/employer defined by, 633
501(c)(6), 14
Form 1040, 658–659
Form 1099, 659
Form SS-8, 635
information booklets, 657, 658
Schedule C, 659
Schedule SE, 659
W-2 forms, 658–659
Internal validity, 128
International Association of Infant Massage (IAIM®), 16
International Classification of Disease, 10th Revision, Clinical Modification (ICD-10-CM), 662
International Council of Reflexologists, 563
International Journal of Therapeutic Massage & Bodywork (IJTMB), 17, 127, 161
Interstitial matrix, 542, 542f
Interstitial space, 542
Intervention model, 106–107
Interviews. *See* Job interviews
Introductions, 57
Intuition, 53
IRS. *See* Internal Revenue Service (IRS)
Ischemia, 141
Ischemic compression, 284, 284f, 530

J
Jitsu, 583, 584f
Job interviews, 641–643
after the interview, 643
illegal interview questions, 642–643
questions to ask during, 641–642
Joint manipulations or adjustments, 291
Joint mobilizing and stretching techniques. *See* Joint movement techniques
Joint movements, 290–309, 295
ankle, 303–304, 303f
at-a-glance, 305t
categories of, 291

Joint movements (*continued*)
cautions and contraindications, 294–295
chest, 300–301, 300*f*, 301*f*
comparing techniques, 291*t*
elbow, 298, 299*f*
foot, 304–305, 304*f*
guidelines for, general, 295
hand, 299–300, 300*f*
hip, 301–302, 301*f*, 302*f*
knee, 303, 303*f*
manipulations or adjustments, 291
mobility and flexibility, 134
mobilizing, 291, 291*t*
neck, 295–296, 296*f*
overview of, 291–292
in reflexology, 566
safety in, 292–295
shoulder girdle, 297–298, 297–298*f*
stretching, 291–292, 291*t*, 293*t*
stretching methods, 292, 293*t*
synovial joints and, 292, 293*t*
wrist, 299, 299*f*
Joint movement techniques, 291–305.
    See also Stretching
ankle, 303–304
chest, 300–301
comparison of, 291*t*
elbow, 298
foot, 304–305
guidelines for, 295
hand, 299–300
hips and buttocks, 301–302, 378
knee, 303
neck, 295–296
shoulder girdle, 297–298
stretching methods, 292, 293*t*
wrist, 299
Jojoba, 236
Jostling, 283, 283*f*
Journal of Bodywork and Movement Therapies, The, 17
Juhan, Deane, 110
Jumping Round acupoint, 581*t*
Jump sign, 530

K
Kapha, 610, 610*t*
Kellogg, J. Harvey, 37, 401
Kidneys
acupoint, 582*f*
as endangerment site, 171
tapotement over, 171, 171*f*
Knee
cold applications for, 410–412
joint movements to, 303, 303*f*
Knee to chest flexion, 302, 302*f*
Kneipp, Sebastian, 401
Knowledge, in intellectual skills, 51, 51*t*
Knowledge of effects, 124–125
Knuckling effleurage, 273, 273*f*
Ko cycle, 579, 580, 580*f*
Koshas, 609–611, 609*f*, 609*t*
innermost, 611
physical body, 609–610
pranamaya, 609*f*, 610
subtle energy, 610
Krieger, Dolores, 160–161
Kunlun Mountain acupoint, 581*t*
Kyo, 583, 584*f*

L
Labor, delivery, and recovery, 435
Large breasts, 458
Large intestine acupoint, 582*f*
Latent TrPs, 527, 527*t*
Lateral flexion, 296
Lateral pelvis/hip, in reflexology sessions, 569

Lavender, 486*t*
Law, ethics and, 95–96
Legal issues in documentation, 219
Legal structure of business, 648, 649
Leg pull, 620
Leg toss, 303
Length of sessions, 258
LF. *See* Lymphatic facilitation (LF)
Libel, 676
Licensed Massage Therapist (LMT), 670
Licenses and insurance, 652
Lief, Stanley, 527
Ligaments, 130, 131*f*
Light effleurage with vibration, 282
Lighting, 238
Limbic structures of brain, 53–54
Limbic system
effects of massage on, 143–144
essential oils and, 482, 483*f*
Linens, for spa treatments, 467
Ling, Pehr Henrik, 28, 33–35
Liniments, 236
Listening, 62–63
active, 62–63
affirmative, 62
defined, 62
Liver acupoint, 583*f*
LMT. *See* Licensed Massage Therapist (LMT)
Local contraindications, 173
Local regulations, 668
Local twitch response, 530
Logo, 637
Longitudinal tendon guideline, in zone therapy, 562, 562*f*
Long stroke, 546–547, 547*f*
Long-term effects, 121
Long-term planning, 199–200
Loss of structural integrity, 173–174
Lotions
scented, 487
uses of, 236
Love, in polarity therapy, 618
Low blood pressure, 176
Lower body regions, 376–399, 377
hips and buttocks, 377–383
lower extremities, 383–396
Lower extremities
anatomy of, 383–385
cautions, 385
enhancing mobility, 386–396
feet, 384, 385*f*
lower leg, 383, 384*f*
massage applications for, 386–396
thigh and lower leg, 383, 384*f*, 386–392
Lower leg, 383, 384*f*, 386–392
L stroke, 546, 546*f*
Lubricating substances, 3
amount to use, 260–261
Lung acupoint, 582*f*
Lust, Benedict, 37
Lymph, 541
Lymphangion, 543
Lymphangitis (blood poisoning), 176
Lymphatic drainage on dorsum with ankle rotation, in reflexology sessions, 569
Lymphatic facilitation (LF), 3, 539–557. *See also* Lymphatic system
applications, 547–553
contraindications for, 544–545
indications for, 544
integration of, into massage session, 553
manual lymphatic drainage compared to, 540
overview of, 540

practice sequence for lower extremity, 547–550
stroke in, 545–547, 546*f*, 547*f*
Lymphatic massage, history of, 540
Lymphatic system, 138–139, 138*f*, 540–545. *See also* Lymphatic facilitation (LF)
clinical massage and, 156
drainage patterns in (watersheds), 544, 545*f*
homeostasis, 540–541
immunity, 138–139
immunity and, 138–139
interstitial matrix, 542, 542*f*
lymph, 541
lymph fluid movement, 138, 138*f*
lymph nodes, 541*f*, 544, 544*f*
overview of, 540, 541*f*
Lymphatic system vessels, 542–544, 542*f*
cisterna chyli, 541*f*, 543
collector vessels, 543
initial/terminal (I/T) lymph vessels, 542–543, 543*f*
terminus, 543–544
transport vessels, 542*f*, 543
Lymphedema, 155, 540
Lymph fluid movement, 138, 138*f*
Lymph nodes, 541, 541*f*, 544, 544*f*

M
Macfadden, Bernarr, 37, 527
Machines that mimic massage techniques, 3
Maintenance schedule, 237–238, 239
Maintenance sports massage, 421, 422
Major conflicts, in conflict resolution, 58
Major veins in extremities, endangerment sites, 171, 172*f*
Management, 651–655
appointments, 654–655
client records, 655
contracts, 652–653
licenses and insurance, 652
massage practice office space, 654
practice policies, 653
Manipulators, 33
Manipura (Solar Plexus Chakra), 610, 610*f*
Manners, 56
Manomaya, 609*f*, 611
Manual exfoliation, 469–472
body polishes in, 471–472, 471*f*
dry brushing in, 469–470, 470*f*
half-moon stroke used in, 470, 470*f*
scrubs in, 470–471, 471*f*
tools for, 467
Manual for Students of Massage, A (Ellison), 33
Manual lymphatic drainage (MLD), 138, 156, 540. *See also* Lymphatic facilitation (LF)
Vodder Method®, 540
Manual therapeutics, 3, 33
Marjoram, 486*t*
Marketing, 649–651
advertising and promotions, 651–652
client base, building, 650, 652
defined, 649
market research, 650
Market research, 650
Marma point massage, 614
Marma points, 611, 612*f*
Massage
defined, 3
effects of (*See* Effects of massage)
origin of word, 33

physical side of (*See* Physical skills)
Swedish, 3
Massage as a vocation, history of, 25–44
health care, 31–36
massage therapists and bodyworkers, 38–40
natural healing and drugless doctors, 36–37
in natural healing tradition, 36–37
personal grooming and rejuvenation, 26–29
sports and fitness, 29–31
in United States, 37–38
Massage & Bodywork (ABMP), 17
Massage & Bodywork Licensing Examination (MBLEx), 13
Massage chair, 231–233, 232*f*
adjustments, 499–500
history of first, 497
Massage establishment ordinances, 668
Massage guidelines, 258
amount of lubricant, 260–261
length of sessions, 258
pacing, 262
pressure, 262
rhythm, 262
sequence of techniques and routines, 261
specifity and direction, 261
summary of, 263*t*
Massage magazine, 17
Massage oils
in Ayurvedic massage, 613
essential, in aromatherapy, 482–487
scented, 487
for stone massage, 489
uses of, 236
Massage operator, 29
Massage Operator, The (Puderbach), 36
Massage tables, 230–231, 230*f*
alternatives to, 233
checklist for choosing, 231–232*t*
portable, 230, 234*f*
Massage therapists and bodyworkers, 38–40. *See also* Massage therapy profession
physical therapists compared to, 35
sexual misconduct by, 104–106
Massage therapy
claims for, 671–672
in complementary and alternative medicine, 4
defined, 3
goals of, in WMP, 3–4, 4*f*
intimacy in, 99
modern, timeline of, 39*f*
origin of term, 39
professionalism in (*See* Professionalism in massage therapy)
professionalizing, 9 (*See also* Massage therapy profession)
public acceptance of, 17–18
research in, 17
revived in United States, 37–38
trends in, 4–5
unified profession of, 40
as wellness profession, 4
Massage Therapy Foundation (MTF), 10*t*, 17, 40, 127, 161
Massage Therapy Journal (AMTA), 17
Massage therapy office or clinic, 6*t*, 8
Massage therapy profession
becoming, 8–10
benchmarks of, 8–9, 10

body of knowledge and skills that defines, 10
credentials in, 12–14, 13*t*
education in, 10–12
ethical standards in, 9, 17
organizations in, 9, 10*t,* 14–16
publications in, 16–17
recognition of, from other professionals, 17–18
scholarship in, 16–17
stereotypes of, 17
work settings for, 6–8
Massage Today, 17
Masseurs/masseuses
hints for, 34*f*
history of, 28, 28*f,* 33
Massotherapy, 33
MBLEx. *See* Massage & Bodywork Licensing Examination (MBLEx)
McKenzie, R. Tait, 30
Mechanical effects, 144
Mechanisms of massage, 144–145, 144*t*
energetic effects, 145
mechanical effects, 144
mind-body effects, 144, 145
physiological effects, 144
reflex effects, 144
Medial pelvis/hip, in reflexology sessions, 569
Medical gymnast, 28, 33–35, 35*f*
Medical reasons for massage, 3, 5
Medical Reports on the Effects of Water, Both Warm and Cold, as a Remedy in Fevers and Other Diseases (Currie), 402
Medical rubbing, 32–33
Medical spas, 6
Medical terminology, 189–197
abbreviations and symbols, 195, 195–197*t*
prefixes, 189, 189–191*t*
singular and plural endings, 191, 195, 195*t*
suffixes, 191, 193–195*t*
word roots/combining forms, 191, 192–193*t*
Medications, 178–182
guidelines for, 178, 179
pharmacology, 178, 179–182*t*
spa applications and, 468
Medicina Gymnastica (Fuller), 33
Medieval Europe, public baths in, 27
Meditation, 81–82, 81*f*
Melting, 515
Member services organizations, 15
Memos, 64, 65*f*
Mennell's superficial stroking, 270, 270*f*
Mental clarity, 142
Mercurialis, 33
Meta-analysis, 127
Metal element, 579
Mezger, Johann, 33, 35
Mind-body effects, 144, 145
Mineral water hospitals, 402
Minor conflicts, in conflict resolution, 58
Mission statement, 636, 637
Mitchell, Weir, 33
MLD. *See* Manual lymphatic drainage (MLD)
Mobility
challenges, 458–459, 459*f*
of joints, 134
restrictions, 386
Mobilizing techniques, 295
Modern professional reflexology, 561
Moles, 176, 176*f*
Moor mud, 476–477, 477*f*

Mothers with infants and toddlers, 436
Moxibustion, 584
MRSA (methicillin-resistant staphylococcus aureus), 240
MTF. *See* Massage Therapy Foundation (MTF)
Muds and clays, 475–477
differentiating, 475
examples of, 476*t*
Moor mud, 476–477, 477*f*
peat, 476
seaweed and sea mud, 477
therapeutic effects of, 475–476
Muladhara (Root Chakra), 610, 610*f*
Multiple-choice questions, 204
Multiple-dose effects, 121
Multitasking, 53
Muscle approximation, 134
Muscle relaxation, 133–134, 133*f*
Muscle spindles, 134, 134*f*
Muscular strength and endurance, 77
Muscular system, 132–135
applications, 154–155
cellular level activity, 133
clinical massage and, 154–155
fibromyalgia syndrome, 154, 155*f*
Golgi tendons, 134, 135*f*
increased joint mobility and flexibility, 134
joint mobility and flexibility, 134
muscle relaxation, 133–134, 133*f*
muscle spindles, 134, 134*f*
posture, 135
Music, 238
Music therapy, 4, 5*f,* 123
Myofascial massage, 3, 512–525
contraindications for, 515–516
fascia and, 513–514, 513*f*
fascial restrictions, 513, 515
fascial structures and, 514, 514*f*
guidelines for, 515–516
history of, 513
overview of, 513
trigger points, 141
Myofascial massage techniques, 516–518
back, 518–521
fascial mobilizations, 517–518, 517*f*
fascial stretching, 516–517, 516*f*
resting after, 518, 518*f*
skin lifting, 516, 516*f*
Myofascial Pain and Dysfunction: The Trigger Point Manual (Travell and Simons), 527
Myofascial trigger points, 141
Myotherapy (Prudden), 527
MyPlate, 84, 84*f,* 86
My Water Cure (Kneipp), 401

N

NACCAS. *See* National Accrediting Commission of Cosmetology Arts and Sciences (NACCAS)
Nanamaya, 609*f,* 611
NATA. *See* National Athletic Training Association (NATA)
National Accrediting Commission of Cosmetology Arts and Sciences (NACCAS), 11
National Association for Holistic Therapy, 481
National Athletic Training Association (NATA), 30
National Certification Board for Therapeutic Massage and Bodywork (NCBTMB), 10*t,* 12, 39, 670
Code of Ethics, 92, 93, 101, 103, 111
Standards of Practice, 104, 105, 106

National Certification Commission for Acupuncture and Oriental Medicine (NCCAOM), 12, 584
National Certification Examination for Therapeutic Massage and Bodywork, 39–40
National Commission for Certifying Agencies (NCCA), 12
National Health Interview Survey, 5
National Institutes of Health (NIH), 18, 40, 80, 127, 563
Native practices, 3
Natural healing, history of, 36–37
complementary and alternative medicine in, 37
massage in, 36–37
timeline, 37
Natural healing centers, 37
Nature of ethics, 92
Naturopath, The, 36
Naturopathic clinics, 6*t,* 8
Naturopathic medicine, 4
Naturopathic offices, 7, 8
Naturopathic physician, 8, 36, 677
Naturopathic Society of America, 36
Naturopaths, 36–37
Navel-third eye, 623
NCBTMB. *See* National Certification Board for Therapeutic Massage and Bodywork (NCBTMB)
NCBTMB Code of Ethics, 92, 93, 101, 103, 111
NCBTMB Standards of Practice, 104, 105, 106
NCCA. *See* National Commission for Certifying Agencies (NCCA)
NCCAOM. *See* National Certification Commission for Acupuncture and Oriental Medicine (NCCAOM)
Neck, 347–352
alignment, 585
anatomy of, 347–348, 348–349*f*
joint movements to, 295–296, 296*f*
massage applications for, 348, 349–352
in reflexology sessions, 569
stretch, 620
Neck-head-face, AMI for, 585–586, 586*f,* 599–606
Neck/shoulder guideline, in zone therapy, 562, 562*f*
Negative transference, 100
Neocortex, 53–54
Nerve strokes, 273
Nervous system, 135–136
Neural-gating mechanism, 141
Neuromuscular therapy (NMT), 527
Neutral position of wrist, 247, 248*f*
Neutral zone, in WMP, 3, 4*f*
Neutrotherapy, 402, 402*t. See also* Hydrotherapy
NH-PA. *See* Nurse Healers-Professional Associates (NH-PA)
NIH. *See* National Institutes of Health (NIH)
NMT. *See* Neuromuscular therapy (NMT)
Nondiscrimination, 92
Nonmaleficence, 94
Nonprofit community centers, massage offered in, 6*t,* 7
Nonspecific movements, 291
Notes, essential oils classified by, 484, 485*t*
Nuad boran. *See* Thai massage
Nurse Healers-Professional Associates (NH-PA), 161
Nursing mothers, 436
Nutrients, 84

Nutrition, 84–86
calories, 84, 85
defined, 84
food groups, 84, 85*t*
ideal weight, 85–86
MyPlate, 84, 84*f,* 86
nutrients, 84

O

Obesity, 458
Objective information, 205–212
biomechanical analysis, 210–211
gait analysis, 211, 211*f,* 212*t*
general observations, 205
observations, general, 205
orthopedic tests, 211
palpation, 205–206
posture analysis, 208–210, 210*f*
range of motion evaluation, 206–208, 207–208*f*
Observations, general, 205
Occipital press, 623
Occipital ridge, in reflexology sessions, 569
Occupational licensing, 13–14, 13*t,* 14*f,* 668
Office of Alternative Medicine, 40
Office of Civil Rights (OCR), 111
Office space for massage practice, 654
One-handed kneading, 275, 275*f*
On-site chair massage, 6*t,* 8
On-site massage, 8, 497
Open-ended questions, 203
Opening technique, 312
Organism level, 140–141
growth and development, 140
pain reduction, 140–141
stress reduction, 141
summary of, 123*t*
Organizations, 14–16
guide to, 10*t*
importance of, 9
member services organizations, 15
professional associations, 14–15
specialty associations, 16
Organ system level, 131–140
cardiovascular system, 136–138
digestive system, 139
endocrine system, 136
integumentary system, 131–132
lymphatic system and immunity, 138–139
muscular system, 132–135
nervous system, 135–136
reproductive system, 140
respiratory system, 139
skeletal system, 132
summary of, 122*t*
urinary system, 139
Organ systems, 131–140
cardiovascular system, 136–138
digestive system, 139, 139*f*
endocrine system, 136
integumentary system, 131–132, 132*f*
lymphatic system, 138–139, 138*f*
muscular system, 132–135
nervous system, 135–136
reproductive system, 140
respiratory system, 139
skeletal system, 132, 133*f*
urinary system, 139
Origin and insertion technique, 134
Orthopedic tests, 211
Osteoporosis, 177, 178*f*
Outcomes, 153–154
Outer Gate acupoint, 581*t*
Outside ankle press, 621
Overactivity, 133
Overhead stretch, 298, 299, 301

P

Pacemakers, 460
Pacing
   in full-body Swedish massage, 313
   guidelines, 262
Paidotribes, 29
Pain
   reduction, 140–141
   during reflexology, 563–564
Pain Erasure (Prudden), 527
Palliative care, 153, 451
Palmer, David, 497
Palpation, 76, 205–206
   skills, 292, 294
   in trigger point therapy, 530
Palpatory sensitivity, 378
Parallel friction, 278
Part-time *vs.* full-time work, 633
Passive movements, 291
Passive shoulder roll, 297
Passive stretching, 130, 133*f*
Passive touch, 283, 283*f*
Patents, 672–673
Peaceful abiding, 82
Peat, 476
Pediatric applications, 158–159. *See also* Infant massage
   additional, 159
   preterm infants, 158–159
Peer-reviewed journals, 127
Pelvic guideline, in zone therapy, 562, 562*f*
Pelvic rock, 622
Pelvis and knee rock, 621
Peppermint, 485*t*
Percussion. *See* Tapotement
Pericardium acupoint, 583*f*
Perpendicularity, 585
Personal appliances, 178
Personal boundary, 101
Personal care settings, 6, 6*f*, 6*t*
Personal grooming and rejuvenation, 26–29
   in ancient civilizations, 26–28
   public baths, 27–28
   salons and spas, 28–29
   shampooing, 26
   timeline, 29
Personal hygiene, 227. *See also* Personal grooming and rejuvenation
Personal temptations, 96
Person-centered massage, 182–183
Persuasion, 64
Petrissage, 3, 274–277
   alternating one-handed kneading, 275, 275*f*
   basic two-handed kneading, 274–275, 275*f*
   circular two-handed, 275–276, 276*f*
   compression techniques, 276–277, 277*f*
   fingers-to-thumb, 276, 276*f*
   one-handed kneading, 275, 275*f*
   overview of, 274
   rolling, 277, 277*f*
   skin lifting, 276, 276*f*
Pet therapy, 5*f*
Pharmacology, 178, 179–182*t*
Phlebitis, 173
Physcultopathists, 37
Physical body kosha, 609–610
   Kapha, 610
   Pitta, 609
   Vata, 609
Physical boundaries, 49
Physical culture, 37
Physical Culture Training School, 37

Physical environment for massage, 237–239
   color, 238
   floors, 237
   fresh air, 238
   humidity, 238
   lighting, 238
   maintenance schedule, 237–238, 239
   music, 238
   room setup, 237
   safety, 238–239
   sound, 238
   temperature, 238
   walls, 237
   windows, 237
Physical fitness, 76–80. *See also* Self-care
   body composition, 80
   cardiovascular fitness, 76–77, 77*f*, 78*f*
   flexibility, 77–79, 78–79*f*
   muscular strength and endurance, 77
   profile, 76, 77*f*
Physical impairments, 456. *See also* Impairments and disabilities
Physical skills, 74–76. *See also* Physical fitness
   body awareness, 74–75
   skilled touch, 75–76
Physical therapists
   history of, 35
   licensing for, 35
Physical therapy, history of, 35
Physiological age, 442
Physiological effects of massage, 129–140. *See also individual levels*
   defined, 144
   organism level, 140–141
   organ system level, 131–140
   tissue level, 129–131
Pilates, 81, 81*f*
Pillows, 235, 235*f*
Pilot studies, 125
Pincement, 281, 281*f*
Pincer technique, 530, 531, 532*f*
Pitta, 609, 610*t*
Pity, 55
Place of service codes, 662
Planning, 197. *See also* Documentation
   goal-oriented, 197–199
   importance of, 197
   individual session, 200–201
   information for, collecting, 202–211
   long-term, 199–200
   treatment, 201
Plan of care, 106
Plantar flexion, 303, 304
Plutarch, 26
PNI. *See* Psychoneuroimmunology (PNI)
Polarity movements, 619–625
   arm-shoulder rotations, 622
   brushing off to finish-back/front, 624
   cradle, 619–620
   cranial polarization, 623
   elbow milk-abdomen rock, 622
   inside ankle press, 621
   leg pull, 620
   navel-third eye, 623
   neck stretch, 620
   occipital press, 623
   outside ankle press, 621
   pelvic rock, 622
   pelvis and knee rock, 621
   practice sequence, 625
   preliminary instructions, 619

   thumb web-forearm stimulation, 622
   tummy rock, 620
Polarity therapy, 3, 615, 618–625
   defined, 615
   energy in, 618
   love in, 618
   overview of, 615
   principles of, 618–619
   removing obstructions in, 618
   techniques (*See* Polarity movements)
   theory, 615
   understanding in, 619
Poor speech habits, 59
Popliteal area, endangerment sites, 171, 172*f*
Portable massage tables, 230, 234*f*
Positioning, 254–256
   defined, 254
   for elderly, 442–443
   face cradle adjustment, 254–255, 255*f*
   pregnant women, 430–431
   prone, 254, 254*f*
   in reflexology, 564, 564*f*
   seated, 256, 256*f*, 257*f*
   for seated massage, 499–500
   semireclining, 256, 256*f*
   side-lying, 255, 256*f*
   supine, 254, 254*f*
Positive attitude, 46
Positive transference, 100
Postevent massage, 422–423
Posttraumatic stress disorder, children with, 159
Posture, 48, 60, 135
Posture analysis, 208–210, 210*f*
Post-White, Janice, 158
Power differential, 99
Practice identity, 637–640
   brochures and websites, 640
   business cards and stationery, 639–640, 639*f*
   business name and logo, 637
   credentials, 637–638
   defined, 637
   résumé, 638–639, 638*f*
Practice policies, 653
Pranamaya, 609*f*, 610
Preevent massage, 422
Pregnant women, 429–436
   cautions and adaptations, 431–432
   contraindications for, 429–430
   environment for massage, 430
   fetal position, 430, 430*f*
   labor, delivery, and recovery, 435
   positioning options, 430–431
   practice sequence, 433–435
   table height, 431
   trimester considerations, 432
Prelymphatic channel, 542
Preparation for massage therapy, 227–244
   equipment, 230–233
   hand washing, 227–230
   infection control, 239–240
   introduction to, 227
   personal hygiene, 227
   physical environment for massage, 237–239
   supplies, 233, 235–236
   topical substances, 236–237
Prescriptions (Rx), 110–111
Presentations, 63–64
Press-and-flex, 565, 566*f*
Pressure
   in full-body Swedish massage, 313
   guidelines, 262
Preterm infants, 158–159

Prices and bait advertising, 671
Pricing, 673
Priessnitz, 401
Primary TrPs, 527, 527*t*
Principle-based therapy, 153
Privacy, right to, 93
Private practice, 647–666. *See also* Business ethics; individual headings
   business plan overview, 648
   defined, 648
   description of business, 648–649
   employment in, 633, 634–635, 636*t*
   finances, 655–661
   health insurance billing and reimbursement, 661–663
   management, 651–655
   marketing, 649–651
   settings, 6*t*, 8, 8*f*
Problem solving, 52, 52*t*
Professional associations, 14–15
Professional boundaries, 48–49, 50
Professional ethics, 92
Professional image, 46–48
   in advertising, 669–670
   dress, 47
   grooming, 48
   image detractors, 48
   posture, 48
Professionalism in massage therapy, 46–72
   communication skills in, 59–66
   emotional intelligence in, 53–55
   ethics for massage student, 49–50
   intellectual skills, 50–53
   intuition in, 53
   of massage student, 49–50
   professional boundaries in, 48–49
   professional image in, 46–48
   service in, 46
   social skills in, 55–59
   work ethic in, 46
Progressive relaxation, 5*f*, 141
Progress notes, 213
Projection, 100
Promotions, 651–652
Pronation, 298, 303
Prone position, 254, 254*f*
Prosthesis, amputees and, 459–460
Prudden, Bonnie, 527
Psoriasis, 176, 176*f*
Psychological clinical applications, 160
Psychological effects of massage, 141–144
   anxiety and depression, reduced, 142
   character armor, 142
   emotional release, 142–143
   limbic system, 143–144
   mental clarity, 142
   summary of, 123*t*
   well-being, feelings of, 143
Psychological factors, in therapeutic relationship, 100
Psychoneuroimmunology (PNI), 144, 145
Public baths, 27–28
   Chinese, 27
   Medieval Europe, 27
   Roman, 27
   Turkish, 27
PubMed, 127, 563
Puderbach, P., 36–37

Q

Qi, 81, 578
Qi deficiency (Kyo), 583, 584*f*
Qi excess (Jitsu), 583, 584*f*
Qi gong, 81, 607–609

breathing in, 609
forms of, 607
Gliding Phoenix, 607f
meaning of, 607
Spring for the Crane and Deer, 606f
Quacking, 281, 281f
Qualified business expenses, 658
Qualifying statements, 672
Qualities of touch, 76
Quiet sitting, 82

R

Randomized control trial (RCT), 125, 127
Range of motion (ROM)
active, 208, 209f
evaluation, 206–208, 207–208f
Rapping, 280, 280f
Rashes, 174
Rating scales, 204
Rational Hydrotherapy (Kellogg), 401
RBCs. *See* Red blood cells (RBCs)
RCT. *See* Randomized control trial (RCT)
Recipe-based massage, 153
Reciprocal inhibition, 292, 293t
Reclining hand to foot pose (sputa padangushtasana), 617f
Reconstruction aides, 35
Recovery sports massage, 421, 422
Recreation
activities, 82
settings for massage, 6–7, 6t, 7f
Red blood cells (RBCs), 138
Reducing massage, 28
Reference zones, in trigger point therapy, 528–529, 529f
Referrals, 675
Reflex effects, 144
Reflexology, 3, 558–575
in America, 561
ancient roots of, 559
body mechanics in, 564
chart, 559, 560f
in Europe, 559
foot, 559
history of, 559–561
modern professional, 561
overview of, 559
positioning in, 564, 564f
research and application, 563
sessions during and after, 563–564, 567–571
tenderness and pain during, 563–564
theories about, 562–563
zone therapy and guidelines, 561–562
Reflexology session
during and after, 563–564
bidirectional thumb pressure on plantar surface, 569
diaphragm, 569
ending, 571
lateral pelvis/hip, 569
lymphatic drainage on dorsum with ankle rotation, 569
medial pelvis/hip, 569
neck and occipital ridge, 569
preliminary instructions, 568
spinal reflex, 569
spinal twist, 568
toe rotations, 569
warm-up, 568
Reflexology techniques, 564–567
adjuncts to, 567
diaphragm relaxation technique, 566, 567f

direct pressure and friction, 565–566, 566f
dorsal fulling, 566, 566f
hook-and-backup, 565, 566f
joint movements, 566
press-and-flex, 565, 566f
walk and roll, 565, 565f
Regeneration, 129
Regional massage
defined, 340
human meaning in, 340
interconnections in, 340
lower body, 376–399 (*See also* Lower body regions)
regional practice sequences, overview of, 340
upper body, 339–375 (*See also* Upper body regions)
Registered Massage Therapist (RMT), 38, 670
Regulations, local and state, 668
Rehabilitation
facilities, 6t, 7
friction in, 279
massage, 421, 422
Reich, Wilhelm, 142
Reiki, 5f, 145, 206
Rejuvenation. *See* Personal grooming and rejuvenation
Relationships
with classmates, 50
interpersonal, handling, 55
with school, 50
therapeutic, 55
Relaxation response, 141
Relaxation training, 5f
Reliability, 46
Remedial sports massage, 421, 422
Remodeling, 129
Removing obstructions, 618
Reparations, 94
Repetitive strain injuries (RSIs), 498
Repression, 101
Reproductive system, 140
Research
basic, 124
overview of, 124–125
terminology, 126t
Research Analysis Document, 563
Research literacy, 125–129
defined, 125
evidence in, levels of, 125, 126–127
research reports, reading, 127–129, 128t
research studies, locating, 127
scientific method, 125
Research report
evaluation worksheet, 128t
reading, 127–129
sections of, 128t
Research studies, locating, 127
Resistance, 101
Resisted movements, 291
Resort and hotel spas, 6
Resources for practitioner, 183
Respiratory system, 139
clinical massage and, 156–157
complications, tapotement for, 156
Responsibilities, 93–94
Rest Cure, 33
Resting heart rate (RHR), 76–77
Résumé, 638–639
building, 639
design, 639
elements of, 638–639
sample, 638f
Retinaculae, 514
Rheumatoid arthritis, 173
RHR. *See* Resting heart rate (RHR)

Rhythm, in full-body Swedish massage, 313
Rhythm guidelines, 262
Rights, 93
Riley, Shelby, 561
Ringworm, 174, 175f
RMT. *See* Registered Massage Therapist (RMT)
Robust elders, 442
Rocking, 300–301, 300–301f
Roles, in therapeutic relationship, 101
Rolfing®, 38
Rolf Institute® of Structural Integration, 16, 670
Rolling, 277, 277f, 565
Roman baths, 27, 27f
Room setup, 237
Root Chakra (Muladhara), 610, 610f
Rosemary, 486t
Rotation, 296
Royal Gymnastic Central Institute, 34
RSIs. *See* Repetitive strain injuries (RSIs)
Rubbers, 29–30

S

Sacral Chakra (Svadhisthana), 610, 610f
Safety, 238–239
and of clients, 677
in joint movement techniques, 292–295
in physical environment for massage, 238–239
right to, 93
Sahasrar (Crown Chakra), 610f, 611
Salary draw, 657
Salons and spas, history of, 28–29
Salt, 470–471
Sama, 610
Sanitation
defined, 227
topical substances and, 237
Sanitation, in spa treatments, 467
Satellite TrPs, 527
Sauna, 3, 404
Savasana (corpse pose), 614, 615f
Sawing friction, 277, 278f
Scapula mobilizing, 297
Schedule C, 659
Schedule SE, 659
School, relationship with, 50
School diploma, 12, 13, 13t
School of Health Service and Massage, 31
Schools, relationships in, 107–108
Scientific method, 125
Scissoring, 300, 300f, 304
Scope of practice, 108–111
defined, 108–109
education and home care, 110–111
prescriptions, 110–111
staying in bounds, 109–110
Screening interview, 498–499
Scrubs, in aroma therapy, 487
Scrub treatment, 472–474
dry room sheet removal techniques, 474
performing, 473–474, 473f, 474f
preparing for, 472
Sea mud, 477
Seated/chair massage, 496–509
benefits of, 497–498
body and hand mechanics used in, 498
in different venues, preparing for, 505–506
hand and body mechanics for, 251–252
history of, 497

on-site, 497
overview of, 497
popularity of, 498
positioning for, 256, 499–500
practice sequence, 501–505
in public places and events, 497
for repetitive strain injuries, 498
screening for, 498–499
sessions, 500
in workplace wellness programs, 498
Seated position, 256, 256f, 257f, 431, 442, 442f
Seaweed, 477
Secondary TrPs, 527
Second trimester considerations, 432
Sedating effleurage, of back, 354
Self-awareness, 54
Self-care, 80–86
body–mind practices, 80–82
defined, 80
holistic, 86, 86f
nutrition, 84–86
stress-control strategies, 82
of terminally ill, 456
time management, 82–84, 83f
Self-determination, right to, 93
Self-efficacy, 55
Self-employed, 633, 634–635, 636t
Self-employment (SE) tax, 659
Self-employment settings, 6t, 8, 8f
Selfless service, 92
Self-regulation, 95
Selling products, 674–675
Semireclining position, 256, 256f, 431, 444–445
Sen lines, 615, 617f
Sensation, decreased, 176
Sensitivity to touch, increased, 176
Sequence of techniques and routines, 261
Service, 46
Sessions, length of, 258
SE tax. *See* Self-employment (SE) tax
Severe distress, 173
Sexual boundaries, 49
Sexual misconduct, 104–107
appropriate touch, 105
categories of, 104
by client, 106
common forms of, 105
defined, 104
degree of severity of, 105
illegal forms of, 106
informed voluntary consent, 105–106
intervention model, 106–107
by massage therapist, 104–106
Sexual relationships, 103–104
Shaking, 282, 283f, 297
Sham treatment, 125
Shared knowledge, 10
Sheets, 235–236, 235f
Sheng cycle, 579–580, 580f
Shiatsu, 8, 38, 40, 140, 583
Shingles effleurage, 271, 271f
Shirodhara (pouring herbal oil over forehead), 612
Short-term effects, 121
Shoulder
endangerment sites, 169, 170f
joint movements to, 297–298, 297–298f
Shoulder Bone acupoint, 581t
Shoulder Well acupoint, 581t
Showers, 404
Side-lying position, 255, 256f, 431, 431f
Side-to-side mobilizing, 304

Signature massage, 313
Simons, David, 527
Simple mobilizing movements, 295
Simple static stretch, 292, 293*t*
Simplified documentation, 216, 217, 218*f*
Single-dose effects, 121
Single-tasking, 53
Skeletal system, 132, 133*f*, 154–155. *See also* Joint movements
Skilled nursing facilities, 6*t*, 7
Skilled touch, 75–76
  communication through touch, 76
  contact, 75–76, 75*f*
  palpation, 76
  qualities of touch, 76
Skin cancer, 175, 175*f*
Skin conditions, 174–176, 175*f*, 304*f*, 304
Skin lifting, 276, 276*f*, 516, 516*f*
Skin rolling, 277, 277*f*
Slander, 676
Slapping, 281
Small intestine acupoint, 582*f*
Smile, 61
SOAP notes, 212–216
  chart with body diagram, example of, 217*f*
  content of, 213–214, 215*t*
  entries, example of, 216*f*
  format of, 213
  overview of, 212–213
  writing, 214–215
Sobardoras, 32
Social Security and Medicare tax (FICA), 633, 659
Social skills, 55–59
  conflict resolution, 57–59
  courtesy and good manners, 56
  defined, 56
  first impressions, 56
  greeting first-time client, 56–57, 57*f*
  introductions, 57
Society of Trained Masseuses, 33
Soft tissue
  manipulation, specialized systems of, 3
  technique applications, history of, 32
Solar Plexus Chakra (Manipura), 610, 610*f*
Sole proprietor, 634
Somatic therapy, 4, 15, 18, 39
SOTAP note, 213
Sound, 238
Spas
  club, 6
  cruise ship, 6
  day, 6
  destination, 6
  history of, 28–29
  medical, 6
  overview of, 6, 6*t*
  resort and hotel, 6
  services offered in, 6
Spa treatments, 465–495
  aromatherapy, 481–487
  body wraps, 475–481
  clients' choice of, 467–469
  equipment for, 466
  exfoliation, 469–475
  health and medical considerations in choosing, 468
  other considerations in choosing, 468–469
  overview of, 466
  practitioner's role in choosing, 467–468
  sanitation in, 467
  stone massage, 488–490

supplies for, 466–467
Special exercise studios, massage offered in, 6*t*, 7
Specialized systems of soft tissue manipulation, 3
Special populations, 420–464. *See also* Impairments and disabilities
  athletes, 421–429
  defined, 421
  elderly, 441–451
  infants, 436–441
  introduction, 421
  pregnant women, 429–436
  rewards and challenges in, 461
  terminally ill, 451–456
Specialty associations, 16
Specialty certifications, 12–13, 13*t*
Specificity
  in full-body Swedish massage, 313
  guidelines, 261
  in lower body massage, 377
  in upper body massage, 340
Speech impairment, 457
Speed of talk, 59
Spinal reflex, in reflexology sessions, 569
Spinous processes, tapotement over, 169
Spleen acupoint, 582*f*
Sports and fitness, history of, 29–31
  athletic masseur, 29–30
  expert masseuses, 31
  health service operators, 31, 31*f*
  rubbers, 29–30
  timeline, 31
  trained massage therapists, 30
  trainers, 30
  YMCA, 30–31
Sports clubs or teams, massage offered in, 6*t*, 7
Sports massage, 30, 421–428
  applications of, 421–423
  events, 421, 422–428
  maintenance, 421, 422
  recovery, 421, 422
  remedial massage and rehabilitation, 421, 422
  settings for, 6–7, 6*t*, 7*f*
  techniques and knowledge, 421–422
Spreading disease by circulation, 176
Spring for the Crane and Deer, 606*f*
Sputa padangushtasana (reclining hand to foot pose), 617*f*
Squishes, 281
Stacking the joints, 247, 247*f*, 585, 585*f*
Standardized forms and billing codes, 662–663
Standards of practice, 94–95
Standards of Practice (NCBTMB), 104, 105, 106
Starling, Ernst Henry, 541
Startup costs, 658
State regulations, 668
States that require licensing or certification, 14, 14*f*
Static pressure, 284, 284*f*
Stationery, 639–640
Steam rooms, 3, 404
Sternocleidomastoid (SCM), 529*f*, 531, 532*f*
Stoma, 460
Stomach acupoint, 582*f*
Stone massage, 488–490
  benefits of and contraindications for, 488, 488*t*
  cold, 490
  hot, 489, 489*f*, 490*f*

oil for, 489
  overview of, 488
  preparing for, 488–489
  stones used in, 488, 488*f*
Storefront businesses, massage offered in, 6*t*, 8
Strabo, 26
Straight leg flexion, 302, 302*f*
Straight leg hyperextension, 302
Street slang, 59–60
Stress-control strategies, 82
Stress reduction, 3, 5, 141
Stretching
  defined, 291
  hips and buttocks, 378
  methods, 291*t*, 292, 293*t*
Stripping, 271, 271*f*
Stroke, contraindications and cautions for, 176
Stroke, in lymphatic facilitation, 545–547, 546*f*, 547*f*
  applied in the direction of lymph flow, 546
  light, 545
  long stroke, 546–547, 547*f*
  L stroke, 546, 546*f*
  rhythmic, 546
  skin stretches and releases, 546
  slow, 546
Structural integrity, loss of, 173–174
Subcutaneous fascia, 513–514, 514*f*
Subjective information, 202–205
  health/medical history, 202–203
  intake interview, 203–205
Suboccipital release, 295
Subserous fascia, 514
Substances, for spa treatments, 467
Sugar, 470–471
Sunny Side of Mountain acupoint, 581*t*
Sun Salutation (Surya Namaskar), 614, 616*f*
Superficial warming friction, 277, 277*f*
Supination, 298, 303
Supine position, 254, 254*f*
Supplies, for massage, 233, 235–236
  blankets, 235
  bolsters, 233, 235, 235*f*
  pillows, 235, 235*f*
  sheets, 235–236, 235*f*
  towels, 235–236, 236*f*
Supplies, for spa treatments, 466–467
  cleaning supplies, 467
  disposables, 467
  linens, 467
  purchasing, 467
  substances, 467
  toiletries, 467
Surgery, recent, 173
Surya Namaskar (Sun Salutation), 614, 616*f*
Svadhisthana (Sacral Chakra), 610, 610*f*
Swedana (herbal steam bath), 612
Swedish massage, 3, 269
Swedish massage techniques, 268–289. *See also* Joint movements
  effleurage, 270–274
  friction, 277–279
  overview of, 269–270, 269–270*t*
  petrissage, 274–277
  tapotement, 279–282
  touch without movement, 283–284
  vibration, 282–283
Swedish movement cure institutions, 35
Swiss shower, 404
Swollen glands, 176

Sympathy, 55
Synovial joints, 292, 293*t*
Synthesis, in intellectual skills, 51, 51*t*
Systematic review, 127
Systolic pressure, 76

T
Table massage
  assistance getting onto and off of table, 253–254
  assistance in turning over, 254
  hand and body mechanics for, 248–251
  portable massage table, 230, 256, 257*f*
  positioning for, 254–256
  skills, 253–254
  table height, for pregnant women, 431
Tai chi, 74, 74*f*, 81, 248
Tapotement, 3, 279–282
  cupping and clapping, 280–281, 280*f*
  effect of, 121
  hacking, 280, 280*f*
  history of, 26, 27, 27*f*
  over kidneys, 171, 171*f*
  over spinous processes, 169
  overview of, 270*t*, 279–280
  pincement, 281, 281*f*
  quacking, 281, 281*f*
  rapping, 280, 280*f*
  for respiratory complications, 156
  slapping, 281
  squishes, 281
  tapping, 281, 281*f*
Tapping, 281, 281*f*
Taxable income, 657, 673–674
Taxes. *See* Income taxes
Tax preparation professionals, 662
Tax year, 657
Taylor, George, 35
Tea tree, 485*t*
Telephone use, 60, 61*f*
Telltack, 27
Temezcalli, 401
Temperament, 54
Temperature
  in physical environment for massage, 238
  ranges, in hydrotherapy, 403, 403*t*
  sensations, in hydrotherapy, 402, 402*t*
  tolerance, spa applications and, 468
Temperature therapy, 401. *See also* Hydrotherapy
Tenderness, during reflexology, 563–564
Tendons, 130, 131*f*
Tension headaches, trigger point therapy for, 532–535
Tenting, 254
Terminally ill, 451–456
  adaptations for, 452
  overview of, 451–452
  palliative care, 451
  practice sequence for, 452–455
  self-care, 456
Terminus, 543–544
Thai chop, 281, 281*f*
Thai massage, 614–615
Therapeutic massage and bodywork, 3. *See also* Massage therapy
Therapeutic outcomes, 153–154
Therapeutic relationship, 55, 99–112. *See also* Ethics
  confidentiality and, 111
  countertransference in, 100
  defense mechanisms in, 100–101

defined, 99
dual relationships in, 102–103
explicit and implicit agreements in, 99–100
fiduciary responsibility in, 99
power differential in, 99
psychological factors in, 100
roles and boundaries in, 101
in schools, 107–108
scope of practice, 108–111
sexual misconduct in, 104–107
sexual relationships in, 103–104
transference in, 100
Therapeutic Touch (TT), 5f, 160–161
Therm-Aire Corporation, 37
Thermotherapy, 402, 402t. See also Hydrotherapy
contraindications for, 404
vs. cryo-hydrotherapy, 403, 403t
guidelines for safe use of, 405
Thigh, 383, 384f, 386–392
Third Eye Chakra (Ajna), 610f, 611
Third trimester considerations, 432
Thixotropy, 130, 513
Thoracic cage, endangerment sites, 169
Three-count stroking of the trapezius, 272–273, 272f
3 Mile Point acupoint, 581t
Throat Chakra (Vishuddha), 610f, 611
Thumbwalking, 565, 565f
Thumb web-forearm stimulation, 622
Tiger's Mouth acupoint, 581t
Time management, 82–84, 83f
Time wasters, 83
Tips, 657, 673–674
Tissot, Clement, 33
Tissot, Simon Andre, 32
Tissue level, 129–131
connective tissue, 130–131, 131f
summary of, 122t
tissue repair, 129–130, 129f
wound and tissue repair, 129–130, 130f
Tissue repair, 129–130, 129f
Toe
effleurage of, 304
rotations, in reflexology sessions, 569
Toiletries, for spa treatments, 467
Topical substances, 236–237
sanitation and, 237
uses of, 236–237
Torso, endangerment sites, 169, 171, 171f
Touch, appropriate/inappropriate, 105
Touch Research Institute (TRI), 17, 40, 127, 142, 156, 158, 159
Touch therapy, 39
Touch Therapy (Field), 152
Touch without movement, 3, 283–284
defined, 283
direct (static) pressure, 284, 284f
passive touch, 283, 283f
Towels, 235–236, 236f
Trademarks, 672–673
Traditional Chinese medicine (TCM), 577–584
acupoints, 580, 581t, 583
assessment and treatment in, 583–584
defined, 577
energy channels, 580, 582–583f
energy imbalances in, 584
Five Elements, 578–580
Qi, 578
Yin and Yang, 577–578, 578f
Traditions of manual therapy, 3

Trager® approach, 38, 291
Trained masseuses, 33
Transference, 100
Transition techniques, 312
Transport vessels, 542f, 543
Traveling massage practice, 8
Travell, Janet, 527
Treatise on Massage, A (Graham), 32
Treatment planning, 201
TRI. See Touch Research Institute (TRI)
Trigger points (TrPs), 527–532
contraindications and cautions, 530
deactivation techniques, 530–532
defined, 527
direct pressure, 530–532, 531f, 532f
locating, 529–530
origins of, 528
palpation of, 530
reference zones, 528–529, 529f
varieties of, 527, 527t, 528f
Trigger point therapy, 3, 526–538. See also Trigger points (TrPs)
history of, 527
overview of, 527
for tension headaches, 532–535
Trimester considerations, 432
Triple warmer acupoint, 583f
Triptai, 32
TrPs. See Trigger points (TrPs)
Trustworthy, 92
TT. See Therapeutic Touch (TT)
Tuina, 8, 38, 584
Tummy rock, 620
Turkish baths, 27

U

Udvartana (herbal paste and exfoliating lymphatic massage), 612
Ulnar friction, 277, 278f
Umbilicus, endangerment sites, 169
Unconditional regard for others, 93
Underactivity, 133
Understanding, in polarity therapy, 619
Unethical behavior
reporting, 677
vulnerability to, 94
United States
reflexology in, 561
revival of massage in, 37–38
trigger point therapy popularized in, 527
U.S. Department of Agriculture (USDA), 84, 86
U.S. Department of Education (USDE), 10t, 11
U.S. Department of Health & Human Services (DHHS), 111
Office of Civil Rights, 111
U.S. Department of Labor, 5
Universal precautions, 239–240
Upavistha konasana (wide angle pose), 617f
Upper body regions, 339–375
back, 353–359
chest and abdomen, 367–372
head and face, 340–347
neck, 347–352
upper extremities, 359–366
Upper extremities, 359–366
anatomy of, 359–360, 360f
massage applications for, 361–366
Urinary system, 139
USDA. See U.S. Department of Agriculture (USDA)
USDE. See U.S. Department of Education (USDE)

V

VA. See Veteran's Administration (VA)
Values, 92–93
Variable costs, 657
Varicose veins, 176, 177f
Vata, 609, 610t
Venous return, 137
Veracity, 94
Verbal skills, 59–60
hearing challenges, 59
poor speech habits, 59
speed of talk, 59
street slang, 59–60
telephone use, 60, 61f
voice quality, 59
Vertebral column, endangerment sites, 167, 169, 170f
Vertical position, 499
Veteran's Administration (VA), 157
Vibration, 3, 282–283
deep, 282, 282f
electronic vibration devices, 282
jostling, 283, 283f
light effleurage with, 282
overview of, 282
shaking, 282, 283f
Vichy shower, 404, 466, 466f
Vishuddha (Throat Chakra), 610f, 611
Vision, 633–637
defined, 633
employment vs. self-employment, 633, 634–635, 636t
income goal, 636, 637
mission statement, 636, 637
part-time vs. full-time work, 633
worksheet, 633, 634f
Visual impairment, 456–457
Vocation, history of, 25. See also Massage as a vocation, history of
Vodder Method®, 540
Voice quality, 59

W

Wagging, 297, 298
Waist guideline, in zone therapy, 562, 562f
Walk and roll, 565, 565f
Walls, 237
Warming friction, 277, 277f
Warming technique, 312
Water, healing properties of, 402–403
Water element, 579
Watersheds (drainage patterns), 544, 545f
Wave movement, 295–296, 299
Weber, Tammy, 561
Websites, 640
Weight transfer, 585
Welcome Fragrance acupoint, 581t
Welfare of clients, 677
Well-being, feelings of, 143
Wellness massage, benefits of, 145
Wellness Massage Pyramid (WMP), 3–4, 4f, 10, 198
Wellness profession, 3–4
Western medicine, history of, 32–35
anatriptic art, 32
Hippocrates, 32
medical gymnast, 33–35, 35f
medical rubbing, 32–33
soft tissue technique applications, 32
trained masseuses, 33
triptai, 32
Wet room, 466

Wet table, 466, 466f
WHCCAMP. See White House Commission on Complementary and Alternative Medicine Policy (WHCCAMP)
Whiplash, 177
Whirlpool bath, 3, 403–404
White House Commission on Complementary and Alternative Medicine Policy (WHCCAMP), 4, 14–15, 18
WHO. See World Health Organization (WHO)
Wide angle pose (upavistha konasana), 617f
Widening the foot at the metatarsals, 305, 305f
Windows, 237
Wind Pond acupoint, 581t
Winternitz, Wilhelm, 402
WMP. See Wellness Massage Pyramid (WMP)
Wood element, 579
Work ethic, 46
Workplace wellness programs, 498
Work settings, for massage therapists, 6–8, 6t
health care settings, 7–8, 8f
personal care settings, 6, 6f
private practice settings, 8, 8f
sports, fitness, and recreation settings, 6–7, 7f
Work-site acupressure massage, 498
World Health Organization (WHO), 662
"Worst-case" exercises, 102–103
Wound and tissue repair, 129–130, 129f
Wringing, 273
Wrist
care, 246–247
endangerment sites, 169, 170f
joint movements to, 299, 299f
Written communication, 64–66
business letter, 64, 66f
email, 64
guidelines, 65
memos, 64, 65f
W-2 forms, 658–659

X

Xiphoid process, 169, 170f

Y

Yellow Emperor's Classic of Internal Medicine, 577
Yin and Yang, 577–578, 578f. See also Five Elements
body in terms of, 578
overview of, 577–578
principles of, 578
Yin Intersection acupoint, 581t
YMCA, 7, 30–31, 38, 650
Yoga, 80
Yungborn, 37

Z

Zabludowski, J. B., 32, 32f
Zen, 82
Zone, being in, 55
Zone therapy and guidelines, in reflexology, 561–562, 562f
diaphragm, 562, 562f
longitudinal tendon, 562, 562f
neck/shoulder, 562, 562f
pelvic, 562, 562f
waist, 562, 562f
Zone Therapy (Fitzgerald), 561

Human Skeleton, Anterior View

Frontal bone

Nasal bone

Zygomatic
bone

Orbit

Maxilla

Mandible

Clavicle

Manubrium

Scapula

Sternum

Costal
cartilage

Xiphoid
process

Ribs

Vertebral
column

Humerus

Coxal
(hip) bone

Radius

Ilium

Ulna

Sacrum

Coccyx

Carpals

Metacarpals

Phalanges

Pubis

Ischium

Greater
trochanter

Femur

Patella

Tibia

Fibula

Tarsals

Metatarsals

Phalanges